Precision Cancer Therapies

Precision Cancer Therapies

Volume 1

Targeting Oncogenic Drivers and Signaling Pathways in Lymphoid Malignancies

From Concept to Practice

Edited by

Owen A. O'Connor
Stephen M. Ansell
John F. Seymour

WILEY Blackwell

This edition first published 2023

Registered Office(s)
John Wiley & Sons, Inc., 111 River Street, Hoboken, NJ 07030, USA
John Wiley & Sons Ltd, The Atrium, Southern Gate, Chichester, West Sussex, PO19 8SQ, UK

For details of our global editorial offices, customer services, and more information about Wiley products visit us at www.wiley.com.

Wiley also publishes its books in a variety of electronic formats and by print-on-demand. Some content that appears in standard print versions of this book may not be available in other formats.

A catalogue record for this book is available from the Library of Congress

Hardback ISBN: 9781119819929; ePub ISBN: 9781119819943; ePDF ISBN: 9781119819936; oBook ISBN: 9781119819950

Cover Image: © Jorg Greuel/Getty Images
Cover Design: Wiley

Set in 9.5/12.5pt STIXTwoText by Integra Software Services Pvt. Ltd, Pondicherry, India
Printed and bound by CPI Group (UK) Ltd, Croydon, CR0 4YY

C9781119819929_030323

Contents

List of Contributors

Inhye E. Ahn
Dana-Farber Cancer Institute
Harvard Medical School
Boston, MA, USA

Kenneth C. Anderson
LeBow Institute for Myeloma Therapeutics and Jerome Lipper Multiple Myeloma Center
Department of Medical Oncology, Dana Farber Cancer Institute, Harvard Medical School
Boston, MA, USA

Julia Aronson
Memorial Sloan Kettering Cancer Center
New York, NY, USA

Francesco Bertoni
Institute of Oncology Research
Faculty of Biomedical Sciences
USI, Bellinzona, Switzerland

Oncology Institute of Southern Switzerland
Ente Ospedaliero Cantonale
Bellinzona, Switzerland

Giada Bianchi
Amyloidosis Program, Division of Hematology
Department of Medicine, Brigham and Women's Hospital
Harvard Medical School
Boston, MA, USA

Noa Biran
John Theurer Cancer Center at HMH and Hackensack Meridian School of Medicine
Hackensack, NJ, USA

Alessandro Broccoli
IRCCS Azienda Ospedaliero-Universitaria di Bologna
Bologna, Italy

Istituto di Ematologia "Seràgnoli"
Dipartimento di Medicina Specialistica
Diagnostica e Sperimentale
Università degli Studi
Bologna, Italy

Jennifer R. Brown
Dana-Farber Cancer Institute
Harvard Medical School
Boston, MA, USA

Jan A. Burger
Department of Leukemia
The University of Texas MD Anderson Cancer Center
Houston, TX, USA

Catherine C. Coombs
University of North Carolina
Chapel Hill, NC, USA

Sandeep S. Dave
Department of Medicine and Center for Genomic and Computational Biology
Duke Cancer Institute, Duke University
Durham, NC, USA

Matthew S. Davids
Dana-Farber Cancer Institute
Harvard Medical School
Boston, MA, USA

Andrew Davies
Southampton Cancer Research UK Centre
Cancer Sciences Unit, Faculty of Medicine
University of Southampton, Centre for Cancer Immunology
Southampton General Hospital
Southampton SO16 6YD, Hampshire, UK

Qing Deng
Department of Lymphoma & Myeloma
University of Texas MD Anderson Cancer Center
Houston, TX, USA

Michael Dickinson
Peter MacCallum Cancer Centre
Melbourne, Victoria, Australia

Sir Peter MacCallum Department of Oncology
University of Melbourne
Melbourne, Victoria, Australia

Sarah T. Diepstraten
The Walter and Eliza Hall Institute of Medical Research
Melbourne, Victoria, Australia

The Department of Medical Biology
The University of Melbourne
Melbourne, Victoria, Australia

Omar Elghawy
University of Virginia Cancer Center
University of Virginia School of Medicine
Charlottesville, VA, USA

Department of Medicine
Division of Hematology/Oncology
University of Virginia School of Medicine
Charlottesville, VA, USA

Toby Eyre
University of Oxford
Oxford, UK

David J. Feith
University of Virginia Cancer Center
University of Virginia School of Medicine
Charlottesville, VA, USA

Department of Medicine
Division of Hematology/Oncology
University of Virginia School of Medicine
Charlottesville, VA, USA

Georgia Alice Galimberti
Laboratory of Experimental Hematology
Institute of Oncology Research
Bellinzona, Switzerland

Philippe Gaulard
Département de Pathologie
Groupe Hospitalier Henri Mondor
AP-HP, Créteil, France

Université Paris-Est
INSERM U955, Créteil, France

Michael R. Green
Department of Lymphoma & Myeloma
University of Texas MD Anderson Cancer Center
Houston, TX, USA

Department of Genomic Medicine
University of Texas MD Anderson Cancer Center
Houston, TX, USA

Ashwin Gollerkeri
Kymera Therapeutics
Watertown, MA, USA

Jared Gollob
Kymera Therapeutics
Watertown, MA, USA

Andre Goy
John Theurer Cancer Center at HMH and Hackensack
Meridian School of Medicine
Hackensack, NJ, USA

John G. Gribben
Centre for Haemato-Oncology, Barts Cancer Institute
Queen Mary University of London
London, UK

Emily Gruber
The Peter MacCallum Cancer Centre
Melbourne, Victoria, Australia

Sean Harrop
Peter MacCallum Cancer Centre
Melbourne, Victoria, Australia

Matthew Ho
Department of Internal Medicine
Mayo Clinic, Rochester, MN, USA

David C.S. Huang
The Walter and Eliza Hall Institute of Medical Research
Melbourne, Victoria, Australia

The Department of Medical Biology
The University of Melbourne
Melbourne, Victoria, Australia

Prioty Islam
Levine Cancer Center
Raleigh, NC, USA

Yusuke Isshiki
Division of Hematology and Oncology
Joan and Sanford I Weill Department of Medicine
Weill Cornell Medicine
New York, NY, USA

Ricky Johnstone
Peter MacCallum Cancer Centre
Melbourne, Victoria, Australia

Sir Peter MacCallum Department of Oncology
University of Melbourne
Melbourne, Victoria, Australia

Matko Kalac
Precision Immunology Institute
Tisch Cancer Center, Icahn School of Medicine at Mount Sinai
New York, NY, USA

Lev M. Kats
The Peter MacCallum Cancer Centre
Melbourne, Victoria, Australia

The Sir Peter MacCallum Department of Oncology
University of Melbourne
Parkville, Victoria, Australia

Gemma L. Kelly
The Walter and Eliza Hall Institute of Medical Research
Melbourne, Victoria, Australia

The Department of Medical Biology
The University of Melbourne
Melbourne, Victoria, Australia

John Kuruvilla
Princess Margaret Cancer Centre
University of Toronto
Canada

Rob C. Laister
Princess Margaret Cancer Centre
University of Toronto
Canada

Laurence de Leval
Institute of Pathology
Department of Laboratory Medicine and Pathology
Lausanne University Hospital and Lausanne University
Lausanne, Switzerland

Thomas E. Lew
Department of Haematology
The Royal Melbourne Hospital and Peter MacCallum Cancer Centre
Melbourne, Victoria, Australia

Blood Cells and Blood Cancer Division
Walter and Eliza Hall Institute of Medical Research
Parkville, Victoria, Australia

Alexander C. Lewis
The Peter MacCallum Cancer Centre
Melbourne, Victoria, Australia

Jennifer K. Lue
Memorial Sloan Kettering Cancer Center
Lymphoma Service
New York, NY, USA

Jemma Longley
Southampton Cancer Research UK Centre, Cancer Sciences Unit, Faculty of Medicine
University of Southampton, Centre for Cancer Immunology
Southampton General Hospital
Southampton SO16 6YD, Hampshire, UK

Thomas P. Loughran Jr
University of Virginia Cancer Center
University of Virginia School of Medicine
Charlottesville, VA, USA

Department of Medicine, Division of Hematology/Oncology
University of Virginia School of Medicine
Charlottesville, VA, USA

Ralitsa R. Madsen
University College London Cancer Institute
Paul O'Gorman Building
University College London
London, UK

Nello Mainolfi
Kymera Therapeutics
Watertown, MA, USA

John Sanil Manavalan
Division of Hematology-Oncology
Department of Medicine, University of Virginia
Comprehensive Cancer Center
VA, USA

Farheen Manji
Princess Margaret Cancer Centre
University of Toronto
Canada

John E. La Marca
The Walter and Eliza Hall Institute of Medical Research
Melbourne, Victoria, Australia

The Department of Medical Biology
The University of Melbourne
Melbourne, Victoria, Australia

Enrica Marchi
Division of Hematology-Oncology
Department of Medicine
University of Virginia Comprehensive Cancer Center
VA, USA

Anthony R. Mato
Memorial Sloan Kettering Cancer Center
New York, NY, USA

Joel McCay
Centre for Haemato-Oncology, Barts Cancer Institute
Queen Mary University of London
London, UK

Ari Melnick
Division of Hematology and Oncology
Joan and Sanford I Weill Department of Medicine
Weill Cornell Medicine
New York, NY, USA

Anjali Mishra
Division of Hematologic Malignancies and Hematopoietic Stem Cell Transplantation
Department of Medical Oncology and Department of Cancer Biology, Sydney Kimmel Cancer Center
Thomas Jefferson University
Philadelphia, PA, USA

Owen A. O'Connor
Department of Medicine, Division of Hematology and Medical Oncology
T-Cell Malignancies Program University of Virginia Comprehensive Cancer Center Department of Microbiology Immunology and Cancer Biology University of Virginia
Charlottesville, VA, USA

Robert Z. Orlowski
Departments of Lymphoma & Myeloma, and Experimental Therapeutics
The University of Texas MD Anderson Cancer Center
1515 Holcombe Blvd., Unit 429, Houston, TX 77030, USA

Ipsita Pal
Division of Hematology-Oncology, Department of Medicine
University of Virginia Comprehensive Cancer Center
VA, USA

Deborah Piffaretti
Laboratory of Experimental Hematology
Institute of Oncology Research
Bellinzona, Switzerland

Pooja Phull
John Theurer Cancer Center at HMH and Hackensack Meridian School of Medicine
Hackensack, NJ, USA

Henry Miles Prince
Peter MacCallum Cancer Centre
Melbourne, Victoria, Australia

Sir Peter MacCallum Department of Oncology
University of Melbourne
Melbourne, Victoria, Australia

Epworth Healthcare, Sir Peter MacCallum Department of Oncology
University of Melbourne
Victoria, Australia

Craig A. Portell
Hematology/Oncology Division, University of Virginia Cancer Center, Charlottesville
VA, USA

Lindsey E. Roeker
Memorial Sloan Kettering Cancer Center
New York, NY, USA

Davide Rossi
Laboratory of Experimental Hematology
Institute of Oncology Research
Bellinzona, Switzerland

Clinic of Hematology
Oncology Institute of Southern Switzerland, Ente Ospedaliero Cantonale, Bellinzona
Bellinzona, Switzerland

Faculty of Biomedical Sciences
Università della Svizzera Italiana
Lugano, Switzerland

Nicholas J. Schmidt
Hematology/Oncology Division, University of Virginia Cancer Center, Charlottesville
VA, USA

John F. Seymour
Department of Haematology
The Royal Melbourne Hospital and Peter MacCallum Cancer Centre
Melbourne, Victoria, Australia

Faculty of Medicine, Dentistry and Health Sciences
The University of Melbourne
Parkville, Victoria, Australia

Jennifer Shingleton
Department of Medicine and Center for Genomic and Computational Biology
Duke Cancer Institute, Duke University
Durham, NC, USA

Pierre Sujobert
Service d'hématologie biologique Hospices Civils de Lyon, Hôpital Lyon Sud
France

Université Lyon, Faculté de médecine et de maïeutique, Lyon Sud
France

Charles Mérieux, Lymphoma Immunobiology Team
Pierre Bénite
France

Chiara Tarantelli
Institute of Oncology Research
Faculty of Biomedical Sciences
USI, Bellinzona, Switzerland

Kyla Trkulja
Princess Margaret Cancer Centre
University of Toronto
Canada

James Turkson
Department of Medicine
Cedars-Sinai Medical Center
Los Angeles, CA, USA

Johnson Ung
University of Virginia Cancer Center
University of Virginia School of Medicine
Charlottesville, VA, USA

Department of Medicine
Division of Hematology/Oncology, University of Virginia School of Medicine
Charlottesville, VA, USA

William G. Wierda
D.B. Lane Cancer Research Distinguished Professor of Medicine Section Head
CLL Department of Leukemia Division of Cancer Medicine
Holcombe Blvd
Unit 428, Houston, TX, USA

Thomas E. Witzig
Division of Hmeatology
Mayo Clinic, Rochester, MN, USA

Michael E. Williams
Hematology/Oncology Division
University of Virginia Cancer Center
VA, USA

Peibin Yue
Department of Medicine
Cedars-Sinai Medical Center
Los Angeles, CA, USA

Pier Luigi Zinzani
IRCCS Azienda Ospedaliero-Universitaria di Bologna
Bologna, Italy

Istituto di Ematologia "Seràgnoli"
Dipartimento di Medicina Specialistica, Diagnostica e Sperimentale, Università degli Studi
Bologna, Italy

Volume Foreword

The past two decades have seen the emergence of remarkable new insights into basic cancer biology, with the result that principles governing the approach to cancer treatment have undergone fundamental revision and reorganization. Recognizing the need to address this evolution in our understanding of how cancer treatment works, the editors and authors of ***Precision Cancer Therapies*** have set themselves the daunting task of providing clinicians and researchers with a basic guide to the underlying biology of cancer and, in particular, a guide to how this understanding can rationalize treatment. The first volume explores the biology of lymphoid cancer, one of the cancer types that has seen the most rapid accumulation of new agents and approaches, with particular attention to the role of small molecules and targeted agents and the nature of those agents' specific biological targets and associated pathways. Volume 2 focuses on immunotherapy, tracing how steadily accumulating insight into how the extraordinarily complex human immune system works and how, in recent years, that expanding insight has exploded with increasingly specific methods to manipulate passive and active immunity for cancer treatment. The editors' and authors' timing are impeccable. Clinicians, researchers, students, trainees, and representatives of funding and regulatory agencies will all find ***Precision Cancer Therapies*** the timely, in-depth resource they need to guide them through the blizzard of emerging data, trial results, drug approvals, and regulatory decisions as cancer therapy becomes ever more precise.

Throughout a century of modest steps beginning in the late 1800s, improvements in cancer treatment were slowly achieved employing surgery, radiation therapy, supportive care, diagnostic tests, and microscopic pathology. The contribution of systemic therapy to cancer treatment began during the latter half century of the 1900s with empiric interventions employing nonspecific, cytotoxic agents such as corticosteroids, alkylating agents, plant-based toxins, antimetabolites, hormonal agents, and disruptors of nucleic acid metabolism. It is only in retrospect that we have come to understand that these nonspecific interventions fundamentally rested on differential induction of apoptosis, the programmed self-destruction to which cancer cells are often more susceptible than healthy normal cells. Although much was achieved employing these cytotoxic agents in the treatment of a short list of cancers such as Hodgkin's lymphoma, childhood leukemia, testicular cancer, and choriocarcinoma, the systemic treatment of cancer had largely stalled by the end of the century. Genuine progress required improved understanding of the fundamental biology of cancer and more precise dissection of how the immune system works. Everything that happens in every cell in the body, including normal and cancer cells, and, therefore, in every tissue of which these cells are assembled, is directed by signals that originate in the cellular genome ramified through enormously complex signaling pathways. Precision in cancer treatment thus awaited progress in genomics, which is now rapidly transforming all of medicine, especially cancer medicine. In multicellular organisms, including humans, complex signaling pathways guide pluri-potential stem cells through stepwise differentiation to finalized effector cells and then govern how these cells and the tissues which they constitute accomplish all the tasks of living including nutrition, energy metabolism, and cellular repair and replacement. These signaling pathways tell cells what to do, where to stay, how to interact with other cells, how to procreate, and when to die. When mutations, regulatory pathway disruptions, and signaling errors, lead cells to stray from their assigned tasks, move haphazardly to inappropriate locations, linger despite obsolescence, and reproduce when not needed, cancer arises. The modern era of precision medicine focuses tightly on these signaling errors, suggesting interventions that are specific to the individual signaling error and, therefore, having the potential to exert their effect solely on the broken cells and broken pathways leaving normal cells, which are not making the signaling errors, untouched. Volume 1 of ***Precision Cancer Therapies*** focuses on the signaling pathways prominent in lymphomas with particular attention to the drivers of lymphomagenesis, phosphoinositide 3-kinase (PI3 kinase) pathways, regulatory control of programmed cell death (apoptosis), the B-cell receptor pathways, proteosome function and regulation, and epigenetic control of these pathways, identifying promising targets within them and what has been achieved clinically by targeting them.

After its focus on signaling pathways and targets for lymphoid cancer treatment in Volume 1, Volume 2 of ***Precision Cancer Therapies*** shifts focus to the equally remarkable progress that has occurred mimicking and recruiting the immune system for cancer treatment. After decades of disappointment in clinicians' ability to manipulate the human immune system to attack cancers effectively, the past two decades have seen an unprecedented transformation. Passive immunotherapy employing monoclonal antibodies and, later, radioimmunoconjugates and antibody drug conjugates have now been shown to be powerful, precise ways to attack cancer cells directly while largely sparing normal cells. Immune checkpoint inhibition employing antibodies to programmed death ligand signaling molecules now allows clinicians to cancel cancer cells' ability to paralyze immune effector cells. By neutralizing the immune destruction blockers that cancer cells employ to escape detection and destruction by cytotoxic cells of the immune system, first-generation FDA-approved checkpoint inhibitors such as pembrolizumab and nivolumab, and an array of second-generation monoclonal antibodies currently in development, have demonstrated the ability of such agents to bring the highly potent but equally highly specific destructive power of the immune system into play to attack cancer cells. The success of these agents has encouraged wider exploration of the potential to recruit immune effector cells by targeting tumor-associated antigens that are intrinsic to lymphoid cancers or are expressed in lymphoid cells whose behavior has been distorted or hijacked by Epstein–Barr virus. Complementing the descriptions of passive immunologic intervention offered by monoclonal antibodies, checkpoint inhibitors, radioimmunotherapy, and antibody drug conjugates, Volume 2 of ***Precision Cancer Therapies*** also includes several sections devoted to active cell-based immunotherapy. Building on older experience with allogeneic hematopoietic stem cell transplantation, these sections explore the potential of chimeric antigen receptor T-cells (CAR-T cells) to knit together the two remarkable characteristics of the effector cells of the immune system: precise specificity and extraordinary potency. This technique utilizes autologous T-cells that have been equipped in the laboratory with cell surface receptors specific for lymphoid cancer cell antigens and then clonally expanded to large numbers before being re-infused into the patient. This use of crafted "hunter-killer" cells thus brings specificity by employing antigen receptors tailored to bind to potentially unique antigens on the lymphoid cancer cells and power by employing the most potent cytotoxic cells of the immune system.

Systemic cancer treatment is currently in the midst of profound transformation. Although much was accomplished previously utilizing nonspecific interventions in which the therapeutic agents employed induce broad cell injury with the intention that the cancer cells be irreversibly damaged but normal healthy cells allowed to recover, the limits of this overall approach have become apparent. Going forward it has become clear that the key to progress in cancer treatment is precision. In ***Precision Cancer Therapies***, the editors and authors provide essential guidance to how this precision is being achieved. Volume 1 addresses the way in which novel agents target key signaling pathways in lymphoid cancer cells, providing precision by focusing on unique vulnerabilities in the malignant cells. Volume 2 explores the ways in which the specificity and power of the human immune system can be employed to focus treatment precisely. Together these two volumes provide clinicians, researchers, and regulators essential insight in this exciting new era of cancer treatment.

Joseph M. Connors, MD, CM
Emeritus Professor
BC Cancer Centre for Lymphoid Cancer
University of British Columbia
Vancouver, BC, Canada

Volume Preface

What does the future hold?

Treatment for patients with lymphoid malignancies has changed dramatically in the past 20 years. Two decades ago, treatment approaches for patients with various lymphomas typically constituted the use of non-crossresistant chemotherapy drugs. These agents were used in combination and were effective in a subset of patients. However, in relapsing patients, responses to additional chemotherapy treatments were typically dramatically shorter than the benefits seen with the initial regimen, while the subset of patients who durably benefited from more chemotherapy was typically limited to those who underwent autologous stem cell transplantation. Since then, a greater understanding of the biology of lymphoid malignancies has led to to the development of multiple classes of highly active new drugs. As outlined in this book, most classes of these novel agents have now been established as very effective. However, most novel therapies are not curative even though patients may benefit with extended durations of remission. As one looks to the future, rational combination approaches using these novel treatments will clearly be the next logical step.

In determining the most optimal combination, a number of approaches can be considered. Firstly, one could consider a "depletion" approach where the primary focus is to suppress or eradicate the malignant clone or other cells that are facilitating the growth of the malignant cell. Clearly, if every malignant cell was eradicated, the patient would be cured of the disease and treatments that kill every malignant cell would be favored. Furthermore, the malignant cell often dictates the composition of the tumor microenvironment creating an immune niche that favors the growth and survival of the cancer cell. Lymphoma cells may also directly suppress immune cells preventing their ability to lyse the malignant clone. Additionally, cells such as monocytes and macrophages present in the tumor microenvironment, may directly support and nurture the growth of the malignant cells. Therapeutically, those populations of cells supporting the cancer clone can also be targeted and depleted, theortically leading to an improvement in patient outcome. Clearly, this approach has met with limited success and needs to be improved. Strategies that may improve a "depletion" approach could include utilizing targeted therapy such as antibody drug conjugates in combination with chemotherapy, or by adding immune depleting agents targeting macrophages or T regulatory cells to chemotherapy, or sequencing chemotherapy before adding immunotherapy to first suppress the malignant clone and then allow for optimal immune activation.

A second combination strategy that could be considered would be an "inhibition" approach. This approach would focus on critical intracellular pathways that support the survival of the malignant cell. A rational approach to inhibition would include potentially targeting multiple different pathways that are important to the survival of the cancer cell or alternatively targeting the same dominant pathway at multiple levels. One potential risk of this approach may be upregulation of alternative pathways when one or more critical pathways are suppressed. Furthermore, novel agents could be used to specifically upregulate particular pathways that create an additional vulnerability for the malignant cell. An example of this could be the use of HDAC inhibitors which upregulate PD-L1 expression, potentially making a cell more vulnerable to immune checkpoint therapy when given in combination. Additionally, pathway inhibitors may have off target effects that may be of significant benefit. This could include the immunological effects of BTK inhibitors, mTOR inhibitors or PI3K inhibitors, all of which have both direct effects on the malignant B-cells but also effects on immune cells including normal T-cells.

A third strategy could be an "immune optimization" approach. While not the primary focus of this book, Volume 2 of the Precision Cancer Therapies series will exclusively focus on many of the agents that mediate lymphoma cell kill through a variety of immunologic mechanisms. Specific strategies to optimize immune function could include direct activation of immune cells using small molecules, immune checkpoint targeted therapy or the use of bispecific antibodies. Additional strategies that could be used in an "immune optimization" approach could specifically suppress cells that inhibit the immune response such as regulatory T-cells or suppressive monocytes, thereby improving the antitumor response. The challenge of utilizing single agent therapy to achieve immune optimization has been the development of immune exhaustion when cells are non-specifically stimulated. Strategies to improve this "immune optimization" approach would be to intermittently stimulate the immune system and thereby avoid exhaustion or to block inhibitory signals associated with immune exhaustion at a time when the immune system is activated. All of these strategies are being evaluated in the laboratory and in patients, though most have met with mixed results.

Possibly the optimal strategy for the future might be a "reprogramming" approach that incorporates all of the elements outlined above. This "reprogramming" strategy would potentially focus not only on directly depleting the malignant cell, but also on inhibiting specific pathways on which the cell is dependent, as well as activating the immune system. These strategies would be employed all at the same time. Just as in the past, combination non-cross-resistant chemotherapy approaches have been our most successful therapies, future approaches should utilize the varied tools we have in combination to optimize patient management. Aside from utilizing agents with different mechanisms of action in combination, future studies will also focus on whether combination treatment should be given at the same time or sequenced in an optimal order of administration. Furthermore, it may also be necessary to determine whether some therapies may be required as longer term maintenance treatment.

All told, the future for treatment of lymphoid malignancies has many opportunities. Using new drugs and with a greater understanding of the tumor biology, we have an opportunity to impact the clinical outcome of many patients. Not only is the opportunity to increase response rates and durability of clinical benefit, but also to utilize targeted therapy and minimize toxicities. However, our challenge is to continue the research and drug development until every patient with a malignancy can be cured.

Stephen M. Ansell, MD, PhD
Dorotha W. and Grant L. Sundquist Professor in
Hematologic Malignancies Research
Chair, Division of Hematology
Mayo Clinic

Series Preface

The pace of growth in scientific literature has been a subject for scientists who like to study bibliometric data, for decades. As early as 1951, Derek John de Solla Price, often regarded as one of the pioneers in studying rates of change in scientific literature, noted that the development of scientific information follows the law of exponential growth (de Solla Price 1951). In 1976, Price concluded that "at any time the rate of growth is proportional to the ... total magnitude already achieved – the bigger a thing is, the faster it grows" (de Solla Price 1976). More recently, in 2018, Fortunato et al. concluded that "early studies discovered an exponential growth in the volume of scientific literature ... a trend that continues with an average doubling period of 15 years" (Fortunato et al. 2018). Barabási and Wang suggested that if the scientific literature doubles every 15 years, "the bulk of knowledge remains always at the cutting edge" (Barabási and Wang 2021). That means, that the bulk of what a typical physician learns in undergraduate, graduate, or medical school is potentially obsolete by the time they assume responsibility for the care of patients, or that the information they rely on today was not yet in the textbooks that laid the foundation for their career.

For practicing oncologists, there in lies the problem. How does one stay abreast of these incomprehensible changes in scientific knowledge, much less understand it in a manner that can be used to help their patients. Cancer medicine has become a field where the need to appreciate basic science, and I emphasize "appreciate" not "comprehensively understand," has become indispensable. Cancer medicine has become the place where fundamental cellular biology, pharmacology, and clinical medicine all collide, as physicians struggle to understand how they should integrate and evaluate diverse streams of information in order to arrive at the best solution for the patient sitting before them. It has become a field where translating the details of science has taken on larger and larger roles as physicians consider how to cure a disease, palliate pain, or improve the status quo, using only the information they have at their disposal.

Precision Cancer Therapies is designed to try and meet that very need. The volumes that will be produced in the series, the first two of which are devoted to the lymphoid malignancies, are developed around categories of diseases that share common themes in their pathogenesis, and, potentially, the strategies one might consider in targeting their dysregulated biology. Sections are organized around select mechanistic themes in disease biology established as being potentially important in disease pathogenies, followed by a chapter on the pharmacology of drugs identified as effective in nullifying that abnormal biology. Subsequent chapters in each section are focused on the translational aspects: how does one use the drugs at hand to alter the pathology in a therapeutically meaningful manner. Succeeding chapters highlight actual clinical data with specific drugs as both monotherapies and in "rational" combination. The sections within a volume are designed to share information using the same kind of logic a clinician might invoke in thinking about their patient. Here are some pertinent questions:

i) What is the disease biology causing the problem?
ii) What are the drugs at my disposal?
iii) What is the data for the use of these drugs?
iv) Are there ways to improve on these drugs' efficacy by considering combination effects?

The sections take a decidedly translational approach to the problem.

With the advent of so much web-based learning and now the passion around how artificial intelligence (AI) might transform our approach, some might suggest, why another book, let alone a series of books. The answer lies in the simple fact that there is no substitute or singular surrogate that can replace your very own fund of knowledge. Perhaps the most widely recognized and touted AI approach ever to come to our attention did so in 2011, when we watched, with complete astonishment I might add, IBMs Watson beat the famed Ken Jennings and Brad Rutter in Jeopardy. Jennings and Rutter were the greatest Jeopardy champions of all time: more wins and more money than any other contestants in the history of the show. But, despite their intellectual prowess, they were no match for a computer that had intensely trained for years and "learned" how to beat Jennings and Rutter by playing simulated games against 100 of the best Jeopardy contestants ever. Yes, Watson too had to learn, and read, and assimilate years of information to compete with the human brain. While Jeopardy may be the most widely recognized and successful adventures for a room-sized computer, other forays of AI – and Watson in particular – in the field of oncology have, thus far at least, fallen short. IBM's Watson for Oncology has been in development since 2012. It is being developed to provide state-of-the-art personalized treatment recommendations for patients with very specific kinds of malignant disease. Watson has undergone extensive "learning" at some of the most prestigious cancer centers in the world, being nurtured on the nuances of cancer medicine. Comprehensive details around the interpretation of blood tests, pathology, genetics, imaging data, and patient-oriented detail get fed into the computer. Then, the computational prowess of Watson combs through the vast medical literature we discussed above, to generate an evidence-based treatment recommendation for that specific patient. Why did Watson outperform on Jeopardy and underperform in oncology? One reason may be obvious. The state of cancer research and its impact on the practice of cancer medicine is extremely dynamic and in constant flux, at times it relies on instinct and experience, apparently making an appearance on Jeopardy look easy. Encyclopedic facts about the real world change slowly, if at all. Acknowledging that this type of AI technology is in its infancy (though most of us completed medical school, residency, and fellowship in the time Watson has been in development), the decade-long experience of Watson in cancer medicine has to date been less than flattering. The lay press has taken a decidedly negative impression of Watson's first steps (watson-ibm-c), suggesting that while AI may have enormous appeal to the average observer, it is likely to never replace the intellectual prowess – and instinct – of that physician sitting in front of a patient. It re-enforces a centuries-old and fundamental truth, "knowledge itself is power," at least as Sir Francis Bacon understood it.

And so, with some data in hand, and curiosity in endless supply, Precision Cancer Therapies intends to help keep physicians, scientists, health care providers, and the motivated reader stay up to date on the dynamic and every growing state of information in our fascinating profession. Sure, Watson and PubMed and Society Guidelines can aid us in our decision-making. However, there is nothing that can replace a good old-fashioned education nor the instinct of an informed practitioner of this most rewarding of crafts.

Owen A. O'Connor, MD, PhD
American Cancer Society Research Professor
Professor of Medicine
University of Virginia Comprehensive Cancer Center

References

Barabási, A.-L. and Wang, D. (2021). The Science of Science, Cambridge University Press.

de Solla Price, D.J. (1951). Quantitative Measures of the development of science. Archives Internationales d'Histoire des Sciences 4(14): 85–93, http://garfield.library.upenn.edu/price/pricequantitativemeasures1951.pdf

de Solla Price, D.J. (1976). General theory of bibliometric and other cumulative advantage processes. J. Am. Soc. Inf. Sci. 27 (5–6): 292–306, http://garfield.library.upenn.edu/price/pricetheory1976.pdf

Fortunato, S., Bergstron, C.T., Borner, K. et al. (2018) Science of science. Science 359 (6379): eaao0185. doi: 10.1126/science.aao0185.

IBM pitched Watson as a revolution in cancer care. It's available at: https://www.statnews.com/2017/09/05/watson-ibm-cancer/

Section I

Biological Basis of the Lymphoid Malignancies

1

Fundamental Principles of Lymphomagenesis

Pierre Sujobert[1], Philippe Gaulard[2], and Laurence de Leval[3]

[1] *Service d'hématologie biologique Hospices Civils de Lyon, Hôpital Lyon Sud, France; Université Lyon, Faculté de médecine et de maïeutique, Lyon Sud, France; Charles Mérieux, Lymphoma Immunobiology Team, Pierre Bénite, France*
[2] *Département de Pathologie, Groupe Hospitalier Henri Mondor, AP-HP, Créteil, France; Université Paris-Est, INSERM U955, Créteil, France*
[3] *Institute of Pathology, Department of Laboratory Medicine and Pathology, Lausanne University Hospital and Lausanne University, Lausanne, Switzerland*

Take Home Messages

- Lymphomagenesis is a complex process involving environmental and genetic drivers.
- There is a continuum between preneoplastic lesions and overt lymphomas.
- Lymphoid neoplasms are defined and classified according to the concept of cell of origin reflecting the resemblance of lymphoma cells to their normal counterparts.
- The research for new treatment largely relies on the concept of hallmarks of cancer highlighting the targetable pathways specific to transformed cells.

Introduction

If one asks a cancer scientist a seemingly naive question such as "what are the hallmarks of cancer cells," they will probably cite at first somatic mutations and genomic rearrangement, leading to excessive proliferation, resistance to apoptosis, and dissemination potential (Hanahan and Weinberg 2011). Intriguingly, all of these hallmarks are physiological properties of B- and T-lymphocytes, selected by evolution because they ensure an efficient immune response against pathogens. So, it is a fascinating paradox to observe that lymphoma remains a relatively rare cancer as compared to epithelial cancers. Hence, understanding the tumor suppressor mechanisms that mitigate lymphomagenesis or eradicate lymphoma cells at preclinical stages appears an extraordinary challenge. After a short overview of the current models used to analyze lymphomagenesis, we will highlight that the frontier between reactive lymphoproliferation and overt lymphoma is not always clear. Then, we will present how the classification of lymphomas based on the concept of cell of origin might reveal important phenotypical properties of lymphoma subtypes. Finally, we propose an overview of the main hallmarks of lymphomas and discuss their contribution in the most frequent subtypes of lymphomas.

How to Study Lymphomagenesis

As in other scientific fields, the nature of our knowledge of lymphomagenesis is tightly linked to the tools used to produce this knowledge. Hence, it seems interesting to start this review with a methodological perspective, providing a brief overview of the different scientific approaches which have brought major contributions to our understanding of lymphomagenesis.

Epidemiology was the first approach which shed light on the mechanisms of lymphomagenesis, by deriving statistical correlations from direct observation of cohorts of patients. First, epidemiology has established the link between lymphoma incidence and aging. The incidence of most lymphomas follows an exponential growth after the fifth decade as observed for most cancers, suggesting that common processes are shared with solid tumors (Rozhok and DeGregori 2016; Sarkozy et al. 2015). In the case of Hodgkin's lymphomas, the bimodal distribution of incidence suggests that specific mechanisms are occurring in young patients, which have not been fully elucidated to date. Second, epidemiology has also proven a counterintuitive association of lymphomas with immunosuppression, either inherited (common variable immunodepression for example) or acquired after HIV infection, or immunosuppressive drugs (Kaplan 2012;

Precision Cancer Therapies: Targeting Oncogenic Drivers and Signaling Pathways in Lymphoid Malignancies: From Concept to Practice, Volume 1, First Edition. Edited by Owen A. O'Connor, Stephen M. Ansell, and John F. Seymour.

van Leeuwen et al. 2009). This association revealed the role of the immune system in repressing the growth of transformed lymphocytes, for example by active eradication of tumor cells or by exerting a competition for resources. Third, the analysis of the geographic distribution of lymphoma subtypes also shows striking differences, such as the higher incidence of T-cell lymphoma in Asia as compared to Western countries (Perry et al. 2016). These differences suggest two non-mutually exclusive hypotheses, related to environmental or genetic differences. The fourth major insight from epidemiological studies was to shed light on the role of pathogens such as *Helicobacter pylori*, hepatitis C virus (HCV), Epstein–Barr virus (EBV), or human T-cell lymphotropic virus 1 (HTLV-1) in specific subtypes of lymphoma (Couronné et al. 2018; Lecuit et al. 2004; Suarez et al. 2006), which has been then confirmed experimentally. Besides pathogens, epidemiological studies have also demonstrated the role of environmental exposures such as herbicides in lymphomagenesis, which might have important consequences for health policies (Weisenburger 2021). More recently, molecular epidemiology based on genome-wide association studies has demonstrated the association of host genetic polymorphisms with the risk of specific lymphoma subtypes (Cerhan et al. 2014), highlighting unsuspected pathways which can then be experimentally explored.

The other descriptive approach is based on so-called "-omics" approaches, which have generated much data during the past two decades thanks to the technological outbreaks of next-generation sequencing. The principle of these studies is to characterize genomic and/or transcriptomic profiles of hundreds of cases, in order to discover recurrent events or associations, to examine the clustering of similar cases, and to evaluate their correlation with clinical presentation, response to therapy or prognosis. For example, these approaches were successfully applied to diffuse large B-cell lymphomas (DLBCL), which have been classified into germinal center B-cell (GC), activated B-cell (ABC), and unclassified subtypes after transcriptomic profiling (Alizadeh et al. 2000; Rosenwald et al. 2002), and are now being divided into genomic subtypes with partial overlap with former transcriptomic classes (Chapuy et al. 2018; Schmitz et al. 2018; Wright et al. 2020). Importantly, preclinical data has demonstrated that the transcriptomic subtypes rely on specific pathways related to proliferation, immune escape, and apoptosis, making them more or less sensitive to targeted therapies (Yang et al. 2012). However, the clinical trials based on these observations have not been successful so far (Davies et al. 2019; Younes et al. 2019), highlighting the need to further refine our experimental approaches to increase the translational impact of these descriptive approaches.

Beyond these two descriptive approaches, experimental models have been developed which enable direct testing of hypotheses. An exhaustive description of all the experimental models available to study lymphoma biology is beyond the scope of this chapter, but we will briefly describe three models which have been widely used. The first one is cell lines, which are derived from primary samples and can be maintained and expanded *in vitro*. These are a very important resource for research, which enables the modulation of the expression of a gene of interest or to perform whole genome screens, to test the effects of drugs, and to assess a variety of phenotypic characteristics (proliferation, apoptosis, etc.). Accordingly, this is a model of choice to provide preclinical data supporting personalized medicine approaches, which aim at choosing the treatment according to the specific features of the neoplastic cells. Of note, the cell line model has many limitations such as genetic drift or contaminations (Drexler et al. 2003). Even more problematic is the fact that the cells grow in suspension and without interaction with other cell types, in a stereotyped metabolic environment (glucose and amino-acids concentration, or oxygen concentration for example) which is far from the real *in vivo* conditions of growth of lymphoma cells. Refinements of culture conditions might improve some of these limitations, by reconstitution of cell–cell interaction with a stroma layer and/or a three-dimensional structure such as spheroids (Lamaison et al. 2021).

The second major group of experimental models is represented by lymphomas developed in genetically engineered mice. After the recognition of recurrent genetic hits in lymphomas, various models have been proposed where the genome of the mice is modified to mimic what is observed in patients. For example, BCL2 overexpression, which is a hallmark of follicular lymphomas due to the t(14;18) translocation, can drive an oligoclonal lymphoproliferation in irradiated mice reconstituted with bone marrow cells expressing the Vav-P *BCL2* transgene (Egle 2004). This model has also served as a platform to assess the oncogenic role of other somatic mutations such as those occurring in *KMT2D*, *CREBBP*, *TBL1XR1*, or *BTG1* (Boice et al. 2016; Delage et al. 2022; Ortega-Molina et al. 2015; Venturutti et al. 2020; Zhang et al. 2015), which are not sufficient to drive lymphomagenesis by themselves.

The third major experimental model of lymphomagenesis is the xenografting of primary human lymphoma samples into immunodeficient recipients, usually NSG (NOD.Cg-Prkdc^{scid} Il2rg^{tm1Wjl} / SzJ) mice (Townsend et al. 2016). These strategies enable the analysis of primary cells in a microenvironment that recapitulates some of the features of the human microenvironment. However, the establishment of such models is even more difficult for lymphomas than for other hematological malignancies like acute leukemias, and many key aspects of lymphoma biology such as the role of the immune system are not captured. Alternative recipients might warrant further evaluation such as zebrafish or chicken embryos (Delloye-Bourgeois et al. 2017), but none of them will eventually capture all the features of human lymphoma biology.

Finally, one should be reminded that every model of lymphoma describes only a fraction of the disease, and the overall picture requires the integration of all the data. The main role of lymphoma models is to generate hypotheses, which should ideally be tested in clinical trials when possible.

Before Lymphoma: The Gray Frontier Between Physiology and Pathology

Lymphoma could be defined by a clonal proliferation of B-, T-, or natural killer (NK)-lymphocytes with tissue involvement and clinical manifestations, that is, symptoms related to lesions involving lymph nodes and/or extranodal sites. Similar to the paradigm proposed for colorectal carcinoma (Fearon and Vogelstein 1990), the development of lymphoid malignancies is believed to follow a multistep process with progressive accumulation of genetic events. Accordingly, it is not surprising that early lesions preceding lymphomas have been observed in healthy individuals. Early steps of lymphomagenesis may manifest as "reactive" lymphoproliferations; *in situ* lymphomas, – better designated as *in situ* neoplasms in view of their limited potential to develop into an overt lymphoma, and lymphomas with low tumor burden and no clinical impact. Even more frequent is the identification of oncogenic translocations associated with lymphoma by sensitive molecular techniques in healthy adults, which will only rarely give rise to overt lymphomas. In the following section, we will describe some of these pre-lymphomatous lesions, which challenge our understanding on how to define lymphoma.

Driver Without Disease

Chromosomal translocations are hallmark features of several lymphoid malignancies that result in the deregulated expression of oncogenes or in the generation of novel fusion genes. Using sensitive molecular studies to screen healthy individuals, translocations such as the t(14;18)(q32;q21), the t(11;14)(q13;q32), as well as the t(2;5)(p23;q35) resulting in *NMP1:ALK* fusion transcript – the hallmark driver events for follicular lymphoma (FL), mantle cell lymphoma (MCL), and Anaplastic Lymphoma Kinase (ALK)-positive anaplastic large cell lymphoma, respectively – have been detected, though at a low rate, in circulating cells of healthy individuals (Laurent et al. 2012; Lecluse et al. 2009; Roulland et al. 2014; Trümper et al. 1998). The best example is given by the observation that the t(14;18)(q32;q21) is detectable in the peripheral blood of two-thirds of healthy adults at a detection threshold of ~ 1 cell per million B-cells (Roulland et al. 2014). Given that the vast majority of these patients will never progress to overt FL, it suggests that such progression requires additional genetic events (Milpied et al. 2015; Sungalee et al. 2014), and/or an escape from immunological control of lymphoma outgrowth.

From *In Situ* Neoplasms to Asymptomatic Lymphomas

A tissue equivalent of the detection of driver translocations in the blood of healthy people are the limited lymphoma lesions discovered incidentally. The best described is "*in situ follicular neoplasm*," which is characterized by scattered follicles occupied by clonal B-cells with both t(14;18) as well as BCL2 and CD10 co-expression (Cong et al. 2002). Similarly, though at a lower prevalence, "*in situ mantle cell neoplasm*" due to the incidental observation of accumulating cyclin D1+ cells in the mantle zone of otherwise morphologically reactive lymph nodes has been recognized, which can antedate the occurrence of overt MCL.

Another early histological lesion is represented by the tissue equivalent of monoclonal B-cell lymphocytosis (MBL) (Gibson et al. 2011; Rawstron et al. 2008). The latter is defined as the presence of less than 5×10^9/L clonal B-cells in the peripheral blood which share the phenotypic and genetic characteristics of patients with chronic lymphocytic leukemia (CLL), or less commonly display a "non-CLL" phenotype. The absence of clear clinical or biological parameters that clearly distinguishes MBL from CLL indicates a continuum between both conditions without sharp delineation (Barrio et al. 2017). This also means that CLL develops slowly following a prolonged prodromal phase without clinical symptoms and obvious lymphocytosis, and this asymptomatic phase may also persist many years in a proportion of patients with overt CLL. Similarly, monoclonal gammopathy of unknown significance is the subclinical precursor lesion to plasma cell myeloma (Scarfò and Ghia 2016).

Chronic Antigenic Stimulation as an Early Step of Lymphomagenesis

There is evidence that gastric extranodal marginal zone lymphoma arises from a mucosa-associated lymphoid tissue (MALT) that has been acquired because of *Helicobacter pylori* infection. First, *H. pylori* is present in most gastric MALT lymphomas. Second, the therapeutic efficacy of antibiotics on gastric MALT lymphomas demonstrates the addiction of lymphoma cells to chronic antigenic stimulation (Steinbach et al. 1999). Third, *in vitro* studies also showed that lymphoma growth could be stimulated by *H. pylori* strain-specific T-cells (Wotherspoon et al. 1991). Therefore, *H. pylori*-induced chronic gastritis can be regarded as a preneoplastic lesion in which the lymphoma B-cell clone can be detected preceding the occurrence of MALT lymphoma, emphasizing a continuum between *H. pylori* chronic inflammation and MALT lymphoma without sharp delineation (Isaacson et al. 1999).

Regarding the T-cell system, intolerance to gliadin in a specific HLA context causes celiac disease. Celiac disease is characterized by chronic antigen stimulation and expansion of intestinal intraepithelial T lymphocytes (IEL) which subsequently favors the development of enteropathy-associated T-cell lymphomas (EATL). Overt EATL with intestinal tumors is often associated with mesenteric lymph node involvement may be preceded by early lesions composed of morphologically non-transformed IEL which are already clonal with an aberrant phenotype and genetic lesions, a condition referred to as refractory celiac disease. Therefore, lymphoma development in this setting follows a multistep process from celiac disease to refractory celiac disease – regarded as a preneoplastic condition or *in situ* lymphoma – to EATL, following early acquisition of gain-of-function mutations in genes of the *JAK1/STAT3* pathway (Cording et al. 2021; Ettersperger et al. 2016).

EBV-associated B-cell lymphoproliferative disorders (LPDs) that occur in immunocompromised patients constitute another illustration of the first steps of lymphomagenesis. These disorders constitute a heterogeneous group of lesions ranging from polyclonal polymorphic proliferations to clonal monomorphic lesions which share common oncogenic and biological features. In these diseases, EBV is an important oncogenic driver and the balance between viral oncogenic proteins, defective immune surveillance, and genetic background likely explains the clinical manifestations, and their potential response to reduction or withdrawal of immune-suppression whenever possible (Natkunam et al. 2018).

Another intriguing condition, probably secondary to chronic antigenic stimulation, is persistent polyclonal B-cell lymphocytosis (PPBL). This infrequent disorder occurring mostly in middle-aged smoking women is characterized by an expansion of dysplastic – binucleated – B-cells which are polytypic (as assessed by kappa or lambda light chain expression) but clonal as demonstrated by recurrent cytogenetic abnormalities such as isochromosome 3q (Callet-Bauchu et al. 1999). However, this condition is not driven by gene mutations (Tesson et al. 2017), and the reason why around 10% of PPBL patients develop overt lymphomas remains to be determined (Lesesve and Troussard 2011).

Another way to tackle the problematic definition of lymphomas relies on the cell of origin concept, which is presented in the next section.

The Cell of Origin Concept: A Classification Based on Physiology

Lymphomas derive from B-cells, T-cells, or NK-cells at various stages of differentiation possess many features of their normal counterparts. These features – including physiological antigen receptor gene editing, gene expression, immunophenotype, morphology, homing patterns, and proliferation capacities – in large part dictate the clinical behavior of these diseases. Thus, understanding the normal counterpart of neoplastic cells provides a useful framework for understanding the biology of the lymphomas, and to a large extent constitutes the basis for lymphoma classification (Alaggio et al. 2022; Campo et al. 2022; Swerdlow et al. 2016). Two major categories of lymphoid neoplasms are recognized: precursor (lymphoblastic) neoplasms, corresponding to the earliest stages of differentiation, and peripheral or mature neoplasms, corresponding to later stages of differentiation. Lymphoblastic neoplasms tend to be more common in children who have large pools of precursor cells, while those corresponding to mature effector cells tend to be seen more often in adults; for example, plasma cell myeloma is common in older adults with large pools of post-germinal center antigen-exposed plasma cells, as is mycosis fungoides which is a neoplasm derived from effector CD4+ T-cells. Tumors corresponding to proliferating normal cells such as lymphoblasts or centroblasts are likely to be rapidly growing and clinically aggressive, while those that correspond to resting stages, such as small lymphocytic lymphoma/CLL, are more likely to be indolent. Lymphoid neoplasms also reflect their normal counterpart in their growth and homing pattern; tumors of bone marrow-derived precursors become acute leukemias and those of marrow-homing plasma cells multiple myeloma; tumors derived from cells of MALT tend to involve MALT sites; FL cells which represent the neoplastic counterpart to germinal center centroblasts and centrocytes populate the follicles of lymphoid tissues throughout the body.

The correspondence of lymphoma entities to normal lymphoid subsets or to a specific stage of normal lymphoid differentiation is particularly well established for mature B-cell neoplasms. The germinal center reaction which is pivotal in normal immune responses also plays a major role in lymphomagenesis since mutations in many oncogenes are acquired as a secondary effect of the activation of the somatic mutation and immunoglobulin heavy chain (IGH) locus class-switch recombination machinery which physiologically occurs during T-cell-dependent germinal center reaction and is mediated by AID (activation-induced cytidine deaminase) (Robbiani and Nussenzweig 2013). In addition, the analysis of somatic hypermutations in the variable regions of the immunoglobulin genes which constitute definitive genomic imprints of the germinal center reaction has been a major tool to characterize the cellular origin of various mature B-cell lymphomas, into naïve or pre-germinal center, germinal center, or post-germinal center neoplasms. Moreover, the presence of ongoing somatic hypermutations in tumors is considered a feature of germinal center neoplasms. In CLL, immunogenetic analysis has proven instrumental in delineating two subgroups of the disease according to their hypermutation status, which translate into differing clinical courses and are taken into account for patient risk stratification and the choice of treatment modalities (Fabbri and Dalla-Favera 2016).

Interestingly, while the notion of cellular origin is usually used interchangeably with that of "normal cell counterpart," in fact it is established that in several instances the oncogenic process starts at an earlier stage of differentiation. For example, the translocations involving *BCL1* and *BCL2* in MCL and FL, respectively, occur in bone marrow lymphoid progenitors where they are mediated by the recombination activating gene (RAG) complex normally involved in VDJ recombination of immunoglobulin and T cell receptor (TCR) genes in immature lymphoid cells (Lieber 2016). In the case of T-cell lymphomas with a follicular helper T-cell phenotype, the mutations in epigenetic modifiers *TET2* and *DNMT3A* target hematopoietic stem cells not yet committed to the lymphoid lineage (Lemonnier et al. 2018a).

For T-cell lymphomas, the significance of cell lineage or cellular counterpart is variably established for the many different entities (Gaulard and de Leval 2014). In the case of lymphomas derived from the innate immune system, for example EBV-associated extranodal NK/T-cell lymphomas, it appears that the derivation from NK versus gamma–delta (or alpha–beta) T-cells is essentially not relevant clinically or biologically, and the same applies to primary intestinal or hepatosplenic T-cell lymphomas, which may express the alpha–beta or gamma–delta isoform of the TCR, or neither or both, with no established correlation to biology or outcome (Travert et al. 2012). Conversely, a neoplastic phenotype resembling that of follicular helper T-cells defines a relatively large group of diseases which have in common other genotypic and clinical traits (Dobay et al. 2017). The possibility to identify subgroups among peripheral T-cell lymphomas, not otherwise specified (PTCL-NOS), based on expression signatures resembling those of normal T helper (Th)1 or Th2 cells, appears promising (Amador et al. 2019; Iqbal et al. 2014).

Of note, the cell of origin concept highlights the similarities between normal and cancer cells. On the other hand, the concept of cancer hallmarks shed light on the biological properties that are specific to cancer cells and might be targeted without excessive toxicity against their normal counterpart (Figure 1.1).

What Are the Hallmarks of Lymphoma?

Taking into account the considerations proposed above, it is tempting to adapt the concept of hallmarks of oncogenesis to B- and T-cell lymphomas. Based on the analysis of epidemiological data, pathological features, characteristic molecular drivers, and experimental models, we can propose a panel of seven hallmarks of lymphomagenesis which are contributing to various extents to the development of the main lymphoma subtypes.

Epigenetics and Metabolism

Beyond the coding sequence, the structure of chromatin is a strong determinant of cell phenotype, which connects the global control of transcription with the metabolic state (Goldberg et al. 2007). The most described epigenetic modifications relate to the DNA molecule itself (cytosine methylation/demethylation, involving genes such as *IDH1* and *2*, *TET2*, or *DNMT3A*) and the modifications of the histone proteins (including among others acetylation [mediated by *CREBBP*, *EP300*] and methylation [mediated by *KMT2D*, EZH2]). As in myeloid malignancies, mutations of the genes encoding the epigenetic machinery are highly recurrent in specific subtypes of lymphomas, such as FL (*KMT2D, CREBBP, EP300*, EZH2) or angioimmunoblastic T-cell lymphomas (*TET2, IDH2, DNMT3A*) (García-Ramírez et al. 2017; Lemonnier et al. 2012; Ortega-Molina et al. 2015; Zhang et al. 2015). An interesting hypothesis is that epigenetic marks might represent a barrier against the transformation of hematological cells just as spatial organization of tissues acts against the development of epithelial cancers (Nam et al. 2021). Of note, epigenetics is now recognized as a therapeutic target with EZH2 inhibitors in B-cell malignancies (Morschhauser et al. 2020), or histone deacetylase (HDAC) inhibitors and hypomethylating agents in T-cell lymphomas (Falchi et al. 2021; Lemonnier et al. 2018b; O'Connor et al. 2019).

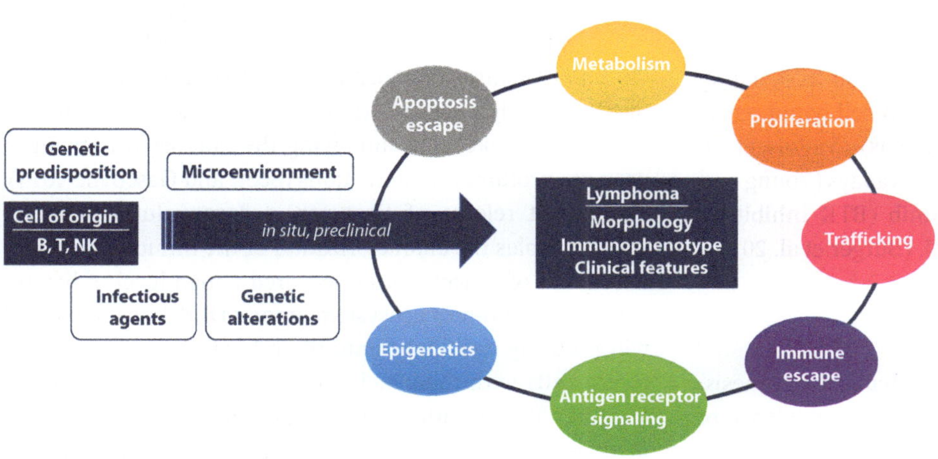

Figure 1.1 Overview of the main hallmarks of lymphomas.

Apoptosis Escape

As in other malignancies, escape from apoptosis is an essential step in lymphomagenesis. Alterations of the *TP53* pathway are highly prevalent in most of the lymphoma subtypes and are generally associated with poor response to chemotherapy. Alternatively, overexpression of the *BCL2* gene, for example as a consequence of the t(14;18) translocation in FL or of a gene amplification in some DLBCL (Chapuy et al. 2018), inhibits the mitochondrial outer membrane permeabilization induced by most pro-apoptotic signals. Here again, resistance to apoptosis is now targetable by BCL2 inhibitors such as venetoclax.

Proliferation

Escaping apoptosis is probably not sufficient to explain the outgrowth of large tumor masses as observed in lymphoma patients. Somatic alterations of the genetic machinery that controls the cell cycle are very frequent in lymphomas, with the paradigmatic example of cyclin D1 overexpression in MCL, resulting from the pathognomonic t(11;14) translocation. More indirectly, constitutive expression of c-MYC (for example in Burkitt's lymphoma as a consequence of transcriptional deregulation related to the rearrangement of the *MYC* gene with the promoter of the *IGH* gene) or constitutive activation of the NF-κB pathway in ABC-DLBCL also promotes the entry into cell cycle.

TCR/BCR Signaling

Unique to B- and T-lymphocytes is the expression of a specific antigenic receptor, respectively the B-cell receptor (BCR) and the T-cell receptor (TCR). These receptors transduce survival signals and promote proliferation, which is critical to amplify the immune response in physiological conditions when the lymphocytes encounter their cognate antigen. However, these signals are also strongly oncogenic, and many mechanisms are now well described which result in their constitutive activation such as chronic antigenic stimulation due to HCV, *H. pylori*, antigen-independent signaling in CLL, (Dühren-von Minden et al. 2012), and mutations in signaling genes (for example *CD79A* and *CD79B* in B-cell lymphomas, or *PLCG1* and *CD28* in T-cell lymphomas) (Vallois et al. 2016). This hallmark is also targetable nowadays (Young and Staudt 2013), for example with ibrutinib (BTK inhibitor), which shows impressive efficacy in CLL (Burger et al. 2015).

Immune Escape

Immune evasion plays a critical role in lymphomagenesis, which is negatively illustrated by the increased incidence of lymphomas in immunocompromised patients. This mechanism is especially important in Hodgkin's lymphoma or primary mediastinal B-cell lymphomas, where 9p24.1 amplification leads to overexpression of PDL1 and promotes anergy of cytotoxic T-cells (Green et al. 2010). Other strategies are observed such as decrease antigen presentation after *CREBBP* inactivation by somatic mutations in FL (Green et al. 2015), inhibition of HLA expression after B2 microglobulin (*B2M*) mutation/deletion in DLBCL (Challa-Malladi et al. 2011), among others. The escape from the immune system has been successfully targeted with checkpoint inhibitors (such as PD1 or PDL1 inhibitors in Hodgkin's lymphoma), or with chimeric antigen receptor T-cells.

Trafficking

At the time of diagnosis, lymphoma has often spread to multiple locations in the body, including distant lymph nodes or extranodal sites such as bone marrow, central nervous system, skin, and virtually all organs. This dissemination is associated with a poor prognosis and is incorporated into clinical staging systems. Trafficking is a property of lymphocytes, which is essential for their immune functions. However, lymphoma cells can also enhance their ability to migrate through mutations of genes involved in germinal center confinement such as *Gα13* or *S1PR2* (Muppidi et al. 2014). In DLBCL, extranodal dissemination is highly frequent is the MCD/C5 subtype (Chapuy et al. 2018; Schmitz et al. 2018; Wright et al. 2020), which is associated with recurrent mutations of BTG1, and recent works demonstrated a link between BTG1 inactivation and lymphoma dissemination through the activation of the BCAR1 pathway (Delage et al. 2022).

Microenvironment

Even if lymphomas are aggressive *in vivo*, they are very difficult to maintain and grow *in vitro*, revealing their dependency on signals from the microenvironment. Of note, the interaction of lymphomas with their microenvironment is heterogeneous, with some lymphomas recruiting various cellular subtypes – the prototype being Hodgkin's lymphoma where the neoplastic cells are typically outnumbered by an abundant and usually polymorphous reactive infiltrate; others – like Burkitt's lymphoma – destroying the microenvironment, and others – like FL – modifying the microenvironment to promote protumoral interactions (Scott and Gascoyne 2014). The recent release of Ecotyper, a deconvolution method which enables the characterization of the immune microenvironment of cancers, has uncovered a high level of heterogeneity of the tumor ecosystem among DLBCL patients, and will probably shed light onto the role of the interactions of tumor cells with their niche in other lymphomas (Steen et al. 2021). Therapeutic approach targeting the microenvironment is an appealing strategy, because normal cells are far more homogeneous than cancer cells, and accordingly less prone to resist to treatment. But obviously, targeting normal cells without excessive toxicities is challenging, even if not impossible (rituximab for example).

Conclusion

Lymphomas constitute a heterogeneous group of diseases, which are not always easy to distinguish from physiological conditions resulting from chronic antigenic stimulation. The last decades have enabled an extraordinary accumulation of knowledge which translates into clinical benefits, even if the road is still long to cure the majority of patients. Understanding the fundamental principles of lymphomagenesis is a never-ending process, where our established knowledge is constantly challenged by technological advances, clinical observations, and therapeutic innovations. We cannot overemphasize the importance of collaborations between scientists and medical doctors to tackle this challenge.

Must Read References

Alizadeh, A.A., Eisen, M.B., Davis, R.E. et al. (2000). Distinct types of diffuse large B-cell lymphoma identified by gene expression profiling. *Nature* 403: 503–511.

Lemonnier, F., Gaulard, P., and de Leval, L. (2018a). New insights in the pathogenesis of T-cell lymphomas. *Curr. Opin. Oncol.* 30: 277–284.

Chapuy, B., Stewart, C., Dunford, A.J. et al. (2018). Molecular subtypes of diffuse large B cell lymphoma are associated with distinct pathogenic mechanisms and outcomes. *Nat. Med.* 24: 679–690.

O'Connor, O.A., Falchi, L., Lue, J. et al. (2019). Oral 5-azacytidine and romidepsin exhibit marked activity in patients with PTCL: a multicenter phase 1 study. *Blood* 134 (17): 1395–1405.

Scott, D.W. and Gascoyne, R.D. (2014). The tumour microenvironment in B cell lymphomas. *Na. Rev. Cancer* 14: 517–534.

References

Alaggio, R., Amador, C., Anagnostopoulos, I. et al. (2022). The 5th edition of the World Health Organization Classification of haematolymphoid tumours: lymphoid neoplasms. *Leukemia* 36: 1720–1748.

Alizadeh, A.A., Eisen, M.B., Davis, R.E. et al. (2000). Distinct types of diffuse large B-cell lymphoma identified by gene expression profiling. *Nature* 403: 503–511.

Amador, C., Greiner, T.C., Heavican, T.B. et al. (2019). Reproducing the molecular subclassification of peripheral T-cell lymphoma-NOS by immunohistochemistry. *Blood* 134: 2159–2170.

Barrio, S., Shanafelt, T.D., Ojha, J. et al. (2017). Genomic characterization of high-count MBL cases indicates that early detection of driver mutations and subclonal expansion are predictors of adverse clinical outcome. *Leukemia* 31: 170–176.

Boice, M., Salloum, D., Mourcin, F. et al. (2016). Loss of the HVEM tumor suppressor in lymphoma and restoration by modified CAR-T cells. *Cell* 167: 405–418.e13.

Burger, J.A., Tedeschi, A., Barr, P.M. et al. (2015). Ibrutinib as initial therapy for patients with chronic lymphocytic leukemia. *N Engl J Med* 373: 2425–2437.

Callet-Bauchu, E., Gazzo, S., Poncet, C. et al. (1999). Distinct chromosome 3 abnormalities in persistent polyclonal B-cell lymphocytosis. *Genes Chromosom. Cancer* 26: 221–228.

Campo, E., Jaffe, E.S., Cook, J.R. et al. (2022). The international consensus classification of mature lymphoid neoplasms: a report from the clinical advisory committee. *Blood* 140 (11): 1229–1253.

Cerhan, J.R., Berndt, S.I., Vijai, J. et al. (2014). Genome-wide association study identifies multiple susceptibility loci for diffuse large B cell lymphoma. *Nat. Genet.* 46: 1233–1238.

Challa-Malladi, M., Lieu, Y.K., Califano, O. et al. (2011). Combined genetic inactivation of beta2-microglobulin and CD58 reveals frequent escape from immune recognition in diffuse large B-cell lymphoma. *Cancer Cell* 20: 728–740.

Chapuy, B., Stewart, C., Dunford, A.J. et al. (2018). Molecular subtypes of diffuse large B cell lymphoma are associated with distinct pathogenic mechanisms and outcomes. *Nat. Med.* 24: 679–690.

Cong, P., Raffeld, M., Teruya-Feldstein, J. et al. (2002). In situ localization of follicular lymphoma: description and analysis by laser capture microdissection. *Blood* 99: 3376–3382.

Cording, S., Lhermitte, L., Malamut, G. et al. (2021). Oncogenetic landscape of lymphomagenesis in coeliac disease. Gut gutjnl-2020-322935.

Couronné, L., Bachy, E., Roulland, S. et al. (2018). From hepatitis C virus infection to B-cell lymphoma. *Ann. Oncol.* 29: 92–100.

Davies, A., Cummin, T.E., Barrans, S. et al. (2019). Gene-expression profiling of bortezomib added to standard chemoimmunotherapy for diffuse large B-cell lymphoma (REMoDL-B): an open-label, randomised, phase 3 trial. *Lancet Oncol* 20 (5): P649–662.

Delage, L., Lambert, M., Bardel, E. et al. (2022). BTG1 inactivation drives lymphomagenesis and promotes lymphoma dissemination through activation of BCAR1. *Blood* 202201694.

Delloye-Bourgeois, C., Bertin, L., Thoinet, K. et al. (2017). Microenvironment-driven shift of cohesion/detachment balance within tumors induces a switch toward metastasis in neuroblastoma. *Cancer Cell* 32 (427–443): e8.

Dobay, M.P., Lemonnier, F., Missiaglia, E. et al. (2017). Integrative clinicopathological and molecular analyses of angioimmunoblastic T-cell lymphoma and other nodal lymphomas of follicular helper T-cell origin. *Haematologica* 102: e148–e151.

Drexler, H.G., Dirks, W.G., Matsuo, Y. et al. (2003). False leukemia–lymphoma cell lines: an update on over 500 cell lines. *Leukemia* 17: 416–426.

Dühren-von Minden, M., Übelhart, R., Schneider, D. et al. (2012). Chronic lymphocytic leukaemia is driven by antigen-independent cell-autonomous signalling. *Nature* 489: 309–312.

Egle, A. (2004). VavP-Bcl2 transgenic mice develop follicular lymphoma preceded by germinal center hyperplasia. *Blood* 103: 2276–2283.

Ettersperger, J., Montcuquet, N., Malamut, G. et al. (2016). Interleukin-15-dependent T-cell-like innate intraepithelial lymphocytes develop in the intestine and transform into lymphomas in celiac disease. *Immunity* 45: 610–625.

Fabbri, G. and Dalla-Favera, R. (2016). The molecular pathogenesis of chronic lymphocytic leukaemia. *Nat. Rev. Cancer* 16: 145–162.

Falchi, L., Ma, H., Klein, S. et al. (2021). Combined oral 5-azacytidine and romidepsin are highly effective in patients with PTCL: a multicenter phase 2 study. *Blood* 137: 2161–2170.

Fearon, E.R. and Vogelstein, B. (1990). A genetic model for colorectal tumorigenesis. *Cell* 61: 759–767.

García-Ramírez, I., Tadros, S., González-Herrero, I. et al. (2017). Crebbp loss cooperates with Bcl2 over-expression to promote lymphoma in mice. *Blood*. 129 (19): 2645–2656.

Gaulard, P. and de Leval, L. (2014). Pathology of peripheral T-cell lymphomas: where do we stand? *Semin. Hematol.* 51: 5–16.

Gibson, S.E., Swerdlow, S.H., Ferry, J.A. et al. (2011). Reassessment of small lymphocytic lymphoma in the era of monoclonal B-cell lymphocytosis. *Haematologica* 96: 1144–1152.

Goldberg, A.D., Allis, C.D., and Bernstein, E. (2007). Epigenetics: a landscape takes shape. *Cell* 128: 635–638.

Green, M.R., Kihira, S., Liu, C.L. et al. (2015). Mutations in early follicular lymphoma progenitors are associated with suppressed antigen presentation. *PNAS* 112: E1116–E1125.

Green, M.R., Monti, S., Rodig, S.J. et al. (2010). Integrative analysis reveals selective 9p24.1 amplification, increased PD-1 ligand expression, and further induction via JAK2 in nodular sclerosing Hodgkin lymphoma and primary mediastinal large B-cell lymphoma. *Blood* 116: 3268–3277.

Hanahan, D. and Weinberg, R.A. (2011). Hallmarks of cancer: the next generation. *Cell* 144: 646–674.

Iqbal, J., Wright, G., Wang, C. et al. (2014). Gene expression signatures delineate biological and prognostic subgroups in peripheral T-cell lymphoma. *Blood* 123: 2915–2923.

Isaacson, P.G., Diss, T.C., Wotherspoon, A.C. et al. (1999). Long-term follow-up of gastric MALT lymphoma treated by eradication of H. pylori with antibodies. *Gastroenterology* 117: 750–751.

Kaplan, L.D. (2012). HIV-associated lymphoma. *Best Pract. Res. Clin. Haematol.* 25: 101–117.

Lamaison, C., Latour, S., Hélaine, N. et al. (2021). A novel 3D culture model recapitulates primary FL B cell features and promotes their survival. *Blood Adv.* 5 (23): 5372–5386.

Laurent, C., Lopez, C., Desjobert, C. et al. (2012). Circulating t(2;5)-positive cells can be detected in cord blood of healthy newborns. *Leukemia* 26: 188–190.

Lecluse, Y., Lebailly, P., Roulland, S. et al. (2009). t(11;14)-positive clones can persist over a long period of time in the peripheral blood of healthy individuals. *Leukemia* 23: 1190–1193.

Lecuit, M., Abachin, E., Martin, A. et al. (2004). Immunoproliferative Small Intestinal Disease Associated with *Campylobacter jejuni*. *N. Engl. J. Med.* 350: 239–248.

van Leeuwen, M.T., Grulich, A.E., Webster, A.C. et al. (2009). Immunosuppression and other risk factors for early and late non-Hodgkin lymphoma after kidney transplantation. *Blood* 114: 630–637.

Lemonnier, F., Couronné, L., Parrens, M. et al. (2012). Recurrent TET2 mutations in peripheral T-cell lymphomas correlate with TFH-like features and adverse clinical parameters. *Blood* 120: 1466–1469.

Lemonnier, F., Dupuis, J., Sujobert, P. et al. (2018b). Treatment with 5-azacytidine induces a sustained response in patients with angioimmunoblastic T-cell lymphoma. Blood *blood*-2018-04-840538.

Lemonnier, F., Gaulard, P., and de Leval, L. (2018a). New insights in the pathogenesis of T-cell lymphomas. *Curr. Opin. Oncol.* 30: 277–284.

Lesesve, J.F. and Troussard, X. (2011). Persistent polyclonal B-cell lymphocytosis. *Blood* 118: 6485.

Lieber, M.R. (2016). Mechanisms of human lymphoid chromosomal translocations. *Nat. Rev. Cancer* 16: 387–398.

Milpied, P., Nadel, B., and Roulland, S. (2015). Premalignant cell dynamics in indolent B-cell malignancies. *Curr. Opin. Hematol.* 22: 388–396.

Morschhauser, F., Tilly, H., Chaidos, A. et al. (2020). Tazemetostat for patients with relapsed or refractory follicular lymphoma: an open-label, single-arm, multicentre, phase 2 trial. *Lancet Oncol.* 21: 1433–1442.

Muppidi, J.R., Schmitz, R., Green, J.A. et al. (2014). Loss of signalling via Gα13 in germinal centre B-cell-derived lymphoma. *Nature* 516: 254–258.

Nam, A.S., Chaligne, R., and Landau, D.A. (2021). Integrating genetic and non-genetic determinants of cancer evolution by single-cell multi-omics. *Nat. Rev. Genet.* 22: 3–18.

Natkunam, Y., Gratzinger, D., Chadburn, A. et al. (2018). Immunodeficiency-associated lymphoproliferative disorders: time for reappraisal? *Blood* 132: 1871–1878.

O'Connor, O.A., Falchi, L., Lue, J. et al. (2019). Oral 5-azacytidine and romidepsin exhibit marked activity in patients with PTCL: a multicenter phase 1 study. *Blood* 134 (17): 1395–1405.

Ortega-Molina, A., Boss, I.W., Canela, A. et al. (2015). The histone lysine methyltransferase KMT2D sustains a gene expression program that represses B cell lymphoma development. *Nat. Med.* 21: 1199–1208.

Perry, A.M., Diebold, J., Nathwani, B.N. et al. (2016). Non-Hodgkin lymphoma in the developing world: review of 4539 cases from the International Non-Hodgkin Lymphoma Classification Project. *Haematologica* 101: 1244–1250.

Rawstron, A.C., Bennett, F.L., O'Connor, S.J.M. et al. (2008). Monoclonal B-cell lymphocytosis and chronic lymphocytic leukemia. *N. Engl. J. Med.* 359: 575–583.

Robbiani, D.F. and Nussenzweig, M.C. (2013). Chromosome translocation, B cell lymphoma, and activation-induced cytidine deaminase. *Annu. Rev. Pathol.* 8: 79–103.

Rosenwald, A., Wright, G., Chan, W.C. et al. (2002). The use of molecular profiling to predict survival after chemotherapy for diffuse large-B-cell lymphoma. *N. Engl. J. Med.* 346: 1937–1947.

Roulland, S., Kelly, R.S., Morgado, E. et al. (2014). *T(14;18) Translocation: A Predictive Blood Biomarker for Follicular Lymphoma*. JCO. JCO.2013.52.8190.

Rozhok, A.I. and DeGregori, J. (2016). The evolution of lifespan and age-dependent cancer risk. *Trends Cancer* 2: 552–560.

Sarkozy, C., Salles, G., and Falandry, C. (2015). The biology of aging and lymphoma: a complex interplay. *Curr. Oncol. Rep.* 17: 32.

Scarfò, L. and Ghia, P. (2016). What does it mean I have a monoclonal B-cell lymphocytosis?: recent insights and new challenges. *Semin. Oncol.* 43: 201–208.

Schmitz, R., Wright, G.W., Huang, D.W. et al. (2018). Genetics and Pathogenesis of Diffuse Large B-Cell Lymphoma. *N. Engl. J. Med.* 378: 1396–1407.

Scott, D.W. and Gascoyne, R.D. (2014). The tumour microenvironment in B cell lymphomas. *Na. Rev. Cancer* 14: 517–534.

Steen, C.B., Luca, B.A., Esfahani, M.S. et al. (2021). The landscape of tumor cell states and ecosystems in diffuse large B cell lymphoma. *Cancer Cell* 39: 1422–1437.e10.

Steinbach, G., Ford, R., Glober, G. et al. (1999). Antibiotic treatment of gastric lymphoma of mucosa-associated lymphoid tissue: an uncontrolled trial. *Ann. Intern. Med.* 131: 88.

Suarez, F., Lortholary, O., Hermine, O. et al. (2006). Infection-associated lymphomas derived from marginal zone B cells: a model of antigen-driven lymphoproliferation. *Blood* 107: 3034–3044.

Sungalee, S., Mamessier, E., Morgado, E. et al. (2014). Germinal center reentries of BCL2-overexpressing B cells drive follicular lymphoma progression. *J. Clin. Investig.* 124: 5337–5351.

Swerdlow, S.H., Campo, E., Pileri, S.A. et al. (2016). The 2016 revision of the World Health Organization classification of lymphoid neoplasms. *Blood* 127: 2375–2390.

Tesson, B., Huet, S., Grange, B. et al. (2017). Absence of driver mutations in persistent polyclonal B-cell lymphocytosis with binucleated lymphocytes. *Blood* 130: 1267–1269.

Townsend, E.C., Murakami, M.A., Christodoulou, A. et al. (2016). The public repository of xenografts enables discovery and randomized phase II-like trials in mice. *Cancer Cell* 30: 183.

Travert, M., Huang, Y., de Leval, L. et al. (2012). Molecular features of hepatosplenic T-cell lymphoma unravels potential novel therapeutic targets. *Blood* 119: 5795–5806.

Trümper, L., Pfreundschuh, M., Bonin, F.V. et al. (1998). Detection of the t(2;5)-associated NPM/ALK fusion cDNA in peripheral blood cells of healthy individuals. *Br. J. Haematol.* 103: 1138–1144.

Vallois, D., Dobay, M.P.D., Morin, R.D. et al. (2016). Activating mutations in genes related to TCR signaling in angioimmunoblastic and other follicular helper T-cell-derived lymphomas. Blood blood-2016-02-698977.

Venturutti, L., Teater, M., Zhai, A. et al. (2020). TBL1XR1 mutations drive extranodal lymphoma by inducing a pro-tumorigenic memory fate. *Cell* 182: 297–316.e27.

Weisenburger, D.D. (2021). A review and update with perspective of evidence that the herbicide glyphosate (Roundup) is a cause of non-Hodgkin lymphoma. *Clin. Lymphoma. Myeloma. Leuk.* 21: 621–630.

Wotherspoon, A.C., Ortiz-Hidalgo, C., Falzon, M.R. et al. (1991). Helicobacter pylori-associated gastritis and primary B-cell gastric lymphoma. *Lancet* 338: 1175–1176.

Wright, G.W., Huang, D.W., Phelan, J.D. et al. (2020). A probabilistic classification tool for genetic subtypes of diffuse large B cell lymphoma with therapeutic implications. *Cancer Cell* 37: 551–568.e14.

Yang, Y., Shaffer, A.L., Emre, N.C.T. et al. (2012). Exploiting synthetic lethality for the therapy of ABC diffuse large B cell lymphoma. *Cancer Cell* 21: 723–737.

Younes, A., Sehn, L.H., Johnson, P. et al. (2019). Randomized phase iii trial of ibrutinib and rituximab plus cyclophosphamide, doxorubicin, vincristine, and prednisone in non-germinal center b-cell diffuse large b-cell lymphoma. *J. Clin. Oncol* 37 (15): 1285–1295.

Young, R.M. and Staudt, L.M. (2013). Targeting pathological B cell receptor signalling in lymphoid malignancies. *Nat. Rev. Drug Discov.* 12: 229–243.

Zhang, J., Dominguez-Sola, D., Hussein, S. et al. (2015). Disruption of KMT2D perturbs germinal center B cell development and promotes lymphomagenesis. *Nat. Med.* 21: 1190–1198.

2

Identifying Molecular Drivers of Lymphomagenesis

Jennifer Shingleton and Sandeep S. Dave

Department of Medicine and Center for Genomic and Computational Biology, Duke Cancer Institute, Duke University, Durham, NC, USA

Take Home Messages

- Next-generation sequencing has enabled tremendous progress in identifying the molecular drivers of lymphoma.
- Identification of molecular drivers has led to development of many targeted therapies, but several barriers to clinical translation remain.
- Barriers to translation include limited sequencing of very rare lymphoma types, inadequate representation of most ethnic groups in sequencing studies, and limitations of preclinical and early phase studies.
- "Basket" clinical trials that enroll patients based on specific genetic lesions, rather than specific diagnoses, can help inform the tailoring of drug regimens to the biology of the disease.

Introduction

Lymphoma drivers confer survival or proliferative advantage to tumors. These advantages include uncontrolled cell proliferation, avoiding cell death or senescence, and evasion of the immune system (Hanahan and Weinberg 2011). A driver can be defined as a genetic alteration that contributes to one or more of these advantages and helps propel cells along the path to malignant transformation.

Early cytogenetic research helped identify characteristic translocations and gene fusions that were clear genetic drivers in different lymphomas (e.g. *MYC* and *BCL2* translocations in Burkitt's lymphoma [BL] and follicular lymphoma [FL], respectively). Unfortunately, not all molecular drivers have been as easy to identify, especially given the high degree of genetic heterogeneity of not just the drivers but also the genetic mechanisms in most lymphomas. The advent of genomic technologies, particularly next-generation sequencing (NGS), has given us more sophisticated and powerful techniques to identify these genetic drivers and their mechanisms. However, these advanced techniques are a double-edged sword as they require greater sophistication to analyze and interpret results. For instance, the increased sensitivity of NGS allows detection of potential genetic drivers occurring at very low frequency, which may represent passenger mutations that have no effect on lymphomagenesis.

The ever-decreasing cost of NGS has allowed unbiased whole exome sequencing and whole genome sequencing of different lymphoma cohorts, which have identified recurrently mutated genes and pathways. These studies have been invaluable for revealing mutation patterns that point to mechanisms of lymphomagenesis and for informing patient prognosis. Nearly every lymphoma subtype has been the subject of such studies. However, the rarity of many subtypes precludes large cohort sizes, and remains a limiting factor for defining infrequent or subtle mechanisms implicating new drivers.

Identifying molecular drivers of lymphomagenesis comprises two separate but related issues: which variants have an effect on downstream function and which mutated genes actually drive malignant transformation? Not every genetic variant will have a significant effect on protein function, and not every altered gene can functionally contribute to lymphomagenesis. Discerning molecular drivers remains an important problem in drug development since a therapy that targets a passenger gene will likely have minimal impact on the disease. In addition, molecular drivers can vary between different subtypes or lineages, so drug development and clinical trials may need to be designed in a subtype- or lineage-specific fashion.

In this chapter, we describe our current knowledge and methodologies for defining the genetic landscapes of lymphomas,

Precision Cancer Therapies: Targeting Oncogenic Drivers and Signaling Pathways in Lymphoid Malignancies: From Concept to Practice, Volume 1, First Edition. Edited by Owen A. O'Connor, Stephen M. Ansell, and John F. Seymour.

noting both common themes and lineage-specific drivers. We will also cover the various classes of targeted therapies and how identification of molecular drivers guides therapeutic development.

Sequencing and Bioinformatics Methods

Many tools have been developed to distinguish molecular drivers from passengers. Some of these tools identify putative driver mutations by predicting the functional impact of identified amino acid changes (Reva et al. 2011; Shihab et al. 2013). For example, if a protein is normally activated upon phosphorylation of a tyrosine residue, then mutation of that tyrosine to phenylalanine can lead to constitutive activation. Nonsense mutations that truncate a protein or frameshift mutations that alter long stretches of amino acid sequence are highly likely to abolish protein function. Hotspot mutations targeting the same amino acid repeatedly across cases are typically gain-of-function and are highly likely to be drivers. Investigators can also compare sequencing results to databases of driver genes and variants in other cancers (e.g. The Cancer Genome Atlas, COSMIC [Forbes et al. 2011, 2015]).

The frequency at which a particular genetic variant is found within a tumor (expressed as variant allele frequency, VAF) may also serve as a clue. A high VAF signifies that a high percentage of tumor cells express that variant; therefore, there is a higher likelihood that variant is a molecular driver. However, VAF is not a perfect indicator as a high VAF can also occur with a neutral mutation that arose early. Other methods take background mutation rates into account and give weight to genes with significantly higher mutation frequencies (Hodis et al. 2012; Lawrence et al. 2013). When feasible, consecutive biopsies of the same patient can allow construction of phylogenetic trees of mutations, which can help pinpoint drivers. This strategy will become more feasible with continual improvement in techniques to analyze circulating tumor DNA from the blood, allowing for frequent, non-invasive sampling.

Another approach analyzes the spatial distribution of variants within a gene. Variants should occur by random chance equally along the length of a gene. If a gene is not a driver, then variants will display an even distribution when assessed across a cohort of tumors. On the other hand, driver gene variants that confer an advantage will exhibit clusters, usually in functional domains.

Numerous methods leverage pathway-based or network-based approaches to identify cancer driver modules that consist of many genes crucial to cancer development (Babaei et al. 2013; Gao et al. 2017; Jia and Zhao 2014; Leiserson et al. 2015). This approach is useful in settings where any one of many genes in a pathway could be mutated to achieve the same effect (e.g. JAK/STAT pathway).

"Meta-predictor" methods and pipelines (Bertrand et al. 2018; Dees et al. 2012; Gonzalez-Perez et al. 2013) rank the candidate genes based on the ranking results of several computational tools that have complementary approaches and analyses. New techniques are continually under development to improve performance, including machine-learning approaches using datasets available from large sequencing studies.

The combination of approaches described above has been the cornerstone of genomic studies that have collectively served to define the drivers of most lymphomas.

Functional Validation of Drivers

Functional validation remains the definitive way to establish whether a particular variant is oncogenic. Such validation studies can take many forms. These include cell-free biochemical assays that are able to confirm changes in protein function, but not necessarily effects on larger cellular processes. These effects must be measured in cell culture-based assays involving primary or immortalized cell lines. Specific variants of interest may be expressed, or genes knocked out to model loss-of-function mutations. Investigators can then measure changes in cell proliferation, cell death, gene expression, or other relevant cellular processes. These types of assays are relatively rapid, cost-effective, and simple to interpret, but phenotypes are restricted to those that are independent of the microenvironment. In addition, it can be challenging to investigate the effects of oncogenic variants in transformed cell lines because they are already selected to proliferate rapidly. Patient-derived xenografts maintain the original genotype(s) of the tumor, but do not always propagate faithfully and lack critical interactions with the microenvironment. Organoid-based assays have been utilized as a way to overcome some of these obstacles while avoiding the complexities of animal models.

Transgenic animal models can be used to investigate effects of molecular drivers in a broader physiological context. This physiological context is particularly important in lymphomas, where malignant cells communicate with and are affected by many different cell types in the microenvironment including other immune cells. Conditional alleles allow tissue-specific or temporal control of increased gene expression or gene knockout. Importantly, the tumorigenic process begins with normal cells within a relevant microenvironment, so investigators can observe the transformative effects of molecular drivers in a context that more closely resembles a human patient.

Genome-wide screens can also be used to functionally identify molecular drivers. Screens can model genetic variants by insertional mutagenesis, transposons, RNA interference, or clustered regularly interspaced short palindromic repeats (CRISPR)-mediated editing. These screens are valuable as an orthogonal method to validate results from genomic studies in patient tumors.

Each of these approaches carries its own significant tradeoffs in terms of ease of use, representativeness of the human tumors, and the ability to test different perturbations including the effects of targeted therapies. The development of new models that reflect the molecular spectrum remains an important and open research question.

Common Themes in B- and T-cell Lymphoma

While Chapter 1 gave a good high-level view of lymphomagenesis, there are a number of important and recurring themes worth emphasizing in the context of identifying important "drivers" of the pathophysiology. As a whole, lymphomas exhibit a high degree of genetic heterogeneity. Lymphoma cells are susceptible to several mutagenic processes that are part of normal lymphocyte development: B/T-cell receptor rearrangement, class-switch recombination and somatic hypermutation. Each time these processes occur, there is a risk of incurring an oncogenic mutation.

Lymphomas that arise from various stages along the B- or T-cell development path have different characteristics including morphology, surface marker expression, immunoglobulin (IG) status, and genetic features. Clinicians use these characteristics to classify lymphomas based on the normal cell type that they originate from ("cell of origin") (Figures 2.1 and 2.2).

There are genetic patterns in lymphomas that reflect differentiation processes that occurred in the cell of origin. B-cell precursors undergo V(D)J recombination to assemble exons that code for the antibody variable region. This process involves creation of double-stranded breaks at the IG locus, which can result in translocations that overexpress oncogenes. Such translocations involving an IG locus can also be a consequence of class-switch recombination (which also involves creation of double-stranded breaks) or somatic hypermutation. These lesions characterize many types of B-cell lymphoma (see Table 2.1).

Activated mature B-cells undergo several rounds of somatic hypermutation in germinal centers to increase antigen affinity. These B-cells also undergo class-switch recombination to alter the antibody isotype and function. The key enzyme (activation-induced cytidine deaminase, or AID) involved in both somatic hypermutation and class-switch recombination can act aberrantly, leading to accumulation of both driver and passenger mutations. There is a recognizable AID mutational signature in these tumors.

Many lymphoma driver genes are related to lymphocyte development and function. *PAX5* and *EBF1* are important transcription factors in normal B-cell lymphocyte development. Both of these genes are genetically altered in B-cell malignancies. T-cell malignancies, on the other hand,

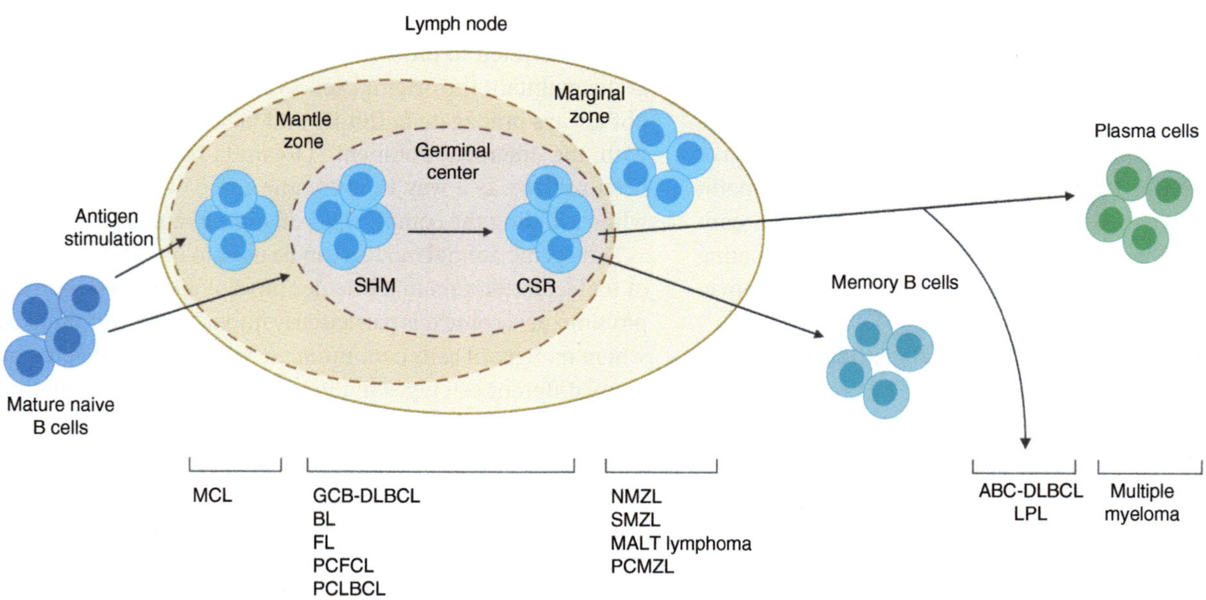

Figure 2.1 B-cell lymphomas and normal cells of origin. Upon antigen stimulation, mature B-cells home to germinal centers where they undergo somatic hypermutation (SHM) and class-switch recombination (CSR) before terminal differentiation into plasma or memory B-cells. Examples of lymphomas that can arise at each B-cell stage are noted. MCL, mantle cell lymphoma; GCB-DLBCL, germinal center B-cell diffuse large B-cell lymphoma; BL, Burkitt's lymphoma; FL, follicular lymphoma; PCFCL, primary cutaneous follicle center lymphoma; PCLBCL, primary cutaneous large B-cell lymphoma; NMZL, nodal marginal zone lymphoma; SMZL, splenic marginal zone lymphoma; MALT, mucosa-associated lymphoid tissue; PCMZL, primary cutaneous marginal zone lymphoma; ABC-DLBCL, activated B-cell like DLBCL; LPL, lymphoplasmacytic lymphoma.

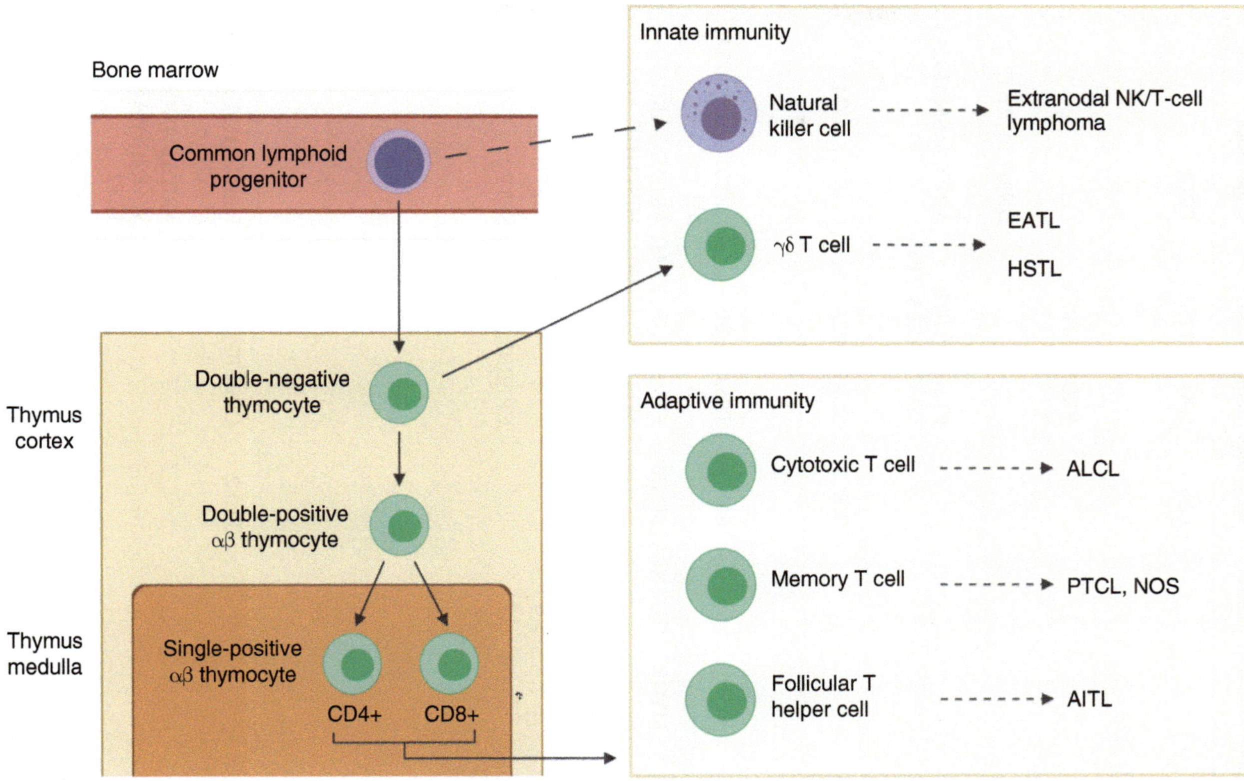

Figure 2.2 T-cell lymphomas and normal cells of origin. T-cell lymphomas can arise at various stages of development and from differentiated T-cells of both innate and adaptive immunity. Examples of these lymphomas are noted. NK, natural killer; EATL, enteropathy-associated T-cell lymphoma; HSTL, hepatosplenic T-cell lymphoma; ALCL, anaplastic large cell lymphoma; PTCL-NOS, peripheral T-cell lymphoma-not otherwise specified; AITL, angioimmunoblastic T-cell lymphoma.

have more frequent genetic events in *LEF1* and *PHF6*, which are important in T-cell lineage commitment.

Components of B- or T-cell receptor signaling are often mutated or activated, triggering survival and proliferation programs that are normally only activated during an immune response. Some of these mutations are specific to lymphomas of either the B- or T-cell lineage. For example, *PLCG1* and CD28 mutations are found in T-cell lymphomas, while *BTK* and CD79B mutations are found in B-cell lymphomas. On the other hand, several genes involved in these pathways are frequently mutated in both lineages indicating shared components of lymphocyte signaling in both lineages.

Lymphocyte receptor signaling feeds into multiple pathways including MAPK, NF-κB, and AKT signaling. Components of these pathways are also frequently mutated in lymphomas and can exhibit a lineage-specific pattern. Several B-cell lymphoma subtypes exhibit mutations in *CARD11*, *TNFAIP3*, and the *MYD88* L265P hotspot mutation. These mutations are rarely found in T-cell lymphomas. On the other hand, *TNFR2* and *NFKB2* are frequently mutated in T- but not B-cell lymphomas. In the MAPK pathway, *KRAS* and *NRAS* are mutated frequently in some T-cell lymphomas subtypes, but plasma cell myeloma is the only B-cell lymphoma that frequently exhibits mutations in these genes.

Lymphocyte migration within germinal centers plays a critical role in the adaptive immune response. Deregulated cell motility can lead to blocks in lymphocyte differentiation or activation that lay the groundwork for acquisition of further driver mutations. Cell motility genes that are frequently mutated in lymphomas include *RHOA* and *GNA13*.

Mutations affecting the Notch pathway are found in both B- and T-cell lymphomas that arise from many stages of lymphocyte development. On the other hand, mutations activating the JAK/STAT pathway are found in nearly all T-cell lymphoma subtypes but are found less frequently in B-cell lymphomas.

Many enzymes involved in epigenetic modifications are mutated in lymphomas. Some of these are involved in DNA methylation (e.g. DNA methyltransferases and TET2), while others modify histones (e.g. SETD2 and histone deacetylases). Loss of these enzymes can lead to widespread disruption of gene regulation and lymphocyte differentiation. It is thought that these mutations occur early in the hematopoietic lineage, impair normal differentiation, and set the stage for successive genetic events that drive lymphomagenesis.

Commonalities in driver genes and pathways can unite rare lymphoma subtypes for basket trials of targeted therapies. Separately, investigators would not be able to accrue sufficient numbers of patients for clinical trials.

Table 2.1 Common translocations and frequently mutated genes in lymphomas.

Subtype	Translocations	B/T-cell receptor signaling	NF-κB signaling	JAK/STAT signaling	Notch signaling	MAPK signaling	AKT signaling	Cell cycle control	Apoptosis	Transcription	Epigenetics	DNA repair
Adult T-cell lymphoma	CTLA4/CD28 fusion ICOS/CD28 fusion	CARD11; CCR4; CCR7; IRF4; PLCG1; PRKCB; VAV1	CARD11; IRF4; PRKCB	STAT3	NOTCH1				FAS	GATA3; TP53	TET2	TP53
Anaplastic large cell lymphoma	t(2;5)(ALK/NPM1)			JAK1; STAT3						PRDM1; TP53		TP53
Angioimmunoblastic T-cell lymphoma	CTLA4/CD28 fusion	CD28; FYN				FYN					DNMT3A; TET2	
Burkitt's lymphoma	t(2;8)(IGK/MYC) t(8;14)(MYC/IGH) t(8;22)(MYC/IGL)				NOTCH1					CREBBP; ID3; MYC; SALL3; TP53	ARID1A; SMARCA4	
Chronic lymphocytic leukemia/Small lymphocytic lymphoma	t(14;18)(IGH/BCL2) t(14;19)(IGH/BCL3)		MYD88; NFKBIE		NOTCH1	BRAF; MAPK1			BIRC3	EGR2; MGA; TP53	CHD2; ZMYM3	ATM; POT1; TP53
Cutaneous T-cell lymphoma		CD28; PLCG1	NFKB2	JAK3; STAT5B					FAS	TP53; ZEB1	ARID1A; DNMT3A; SMARCA4	TP53
Diffuse large B-cell lymphoma (ABC)	BCL2, BCL6, MYC rearrangements	CARD11, CD79B	MYD88		NOTCH2		MTOR	CDKN2A	BIRC6	ETV6; MGA; PIM1; SPEN; TP53; ZEB2	ARID1A; ARID1B; HIST1H1E; MLL2	ATM, TP53
Diffuse large B-cell lymphoma (GCB)	BCL2, BCL6, MYC rearrangements	CARD11, IRF8	TNFRSF14	SOCS1; STAT6	NOTCH2		MTOR		BCL2, BIRC6	CREBBP; EBF1; SPEN; TP53	ARID1A; ARID1B; BCL7A; EZH2; HIST1H1E; MLL2	ATM, TP53
Enteropathy-associated T-cell lymphoma				JAK1; JAK3; SOCS1; STAT3; STAT5B		KRAS; NRAS				CREBBP; TP53	SETD2	TP53
Extranodal marginal zone lymphoma	t(1;14)(BCL10/IGH) t(14;18)(IGH/MALT1) t(11;18)(BIRC3/MALT1)		TNFAIP3									
Follicular lymphoma	t(14;18)(IGH/BCL2)		TNFRSF14	STAT6					BCL2	CREBBP	HIST1H1C-E; EZH2; KMT2D	
Hepatosplenic T-cell lymphoma				STAT3; STAT5B			PIK3CD				ARID1B; INO80; SETD2; SMARCA2; TET3	
Hodgkin's lymphoma			TNFAIP3	PTPN1; SOCS1						EEF1A1	HIST1H1E	

Mantle cell lymphoma	t(2;11)(IGK/CCND1) t(3;14)(BCL6/IGH) t(8;14)(MYC/IGH) t(11;14)(CCND1/IGH) t(11;22)(CCND1/IGL)				NOTCH1; NOTCH2			BIRC3; CCND1; RB1	RB1; TP53	MLL2; MLL3; SMARCA4; WHSC1	ATM; TP53
Mycosis fungoides			TNFR2	JAK3; STAT3		MAPK1			NCOR1		
Natural killer/T-cell lymphoma				JAK3; STAT3; STAT5B		KRAS; NRAS			ASXL3; MGA	ARID1A; EP300; MLL2	TP53
Peripheral T-cell lymphoma										DNMT3A; TET2; TET3	
Plasma cell myeloma	t(4;14)(FGFR3/IGH) t(11;14)(CCND1/IGH)					BRAF; KRAS; NRAS			TP53		TP53
Primary CNS lymphoma	BCL6, MYC, IG rearrangements	CARD11; CD79B; IRF2BP2; IRF4; PRKCD	CARD11; IRF4; MYD88; PRKCD; TNFAIP3				CDKN2A		EBF1; ETV6; PIM1		
Primary cutaneous marginal zone lymphoma	t(3;14)(FOXP1/IGH) t(14;18)(IGH/MALT1) t(11;18)(BIRC3/MALT1)										
Sezary's syndrome	t(12;18)	CARD11; PLCG1	CARD11; TNFR2	JAK1; JAK3; STAT3; STAT5B			CDKN1B			ARID1A; ARID3A; DNMT1; DNMT3A; DNMT3B; SETD family; TET1; TET2	TP53; POT1
Splenic marginal zone lymphoma	t(1;14)(BCL10/IGH) t(2;7)(IGK/CDK6) t(11;14)(CCND1/IGH) t(11;18)(BIRC3/MALT1) t(14;18)(IGH/BCL2) t(14;18)(IGH/MALT1)	CARD11	CARD11; IKBKB; MYD88; TNFAIP3		NOTCH1; NOTCH2		BIRC3		SPEN; TP53	ARID1A; EP300; MLL2; SIN3A	TP53
T-lymphoblastic lymphoma					NOTCH1				NFIL3; PHF6; PRDM2; ZNF91		
Waldenstrom's macroglobulinemia			MYD88							ARID1A; MLL2	

Genetic Landscapes of Lymphomas

Mature B-cell Lymphomas

These lymphomas comprise the majority of B-cell lymphomas. Mantle cell lymphoma (MCL) is characterized by the t(11;14) translocation, which situates *CCND1* next to the IG locus and leads to its overexpression. Genetic studies in MCL also identified frequent mutations in *ATM*, *CCND1*, and *TP53* (Bea et al. 2013; Kridel et al. 2012; Zhang et al. 2014). Notch signaling pathway mutations are also common and have been found to be associated with poor survival in MCL.

Diffuse large B-cell lymphoma (DLBCL) is the most common form of lymphoma in adults. The genetics of DLBCL have been studied extensively and reveal a striking heterogeneity underlying the disease (Lohr et al. 2012; Morin et al. 2011; Pasqualucci et al. 2011; Reddy et al. 2017; Zhang et al. 2013). The disease has been shown to comprise at least two different subtypes that have different underlying biology and responses to therapy: the germinal center B-cell-like (GCB) and activated B-cell-like (ABC) subtypes (Alizadeh et al. 2000; Rosenwald and Staudt 2002; Wright et al. 2003).

Most driver genes are mutated at similar frequencies in the two subtypes, with a few notable exceptions. Genes associated with the GCB subtype include EZH2, *STAT6*, and *BCL2*. Recurring mutations are found in the B-cell development genes *PAX5*, *IKAROS*, and *EBF1*. Activating mutations implicate the JAK/STAT pathway in a subset of DLBCLs.

A subset of cases (of both subtypes) present with chromosomal translocations involving *BCL2*, *BCL6*, and/or *MYC*. While the classification of these tumors may change in the future iterations of the WHO Classification, they are presently referred to as "double-hit" or "triple-hit" lymphomas and are associated with a particularly poor prognosis.

BL is a highly aggressive B-cell lymphoma, characterized by the t(8;14) translocation of *MYC* to the IG locus, which results in high constitutive MYC expression (Swerdlow et al. 2017). Several genomic studies have characterized the genomic somatic mutation landscape in BL (Love et al. 2012; Panea et al. 2019; Richter et al. 2012; Schmitz et al. 2012), implicating mutations in focal adhesion signaling genes *RHOA* and *GNA13*, PI3K pathway genes, as well as mutations in *MYC*, *ID3*, *NOTCH1*, and several chromatin modifiers.

FL is the second most common lymphoma in adults. FL is considered an indolent lymphoma but can undergo transformation into an aggressive disease that appears similar to DLBCL. Most cases of FL carry the t(14;18) translocation of *BCL2* to the IG locus, resulting in overexpression of this oncogene (Swerdlow et al. 2017). High BCL2 expression is usually observed even in translocation-negative cases (Leich et al. 2016).

The various subtypes of marginal zone lymphomas (MZL) differ in their mutational landscapes. Mutations in PTPRD that activate JAK/STAT signaling are frequently found in nodal MZL but are rare in other types. Extranodal MZL and primary cutaneous MZL feature t(14;18) and t(11;18) translocations that activate the NF-κB pathway (Cho-Vega et al. 2006; Du 2017).

The ABC subtype of DLBCL is characterized by mutations in CD79B, MYD88, and other genes involved in B-cell receptor signaling. The mutational landscape of ABC-DLBCL reflects its dependence on B-cell receptor signaling.

Waldenstrom's macroglobulinemia (WM) commonly exhibits the MYD88 L265P hotspot mutation. This variant results in constitutive MYD88 activity and activation of JAK/STAT3 and NF-κB signaling (Bruno et al. 2014). MYD88 L265P is a favorable indicator of ibrutinib response, but accompanying mutations in CXCR4 can lead to resistance (Treon et al. 2015).

Plasma cell (multiple) myeloma is highly dependent on MAPK signaling, with up to 50% of patients exhibiting a mutation in either KRAS or NRAS, or BRAF (Walker et al. 2015). The t(11;14) translocation that results in CCND1 overexpression is also a characteristic driver.

Primary mediastinal B-cell lymphoma (PMBCL) is an aggressive B-cell lymphoma derived from thymic medullary B-cells. PMBCL shows both clinical and genetic similarities to Hodgkin's lymphoma. Both have recurring mutations in B2M, TNFAIP3, and PTPN1. PMBCL also exhibits frequent JAK/STAT pathway mutations in SOCS1 and STAT6 (Gunawardana et al. 2014).

Classic Hodgkin's lymphoma (cHL) has traditionally been classified separately from the non-Hodgkin's lymphomas, but it shares some genetic features with other B-cell lymphomas. Studies have described frequent PTPN1 mutations in cHL, leading to increased activity of JAK/STAT signaling (Gunawardana et al. 2014; Reichel et al. 2015).

T-cell Lymphomas

T-cell lymphoblastic lymphoma (T-LBL) is derived from early T-cell precursors and features frequent mutations in NOTCH1 and genes involved in transcription.

Two T-cell lymphomas are derived from gamma/delta T-cells of the innate immune system: hepatosplenic T-cell lymphoma (HSTL) and enteropathy-associated T-cell lymphoma (EATL). Both exhibit frequent mutations in JAK/STAT pathway genes and the chromatin modifier SETD2. EATL also features frequent KRAS and NRAS mutations. Extranodal NK/T-cell lymphoma is also derived from the innate immune system and features frequent JAK/STAT pathway mutations as well as mutations in MLL2.

The T-cell lymphomas that are derived from T-cells of the adaptive immune response vary widely in their genetic landscapes. Anaplastic large cell lymphoma (ALCL) is derived from cytotoxic T-cells and features recurring mutations in TP53 and the JAK/STAT pathway. ALK gene fusions define a clinically relevant subset.

Peripheral T-cell lymphoma-not otherwise specified (PTCL-NOS), derived from memory T-cells, is the most common form of T-cell lymphoma. PTCL-NOS exhibits frequent mutations in chromatin modifiers and the *RHOA* gene that regulates cell motility.

Angioimmunoblastic T-cell lymphoma (AITL) is derived from T follicular helper cells. AITL also features frequent mutations in chromatin modifiers and RHOA, but also exhibit mutations in T-cell receptor signaling genes. Some cases feature the CTLA4-CD28 gene fusion that promotes T-cell activation.

Adult T-cell lymphoma (ATL) is caused by human T-cell lymphotropic virus (HTLV-1) infection, which leads to constitutively active NF-κB signaling.

Genomic Subgrouping Approaches in DLBCL

DLBCL is the most common form of lymphoma and is characterized by a high degree of both genetic and clinical heterogeneity. While many patients respond well to immunochemotherapy, others relapse quickly or have drug-resistant tumors and require more intensive treatment. The high degree of clinical heterogeneity observed in DLBCL has led to great interest in defining genetic subgroups of this disease to allow more refined prognosis. The aim is to create a system that allows clinicians to classify patients into high- or low-risk categories through genetic characterization of the tumor. The patient's risk level would then inform the most appropriate course of treatment.

Genetic subgroups can also shed light on molecular drivers. Identification of mutated genes that are mutually exclusive or frequently co-occurring can enable a better understanding of the mechanisms underlying lymphomagenesis.

Several investigators have undertaken extensive genomic characterization of DLBCL to define subgroups and refine molecular correlates of prognosis (Chapuy et al. 2016; Reddy et al. 2017; Wright et al. 2020). Because DLBCL is so heterogeneous, a daunting number of samples are needed to discern the prognostic power of various mutations or identify patterns of mutual exclusivity or co-occurrence.

The most commonly utilized classification scheme was defined two decades ago (Alizadeh et al. 2000). This approach classifies DLBCL tumors into two subtypes based on the presumed normal cell of origin whose gene expression profile correlates closely with the tumor. These subtypes are the GCB type, originating from GC B-cells, and an ABC type, derived from a still undetermined post-GC B cell. The GCB subtype has a better prognosis compared to the ABC subtype, so determining a DLBCL patient's subtype by way of sequential immunohistochemistry (the Hans's algorithm [Hans et al. 2004]) has become part of routine clinical workup. However, there still remains a good deal of heterogeneity with respect to clinical outcome and genetic alterations within each of these two groups. Additionally, nearly a third of cases have gene expression profiles intermediate between the GCB and ABC subtypes, so remain unclassified.

Recent efforts to identify molecular subtypes based on genetic alterations have resulted in more complex classification schemes with more groupings (Chapuy et al. 2016; Wright et al. 2020). The results of these studies have highlighted genetic events that likely serve as the molecular drivers of disease (e.g. MYD88 L265P, *BCL2*/*BCL6* translocations, and *TP53* mutations). These classification schemes have potential for identifying effective targeted therapies or promising drug targets for future therapeutic development.

However, there is still a good deal of molecular and clinical heterogeneity within each group. Established survival factors such as *BCL2* and *MYC* expression, Epstein–Barr virus infection, and cell of origin subtype (ABC vs. GCB) still retain prognostic power within these groups. Classification into one group or another still does not fully characterize a patient's risk category. Also, the genetic events that characterize each subgroup are not mutually exclusive. This genetic overlap between subgroups would complicate efforts to classify individual patients in a clinical setting if only a small number of genes were sequenced. On the other hand, the Wright classification scheme failed to assign nearly 40% of tumors to a subgroup. The subgroups defined in these systems are also not completely overlapping, so there remains a lack of consensus on patient stratification.

An alternative approach is to treat patient risk as a continuous variable, with combinations of individual genetic events and gene expression profiles strongly affecting patient survival (Reddy et al. 2017). This approach has the advantage of distilling clinical risk into a smaller number of molecular features, making it simpler to assess in the clinic. However, this approach is limited by the low incidence of individual drivers and the complexity of risk-stratification.

Challenges of Incorporating Genomic Subgrouping Approaches in Clinical Trials

There has been widespread interest in the clinical translation of DLBCL subgroups and their distinct responses to targeted therapies. The largest trials in DLBCL are summarized in Table 2.2. While these trials were supported by seemingly robust preclinical and promising early clinical results, they nevertheless failed to prove that incorporation of a targeted agent was superior to standard therapy.

These trials have provided important lessons in several aspects of clinical trial design. First, the trials identified limitations with existing assays that are used to identify subgroup-based effects. These limitations include assay failures and prolonged turnaround times that can confound upfront

Table 2.2 Recent major clinical trials of targeted therapies in DLBCL.

Trial	Trial design	Subgroup	Improvement over standard therapy?
REMoDL-B (Davies et al. 2019)	R-CHOP + Bortezomib	All DLBCL	No
PHOENIX (Younes et al. 2019)	R-CHOP + Ibrutinib	ABC DLBCL	No
ROBUST (Nowakowski et al. 2016)	R-CHOP + Lenalidomide	ABC DLBCL	No
CAVALLI (Zelenetz et al. 2019)	R-CHOP/G-CHOP + Venetoclax	High risk	PFS potentially improved in BCL2 IHC+

Abbreviations: IHC = immunohistochemistry; PFS = progression-free survival

patient selection. Newer assays that provide robust and timely patient selection strategies are urgently needed. Second, these trials also exposed our limited understanding of the connections between molecular features and targeted therapies.

Shortcomings of preclinical models, the complex biology of patient tumors, and limitations in the design of early phase studies may all have contributed to the observed negative effects in larger trials. While these trials may have interesting subgroup effects, those effects need to be evaluated prospectively. Overall, these findings should nevertheless provide a note of caution in the interpretation of preclinical results and early phase trials.

Leveraging Underlying Pathophysiology to Inform Therapeutic Consideration

The early development in lymphomas was characterized by the combination of different chemotherapy agents. These approaches culminated in a number of different treatment regimens (e.g. CHOP comprising cyclophosphamide, doxorubicin, vincristine, and prednisone) that remain the backbone of upfront treatment of most lymphomas to this day.

With the advent of targeted therapies, there are two main approaches that account for nearly all the new developments in lymphomas in the past two decades:

1) Therapies based on lineage/surface markers
2) Therapies based on inhibiting molecular targets

Genomic studies that can identify both genetic alterations as well as expression have been helpful in development of both approaches. Unlike conventional chemotherapy, patient tumors are generally tested for expression of the surface marker or molecular target before assigning one of these therapies. Variants can be assessed by NGS panels, surface marker expression by immunohistochemistry, and translocations or gene fusions by fluorescence *in situ* hybridization.

In general, surface marker-based therapies take advantage of a protein that is expressed on the surface of tumor cells. In many instances, these proteins reflect the lineage of the tumors (e.g. CD20 in tumors derived from mature B-cells). These therapies generally elicit an immune or microenvironment anti-tumor response, but some treatments can induce direct cell killing. This category comprised such diverse therapies as monoclonal antibodies, antibody–drug conjugates, chimeric antigen receptor (CAR) T-cell therapies, and bi-specific T-cell engagers (BiTE) (Table 2.3). These therapies target all cells that express that particular surface marker and many of these therapies have been highly successful in the clinic. One monoclonal antibody (rituximab) has been such a profound game-changer in the treatment of B-cell lymphoma that the time period following its approval by the FDA in 1997 has been termed "the rituximab era."

Other than rituximab (given as frontline in combination with chemotherapy), these therapies usually do not have established efficacy in the front-line and therefore tend to be used as salvage therapies for relapsed or refractory disease. In addition, some of these treatments remain extremely expensive, and treatments such as CAR-T cell therapy require specialized medical centers to administer and manage side effects.

Genomic studies have also informed the development of inhibitors of molecular targets (Table 2.3). These targets comprise genes frequently mutated in lymphomas (e.g. BCL2 and BRAF) or components of pathways driving tumor growth (e.g. BTK and JAK). In the first case, the variant or activated gene is considered a biomarker for drug efficacy. In the second case, the driver pathway may be activated by one of several mechanisms (e.g. gene copy number changes, genetic variants, and gene fusions) affecting any one of the signaling components, and the effect of the drug is to decrease overall pathway activity. Inhibitors of molecular targets tend to be variably effective and tissue-agnostic, which can lead to systemic side effects. In addition, acquired resistance is nearly always a major problem. Resistance often arises through activation of alternative, compensatory pathways, or acquisition of mutations at the target site that preclude binding of the inhibitor.

This combined understanding of the genetic drivers of lymphomagenesis and the ability to target these lesions remains the most pressing problem of therapeutic development in lymphomas. The solution to this problem will likely occur in the form of many different therapies of incremental improvements that are highly effective for the patients whose tumors harbor those targets.

Table 2.3 Current lymphoma therapeutics and their targets.

Broad therapeutic class		Target(s)	Examples	Lymphoma indications
Cell Surface/ Lineage-expressed proteins	Monoclonal antibodies	CD20	Rituximab, obinutuzumab, ofatumumab	B-cell lymphomas
		CCR4	Mogamulizumab	ATL, PTCL, CTCL
		CD52	Alemtuzumab	PTCL, CTCL, NKTCL
		CD38	Daratumumab, isatuximab	MM, NKTCL, PTCL, DLBCL
		SLAMF7	Elotuzumab	MM
		CD40	Dacetuzumab*	DLBCL, MM, MZL
		ROR1	Cirmtuzumab*	B-cell lymphomas, SLL
	Antibody–drug conjugates	CD79b	Polatuzumab vedotin	DLBCL, other B-cell lymphomas
		CD22	Pinatuzumab vedotin*, inotuzumab ozogamicin	B-cell lymphomas
		CD19	Coltuximab ravtansine*, denintuzumab mafodotin*	B-cell lymphomas
		CD37	IMGN529*	B-cell lymphomas
		B7H3 (CD276)	Mirzotamab clezutoclax*	
		BCMA	Belantamab mafodotin	MM
		CD30	Brentuximab vedotin	CD30+ PTCL, CD30+ CTCL, ALCL, NKTCL, cHL
		ROR1	Zilovertamab vedotin*	B-cell lymphomas, T-cell lymphomas
	Bi-specific T-cell engagers (BiTE)	CD3xBCMA	Elranatamab*, teclistamab*, pavurutamab*	MM
		CD3xCD20	Mosunetuzumab*, glofitamab* Epcoritamab*	B-cell lymphomas
		CD3xFcRH5	Cevostamab*	MM
		CD3xCD19	Blinatumomab	B-cell lymphomas
		CD47xCD20	IMM0306*	B-cell lymphomas
		CD47xCD19	TG-1801*	B-cell lymphomas
	Chimeric antigen receptor (CAR) T cells	CD19	Axicabtagene ciloleucel, brexucabtagene autoleucel, lisocabtagene maraleucel	DLBCL, PMBCL, FL, MCL
		ROR1	ONCT-808**	MCL
		BCMA	Idecabtagene vicleucel	MM
		CD30	CD30 CAR T-cells*	CD30+ ALCL, cHL
Signaling/targeted inhibitors	Single gene/ protein	BTK	Ibrutinib, acalabrutinib Zanubrutinib, and many others	MCL, SLL, MZL, WM
		HDAC6	Ricolinostat*	Lymphomas
		BRAF	Vemurafenib, dabrafenib	MM, non-Hodgkin's lymphomas
	Multigene/ protein	BCL2	Venetoclax	SLL, MCL, MM
		PI3K alpha/delta	Copanlisib, idelalisib, and many others	FL, SLL, DLBCL, MCL
		JAK1/2	Ruxolitinib	PTCL, MF, cHL, MM
		EZH1/2	Tazemetostat, valemetostat*	PTCL, ATL, B-cell lymphomas
		HDAC	Vorinostat, romidepsin, belinostat, panobinostat	CTCL, PTCL, MM
		ALK	Crizotinib, and many others	ALK+ ALCL
		MEK1/2	Cobimetinib	MM, NHL

*Investigative drug.
**Drug in preclinical development.Abbreviations: ALCL = anaplastic large cell lymphoma; ALK = anaplastic lymphoma kinase; ATL= adult T-cell lymphoma; cHL = classic Hodgkin's lymphoma; CTCL = cutaneous T-cell lymphoma; DLBCL = diffuse large B-cell lymphoma; FL = follicular lymphoma; MCL = mantle cell lymphoma; MM = multiple myeloma; MZL = marginal zone lymphoma; MF = mycosis fungoides; NHL = non-Hodgkin's lymphomas; NKTCL = natural killer/T-cell lymphoma; PMBCL = primary mediastinal B-cell lymphoma; PTCL = peripheral T-cell lymphoma; SLL = small lymphocytic lymphoma; WM = Waldenstrom's macroglobulinemia.

Conclusion

Here we have discussed the genetics and major genetic drivers that affect lymphomas. These driver genes and pathways can potentially inform diagnosis, prognosis, and therapeutic decisions. Our understanding of these drivers has been greatly accelerated by the advent of genomic technologies, particularly NGS.

However, there remain gaps in our knowledge of the complete spectrum of genetic drivers in lymphomas. First, many rare lymphoma types have been studied very little or not at all. A comprehensive approach is needed to understand how each different pathologically defined lymphoma type or subtype is similar or different from all others. Second, many racial and ethnic groups have not been adequately represented in previous genomic studies. Thus, there are gaps in our knowledge of how lymphoma drivers differently affect individuals of African, Asian, and other ethnic/racial groups. We need comprehensive and inclusive efforts that develop a systematic understanding of lymphoma drivers. Such approaches would greatly enable diagnostic and therapeutic development across the entire spectrum of lymphomas.

In some ways, the advent of NGS has been a mixed blessing for clinical applications. While NGS has undeniably advanced our understanding of the drivers of lymphomas, this understanding has not kept pace with our ability to connect these drivers with new therapies. Further, the extensive classification and subclassification has also made it challenging to perform well-powered and timely clinical trials.

The tools for translating NGS also remain somewhat limited. While most discovery studies utilize exome-wide or genome-wide DNA and RNA sequencing, the application of NGS in the clinic remains, for the most part, limited to small panels of mostly DNA sequencing. This gulf between discovery tools and clinical assays remains wide, and the process of clinical translation for even seemingly minor findings (e.g. a new driver gene) can take months or years. Reimbursement for these tests can be uncertain, further disincentivizing the process of clinical translation.

For these reasons, the clinical application of our knowledge of lymphoma drivers continues to remain a work in progress. These steps can be collectively addressed through the development of well-powered "basket" clinical trials where enrollment of patients is determined based on the specific genetic lesion(s) or subgroup identified alongside carefully chosen controls who receive standard-of-care.

The rarity of many lymphomas renders it nearly impossible for a single institution to accumulate sufficient numbers of patient samples. Fortunately, emerging data has begun to identify shared common driver pathways that can enable clinical trials and treatment strategies that go beyond histological classification and deliver new therapies where they are urgently needed.

The past decade has witnessed an explosion in our understanding of the genetic drivers of lymphoma in a manner that would have likely been unimaginable in the decade prior. The main task of the upcoming years is to translate those discoveries into effective therapies and develop the tools to ensure that the gains of those discoveries are spread effectively and equitably for all patients with lymphomas.

Must Read References

These papers describe driver discovery approaches that have been utilized across the spectrum of lymphomas.

Reddy A., Zhang J., Davis N.S. et al. (2017). Genetic and functional drivers of diffuse large B cell lymphoma. *Cell* 171 (2): 481–494.e15.

This paper describes comprehensive genetic driver discovery, as well as a functional genomics approach that demonstrates the downstream effects of molecular drivers.

Chapuy B., Cheng H., Watahiki A. et al. (2016). Diffuse large B-cell lymphoma patient-derived xenograft models capture the molecular and biological heterogeneity of the disease. *Blood* 127 (18): 2203–2213.

This paper describes genetic subgroupings of DLBCL and correlates of patient outcome.

Schmitz R., Wright G.W., Huang D.W. et al. (2018). Genetics and pathogenesis of diffuse large B-cell lymphoma. *N. Engl. J. Med.* 378 (15): 1396–1407.

This paper describes genetic subgroupings of DLBCL and correlates of patient outcome.

References

Alizadeh, A.A., Eisen, M.B., Davis, R.E. et al. (2000). Distinct types of diffuse large B-cell lymphoma identified by gene expression profiling. *Nature* 403: 503–511.

Babaei, S., Hulsman, M., Reinders, M. et al. (2013). Detecting recurrent gene mutation in interaction network context using multi-scale graph diffusion. *BMC Bioinform.* 14: 29.

Bea, S., Valdes-Mas, R., Navarro, A. et al. (2013). Landscape of somatic mutations and clonal evolution in mantle cell lymphoma. *Proc. Natl. Acad. Sci. U.S.A.* 110 (45): 18250–18255.

Bertrand, D., Drissler, S., Chia, B.K. et al. (2018). ConsensusDriver improves upon individual algorithms for predicting driver alterations in different cancer types and individual patients. *Cancer Res.* 78 (1): 290–301.

Bruno, A., Boisselier, B., Labreche, K. et al. (2014). Mutational analysis of primary central nervous system lymphoma. *Oncotarget* 5 (13): 5065–5075.

Chapuy, B., Cheng, H., Watahiki, A. et al. (2016). Diffuse large B-cell lymphoma patient-derived xenograft models capture the molecular and biological heterogeneity of the disease. *Blood* 127 (18): 2203–2213.

Cho-Vega, J.H., Vega, F., Rassidakis, G. et al. (2006). Primary cutaneous marginal zone B-cell lymphoma. *Am. J. Clin. Pathol.* 125 Suppl: S38–49.

Davies, A., Cummin, T.E., Barrans, S. et al. (2019). Gene-expression profiling of bortezomib added to standard chemoimmunotherapy for diffuse large B-cell lymphoma (REMoDL-B): an open-label, randomised, phase 3 trial. *Lancet Oncol.* 20 (5): 649–662.

Dees, N.D., Zhang, Q., Kandoth, C. et al. (2012). MuSiC: identifying mutational significance in cancer genomes. *Genome Res.* 22 (8): 1589–1598.

Du, M.Q. (2017). MALT lymphoma: genetic abnormalities, immunological stimulation and molecular mechanism. *Best Pract. Res. Clin. Haematol.* 30 (1–2): 13–23.

Forbes, S.A., Beare, D., Gunasekaran, P. et al. (2015). COSMIC: exploring the world's knowledge of somatic mutations in human cancer. *Nucleic Acids Res.* 43 (Database issue): D805–11.

Forbes, S.A., Bindal, N., Bamford, S. et al. (2011). COSMIC: mining complete cancer genomes in the Catalogue of Somatic Mutations in Cancer. *Nucleic Acids Res.* 39(Database issue): D945–50.

Gao, B., Li, G., Liu, J. et al. (2017). Identification of driver modules in pan-cancer via coordinating coverage and exclusivity. *Oncotarget* 8 (22): 36115–36126.

Gonzalez-Perez, A., Perez-Llamas, C., Deu-Pons, J. et al. (2013). IntOGen-mutations identifies cancer drivers across tumor types. *Nat. Methods* 10 (11): 1081–1082.

Gunawardana, J., Chan, F.C., Telenius, A. et al. (2014). Recurrent somatic mutations of PTPN1 in primary mediastinal B cell lymphoma and Hodgkin lymphoma. *Nat. Genet.* 46 (4): 329–335.

Hanahan, D. and Weinberg, R.A. (2011). Hallmarks of cancer: the next generation. *Cell* 144 (5): 646–674.

Hans, C.P., Weisenburger, D.D., Greiner, T.C. et al. (2004). Confirmation of the molecular classification of diffuse large B-cell lymphoma by immunohistochemistry using a tissue microarray. *Blood* 103 (1): 275–282.

Hodis, E., Watson, I.R., Kryukov, G.V. et al. (2012). A landscape of driver mutations in melanoma. *Cell* 150 (2): 251–263.

Jia, P. and Zhao, Z. (2014). VarWalker: personalized mutation network analysis of putative cancer genes from next-generation sequencing data. *Plos Comput. Biol.* 10 (2): e1003460.

Kridel, R., Meissner, B., Rogic, S. et al. (2012). Whole transcriptome sequencing reveals recurrent NOTCH1 mutations in mantle cell lymphoma. *Blood* 119 (9): 1963–1971.

Lawrence, M.S., Stojanov, P., Polak, P. et al. (2013). Mutational heterogeneity in cancer and the search for new cancer-associated genes. *Nature* 499 (7457): 214–218.

Leich, E., Hoster, E., Wartenberg, M. et al. (2016). Similar clinical features in follicular lymphomas with and without breaks in the BCL2 locus. *Leukemia* 30 (4): 854–860.

Leiserson, M.D., Vandin, F., Wu, H.T. et al. (2015). Pan-cancer network analysis identifies combinations of rare somatic mutations across pathways and protein complexes. *Nat. Genet.* 47 (2): 106–114.

Lohr, J.G., Stojanov, P., Lawrence, M.S. et al. (2012). Discovery and prioritization of somatic mutations in diffuse large B-cell lymphoma (DLBCL) by whole-exome sequencing. *Proc. Natl. Acad. Sci. U.S.A.* 109 (10): 3879–3884.

Love, C., Sun, Z., Jima, D. et al. (2012). The genetic landscape of mutations in Burkitt lymphoma. *Nat. Genet.* 44 (12): 1321–1325.

Morin, R.D., Mendez-Lago, M., Mungall, A.J. et al. (2011). Frequent mutation of histone-modifying genes in non-Hodgkin lymphoma. *Nature* 476 (7360): 298–303.

Nowakowski, G.S., Chiappella, A., Witzig, T.E. et al. (2016). ROBUST: lenalidomide-R-CHOP versus placebo-R-CHOP in previously untreated ABC-type diffuse large B-cell lymphoma. *Future Oncol.* 12 (13): 1553–1563.

Panea, R.I., Love, C.L., Shingleton, J.R. et al. (2019). The whole genome landscape of Burkitt lymphoma subtypes. *Blood 134 (19): 1598–1607.*

Pasqualucci, L., Trifonov, V., Fabbri, G. et al. (2011). Analysis of the coding genome of diffuse large B-cell lymphoma. *Nat. Genet.* 43 (9): 830–837.

Reddy, A., Zhang, J., Davis, N.S. et al. (2017). Genetic and functional drivers of diffuse large B cell lymphoma. *Cell* 171 (2): 481–94.e15.

Reichel, J., Chadburn, A., Rubinstein, P.G. et al. (2015). Flow sorting and exome sequencing reveal the oncogenome of primary Hodgkin and Reed-Sternberg cells. *Blood* 125 (7): 1061–1072.

Reva, B., Antipin, Y., and Sander, C. (2011). Predicting the functional impact of protein mutations: application to cancer genomics. *Nucleic Acids Res.* 39 (17): e118.

Richter, J., Schlesner, M., Hoffmann, S. et al. (2012). Recurrent mutation of the ID3 gene in Burkitt lymphoma identified by integrated genome, exome and transcriptome sequencing. *Nat. Genet.* 44 (12): 1316.

Rosenwald, A. and Staudt, L.M. (2002). Clinical translation of gene expression profiling in lymphomas and leukemias. *Semin. Oncol.* 29 (3): 258–263.

Schmitz, R., Young, R.M., Ceribelli, M. et al. (2012). Burkitt lymphoma pathogenesis and therapeutic targets from structural and functional genomics. *Nature* 490 (7418): 116–120.

Shihab, H.A., Gough, J., Cooper, D.N. et al. (2013). Predicting the functional consequences of cancer-associated amino acid substitutions. *Bioinformatics (Oxford, England)* 29 (12): 1504–1510.

Swerdlow, S.H., Campo, E., Harris, N.L. et al. (2017). *WHO Classification of Tumours of Haematopoietic and Lymphoid Tissues*, Revised 4e. Lyon France: IARC Press.

Treon, S.P., Tripsas, C.K., Meid, K. et al. (2015). Ibrutinib in previously treated Waldenstrom's macroglobulinemia. *N. Engl. J. Med.* 372 (15): 1430–1440.

Walker, B.A., Boyle, E.M., Wardell, C.P. et al. (2015). Mutational spectrum, copy number changes, and outcome: results of a sequencing study of patients with newly diagnosed myeloma. *J. Clin. Oncol.* 33 (33): 3911–3920.

Wright, G., Tan, B., Rosenwald, A. et al. (2003). A gene expression-based method to diagnose clinically distinct subgroups of diffuse large B cell lymphoma. *Proc. Natl. Acad. Sci. U.S.A.* 100 (17): 9991–9996.

Wright, G.W., Huang, D.W., Phelan, J.D. et al. (2020). A probabilistic classification tool for genetic subtypes of diffuse large B cell lymphoma with therapeutic implications. *Cancer Cell* 37 (4): 551–68.e14.

Younes, A., Sehn, L.H., Johnson, P. et al. (2019). Randomized phase III trial of ibrutinib and rituximab plus cyclophosphamide, doxorubicin, vincristine, and prednisone in non-germinal center B-cell diffuse large B-cell lymphoma. *J. Clin. Oncol.* 37 (15): 1285–1295.

Zelenetz, A.D., Salles, G., Mason, K.D. et al. (2019). Venetoclax plus R- or G-CHOP in non-Hodgkin lymphoma: results from the CAVALLI phase 1b trial. *Blood* 133 (18): 1964–1976.

Zhang, J., Grubor, V., Love, C.L. et al. (2013). Genetic heterogeneity of diffuse large B-cell lymphoma. *Proc. Natl. Acad. Sci. U.S.A.* 110 (4): 1398–1403.

Zhang, J., Jima, D., Moffitt, A.B. et al. (2014). The genomic landscape of mantle cell lymphoma is related to the epigenetically determined chromatin state of normal B cells. *Blood 123 (19): 2988–2996.*

3

Characterizing the Spectrum of Epigenetic Dysregulation Across Lymphoid Malignancies

Sean Harrop[1], Michael Dickinson[1,2], Ricky Johnstone[1,2], and Henry Miles Prince[1,2,3]

[1] *Peter MacCallum Cancer Centre, Melbourne, Victoria, Australia*
[2] *Sir Peter MacCallum Department of Oncology, University of Melbourne, Melbourne, Victoria, Australia*
[3] *Epworth Healthcare, Sir Peter MacCallum Department of Oncology, University of Melbourne, Victoria, Australia*

Take Home Messages

- Epigenetic regulation is necessary for normal lymphocyte development, cellular differentiation, and immune response.
- Epigenetic alterations play a significant role in lymphomagenesis, largely through DNA methylation and histone modification that result in changes in gene expression.
- Mutations resulting in gain- and loss-of-function of epigenetic proteins are seen in varying frequency and different combinations across the different lymphoid malignancies.
- These aberrations are attractive therapeutic targets with epigenetic targeted therapies becoming established in T-cell disorders and emerging in certain B-cell malignancies.

Introduction: Epigenetics and Lymphoid Malignancies

Cancers have a distinct pattern of disrupted cell signaling pathways, which are the result not only of genetic alterations but also of disrupted gene regulation. Epigenetics describes the regulation of the transcription of this genetic information independent of DNA sequence usually via DNA methylation or histone modification. The epigenome is critical for normal lymphocyte development and in mediating cell differentiation and immune response via selective gene suppression. Distinct patterns of DNA methylation have been shown to involve in immune cell growth including T-cell activity and B-cell development (Béguelin et al. 2013; Lee et al. 2001; Shaknovich et al. 2011). Alterations in DNA methylation patterns, either DNA global hypomethylation or promoter-localized hypermethylation, often result in silencing of tumor suppressor genes and affect a plethora of cellular functions leading to changes in the microenvironment and immune response (Marks et al. 2016; Nishida et al. 2020).

Epigenetic dysregulation has been shown to have a role in the pathogenesis of most hematological malignancies although epigenetic variability, which is central to tumor heterogeneity, has made it difficult to establish epigenetic alterations as key drivers of oncogenesis (Easwaran et al. 2014). There is recognition that the deregulated epigenome is reflective of the underlying lymphoid maturation stage and these epimutations are now regarded as hallmark features of certain lymphoid cancers. These epigenetic mutations have been utilized to define clinically relevant subtypes within existing entities. Furthermore, these "epigenetic vulnerabilities" can be exploited therapeutically.

The implications of epigenetic mutations across lymphoproliferative diseases are variable. In B-cell malignancies for example, and particularly for follicular lymphoma (FL), these clonal epimutations are often early in cellular development and usually lead to transcriptionally repressive mutations affecting histone post-translational modification. This subsequently impairs normal differentiation and promotes lymphomagenesis by altering the expression of genes critical for B-cell signaling while cooperating with anti-apoptotic proteins. On the other hand, the T-cell malignancies are increasingly being seen as "epigenetic diseases" that are becoming defined by their epimutational profile which is seemingly distinct from the B-cell disorders. There are frequent loss-of-function mutations in proteins active in DNA methylation pathways which lead to global changes in the methylation profile. Indeed, many of the epigenetic gene variants seen in

Precision Cancer Therapies: Targeting Oncogenic Drivers and Signaling Pathways in Lymphoid Malignancies: From Concept to Practice, Volume 1, First Edition. Edited by Owen A. O'Connor, Stephen M. Ansell, and John F. Seymour.

T-cell lymphomas are analogous to those associated with the prototypical epigenetic myeloid disorders such as the myelodysplastic syndromes. This reliance on epigenetic disruption has proven useful clinically with "epigenetically active" agents proving potent across many subtypes of T-cell lymphomas.

Dysregulation of DNA Methylation and Modification of Histone Proteins

In normal cellular development and homeostasis, the methylation of cytosine residues mediates gene imprinting and tissue-specific gene expression. The aberrant hypermethylation of cytosine residues in CpG dinucleotides or "CpG Islands" near promoter regions of DNA is a common feature seen among many types of cancer (McCabe et al. 2009; Pike et al. 2008). The DNA of cancer cells contains hypomethylated areas with deregulation of the distinction between methylated and unmethylated genomic regions. Characteristic of the cancer epigenome is the modification of enzymes that catalyze this aberrant DNA methylation (Table 3.1). These enzymes bind methylated DNA at promoter sites and contribute to tumor suppressor gene silencing (McCabe et al. 2009). Histone proteins are the central component of nucleosomal subunits which themselves compose key building blocks of chromatin, a dynamic structure that packages DNA. There are four core histone proteins (H2A, H2B, H3, and H4), each with a side chain that is subject to extensive post-translational modification that alters the chromatin conformational structure, which in turn affects transcriptional processing. The H1 histone protein binds to the nucleosome and the entry and exit sites of DNA acting as a linker (Bannister and Kouzarides 2011). Aberrancies of histone post-translational modification, both at a global genomic level and at specific gene loci, can result in silencing of tumor suppressors or activation of oncogenes and are frequently seen in human cancers (Table 3.1) (Audia and Campbell 2016).

Table 3.1 Frequent epigenome and chromatin modifier gene variants in lymphoid malignancies.

Gene abbreviation	Gene name	Function of wild-type gene	Lymphoid malignancies with recurrent variants
KMT2D	Lysine (K)-specific methyltransferase 2D	H3K4 methylase: activator	FL (76–89%), DLBCL (30%), MCL (30%), MZL (11%)
KMT2A	Lysine (K)-specific methyltransferase 2A	H3K4 methylase: activator	ALL (33–80%)
EZH2	Enhancer of zeste 2 polycomb repressive complex 2 subunit	H3K27 methylase: repressor	FL (7–27%), DLBCL GCB (22%)
CREBBP	CREB binding protein	H3K27 and H3K18 acetylase: activator	FL (33–68%), DLBCL GCB (32%), DLBCL ABC (13%), MZL (~5%)
EP300	E1A binding protein p300	H3K27 and H3K18 acetylase: activator	FL (9%), DLBCL (10%)
DMT3A	DNA methyltransferase 3A	DNA methylation of specific CpG structures	AITL (25–33%), PTCLNOS (27%), SS (8%)
IDH2	Isocitrate dehydrogenase 2	Decarboxylation of isocitrate to 2-oxoglutarate	AITL (20%), PTCLNOS (7%)
TET2	Ten-Eleven Translocase 2	Catalyzes methylcytosine to 5-hydroxymethylcytosine.	AITL (80%), SS (10%)
ARID1A	AT-rich interactive domain 1A (SWI-like)	SWI/SNF chromatin remodeling complex	BL (30%), FL (9–11%)
SMARCA4	SWI/SNF related, matrix-associated, actin-dependent regulator of chromatin, subfamily A, member 4		
CHD2	Chromodomain helicase DNA binding protein 2	Chromatin remodeling	CLL (5%)
SETD2	SET domain containing 2	H3K36 methylase: activator	EATL (32%), ALL (12%), CLL (2%)

Abbreviations: FL = follicular lymphoma; DLBCL = diffuse large B-cell lymphoma germinal center subtype; DLBCL ABC = DLBCL activated B-cell type; MCL = mantle cell lymphoma; MZL = marginal zone lymphoma; CLL = chronic lymphocytic leukemia; BL = Burkitt's lymphoma; ALL = acute lymphoblastic leukemia; PTCL = peripheral T-cell lymphoma – not otherwise specified; AITL = angioimmunoblastic lymphoma; SS = Sezary's syndrome.

Genes Involved in Histone Modification Implicated in Lymphomagenesis

Enhancer of Zeste Homolog 2 (EZH2)

The polycomb repressive complex 2 (PCR2) has histone methyltransferase activity and methylates histone H3 on lysine 27 (H3K27me3) leading to gene suppression. The enzymatic subunit of the PCR2 is the enhancer of zeste homolog 2 (EZH2). Expression of mutant EZH2 hampers germinal center differentiation, downregulates MHC Class I/II, and drives aberrant proliferation (Béguelin et al. 2013; Ennishi et al. 2019). EZH2 has been shown to be mutated and overexpressed in several lymphoma subtypes and was the first epigenetic regulator mutation to be reported in FL (Morin et al. 2010). In most lymphoid malignant contexts, EZH2 is overexpressed and tumorigenic, yet it is repressed and acts as a tumor suppressor in T-cell acute lymphoblastic leukemia (T-ALL) (León et al. 2020). Gain-of-function somatic mutations of EZH2 at Y641 in the catalytic SET domain are frequently detected in FL (15–25%) and GCB subtype diffuse large B-cell lymphomas (DLBCL) (20%) where it is linked to lymphomagenesis and large-cell transformation (see Section "Follicular Lymphoma") (Bödör et al. 2013; Bouska et al. 2017; Morin et al. 2011). EZH2 mutations also repress anti-tumor immunity via suppression of the CXCL10-CXCR3 axis, which is important in T-cell migration in inflammatory conditions and the peripheral T-cell lymphomas (PTCL) such as adult T-cell lymphoma (ATLL) (Fujikawa et al. 2016; Peng et al. 2015).

CREB-binding Protein (CREBBP) and Histone Acetyltransferase P300 (EP300)

CREBBP and *EP300* belong to the KAT3 family of histone/protein lysine acetyltransferases. *CREBBP* is regarded as a tumor suppressor and codes for the cAMP response element-binding protein (CREB) which catalyzes histone acetylation. Mutations are highly recurrent in B-cell lymphomas and either inactivate its histone acetyltransferase domain or truncate the protein (Pasqualucci et al. 2011). *CREBBP* knock-out mice lose their MHCII expression and form hyperproliferative germinal center B-cells leading to lymphoma development. This loss of *CREBBP* has been demonstrated to cooperate with *Bcl2* overexpression to promote lymphomagenesis (García-Ramírez et al. 2017; Hashwah et al. 2017). *CREBBP* is functionally opposed by the BCL6/HDAC3 oncorepressor complex. In fact, HDAC3 selective inhibitors have reversed *CREBBP* mutant aberrant epigenetic programming *in vitro* (Jiang et al. 2017). *CREBBP* also plays a critical role in supporting p53 dependent tumor suppressor functions and is inhibited by viral basic leucine zipper transcription factor HBZ encoded by HTLV-1 (human T-cell lymphotropic virus) (Grossman 2001; Wurm et al. 2012). Histone acetyltransferase p300 (*EP300*) is closely related to *CREBBP* and plays a similar role by modifying lysine residues on both histone and non-histone nuclear proteins. *EP300* mutations have also been identified as a major oncogenic pathway in DLBCL and FL (Pasqualucci et al. 2011).

The H3K4 Methyltransferase Family

Histone lysine methyltransferase 2 (KMT2) proteins form complexes that methylate lysine 4 on histone H3 (H3K4) and are among the most frequently mutated in human cancers (Rao and Dou 2015). *KMT2A* (previously known as mixed lineage leukemia 1, MLL1) rearrangements are pathogenic drivers of pediatric acute lymphoblastic leukemia and associated with a poorer survival (Andersson et al. 2015). *KMT2D* (*MLL2*) and *KTM2C* (*MLL3*) are some of the most frequently mutated genes in FL (~70% of cases) and to a lesser extent DLBCL (~25% of cases) (Green 2018; Solène et al. 2019); KMT2D functions as a tumor suppressor and deficiency impedes B-cell differentiation and signaling pathways (Ortega-Molina et al. 2015; Zhang et al. 2015). *KMT2C* and *KMT2D* mutations are not mutually exclusive, suggesting that these genes may have non-redundant functioning. Mutations have also been seen in T-cell lymphomas, with up to 36% of patients with PTCL-NOS (peripheral T-cell lymphoma – not otherwise specified) subtype carrying the mutation (Ji et al. 2018).

The Bromodomain and Extra-Terminal Domain (BET) Family

The bromodomain and extra-terminal (BET) protein family (BRD2, BRD3, BRD4, and BRDT) recognize epigenetic modifications and regulate gene expression by binding to acetylated lysine residues on histones. After binding, BET proteins recruit other transcriptional regulators such as pTEFb generally leading to an increase in transcriptional output. The BET family is known to activate key oncogenes such as *MYC*, *CCND1*, and *CCN1*. Commonly upregulated in many cancers it is currently unclear what contribution they play in the development of malignancy. While a mechanistically attractive target preclinically, trials of small molecule inhibitors that competitively bind the bromodomain have been somewhat disappointing for the treatment of lymphoma to date (Fujisawa and Filippakopoulos 2017; Mita and Mita 2020).

Genes Involved in DNA Methylation Implicated in Lymphomagenesis

DNA Methyltransferase 3A (DNMT3A)

DNMT3A functions as a DNA methyltransferase catalyzing cytosine methylation of CpG islands in promoters leading to transcriptional silencing. *DNMT3A* is critical for hematopoietic stem cell differentiation and mutations in lymphoid malignancies are thought to be early events (Challen et al. 2011). Mutations in *DNMT3A* have also been identified in about 11–33% of PTCL patients due to missense or nonsense mutation and frequently coexist with mutated *TET2*. The interaction between mutated *DNMT3A* (thought to decrease global DNA methylation levels) and loss of *TET2* (thought to increase global DNA methylation levels) generates a complex methylation landscape with increased DNA methylation and reduced expression of several tumor suppressors and hypomethylation and overexpression of important T-cell genes such as *Notch1* (Couronné et al. 2012). In T-cell acute lymphoblastic leukemia (T-ALL), biallelic mutations are more common than in myeloid cancers suggesting *DNMT3A* is a tumor suppressor in this disease (Roller et al. 2013). *DNMT3A* mutations in T-ALL are associated with poorer outcomes (Van Vlierberghe et al. 2013)

Ten-Eleven Translocation 1/2 (TET1/2)

The ten-eleven translocation 2 (*TET2*) gene encodes an alpha-ketoglutarate dependent dioxygenase, which converts 5-methylcytosine (5mC) to 5-hydroxymethylcytosine (5hmC), 5-formylcytosine (5fC), and 5-carboxylcytosine (5caC) (He et al. 2011; Ito et al. 2011; Tahiliani et al. 2009). Oxidation of 5mC is part of a demethylation pathway that influences transcriptional activation, where hypermethylation leads to silencing of gene expression, while hypomethylation leads to gene expression (François et al. 2018). The TET family of proteins is also known to be important in T-cell differentiation, where loss-of-function mutations can lead to T-cell lymphoma with follicular helper cell-like features (Lemonnier et al. 2012). *TET2* mutations are seen in up to 70% of PTCL patients. Specifically, it is estimated that *TET* mutations are found in 42–83% of patients with angioimmunoblastic T-cell lymphoma (AITL), 28–48.5% of patients with PTCL-NOS, and 10% of patients with adult T-cell leukemia and lymphoma (ATLL) (Couronné et al. 2012; Nagata et al. 2016; Odejide et al. 2014). TET2 function has also been shown to be critical for germinal center and plasma cell differentiation, and its deficiency has been associated with the development of GC-subtype DLBCL (Rosikiewicz et al. 2020). Moreover, there can be interactions between the various epigenetic modulators. For example, wild-type *DNMTA3* binding occurs when there is less CpG density compared to *TET1* binding, which occurs at a relatively higher CpG density. Both affect the PCR2-mediated methylation of lysine 27 of histone H3 (H3K27), which leads to enrichment of trimethylation at H3K27 which ultimately influences gene expression (Gu et al. 2018).

Isocitrate Dehydrogenase 2 (IDH2)

Mutations in isocitrate dehydrogenase 2 (*IDH2*), especially at the R172 residue, are frequently identified in AITL (Cairns et al. 2012). Mutations in *IDH2* alter the catalytic reactions of the Krebs cycle. Wild-type IDH converts isocitrate to a-ketoglutarate, a key cofactor in the oxidative demethylase reactions which remove methyl-groups from DNA. Mutant *IDH2* converts isocitrate to 2-hydroxyglutarate (2HG), which is an oncogenic metabolite that cannot function as an obligatory cofactor of TET catalytic functions (Figueroa et al. 2010). Mutations in *IDH2* and *TET2* reduce 5hmC levels due to global hypermethylation of promoters and CpG islands (leading to transcriptional repression and gene silencing), likely contributing to lymphomagenesis (François et al. 2018).

The Epigenetic Landscape of Specific Lymphoid Malignancies

Oncogenesis is a complex process composed of distinct "Hallmarks" many of which result in the dysregulation of signaling pathways intrinsic to malignant cells, while others involve the interplay between the malignant cell and the non-neoplastic tumor microenvironment (Hanahan and Weinberg 2011). Lymphomagenesis has many of these characteristics and in addition, in select subtypes, the neoplastic transformation can be driven by viruses and chronic immunoinflammation (Coussens and Werb 2002). The level of epigenetic activity and dysregulation is reflective of not only a consequence of lymphomagenesis but also of the distinct stage of differentiation, for example the acquirement of somatic alterations in B-cell lymphomas is a critical determinant of the B-cell stage at point of malignant transformation.

Follicular Lymphoma

Follicular lymphoma (FL) is defined genetically by the t(14;18) translocation leading to constitutive overexpression of the anti-apoptotic BCL2 protein; however, it is recognized that despite the survival advantage conveyed by the translocation it is not sufficient in itself for lymphomagenesis (Kridel et al. 2012; Tsujimoto et al. 1985). Aberrancies in epigenetic regulation are now recognized as a hallmark of FL with mutations seen in almost all patients (>90%) and have emerged as a key feature in the pathogenesis of FL. The histone transferases *KMT2D* (80%), EZH2 (25%), *CREBBP* (33–68%), and *EP300* (9%) are frequently mutated and clonal evolution studies have demonstrated that these mutations occur early in oncogenesis and result in a pattern of gene repression centering on key lysine residues, H3K4 and H3K27 (Bödör et al. 2013; Morin et al. 2010, 2011; Pasqualucci et al. 2011). This epigenetic landscape has been found to overlap substantially with germinal center cell of origin diffuse large B-cell lymphoma (GCB DLBCL) (Morin et al. 2010). Loss of *KMT2D* alters the expression of genes responsible for B-cell and JAK/STAT signaling leading to impairment of B-cell differentiation. The loss of *CREBBP* function also impacts terminal differentiation and cooperates with BCL2 to contribute to MHCII downregulation and avoidance of immune surveillance. *EP300* and *CREBBP* are similar structurally with distinct but overlapping functions (Hashwah et al. 2017). Most histone modifiers are subject to loss-of-function mutations in FL with the notable exception of EZH2 which are gain-of-function in FL and lead to increased marking of H3K27me3 associated with differentiation block.

These epigenetic aberrations have prognostic implications, and several have been incorporated in the clinicogenetic risk model which combines clinical factors with mutations in seven genes that include several that are important for epigenetic modification of the genome – EZH2, CREBBP, ARID1A, and EP300 (Pastore et al. 2015). With respect to standard chemoimmunotherapy, the M7-FLIPI (Table 3.2) was validated in the GALLIUM cohort which compared obinutuzumab-based chemotherapy to rituximab-based chemotherapy. Moreover, mutations in EZH2 were associated with superior progression-free-survival in patients treated with CHOP or CVP-based regimens but not bendamustine based (Jurinovic et al. 2019).

Beyond standard chemoimmunotherapy, the enrichment of epigenetic mutations in FL has led to the pursuit of therapeutics that exploit these genetic variants for more targeted therapies. Therapies with broad epigenomic activity such as the histone deacetylase (HDAC) inhibitors have been evaluated in FL with modest activity (Ogura et al. 2014). The efficacy of targeted EZH2 inhibitors such as tazemetostat, which the US Food and Drug Administration (FDA) approved in 2020 for use in relapsed/refractory FL, has been more promising. Tazemetostat inhibits both mutant and wild-type EZH2 via inhibition of cofactor S-adenosyl-L-methionine (SAM) which is required for EZH2 function. A phase two trial reported durable responses in a heavily pretreated population of 99 patients. Mutations in EZH2 were associated with superior overall response rates (69% ORR) compared to EZH2 wild-type patients (35% ORR) (Morschhauser et al. 2020).

Table 3.2 M7 FLIPI prognostic score for follicular lymphoma. The m7-FLIPI is calculated by summing the predictor values calculated by Lasso coefficients. A total score >0.8 defines a high-risk cohort.

m7-FLIPI predictor values	Lasso coefficients (βLasso)
High-risk FLIPI	+0.79
ECOG > 1	+0.38
Non-silent mutations in:	
EZH2*	−0.53
ARID1A*	−0.40
EP300*	+0.33
FOX01	+0.26
MEF2B	−0.07
CREBBP*	+0.05
CARD11	+0.04

*Epigenetic mutations.

Diffuse Large B-cell Lymphoma

Diffuse large B-cell lymphoma (DLBCL) is an aggressive non-Hodgkin's lymphoma (NHL) derived from mature B-cells that have undergone, or are undergoing, the germinal center (GC) reaction in response to antigen and helper T-cell stimulation. While there is significant clinical and molecular heterogeneity, gene expression profiling (GEP) studies have been used to define two main subtypes based on cell of origin (COO): germinal center B-cell-like (GCB) and activated B-cell-like (ABC). Exome and transcriptome sequencing has demonstrated key differences in genetic signals between GCB- and ABC-subtype DLBCL (Meyer et al. 2011; Schmitz et al. 2018; Scott et al. 2015). The ABC subtype is enriched with mutations altering B-cell signaling pathways, while GCB subtype, which aligns with FL in germinal center stage of differentiation, predominately exhibits alterations of chromatin modifying genes (Morin et al. 2011). These epigenetic regulatory genes are among the most common mutations, with the histone methyltransferase *KMT2D* being the most frequently (25%) altered in the series while *CREBBP* (11%) and *EP300* (6%) were also well represented. EZH2 mutations were frequent in GCB subtype (22%) but were not seen in other subtypes (Reddy et al. 2017).

The frequency of epigenetic aberrancies in DLBCL may, in part, explain the variability in clinical outcomes with high levels of epigenetic dysregulation associated with a poorer prognosis (Chambwe et al. 2014; Schmitz et al. 2018). These differences have provided rationale for further stratification by the LymphGen classification tool that can separate patient's tumors into six distinct genomic subtypes (EZB, ST2, BN2, A53, N1, MCD). This classification tool utilizes the mutational profile to highlight similarities between specific subtypes and other various indolent lymphoma types which share common deregulated growth and cell signaling pathways (Table 3.2). It has prognostic implications and the EZB subtype, which is based on EZH2 mutations and BCL2 translocations, has a generally good prognosis in the absence of "double-hit" or "triple-hit" rearrangements. The EZB subtype is enriched for epigenetic pathway dysregulation with frequent gene mutations that have been associated with the GCB subtype while sharing genetic similarities with FL. This demonstration of subtype defining genetic hallmarks has provided a potential pathway to the realization of "precision medicine" (Schmitz et al. 2018; Wright et al. 2020).

Attempts to utilize these recurring epigenetic defects therapeutically, however, have so far been disappointing to date with trials of the HDAC-, EZH2-, and Bromodomain (BET)-inhibitors reporting only modest single-agent activity.

Table 3.3 LymphGen classification of diffuse large B-cell lymphoma with corresponding molecular features.

LymphGen classification	Associated cell of origin	Frequent genetic variants	Biologic pathways affected
EZB	**Germinal center B-cell-like**	*BCL2*, EZH2*, *TNFSFR14*, *CREBBP**, *KMT2D**	Epigenetic; PI3K signaling Cell migration; immune cell Interactions
ST2		*TET2**, *SGK1*, *DUSP2*, *ZFP36L1*, *ACTG1*, *ACTB*, *ITPKB*, *NFKBIA*	JAK/STAT
BN2	**Activated B-cell-like**	*BCL6*, *NOTCH2*, *TNFAIP3*, *DTX1*	NOTCH2 signaling Immune evasion
A53		*TP53*, Aneuploidy	Genetic instability Immune evasion
N1		*NOTCH1*, *IRF2BP2*	NF-κB activation
MCD		*MYD88*, *CD79B*, *PIM1*, *HLA-B*, *BTG1*, *CDKN2A*, *ETV6*, *SPIB*, *OSBPL10*	B-cell receptor and NF-κB signaling

*Epigenetically active mutations.

Ongoing combination trials have proven more promising with BET inhibition in combination with the BH3 mimetic venetoclax demonstrating in vitro synergism and early data suggesting clinically meaningful responses in a phase 1b trial (Crump et al. 2008; Cummin et al. 2020; Dickinson et al. 2018, 2021; Italiano et al. 2018).

Marginal Zone Lymphoma

A group of rare indolent lymphomas thought to be derived from B-cell in the marginal zone of the lymph nodes, three distinct types of marginal zone lymphoma (MZL) have been recognized in the 2016 World Health Organization classification, including splenic MZL, extranodal MZL, and nodal MZL. Recurrent mutations in *KMT2D* (11%) and *CREBBP* (~5%) have been reported in splenic MZL (Parry et al. 2015; Swerdlow et al. 2016). Genome-wide DNA-promoter methylation profiling and GEP of splenic marginal lymphoma have demonstrated two distinct subtypes differing in the degree of promoter methylation. Tumors with a high degree of promoter methylation were associated with poorer overall patient survival with repression of tumor suppressor genes such as *KLF4*, *DAPK1*, *CDKN1C*, and *CDKN2A* seen. Demethylating therapy with decitabine caused *in vitro* inhibited proliferation in the hypermethylated group but further research beyond the preclinical setting is needed (Arribas et al. 2015).

Burkitt's Lymphoma

Burkitt's lymphoma (BL) is a highly aggressive B-cell NHL characterized by the presence of the *MYC*-associated translocation, typically the t(8;14) involving the translocation of *MYC* to the partner gene of the immunoglobulin heavy chain (~80% of patients) or the kappa or lambda light chain gene locus on chromosome 2 or 22 (~10% of patients each), respectively (Dalla-Favera et al. 1982; Molyneux et al. 2012). The activation of c-MYC is clearly a critical event in BL leading to lymphomagenesis with the consequences of the translocation including a general growth-promoting effect and stimulation of cell cycle progression. However, genomic analyses have revealed additional oncogenic pathways in BL which suggest that translocation of *MYC* alone is insufficient for oncogenesis and epigenetic silencing of tumor suppressor genes may be important (Giulino-Roth et al. 2012; Schmitz et al. 2012). Mutations in epigenetic regulatory genes and chromatin modifiers are seen in approximately one-third of BL tumors. Despite the disparity in clinical behavior, BL cells are derived from the same germinal B-cells as FL with recurrent mutations in *CREBBP*, EZH2, and *KMTD* reported although much less frequently than in FL and GCB DLCBL. ARID1A is an ATP-dependent SWI/SNF complex involved in chromatin remodeling which is mutated in BL around 30% of cases in some series (Giulino-Roth et al. 2012; Love et al. 2012)

Acute Lymphoblastic Leukemia

Acute lymphoblastic leukemia (ALL) is the most common malignancy in children but is uncommon in adults with an estimated incidence of 1.6 per 100 000 population (Terwilliger and Abdul-Hay 2017). ALL is classified into genetic subtypes based on recurrent chromosomal abnormalities that are understood to lead to leukemogenesis. DNA methylation studies have demonstrated subtype-specific signatures, though recurrent DNA hypermethylation of CpG islands are seen across all subtypes of the disease, suggesting that epigenetic alteration contributes to leukemogenesis (Kuang et al. 2008; Taylor et al. 2007). The degree of methylation appears to be similar between childhood and adult ALL although aberrant methylation of different specific pathways is seen and may contribute to the difference in prognosis (Garcia-Manero et al. 2003). The cyclin-dependent kinase inhibitor p57KIP2 is almost exclusively methylated in adult ALL and associated with a poorer outcome (Canalli et al. 2005; Shen et al. 2003). Chromatin modifier genes are enriched in ALL with frequent somatic point mutations in *PRC2*, *KMT2A*, *KMT2D*, *CREBBP*, *EP300*, and *SETD2*, while DNA methyltransferase mutations are rare (Janczar et al. 2017; Lindqvist et al. 2015; Mar et al. 2014; Mullighan et al. 2011). These mutations are seemingly not specific to a particular subtype except for PRC2 which is more frequently aberrant in T-ALL (Huether et al. 2014). In particular, *KMT2A* rearrangements are recognized as potent drivers of leukemogenesis in infant ALL, and KMT2A fusion proteins are often seen in the absence of additional mutations while EZH2 loss-of-function is sufficient to cause T-ALL in mouse models (Andersson et al. 2015; Ding et al. 2017; Ntziachristos et al. 2012; Schäfer et al. 2016; Simon et al. 2012).

Chronic Lymphocytic Leukemia

A malignancy of mature B-cells with well-characterized pathways of differentiation and maturation, the biology of chronic lymphocytic leukemia (CLL) is highly heterogeneous and influenced by genomic, epigenetic, and immunogenetic factors. The mutational burden within the immunoglobulin heavy chain variable (IGHV) region has been used to dichotomously classify CLL into two key subtypes, mutated and unmutated IGHV, each with its own unique biological and clinical behavior (Damle et al. 1999; Hamblin et al. 1999). Whole genome analysis of the methylation patterns of CLL has demonstrated that mutated CLL and unmutated CLL maintain the epigenetic profile of memory B-cells and naïve B-cells, respectively. Furthermore, DNA methylation analysis has identified three distinct subgroups: memory-like CLL (m-CLL) which comprises mostly mutated IGHV and intermediate CLL (i-CLL) and naïve-like CLL (n-CLL) which are mostly unmutated IGHV (Kulis et al. 2012; Queirós et al. 2015). The epigenetic profile of these subgroups represents a stable epigenetic mark from their cellular origin and has different clinicobiological features, varies in therapy response, and has prognostic value supported by analysis of population and clinical trial cohorts (Queirós et al. 2015; Tsagiopoulou et al. 2019; Wojdacz et al. 2019).

The chromatin modifier chromodomain helicase DNA binding protein 2 (*CHD2*) is the most frequently mutated gene in IGHV-mutated CLL where it likely acts as a driver of malignancy (Rodríguez et al. 2015). Recurrent early loss-of-function of the histone methyltransferase *SETD2* has been reported and associated with poor prognosis disease (Parker et al. 2016). EZH2 overexpression is also associated with an aggressive clinical phenotype and appears to be regulated by signals from the CLL microenvironment with EZH2 inhibitors demonstrating *ex vivo* efficacy in reduction of H3K27me3 levels (Chartomatsidou et al. 2019).

Mantle Cell Lymphoma

Mantle cell lymphoma (MCL) is characterized by the t(11;14)(q13;q32) translocation which leads to *CCND1* overexpression. There are two recognized subtypes that differ in their clinical and biological behavior. The most common conventional MCL derives from naive-like mature B-cells, expresses the transcription factor SOX11, and accumulates genetic alterations. It is associated with lymphadenopathy and a poorer prognosis. Leukemic non-nodal MCL originates from memory-like B-cells and is negative for SOX11.

KMT2D is the most frequent recurrent mutation present in approximately 20% of MCL, and has been associated with a poorer prognosis, but the epigenetic landscape of MCL is otherwise remarkably heterogeneous. There are high levels of variation between levels of DNA methylation and infrequent recurrently mutated epigenetic drivers which often reflect the underlying naïve B-cell of origin (Beà et al. 2013; Ferrero et al. 2020; Queirós et al. 2016; Zhang et al. 2014).

Hodgkin's Lymphoma

Classical Hodgkin's lymphoma (cHL) is usually composed of a small number of mononuclear Hodgkin cells and multinucleated Reed–Sternberg (RS) cells residing in an extensive inflammatory background and derived from (post-) germinal center B-cells in almost all instances. A key feature that distinguishes cHL from other B-cell lymphomas is the almost complete absence of B-cell markers from the HRS (Hodgkin and Reed–Sternberg) cells and the upregulation of non-B-cell lineage genes. This loss of "B-cell identity" is pivotal in the lymphomagenesis of cHL, and recent evidence suggests that epigenetic alterations via promoter methylation and chromatin modification have been implicated in the silencing of B-cell specific genes (Ushmorov et al. 2006). Sharing a common origin with FL and GCB DLBCL, there is mutational overlap with mutations in *CREBBP*, *EP300*, and *KMT2D* reported; however, despite this there is a heterogeneity suggestive of distinct events leading to lymphomagenesis (Liu et al. 2014; Mata et al. 2017). The import of this biology and the natural history of the disease or its response to various therapies is still a matter of translational research.

Multiple Myeloma

Multiple myeloma (MM) is a clonal expansion of plasma cells usually accompanied by a monoclonal paraprotein and associated with end-organ damage. It is usually preceded by a premalignant disease, monoclonal gammopathy of unclear significance (MGUS), which develops into MM through interactions with the bone marrow microenvironment and acquisition of molecular abnormalities. MM is one of the most biologically complex lymphoid malignancies with significant heterogeneity of genetic alterations. Genome-wide methylation microarray has demonstrated distinct methylation patterns between normal plasma cells and MGUS cells, while gene-specific hypermethylation was seen at the transition point of MGUS to myeloma (Walker et al. 2011). Mutations in epigenetic regulators are seen in around 24% of cases but do not appear to be prognostically significant and the frequency of individual recurrent mutations is low (~2%) (Alzrigat et al. 2018; Walker et al. 2018). Whole genome sequencing has demonstrated alterations in epigenetic regulators including *CREBBP*, *TET2*, *IDH1*, *DNMT3A*, *ARID1A*, *KMT2D*, *KMT2C*, *EP300*, *UTX*, and *WHSC1* resulting in increased expression of HOX9 (Chapman et al. 2011; Pawlyn et al. 2016; van Haaften et al. 2009; Walker et al. 2018). Interleukin-6 mediates upregulation of EZH2 in MM which leads to increased silencing of PRC2-target genes via H3K27me3. The frequent t(4;14) translocation in MM is a predictor of adverse prognosis. The MMSET (multiple myeloma SET domain) is upregulated in all cases of t(4:14) MM where it catalyzes methylation of H3K36, enhances the function of HDAC enzymes, and promotes activation of the NF-κB pathway (Walker et al. 2011). Therapeutic agents targeting epigenetic pathways such as the HDAC inhibitors romidepsin and panobinostat have demonstrated clinically relevant activity without significant tumor regression possibly reflective of the underlying genetic heterogeneity driving myeloma growth. The PANORAMA-1 trial demonstrated a modest overall survival benefit with the addition of panobinostat to bortezomib and dexamethasone leading to FDA approval for use in relapsed/refractory MM (Harrison et al. 2011; Laubach et al. 2015; Niesvizky et al. 2011; San-Miguel et al. 2016).

Peripheral T-cell Lymphoma – Not Otherwise Specified

Epigenetic mutations are less frequent in PTCL-NOS than in other subtypes such as AITL. Mutations in epigenetic regulators including *KMT2D*, *TET2*, and *DNMT3* which control genes involved in various signaling pathways including *ZAP70*, *CHD8*, *APC*, and *TRAF3* have been reported. A subgroup of PTCL is now defined as PTCL with T follicular helper (TFH) cell phenotype and is now a separate category to PTCL-NOS as defined by the WHO classification and is particularly enriched with epigenetic alterations.

Angioimmunoblastic T-cell Lymphoma and PTCL with TFH Phenotype

The clinical presentation of AITL and PTCL with TFH phenotype is often associated with skin rashes and autoimmune phenomena explained by the role of TFH cells in the regulation of B-cells. They share a common COO in the TFH cell and are distinguished histologically by the presence (AITL) or absence (PTCL with TFH phenotype) of abundant endothelial venules in the tumor sample and both subtypes require express at least two or more markers of TFH cells such as PD-1, BCL6, CXCL13, and CD10 (Gaulard and de Leval 2011).

AITL and PTCL-TFH are characterized by a dysregulated epigenome with classic hallmark mutations in *TET2*, *IDH2*, and *RHOA* that define them as epigenetic disorders. Mutations in *IDH2* are identified in about a third of AITL cases (Cairns et al. 2012), while *TET2* mutations have been reported in up to 76% of AITL resulting in DNA hypermethylation which also appears to have effects on other proteins including HDAC1/2 (Couronné et al. 2012). Only *IDH2* codon 172 mutations have been observed in AITL and occur with *TET2* mutations. *DNMT3* loss-of-function is reported in 10–25% cases of AITL, 80% of which also have *TET2* mutations confirming a dysregulated and complex epigenome (Odejide et al. 2014). Epigenetic mutations in *TET2* and *IDH2* are strongly associated with the *RHOA* G17V mutation and the *RHOA* G17V mutation is seen exclusively in the background of *TET2* mutations with or without *IDH2* mutations in 70% of AITL patients (Nguyen et al. 2021). These mutants do not bind GTP and disrupt the important RhoA signaling. The *RHOA* G17V mutation results in increased AKT activity through several interactions that include VAV1, ROCK1 and 2, and PTEN. A subset of *IDH2* mutated cases harbor both *TET2* and *RHOA* (Nguyen et al. 2021). This extensive epigenomic dysfunction in these subtypes appears to be particularly vulnerable to exploitation with epigenetically active therapeutics such as the HDAC inhibitors and hypomethylating agents. Prospective trials have demonstrated high response rates in these subtypes when compared to other T-cell lymphomas albeit with small sample size. Combination therapy appears to be particularly effective and clinical trials are ongoing.

Anaplastic Large Cell Lymphoma

ALCL is characterized by sheets of large anaplastic cells that are CD30 positive and an absence of surface expression of typical T-cell markers. The three different types of ALCL can be differentiated based on clinical presentation: systemic ALCL, primary cutaneous ALCL, and breast implant associated ALCL. Systemic ALCL has a primarily nodal presentation and the presence of anaplastic lymphoma kinase (ALK) protein detected by immunohistochemistry (IHC) in tumor samples can differentiate between ALK-positive and ALK-negative ALCL, each carrying a distinctly different prognosis. Extranodal manifestations including skin involvement are common among the nodal ALCL irrespective of the ALK status (Giulino-Roth et al. 2012). *DNMT3* and *TET2* mutations have been identified in some cases of systemic ALCL, albeit comparatively few compared to AITL and PTCL-TFH (Love et al. 2012). Whole exome sequencing of Breast implant-associated ALCL has demonstrated recurrent alterations of epigenetic mutations with recurrent mutations seen in *KMT2C, KMT2D, CHD2*, and *CREBBP* (Laurent et al. 2020).

Adult T-cell Leukemia/Lymphoma

Adult T-cell leukemia/lymphoma is etiologically linked to the HTLV-1 and alterations of methylation pathway genes (TET2, DNMT3, and IDH2) are reported although less frequently than AITL. Gene expression in ATLL is influenced by trimethylation of H3K27me3 leading to polycomb-dependent repression. The HTLV-1 viral protein *Tax* regulates viral gene expression and is a potent activator of NF-κB and various cell signaling pathways. Silencing of *Tax* via DNA methylation has been demonstrated in ATLL (Takeda et al. 2004). KDM6B, a gene that encodes a lysine-specific demethylase that specifically demethylates di- or tri-methylated lysine 27 of histone H3 is considered a repressive histone mark controlling chromatin condensation. The gene is downregulated in ATLL, locking in the effects initiated by Tax even when Tax expression is lost during disease progression (Fujikawa et al. 2016). EZH2 and other components of the PRC2 complex are upregulated in ATLL. The oral EZH1/2 dual inhibitor valemetostat has demonstrated a promising overall response rate in a recent phase 1 trial (Morishima et al. 2019).

Intestinal T-cell Lymphoma

The intestinal T-cell lymphomas are derived from intestinal intraepitheliod lymphocytes and there are at least three clinical variants. Enteropathy-associated T-cell lymphoma (EATL) is associated with celiac disease and an aggressive clinical course. Monomorphic epitheliotropic intestinal T-cell lymphoma (MEITL) was formerly known as EATL type II and is similarly aggressive with the majority of cases being γ/δ subtype. The third subtype, indolent T-cell lymphoproliferative disorder, of the gastrointestinal tract has a more indolent course. The JAK/STAT pathway is the most frequently mutated pathway with mutations in *KRAS, TP53, TERT11* also reported. *SETD2* is the most frequently mutated gene in EATL (32% of cases) and is a histone methyltransferase that is specific for lysine-36 of histone H3, methylation of this residue is associated with active chromatin. The trimethylation of lysine-36 of histone H3 (H3K36me3) is required in human cells for homologous recombinational repair and genome stability. Depletion of *SETD2* increases the frequency of deletion mutations that arise by the alternative DNA repair process of microhomology-mediated end joining (Taylor et al. 2007).

Hepatosplenic T-cell Lymphomas

This rare entity is associated with prior immunosuppression and occurs more commonly in young males with a median age of around 35 years. Most patients have a γ/δ histological subtype although α/β subtype has also been reported. Recurrent isochromosome 7q and trisomy 8 has also been noted on cytogenetic studies, while *STAT5B* is mutated in up to 31% of cases (Nicolae et al. 2014). Dysregulation of various epigenetic pathways has been reported with comprehensive genomic studies of hepatosplenic T-cell lymphomas (HSTCL) identifying chromatic modifying gene mutations in a variety of genes including *SETD2* and *ARID1B* in up to 62% of cases. The *ARID1B* gene (AT-rich interactive domain containing protein 1B) encodes for a protein that binds to DNA helping to target SWI/SNF complexes which regulate gene expression by modulating chromatin remodeling (McKinney et al. 2017).

NK/T Cell Lymphoma

NK/T cell lymphomas arise from natural killer (NK)-cells and are divided into three different subtypes: extranodal ENK/T cell lymphoma nasal type (ENKTL), aggressive NK cell leukemia (ANKL), and chronic lymphoproliferative disorder of NK cells. WES (whole exome sequencing) has described the mutational landscape of ENKTCL. Most frequent mutations involve DDX3X which is also highly methylated. The mutants reduce RNA helicase activity but its role in pathogenesis is unclear. Genome-wide studies have shown that there is global hypermethylation in ENKTCL, and that several important genes including *TP53, SHP1*, and *TP73* are affected. TP73 is a TP53 family member which may also be a negative regulator of NK-cell activation. SHP1 regulates STAT3 activation, and its loss may contribute to the aberrant activation of the JAK/STAT3 pathway. There is frequent methylation of ASNS which encodes asparaginase synthetase which may explain the sensitivity of ENKTCL to L-asparaginase therapy. Mutations in *KMT2D* and *TET2* have been reported and are associated with a poorer prognosis (Gao et al. 2019).

Mycosis Fungoides and Sezary's Syndrome

Mycosis fungoides (MF) is the most common primary cutaneous T-cell lymphoma (CTCL) variant and is closely related to a rare leukemic variant, Sezary's syndrome (SS). Recurrent loss-of-function mutations in *ARID1A* (62%) and *DNMT3A* (42%) have been demonstrated in CTCL, and SS has a significantly higher prevalence of methylation abnormalities when compared to other malignancies, suggestive that DNA methylation plays a critical role in oncogenesis (Choi et al. 2015; Weinstein et al. 2013). Recurrent genes with hypermethylation of CpG-rich promoters as candidates for transcriptional repression have been identified and may play a potential causal role in the pathogenesis of SS (Choi et al. 2015; da Silva Almeida et al. 2015). This hypermethylation notably involves methylation of the CMTM2 gene, which encodes a chemokine-like factor and appears to be distinct to SS (van Doorn et al. 2016). Furthermore, many of the highly expressed genes identified in SS, such as those for CD158, DNMT3, PLS3, and TWIST1, have large CpG islands suggesting that changes in methylation may be a mechanism for the activation of these genes (Kiel et al. 2015; Michel et al. 2013). This enrichment of epigenetic dysregulation provides rationale for the use of epigenetically active agents such as HDAC inhibitors which have demonstrated clinically relevant activity in both MF and SS (Papps et al. 2020)

Summary

The epigenome facilitates the maturation and activity of lymphoid cells necessary for a functional immune system. Characterization of the dysregulated epigenetic landscape of the lymphoid malignancies has provided insight into the mechanisms contributing to lymphomagenesis, and further recognition of distinct clinicogenetic subgroups within entities has led to an understanding of the heterogeneous clinical behavior and the refinement of prognostic tools. The B-cell disorders, FL, and the genetically related DLBCL GCB subtype are particularly enriched with epigenetic aberrancies. The T-cell disorders have a frequently dysregulated epigenome to the extent that some disorders, such as AITL, are being recognized as epigenetic diseases. The recognition of this reliance on epigenetic dysregulation in specific lymphoid disorders has led to the promise of novel therapeutics with encouraging results thus far.

Must Read References

Morin, R.D., Mendez-Lago, M., Mungall, A.J. et al. (2011). Frequent mutation of histone-modifying genes in non-Hodgkin lymphoma. *Nature* 476 (7360): 298–303.

Wright, G.W., Huang, D.W., Phelan, J.D. et al. (2020). A probabilistic classification tool for genetic subtypes of diffuse large B cell lymphoma with therapeutic implications. *Cancer Cell* 37 (4): 551–68.e14.

Odejide, O., Weigert, O., Lane, A.A. et al. (2014). A targeted mutational landscape of angioimmunoblastic T-cell lymphoma. *Blood* 123 (9): 1293–1296.

References

Alzrigat, M., Jernberg-Wiklund, H., and Licht, J.D. (2018). Targeting EZH2 in multiple myeloma-multifaceted anti-tumor activity. *Epigenomes* 2 (3): 16.

Andersson, A.K., Ma, J., Wang, J. et al. (2015). The landscape of somatic mutations in infant MLL-rearranged acute lymphoblastic leukemias. *Nat. Genet.* 47 (4): 330–337.

Arribas, A.J., Rinaldi, A., Mensah, A.A. et al. (2015). DNA methylation profiling identifies two splenic marginal zone lymphoma subgroups with different clinical and genetic features. *Blood* 125 (12): 1922–1931.

Audia, J.E. and Campbell, R.M. (2016). Histone modifications and cancer. *Cold Spring Harb. Perspect. Biol.* 8 (4): a019521–a.

Bannister, A.J. and Kouzarides, T. (2011). Regulation of chromatin by histone modifications. *Cell Res.* 21 (3): 381–395.

Beà, S., Valdés-Mas, R., Navarro, A. et al. (2013). Landscape of somatic mutations and clonal evolution in mantle cell lymphoma. *Proc. Natl. Acad. Sci. U.S.A.* 110 (45): 18250–18255.

Béguelin, W., Popovic, R., Teater, M. et al. (2013). EZH2 is required for germinal center formation and somatic EZH2 mutations promote lymphoid transformation. *Cancer Cell* 23 (5): 677–692.

Bödör, C., Grossmann, V., Popov, N. et al. (2013). EZH2 mutations are frequent and represent an early event in follicular lymphoma. *Blood* 122 (18): 3165–3168.

Bouska, A., Zhang, W., Gong, Q. et al. (2017). Combined copy number and mutation analysis identifies oncogenic pathways associated with transformation of follicular lymphoma. *Leukemia* 31 (1): 83–91.

Cairns, R.A., Iqbal, J., Lemonnier, F. et al. (2012). IDH2 mutations are frequent in angioimmunoblastic T-cell lymphoma. *Blood* 119 (8): 1901–1903.

Canalli, A.A., Yang, H., Jeha, S. et al. (2005). Aberrant DNA methylation of a cell cycle regulatory pathway composed of P73, P15 and P57KIP2 is a rare event in children with acute lymphocytic leukemia. *Leuk. Res.* 29 (8): 881–885.

Challen, G.A., Sun, D., Jeong, M. et al. (2011). Dnmt3a is essential for hematopoietic stem cell differentiation. *Nat. Genet.* 44 (1): 23–31.

Chambwe, N., Kormaksson, M., Geng, H. et al. (2014). Variability in DNA methylation defines novel epigenetic subgroups of DLBCL associated with different clinical outcomes. *Blood* 123 (11): 1699–1708.

Chapman, M.A., Lawrence, M.S., Keats, J.J. et al. (2011). Initial genome sequencing and analysis of multiple myeloma. *Nature* 471 (7339): 467–472.

Chartomatsidou, E., Ntoufa, S., Kotta, K. et al. (2019). Inhibition of EZH2 and immune signaling exerts synergistic antitumor effects in chronic lymphocytic leukemia. *Blood Adv.* 3 (12): 1891–1896.

Choi, J., Goh, G., Walradt, T. et al. (2015). Genomic landscape of cutaneous T cell lymphoma. *Nat. Genet.* 47 (9): 1011–1019.

Couronné, L., Bastard, C., and Bernard, O.A. (2012). TET2 and DNMT3A mutations in human T-cell lymphoma. *N. Engl. J. Med.* 366 (1): 95–96.

Coussens, L.M. and Werb, Z. (2002). Inflammation and cancer. *Nature* 420 (6917): 860–867.

Crump, M., Coiffier, B., Jacobsen, E.D. et al. (2008). Phase II trial of oral vorinostat (suberoylanilide hydroxamic acid) in relapsed diffuse large-B-cell lymphoma. *Ann. Oncol.* 19 (5): 964–969.

Cummin, T.E.C., Cox, K.L., Murray, T.D. et al. (2020). BET inhibitors synergize with venetoclax to induce apoptosis in MYC-driven lymphomas with high BCL-2 expression. *Blood Adv.* 4 (14): 3316–3328.

da Silva Almeida, A.C., Abate, F., Khiabanian, H. et al. (2015). The mutational landscape of cutaneous T cell lymphoma and Sézary syndrome. *Nat. Genet.* 47 (12): 1465–1470.

Dalla-Favera, R., Bregni, M., Erikson, J. et al. (1982). Human c-myc onc gene is located on the region of chromosome 8 that is translocated in Burkitt lymphoma cells. *Proc. Natl. Acad. Sci. U.S.A.* 79 (24): 7824–7827.

Damle, R.N., Wasil, T., Fais, F. et al. (1999). Ig V gene mutation status and CD38 expression as novel prognostic indicators in chronic lymphocytic leukemia. *Blood* 94 (6): 1840–1847.

Dickinson, M., Kamdar, M., Huntly, B.J.P. et al. (2018). A phase I study of molibresib (GSK525762), a selective bromodomain (BRD) and extra terminal protein (BET) inhibitor: results from part 1 of a phase I/II open label single agent study in subjects with non-Hodgkin's lymphoma (NHL). *Blood* 132: 1682.

Dickinson, M., Mejjide, J.B., Herrera, A.F. et al. (2021). Phase Ib study of BET protein inhibitor RO6870810 with venetoclax and rituximab in patients with diffuse large B-cell lymphoma. *Blood Adv.* 5(22):4762–4770.

Ding, L.-W., Sun, Q.-Y., Tan, K.-T. et al. (2017). Mutational landscape of pediatric acute lymphoblastic leukemia. *Cancer Res.* 77 (2): 390.

Easwaran, H., Tsai, H.-C., and Baylin, S.B. (2014). Cancer epigenetics: tumor heterogeneity, plasticity of stem-like states, and drug resistance. *Mol. Cell* 54 (5): 716–727.

Ennishi, D., Takata, K., Béguelin, W. et al. (2019). Molecular and genetic characterization of MHC deficiency identifies EZH2 as therapeutic target for enhancing immune recognition. *Cancer Discov.* 9 (4): 546.

Ferrero, S., Rossi, D., Rinaldi, A. et al. (2020). KMT2D mutations and TP53 disruptions are poor prognostic biomarkers in mantle cell lymphoma receiving high-dose therapy: a FIL study. *Haematologica* 105 (6): 1604–1612.

Figueroa, M.E., Abdel-Wahab, O., Lu, C. et al. (2010). Leukemic IDH1 and IDH2 mutations result in a hypermethylation phenotype, disrupt TET2 function, and impair hematopoietic differentiation. *Cancer Cell* 18 (6): 553–567.

François, L., Elsa, P., Aurélie, D. et al. (2018). Loss of 5-hydroxymethylcytosine is a frequent event in peripheral T-cell lymphomas. *Haematologica* 103 (3): e115–e8.

Fujikawa, D., Nakagawa, S., Hori, M. et al. (2016). Polycomb-dependent epigenetic landscape in adult T-cell leukemia. *Blood* 127 (14): 1790–1802.

Fujisawa, T. and Filippakopoulos, P. (2017). Functions of bromodomain-containing proteins and their roles in homeostasis and cancer. *Nat. Rev. Mol. Cell Biol.* 18 (4): 246–262.

Gao, L.M., Zhao, S., Zhang, W.Y. et al. (2019). Somatic mutations in KMT2D and TET2 associated with worse prognosis in Epstein-Barr virus-associated T or natural killer-cell lymphoproliferative disorders. *Cancer Biol. Ther.* 20 (10): 1319–1327.

Garcia-Manero, G., Jeha, S., Daniel, J. et al. (2003). Aberrant DNA methylation in pediatric patients with acute lymphocytic leukemia. *Cancer* 97 (3): 695–702.

García-Ramírez, I., Tadros, S., González-Herrero, I. et al. (2017). Crebbp loss cooperates with Bcl2 overexpression to promote lymphoma in mice. *Blood* 129 (19): 2645–2656.

Gaulard, P. and de Leval, L. (2011). Follicular helper T cells: implications in neoplastic hematopathology. *Semin. Diagn. Pathol.* 28 (3): 202–213.

Giulino-Roth, L., Wang, K., MacDonald, T.Y. et al. (2012). Targeted genomic sequencing of pediatric Burkitt lymphoma identifies recurrent alterations in antiapoptotic and chromatin-remodeling genes. *Blood* 120 (26): 5181–5184.

Green, M.R. (2018). Chromatin modifying gene mutations in follicular lymphoma. *Blood* 131 (6): 595–604.

Grossman, S.R. (2001). p300/CBP/p53 interaction and regulation of the p53 response. *Eur. J. Biochem.* 268 (10): 2773–2778.

Gu, T., Lin, X., Cullen, S.M. et al. (2018). DNMT3A and TET1 cooperate to regulate promoter epigenetic landscapes in mouse embryonic stem cells. *Genome Biol.* 19 (1): 88.

Hamblin, T.J., Davis, Z., Gardiner, A. et al. (1999). Unmutated Ig V(H) genes are associated with a more aggressive form of chronic lymphocytic leukemia. *Blood* 94 (6): 1848–1854.

Hanahan, D. and Weinberg, R.A. (2011). Hallmarks of cancer: the next generation. *Cell* 144 (5): 646–674.

Harrison, S.J., Quach, H., Link, E. et al. (2011). A high rate of durable responses with romidepsin, bortezomib, and dexamethasone in relapsed or refractory multiple myeloma. *Blood* 118 (24): 6274–6283.

Hashwah, H., Schmid, C.A., Kasser, S. et al. (2017). Inactivation of CREBBP expands the germinal center B cell compartment, down-regulates MHCII expression and promotes DLBCL growth. *Proc. Natl. Acad. Sci. U.S.A.* 114 (36): 9701–9706.

He, Y.F., Li, B.Z., Li, Z. et al. (2011). Tet-mediated formation of 5-carboxylcytosine and its excision by TDG in mammalian DNA. *Science* 333 (6047): 1303–1307.

Huether, R., Dong, L., Chen, X. et al. (2014 April). The landscape of somatic mutations in epigenetic regulators across 1,000 paediatric cancer genomes. *Nat. Commun. [Internet]* 5: 3630 p.

Italiano, A., Soria, J.-C., Toulmonde, M. et al. (2018). Tazemetostat, an EZH2 inhibitor, in relapsed or refractory B-cell non-Hodgkin lymphoma and advanced solid tumours: a first-in-human, open-label, phase 1 study. *Lancet Oncol.* 19 (5): 649–659.

Ito, S., Shen, L., Dai, Q. et al. (2011). Tet proteins can convert 5-methylcytosine to 5-formylcytosine and 5-carboxylcytosine. *Science* 333 (6047): 1300–1303.

Janczar, S., Janczar, K., Pastorczak, A. et al. (2017). The role of histone protein modifications and mutations in histone modifiers in pediatric B-cell progenitor acute lymphoblastic leukemia. *Cancers* 9 (1): 2.

Ji, M.M., Huang, Y.H., Huang, J.Y. et al. (2018). Histone modifier gene mutations in peripheral T-cell lymphoma not otherwise specified. *Haematologica* 103 (4): 679–687.

Jiang, Y., Ortega-Molina, A., Geng, H. et al. (2017). CREBBP inactivation promotes the development of HDAC3-dependent lymphomas. *Cancer Discov.* 7 (1): 38–53.

Jurinovic, V., Passerini, V., Oestergaard, M.Z. et al. (2019). Evaluation of the m7-FLIPI in patients with follicular lymphoma treated within the gallium trial: EZH2 mutation status may be a predictive marker for differential efficacy of chemotherapy. *Blood* 134 (Supplement_1): 122.

Kiel, M.J., Sahasrabuddhe, A.A., Rolland, D.C.M. et al. (2015). Genomic analyses reveal recurrent mutations in epigenetic modifiers and the JAK–STAT pathway in Sézary syndrome. *Nat. Commun.* 6 (1): 8470.

Kridel, R., Sehn, L.H., and Gascoyne, R.D. (2012). Pathogenesis of follicular lymphoma. *J. Clin. Invest.* 122 (10): 3424–3431.

Kuang, S.Q., Tong, W.G., Yang, H. et al. (2008). Genome-wide identification of aberrantly methylated promoter associated CpG islands in acute lymphocytic leukemia. *Leukemia* 22 (8): 1529–1538.

Kulis, M., Heath, S., Bibikova, M. et al. (2012). Epigenomic analysis detects widespread gene-body DNA hypomethylation in chronic lymphocytic leukemia. *Nat. Genet.* 44 (11): 1236–1242.

Laubach, J.P., Moreau, P., San-Miguel, J.F. et al. (2015). Panobinostat for the treatment of multiple myeloma. *Clin. Cancer Res.* 21 (21): 4767–4773.

Laurent, C., Nicolae, A., Laurent, C. et al. (2020). Gene alterations in epigenetic modifiers and JAK-STAT signaling are frequent in breast implant-associated ALCL. *Blood* 135 (5): 360–370.

Lee, P.P., Fitzpatrick, D.R., Beard, C. et al. (2001). A critical role for Dnmt1 and DNA methylation in T cell development, function, and survival. *Immunity* 15 (5): 763–774.

Lemonnier, F., Couronné, L., Parrens, M. et al. (2012). Recurrent TET2 mutations in peripheral T-cell lymphomas correlate with TFH-like features and adverse clinical parameters. *Blood* 120 (7): 1466–1469.

León, T.E., Rapoz-D'Silva, T., Bertoli, C. et al. (2020). EZH2-deficient T-cell acute lymphoblastic leukemia is sensitized to CHK1 inhibition through enhanced replication stress. *Cancer Discov.* 10 (7): 998–1017.

Lindqvist, C.M., Nordlund, J., Ekman, D. et al. (2015). The mutational landscape in pediatric acute lymphoblastic leukemia deciphered by whole genome sequencing. *Hum. Mutat.* 36 (1): 118–128.

Liu, Y., Abdul Razak, F.R., Terpstra, M. et al. (2014). The mutational landscape of Hodgkin lymphoma cell lines determined by whole-exome sequencing. *Leukemia* 28 (11): 2248–2251.

Love, C., Sun, Z., Jima, D. et al. (2012). The genetic landscape of mutations in Burkitt lymphoma. *Nat. Genet.* 44 (12): 1321–1325.

Mar, B.G., Bullinger, L.B., McLean, K.M. et al. (2014). Mutations in epigenetic regulators including SETD2 are gained during relapse in paediatric acute lymphoblastic leukaemia. *Nat. Commun.* 5: 3469-.

Marks, D.L., Olson, R.L., and Fernandez-Zapico, M.E. (2016). Epigenetic control of the tumor microenvironment. *Epigenomics* 8 (12): 1671–1687.

Mata, E., Díaz-López, A., Martín-Moreno, A.M. et al. (2017). Analysis of the mutational landscape of classic Hodgkin lymphoma identifies disease heterogeneity and potential therapeutic targets. *Oncotarget* 8 (67): 111386–111395.

McCabe, M.T., Brandes, J.C., and Vertino, P.M. (2009). Cancer DNA methylation: molecular mechanisms and clinical implications. *Clin. Cancer Res.* 15 (12): 3927–3937.

McKinney, M., Moffitt, A.B., Gaulard, P. et al. (2017). The genetic basis of hepatosplenic T-cell lymphoma. *Cancer Discov.* 7 (4): 369.

Meyer, P.N., Fu, K., Greiner, T.C. et al. (2011). Immunohistochemical methods for predicting cell of origin and survival in patients with diffuse large B-cell lymphoma treated with rituximab. *J. Clin. Oncol.* 29 (2): 200–207.

Michel, L., Jean-Louis, F., Begue, E. et al. (2013). Use of PLS3, Twist, CD158k/KIR3DL2, and NKp46 gene expression combination for reliable Sézary syndrome diagnosis. *Blood* 121 (8): 1477–1478.

Mita, M.M. and Mita, A.C. (2020). Bromodomain inhibitors a decade later: a promise unfulfilled? *Br. J. Cancer* 123 (12): 1713–1714.

Molyneux, E.M., Rochford, R., Griffin, B. et al. (2012). Burkitt's lymphoma. *Lancet* 379 (9822): 1234–1244.

Morin, R.D., Johnson, N.A., Severson, T.M. et al. (2010). Somatic mutations altering EZH2 (Tyr641) in follicular and diffuse large B-cell lymphomas of germinal-center origin. *Nat. Genet.* 42 (2): 181–185.

Morin, R.D., Mendez-Lago, M., Mungall, A.J. et al. (2011). Frequent mutation of histone-modifying genes in non-Hodgkin lymphoma. *Nature* 476 (7360): 298–303.

Morishima, S., Ishitsuka, K., Izutsu, K. et al. (2019). First-in-human study of the EZH1/2 dual inhibitor valemetostat in relapsed or refractory Non-Hodgkin Lymphoma (NHL) – updated results focusing on adult T-cell leukemia-lymphoma (ATL). *Blood* 134 (Supplement_1): 4025-.

Morschhauser, F., Tilly, H., Chaidos, A. et al. (2020). Tazemetostat for patients with relapsed or refractory follicular lymphoma: an open-label, single-arm, multicentre, phase 2 trial. *Lancet Oncol.* 21 (11): 1433–1442.

Mullighan, C.G., Zhang, J., Kasper, L.H. et al. (2011). CREBBP mutations in relapsed acute lymphoblastic leukaemia. *Nature* 471 (7337): 235–239.

Nagata, Y., Kontani, K., Enami, T. et al. (2016). Variegated RHOA mutations in adult T-cell leukemia/lymphoma. *Blood* 127 (5): 596–604.

Nguyen, P.N., Tran, N.T.B., Nguyen, T.P.X. et al. (2021). Clinicopathological implications of RHOA mutations in angioimmunoblastic T-cell lymphoma: a meta-analysis: RHOA mutations in AITL. *Clin. Lymphoma Myeloma Leuk.* 21 (7): 431–438.

Nicolae, A., Xi, L., Pittaluga, S. et al. (2014). Frequent STAT5B mutations in γδ hepatosplenic T-cell lymphomas. *Leukemia* 28 (11): 2244–2248.

Niesvizky, R., Ely, S., Mark, T. et al. (2011). Phase 2 trial of the histone deacetylase inhibitor romidepsin for the treatment of refractory multiple myeloma. *Cancer* 117 (2): 336–342.

Nishida, J., Momoi, Y., Miyakuni, K. et al. (2020). Epigenetic remodelling shapes inflammatory renal cancer and neutrophil-dependent metastasis. *Nat. Cell Biol.* 22 (4): 465–475.

Ntziachristos, P., Tsirigos, A., Van Vlierberghe, P. et al. (2012). Genetic inactivation of the polycomb repressive complex 2 in T cell acute lymphoblastic leukemia. *Nat. Med.* 18 (2): 298–301.

Odejide, O., Weigert, O., Lane, A.A. et al. (2014). A targeted mutational landscape of angioimmunoblastic T-cell lymphoma. *Blood* 123 (9): 1293–1296.

Ogura, M., Ando, K., Suzuki, T. et al. (2014). A multicentre phase II study of vorinostat in patients with relapsed or refractory indolent B-cell non-Hodgkin lymphoma and mantle cell lymphoma. *Br. J. Haematol.* 165 (6): 768–776.

Ortega-Molina, A., Boss, I.W., Canela, A. et al. (2015). The histone lysine methyltransferase KMT2D sustains a gene expression program that represses B cell lymphoma development. *Nat. Med.* 21 (10): 1199–1208.

Papps, T., McCormack, C., Buelens, O. et al. (2020). A comparative analysis of histone deacetylase inhibitors for the treatment of mycosis fungoides and Sézary syndrome. *Br. J. Dermatol.* 182 (2): 497–498.

Parker, H., Rose-Zerilli, M.J., Larrayoz, M. et al. (2016). Genomic disruption of the histone methyltransferase SETD2 in chronic lymphocytic leukaemia. *Leukemia* 30 (11): 2179–2186.

Parry, M., Rose-Zerilli, M.J., Ljungström, V. et al. (2015). Genetics and prognostication in splenic marginal zone lymphoma: revelations from deep sequencing. *Clin. Cancer Res.* 21 (18): 4174–4183.

Pasqualucci, L., Dominguez-Sola, D., Chiarenza, A. et al. (2011). Inactivating mutations of acetyltransferase genes in B-cell lymphoma. *Nature* 471 (7337): 189–195.

Pastore, A., Jurinovic, V., Kridel, R. et al. (2015). Integration of gene mutations in risk prognostication for patients receiving first-line immunochemotherapy for follicular lymphoma: a retrospective analysis of a prospective clinical trial and validation in a population-based registry. *Lancet Oncol.* 16 (9): 1111–1122.

Pawlyn, C., Kaiser, M.F., Heuck, C. et al. (2016). The spectrum and clinical impact of epigenetic modifier mutations in myeloma. *Clin. Cancer Res.* 22 (23): 5783–5794.

Peng, D., Kryczek, I., Nagarsheth, N. et al. (2015). Epigenetic silencing of TH1-type chemokines shapes tumour immunity and immunotherapy. *Nature* 527 (7577): 249–253.

Pike, B.L., Greiner, T.C., Wang, X. et al. (2008). DNA methylation profiles in diffuse large B-cell lymphoma and their relationship to gene expression status. *Leukemia* 22 (5): 1035–1043.

Queirós, A.C., Beekman, R., Vilarrasa-Blasi, R. et al. (2016). Decoding the DNA methylome of mantle cell lymphoma in the light of the entire B cell lineage. *Cancer Cell* 30 (5): 806–821.

Queirós, A.C., Villamor, N., Clot, G. et al. (2015). A B-cell epigenetic signature defines three biologic subgroups of chronic lymphocytic leukemia with clinical impact. *Leukemia* 29 (3): 598–605.

Rao, R.C. and Dou, Y. (2015). Hijacked in cancer: the KMT2 (MLL) family of methyltransferases. *Nat. Rev. Cancer* 15 (6): 334–346.

Reddy, A., Zhang, J., Davis, N.S. et al. (2017). Genetic and functional drivers of diffuse large B cell lymphoma. *Cell* 171 (2): 481–94.e15.

Rodríguez, D., Bretones, G., Quesada, V. et al. (2015). Mutations in CHD2 cause defective association with active chromatin in chronic lymphocytic leukemia. *Blood* 126 (2): 195–202.

Roller, A., Grossmann, V., Bacher, U. et al. (2013). Landmark analysis of DNMT3A mutations in hematological malignancies. *Leukemia* 27 (7): 1573–1578.

Rosikiewicz, W., Chen, X., Dominguez, P.M. et al. (2020). TET2 deficiency reprograms the germinal center B cell epigenome and silences genes linked to lymphomagenesis. *Sci. Adv.* 6 (25): eaay5872.

San-Miguel, J.F., Hungria, V.T.M., Yoon, -S.-S. et al. (2016). Overall survival of patients with relapsed multiple myeloma treated with panobinostat or placebo plus bortezomib and dexamethasone (the PANORAMA 1 trial): a randomised, placebo-controlled, phase 3 trial. *Lancet Haematol.* 3 (11): e506–e15.

Schäfer, V., Ernst, J., Rinke, J. et al. (2016). EZH2 mutations and promoter hypermethylation in childhood acute lymphoblastic leukemia. *J. Cancer Res. Clin. Oncol.* 142 (7): 1641–1650.

Schmitz, R., Wright, G.W., Huang, D.W. et al. (2018). Genetics and pathogenesis of diffuse large B-cell lymphoma. *N. Engl. J. Med.* 378 (15): 1396–1407.

Schmitz, R., Young, R.M., Ceribelli, M. et al. (2012). Burkitt lymphoma pathogenesis and therapeutic targets from structural and functional genomics. *Nature* 490 (7418): 116–120.

Scott, D.W., Mottok, A., Ennishi, D. et al. (2015). Prognostic significance of diffuse large B-cell lymphoma cell of origin determined by digital gene expression in formalin-fixed paraffin-embedded tissue biopsies. *J. Clin. Oncol.* 33 (26): 2848–2856.

Shaknovich, R., Cerchietti, L., Tsikitas, L. et al. (2011). DNA methyltransferase 1 and DNA methylation patterning contribute to germinal center B-cell differentiation. *Blood* 118 (13): 3559–3569.

Shen, L., Toyota, M., Kondo, Y. et al. (2003). Aberrant DNA methylation of p57KIP2 identifies a cell-cycle regulatory pathway with prognostic impact in adult acute lymphocytic leukemia. *Blood* 101 (10): 4131–4136.

Simon, C., Chagraoui, J., Krosl, J. et al. (2012). A key role for EZH2 and associated genes in mouse and human adult T-cell acute leukemia. *Genes Dev.* 26 (7): 651–656.

Solène, M.E., Sarah, P., David, G. et al. (2019). Targeted next generation sequencing reveals high mutation frequency of CREBBP, BCL2 and KMT2D in high-grade B-cell lymphoma with MYC and BCL2 and/or BCL6 rearrangements. *Haematologica* 104 (4): e154–e7.

Swerdlow, S.H., Campo, E., Pileri, S.A. et al. (2016). The 2016 revision of the World Health Organization classification of lymphoid neoplasms. *Blood* 127 (20): 2375–2390.

Tahiliani, M., Koh, K.P., Shen, Y. et al. (2009). Conversion of 5-methylcytosine to 5-hydroxymethylcytosine in mammalian DNA by MLL partner TET1. *Science* 324 (5929): 930–935.

Takeda, S., Maeda, M., Morikawa, S. et al. (2004). Genetic and epigenetic inactivation of tax gene in adult T-cell leukemia cells. *Int. J. Cancer* 109 (4): 559–567.

Taylor, K.H., Pena-Hernandez, K.E., Davis, J.W. et al. (2007). Large-scale CpG methylation analysis identifies novel candidate genes and reveals methylation hotspots in acute lymphoblastic leukemia. *Cancer Res.* 67 (6): 2617–2625.

Terwilliger, T. and Abdul-Hay, M. (2017). Acute lymphoblastic leukemia: a comprehensive review and 2017 update. *Blood Cancer J.* 7 (6): e577–e.

Tsagiopoulou, M., Papakonstantinou, N., Moysiadis, T. et al. (2019). DNA methylation profiles in chronic lymphocytic leukemia patients treated with chemoimmunotherapy. *Clin. Epigenetics* 11 (1): 177.

Tsujimoto, Y., Gorham, J., Cossman, J. et al. (1985). The t(14;18) chromosome translocations involved in B-cell neoplasms result from mistakes in VDJ joining. *Science* 229 (4720): 1390–1393.

Ushmorov, A., Leithäuser, F., Sakk, O. et al. (2006). Epigenetic processes play a major role in B-cell-specific gene silencing in classical Hodgkin lymphoma. *Blood* 107 (6): 2493–2500.

van Doorn, R., Slieker, R.C., Boonk, S.E. et al. (2016). Epigenomic analysis of Sézary syndrome defines patterns of aberrant DNA methylation and identifies diagnostic markers. *J. Invest. Dermatol.* 136 (9): 1876–1884.

van Haaften, G., Dalgliesh, G.L., Davies, H. et al. (2009). Somatic mutations of the histone H3K27 demethylase gene UTX in human cancer. *Nat. Genet.* 41 (5): 521–523.

Van Vlierberghe, P., Ambesi-Impiombato, A., De Keersmaecker, K. et al. (2013). Prognostic relevance of integrated genetic profiling in adult T-cell acute lymphoblastic leukemia. *Blood* 122 (1): 74–82.

Walker, B.A., Mavrommatis, K., Wardell, C.P. et al. (2018). Identification of novel mutational drivers reveals oncogene dependencies in multiple myeloma. *Blood* 132 (6): 587–597.

Walker, B.A., Wardell, C.P., Chiecchio, L. et al. (2011). Aberrant global methylation patterns affect the molecular pathogenesis and prognosis of multiple myeloma. *Blood* 117 (2): 553–562.

Weinstein, J.N., Collisson, E.A., Mills, G.B. et al. (2013). The cancer genome atlas pan-cancer analysis project. *Nat. Genet.* 45 (10): 1113–1120.

Wojdacz, T.K., Amarasinghe, H.E., Kadalayil, L. et al. (2019). Clinical significance of DNA methylation in chronic lymphocytic leukemia patients: results from 3 UK clinical trials. *Blood Adv.* 3 (16): 2474–2481.

Wright, G.W., Huang, D.W., Phelan, J.D. et al. (2020). A probabilistic classification tool for genetic subtypes of diffuse large B cell lymphoma with therapeutic implications. *Cancer Cell* 37 (4): 551–68.e14.

Wurm, T., Wright, D.G., Polakowski, N. et al. (2012). The HTLV-1-encoded protein HBZ directly inhibits the acetyl transferase activity of p300/CBP. *Nucleic Acids Res.* 40 (13): 5910–5925.

Zhang, J., Dominguez-Sola, D., Hussein, S. et al. (2015). Disruption of KMT2D perturbs germinal center B cell development and promotes lymphomagenesis. *Nat. Med.* 21 (10): 1190–1198.

Zhang, J., Jima, D., Moffitt, A.B. et al. (2014). The genomic landscape of mantle cell lymphoma is related to the epigenetically determined chromatin state of normal B cells. *Blood* 123 (19): 2988–2996.

4

Animal Models of Lymphoid Malignancies

Anjali Mishra

Division of Hematologic Malignancies and Hematopoietic Stem Cell Transplantation, Department of Medical Oncology and Department of Cancer Biology, Sydney Kimmel Cancer Center, Thomas Jefferson University, Philadelphia, PA, USA

Take Home Messages

- The use of non-mammalian models such as zebrafish to study lymphoid malignancies has increased in recent years due to the conservation of key genes and developmental processes with humans. The improved genetic tractability, high-throughput screening, and reduced experimental costs make these models superior to traditional murine models.
- Genetically engineered mouse models (GEMMs) of lymphoid neoplasia are important for validating gene function and discovering novel biomarkers. The GEMMs have provided valuable insights into the molecular and cellular processes of cancer development.
- The second generation of human lymphoid neoplasm models, using conditional knockout and regulatable oncogenes, has improved the accuracy and consistency of mouse models that closely mirror the disease in humans.
- The humanized patient-derived xenograft (Hu-PDX) mouse model is emerging as the most reliable method for assessing the effectiveness of immunotherapies. These can be utilized for studying both cell-mediated and immune checkpoint blockade-based approaches.

Introduction

Lymphoid neoplasms are a heterogeneous group of cancer with various clinical presentations and therapeutic responses (Swerdlow et al. 2016). They can be grouped into five major diagnostic categories: Hodgkin's lymphoma, non-Hodgkin's lymphoma, acute and chronic lymphocytic leukemias, and plasma cell neoplasms. Despite the progress in treating these neoplasms, in aggregate they remain the sixth leading cause of cancer-related deaths in the United States (Morton et al. 2007). Currently, there is a need for further studies on the pathogenesis of various types of lymphoid malignancies to develop more effective treatment strategies. The development of precision cancer care relies on the use of animal models. Creating *in vivo* models for cancer therapy is a significant step in drug development (Collins and Workman 2006). Through currently available animal models, we have been able to gain a deeper understanding of how cancer develops, which has dramatically impacted the way we treat patients.

It is believed that the use of animals for scientific purposes started in ancient Greece (Ericsson et al. 2013). The earliest references to the concept of animal experimentation can be found in the writings of Aristotle and Erasistratus, Greek philosophers who were involved in numerous experiments with animals as models for human physiology and anatomy. Animal models to study cancers became more prevalent during the twentieth century. Researchers can study the biological mechanisms involved in cancer initiation, progression, and treatment through these models. While it was initially criticized for its unethical use, animal models eventually became known for their biological and clinical significance. The importance of conducting human clinical trials is still considered essential to developing effective treatment strategies. A recent study revealed that about a third of the animal studies published in scientific journals were translated to human trials, and one-tenth were approved for use in patients (Hackam and Redelmeier 2006). The selection of suitable animal species for a particular disease is also challenging since it involves factors such as the disease prevalence and characteristics.

The evolution of cancer models has been widely influenced by the development of new technologies and the integration of clinical data from patients. Each animal model should replicate the various characteristics of the disease, including its clinical behavior and therapeutic response. This chapter highlights the potential of small and large animal platforms to bridge the gap between clinical and basic research in lymphoid neoplasms.

Precision Cancer Therapies: Targeting Oncogenic Drivers and Signaling Pathways in Lymphoid Malignancies: From Concept to Practice, Volume 1, First Edition. Edited by Owen A. O'Connor, Stephen M. Ansell, and John F. Seymour.

Optimal Animal Models to Study Lymphoid Neoplasms

Since rodents have a close evolutionary relationship with humans, they have been the preferred models for studying blood cancers. Depending on the scientific inquiry, non-rodent models may be preferred over rodents. The following sections aim to identify the utility of rodent and non-rodent models in lymphoid malignancies. In this chapter, we discuss the four model species (zebrafish, fruit fly, non-human primates, and mouse) that can be used for studying human lymphoid tumors pathogenesis treatment (Figure 4.1).

Zebrafish Model

The zebrafish (*Danio rerio*) has emerged as a promising model for cancer research due to its numerous advantages (Stoletov and Klemke 2008; White et al. 2013). Its low cost, high fecundity, and optical translucency make it an excellent platform for studying cancer. In particular, they make an ideal model to study human blood disorders due to a high degree of functional homology with humans, with the presence of equivalent blood cell types of erythroid, myeloid, and lymphoid lineages (Davidson and Zon 2004; Gore et al. 2018). The conserved genes and pathways that regulate hematopoiesis between zebrafish and humans have made this model an ideal system for studying hematological malignancies.

Zebrafish Model of T-cell Neoplasms

- ***Myc-driven model of T-cell acute lymphoblastic leukemia (T-ALL)***: The first genetically engineered zebrafish model of leukemia was made by induction of mouse proto-oncogene "Myc" in T- and B-cells using the zebrafish *Rag2* promoter to create transgenic line *Rag2:cMyc* (Langenau et al. 2003). The fusion of the Myc and green fluorescent protein (GFP) transgene led to the induction of T-ALL in the thymus of zebrafish. The T-ALL cells from the primary zebrafish were then transferred into the secondary fish. In the irradiated recipient fish, the transplanted GFP+ T-ALL cells colonized the thymus. This was the first study that showed that transgenic zebrafish could be used as a platform for large-scale drug screens for the treatment and prevention of acute lymphoblastic leukemia (ALL). In a subsequent study using *Rag2:EGFP-mMyc*, zebrafish developed highly aggressive T-ALL with a short latency of only 44–52 days (Langenau et al. 2005). Leukemia cells show T-cell receptor α (TCR-α) gene rearrangements, clonal expansion, and upregulation of the two genes, *scl* and *lmo2*, commonly seen overexpressed

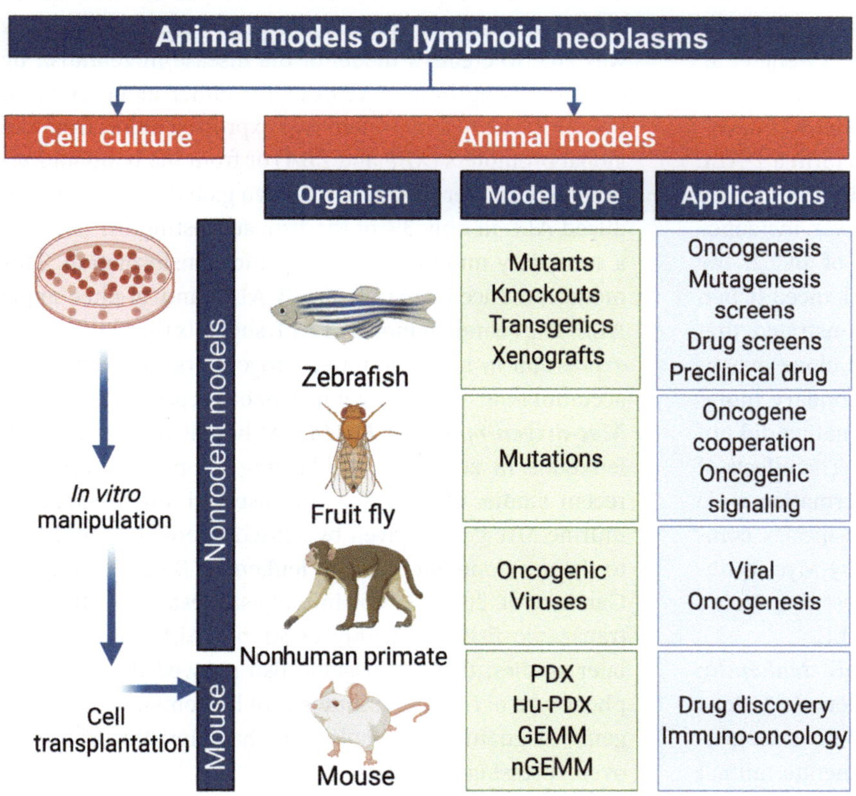

Figure 4.1 Schematic representation of animal models of lymphoid neoplasms: Summary of characteristics of select animal models that could be used to investigate initiation and progression of lymphoid cancers. The potential of these animal models for therapeutic discoveries is essential to bridging the gap between basic and translational medicine.

in the treatment-resistant subgroup of T-ALL patients (La Starza et al. 2014). The T-ALL cells could rapidly grow new tumors after being injected into irradiated recipients. However, leukemia in this model progressed at an accelerated pace, and most of the F1 progeny were diagnosed with the advanced disease before reaching sexual maturity. This limitation prompted the development of a conditional transgenic zebrafish using Cre/lox technology. There are now three inducible approaches that can be used to create germline models of Myc-driven T-ALL. These include: (i) injecting Cre mRNA into the embryos of transgenic fish (*Rag2-lox-dsRED-lox-EGFP-mMyc*) (Langenau et al. 2005), (ii) crossing the two transgenic lines (*Rag2:LDL-EGFP-mMyc* x *hsp70:Cre*) (Feng et al. 2007), and (iii) treating the *Rag2:hMyc-ER* (Gutierrez et al. 2011) fish with 4-hydroxytamoxifen. The increased tumor penetrance and reproducibility of these refined models have allowed the discovery of new genes and pathways that promote or inhibit the growth and survival of T-ALL. Studies involving single-cell transplantation have shown that T-ALLs can self-renew and produce tumor-initiating characteristics (Smith et al. 2010). In this model, T-ALLs can also be introduced into other animals and, in some cases, can be transplanted into mixed genetic backgrounds, to generate large numbers of zebrafish to interrogate the self-renewal gene pathways in the treatment of cancer.

- ***Notch1 driven T-ALL model***: The activated Notch signaling pathway is associated with over 60% of T-ALL cases and can promote T-ALL tumorigenesis (Weng et al. 2004). Considering the high incidence of *NOTCH1* activating mutations in patients, a zebrafish model was developed by combining the *hICN1* with EGFP to form a T-ALL line (*Rag2:EGFP-ICN1*) (Blackburn et al. 2012). This line is consistent with T-ALL but exhibits a lower incidence than Myc-driven T-ALL. In the presence of BCL2, the latency and incidence were significantly enhanced (Chen et al. 2007). Blackburn et al. (2012) demonstrated that the Notch signaling activates pre-leukemic clone expansions, which require the acquisition of secondary mutations. In addition, the presence of Notch signaling did not affect the frequency of leukemia stem cells. The effects of this signaling on pre-leukemic clone transformation were not significant. They also performed cross-species comparisons to identify novel genes regulated by Myc in humans and mouse T-ALL. The studies suggest that Notch activation alone is not enough to induce T-ALL.
- ***Mutagenesis models of heritable T-cell leukemia***: Zebrafish can be used to identify novel genetic lesions that are not yet known to cause T-ALL. With mutagenesis screens in transgenic fish, one can generate animal models with a heritable predisposition to cancer. For example, using a zebrafish line where the native $p56^{lck}$ promoter directs T cell-specific expression of GFP (*lck:EGFP*), several mutant lines were discovered using an *N*-ethyl-*N*-nitrosourea (ENU)-mediated mutagenesis screen (Frazer et al. 2009). The screen detected three mutant lines (*srk*, *hlk*, and *otg*) that showed clinical and molecular characteristics of human T-ALL and T-lymphoblastic lymphoma (T-LBL). Two of the lines, Shrek (srk) and hulk (hlk), had dominant mutations while the other one, Oscar-the-grouch (otg), had a recessive mutation. The average time to tumor induction in each of these lines was around six to eight months. Leukemia cells could be transplanted and produce large numbers of new malignant cells with high engraftment rates. The screens show the potential for identifying genes that cause different types of leukemias. Using the same approach, these models were able to screen over 26 400 molecules for their activity against leukemic T-cells (Ridges et al. 2012). The team then identified a compound called Lenaldekar that can eliminate the immature T-cell blasts *in vivo*.

Zebrafish Model of B-cell Neoplasms

- ***TEL-AML1 driven B-ALL model***: ALL is a clonal disease that develops through the accumulation of genetic modifications and/or mutations in the dominant clone. The most common type of genetic alteration in childhood ALL is the TEL-AML1(ETV6/CBFA2) fusion. An attempt to develop a B-ALL model from this fusion gene was unsuccessful in mice (Andreasson et al. 2001). In 2006, a group of scientists was able to create a model of the disease in zebrafish by overexpressing human TEL-AML1, either alone or fused to EGFP. The fusion protein was expressed either from the global promoters (*XEF* and *ZBA*) or from the lymphoid zebrafish promoter (*ZRAG2*). The two global promoters produced ALL in only 3% of the fish, suggesting the need for a secondary mutation for oncogenic transformation. This model produced T-ALLs, pro-B ALL, and bi-phenotypic ALL. The zebrafish model of ALL suggests that TEL-AML1 expression in non-committed progenitors can lead to the accumulation of pre-leukemic clone precursors.
- ***Myc-driven model of B-ALL***: Although modeling B-cell leukemia in zebrafish was lagging for many years, two recent studies showed that the use of human *c-MYC* or murine *Myc* genes driven by *ZRAG2* promoter could lead to the development of B-cell leukemia (Borga et al. 2019; Garcia et al. 2018). It was initially suggested that the Myc transgenic fish could only develop T-ALL. However, in later studies, these transgenic fish showed the immunophenotype of four different types of leukemia, with unique genetic signatures and molecular characteristics. The *MYC* overexpressing zebrafish develop T-ALL, bi-phenotypic B/T-ALL, ighm+ B-ALL, and ighz+ B-ALL. The authors of this study show that these models are highly penetrant B-ALLs that resemble human pre-B-ALL. The GFP

expressing leukemia cells could engraft when injected into irradiated wild-type, showing that hMYC B-ALL cells were truly malignant. The leukemia cells could be engrafted in the recipient fish; however, B-ALL exhibited lower numbers of leukemia-initiating cells in comparison to T-ALL. The MYC/hMYC zebrafish model develops mixed ALLs that are not bi-phenotypic but rather simultaneous cases that develop both T- and B-ALL (Borga et al. 2019; Garcia et al. 2018). Their study highlights the distinct molecular aberrancies that can activate both T- and B-ALL oncogenic pathways. Although overexpressing *MYC* can induce T-ALL or B-ALL, both require different cofactors to develop. The model is also sensitive to the various frontline human treatments, such as dexamethasone and radiotherapy, suggesting their potential clinical relevance to improving the treatment for B-ALL patients.

Zebrafish Model of NK-cell Neoplasms

Aggressive NK cell leukemias (ANKLs) are rare lymphoproliferative disorders of natural killer (NK) cells with a poor prognosis for patients. There have been numerous studies suggesting that the human ANKL could be caused by the *TP53* gene aberration (Huang et al. 2018). Both point mutations and deletions have also been identified in human ANKL cells, which suggest a role for TP53 in the pathogenesis of this disease. To study the effects of *TP53* on the development of leukemia, $tp53^{del/del}$ zebrafish model was generated in syngeneic CG1-strain zebrafish using TALEN endonucleases (Ignatius et al. 2018). The loss of *tp53* resulted in the development of several types of tumors, including malignant peripheral nerve-sheath tumors, germ cell tumors, angiosarcomas, and an NK cell leukemia. The $tp53^{del/del}$ zebrafish is the first animal model to describe the role of the Tp53 protein in the development of aggressive NK cell-like leukemias. Single-cell transcriptomic analysis of zebrafish blood lineages suggested that the $tp53^{del/del}$ ANKL exhibits the same characteristics as human NK cells. The large, vacuolated cytoplasm and prominent nucleoli of the leukemic cells indicated that these cells are high-grade aggressive NK cell cancers. This model was also used to perform large-scale transplantation of primary ANKL and visualize the growth of leukemia in live animals.

Patient-Derived Xenograft Models in Zebrafish

Several strains of zebrafish have been developed that can robustly engraft various human cancer cells (Hess et al. 2013; Moore et al. 2016; Tang et al. 2014). Furthermore, an improved Casper-strain was discovered with a homozygous compound mutation in *prkdc* and *il2rga* that does not have T, B, and NK cells (Yan et al. 2019). The development of *prkdc-/-;il2rga-/-* zebrafish strain has allowed robust long-term human patient-derived xenograft (PDX) engraftment with the same survival and proliferation characteristics as those observed in tumor-matched mouse models. The immune-deficient fish can survive at 37°C and engraft numerous human cancers for up to 28 days. The effects of prolonged exposure on the cell proliferation and growth rates of the fish are similar to those of mice. The zebrafish xenotransplant platform can also measure and analyze drug response in real time on patient-derived biopsy material. These models have been developed for a variety of lymphoid neoplasms (Bentley et al. 2015; Gacha-Garay et al. 2019; Somasagara et al. 2021).

Fruit Fly Model

The fruit fly, known as *Drosophila melanogaster*, serves as a model organism for studying various aspects of fundamental biology. The *Drosophila* genome is homologous to that of humans. Around 75% of the genes that cause diseases in humans have homologs in *Drosophila*, making it a natural target for studies in cancers (Ugur et al. 2016). The fruit fly can be used to study complex biological pathways relevant to cancer research. Its brief generation time and low maintenance costs make it an attractive candidate for biomedical research (Mirzoyan et al. 2019). The hematopoietic system of Drosophila plays a critical role in suppressing pathogenic invaders and in regulating the development and differentiation of hematopoietic cells (Banerjee et al. 2019). The mature blood cells of Drosophila are called hemocytes and can be divided into three cell types: the plasmatocytes, crystal cells, and lamellocytes (Evans et al. 2003). The plasmatocytes are specialized cells (the equivalent of human monocytes, macrophages, and neutrophils) that are capable of engulfing small pathogens and apoptotic cells, and they are also involved in the innate immune response (Letourneau et al. 2016).

For example, adult T-cell leukemia/lymphoma (ATL) is caused by the human T-cell lymphotropic virus type 1 (HTLV-1) following the activation of the Tax-1 transactivator (Giam and Semmes 2016). Transgenic flies with the Tax-1 gene show significantly higher numbers of circulating hemocytes (Shirinian et al. 2015). A study using both hematopoietic and non-hematopoietic tissues to study the transformative phenotype of Tax-1 *in vivo*. The fly eye was used as non-hematopoietic tissue to study the interactions between Tax-1 and its interacting partners. The knockdown of Relish, the Drosophila NF-κB family member, and Kenny, the Drosophila ortholog of IKKγ/NEMO, was then analyzed for a genetic screen to identify potential Tax-1 interactors. UBL-molecule Urm1, which is known to be a key component of the viral oncoprotein tax, has been shown to play a role in the subcellular signaling and targeting of Tax. This study shows that the Tax-1 mutant can transform cells in Drosophila by increasing the level of activated NF-κB. It provides a valuable model to study how this process works. The ability of non-hematopoietic tissue of Drosophila to generate robust phenotypes due to the expression of oncogene proteins can help elucidate the activity of human leukemic proteins.

Another approach to study the function of the human leukemogenic protein in Drosophila employs the fly hematopoietic system. One example would be RUNX1, which plays a crucial role in the development of blood cells. RUNX1 is a regulator of several steps in the development of blood cells. Recurrent point mutations or translocations in the *RUNX1* gene are known to cause human leukemia. The most notable example of a melanotic tumor gene that has been linked to human leukemia is hopscotch. Hop gene encodes the Drosophila homolog for the JAK kinase, which is a key component of the signaling pathway between cytokines (Hou et al. 1996). Early studies linked the JAK/STAT signaling to the development of fly leukemias (Yan et al. 1996). The level of JAK/STAT signaling can regulate the size of the adult eye and required to generate melanotic tumors in lymph gland-derived hemocytes (Amoyel et al. 2014).

Non-human Primate Model

Although the mouse is widely used for research in various fields, the advantages of using a non-human primate over rodents are many. One of these is that they have a closer physiological relationship to man and are more like man in terms of their drug metabolism. The length of the non-human primate's life span allows for long-term studies of carcinogenesis and potential relapse of the tumor. It also allows for the evaluation of the effects of various treatment modalities on the neoplastic process.

The non-human primates have been instrumental in our understanding of virus-induced oncogenesis. Viral infections are known to cause many types of human cancer (Schiller and Lowy 2014). In 2002, the WHO estimated that about 1.9 million cancer cases were caused by viral infections (Parkin 2006). The majority of these were caused by HPVs, lymphotropic viruses (human immunodeficiency virus [HIV] and HTLV-1), and hepatitis B and C viruses. The simian herpesvirus saimiri (HSV) and the herpesvirus ateles (HAV) are known to cause no disease in humans (Estep et al. 2010). However, they can cause cancer in other primates. In primates, such as tamarins and marmosets, exposure to HVS caused acute peripheral T-cell lymphomas (Fleckenstein et al. 1978). Type C wild-type HVS caused acute peripheral T-cells lymphomas in marmosets and cotton-top tamarins within only a few weeks (Knappe et al. 1998).

Similarly, Epstein–Barr virus (EBV), one of the five known human herpesviruses, is known to cause various cancers and lymphoproliferative disorders. The cotton-top tamarin, a new-world monkey, is an example of an animal that can be infected with EBV and develop B-cell lymphomas (Shope et al. 1973). Experiments in this animal were also conducted to evaluate the efficacy of an experimental vaccine (Epstein et al. 1985). Other new-world primates, such as the common marmoset and the owl monkey, can also be infected with EBV (Epstein 1975; Johannessen and Crawford 1999). Thus, the monkey models are suitable analogs for the lymphomas that arise in human organ graft recipients and support a direct role for EBV in tumorigenesis *in vivo*.

Non-Hodgkin's lymphoma is the second most common type of cancer among people with (HIV) infection (Grogg et al. 2007). It affects about 10% of patients with AIDS. Simian immunodeficiency virus infection has been linked to an increased risk of AIDS-associated lymphoma (AAL) (Grogg et al. 2007). This animal model is an appropriate animal study tool to study the pathogenesis of AAL. Another important pathogen that can cause chronic infection leading up to the development of adult T-cell leukemia or lymphoma is HTLV-1. In certain geographic regions, high cases of HIV/HTLV-1 coinfection are reported. The simian T-cell leukemia virus (STLV-1) is known to infect Old World monkeys and cause various immunological and morphological features to appear similar to the human variant of the virus known as HTLV-1 (Courgnaud et al. 2004). The simian ancestor of HTLV-1 is the so-called STLV-1. It is believed that this virus was caused by cross-species transmission among humans and non-human primates. The SIV infection of rhesus monkeys with the HTLV-1 led to the upregulation of its expression and the emergence of flower cells within the peripheral circulation (Traina-Dorge et al. 2007). After SIV coinfection, significant increases in circulating CD8+ T cells, as well as the proviral loads, were noticed. The pattern of recurrent episodes of smoldering and chronic ATLL is consistent with the characteristics of this disease. Also, peripheral blood smears of non-carriers of HTLV-1 rarely show flower cells. In the first macaque that died of AIDS after being coinfected with the virus, the researchers proposed that a pre-leukemic condition might have been caused by the SIV/STLV-1 combination. The SIV/STLV-1 model is a useful tool for studying the effects of coinfection on the development of leukemia. It can also be used to test the efficacy of various anti-neoplastic agents. Therefore, the SIV/HTLV-1 model of coinfection is a useful tool for studying the pathogenesis of HTLV-1 mediated T-cell leukemogenesis. These models can also be used to test the efficacy of various anti-neoplastic agents.

Mouse Models of Lymphoid Neoplasia

The laboratory mouse is a highly effective model system for lymphoid malignancies due to its small size and the significant physiological and molecular similarities between humans and mice. Since the advent of the nude mouse model in the 1960s, various types of genetically engineered and transplantation-based cancer models have been introduced (Flanagan 1966; Pantelouris and Hair 1970). Several different approaches have been used to develop *Mus musculus* tumor models, including the use of explant and chemical carcinogens, the use of genetically engineered mice, and the development of xenograft tumors (Kohnken et al. 2017).

- ***Cell line transplant model***: Allografting human tumor cells are commonly used in cancer research (Voskoglou-Nomikos et al. 2003). The use of cell line allograft models for drug testing allows for the fast evaluation of potential cancer-related genes and their immunological effects (Voskoglou-Nomikos et al. 2003). These models have provided the foundation for the development of cancer immunotherapies. Although cancer cell lines can contain multiple mutations during their early stages, they can also acquire additional aberrations after being inactivated for extended periods. This suggests that these models are not very accurate predictors of clinical response. While allografting mouse cancer cell lines can be done in immunoproficient hosts, the transplant of human material is frequently performed in immunocompromised mice to prevent rejection; therefore, this system is not suitable for studying the role of the immune system in cancer development (Table 4.1).
- ***PDX model***: PDX models are derived from human tumor samples that are removed from their primary host and then introduced to mice (Bhimani et al. 2020). Unlike cell lines, they maintain the molecular, genetic, as well as histologic properties of their primary tumors. These models can be used to evaluate the safety and effectiveness of targeted drugs in combination with standard treatment regimens. Using PDX models, large-scale studies can be carried out to predict the clinical response of drug candidates. While the initial series of PDX models have served as an important tool toward personalized treatment, the lack of translational models that describe the interaction between the human immune system and cancer had initially hindered the development of human immunotherapeutics for cancers.

It is widely believed that the immune system plays a significant role in the development of cancer. The increasing number of new therapeutic regimens based on the concept of immunological blockades has highlighted the importance of the human immune system in the treatment of cancer. Humanized mice are expected to aid in the study of the interactions between cancer and human immune systems. Various humanized mouse models, such as the Hu-PBL (human-peripheral blood leukocytes), SRC (SCID-repopulating cell), and Thy/HSC, are often used in human oncology studies (Abuljadayel et al. 2004; Duchosal et al. 1992; Lan et al. 2006; Traggiai et al. 2004). The Hu-PBL-SCID model is created by the introduction of human peripheral blood cells into immunodeficient mouse models that allows for multi-lineage human immune subpopulations in mice. However, the lack of hematopoietic stem/progenitor cells to replace existing immune cells makes this model difficult to replicate. The SRC-Hu model is a strategy used to develop human immunity by transferring human

Table 4.1 Cell transplant models of lymphoid neoplasms.

	Cell lines	Diseases
B-cells	L1210, Raji, Jijoye, Daudi, Ramos, BJAB, SU-DHL-4, 38C13, BCL1, A20, CA46, MC116, 4TOO, L3055, SC-1, CH44, DoHH-2, S11, LY-ar/LY-as, Granta 519, Pi-BCL1, 38C13 Her2/neu, Myc5-M5, FL5.12, 38C13 CD20+, Z138, HKBML, NALM6, 697, KOPN-8, SEM, VAL, HG-3, JVM-3, JVM-13, MEC-1, PGA-1, NU-DHL-1, OCI-LY3, RI-1, U-2932, U-2946, OCI-LY7, OCI-LY19, SU-DHL-6, WSU-DLCL2, BONNA-12, HAIR-M, HC-1, GRANTA-519, JEKO-1, JVM-2, MINO, REC-1, BC-3, BCBL-1, CRO-AP2, CRO-AP5, U-2940	Pre-B-ALL B-NHL: Burkitt/B-ALL B-NHL: CLL/PLL B-NHL: DLBCL ABC B-NHL: DLBCL GC B-NHL: HCL B-NHL: MCL B-NHL: PEL B-NHL: PMBL
T-cells	T-ALL-1, KOPTK1, DND41, HPB-ALL, RPMI-8402, CEM, PF382, HSB2, BE-13, SUP-T11, Jurkat, Loucy, Molt-4, Molt-16, SKW-3, MyLa, Hut78, HH, MAC2A, MAC2B, FE-PD, MAC1, SeAx, Sez4, L929, C127, EL4, RMA, Yac-1, DERL-2, DERL-7, SUP-T1, SR-786, HDLM-2, CCRF-CEM, DND-41, HPB-ALL, MOTN-1, DEL, SR-786, SU-DHL-1, SUP-M2	Hodgkin's lymphoma T-ALL/T-LL Mature T-malignancy CTCL ALCL
NK-cells	NK-92, KHYG-1, YT	NK malignancy
Plasma cells	KMS-12-BM, L-363, LP-1, OPM-2, RPMI-8226, U-266	Multiple myeloma/PCL
Non-T- and non-B-cells	Reh	ALL

hematopoietic stem/progenitor cells into adult or neonatal Il2rg knockout recipients. The Thy/HSC model was developed by the co-transplantation of human liver and thymic tissues into a renal capsule and the administration of CD34+ human fetal cells. The engrafted mice showed the robust reconstitution of various human hematopoietic cells, including T-, B-, and dendritic cells.

- ***Genetically engineered mouse model (GEMM) of de novo cancer***: The first cloned oncogene was used in the development of transgenic mice during the early 1980s (Brinster et al. 1984). This *OncoMouse*, which was a GEMM, exhibited the activation of a specific oncogene, which could cause mammary tumors. The study established the possibility that the expression of oncogenes in normal cells could lead to the formation of tumors. The development of gene-targeting technology in 1992 opened the possibility of studying the link between cancer and the tumor suppressor gene (TSG) (Finlay 1992). The oncogene transgenic model and the tumor suppressor knockout mouse have provided insight into the molecular basis of a variety of human cancer. However, these models are no match for the sporadic nature of cancer. A more sophisticated mouse model can be used to enable the expression of tumor suppressors and oncogenes in a conditional GEMM. The use of conditional knock-out alleles has been successfully utilized to study the *in vivo* role of several B-cell lymphomas associated tumor suppressors such as EZH2, *TET2*, *CREBBP*, and *BLIMP1* (Meyer et al. 2021; Ogilvy et al. 1999). Similarly, the conditional activation of the gain-of-function (BCL2) alleles can allow to study of the role of these genes in tumor development (McDonnell et al. 1989). Through the introduction of certain genetic mutations, one can generate mouse models with the same characteristics of tumors in patients (Table 4.2).

  Genetically engineered mice are often used for studying human diseases due to their similarities in pathophysiology. A Cre-loxP system is a tool used for generating the conditional expression of genes that are relevant to a tissue or cell's spatial control (Kim et al. 2018). Although the Cre-LoxP system can modify the expression of multiple genes simultaneously, it does not fully replicate the sequential accumulation of mutational events in multistep carcinogenesis. This system can be used to allow the sequential generation of mutations that can be used to target specific cancer cells. In 2014, a dual-recombination system was developed, which allows the sequential manipulation of gene expression through two independent recombination systems (Schonhuber et al. 2014). This approach aims to identify and develop therapeutic targets for autochthonous tumors through the sequential induction of mutations in non-autonomous pathways or processes. Similarly, an intricate induction of somatic mutation at a chosen time and in a specific tissue can be achieved through the fusion of a mutated hormone-binding domain of estrogen receptor (ERT) with the Cre-recombinase (Whitfield et al. 2015). The inducible Cre-ERT pathway generates a Cre-recombinase activation response after administration of tamoxifen.
- **Non-germline genetically engineered mouse models (GEMM):** Although the use of germline GEMMs has been valuable in cancer research, their validation and development are still hampered by time and expense. The increasing number of cancer mutations identified in sequencing studies has raised the prospect of accelerating *in vivo* evaluation of cancer candidate genes and the known cancer genes in nGEMMs (Heyer et al. 2010). For example, in a well-characterized Eμ-Myc mouse lymphoma model, a complex pool of shRNAs was then introduced to identify genes that promote tumorigenesis (Bric et al. 2009). The resulting pool of shRNAs revealed various tumor suppressors, such as Sfrp1, Numb, and Mek1. The study also identified other components of the DNA damage response machinery, such as Rad17. The loss of Rad17 is associated with a poor prognosis in humans (Bric et al. 2009; Heyer et al. 2010).

Over the past decades, various approaches for genome editing were developed, such as the Zinc-finger nucleases and the transcription activator-like nucleases. The advent of CRISPR/Cas9 (clustered regularly interspaced short palindromic repeats/Cas9) technology has allowed us to utilize these approaches more effectively. The CRISPR/Cas9 system was first observed as a prokaryotic system that confers resistance to genetic elements (Lander 2016). It is now widely used to develop effective gene editing. The system can be directed to any genomic region by using single-guide RNAs, and Cas9 nucleases can trigger double-stranded cleavage of target DNA sequences. The use of CRISPR/Cas9 technology for rapid cancer modeling has shown to be an efficient method for introducing human genetic alterations into the mouse germline (Ishio et al. 2021; van der Weyden et al. 2021). These changes can be rapidly introduced using a variety of methods, including point mutations, deletions, and translocations.

Misidentified germline and somatic mutations in human tissue samples can result in the production of defective proteins with residual activity. It has been shown that patient-relevant TSG mutations can induce different phenotypes in mice. These studies provide important information about the contribution of these mutations to tumorigenesis and the therapy response. For example, the presence of Trp53 hotspots in mice has been associated with enhanced oncogenic activity when compared to the Trp53 knockout mice. This method can identify the causal link between introducing germline or somatic mutations into GEMMs and improving therapy responsiveness.

Table 4.2 Genetically engineered mouse models of lymphoid neoplasms.

Model	Lineage	Diseases	Secondary mutations
B10 H-2^a H-4^bp/Wts	B-cells	CLL	
SL/KH	B-cells	Pre-B lymphoma	
Eμ-N-myc *transgenic mice*	B-cells	Indolent B-NHL	
NFS.V+	B-cells	Marginal zone lymphoma	
NMRI/RFB-MuLV	B-cells		
B6-l-MYC	B-cells	Burkitt-like lymphoma	
VavP-Bcl2	B-cells	Follicular lymphoma	
Lig4/p53 KO	B-cells	Pro/Pre-B lymphoma	
Eμ-BRD2	B-cells	DLBCL	
Bcl6 Knock in	B-cells	DLBCL	
Bcl6/Myc transgenic	B-cells	DLBCL	
IL-14aTGxc-Myc transgenic	B-cells	Mantle cell lymphoma	
Myc/BCR^{HEL}/HEL	B-cells	Burkitt-like lymphoma	
Eμ-myc	B-cells	DLBCL	
RzCD19Cre	B-cells	Non-Hodgkin's lymphoma	
UVB induced $p53^{+/-}$	B-cells	Mature B-cell lymphoma	
ETV-RUNX1; t(12:21) (p13;q22)	B-cells	B-ALL	$Cdkn2a^{-/-}$
E2A-PBX1; t(1;19)(q23;p13)	T- and B-cells	Mixed lineage ALL	Pim1, Notch1
E2A-HLF; t(17;19)(q22;p13)	T-cells	T-ALL	
BCR-ABL; t(9;22)(q34;q11)	T-, B-, and myeloid cells	AML, T-ALL, and B-ALL	
MLL-AF4; t(4;11)(q21;q23)	B- and myeloid cells	BCL, B-ALL, and AML	
MLL-ENL; t(9;11)(p22;q23)	T-, B-, and myeloid cells	B-ALL, mixed lineage ALL	
$Pax5^{+/-}$	B-cells	B-ALL	STAT5b
IGH-Myc	B-cells	BCL, B-ALL	
NOTCH1	T-cells	T-ALL	KRasG12D
TAL1 mutation	T-cells	TCL and T-ALL	
LMO2	*T-cells*	*TCL and T-ALL*	
mir-15a/16–1$^{-/-}$ and *mir-15a/16-1*^{floxed}CD19-Cre	B-cells	MBL and CLL	
14qC3 minimal deleted region (MDR)$^{-/-}$ and *MDR*^{floxed}CD19-Cre	B-cells	MBL, CLL, and NHL	
14qC3 common deleted region (CDR)^{floxed}CD19-Cre	B-cells	MBL, CLL, and NHL	
Eμ-TCL1	B-cells	CLL	
APRIL	B-cells	CLL	
BCL2 × traf2dn	B-cells	CLL	
ROR1	B-cells	CLL	
Eμ-mir-29	B-cells	CLL	
Vh11 × irf4$^{-/-}$	B-cells	CLL	
IgH.T and IgH.TEμ	B-cells	CLL	
5T2MM	Plasma cells	MM	
5T33MM	Plasma cells	MM	
5TGM1	Plasma cells	MM	
MOPC315.BM	Plasma cells	MM	
Vk12653	Plasma cells	MM	

(Continued)

Table 4.2 (Continued)

Model	Lineage	Diseases	Secondary mutations
Vk12598	Plasma cells	MM	
Myc/Bcl-X_L double	Plasma cells	MM	
Eμ-XBP-1	Plasma cells	MM	
LTR-Tax	T-cells	ATL	
Lck-Tax	T-cells	ATLL	
CD4-HBZ	T-cells	ATL	
Lck^d-Tax	T-cells	ATLL	
HTLV-1 Tax x IFN-$\gamma^{-/-}$	T-cells	Large granular leukemia/ lymphoma	
EμSRα-tTA/Tet-o-wt/M22/M47 Tax	T-cells	Cutaneous ATL	
Lck-HTLV-1 Tax	T-cells	Leukemia and lymphoma	
huGMZB-Tax	T-cells	LGLL	
HTLV-I LTR/c-myc x Ig/tax	T-cells	ATL	
$hSTAT5B^{N642H}$	T-cells	LGLL	
Lck^{pr}-hTCL1A	T-cells	T-PLL	
Eμ-B29-TCL1	T-cells	T-PLL	
CD2-p13(MTCP1)	T-cells	T-PLL	
$Roquin^{san/+}$	T-cells	AITL	
Vav-Lin28 transgenic mice	T-cells	PTCL-NOS	
CD4-and Lck^{pr}-Snf5 fl/fl	T-cells	PTCL-NOS	
ITK-SYK-CD4-Cre transgenic mice	T-cells	PTCL-NOS	
Lck^{pr}-BCL2 transgenic mice	T-cells	LCL and/or SLL	

Use of Animal Models in Translational Research

- **Drug discovery**: Despite the large number of new drug targets identified during the Human Genome Project, the success rate for drugs during the development stage remains low (Takebe et al. 2018). The high attrition rate of potential cancer drugs during preclinical testing reflects the inefficient nature of the drug discovery and development process (Arrowsmith 2011; Arrowsmith and Miller 2013). This high rate of failure underscores the need for more accurate modeling to predict the effectiveness of compounds before they are launched in human trials. Animal models have become increasingly popular in the field of medical research due to their ability to provide insight into the complexity of human diseases. Having the most successful results during the non-clinical phases of drug development can help minimize the risk of failure. The importance of a well-defined preclinical model is critically important for the development of a drug candidate. A good animal model can support the validation of a potential target, provide insight into the effects of the drug candidate, and help build confidence in the efficacy of the trial (Johnson et al. 2001). To properly utilize an animal model, it is important to first define a question and then select the appropriate model. Most drug discovery programs follow a process that involves identifying a target, validating the compound, and performing a series of tests for safety and efficacy.
- **Personalized medicine**: Patient-derived xenograft, or PDX, models are designed to replicate the characteristics of a particular type of cancer cell (Hidalgo et al. 2014). Serially passaged PDXs have biological consistency with the origin of the tumor and are phenotypically stable over multiple generations (Whittle et al. 2015). Although they are often perceived as slow and variable, these models may help elucidate the dynamics of human tumors. While PDX models are commonly used as research tools, they are also being touted as predictive tools for clinical decisions. Several studies have shown that the models can predict the outcome of a patient's clinical response. These models can identify biomarkers that predict the sensitivity or resistance of a given therapy (Sun et al. 2021). This approach could help identify potential therapeutic

options for future patient populations based on the endpoints of a given disease. For example, in a recent study, the PDX model of B-cell lymphoma recapitulated the various features of the original tumor. DNA sequencing revealed that PDX mice exhibited the same original mutation that caused the tumors (Zhang et al. 2017). The PDX model was also able to mimic the transient lymphocytosis that was observed in patients with relapsed/refractory mantle cell lymphoma. Furthermore, the investigators were able to generate model of primary and acquired resistance to ibrutinib to study the effects of different drug resistance on the development and use of new drug combination regimens. These models successfully guided the therapy of a patient with B-cell lymphoma. The impact of PDX models on precision medicine is likely to be substantial, as they can reveal biomarkers that predict the sensitivity or resistance to a given therapy. Moreover, a diverse portfolio of PDX models could be used to evaluate the therapeutic efficacy of a given drug or combination. The large number of diverse models will identify molecular features that can trigger different responses in different models.

- **Immune checkpoint blockers and combination with immunotherapies:** The success of checkpoint blockers in treating cancer has shown that the immune system is a crucial component of the war against cancer (Darvin et al. 2018). Following the successful treatment of solid tumor patients with immune checkpoint blockade therapy, it has gained momentum as a promising treatment option for lymphoid malignancies. A variety of agents are being studied to improve the level of an immunological response that can trigger the elimination of cancer cells. The goal is to develop effective agents that can activate this process and improve the level of immune response against tumors. The programmed death 1 (PD1) and the cytotoxic T-cell-associated protein 4 (CTLA-4) have emerged as key targets of unprecedented activity in treating various types of lymphoid neoplasms (Ansell et al. 2009; Bashey et al. 2009). As the role of immune checkpoint blockers in the treatment of patients with relapsed/refractory lymphoma evolves, it is important to note that the importance of predicting which patients will benefit from checkpoint blockers is also emphasized. Due to the significant role of the tumor's microenvironment on the development and efficacy of cancer immunotherapies, a more accurate and representative model is needed. Developing animal models with human immune systems is a promising strategy to improve the understanding of the human tumor microenvironment and the therapeutic effects of various immunomodulatory agents. Engrafting human peripheral blood mononuclear cells in mice is a simple and economical method to generate humanized mice. The T-cells, which are a central component of the immune system, have become a focal point of research in the effort to fight cancer. The tumor-infiltrating T-cells commonly fail to kill cancer cells despite carrying out their intended function (Woo et al. 2012). They also often co-express other negative molecules such as LAG-3 and T-cell immunoglobulin (Anderson et al. 2016). The anti-LAG-3 and PD-1 blockades have been shown to reverse T-cell functions in animal models (Sakuishi et al. 2010). A combination of these agents is currently being studied in clinical trials. There are numerous targets and checkpoints in the tumor microenvironment that can be exploited to enhance the level of immune response.

Modeling cancer in animals is a dynamic and continuously evolving experimental pursuit in medical research. As they have evolved to reflect different aspects of human disease, they have become more accurate, though no one model can perfectly recapitulate any human disease. Collective experiences from a variety of different animal models may be one approach to enhance the relevance and informativeness of the research. The next step will be to see if they have predictive value in the development of drugs.

Conclusions

Animal modeling is considered the gold standard in terms of understanding disease pathways. Each of these animal models has greatly impacted the study of lymphoid cancer biology, and its treatment. They allow us to study the mechanisms by which novel mutations can affect the development of cancer cells and their potential treatment. The increasing number of studies related to the use of animal models and the advancements in the field of molecular biology are contributing to the improvement of patients with lymphoid malignancies.

Must Read References

Davidson, A.J. and Zon, L.I. (2004). The 'definitive' (and 'primitive') guide to zebrafish hematopoiesis. *Oncogene* 23: 7233–7246.

Duchosal, M.A., Eming, S.A., McConahey, P.J. et al. (1992). The hu-PBL-SCID mouse model. long-term human serologic evolution associated with the xenogeneic transfer of human peripheral blood leukocytes into SCID mice. *Cell. Immunol.* 139: 468–477.

Mirzoyan, Z. et al. (2019). Drosophila melanogaster: a model organism to study cancer. *Front. Genet.* 10: 51.

Ridges, S. et al. (2012). Zebrafish screen identifies novel compound with selective toxicity against leukemia. *Blood* 119: 5621–5631.

References

Abuljadayel, I.S. et al. (2004). SCID repopulating cells derived from unmobilised adult human peripheral blood. *Curr Med Res Opin* 20: 87–100.

Amoyel, M., Anderson, A.M., and Bach, E.A. (2014). JAK/STAT pathway dysregulation in tumors: a Drosophila perspective. *Semin. Cell Dev. Biol.* 28: 96–103.

Anderson, A.C., Joller, N., and Kuchroo, V.K. (2016). Lag-3, Tim-3, and TIGIT: co-inhibitory receptors with specialized functions in immune regulation. *Immunity* 44: 989–1004.

Andreasson, P., Schwaller, J., Anastasiadou, E. et al. (2001). The expression of ETV6/CBFA2 (TEL/AML1) is not sufficient for the transformation of hematopoietic cell lines in vitro or the induction of hematologic disease in vivo. *Cancer Genet. Cytogenet.* 130: 93–104.

Ansell, S.M. et al. (2009). Phase I study of ipilimumab, an anti-CTLA-4 monoclonal antibody, in patients with relapsed and refractory B-cell non-Hodgkin lymphoma. *Clin. Cancer Res.* 15: 6446–6453.

Arrowsmith, J. (2011). Trial watch: phase II failures: 2008-2010. *Nat. Rev. Drug Discov.* 10: 328–329.

Arrowsmith, J. and Miller, P. (2013). Trial watch: phase II and phase III attrition rates 2011-2012. *Nat. Rev. Drug Discov.* 12: 569.

Banerjee, U., Girard, J.R., Goins, L.M. et al. (2019). Drosophila as a genetic model for hematopoiesis. *Genetics* 211: 367–417.

Bashey, A. et al. (2009). CTLA4 blockade with ipilimumab to treat relapse of malignancy after allogeneic hematopoietic cell transplantation. *Blood* 113: 1581–1588.

Bentley, V.L. et al. (2015). Focused chemical genomics using zebrafish xenotransplantation as a preclinical therapeutic platform for T-cell acute lymphoblastic leukemia. *Haematologica* 100: 70–76.

Bhimani, J., Ball, K., and Stebbing, J. (2020). Patient-derived xenograft models-the future of personalised cancer treatment. *Br. J. Cancer* 122: 601–602.

Blackburn, J.S. et al. (2012). Notch signaling expands a pre-malignant pool of T-cell acute lymphoblastic leukemia clones without affecting leukemia-propagating cell frequency. *Leukemia* 26: 2069–2078.

Borga, C. et al. (2019). Simultaneous B and T cell acute lymphoblastic leukemias in zebrafish driven by transgenic MYC: implications for oncogenesis and lymphopoiesis. *Leukemia* 33: 333–347.

Bric, A. et al. (2009). Functional identification of tumor-suppressor genes through an in vivo RNA interference screen in a mouse lymphoma model. *Cancer Cell* 16: 324–335.

Brinster, R.L. et al. (1984). Transgenic mice harboring SV40 T-antigen genes develop characteristic brain tumors. *Cell* 37: 367–379.

Chen, J. et al. (2007). NOTCH1-induced T-cell leukemia in transgenic zebrafish. *Leukemia* 21: 462–471.

Collins, I. and Workman, P. (2006). New approaches to molecular cancer therapeutics. *Nat. Chem. Biol.* 2: 689–700.

Courgnaud, V. et al. (2004). Simian T-cell leukemia virus (STLV) infection in wild primate populations in Cameroon: evidence for dual STLV type 1 and type 3 infection in agile mangabeys (Cercocebus agilis). *J. Virol.* 78: 4700–4709.

Darvin, P., Toor, S.M., Sasidharan Nair, V. et al. (2018). Immune checkpoint inhibitors: recent progress and potential biomarkers. *Exp. Mol. Med.* 50: 1–11.

Davidson, A.J. and Zon, L.I. (2004). The 'definitive' (and 'primitive') guide to zebrafish hematopoiesis. *Oncogene* 23: 7233–7246.

Duchosal, M.A., Eming, S.A., McConahey, P.J. et al. (1992). The hu-PBL-SCID mouse model. long-term human serologic evolution associated with the xenogeneic transfer of human peripheral blood leukocytes into SCID mice. *Cell. Immunol.* 139: 468–477.

Epstein, M.A., zur Hausen, H., Ball, G. et al. (1975). Pilot experiments with EB virus in owl monkeys (Aotus trivirgatus). III. Serological and biochemical findings in an animal with reticuloproliferative disease. *Int. J. Cancer* 15: 17–22.

Epstein, M.A., Morgan, A.J., Finerty, S. et al. (1985). Protection of cottontop tamarins against Epstein-Barr virus-induced malignant lymphoma by a prototype subunit vaccine. *Nature* 318: 287–289.

Ericsson, A.C., Crim, M.J., and Franklin, C.L. (2013). A brief history of animal modeling. *Mo. Med.* 110: 201–205.

Estep, R.D., Messaoudi, I., and Wong, S.W. (2010). Simian herpesviruses and their risk to humans. *Vaccine* 28 (Suppl 2): B78–84.

Evans, C.J., Hartenstein, V., and Banerjee, U. (2003). Thicker than blood: conserved mechanisms in Drosophila and vertebrate hematopoiesis. *Dev. Cell* 5: 673–690.

Feng, H. et al. (2007). Heat-shock induction of T-cell lymphoma/leukaemia in conditional Cre/lox-regulated transgenic zebrafish. *Br. J. Haematol.* 138: 169–175.

Finlay, C.A. (1992). p53 loss of function: implications for the processes of immortalization and tumorigenesis. *Bioessays* 14: 557–560.

Flanagan, S.P. (1966). 'Nude', a new hairless gene with pleiotropic effects in the mouse. *Genet. Res.* 8: 295–309.

Fleckenstein, B. et al. (1978). Tumour induction with DNA of oncogenic primate herpesviruses. *Nature* 274: 57–59.

Frazer, J.K. et al. (2009). Heritable T-cell malignancy models established in a zebrafish phenotypic screen. *Leukemia* 23: 1825–1835.

Gacha-Garay, M.J. et al. (2019). Pilot study of an integrative new tool for studying clinical outcome discrimination in acute leukemia. *Front. Oncol.* 9: 245.

Garcia, E.G. et al. (2018). Cell of origin dictates aggression and stem cell number in acute lymphoblastic leukemia. *Leukemia* 32: 1860–1865.

Giam, C.Z. and Semmes, O.J. (2016). HTLV-1 Infection and adult T-cell leukemia/lymphoma-A tale of two proteins: tax and HBZ. *Viruses* 8.

Gore, A.V., Pillay, L.M., Venero Galanternik, M. et al. (2018). The zebrafish: a fintastic model for hematopoietic development and disease. *Wiley Interdiscip Rev. Dev. Biol.* 7: e312.

Grogg, K.L., Miller, R.F., and Dogan, A. (2007). HIV infection and lymphoma. *J. Clin. Pathol.* 60: 1365–1372.

Gutierrez, A. et al. (2011). Pten mediates Myc oncogene dependence in a conditional zebrafish model of T cell acute lymphoblastic leukemia. *J. Exp. Med.* 208: 1595–1603.

Hackam, D.G. and Redelmeier, D.A. (2006). Translation of research evidence from animals to humans. *JAMA* 296: 1731–1732.

Hess, I., Iwanami, N., Schorpp, M. et al. (2013). Zebrafish model for allogeneic hematopoietic cell transplantation not requiring preconditioning. *Proc. Natl. Acad. Sci. U S A* 110: 4327–4332.

Heyer, J., Kwong, L.N., Lowe, S.W. et al. (2010). Non-germline genetically engineered mouse models for translational cancer research. *Nat. Rev. Cancer* 10: 470–480.

Hidalgo, M. et al. (2014). Patient-derived xenograft models: an emerging platform for translational cancer research. *Cancer Discov.* 4: 998–1013.

Hou, X.S., Melnick, M.B., and Perrimon, N. (1996). Marelle acts downstream of the Drosophila HOP/JAK kinase and encodes a protein similar to the mammalian STATs. *Cell* 84: 411–419.

Huang, L. et al. (2018). Integrated genomic analysis identifies deregulated JAK/STAT-MYC-biosynthesis axis in aggressive NK-cell leukemia. *Cell Res.* 28: 172–186.

Ignatius, M.S. et al. (2018). tp53 deficiency causes a wide tumor spectrum and increases embryonal rhabdomyosarcoma metastasis in zebrafish. *Elife* 7.

Ishio, T. et al. (2021). Genome-wide CRISPR screen identifies CDK6 as a therapeutic target in adult T-cell leukemia/lymphoma. *Blood* 139 (10): 1541–1556.

Johannessen, I. and Crawford, D.H. (1999). In vivo models for Epstein-Barr virus (EBV)-associated B cell lymphoproliferative disease (BLPD). *Rev. Med. Virol.* 9: 263–277.

Johnson, J.I. et al. (2001). Relationships between drug activity in NCI preclinical in vitro and in vivo models and early clinical trials. *Br. J. Cancer* 84: 1424–1431.

Kim, H., Kim, M., Im, S.K. et al. (2018). Mouse Cre-LoxP system: general principles to determine tissue-specific roles of target genes. *Lab. Anim. Res.* 34: 147–159.

Knappe, A. et al. (1998). T-cell lymphoma caused by herpesvirus saimiri C488 independently of ie14/vsag, a viral gene with superantigen homology. *J. Virol.* 72: 3469–3471.

Kohnken, R., Porcu, P., and Mishra, A. (2017). Overview of the use of murine models in leukemia and lymphoma research. *Front. Oncol.* 7: 22.

La Starza, R. et al. (2014). Genetic profile of T-cell acute lymphoblastic leukemias with MYC translocations. *Blood* 124: 3577–3582.

Lan, P., Tonomura, N., Shimizu, A. et al. (2006). Reconstitution of a functional human immune system in immunodeficient mice through combined human fetal thymus/liver and CD34+ cell transplantation. *Blood* 108: 487–492.

Lander, E.S. (2016). The heroes of CRISPR. *Cell* 164: 18–28.

Langenau, D.M. et al. (2003). Myc-induced T cell leukemia in transgenic zebrafish. *Science* 299: 887–890.

Langenau, D.M. et al. (2005). Cre/lox-regulated transgenic zebrafish model with conditional myc-induced T cell acute lymphoblastic leukemia. *Proc. Natl. Acad. Sci. U S A* 102: 6068–6073.

Letourneau, M. et al. (2016). Drosophila hematopoiesis under normal conditions and in response to immune stress. *FEBS Lett.* 590: 4034–4051.

McDonnell, T.J. et al. (1989). bcl-2-immunoglobulin transgenic mice demonstrate extended B cell survival and follicular lymphoproliferation. *Cell* 57: 79–88.

Meyer, S.N., Koul, S., and Pasqualucci, L. (2021). Mouse models of germinal center derived B-cell lymphomas. *Front. Immunol.* 12: 710711.

Mirzoyan, Z. et al. (2019). Drosophila melanogaster: a model organism to study cancer. *Front. Genet.* 10: 51.

Moore, J.C. et al. (2016). Single-cell imaging of normal and malignant cell engraftment into optically clear prkdc-null SCID zebrafish. *J. Exp. Med.* 213: 2575–2589.

Morton, L.M. et al. (2007). Proposed classification of lymphoid neoplasms for epidemiologic research from the pathology working group of the international lymphoma epidemiology consortium (interlymph). *Blood* 110: 695–708.

Ogilvy, S. et al. (1999). Constitutive Bcl-2 expression throughout the hematopoietic compartment affects multiple lineages and enhances progenitor cell survival. *Proc. Natl. Acad. Sci. U S A* 96: 14943–14948.

Pantelouris, E.M. and Hair, J. (1970). Thymus dysgenesis in nude (nu nu) mice. *J. Embryol. Exp. Morphol.* 24: 615–623.

Parkin, D.M. (2006). The global health burden of infection-associated cancers in the year 2002. *Int. J. Cancer* 118: 3030–344.

Ridges, S. et al. (2012). Zebrafish screen identifies novel compound with selective toxicity against leukemia. *Blood* 119: 5621–5631.

Sakuishi, K. et al. (2010). Targeting Tim-3 and PD-1 pathways to reverse T cell exhaustion and restore anti-tumor immunity. *J. Exp. Med.* 207: 2187–2194.

Schiller, J.T. and Lowy, D.R. (2014). Virus infection and human cancer: an overview. *Recent Results Cancer Res.* 193: 1–10.

Schonhuber, N. et al. (2014). A next-generation dual-recombinase system for time- and host-specific targeting of pancreatic cancer. *Nat. Med.* 20: 1340–1347.

Shirinian, M. et al. (2015). A transgenic drosophila melanogaster model to study human T-lymphotropic virus oncoprotein tax-1-driven transformation in vivo. *J. Virol.* 89: 8092–8095.

Shope, T., Dechairo, D., and Miller, G. (1973). Malignant lymphoma in cottontop marmosets after inoculation with Epstein-Barr virus. *Proc. Natl. Acad. Sci. U S A* 70: 2487–2491.

Smith, A.C. et al. (2010). High-throughput cell transplantation establishes that tumor-initiating cells are abundant in zebrafish T-cell acute lymphoblastic leukemia. *Blood* 115: 3296–3303.

Somasagara, R.R. et al. (2021). Targeted therapy of human leukemia xenografts in immunodeficient zebrafish. *Sci. Rep.* 11: 5715.

Stoletov, K. and Klemke, R. (2008). Catch of the day: zebrafish as a human cancer model. *Oncogene* 27: 4509–4520.

Sun, H. et al. (2021). Comprehensive characterization of 536 patient-derived xenograft models prioritizes candidatesfor targeted treatment. *Nat. Commun.* 12: 5086.

Swerdlow, S.H. et al. (2016). The 2016 revision of the World Health Organization classification of lymphoid neoplasms. *Blood* 127: 2375–2390.

Takebe, T., Imai, R., and Ono, S. (2018). The current status of drug discovery and development as originated in united states academia: the influence of industrial and academic collaboration on drug discovery and development. *Clin. Transl. Sci.* 11: 597–606.

Tang, Q. et al. (2014). Optimized cell transplantation using adult rag2 mutant zebrafish. *Nat. Methods* 11: 821–824.

Traggiai, E. et al. (2004). Development of a human adaptive immune system in cord blood cell-transplanted mice. *Science* 304: 104–107.

Traina-Dorge, V.L., Martin, L.N., Lorino, R. et al. (2007). Human T cell leukemia virus type 1 up-regulation after simian immunodeficiency virus-1 coinfection in the non-human primate. *J. Infect. Dis.* 195: 562–571.

Ugur, B., Chen, K., and Bellen, H.J. (2016). Drosophila tools and assays for the study of human diseases. *Dis. Model. Mech.* 9: 235–244.

van der Weyden, L., Jonkers, J., and Adams, D.J. (2021). The use of CRISPR/Cas9-based gene editing strategies to explore cancer gene function in mice. *Curr. Opin. Genet. Dev.* 66: 57–62.

Voskoglou-Nomikos, T., Pater, J.L., and Seymour, L. (2003). Clinical predictive value of the in vitro cell line, human xenograft, and mouse allograft preclinical cancer models. *Clin. Cancer Res.* 9: 4227–4239.

Weng, A.P. et al. (2004). Activating mutations of NOTCH1 in human T cell acute lymphoblastic leukemia. *Science* 306: 269–271.

White, R., Rose, K., and Zon, L. (2013). Zebrafish cancer: the state of the art and the path forward. *Nat. Rev. Cancer* 13: 624–636.

Whitfield, J., Littlewood, T., Evan, G.I. et al. (2015). The estrogen receptor fusion system in mouse models: a reversible switch. *Cold Spring Harb. Protoc.* 2015: 227–234.

Whittle, J.R., Lewis, M.T., Lindeman, G.J. et al. (2015). Patient-derived xenograft models of breast cancer and their predictive power. *Breast Cancer Res.* 17: 17.

Woo, S.R. et al. (2012). Immune inhibitory molecules LAG-3 and PD-1 synergistically regulate T-cell function to promote tumoral immune escape. *Cancer Res.* 72: 917–927.

Yan, C. et al. (2019). Visualizing engrafted human cancer and therapy responses in immunodeficient zebrafish. *Cell* 177: 1903–1914 e14.

Yan, R., Small, S., Desplan, C. et al. (1996). Identification of a Stat gene that functions in Drosophila development. *Cell* 84: 421–430.

Zhang, L. et al. (2017). B-cell lymphoma patient-derived xenograft models enable drug discovery and are a platform for personalized therapy. *Clin. Cancer Res.* 23: 4212–4223.

Section II

Targeting the PI3 Kinase-AKT-mTOR Pathway

5

Principles of PI3K Biology and Its Role in Lymphoma

Ralitsa R. Madsen

University College London Cancer Institute, Paul O'Gorman Building, University College London, London, UK

Take Home Messages

- Both PI3K signaling quality (interaction partners, effectors) and quantity (strength, kinetics) differ across contexts and are under dynamic regulation.
- Rather than as a simple ON/OFF cellular switch, the PI3K signaling pathway should be viewed as a highly sensitive dial, whose accurate tuning is a prerequisite for a given cell's optimal function.
- Information transmission within the PI3K signaling pathway is not linear but features complex network properties whose understanding is necessary for successful pharmacological targeting in cancer.
- Despite the relatively small number of known (epi)genetic alterations in the PI3K pathway in hematological malignancies, leukemic cells often hijack its functionality for enhanced survival, uncontrolled proliferation, and reprogramming of their microenvironment.

Introduction: Overview

The coordinated phenotypes of mammalian cells rely on complex signaling networks, which are composed of a highly conserved set of signal transduction pathways. The so-called PI3K signaling pathway, featuring activation of class I phosphoinositide 3-kinases (PI3Ks) and the serine/threonine kinases AKT, is among the best studied due to its involvement in numerous human disorders. Originally a primary nutrient storage pathway, it subsequently evolved into a key homeostatic signaling mechanism that senses and integrates myriad external signals, including hormones, growth factors, cytokines, and chemokines (Fruman et al. 2017; Manning and Toker 2017). Far from being a linear information relay, this pathway features complex feedback loops, which ensure response accuracy as well as remarkable robustness in the face of perturbation. While these properties are essential for the high fidelity of information transmission in normal cells, they also make effective pharmacological targeting of PI3K signaling in disease settings very challenging (Madsen and Vanhaesebroeck 2020). This is compounded by the many subtle ways in which the biochemical wiring of the pathway may differ depending on cell type, developmental stage, and environmental input. The aim of this chapter is to provide a flavor of this complexity, with a particular focus on lymphocyte (patho)physiology. Emphasis is put on appreciating the exquisite quantitative regulation of the PI3K signaling pathway, with both "too much" and "too little" activity causing debilitating human disease.

Four Decades of PI3K Signaling Research

Research into the PI3K signaling pathway spans more than three decades and can broadly be subdivided into three phases. The first phase (1980–2000), spurred by the preceding molecular biology revolution, saw the discovery of the basic building blocks of the canonical PI3K pathway, most importantly the different class I PI3K enzymes, as well as phosphatase and tensin homolog (PTEN), AKT, and mammalian target of rapamycin (mTOR). The remarkable phylogenetic conservation of these components hinted at the fundamental importance of the PI3K signaling pathway in metazoans, and its likely evolution from a rudimentary version with key roles in chemotaxis and metabolic remodeling in response to nutrient availability (Kriplani et al. 2015).

With the advent of large-scale DNA sequencing, the second phase of PI3K signaling research (2000–2010) firmly established the PI3K pathway as one of the most commonly perturbed in human cancers, in line with the discovery of

Precision Cancer Therapies: Targeting Oncogenic Drivers and Signaling Pathways in Lymphoid Malignancies: From Concept to Practice, Volume 1, First Edition. Edited by Owen A. O'Connor, Stephen M. Ansell, and John F. Seymour.

many of its basic components in the context of cellular transformation. In parallel, discoveries of monogenic disorders caused by mutations in PI3K pathway components, alongside ever-more sophisticated genetically engineered mouse models, revealed a fundamental requirement for PI3K signaling in organismal growth, metabolic, and immune homeostasis (Madsen et al. 2018; Nunes-Santos et al. 2019).

Enthused by these discoveries and the druggability of key pathway components, many academic and pharmaceutical teams subsequently invested in the development and trialing of chemical compounds targeting one or more nodes in the PI3K network, particularly in the context of cancer. This third phase (2010–2020) of PI3K signaling research was not without disappointments, however. Except for regulatory approval of PI3Kδ-selective inhibition in certain blood cancers, and PI3Kα-selective inhibition in a subset of breast cancers, efforts to target the PI3K pathway in disease settings have often led to underwhelming results due to issues with tolerability and drug resistance (Castel et al. 2021a; Vanhaesebroeck et al. 2021).

Perhaps the most important lesson learned from the first three phases of PI3K signaling research is that successful pharmacological targeting of a fundamental signaling network with pleiotropic organismal functions requires an in-depth understanding not only of the signaling "hardware" (the constituent pathway components) but also of the signaling "software" (the flow of biochemical information between individual components). Different cell types employ the PI3K signaling "hardware" in different ways, giving rise to myriad cell-specific "software" versions, as illustrated by the distinct wiring of the pathway in non-lymphoid versus lymphoid cell types. It is therefore likely that the fourth phase (2020 onward) of PI3K signaling research will feature the systematic disentangling of the context-dependent wiring of the network, with the resulting discoveries used to guide the rational optimization of existing therapeutic modalities (Madsen and Vanhaesebroeck 2020).

Class I PI3K Enzymes

Isoforms

Class I PI3Ks are heterodimeric enzymes characterized by their ability to synthesize the phospholipid second messenger phosphatidylinositol-(3,4,5)-trisphosphate (PIP_3) from phosphatidylinositol-(4,5)-bisphosphate, an event that predominantly occurs at the cytosolic face of the plasma membrane as well as at some endomembranes (Manning and Toker 2017). This class is further divided into two subfamilies, class IA and class IB, based on interactions with different regulatory subunits (Figure 5.1). Class IA enzymes consist of either one of three catalytic p110 isoforms (α, β, and δ encoded by *PIK3CA*, *PIK3CB*, and *PIK3CD*, respectively), coupled to either one of five regulatory subunits (p85α/p55α/p50α, p85β, and p55γ encoded by *PIK3R1*, *PIK3R2*, *PIK3R3*, respectively). Class IB PI3K consists of a single catalytic subunit (p110γ encoded by *PIK3CG*), complexed with either one of two regulatory subunits (p101 and p84 encoded by *PIK3R5* and *PIK3R6*, respectively) (Bilanges et al. 2019).

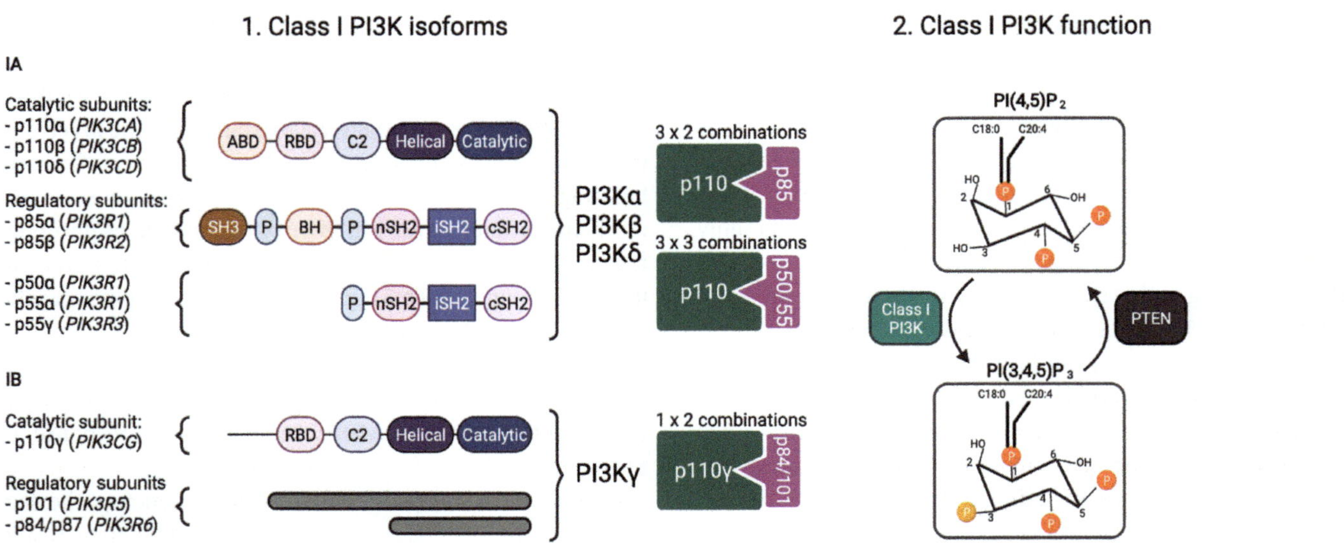

Figure 5.1 On the left: the different class I PI3K subunit isoforms, their structural organization, and the combinatorial diversity arising upon heterodimerization (e.g. there are three catalytic p110 subunits that can heterodimerize with either one of the two regulatory p85 subunits, resulting in 3 × 2 combinations). Note that the regulatory p84 subunit of class IB PI3K is also known as p87; neither p101 nor p84/p87 have a recognizable domain structure and are therefore depicted as gray rods. On the right: the enzymatic reaction catalyzed by class I PI3Ks is phosphorylation of $PI(4,5)P_2$ to $PI(3,4,5)P_3$, with PTEN acting as the opposing phosphatase. Note that these phosphoinositides are embedded in the plasma membrane via their fatty acyl moieties, most commonly stearoyl (C18:0) and arachidonoyl (C20:4). Created with BioRender.com.

Mammalian cells express two additional classes of PI3Ks: class II (PI3K-C2α, β, γ) and the highly evolutionarily conserved, single class III PI3K (VPS34). Classes II and III PI3Ks have important functions in intracellular membrane dynamics, vesicular trafficking, and autophagy, enabling them to influence class I PI3K signaling indirectly (Bilanges et al. 2019). The remainder of this chapter will focus exclusively on signaling downstream of class I PI3Ks (henceforth referred to as PI3K signaling).

Structural Organization

The catalytic p110 subunits share a common domain structure, composed of an N-terminal adaptor binding domain (ABD), a RAS binding domain (RBD), a C2 domain, a helical domain, and a C-terminal kinase domain (Bilanges et al. 2019). Collectively, these domains orchestrate the catalytic activity of the p110 subunit in time and space, both through intramolecular interactions as well as interactions with the regulatory subunits and other cellular components.

The regulatory subunits of class IA PI3Ks contain two SRC homology 2 domains (nSH2 and cSH2), separated by an intervening iSH2 domain that mediates tight binding to the catalytic p110 subunit. The longer regulatory isoforms, p85α and p85β, have additional N-terminal domains, including an SH3 domain, a BAR cluster region homology (BH) domain, and two proline-rich regions (Bilanges et al. 2019). The regulatory subunits of class IA PI3Ks are important for stabilizing the catalytic p110 subunit, for inhibiting its baseline kinase activity, and for coupling the catalytic subunit to sites of receptor activation (Dornan and Burke 2018). In addition, there is evidence for the existence of p110-free regulatory subunits with independent functions as well as indirect effects on class IA PI3K activity (Cheung et al. 2015; Tsolakos et al. 2018).

The different regulatory subunits also shape the functional specificity of individual class I PI3K isoforms through their ability to interact with distinct signaling components, possibly targeting the catalytic p110 subunits to spatially defined signaling domains. This is best illustrated with the two regulatory subunits of class IB PI3K, where loss of p84 in neutrophils leads to selective defects in p110γ-dependent reactive oxygen species (ROS) generation, in contrast to defects in p110γ-dependent migration in neutrophils lacking p101 (Deladeriere et al. 2015).

Isoform-specific Functions

Unique biological functions of the different class I PI3K isoforms are well established based on evidence from targeted gene inactivation in mice, studies with isoform-selective pharmacological inhibitors, and the clinical phenomenology of monogenic disorders caused by mutations in individual PI3K subunits. An appreciation of isoform-specific functions is critical for interpreting the efficacy and on-target toxicity profiles of the numerous PI3K-targeted inhibitors in clinical development.

The differential expression of the catalytic p110 subunits partly explains known isoform-specific functions (Figure 5.2). The p110α and p110β subunits, alongside the regulatory p85α and p85β subunits, are ubiquitously expressed, whereas p110δ and p110γ are enriched in cells of the hematopoietic system. This distinction is not absolute, however, with p110α and p110β contributing to immune cell biology in specific contexts (Okkenhaug 2013). Conversely, p110δ and p110γ can also be expressed in non-hematopoietic cells. Adding to this complexity, the interactions between individual catalytic and regulatory subunits exhibit subtle but important differences (Burke and Williams 2015), which may further determine the selective involvement of a given class I PI3K isoform in a biological process (Dornan and Burke 2018; Tsolakos et al. 2018).

Another factor that contributes to isoform-specific biological functions is the differential ability of class I PI3Ks to be activated downstream of unique combinations of receptor and non-receptor tyrosine kinases (RTKs and nRTKs, respectively), tyrosine-phosphorylated adaptor proteins, G protein-coupled receptors (GPCRs), and small GTPases from the RAS superfamily (Figure 5.3a). The key determinants for individual interaction preferences reside with the specific domains of each regulatory and catalytic isoform. Thus, the SH2 domains of the regulatory subunits enable all class IA PI3K isoforms (α, β, δ) to be activated downstream of tyrosine-phosphorylated YXXM motifs (Bilanges et al. 2019). The RBD of p110α, p110δ, and p110γ couples to RAS family GTPases (mainly RAS), whereas the equivalent domain in p110β enables its activation downstream of RHO family GTPases (mainly RAC1 or CDC42). The various upstream inputs often act in synergy, with both RAS and phosphorylated RTKs contributing to the enhanced membrane interaction and activation of p110α and p110δ. Conversely, p110β integrates inputs from RTKs as well as GPCRs, and p110γ from GPCRs and RAS (Bilanges et al. 2019). The different regulatory subunit isoforms may also couple to upstream receptors in a context-dependent manner (Fos et al. 2008), yet this is less well understood compared to the catalytic subunits. In summary, isoform-specific functions of the different class I PI3Ks are highly dependent on levels of expression, intrinsic catalytic activity, and spatial localization as determined by differential interactions with upstream regulators and downstream effectors.

In the following sections, "PI3K" will be used to refer to class I PI3Ks, and where relevant individual heterodimers will be denoted as PI3Kα, PI3Kβ, PI3Kδ, and PI3Kγ as determined by the catalytic p110 subunit, irrespective of the associate regulatory subunit unless specified.

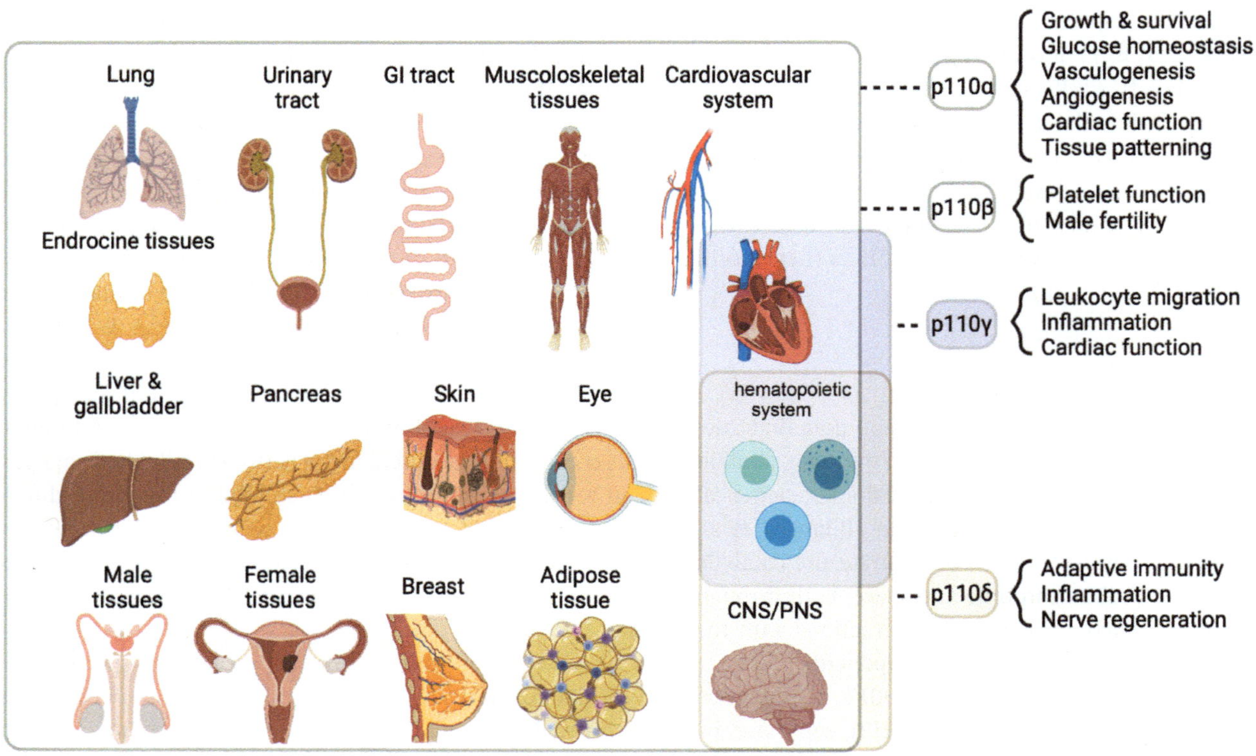

Figure 5.2 Overview of tissue-specific expression and physiological functions of class I PI3K catalytic subunits. Whereas p110α and p110β are ubiquitously expressed (outer box), p110δ and p110γ are enriched for in specific tissues (highlighted inner boxes) and overlap in the hematopoietic lineage. Only the boxes and their colors, not the position of their names with respect to the shown tissues, are used to specify relative expression levels of the catalytic p110 subunits. CNS, central nervous system; PNS, peripheral nervous system. Created with BioRender.com.

The Essential Phospholipid Second Messenger PIP_3

Understanding why PI3Ks are of such fundamental importance to human physiology, and, conversely, why they are so prominent in diverse human disorders requires appreciation of the powerful function of their product: the second messenger PIP_3 (Figure 5.1). This phospholipid is mainly generated at the inner leaflet of the plasma membrane and is estimated to comprise <0.05% of cellular polyphosphoinositides, being almost undetectable in quiescent cells (Dickson and Hille 2019). In physiological settings, PIP_3 synthesis is very rapid and usually transient, attesting to the importance of keeping levels of this second messenger low. In addition to spatial localization, quantitative and temporal differences in PIP_3 are key determinants of downstream biological responses. For example, both B-cell negative selection and anergy depend on the magnitude of the PIP_3 signal (Browne et al. 2009). In most cases, however, the detailed mechanisms whereby these factors contribute to the translation of a given signaling input into a specific biological output remain unknown, yet their importance for the fidelity of cellular information transmission cannot be understated (Madsen and Vanhaesebroeck 2020).

Tight regulation of PIP_3 levels is ensured by several lipid phosphatases, with the tumor suppressor PTEN as the best known. PTEN is a lipid 3-phosphatase that catalyzes the conversion of PIP_3 back to $PI(4,5)P_2$, and acts as the main break to PI3K pathway activation (Figure 5.1b). PIP_3 can also be metabolized into $PI(3,4)P_2$ by 5-phosphatases such as SHIP1 or SHIP2 (Bilanges et al. 2019). As $PI(3,4)P_2$ retains key signaling functions, full inactivation is achieved through its dephosphorylation by PTEN and/or the 4-phosphatases INPP4A and INPP4B (Malek et al. 2017) (Figure 5.3a).

The range of cellular phenotypes regulated by PIP_3, and to some extent $PI(3,4)P_2$, is extraordinary. This is achieved through the ability of this second messenger to recruit proteins with pleckstrin homology (PH) domains (Figure 5.3a). The list of PH-domain-containing proteins is long (>250); however, not all of them bind PIP_3 or $PI(3,4)P_2$. PDK1 and AKT are among the best-known PI3K signaling effectors able to bind both phosphoinositides. The PH domains of TEC family members, including BTK (Bruton's tyrosine kinase) and ITK (interleukin-2-inducible T-cell kinase), have high affinity for PIP_3, whereas other adaptor proteins such as BAM32 (B-cell adapter molecule of 32 kDa) and TAPP1/2 (tandem PH domain-containing protein 1 and 2) exhibit selectivity for $PI(3,4)P_2$ (So and Fruman 2012) (Figure 5.3a).

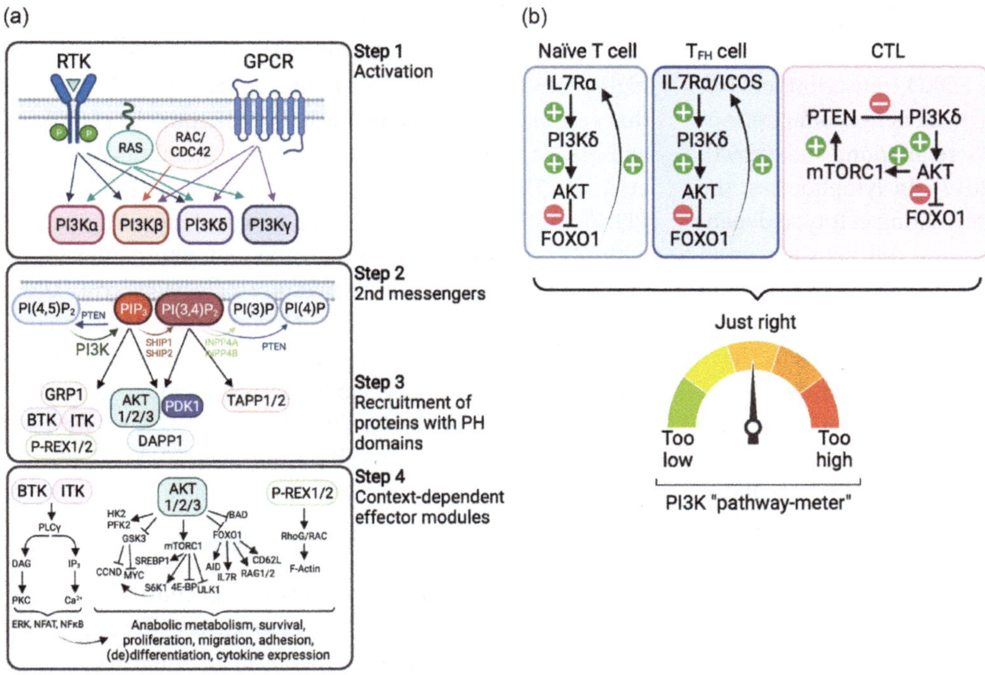

Figure 5.3 (a) Modular overview of the PI3K signaling pathway, emphasizing the combinatorial complexity at the level of upstream regulators and downstream effectors. Generic receptor tyrosine-kinase (RTK) input into class IA PI3Ks is shown, with more specific details related to B-cell receptor (BCR) and T-cell receptor (TCR) signaling included in Figure 5.4. The FOXO1 targets shown are mostly lymphocyte-specific and include components involved in class-switch recombination and somatic hypermutation (AID, RAG1/2) as well as lymphocyte homing (CD62L). For a more general list of FOXO1 targets, the reader is referred to Manning and Toker (2017). Also note the examples of crosstalk with other signaling pathways such as RAS/MAPK (ERK), NFAT, and NF-κB. (b) Non-exhaustive examples of reported negative feedback loops in the PI3K signaling pathway in lymphocytes. Additional negative feedback loops have been studied more extensively in non-lymphoid contexts and are not covered here. Such loops endow the PI3K signaling pathway with remarkable robustness in the face of perturbations, ensuring that the signaling output remains "just right" in physiological settings. Created with BioRender.com.

PI3K Pathway Effectors

Conventionally, textbooks represent the PI3K signaling pathway as a linear signal transduction, originating at the plasma membrane, followed by intracellular information transmission via AKT, mTORC1, and their myriad substrates. However, the relative importance of individual effectors can be highly context-dependent, including numerous non-linear feedback and feedforward loops. Such loops are key to understanding so-called adaptive resistance to PI3K pathway inhibitors, a phenomenon that has been studied mostly in the context of non-lymphoid cancers. This should be borne in mind when reading the following generic outline of PI3K signaling effectors, with lymphocyte-specific examples highlighted where relevant. Cell type-specific differences notwithstanding, activation of the PI3K pathway typically promotes anabolic metabolism, cell proliferation, survival, and migration (Figure 5.3a). Activation of this pathway can also shape cell fate decisions, either promoting or opposing differentiation depending on context (Madsen 2020). Collectively, all these cellular processes are dysregulated in cancer, and thus it is not surprising that PI3K signaling is frequently activated across human malignancies.

AKT, FOXO, and mTORC1

AKT comprised three isoforms – AKT1, 2, and 3 – which exhibit overlapping as well as non-redundant functions. The three isoforms are ubiquitously expressed (Uhlén et al. 2015), though relative levels in any given cell type will differ and thus contribute to reported isoform-specific functions (Manning and Toker 2017). Irrespective of AKT isoform, the PH domain recruits this serine-threonine kinase to sites of PI3K activation, alongside PDK1. The latter is required for AKT activation via direct phosphorylation of T308/T309/T305 (AKT1/AKT2/AKT3) in the activation loop. Maximal activation requires phosphorylation of S473/S474/S472 (AKT1/AKT2/AKT3) in the hydrophobic motif (Manning and Toker 2017), with mammalian target of rapamycin complex 2 (mTORC2) often considered to be the primary kinase although the exact mechanisms, including the potential for AKT autophosphorylation, may differ depending on cell type and context (Baffi et al. 2021; Feng et al. 2004; Toker and Newton 2000).

AKT is suggested to have over 100 substrates and downstream effectors, with the FOXO family of transcription factors and upstream components of mTORC1 among the best studied. Upon AKT-mediated phosphorylation of three conserved residues, FOXO isoforms are excluded from the nucleus and become sequestered by 14-3-3 proteins in the cytosol. AKT thus acts to suppress FOXO transcriptional targets, many of which are involved in induction of apoptosis, cell cycle arrest, catabolism, ROS regulation, and growth inhibition (Manning and Toker 2017). In lymphocytes, the AKT-FOXO axis is important for regulating cell type-dependent differentiation programs, effector cell activation and trafficking. The exact nature of the cellular response often depends on integration of the strength of the upstream stimulus. For example, mechanistic studies in T-cells have revealed that the strength of AKT activation may dictate the pattern of chemokine receptors and adhesion molecules expressed on immune-activated T-cells (Waugh et al. 2009). In B-cells, an important consequence of AKT-mediated FOXO inhibition is suppression of class-switch recombination (Omori et al. 2006; Sander et al. 2015).

AKT leads to activation of the serine/threonine kinase mTOR within mTOR complex 1 (mTORC1), primarily through phosphorylation and inhibition of tuberous sclerosis complex 2 (TSC2, also known as tuberin). This phosphorylation inhibits the GAP activity of the TSC complex toward the small GTPase RHEB. In its GTP-bound form, RHEB promotes mTORC1 activation at lysosomes (Liu and Sabatini 2020). Proline-rich AKT substrate of 40 kDa (PRAS40), a component of the mTORC1 complex, is also an AKT substrate; however, it is often considered less important for mTORC1 activation downstream of AKT (Manning and Toker 2017). Importantly, in lymphocytes, mTORC1 activity can be uncoupled from PI3K/AKT activation and is instead more dependent on nutrient signals such as amino acids (Fruman et al. 2017). Once activated, mTORC1 phosphorylates numerous protein substrates, collectively resulting in upregulation of nutrient uptake, cell proliferation, as well as the associated biosynthetic activities including protein, lipid, and nucleotide synthesis (Hukelmann et al. 2016; Liu and Sabatini 2020). Key mTORC1 substrates include the ribosomal S6 kinases and a family of mRNA translation inhibitors known as eIF4E-binding proteins (4E-BPs) (**Figure 5.3a**). Phosphorylation of the latter by mTORC1 enhances the formation of the eIF4F translational initiation complex required for cap-dependent mRNA translation. Through this mechanism, mTORC1 increases the synthesis of activation-induced cytidine deaminase (AID) in activated B-cells, thereby promoting antibody class switching from IgM to IgG and other isotypes (Chiu et al. 2019). This is opposite to the overall negative effect of PI3K pathway activation on this process (Omori et al. 2006; Sander et al. 2015), and serves as an important example of uncoupling between PI3K/AKT and mTORC1 activity.

TEC Tyrosine Kinases

In lymphocytes, the TEC family of tyrosine kinases is important mediators of PI3K pathway activation, in addition to AKT. Among these, BTK and ITK are key signal transducers in B- and T-cells, respectively. Both contain PH domains that are highly selective for PIP_3, in addition to SH2 and SH3 domains that can aid their recruitment to specific protein complexes and sites of PI3K activation at the plasma membrane (Fruman et al. 2017). Within the B-cell receptor (BCR) signalosome, PI3Kδ and BTK are required for maximal signaling output, with BTK contributing to activation of phospholipase Cγ (PLCγ), which drives the formation of diacylglycerol (DAG) and inositol trisphosphate (IP_3) (**Figure 5.3a**). These second messengers are key for triggering Ca^{2+} mobilization as well as activation of NF-κB, NFAT, and the RAS/MAPK signaling cascade (Fruman et al. 2017). The function of ITK in T-cells is similar to that of BTK in B-cells (Wang et al. 2015).

Network Topology and Signal Robustness

An appreciation of network topology is central to understanding some of the difficulties associated with successfully targeting the PI3K pathway with available pharmacological inhibitors. Network topology is another term for network structure, which in the context of signal transduction refers to individual signaling components and the connections between them. The dynamic properties of signal transduction networks are thus determined by their topologies, and these are often built by recurrent motifs such as positive and negative feedback loops (Kolch et al. 2015). A feedback loop is a network motif in which a downstream molecule (B) affects the activity of its upstream regulator (A). Negative feedback loops, where B inhibits A, are important not only for attenuating the output of a signaling pathway but also for conferring robustness to perturbations such as pharmacological inhibitors (Kolch et al. 2015).

Although the PI3K pathway features numerous negative feedbacks, most of them have been uncovered in non-lymphoid settings and rely on molecules that are not necessarily expressed in lymphocytes. Nevertheless, some observations are likely generalizable. Known negative feedbacks within the PI3K pathway operate across a range of time scales: those mediated by post-translational modifications occur within minutes, whereas those involving transcription and translation take hours and even days to be observed. A detailed understanding of fast and slow feedback loops is therefore critically dependent on temporal studies across the relevant time scales.

A common transcriptional feedback loop within the PI3K pathway involves the AKT-FOXO axis, with inhibition of FOXO leading to reduced expression of genes encoding for upstream activators of PI3K signaling (Figure 5.3b). In naïve T-cells, this negative feedback operates at the level of IL7Rα, and homing receptor expression, and may act as a protective mechanism against avaricious T-cells that would otherwise dominate the peripheral population (Kerdiles et al. 2009; Stone et al. 2015). In T follicular helper (T_{FH}) cells, FOXO1 also controls the expression of inducible T-cell co-stimulator (ICOS) (Stone et al. 2015), a co-receptor that promotes PI3K activation. Similar to their non-lymphoid counterparts (Mukherjee et al. 2021), lymphocytes may also rely on mTORC1 for negative regulation of the upstream PI3K signal via control of PTEN translation – as demonstrated in cytotoxic T lymphocytes (CTLs) (Hukelmann et al. 2016) (Figure 5.3b). The signaling ramifications of breaking this negative feedback loop can be profound. Thus, CTLs treated with an inhibitor of both mTORC complexes initially exhibit decreased phosphorylation of AKT T308 (PDK1 site) and S473 (mTORC2 site) (Hukelmann et al. 2016). This is consistent with the known ability of S473 phosphorylation to promote docking of AKT to PDK1 – as a result, loss of S473 phosphorylation would also decrease phosphorylation at T308. However, inhibition of mTORC1 activity results in reduced PTEN translation, eventually causing a compensatory increase in PIP_3 levels and a resurgence in AKT T308 phosphorylation, paralleled by re-phosphorylation of FOXO1. Accordingly, catalytic mTOR inhibitors are not efficient at curbing AKT activity in this context, with increased PIP_3 synthesis seemingly bypassing the need for mTORC2-mediated S473 phosphorylation (Hukelmann et al. 2016).

In contrast to their negative counterparts, positive feedback loops enable signal amplification and are often important for driving irreversible cell fate decisions. Positive feedback loops within the PI3K pathway remain relatively enigmatic, although recent studies have begun to characterize them, specifically in a lymphoid context. Pending independent validation, the small antiviral membrane protein IFITM3 was recently found to function as a scaffold for PIP_3 and mediator of a PI3K signaling amplification loop in B-cells (Lee et al. 2020). Moreover, a study of $CD8^+$ effector T-cells has also demonstrated a positive feedback loop between PI3K-driven glycolytic activity and subsequent ATP-mediated enhancement of PI3K activation (Xu et al. 2021).

Dynamic PI3K Signaling in Lymphocyte Biology

The following sections contain important examples of dynamic PI3K pathway regulation in B- and T-cells, illustrating how the differential usage and wiring of the PI3K "hardware" translates into a highly specialized cellular "software," appropriate for the task at hand. The attentive reader will not fail to notice that corruption of this software is what underpins the myriad immune system pathologies of aberrant PI3K activity, as well as the challenges faced upon pharmacological targeting of this pathway.

B-cell Development and Survival

The PI3K pathway is essential for the survival of pre-B and mature B-cells (Ramadani et al. 2010; Srinivasan et al. 2009). In murine pre-B cells, both PI3Kα and PI3Kδ have been shown to contribute PI3K activity, with important roles in the dynamic suppression of *Rag* expression and VDJ recombination during B-cell development (Ramadani et al. 2010). Moreover, PI3Kα appears able to substitute for PI3Kδ inactivation in the context of tonic BCR signaling, which is likely to be sufficient to allow the development and survival of follicular B-cells (Srinivasan et al. 2009). In contrast, PI3Kδ is essential where BCR crosslinking is involved (Figure 5.4a), for example in the development of B1 and marginal zone B-cells, and for overall antigen-dependent activation of mature B-cells (Clayton et al. 2002; Fruman et al. 1999; Jou et al. 2002; Oak et al. 2009; Okkenhaug 2002; Ramadani et al. 2010; Suzuki et al. 1999). Thus, peripheral B-cell maturation mainly depends on the p85α-p110δ heterodimer as the predominant PI3K isoform, consistent with the immunodeficiency phenotypes observed in people with pathological PI3Kδ activation, caused either by mutations in *PIK3CD* (p110δ) or *PIK3R1* (p85α/p55α/p50α) (see below and Lucas et al. (2016)).

Adequate regulation of the magnitude and duration of PI3K signaling throughout B-cell development averts the generation, activation, and persistence of abnormal cells, including autoreactive clones. Conversely, sustained PIP_3 signaling during B-cell development converts what is normally a tolerogenic response into a mitogenic response, resulting in impaired tolerance induction (Browne et al. 2009). Moreover, while baseline survival of resting mature B-cells depends on tonic BCR signaling through the PI3K-AKT-FOXO1 branch, on its own this is not sufficient and requires engagement of additional signaling pathways via co-receptors such as BAFFR (Srinivasan et al. 2009). Pathological activation of PI3Kδ enhances the survival of B-cells, likely by amplifying or mimicking such crosstalk (Preite et al. 2019).

The Germinal Center (GC) Reaction

Appropriate B-cell selection is critical during the GC reaction. The GC is the site where B-cells undergo somatic hypermutation (SHM), affinity maturation, and class-switch recombination, ultimately leading to positive selection of B-cells capable of producing high-affinity IgG antibodies. Given its importance for humoral immunity, GC dysregulation is associated with immunodeficiency, autoimmune disease, and cancer. For example, B-cell-derived lymphomas, the most common lymphoid malignancies, typically originate from GC or post-GC B-cells, as indicated by their somatically mutated immunoglobulin genes (Klein and Dalla-Favera 2008). Correct function of the GC depends on its patterning into light zone (LZ) and dark zone (DZ), in addition to exquisite spatiotemporal control of interactions between B-cells and $CD4^+$ T_{FH} cells within these topologically and functionally distinct areas (Figure 5.5).

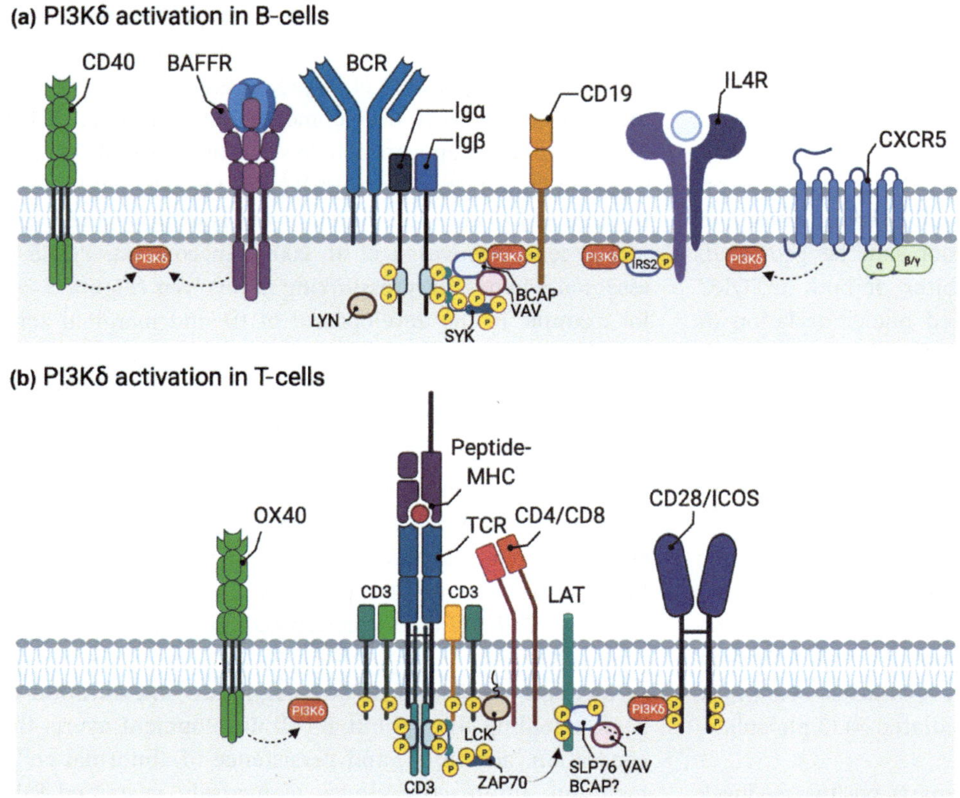

Figure 5.4 In both B (a) and T (b) lymphocytes, PI3Kδ is recruited to signalosomes formed upon clustering of the B-cell receptor (BCR) and T-cell receptor (TCR), respectively. A phosphorylation cascade is triggered by SRC-like non-receptor tyrosine kinases (LYN in B-cells, LCK in T-cells), followed by SYK (B-cells) and ZAP70 (T-cells) – members of the SYK tyrosine kinase family. The BCR co-opts the co-receptor CD19 or the adaptor protein BCAP for recruitment of PI3Kδ via interactions of p85 with YXXM phosphotyrosines within these molecules. How exactly PI3Kδ gets recruited to the TCR signalosome remains under investigation (Luff et al. 2021). In both B- and T-cells, various co-receptors (e.g. CD40 and OX40), cytokine (e.g. IL4R), and chemokine receptors (e.g. CXCR5) also contribute to PI3K pathway activation as indicated. IL2 was previously thought to induce PI3Kδ activation in T-cells; however, more recent work in CTLs has forced a revision of this model, and it has therefore been omitted from this diagram (Ross et al. 2016). While PI3Kδ is shown as the main isoform responsible for PI3K signaling initiation downstream of antigen-dependent receptor activation, other PI3K isoforms can be involved depending on context. For example, chemokine receptors activate PI3Kδ in B-cells but PI3Kγ in T-cells. Created with BioRender.com.

Compared to naïve B-cells, physiological BCR-mediated PI3K signaling is attenuated in GC B-cells, including both lower magnitude and less sustained activation. Moreover, CD40 ligation by T_{FH} cells no longer contributes to PI3K activation in GC B-cells, in contrast to their naïve counterparts. This attenuated PI3K signal is nevertheless sufficient for the selective inactivation of FOXO1 downstream of AKT-mediated phosphorylation (Luo et al. 2018). Its inactivation downstream of PI3K/AKT thus licenses GC B-cells to enter and/or stay in the LZ where they interact with T_{FH} cells and undergo positive selection. Here, dual BCR and CD40 engagement is required for induction of c-MYC expression and S6 phosphorylation (Luo et al. 2018), ultimately coordinating cell cycle reentry and anabolic metabolism for successful positive selection (Ersching et al. 2017). This is a biphasic and transient regulatory phenomenon, with positively selected GC B-cells either undergoing differentiation to plasma and memory cells or re-entering the DZ for another cycle of somatic hypermutation and proliferation. The sequence of these events is critically dependent on the correct spatiotemporal activation of PI3K signaling versus FOXO1 (Dominguez-Sola et al. 2015; Sander et al. 2015) (Figure 5.5). An essential step in the selection of cells expressing high-affinity antibody mutants is their recruitment from the GC LZ back into the DZ. This cyclical process depends on the timely expression of the chemokine receptor CXCR4. In mice, enforced PI3K pathway activation or FOXO1 ablation results in failure to express CXCR4, thus disrupting the GC architecture and impairing positive selection (Dominguez-Sola et al. 2015; Sander et al. 2015). Moreover, CSR and affinity selection but not SHM are selectively hampered in these cells (Dominguez-Sola et al. 2015; Sander et al. 2015). Thus, getting the PI3K signaling balance in GC B-cells right is essential for functional humoral immune responses.

Similarly, the dynamic regulation of PI3K versus FOXO1 activity underpins the successful development of mature, resting B-cells from their pre-B cell counterparts (Okkenhaug 2013). The picture that emerges is one where

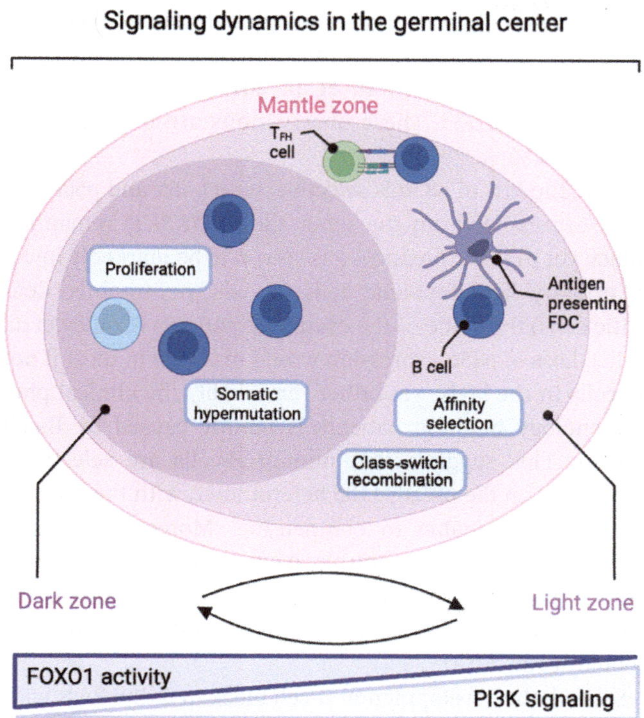

Figure 5.5 The germinal center is a transient microanatomical structure in which mature B lymphocytes under repeated rounds of clonal expansion and genetic diversification of their immunoglobulin genes, ultimately resulting in the generation of high-affinity B-cells, destined to become either memory B-cells or plasma cells. The GC is organized into two topologically and functionally distinct compartments known as the dark zone (DZ) and the light zone (LZ). Proliferative expansion and Ig somatic hypermutation (SHM) occur in the DZ, whereas affinity selection and class-switch recombination take place in the LZ where B-cells expressing high-affinity antibodies interact with follicular dendritic cells (FDCs) and T follicular helper (T_{FH}) lymphocytes. As part of this process, B-cells undergo repeated cycles of LZ–DZ migration, with B-cells in the different zones exhibiting a characteristic PI3K signaling polarity. The transcription factor FOXO1 is essential for the development of the proliferative GC DZ, consistent with low or absent PI3K activity in this area (Dominguez-Sola et al. 2015; Sander et al. 2015). FOXO1 instructs the DZ gene program directly and by licensing the activity of BCL6, a GC master regulator (Dominguez-Sola et al. 2015). Created with BioRender.com.

PI3K pathway activation can promote cellular proliferation, survival, and/or differentiation, depending on the stage of B-cell development and the strength of the stimulus.

T_{FH} Cell Function

Like the BCR in B-cells, the TCR in T-cells is typically the focal point of PI3K activation, augmented further by co-receptors such as CD28 and ICOS (Figure 5.4b). ICOS expression increases on activated T-cells and is particularly important for differentiation of the follicular B helper T (T_{FH}) subtype, a T-cell population that drives and sustains GC formation (Figure 5.5). This function depends on PI3Kδ activation and the timely augmentation of helper cytokine expression, including IL21 and IL4 (Gigoux et al. 2009; Rolf et al. 2010). Consequently, knock-in mice with selective loss of p85 binding to ICOS present with severe defects in T_{FH} cell generation, GC reaction, antibody class switching, and affinity maturation (Gigoux et al. 2009). Moreover, several transcription factors controlling T_{FH} cell differentiation and function are modulated by PI3K signaling. Among these, the master T_{FH} transcription factor, BCL6, is under direct repression by FOXO1, and is upregulated upon PI3K/AKT activation (Stone et al. 2015). Finally, both mTORC2 and mTORC1 are required for T_{FH} cell differentiation downstream of ICOS engagement, enabling the coordination of anabolic metabolism, proliferation, and transcriptional activity in response to immune signals (Yang et al. 2016; Zeng et al. 2016). While these studies support the notion that PI3K activation promotes T_{FH} cell differentiation, it is worth emphasizing some of the parallels to GC B-cells when it comes to balancing FOXO1 activation and inactivation. To initiate T_{FH} cell differentiation, PI3K signaling and FOXO1 inactivation must take place transiently, according to a poorly understood temporal code, whereas final specification of GC-T_{FH} cells appears to occur in a FOXO1-dependent manner (Stone et al. 2015).

Naïve and Effector T-cells

Consistent with the notion that PI3K/AKT activation does not simply function as an ON/OFF switch, its signaling strength has emerged as important in determining the expression pattern of chemokine receptors and adhesion molecules on immune-activated T-cells (Waugh et al. 2009). Whereas relatively weak PI3K/AKT activation is compatible with T-cell survival and proliferation, strong and sustained activation is required to downregulate homing of naïve T-cells to secondary lymphoid tissues *in vivo* (Finlay et al. 2009; Waugh et al. 2009). As a result, loss of PI3Kδ or AKT activity impairs T-cell exit from lymphoid organs and migration to peripheral sites of infection (Liu and Uzonna 2010; Macintyre et al. 2011).

Unbiased comparisons of PI3Kδ signaling in naïve $CD8^+$ T-cells versus CTLs have further emphasized the importance of context. Both the quality and the quantity of the PI3Kδ response differ in these otherwise closely related cell types (Spinelli et al. 2021). For example, naïve $CD8^+$ cells but not their effector cytotoxic counterparts show altered expression of cytolytic effector molecules (decreased) and

ICOS (increased) upon PI3Kδ inhibition. Furthermore, many more TCR-regulated transcripts depend on PI3Kδ activity in naïve T-cells than in CTLs (Spinelli et al. 2021). Among other changes, PI3Kδ inhibition in CTLs enhances gene expression of three important inhibitory receptors: *Ctla4*, *Slamf6*, and *Lag3*. Not all of these and other transcriptional changes in PI3Kδ-inhibited CTLs are mediated by the AKT/FOXO1-axis, with evidence for a substantial contribution by PI3Kδ-dependent activation of the RAS/MAPK signaling pathway (Spinelli et al. 2021). When it comes to understanding the effects of pharmacological PI3K inhibition in cancer, one important conclusion from his work is that the dominant targets for PI3Kδ in both naïve and effector $CD8^+$ T-cells are the secreted molecules and cell surface receptors that orchestrate paracrine communication between $CD8^+$ T lymphocytes and other immune cells (Spinelli et al. 2021).

Other large-scale and in-depth analyses of context-dependent PI3K signaling are also emerging as the required omics technology matures. A recent study looked at differences in the p110δ interactome in murine, primary naïve $CD4^+$ T-cells, and in differentiated T-cell blasts, demonstrating substantial differences in adaptor protein usage and a myriad of previously documented p110δ interactors (Luff et al. 2021), indicating that these complexes might be more extensive than has been appreciated to date. Moving forward, such studies will be instrumental for improving current understanding of how the PI3K pathway fine-tunes immunological responses, a prerequisite for the optimal usage of PI3K-targeted therapies.

Lessons from Monogenic Disorders

While experimental models based on cultured cells and research animals are instrumental for dissecting the detailed cellular and organismal effects of PI3K signaling, their relevance must always be evaluated against direct evidence from human physiology. In contrast to cancers which often harbor numerous genetic and epigenetic changes, human diseases caused by single-gene mutations are powerful experiments of nature, against which to calibrate results from experimental model systems. The importance of quantitative control of PI3K signaling in immune cells is therefore best illustrated by the discovery of human immunodeficiencies caused by either loss- or gain-of-function mutations in the PI3Kδ enzyme (Lucas et al. 2016).

Genetic PI3Kδ Inactivation

Biallelic loss-of-function mutations in either p85α or p110δ have been reported in rare cases of human immunodeficiency. The affected individuals present with B-cell lymphopenia, hypo- or agammaglobulinemia, recurrent infections, and several autoimmunity-related pathologies (Conley et al. 2012; Swan et al. 2019; Tang et al. 2018; Zhang et al. 2013). These observations are important for several reasons.

First, the loss of p85α is selective, with p55α and p50α isoform expression from the same allele (*PIK3R1*) remaining intact, yet p110δ expression was shown to be markedly lower in primary hematopoietic cells (T-cells, neutrophils, dendritic cells) from one of the examined patients (Conley et al. 2012). Loss of p85α expression would manifest in most if not all cells in the body, yet rather remarkably the clinical phenomenology in these patients is mainly caused by B-cell defects. This suggests that human B-cells are selectively dependent on the p85α-p110δ heterodimer, with the remaining isoforms unable to compensate. Moreover, primary B-cells from healthy controls have been shown to only express p85α and not p55α/p50α, which may explain the selective dependence of human B-cells on the p85α isoform (Conley et al. 2012).

Second, the developmental B-cell block in individuals with loss-of-function of PI3Kδ is far more severe than expected from the respective mouse models (Clayton et al. 2002; Fruman et al. 1999; Jou et al. 2002; Oak et al. 2009; Okkenhaug 2002; Ramadani et al. 2010; Suzuki et al. 1999), a clear example of species-specific differences and the need for calibration against human biology. It is worth noting, however, that although the clinical case reports mainly emphasize the primary B-cell defect, the human autoimmunity phenotypes associated with PI3Kδ loss-of-function may be caused by dysfunctional T regulatory (T_{REG}) cells given substantial evidence that PI3K signaling is required for $FOXP^+$ T_{REG} cell homeostasis and function in mice (Patton et al. 2006; So and Fruman 2012). Thus, PI3Kδ-deficient mice develop colitis due to inappropriate suppression of effector T-cells by their regulatory counterparts (Okkenhaug 2002), consistent with colitis being a frequent side effect of PI3Kδ inhibitors tested in the clinic (Lucas et al. 2016).

Genetic PI3Kδ Hyperactivation

Immunodeficiency can also arise from heterozygous mutations that hyperactivate the PI3Kδ enzyme. These mutations are found either in the *PIK3CD* (p110δ) or *PIK3R1* (p85α/p55α/p50α) gene, giving rise to the clinical entities APDS1 and APDS2, respectively. APDS stands for Activated PI3K Delta Syndrome, an autosomal dominant combined immunodeficiency, featuring functional and developmental defects in both T- and B-cells (Angulo et al. 2013; Deau et al. 2014; Lucas et al. 2014a, 2014b). It is notable that these diseases largely phenocopy each other, given that the ubiquitous expression of the *PIK3R1* gene and the ability of p85α/p55α/p50α to pair with all three class IA catalytic subunits would have suggested more widespread organismal dysfunction due to potential activation of all three class IA p110 subunits (Figure 5.1). Structural biology work has demonstrated that p110δ is activated more strongly by the most common APDS2 *PIK3R1* mutation (Dornan et al. 2017), an exon-skip variant resulting in a deletion in the iSH2 domain of p85α/p55α/p50α, thus offering a potential explanation for the selective immune cell defects in this context. Recent quantitative analyses have also shown a preferential association of p110δ with p85α over p85β in mouse embryonic fibroblasts, spleen, and bone marrow extracts (Tsolakos et al. 2018).

Collectively, APDS phenotypes mimic an exaggerated version of the normal biology of PI3Kδ activation in immune cells. Patients often present with recurrent infections, hypogammaglobulinemia (often with increased IgM levels), reduced class-switch memory B-cells and impaired vaccine responses, an increase in transitional B-cells and an increase in effector T-cells (particularly the T_{FH} subset) (Lucas et al. 2016). Freshly isolated peripheral blood cells from APDS patients are prone to apoptosis upon TCR restimulation – in stark contrast to the pro-survival phenotype typically associated with PI3K pathway activation. Moreover, $CD8^+$ T-cells from APDS patients have reduced telomeres and increased expression of senescence markers, suggestive of functional exhaustion. This phenotype is poorly mimicked in available mouse models owing to their long telomeres (Lucas et al. 2016). Finally, benign lymphoproliferation (lymphadenopathy, hepatosplenomegaly, and focal nodular lymphoid hyperplasia) is a common feature of APDS, in addition to increased risk of lymphoma (Lucas et al. 2016). A milder form of APDS-like immunodeficiency has also been observed in patients with Cowden disease, caused by heterozygous loss of the tumor suppressor *PTEN* (Lucas et al. 2016).

Corrupted PI3K Signaling in Cancer

Large-scale, multi-omic molecular profiling by The Cancer Genome Atlas (TCGA) has enabled identification of the most frequently altered cell signaling pathways in malignancy. Consistently, the PI3K signaling pathway tops the list in solid tumors, predominantly due to activating mutations/copy number changes in *PIK3CA* (p110α), or inactivation of *PTEN* (Sanchez-Vega et al. 2018; Zhang et al. 2017). In contrast, genetic PI3K pathway activation is rarely observed in hematological malignancies, with few notable exceptions. Pediatric T-acute lymphoblastic leukemia (T-ALL) features relatively frequent somatic alterations in *PIK3R1*, and less commonly in *PIK3CA* and *PIK3CD* (Ma et al. 2018). Increased PI3K pathway activation in T-ALL is common and may also arise from post-translational inactivation of PTEN lipid phosphatase activity due to high levels of ROS (Silva et al. 2008). Moreover, loss of PTEN expression has been found in over 50% of germinal center B-cell-like (GCB) diffuse large B-cell lymphomas (DLBCL), compared to less than 15% of non-GCB DLBCL patient samples (Pfeifer et al. 2013). Accordingly, GCB DLBCLs are addicted to PI3K pathway activation for their survival (Pfeifer et al. 2013).

Despite the relatively small number of direct (epi)genetic alterations in the PI3K pathway in blood cancers, it is well established that leukemic cells hijack its functionality for enhanced survival, uncontrolled proliferation, and reprogramming of their microenvironment. Similar to their normal counterparts, PI3K signaling in leukemic cells is mainly mediated by PI3Kδ, with a subset of B-cell malignancies showing particular dependence on constitutive BCR signaling via PI3Kδ. It is worth noting that cancer cells may corrupt both positive and negative branches of the PI3K pathway to enhance their survival, with FOXO1 presenting as a prominent example. In contrast to loss-of-function FOXO1 mutations in a variety of solid tumors and Hodgkin's lymphoma, a significant fraction (10–50% depending on subtype) of GC-derived, aggressive variants of B-cell non-Hodgkin's lymphomas (B-NHL) presents with recurrent pro-oncogenic missense mutations that partially disrupt FOXO1 inactivation downstream of PI3K/AKT while also reducing the affinity of FOXO1 for specific target genes (Roberto et al. 2021). Due to transcriptional rewiring and disruption of signaling feedback, mutant B-cells with oncogenic FOXO1 activity also exhibit concomitant hyperactivation of the PI3K/AKT and stress-activated protein kinase (SAPK) pathways, a protective mechanism that promotes cancer cell stress resistance (Roberto et al. 2021). Consistent with FOXO1's critical role in the physiological GC response reaction, expression of the B-NHL-associated oncogenic FOXO1 mutations in mice confers competitive advantage to mutant B-cells by mimicking the positive selection signals that promote GC B-cell expansion (Roberto et al. 2021).

The Success of PI3Kδ Inhibition in Lymphoid Malignancies

The prominent role of PI3K signaling in cancer maintenance and progression inspired the development of numerous PI3K-targed inhibitors (Castel et al. 2021b; Vanhaesebroeck et al. 2021). However, the ubiquitous requirement for this pathway in normal cell biology and organismal function presents a formidable challenge for the successful application of PI3K-targeted therapy in the clinic. While some issues can be addressed by the development of highly isoform-selective inhibitors, there are still substantial toxicity if the targeted isoform is as ubiquitously expressed as the cancer-associated p110α. It is therefore not surprising that most success in this area has been in the context of hematological malignancies and selective inhibitors of p110δ. The anti-cancer efficacy of these agents can be attributed both to cell-intrinsic and cell-extrinsic mechanisms, as demonstrated in studies of chronic lymphocytic leukemia (CLL) and follicular lymphoma (FL)

(Vanhaesebroeck et al. 2021). Thus, in addition to a cancer-selective pro-apoptotic effect, PI3Kδ inhibition also alters cytokine and chemokine production both by CLL cells and the associated stromal cells, thereby influencing the microenvironmental stimuli that support cancer growth (Herman et al. 2010; Hoellenriegel et al. 2011; Okkenhaug and Burger 2016). Consistent with the normal function of the PI3K pathway in lymphocyte migration and homing, PI3Kδ inhibition in CLL triggers an early redistribution of the cancer cells from their protective tissue environment and into the blood, leading to rapid and sustained lymph node size reduction and a transient lymphocytosis (Furman et al. 2010). A similar effect is observed in patients treated with inhibitors of SYK, BTK, and mTOR, in line with a shared signaling mechanism of action (Okkenhaug and Burger 2016). It has also been suggested that some of the beneficial clinical activity of PI3Kδ inhibitors such as idelalisib (Zydelig) may be due to breaking of T_{REG}-mediated immune tolerance, as demonstrated in mouse models of solid tumors (Ali et al. 2014; Lim et al. 2018).

Although PI3Kδ is considered the functionally dominant isoform in lymphocytes, the context-dependent contribution of other PI3K isoforms should not be ignored. For example, inhibition of the other leukocyte-enriched isoform, PI3Kγ, has been shown to reduce CLL cell adhesion to stromal cells to an extent similar to that observed with the PI3Kδ inhibitor idelalisib, with the dual and clinically approved PI3Kδ/γ inhibitor duvelisib giving rise to a greater reduction in CLL migration compared to the use of the respective single isoform-selective inhibitors (Ali et al. 2018). Conversely, PI3Kδ inhibition has been shown to elicit rapid reactivation of BCR signaling via PI3Kα in cell line models of the activated B-cell-like (ABC) subtype of DLBCL, arguing for evaluation of dual PI3Kα/δ inhibition in this context (Pongas et al. 2017). Co-targeting of PI3Kα/δ has also been suggested for a subset of mantle cell lymphomas with increased expression of the p110α protein (Iyengar et al. 2013). Moreover, a subgroup of B-ALL has a gene expression profile similar to normal pre-BCR^+ B-cells (pre-B ALL) and exhibits an exquisite dependence on SYK for PI3K pathway activation and proliferation (Köhrer et al. 2016). Given evidence from mice that normal pre-B cells rely both on PI3Kα and PI3Kδ (Ramadani et al. 2010), dual inhibition of these isoforms may also be relevant in this context. However, in addition to the considerations outlined in the subsequent section, a caveat of this approach relates to the substantial side effects associated with systemic PI3Kα inhibition, with on-target metabolic toxicities as the most prominent (Castel et al. 2021b; Vanhaesebroeck et al. 2021). Finally, primary resistance to PI3Kδ inhibition in CLL has been linked to the emergence of activating mutations in the RAS/MAPK pathway which can be targeted by available pharmacological agents such as trametinib (Murali et al. 2018).

It is rare for cancer cells to be so reliant on a single signaling pathway and PI3K isoform as observed in some of the aforementioned B-cell malignancies. It therefore remains to be established whether PI3Kδ inhibitors will show similar efficacy in the context of other hematological cancers with PI3K pathway hyperactivation, for example ALL (Sanchez et al. 2019). PI3Kδ inhibitors are also receiving attention as potential immunomodulatory agents in solid tumors (Vanhaesebroeck et al. 2021).

Quantitative Biology and Therapeutic Considerations

While it is true that constitutive PI3K pathway activation is a common and often necessary event in malignancy, cancer cells must still ensure control of the exact magnitude and kinetics of this activation for optimal survival. Substantial evidence, particularly in immune cells, suggests that overactivation of oncogenic signaling can be deadly in certain contexts, leading to paradoxical rescue of cancer cells upon treatment with the targeted inhibitors that were designed to kill them (Madsen and Vanhaesebroeck 2020). Thus, pharmacological hyperactivation of pre-BCR signaling components, including SYK, engages the deletional checkpoint for removal of self-reactive B-cells and selectively kills the cancer cells in a mouse model of Ph^+ B-ALL (Chen et al. 2015). Similarly, even modest dose reduction of *Pten* in mouse models of pre-B ALL has been shown to result in rapid cancer cell death and clearance of leukemia from transplant recipient mice. This toxicity is specific to pre-B ALL cells and is attributable to PI3K pathway hyperactivation (Shojaee et al. 2016), consistent with the physiological function of this pathway in determining the outcome of early B-cell selection in the bone marrow. It therefore appears that pre-B ALL cells cannot tolerate PI3K pathway activity beyond a specific threshold, in line with lack of evidence for activating, genetic hits within the PI3K pathway in human pre-B ALL cohorts (Shojaee et al. 2016).

Recent work in mice has also demonstrated that terminally differentiated B-cells, or plasma cells (PCs), with an APDS-related activating PI3Kδ variant have compromised survival due to disrupted endoplasmic reticulum (ER) proteostasis and autophagy (Al Qureshah et al. 2021). Mechanistically, this is caused mainly by increased mTORC1 activity, which promotes protein synthesis and inhibits autophagy. Given their ability to produce and secrete high levels of antibodies, PCs already have a high baseline protein synthesis load, and have developed unique mechanisms to deal with the resulting ER stress in a physiological context. These mechanisms fail in the face of genetic PI3Kδ activation, thus compromising survival upon secondary antigen challenge (Al Qureshah et al. 2021).

The counterintuitive observation that overactivation of an otherwise oncogenic component can elicit cell death is not new, and is best established for the oncoprotein MYC. Within a limited expression range unique to each tumor, MYC appears to have a paradoxical, pro-apoptotic function (Harrington et al. 2021). Given evidence that the PI3K pathway activation can boost MYC protein levels in B-cell malignancies, it has been suggested that transient manipulation of the pathway may allow for MYC stabilization beyond a threshold compatible with cancer cell survival (Harrington et al. 2021).

Finally, the notion of intermittent pharmacological inhibition is gaining traction, with evidence that PI3K-targeted inhibitors administered in this manner lead to fewer adverse effects while retaining their therapeutic efficacy (Vanhaesebroeck et al. 2021). A better quantitative understanding of PI3K signaling dynamics across biological contexts will be necessary to enhance the rational implementation of this therapeutic strategy (Madsen and Vanhaesebroeck 2020).

Concluding Remarks

Studies of PI3K signaling, particularly in immune cells, support the notion that regulation of this pathway must follow the Greek maxim "nothing in excess." Normal cell physiology thus requires a golden mean of PI3K signaling, with both too much and too little resulting in pathology. The challenge now is to determine this golden mean in any given cell type and (patho)physiological context, and to integrate the resulting knowledge in predictive models that can guide the optimal use of PI3K-targeted therapies. While conventional reductionist approaches have been tremendously useful for mapping the individual components of the PI3K pathway, on their own the resulting maps fall short of predicting the extensive non-linear and often unintuitive information transmission that governs PI3K signaling output. Moving forward, such understanding will likely be led by a combination of the new and the old – a symbiotic relationship between emerging computational modeling approaches and unbiased experimental studies of the complex perturbation-response relationship.

Whether studying this pathway in normal or cancer cells, however, two key conclusions apply: (i) both PI3K signaling quality (interaction partners, effectors) and quantity (strength, kinetics) differ across contexts; and (ii) rather than as a simple ON/OFF switch, the PI3K pathway should be viewed as a highly sensitive dial, whose accurate tuning is a prerequisite for a given cell's optimal function.

Acknowledgments

This work was funded by a Sir Henry Wellcome Fellowship (220464/Z/20/Z) to R.R.M. The author would like to thank Professor Bart Vanhaesebroeck and Ms. Emily Erickson for their feedback on the chapter.

Must Read Reference

Fruman, D.A. et al. (2017). The PI3K pathway in human disease. *Cell* 170 (4): 605–635. doi: 10.1016/j.cell.2017.07.029.

References

Al Qureshah, F. et al. (2021). Activated PI3Kδ signals compromise plasma cell survival via limiting autophagy and increasing ER stress. *J. Exp. Med.* 218 (12). Available at: https://rupress.org/jem/article/218/12/e20211035/212672/Activated-PI3K-signals-compromise-plasma-cell.

Ali, A.Y. et al. (2018). Distinct roles for phosphoinositide 3-kinases γ and δ in malignant B cell migration. *Leukemia* Springer US, 32 (9): 1958–1969. doi: 10.1038/s41375-018-0012-5.

Ali, K. et al. (2014). Inactivation of PI(3)K p110δ breaks regulatory T-cell-mediated immune tolerance to cancer. *Nature* 510 (7505): 407–411. doi: 10.1038/nature13444.

Angulo, I. et al. (2013). Phosphoinositide 3-kinase δ gene mutation predisposes to respiratory infection and airway damage. *Science* 342 (6160): 866–871. doi: 10.1126/science.1243292.

Baffi, T.R. et al. (2021). TORC2 controls the activity of PKC and Akt by phosphorylating a conserved TOR interaction motif. *Sci. Signal.* 14 (678): eabe4509. doi: 10.1126/scisignal.abe4509.

Bilanges, B., Posor, Y., and Vanhaesebroeck, B. (2019). PI3K isoforms in cell signalling and vesicle trafficking. *Nat. Rev. Mol. Cell Biol.* Springer US, 20 (9): 515–534. doi: 10.1038/s41580-019-0129-z.

Browne, C.D. et al. (2009). Suppression of phosphatidylinositol 3,4,5-Trisphosphate production is a key determinant of B cell anergy. *Immunity* Elsevier Ltd, 31 (5): 749–760. doi: 10.1016/j.immuni.2009.08.026.

Burke, J.E. and Williams, R.L. (2015). Synergy in activating class I PI3Ks. *Trends Biochem. Sci.* Elsevier Ltd, 40 (2): 88–100. doi: 10.1016/j.tibs.2014.12.003.

Castel, P. et al. (2021a). The present and future of PI3K inhibitors for cancer therapy. *Nat. Cancer* Springer US, 2 (6): 587–597. doi: 10.1038/s43018-021-00218-4.

Castel, P. et al. (2021b). The present and future of PI3K inhibitors for cancer therapy. *Nat. Cancer* Springer US, 180 (5): 428. doi: 10.1038/s43018-021-00218-4.

Chen, Z. et al. (2015). Signalling thresholds and negative B-cell selection in acute lymphoblastic leukaemia. *Nature* 521 (7552): 357–361. doi: 10.1038/nature14231.

Cheung, L.W. et al. (2015). Regulation of the PI3K pathway through a p85α monomer–homodimer equilibrium. *eLife* 4 (20): 9164–9168. doi: 10.7554/eLife.06866.

Chiu, H. et al. (2019). The mTORC1/4E-BP/eIF4E axis promotes antibody class switching in B lymphocytes. *J. Immunol.* 202 (2): 579–590. doi: 10.4049/jimmunol.1800602.

Clayton, E. et al. (2002). A crucial role for the p110delta subunit of phosphatidylinositol 3-kinase in B cell development and activation. *J. Exp. Med.* 196 (6): 753–763. doi: 10.1084/jem.20020805.

Conley, M.E. et al. (2012). Agammaglobulinemia and absent B lineage cells in a patient lacking the p85α subunit of PI3K. *J. Exp. Med.* 209 (3): 463–470. doi: 10.1084/jem.20112533.

Deau, M.-C. et al. (2014). A human immunodeficiency caused by mutations in the PIK3R1 gene. *J. Clin. Invest.* 124 (9): 3923–3928. doi: 10.1172/JCI75746.

Deladeriere, A. et al. (2015). The regulatory subunits of PI3Kγ control distinct neutrophil responses. *Sci. Signal.* 8 (360): 1–13. doi: 10.1126/scisignal.2005564.

Dickson, E.J. and Hille, B. (2019). Understanding phosphoinositides: rare, dynamic, and essential membrane phospholipids. *Biochem. J.* 476 (1): 1–23. doi: 10.1042/BCJ20180022.

Dominguez-Sola, D. et al. (2015). The FOXO1 transcription factor instructs the germinal center dark zone program. *Immunity* Elsevier Inc., 43 (6): 1064–1074. doi: 10.1016/j.immuni.2015.10.015.

Dornan, G.L. et al. (2017). Conformational disruption of PI3Kδ regulation by immunodeficiency mutations in PIK3CD and PIK3R1. *Proc. Natl. Acad. Sci.* 114 (8): 1982–1987. doi: 10.1073/pnas.1617244114.

Dornan, G.L. and Burke, J.E. (2018 March). Molecular mechanisms of human disease mediated by oncogenic and primary immunodeficiency mutations in class IA phosphoinositide 3-kinases. *Front. Immunol.* 9: 1–9. doi: 10.3389/fimmu.2018.00575.

Ersching, J. et al. (2017). Germinal center selection and affinity maturation require dynamic regulation of mTORC1 kinase. *Immunity* Elsevier Inc., 46 (6): 1045–1058.e6. doi: 10.1016/j.immuni.2017.06.005.

Feng, J. et al. (2004). Identification of a PKB/Akt hydrophobic motif Ser-473 kinase as DNA-dependent protein kinase. *J. Biol. Chem.* Â© 2004 ASBMB. Currently published by Elsevier Inc; originally published by American Society for Biochemistry and Molecular Biology, 279 (39): 41189–41196. doi: 10.1074/jbc.M406731200.

Finlay, D.K. et al. (2009). Phosphoinositide-dependent kinase 1 controls migration and malignant transformation but not cell growth and proliferation in PTEN-null lymphocytes. *J. Exp. Med.* 206 (11): 2441–2454. doi: 10.1084/jem.20090219.

Fos, C. et al. (2008). ICOS ligation recruits the p50α PI3K regulatory subunit to the immunological synapse. *J. Immunol.* 181 (3): 1969–1977. doi: 10.4049/jimmunol.181.3.1969.

Fruman, D.A. et al. (1999). Impaired B cell development and proliferation in absence of phosphoinositide 3-kinase p85alpha. *Science (New York, N.Y.)* 283 (5400): 393–397. doi: 10.1126/science.283.5400.393.

Furman, R.R. et al. (2010). CAL-101, an isoform-selective inhibitor of phosphatidylinositol 3-kinase P110δ, demonstrates clinical activity and pharmacodynamic effects in patients with relapsed or refractory chronic lymphocytic leukemia. *Blood* 116 (21): 55–55. doi: 10.1182/blood.V116.21.55.55.

Gigoux, M. et al. (2009). Inducible costimulator promotes helper T-cell differentiation through phosphoinositide 3-kinase. *Proc. Natl. Acad. Sci. U.S.A.* 106 (48): 20371–20376. doi: 10.1073/pnas.0911573106.

Harrington, C.T. et al. (2021). Tilting MYC toward cancer cell death. *Trends Cancer* Elsevier Inc., 1–13. doi: 10.1016/j.trecan.2021.08.002.

Herman, S.E.M. et al. (2010). Phosphatidylinositol 3-kinase-δ inhibitor CAL-101 shows promising preclinical activity in chronic lymphocytic leukemia by antagonizing intrinsic and extrinsic cellular survival signals. *Blood* 116 (12): 2078–2088. doi: 10.1182/blood-2010-02-271171.

Hoellenriegel, J. et al. (2011). The phosphoinositide 3′-kinase delta inhibitor, CAL-101, inhibits B-cell receptor signaling and chemokine networks in chronic lymphocytic leukemia. *Blood* 118 (13): 3603–3612. doi: 10.1182/blood-2011-05-352492.

Hukelmann, J.L. et al. (2016). The cytotoxic T cell proteome and its shaping by the kinase mTOR. *Nat. Immunol.* 17 (1): 104–112. doi: 10.1038/ni.3314.

Iyengar, S. et al. (2013). P110α-mediated constitutive PI3K signaling limits the efficacy of p110δ-selective inhibition in mantle cell lymphoma, particularly with multiple relapse. *Blood* 121 (12): 2274–2284. doi: 10.1182/blood-2012-10-460832.

Jou, S. et al. (2002). Essential, nonredundant role for the phosphoinositide 3-kinase p110δ in signaling by the B-cell receptor complex. *Mol. Cell. Biol.* 22 (24): 8580–8591. doi: 10.1128/MCB.22.24.8580.

Kerdiles, Y.M. et al. (2009). Foxo1 links homing and survival of naive T cells by regulating L-selectin, CCR7 and interleukin 7 receptor. *Nat. Immunol.* 10 (2): 176–184. doi: 10.1038/ni.1689.

Klein, U. and Dalla-Favera, R. (2008). Germinal centres: role in B-cell physiology and malignancy. *Nat. Rev. Immunol.* 8 (1): 22–33. doi: 10.1038/nri2217.

Köhrer, S. et al. (2016). Pre-BCR signaling in precursor B-cell acute lymphoblastic leukemia regulates PI3K/AKT, FOXO1 and MYC, and can be targeted by SYK inhibition. *Leukemia* 30 (6): 1246–1254. doi: 10.1038/leu.2016.9.

Kolch, W. et al. (2015). The dynamic control of signal transduction networks in cancer cells. *Nat. Rev. Cancer* Nature Publishing Group, 15 (9): 515–527. doi: 10.1038/nrc3983.

Kriplani, N. et al. (2015). Class I PI 3-kinases: function and evolution. *Adv. Biol. Regul.* Elsevier Ltd, 59: 53–64. doi: 10.1016/j.jbior.2015.05.002.

Lee, J. et al. (2020). IFITM3 functions as a PIP3 scaffold to amplify PI3K signalling in B cells. *Nature* 588 (7838): 491–497. doi: 10.1038/s41586-020-2884-6.

Lim, E.L. et al. (2018). Phosphoinositide 3-kinase δ inhibition promotes antitumor responses but antagonizes checkpoint inhibitors. *JCI Insight* 3 (11). doi: 10.1172/jci.insight.120626.

Liu, D. and Uzonna, J.E. (2010). The p110δ isoform of phosphatidylinositol 3-kinase controls the quality of secondary anti- leishmania immunity by regulating expansion and effector function of memory T cell subsets. *J. Immunol.* 184 (6): 3098–3105. doi: 10.4049/jimmunol.0903177.

Liu, G.Y. and Sabatini, D.M. (2020). mTOR at the nexus of nutrition, growth, ageing and disease. *Nat. Rev. Mol. Cell Biol.* Springer US, 8. doi: 10.1038/s41580-019-0199-y.

Lucas, C.L. et al. (2014a). Dominant-activating germline mutations in the gene encoding the PI(3)K catalytic subunit p110δ result in T cell senescence and human immunodeficiency. *Nat. Immunol.* 15 (1): 88–97. doi: 10.1038/ni.2771.

Lucas, C.L. et al. (2014b). Heterozygous splice mutation in PIK3R1 causes human immunodeficiency with lymphoproliferation due to dominant activation of PI3K. *J. Exp. Med.* 211 (13): 2537–2547. doi: 10.1084/jem.20141759.

Lucas, C.L. et al. (2016). PI3Kδ and primary immunodeficiencies. *Nat. Rev. Immunol.* Nature Publishing Group, 16 (11): 702–714. doi: 10.1038/nri.2016.93.

Luff, D.H. et al. (2021 March). PI3Kδ forms distinct multiprotein complexes at the TCR signalosome in naïve and differentiated CD4+ T cells. *Front. Immunol.* 12: 1–19. doi: 10.3389/fimmu.2021.631271.

Luo, W., Weisel, F., and Shlomchik, M.J. (2018). B cell receptor and CD40 signaling are rewired for synergistic induction of the c-Myc transcription factor in germinal center B cells. *Immunity* Elsevier Inc., 48 (2): 313–326.e5. doi: 10.1016/j.immuni.2018.01.008.

Ma, X. et al. (2018). Pan-cancer genome and transcriptome analyses of 1,699 paediatric leukaemias and solid tumours. *Nature* Nature Publishing Group, 555 (7696): 371–376. doi: 10.1038/nature25795.

Macintyre, A.N. et al. (2011). Protein kinase B controls transcriptional programs that direct cytotoxic T cell fate but is dispensable for T cell metabolism. *Immunity* Elsevier Inc., 34 (2): 224–236. doi: 10.1016/j.immuni.2011.01.012.

Madsen, R.R. (2020). PI3K in stemness regulation: from development to cancer. *Biochem. Soc. Trans.* 48 (1): 301–315. doi: 10.1042/BST20190778.

Madsen, R.R. and Vanhaesebroeck, B. (2020). Cracking the context-specific PI3K signaling code. *Sci. Signal.* 13 (613): eaay2940. doi: 10.1126/scisignal.aay2940.

Madsen, R.R., Vanhaesebroeck, B., and Semple, R.K. (2018). Cancer-associated PIK3CA mutations in overgrowth disorders. *Trends Mol. Med.* 24 (10): 856–870. doi: 10.1016/j.molmed.2018.08.003.

Malek, M. et al. (2017). PTEN regulates PI(3,4)P2 signaling downstream of class I PI3K. *Mol. Cell* 566–580. doi: 10.1016/j.molcel.2017.09.024.

Manning, B.D. and Toker, A. (2017). AKT/PKB signaling: navigating the network. *Cell* 169 (3): 381–405. doi: 10.1016/j.cell.2017.04.001.

Mukherjee, R. et al. (2021). Regulation of PTEN translation by PI3K signaling maintains pathway homeostasis. *Mol. Cell* Elsevier Inc., 81 (4): 708–723.e5. doi: 10.1016/j.molcel.2021.01.033.

Murali, I. et al. (2018). Activating MAPK pathway mutations mediate primary resistance to PI3K inhibitors in Chronic Lymphocytic Leukemia (CLL). *Blood* American Society of Hematology, 132 (Supplement 1): 587–587. doi: 10.1182/blood-2018-99-115304.

Nunes-Santos, C.J., Uzel, G., and Rosenzweig, S.D. (2019). PI3K pathway defects leading to immunodeficiency and immune dysregulation. *J. Allergy Clin. Immunol.* Elsevier Inc., 143 (5): 1676–1687. doi: 10.1016/j.jaci.2019.03.017.

Oak, J.S. et al. (2009). The p85β regulatory subunit of phosphoinositide 3-kinase has unique and redundant functions in B cells. *Autoimmunity* 42 (5): 447–458. doi: 10.1080/08916930902911746.

Okkenhaug, K. (2002). Impaired B and T cell antigen receptor signaling in p110delta PI 3-kinase mutant mice. *Science* 297: 1–5. doi: 10.1126/science.1073560.

Okkenhaug, K. (2013). Signaling by the phosphoinositide 3-kinase family in immune cells. *Annu. Rev. Immunol.* 31 (1): 675–704. doi: 10.1146/annurev-immunol-032712-095946.

Okkenhaug, K. and Burger, J.A. (2016 October). PI3K signaling in normal B cells and Chronic Lymphocytic Leukemia (CLL). *Curr. Top. Microbiol. Immunol.* 393: 123–142. doi: 10.1007/82_2015_484.

Omori, S.A. et al. (2006). Regulation of class-switch recombination and plasma cell differentiation by phosphatidylinositol 3-kinase signaling. *Immunity* 25 (4): 545–557. doi: 10.1016/j.immuni.2006.08.015.

Patton, D.T. et al. (2006). Cutting edge: the phosphoinositide 3-kinase p110δ is critical for the function of CD4 + CD25 + Foxp3 + Regulatory T cells. *J. Immunol.* 177 (10): 6598–6602. doi: 10.4049/jimmunol.177.10.6598.

Pfeifer, M. et al. (2013). PTEN loss defines a PI3K/AKT pathway-dependent germinal center subtype of diffuse large B-cell lymphoma. *Proc. Natl. Acad. Sci. U.S.A.* 110 (30): 12420–12425. doi: 10.1073/pnas.1305656110.

Pongas, G.N., Annunziata, C.M., and Staudt, L.M. (2017). PI3Kδ inhibition causes feedback activation of PI3Kα in the ABC subtype of diffuse large B-cell lymphoma. *Oncotarget* 8 (47): 81794–81802. doi: 10.18632/oncotarget.20864.

Preite, S. et al. (2019). T and B-cell signaling in activated PI3K delta syndrome: from immunodeficiency to autoimmunity. *Immunol. Rev.* 154–173. doi: 10.1111/imr.12790.

Ramadani, F. et al. (2010). The PI3K isoforms p110alpha and p110delta are essential for pre-B cell receptor signaling and B cell development. *Sci. Signal.* 3 (134): ra60–ra60. doi: 10.1126/scisignal.2001104.

Roberto, M.P. et al. (2021). Mutations in the transcription factor FOXO1 mimic positive selection signals to promote germinal center B cell expansion and lymphomagenesis. *Immunity* Elsevier Inc., 54 (8): 1807–1824.e14. doi: 10.1016/j.immuni.2021.07.009.

Rolf, J. et al. (2010). Phosphoinositide 3-kinase activity in T cells regulates the magnitude of the germinal center reaction. *J. Immunol.* 185 (7): 4042–4052. doi: 10.4049/jimmunol.1001730.

Ross, S.H. et al. (2016). Phosphoproteomic analyses of interleukin 2 signaling reveal integrated JAK kinase-dependent and -independent networks in CD8+ T cells. *Immunity* The Author(s), 45 (3): 685–700. doi: 10.1016/j.immuni.2016.07.022.

Sanchez, V.E. et al. (2019). Targeting PI3K signaling in acute lymphoblastic leukemia. *Int. J. Mol. Sci.* 20 (2). doi: 10.3390/ijms20020412.

Sanchez-Vega, F. et al. (2018). Oncogenic signaling pathways in the cancer genome atlas. *Cell* 173 (2): 321–337.e10. doi: 10.1016/j.cell.2018.03.035.

Sander, S. et al. (2015). PI3 kinase and FOXO1 transcription factor activity differentially control B cells in the germinal center light and dark zones. *Immunity* Elsevier Inc., 43 (6): 1075–1086. doi: 10.1016/j.immuni.2015.10.021.

Shojaee, S. et al. (2016). PTEN opposes negative selection and enables oncogenic transformation of pre-B cells. *Nat. Med.* 22 (4): 379–387. doi: 10.1038/nm.4062.

Silva, A. et al. (2008). PTEN posttranslational inactivation and hyperactivation of the PI3K/Akt pathway sustain primary T cell leukemia viability. *J. Clin. Invest.* 118 (11): 3762–3774. doi: 10.1172/JCI34616.

So, L. and Fruman, D.A. (2012). PI3K signalling in B- and T-lymphocytes: new developments and therapeutic advances. *Biochem. J.* 442 (3): 465–481. doi: 10.1042/BJ20112092.

Spinelli, L. et al. (2021 June). Phosphoinositide 3-kinase p110 delta differentially restrains and directs naïve versus effector CD8+ T cell transcriptional programs. *Front. Immunol.* 12: 1–19. doi: 10.3389/fimmu.2021.691997.

Srinivasan, L. et al. (2009). PI3 kinase signals BCR-dependent mature B cell survival. *Cell* Elsevier Ltd, 139 (3): 573–586. doi: 10.1016/j.cell.2009.08.041.

Stone, E.L. et al. (2015). ICOS coreceptor signaling inactivates the transcription factor FOXO1 to promote Tfh cell differentiation. *Immunity* Elsevier, 42 (2): 239–251. doi: 10.1016/j.immuni.2015.01.017.

Suzuki, H. et al. (1999). Xid -like immunodeficiency in mice with disruption of the p85α subunit of phosphoinositide 3-kinase. *Science* 283 (5400): 390–392. doi: 10.1126/science.283.5400.390.

Swan, D.J. et al. (2019). Immunodeficiency, autoimmune thrombocytopenia and enterocolitis caused by autosomal recessive deficiency of PIK3CD -encoded phosphoinositide 3-kinase δ. *Haematologica* 104 (10): e483–e486. doi: 10.3324/haematol.2018.208397.

Tang, P. et al. (2018). Autosomal recessive agammaglobulinemia due to a homozygous mutation in PIK3R1. *J. Clin. Immunol.* 38 (1): 88–95. doi: 10.1007/s10875-017-0462-y.

Toker, A. and Newton, A.C. (2000). Akt/protein kinase B is regulated by autophosphorylation at the hypothetical PDK-2 site. *J. Biol. Chem.* Â© 2000 ASBMB. Currently published by Elsevier Inc; originally published by American Society for Biochemistry and Molecular Biology, 275 (12): 8271–8274. doi: 10.1074/jbc.275.12.8271.

Tsolakos, N. et al. (2018). Quantitation of class IA PI3Ks in mice reveals p110-free-p85s and isoform-selective subunit associations and recruitment to receptors. *Proc. Natl. Acad. Sci.* 115 (48): 12176–12181. doi: 10.1073/pnas.1803446115.

Uhlén, M. et al. (2015). Tissue-based map of the human proteome. *Science* 347 (6220). doi: 10.1126/science.1260419.

Vanhaesebroeck, B. et al. (2021). PI3K inhibitors are finally coming of age. *Nat. Rev. Drug Discov.* 20 (10): 741–769. doi: 10.1038/s41573-021-00209-1.

Wang, X., Hills, L.B., and Huang, Y.H. (2015 March). Lipid and protein co-regulation of PI3K effectors Akt and Itk in lymphocytes. *Front. Immunol.* 6: 1–11. doi: 10.3389/fimmu.2015.00117.

Waugh, C. et al. (2009). Phosphoinositide (3,4,5)-triphosphate binding to phosphoinositide-dependent kinase 1 regulates a protein kinase B/Akt signaling threshold that dictates T-cell migration, not proliferation. *Mol. Cell. Biol.* 29 (21): 5952–5962. doi: 10.1128/mcb.00585-09.

Xu, K. et al. (2021). Glycolytic ATP fuels phosphoinositide 3-kinase signaling to support effector T helper 17 cell responses. *Immunity* 54 (5): 976–987.e7. doi: 10.1016/j.immuni.2021.04.008.

Yang, J. et al. (2016 September). Critical roles of mTOR complex 1 and 2 for t follicular helper cell differentiation and germinal center responses. *eLife* 5: 1–22. doi: 10.7554/eLife.17936.

Zeng, H. et al. (2016). mTORC1 and mTORC2 kinase signaling and glucose metabolism drive follicular helper T cell differentiation. *Immunity* Elsevier Inc., 45 (3): 540–554. doi: 10.1016/j.immuni.2016.08.017.

Zhang, K. et al. (2013). Identification of a phosphoinositide 3-kinase (PI-3K) p110delta (PIK3CD) deficient individual. *J. Clin. Immunol.* 33 (3): 673–674.

Zhang, Y. et al. (2017). A pan-cancer proteogenomic atlas of PI3K/AKT/mTOR pathway alterations. *Cancer Cell* 31 (6): 820–832.e3. doi: 10.1016/j.ccell.2017.04.013.

6

Pharmacologic Differentiation of Drugs Targeting the PI3K-AKT-mTOR Signaling Pathway

Inhye E. Ahn, Jennifer R. Brown, and Matthew S. Davids

Dana-Farber Cancer Institute, Harvard Medical School, Boston, MA, USA

Take Home Messages

- Pharmacologic targeting of the PI3K-AKT-mTOR signaling pathway in lymphoma has been most successful with inhibition of the proximal component of the pathway through PI3K inhibitors.
- Isoform selectivity and pharmacologic properties of the PI3K inhibitors contribute to the clinical activity and safety of individual agents.
- AKT and mTOR inhibition have been associated with increased toxicity and limited efficacy due to negative feedback mechanisms that reconstitute the upstream signaling.

Introduction

Phosphoinositide 3-kinase (PI3K) and its downstream signaling through AKT and mammalian target of rapamycin (mTOR) govern diverse physiological and disease-related processes. The pathobiology of the PI3K-AKT-mTOR signaling pathway is reviewed in detail in a separate chapter entitled *Principles of PI3K Biology and its Role in Cancer.* Briefly, class I PI3K has four catalytic subunits: p110α, p110β, and p110δ, which link PI3K activity to tyrosine kinases, and p110γ, which is associated with G-protein-coupled receptors. The α and β isoforms are ubiquitously expressed in most human tissues. The γ and δ isoforms are predominantly expressed in hematopoietic cells.

The functional roles of the PI3K isoforms have been extensively characterized in genetic knockout and mutant mouse models (previously reviewed by Vanhaesebroeck et al. 2005). These studies elucidated the immunological and metabolic changes related to each isoform, including regulation of insulin signaling via the α isoform (Knight et al. 2006) platelet adhesion and aggregation via the β isoform (Garcia et al. 2010) innate immune response and macrophage polarization via the γ isoform (Kaneda et al. 2016) and B-cell development and maintenance of mature B-cell survival via the δ isoform (Srinivasan et al. 2009). Notably, the γ- and δ isoforms have complementary and overlapping roles in T-cell development, differentiation, and activity. Genetic models have demonstrated reduced thymocyte survival and defective cytokine production from stimulated T-cells of PI3Kγ null mice (PI3Kγ-/-) (Sasaki et al. 2000) impaired antigen-mediated T-cell activation in PI3Kδ kinase-inactive mice (PI3K$\delta^{D910A/D910A}$) (Okkenhaug et al. 2002) and decreased early T-cell development in PI3Kγ/δ double knockout mice (Webb et al. 2005). The differential tissue expression and distinct functional roles of the isoforms correlate with activity and safety profiles of PI3K inhibitors in the clinic (Lampson and Brown 2021).

Some cancer cells hijack the PI3K signaling pathway for tumorigenesis. Solid tumors frequently utilize genetic mechanisms that upregulate PI3K signaling, which include activating mutations in the gene encoding PI3Kα (*PIK3CA*) and deletion or inactivating mutations in *PTEN*, an antagonist of PI3K signaling (Figure 6.1) (Lawrence et al. 2014; Samuels et al. 2004). Less commonly, activating mutations in *AKT1* (Carpten et al. 2007) and *MTOR* (Grabiner et al. 2014) and inactivating mutations in tuberous sclerosis complex genes (*TSC*) have been reported (Inoki et al. 2005). Unlike solid tumors, lymphoid malignancies infrequently exhibit genetic activation of the PI3K signaling pathway. *PI3KCA* mutations are rare, although *PTEN* inactivation may occur in lymphoma due to deletion or mutations of the gene (Chapuy et al. 2018; Schmitz et al. 2012) or functional suppression of *PTEN* activity through the oncogenic miR-17–92 cluster (Dal Bo et al. 2015). Constitutive upregulation of PI3K signaling in B-cell lymphoma is predominantly driven by increased B-cell receptor (BCR) signaling (Ahn and Brown 2021). PI3K is part of the BCR signaling complex recruited after phosphorylation of the surface BCR. In particular, the δ isoform has a critical role in B-cell lymphoma by being involved in

Precision Cancer Therapies: Targeting Oncogenic Drivers and Signaling Pathways in Lymphoid Malignancies: From Concept to Practice, Volume 1, First Edition. Edited by Owen A. O'Connor, Stephen M. Ansell, and John F. Seymour.

both tonic and chronic activated BCR signaling. PI3K signaling itself can also maintain mature B-cell survival independent of BCR signaling, a finding supported by successful rescue of BCR-ablated B-cells with constitutive activation of PI3K or *PTEN* knockout *in vivo* (Srinivasan et al. 2009). Conversely, genetic inactivation of PI3Kδ causes severe reduction of B-cell numbers and antigen-dependent BCR signaling, which underscores the crosstalk between PI3K and BCR signaling pathways (Okkenhaug et al. 2002). The central role of PI3Kδ in normal B-cell development and tumorigenesis makes it a compelling therapeutic target in lymphoma. Targeting additional PI3K isoforms has biological and clinical relevance to selected lymphoma subtypes. PI3Kα is genetically activated in a subset of mantle cell lymphoma (MCL) and diffuse large B-cell lymphoma (DLBCL) (Abubaker et al. 2007; Psyrri et al. 2009). In T-cell lymphoma, PI3Kδ and PI3Kγ are the primary therapeutic targets due to their known roles in the regulation of T-cell function and chemotaxis (Kaneda et al. 2016; Sasaki et al. 2000). Dual inhibition of the γ and δ isoforms in T-cell lymphoma cell lines with duvelisib led to greater cell killing than sole inhibition of PI3Kδ or the use of the pan-PI3K inhibitor copanlisib, which has less potent activity against PI3Kγ compared to other isoforms (Horwitz et al. 2018). Clinical experiences with PI3K and mTOR inhibitors are discussed in other chapters. Here, we address the pharmacologic properties of molecules targeting the PI3K-AKT-mTOR signaling pathway and their clinical relevance.

PI3K Inhibitors Approved by the US Food and Drug Administration (FDA)

The ATP binding site within the kinase domain of PI3K has a valine residue that is conserved in all PI3K class I isoforms. The valine 882 residue is a critical site for ATP binding by forming a hydrogen bond with the purine ring of the ATP (Vanhaesebroeck et al. 2021). PI3K inhibitors mimic this interaction and compete with ATP at the affinity pocket of PI3K. Early generation PI3K inhibitors (e.g. buparlisib and pictilisib) are characterized by weak hydrogen interactions at the affinity pocket leading to non-selective, weak inhibition of PI3K class I isoforms (Walker et al. 2000; Winkler et al. 2013). Selective PI3K inhibitors (e.g. idelalisib, duvelisib, and umbralisib) differ from the earlier molecules by achieving more potent inhibition of PI3K through stronger interaction at the affinity pocket and obtaining isoform selectivity through additional interactions with non-conserved residues of PI3K (Vanhaesebroeck et al. 2021). Engagement of non-conserved residues, such as methionine 752 and threonine 750, induces conformational changes to the kinase, creating a hydrophobic pocket that selective PI3K inhibitors can intercalate into (also known as a specificity pocket) (Somoza et al. 2015).

Pharmacologic targeting of the PI3K pathway has proven to be challenging due to toxicities that limit tolerance. The mechanism of the toxicity of PI3K inhibitors is not fully understood, though the pharmacologic properties of each agent and isoform selectivity likely contribute. PI3Kδ and/or γ inhibitors are associated with hematologic, infectious, and immune-mediated toxicities. Immune-mediated toxicities manifest clinically as diarrhea/colitis, transaminitis/hepatitis, and interstitial lung disease (ILD)/pneumonitis. While PI3Kδ is involved in the differentiation of various T-cell subsets, regulatory T-cells (Treg) are particularly susceptible to pharmacologic (Hanna et al. 2019) or genetic inactivation of PI3Kδ (Ali et al. 2014; Dong et al. 2019), shifting the balance between Treg and effector T-cells in favor of effector cells. Half-maximal inhibitory concentration (IC_{50}) of a selective PI3Kδ inhibitor idelalisib was substantially lower for Tregs (0.5 μM) than CD4+ (2.0 μM) or CD8+ T cells (6.5 μM) in IL-2 stimulated T-cells from patients with chronic lymphocytic leukemia (CLL) (Chellappa et al. 2019). The immune-modulatory effect of PI3Kδ inhibitors is a key to understanding inflammatory complications and subsequent development of other PI3K inhibitors aimed at improving the safety of this drug class. Inhibition of PI3Kα is associated with hypertension and hyperglycemia. Intriguingly, the metabolic disruption related to PI3Kα inhibition can paradoxically activate PI3K signaling and confer primary resistance to therapy (Figure 6.1). Pivotal to this feedback loop is increased insulin secretion that occurs

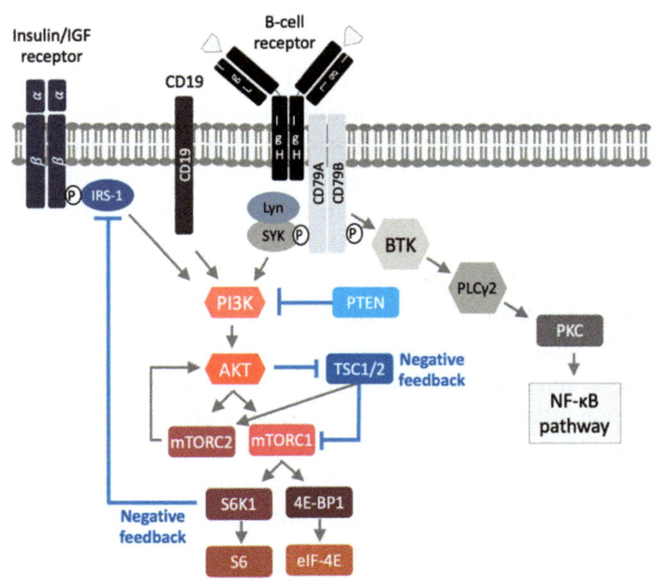

Figure 6.1 Negative regulators of the PI3K-AKT-mTOR signaling pathway.
Abbreviations: BTK, Bruton's tyrosine kinase; eIF-4E, eukaryotic translation initiation factor 4E; IGF, insulin-like growth factor; IRS-1, insulin receptor substrate 1; LYN, Tyrosine-protein kinase Lyn; mTOR, mammalian target of rapamycin; mTORC, mTOR complex; PI3K, phosphoinositide 3-kinase; PKC, protein kinase c; PLCγ2, phospholipase γ2; PTEN, phosphatase and tensin homolog; S6K1, ribosomal protein S6 kinase beta-1; SYK, spleen tyrosine kinase; TSC, tuberous sclerosis complex; 4E-BP1, eIF-4E-binding protein.

in response to hyperglycemia caused by PI3Kα inhibition. This increase in insulin levels has been experimentally shown to be sufficient to partially reconstitute PI3K signaling in the presence of a PI3K inhibitor (Hopkins et al. 2018).

Four PI3K inhibitors have been approved for B-cell malignancies and are utilized in clinical practice, including idelalisib, duvelisib, copanlisib, and umbralisib:

Idelalisib (formerly CAL-101/GS-1101) was the first PI3K inhibitor approved by the FDA and received its initial label in 2014 (Table 6.1). Key structural characteristics of idelalisib include the propeller-shaped structure with the central quinazoline core, which confers selectivity toward the PI3Kδ isoform, and the purine group, which improves the potency of δ inhibition through binding at the hinge region and affinity pocket interactions (Figure 6.2a) (Somoza et al. 2015). The purine group, also found in duvelisib, is thought to contribute to the hepatotoxicity of PI3K inhibitors, affecting up to 40% of patients on idelalisib or duvelisib (Flinn et al. 2019; Sharman et al. 2019). Transaminitis may be relatively less severe and less frequent for the later generation of PI3K inhibitors, although the risk remains elevated. A randomized trial testing umbralisib, a PI3K inhibitor with a pyrazolopyrimidine group instead of purine (Shin et al. 2020), reported a 17% incidence of transaminitis in the umbralisib arm compared to the 4.5% of the control arm treated with chemoimmunotherapy (see below) (Gribben et al. 2020). These data suggest that the structural properties of PI3K inhibitors partially explain the hepatotoxicity of the drug class. Immune-mediated mechanisms and dosing strategies likely contribute to the observed incidences of hepatotoxicity and other adverse events.

Several studies demonstrated strong immune-modulatory effects of idelalisib. In preclinical studies modeling CLL with stromal cell co-culture, idelalisib impaired CLL cell viability by abrogating BCR signaling, disrupting chemokine-mediated crosstalk between CLL cells and the microenvironment (i.e. CCL3, CCL4, and CXCL13), and increasing the priming of CLL cells for apoptosis (Davids et al. 2012; Herman et al. 2010; Hoellenriegel et al. 2011). Idelalisib also induces tissue

Table 6.1 Pharmacologic properties of PI3K inhibitors.

	Idelalisib(CAL-101)	Duvelisib(IPI-145)	Copanlisib(BAY 80-6946)	Umbralisib(TGR-1202)	Parsaclisib (INCB050465)	Zandelisib(ME-401)
Dominant targets	PI3Kδ	PI3Kγ and PI3Kδ	Pan-PI3K inhibitor (greater α and δ inhibition than β and γ)	PI3Kδ and CK-1ε	PI3Kδ	PI3Kδ
IC_{50} (nM)	8 600	1 602	0.5	>10 000	>10 000	1 320
PI3Kα	4 000	85	3.7	1 116	>10 000	18
PI3Kβ	2 100	27	6.4	1 065	>10 000	420
PI3Kγ	19	2.5	0.7	22	1	0.6
PI3Kδ						
FDA approved dose	150 mg PO b.i.d.	25 mg PO b.i.d.	60 mg IV on D1, 8, and 15 of a 28-day cycle	800 mg PO QD	20 mg PO QD#	60 mg PO QD#
$T_{1/2}$ (hours)*	8.2	4.7	39.1	91	8.6–11.5	26
T_{max} (hours)*	1.5	1–2	1	4	0.5–1	5
Comment	First PI3K inhibitor approved by the FDA	Dual inhibitor of PI3Kδ and PI3Kγ. Activity in T-cell lymphoma.	Copanlisib can inhibit mTOR kinase (IC_{50} 45 nM). The M1 metabolite has activity against PI3Kα (IC_{50} 1.5 nM) and PI3Kβ (IC_{50} 5.8 nM)	Inhibits PI3Kδ and CK-1ε	Ongoing phase 2 in DLBCL (NCT02998476)	Ongoing phase 3 in indolent NHL (NCT04745832)
References	(Somoza et al. 2015)	(Winkler et al. 2013)	(Scott et al. 2016)	(Lampson and Brown 2021; Burris et al. 2018)	(Shin et al. 2020; Yue et al. 2019)	(Moreno and Wood 2019; O'Farrell et al. 2012)

Footnote: IC_{50} values are not for comparisons across PI3K inhibitors.

Abbreviations: b.i.d. = twice daily; CK-1ε = casein kinase-1ε; D = day; DLBCL = diffuse large B-cell lymphoma; IC_{50} = half-maximal inhibitory concentration; IV = intravenous; MTD = maximum tolerated dose; NHL = non-Hodgkin's lymphoma; PO = by mouth; QD = once daily; RP2D = recommended phase 2 dose; $T_{1/2}$ = mean elimination half-life; T_{max} = median time to reach peak plasma concentration

* Pharmacokinetic parameters based on FDA-approved doses.

\# Recommended phase 2 dose. Parsaclisib and zandelisib have not been FDA-approved to date.

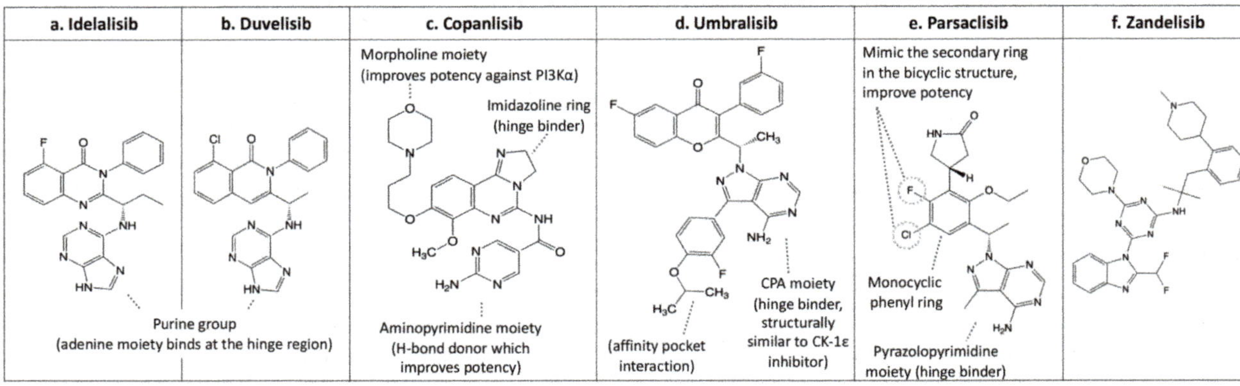

Figure 6.2 Biochemical structures of PI3K inhibitors.
Abbreviations: AA, amino acid; CK-1ε, casein kinase-1ε; CPA: central pyrazolopyrimidine amine.

infiltration of pro-inflammatory CD8+ T cells, supporting the hypothesis of the immune-mediated nature of the adverse events associated with PI3K inhibitors (Lampson et al. 2016; Louie et al. 2015). Diarrhea and transaminitis are the two most common adverse events affecting over half of patients receiving idelalisib as first-line therapy (Lampson et al. 2016; O'Brien et al. 2015) and approximately a third of those treated in the relapsed setting (Furman et al. 2014; Sharman et al. 2019). Pneumonitis is a relatively uncommon adverse event (4–10%) (Furman et al. 2014; Sharman et al. 2019), but fatal events have been reported during idelalisib monotherapy (Brown et al. 2014). The risk of pneumonitis seemingly increases when idelalisib is combined with another BCR signaling pathway inhibitor such as entospletinib (18%) (Barr et al. 2016) or tirabrutinib (14%) (Danilov et al. 2020). The frequency and severity of the immune-mediated toxicities of PI3K inhibitors increase among patients with more competent effector T-cell function, characterized by younger age and without exposure to cytotoxic chemotherapy (Brown et al. 2020; Lampson et al. 2016). Further, fatal cases of opportunistic infection from *Pneumocystis jirovecii* pneumonia (PJP) and cytomegalovirus (CMV) reactivation, as well as typical viral and bacterial infections, have been reported in association with idelalisib (Brown et al. 2014; Furman et al. 2014; Jones et al. 2017; Lampson et al. 2016; Sharman et al. 2019). In a randomized phase 3 study in CLL, opportunistic infection was more frequently observed among patients treated with idelalisib plus bendamustine and rituximab (BR; 2% with PJP, 6% with CMV reactivation) than the control arm treated with BR alone (0% PJP, 1% CMV) (Zelenetz et al. 2017). A pooled analysis of 1391 patients reported similar rates of PJP infection among patients treated with idelalisib plus BR (2.2%) and those treated with idelalisib plus anti-CD20 antibody (3.1%) (Sehn et al. 2016). The pooled analysis did not compare the risk of CMV. However, the 6% rate of CMV reactivation observed among patients receiving idelalisib plus BR (Zelenetz et al. 2017) was numerically higher than 2–4% reported from studies combining idelalisib and anti-CD20 antibody (Brown et al. 2014; Jones et al. 2017; Lampson et al. 2019; Sharman et al. 2019). These data led to recommendations to provide PJP prophylaxis during treatment with all PI3K inhibitors, permanent treatment discontinuation at the onset of PJP, and vigilance in testing for CMV during treatment with PI3K inhibitors. Excess toxicity and deaths associated with idelalisib led to the termination of three randomized trials and a phase 2 study in non-Hodgkin's lymphoma (NHL), including two studies in treatment-naïve CLL (NCT01980888, NCT02044822) (Hillmen et al. 2017). For these reasons, approved indications of idelalisib in the United States have been limited to relapsed NHL and CLL, though notably, the European Medicines Agency (EMA) did approve idelalisib plus rituximab as frontline therapy in CLL.

Duvelisib (formerly IPI-145), a dual inhibitor of PI3Kδ and γ, was FDA-approved in 2018 for the treatment of relapsed CLL and follicular lymphoma (FL) after two prior lines of therapy. Of the two targets of duvelisib, the δ isoform is more potently inhibited than the γ isoform, with about a 10-fold difference in binding affinity and IC_{50}. Duvelisib has a remarkable structural similarity to idelalisib (Figure 6.2b). A notable feature of duvelisib is the use of the *N*-phenyl 8-chloroisoquinolinone core, which substitutes the quinazoline core found in idelalisib and copanlisib. The *N*-phenyl 8-chloroisoquinolinone core determines PI3Kγ selectivity, and this structure is also found in a PI3Kγ inhibitor eganelisib (IPI-549) which is under investigation in solid tumors (Evans et al. 2016). Concurrent inhibition of the δ and γ isoforms has a theoretical advantage over sole inhibition of δ because of the known importance of γ in regulating inflammatory T-cells and macrophage polarization in the microenvironment (Hirsch et al. 2000; Kaneda et al. 2016). Further, *in vitro* studies demonstrated longer target residence time and more potent inhibition of PI3Kδ with duvelisib than idelalisib (Willemsen-Seegers et al. 2017; Winkler et al. 2013). It is unclear whether the potentially favorable pharmacological properties of duvelisib demonstrated preclinically translate to improved outcome and safety in the clinic. There is no head-to-head comparison of idelalisib and duvelisib in patients. The safety profile of duvelisib is similar overall to that of idelalisib. The frequency of high-grade inflammatory and infectious complications is numerically lower in studies using duvelisib than previous studies using idelalisib (Flinn et al. 2018, 2019). Such cross-trial comparison should be interpreted with caution, as these trials differ in terms of the patient populations and the approaches to the management of toxicities. Trials testing duvelisib adopted more proactive approaches in managing infectious toxicities with the mandatory use of prophylactic antimicrobials and growth factors in trials testing combination regimens (Davids et al. 2021; Flinn et al. 2019).

The approved dose of duvelisib is 25 mg taken by mouth (PO) twice daily (b.i.d.). A phase 1 study of duvelisib expanded enrollment of the 25 mg b.i.d. dosing cohort (59 patients) based on favorable safety and additionally expanded the maximum tolerated dose cohort dosed at 75 mg b.i.d. (118 patients) (Flinn et al. 2018). Two patients on duvelisib 100 mg b.i.d. developed increased transaminases and rash, respectively, as dose-limiting toxicities. The rates of adverse events and treatment discontinuation were similar between the two dose expansion cohorts. In B-cell lymphoma, pharmacodynamic markers were also comparable with the 25 mg b.i.d. dose achieving maximal inhibition of phospho-AKT (pAKT) downstream of the PI3K signaling pathway and near-complete reduction of a cellular proliferation marker Ki-67. The steady-state trough of the 25 mg b.i.d. dose is above the 90% inhibitory concentrations for PI3Kδ, suggesting continuous inhibition of PI3Kδ can be achieved by this dose. In clinical practice, patients frequently require dose interruption or reduction of duvelisib down to 15 mg b.i.d. to manage toxicities or drug–drug interactions with strong CYP3A4 inhibitors. None of the published phase 1 studies specified pharmacodynamic effects of the 15 mg b.i.d. dose, raising a question on the clinical efficacy of this dose (Flinn et al. 2018a; Flinn et al. 2018b; O'Brien et al. 2018).

In peripheral T-cell lymphoma, where disease activity is likely more dependent on γ inhibition, a higher overall response rate (ORR) was observed with 75 mg b.i.d. (54%) than 25 mg b.i.d. (35%) during a dose-optimization study (Horwitz et al. 2019). Pharmacokinetics data demonstrated incomplete inhibition of PI3Kγ (steady-state trough $>IC_{50}$ but not $>IC_{90}$) with duvelisib 25 mg b.i.d. unlike excellent PI3Kδ inhibition achieved by this dose (steady-state trough $>IC_{90}$) (Flinn et al. 2018). By increasing the duvelisib dose from 25 mg b.i.d. to 75 mg b.i.d., peak plasma concentration and exposure to duvelisib more than doubled. These data suggest higher doses of duvelisib can achieve more complete inhibition of the PI3Kγ isoform and potentially improve efficacy in peripheral T-cell lymphoma. A clinical trial in T-cell lymphoma has entered the dose-expansion phase which uses duvelisib at 75 mg b.i.d. for the first two cycles to maximize tumor control, followed by 25 mg b.i.d. for maintenance (Pro et al. 2020).

While duvelisib is only approved for the treatment of indolent B-cell lymphoma, it can be a rational strategy for the treatment of T-cell lymphoma and is additionally being tested in a clinical trial to recruit T-cells for anti-tumor activity (Kaneda et al. 2016; Sasaki et al. 2000). In T-cell lymphoma cell lines, dual inhibition of the γ and δ isoforms was more effective than a δ-specific inhibitor or a pan-PI3K inhibitor (Horwitz et al. 2018). A phase 1 study of duvelisib reported ORRs of 50% in peripheral T-cell lymphoma and 32% in cutaneous T-cell lymphoma, confirming the single-agent activity of duvelisib against malignant T-cells (Horwitz et al. 2018). In B-cell lymphoma mouse models, duvelisib can reverse T-cell suppression mediated by myeloid-derived suppressor cells (Davis et al. 2017) and augment the anti-tumor activity of immune checkpoint inhibitors (Pachter and Weaver 2017). Ongoing clinical trials utilize duvelisib for the treatment of T-cell lymphoma (NCT03372057, NCT02783625) or to augment the effects of immune-directed therapy in B-cell lymphoma (NCT03892044, NCT05044039).

Copanlisib (formerly BAY 80–6946) is a pan-PI3K inhibitor approved by the FDA for the treatment of relapsed FL after two lines of systemic therapy. Copanlisib potently inhibits all four PI3K isoforms at relatively lower IC_{50} levels for the α (0.5 nM) and δ (0.7 nM) isoforms compared to β (3.7 nM) and γ (6.4 nM) (Scott et al. 2016). Additionally, copanlisib has activity against mTOR (IC_{50} 45 nM) and has an active metabolite M-1, which also inhibits PI3Kα (IC_{50} 1.5 nM) and β (IC_{50} 5.8 nM). Other than the aforementioned targets within the PI3K-AKT-mTOR pathway, copanlisib does not have significant off-target activity. Additional motifs and amino acid groups attached to the quinazoline core of copanlisib improve potency of the drug and enable PI3Kα inhibition (Figure 6.2c) (Scott et al. 2016). Consistent with its pharmacologic property as a potent inhibitor of PI3Kα, copanlisib blocks AKT phosphorylation in *PIK3CA* mutant breast cancer cell lines more potently than those with *PTEN* mutations (Liu et al. 2013). Idelalisib and copanlisib have comparable potency against PI3Kδ (Paul et al. 2017). Simultaneous inhibition of the α and δ isoforms by copanlisib can enhance anti-tumor activity as demonstrated by a comparative *in vitro* assay of copanlisib and idelalisib resulting in greater cell death and less tumor cell proliferation in a DLCBL cell line treated with copanlisib (Paul et al. 2017).

The tradeoff of targeting the α isoform is the increased incidence of hyperglycemia, which is related to the physiologic function of PI3Kα in regulating insulin receptor signaling. The onset and degree of hyperglycemia associated with copanlisib is dose- and exposure-dependent (Morschhauser et al. 2020). Blood glucose levels peak five to eight hours after the initial dose of copanlisib and normalize in 24–48 hours, which corresponded to the elimination half-life of copanlisib (39 hours) (Patnaik et al. 2016). Hyperglycemia is the most common adverse event of copanlisib, affecting up to 56% of patients (Dreyling et al. 2017; Matasar et al. 2021). Although most hyperglycemia events are self-limited, and rarely result in permanent discontinuation of therapy, grade 3 or greater hyperglycemia is common (30–40%) and patients with preexisting impaired fasting glucose or diabetes often require short-acting insulin. The second most common side effect of copanlisib is hypertension, observed in 30–40% of patients (Matasar et al. 2021; Patnaik et al. 2016). The leading hypothesis for the mechanism of hypertension is the critical role of PI3Kα in regulating voltage-gated calcium channels in cardiac myocytes and vascular smooth muscle cells (Ghigo et al. 2017). Hypertension also occurs in an exposure-dependent manner, with the peak blood pressure at two hours and normalization of the blood pressure in six to eight hours after the start of copanlisib infusion. The blood pressure elevation is usually mild (mean increase in systolic blood pressure: 16.8 mmHg) and medically manageable.

Unlike PI3K inhibitors given as continuous PO therapy, copanlisib is an intermittently dosed intravenous (IV) drug given its long half-life. The approved dosing of copanlisib is 60 mg IV administered weekly for the first three weeks of a 28-day cycle. It has been hypothesized that this intermittent dosing strategy may contribute to the improved tolerability of this PI3K inhibitor. A single-arm phase 2 study of copanlisib in 142 NHL patients did report favorable safety data notable for lower incidence and severity of diarrhea (any grade, 34%), colitis (any grade, 1%), transaminitis (any grade, 23–28%), and pneumonitis (any grade, 8%) compared to studies using daily dosing of idelalisib or duvelisib (Dreyling et al. 2017). The favorable tolerability of copanlisib enables long-term therapy for more patients. Recently published data from studies testing copanlisib in indolent NHL reported a median duration of response of 14 months with copanlisib monotherapy (Dreyling et al. 2020) and 20 months with copanlisib plus rituximab (Matasar et al. 2021). Subsequent trials testing copanlisib-based combination regimens all use the intermittent dosing strategy (NCT02626455: CHRONOS-4 in indolent NHL, NCT04572763: copanlisib plus venetoclax in DLBCL, NCT04685915: copanlisib plus ibrutinib in CLL). Of note, an intermittent dosing strategy is being explored in clinical trials of duvelisib (NCT04038359, NCT03961672) and investigational PI3K inhibitors zandelisib (NCT04745832) and parsaclisib (NCT03126019, NCT03235544).

Umbralisib (formerly TGR-1202) potently inhibits PI3Kδ (IC_{50} 6.2 nM) and less potently inhibits casein kinase-1ε (CK-1ε, IC_{50} 180 nM). The binding of CK-1ε is explained by the unique structure of umbralisib, which has a central pyrazolopyrimidine amine (CPA) moiety (Figure 6.2d). This CPA moiety is a hinge binder for PI3Kδ and also structurally similar to a CK-1ε inhibitor PF4800567 (Deng et al. 2017). CK-1ε is an indispensable component of the non-canonical Wnt signaling pathway, which regulates hematopoietic cell development (Sugimura et al. 2012) and T helper 1-mediated immune response to inflammatory cues (Sato et al. 2015). Several preclinical data highlighted the benefit of targeting CK-1ε for its anti-tumor activity and potentially more favorable safety profile. In Eμ-TCL1 mice, dual inhibition of CK-1δ/CK-1ε blocked interactions between CLL and the microenvironment and slowed CLL growth (Janovska et al. 2018). In humans, human T-cells were treated *ex vivo* with different PI3K inhibitors with relative preservation of the number and the function of Treg during treatment reported with umbralisib compared to profound suppression of the Treg subset after idelalisib and duvelisib therapy (Maharaj et al. 2020). This study also demonstrated that a selective CK-1ε inhibitor can promote the immune-suppressive capacity of normal Treg and mitigate the deleterious effects of idelalisib and duvelisib on Treg, suggesting CK-1ε inhibition can partially offset immune-mediated toxicity of PI3Kδ inhibition.

Clinical data corroborated this finding by showing relatively low frequencies of high-grade immune-mediated toxicities in NHL. These include a pooled safety analysis of 371 patients receiving umbralisib monotherapy (7.3% grade ≥3 diarrhea, 5.7% grade ≥3 transaminitis) (Davids et al. 2021) and a phase 2 study of 208 indolent NHL patients receiving umbralisib monotherapy (10% grade ≥3 diarrhea, 0.5% grade ≥3 colitis, 6–7% grade ≥3 transaminitis, 1% grade ≥3 pneumonitis) (Fowler et al. 2021). A phase 3 study of umbralisib and ublituximab in CLL further highlighted the favorable safety profile of the combination in treatment-naïve and relapsed cohorts (Gribben et al. 2020). However, the study in CLL did show a similar pattern of autoimmune toxicity as seen with the other agents, albeit less commonly. The incidence of grade 3–4 diarrhea was also numerically higher in the treatment-naïve cohort (13.8%) compared to the relapsed cohort (10%) (Gribben et al. 2020). Safety data of umbralisib should be interpreted with some caution considering the relatively short duration of follow-up and a limited number of treatment-naïve patients included in published studies. Umbralisib currently is being actively investigated for the first-line treatment of NHL (NCT03828448 for FL, NCT04692155 for MCL, NCT03801525 for CLL, NCT04508647 for FL and marginal zone lymphoma).

Umbralisib has several other unique pharmacologic properties that distinguish the drug from other PI3K inhibitors. The drug is minimally metabolized by cytochrome P450 (CYP) isoenzymes, unlike other targeted agents. Co-administration of CYP3A4 inhibitors leads to a non-substantial increase (<25%) in the maximum plasma concentration of umbralisib. Intriguingly, a pharmacogenomic study of 50 patients who were intolerant to idelalisib, ibrutinib, or acalabrutinib revealed an overrepresentation of *CYP3A5* and *CYP2D6* poor metabolizer phenotypes (Mato et al. 2021). The vast majority

(86%) of the patients discontinued prior Bruton's tyrosine kinase (BTK) inhibitor therapy most commonly due to rash, arthralgia, atrial fibrillation, or bleeding. Most of these patients tolerated umbralisib well with only four patients (8%) having a reoccurrence of their previous adverse event (AE) at lower severity (bruising and diarrhea, diarrhea, rash, nausea, and fatigue, in one patient each). The study also included seven patients who discontinued idelalisib due to colitis or pneumonitis; none of the patients re-experienced the toxicities during treatment with umbralisib.

The unique metabolism of umbralisib renders it an excellent adjunct for targeted combinations. A phase 1b/2 study of umbralisib and ibrutinib in 42 patients with relapsed or refractory CLL and MCL reported very low rates of high-grade immune-mediated toxicity (only one case with grade 3 transaminitis, none with grade 3/4 colitis or pneumonitis) (Davids et al. 2021). These data contrast with the 14% incidence of pneumonitis reported from relapsed CLL patients treated with idelalisib and the BTK inhibitor tirabrutinib (Danilov et al. 2020). Several studies are testing umbralisib as part of dual BCR targeting strategies (NCT04624633, NCT04783415), with the BCL2 inhibitor venetoclax (NCT03801525, NCT03379051), or in combination with immunomodulatory therapy (NCT04635683) in NHL. Another notable pharmacokinetic profile of umbralisib is its prolonged half-life of 91 hours and the impact of food and formulation on drug exposure. Pharmacokinetic parameters of umbralisib are sensitive to food and are improved by a micronized formulation. In a phase 1 study of umbralisib, maximum plasma concentration (C_{max}) of umbralisib 800 mg PO daily was 71% higher when given with food versus fasting, and 67% higher with the micronized formulation in a fed state versus non-micronized formulation in a fed state (Burris et al. 2018). In February 2021, the FDA granted accelerated approval to umbralisib (manufactured in the micronized formulation) for the treatment of relapsed marginal zone lymphoma after one prior line of therapy with an anti-CD20 antibody-based regimen, and for relapsed FL after three prior lines of systemic therapy. The US prescribing information specifies umbralisib 800 mg PO once daily should be taken with food.

PI3K Inhibitors in Clinical Development

Parsaclisib (formerly INCB050465) is a highly selective orally bioavailable PI3Kδ inhibitor with a unique biochemical structure (Figure 6.2e). Unlike other PI3K inhibitors with a bicyclic core, parsaclisib has a single phenyl ring with fluoro- and chloro- groups attached to the ring (Yue et al. 2019). The phenyl ring is positioned in the specificity pocket of PI3K. The fluoro- and chloro- groups mimic the second ring of the bicyclic structure and markedly improve the potency of the compound. Although the half-life of parsaclisib is relatively short (8–11 hours), C_{max} of parsaclisib 20 mg once daily is 16-fold higher than the IC_{50} for inhibition of pAKT, leading to sustained plasma concentrations above 50% target inhibition for up to five days after a single dose (Forero-Torres et al. 2019). Based on pharmacokinetic and pharmacodynamic data, phases 1 and 2 studies of parsaclisib adopted a dosing strategy of 20 mg once daily for the first eight weeks of therapy followed by 20 mg once weekly (Coleman et al. 2021; Forero-Torres et al. 2019). The once-weekly dosing was well tolerated; none of 26 patients in the phase 2 study stopped therapy due to treatment-emergent adverse events, as opposed to the 29% treatment discontinuation rate observed during the once-daily schedule (Forero-Torres et al. 2019). The median duration of response was 6.2 months in DLBCL (Coleman et al. 2021) and 13.5 months in indolent NHL (Forero-Torres et al. 2019) with the most durable and highest ORR observed in MCL and FL (Forero-Torres et al. 2019). Parsaclisib is being actively investigated in larger studies in indolent NHL including MCL (NCT04849715, a phase 3) and FL (NCT03126019, a phase 2).

Zandelisib (formerly PWT143 and ME-401) is a potent PI3Kδ inhibitor which binds PI3Kδ 37-fold tighter, and remains on target 138-fold longer, than idelalisib, *in vitro* (Moreno and Wood 2019). *In vivo*, oral administration of zandelisib achieved a higher volume of distribution and superior tissue penetration compared to idelalisib (Moreno and Wood 2019). Zandelisib gradually reaches C_{max} in five hours and has a prolonged half-life of 26 hours (Moreno et al. 2018). Similar to other later generation PI3K inhibitors, clinical trials adopted intermittent dosing of zandelisib. For instance, a phase 1b study in FL initiated zandelisib at 60 mg daily for two 28-day cycles followed by seven days of therapy every 28-day cycle (Zelenetz et al. 2020). High-grade immune-related adverse events were uncommon during intermittent dosing (3.5% diarrhea, 3.5% colitis, 2% or one patient each with rash, pneumonitis, and transaminitis) (Zelenetz et al. 2020). Such optimization of pharmacologic properties and dosing of PI3K inhibition translated to improved long-term tolerability and clinical activity of zandelisib. A study in FL reported an ORR of 82% and a promising median duration of response exceeding 17 months in high-risk patients who progressed within 24 months of initial chemoimmunotherapy (Pagel et al. 2021). In March 2020, the US FDA granted zandelisib Fast Track designation for the treatment of relapsed or refractory FL. An international phase 2 study in FL and MCL is ongoing with the goal of obtaining accelerated approval of zandelisib in NHL (NCT03768505). A randomized phase 3 study testing the combination of conventional chemoimmunotherapy and zandelisib in indolent NHL is also ongoing (NCT04745832).

AKT Inhibitors

AKT kinase, also known as protein kinase B, is immediately downstream of PI3K. Constitutive activation of AKT is frequently found in NHL (Wang et al. 2017) and can drive the aggressive histologic transformation of B cells *in vivo* (Kohlhaas et al. 2021). Activation of PI3K leads to AKT phosphorylation at threonine 308 (T308) and serine 473 (S473) residues, a process mediated by phosphoinositide-dependent protein kinase 1 (Stephens et al. 1998) and mTOR complex (mTORC), respectively (Sarbassov et al. 2005). Phosphorylation of both T308 and S473 residues is necessary for AKT activation and downstream signaling (Alessi et al. 1996). Molecular breaks for the growth-promoting activity of AKT are the negative feedback loops centered around mTORC, which will be discussed further in this section.

Pharmacologic inhibition of AKT can be achieved by ATP-competitive or allosteric inhibitors (Table 6.2). Many AKT inhibitors have been tested in clinical trials, but none has received regulatory approval (reviewed in detail by Song et al. 2019). Of the allosteric inhibitors, **MK-2206** is a pan-AKT inhibitor with activity against AKT1 (IC_{50} 5nM) and AKT2 (IC_{50} 12nM) and less potent activity against AKT3 (IC_{50} 65nM). The drug has a long elimination half-life (40–100 hours) and is given every other day (Yap et al. 2011). Pharmacodynamic studies of MK-2206 demonstrated reduction of pAKT S473 and T308 in human DLBCL cell lines (Wang et al. 2017) and in primary samples from solid tumor patients (Yap et al. 2011). However, the clinical activity of this drug was modest, with ORRs of 14% in relapsed lymphoma (Oki et al. 2015), 0% in breast cancer (Xing et al. 2019), and 0–15% in solid tumors of various histology (Doi et al. 2015; Mehnert et al. 2019). In CLL, the ORR was 92% in patients treated with MK-2206 plus bendamustine and rituximab (Larsen et al. 2017). The higher response rate in the CLL study was attributable to the chemoimmunotherapy component of the regimen. Duration of response to the combination was relatively short (median progression-free survival [PFS] 16 months). Clinical development of other allosteric AKT inhibitors has been unsuccessful due to lack of efficacy. Only 1 out of 78 solid tumor patients responded to the allosteric AKT inhibitor **BAY1125976** in a phase 1 study (Schneeweiss et al. 2019). **Perifosine** showed single-agent activity in a phase 1 study for multiple myeloma (Jakubowiak et al. 2012) but failed to improve PFS in a subsequent randomized phase 3 study (Richardson et al. 2013).

Several ATP-competitive AKT inhibitors have been tested in clinical and preclinical settings. **GSK690693** was withdrawn from clinical development due to severe hyperglycemia observed in rodents (NCT00493818) (Rhodes et al. 2008). **Uprosertib** (formerly GSK2141795) and **afuresertib** (formerly GSK2110183) are more potent, orally bioavailable, pan-AKT inhibitors that moved into clinical trials (Dumble et al. 2014). Although hyperglycemia was less severe and less frequent, the later generation of AKT inhibitors showed only minor activity in acute myeloid leukemia (AML) (Ragon et al. 2019) and CLL (NCT01532700, unpublished, data available in ClinicalTrials.gov). Additional dose-limiting toxicities such as diarrhea and hepatotoxicity emerged during single-agent (Aghajanian et al. 2018; Spencer et al. 2014) and combination therapy (Algazi et al. 2018; Blagden et al. 2019). These toxicities are most likely related to off-target activity of ATP-competitive AKT inhibitors (Dumble et al. 2014).

The prevailing hypothesis for the lack of efficacy with AKT inhibition is negative feedback loops within the PI3K-AKT-mTOR pathway (Figure 6.1). AKT inhibition upregulates TSC1/2, which promotes mTORC2 activity (Dalle Pezze et al. 2012). Additionally, ribosomal protein S6 kinase beta-1 downstream of the AKT-mTORC1 axis can recruit insulin receptor substrate-1, which promotes upstream signaling activity

Table 6.2 Pharmacologic properties of AKT inhibitors.

	MK-2206	Perifosine	Uprosertib (GSK2141795)	Afuresertib (GSK2110183)
Binding mechanism	Allosteric AKT inhibitor	Allosteric AKT inhibitor	ATP-competitive AKT inhibitor	ATP-competitive AKT inhibitor
Dominant targets	Pan-AKT inhibitor	Pan-AKT inhibitor	Pan-AKT inhibitor	Pan-AKT inhibitor
Recommended phase 2 dose	60 mg PO on alternate days	150 mg PO day	75 mg PO daily	125 mg PO daily
$T_{1/2}$ (hours)	40–100	81–116	63–85	40.8
T_{max} (hours)	4–6	8–24	3–8	1.5–2.5
Comment	DLT: rash	Inhibits telomerase activity at nanomolar doses	Reversible binding, DLT: hyperglycemia	Reversible binding, DLT: liver function abnormalities
References	(Yap et al. 2011)	(Richardson et al. 2013)	(Dumble et al. 2014; Aghajanian et al. 2018)	(Dumble et al. 2014; Spencer et al. 2014)

Abbreviations: DLT = dose-limiting toxicity; NR = not reported; $T_{1/2}$ = mean elimination half-life; T_{max} = median time to reach peak plasma concentration

(Harrington et al. 2004). In support of this hypothesis, treatment with MK-2206 has been shown to induce compensatory activation of mTORC2 in DLBCL cell lines (Wang et al. 2017) and paradoxical upregulation of cytokines in lymphoma patients (Oki et al. 2015).

mTOR Inhibitors

mTOR is a highly conserved serine-threonine kinase that exists in mutually exclusive complexes: mTORC1 and mTORC2. Commercially available rapamycin analogs inhibit mTORC1 only, allowing mTORC2-mediated upregulation of the signaling activity (Figure 6.1).

Sirolimus is a naturally occurring, orally bioavailable macrolide most commonly used for immunosuppression after solid organ transplant or allogeneic hematopoietic stem cell transplant (HSCT). A retrospective study of lymphoma patients undergoing reduced intensity conditioning HSCT demonstrated improved overall survival when sirolimus was given as part of graft-versus-host disease (GVHD) prophylaxis, suggesting the anti-neoplastic potential of mTORC1 inhibition (Armand et al. 2008). Nevertheless, a subsequent randomized study showed no difference in survival nor reduction of lymphoma relapse between two arms receiving GVHD prophylaxis regimens with or without sirolimus (Armand et al. 2016). Both of these studies were mixed with various histologies including indolent and aggressive NHL limiting the interpretation of the study. Other studies suggested mTOR inhibition to be more effective for the treatment of indolent lymphoma, particularly MCL (Smith et al. 2010). **Temsirolimus** is an IV prodrug of sirolimus that is approved for the treatment of relapsed/refractory MCL in Europe as monotherapy or in combination with rituximab (Ansell et al. 2011; Hess et al. 2009; Witzig et al. 2005). A single 25 mg IV dose of temsirolimus leads to prolonged exposure to sirolimus (half-life 73 hours). Temsirolimus is given 175 mg IV once weekly for the first three weeks followed by 75 mg IV once weekly in MCL. This regimen is based on a three-arm randomized study in MCL, which demonstrated superior PFS associated with the 75 mg once-weekly maintenance dose, but not with the 25 mg once-weekly maintenance dose, compared to investigator's choice of therapy (Hess et al. 2009). Despite the statistically significant improvement in PFS in this randomized study, the clinical benefit of temsirolimus was modest (22% ORR, median PFS five months). The role of temsirolimus is limited in current practice given its IV delivery and toxicities. BTK inhibitors are preferred in MCL given their superior efficacy and more favorable safety profile compared to temsirolimus (Dreyling et al. 2016; Tam et al. 2021; Wang et al. 2018). **Everolimus** is an mTORC1 inhibitor dosed at 10 mg PO once daily for the treatment of breast cancer, renal cell carcinoma, and neuroendocrine tumors. Its mean elimination half-life is 30 hours. Single-agent activity of everolimus in lymphoma is limited with only 8.6% ORR and the median PFS of four months as shown in a phase 2 study in MCL (Wang et al. 2014). Side effect profiles of everolimus are similar to other rapamycin analogs. Another phase 2 study in MCL closed prematurely due to toxicity and reduced quality of life during therapy despite the use of a lower dose of everolimus (5 mg PO daily) (Schreiber et al. 2015).

Key toxicities of commercially available mTOR inhibitors include hyperglycemia, hyperlipidemia, cytopenia, and pulmonary toxicity. Hematologic toxicities are common with up to 80% of patients on temsirolimus or everolimus developing thrombocytopenia (Ansell et al. 2011; Hess et al. 2009; Witzig et al. 2005). Hyperlipidemia occurs in 50–56% and a small fraction (2–6%) of patients develops grade 3 or higher events. Pulmonary toxicity, which presents as pneumonitis or ILD, is less common but can be fatal. A large meta-analysis of 2233 solid tumor patients on various mTOR inhibitors reported 10% overall incidence of any grade pulmonary toxicity including 2% with grade 3 or higher events (Iacovelli et al. 2012).

Conclusions

Pharmacologic targeting of the PI3K-AKT-mTOR signaling pathway in lymphoma has been most successful with inhibition of the proximal components of the pathway through PI3K inhibitors. AKT and mTOR inhibition are associated with increased toxicity and limited efficacy due to negative feedback mechanisms that reconstitute upstream signaling. Four PI3K inhibitors are commercially available for the treatment of lymphoma: idelalisib (PI3Kδ inhibitor), duvelisib (dual PI3Kδ/γ inhibitor), copanlisib (potent PI3Kα/δ inhibitor), and umbralisib (PI3Kδ and CK-1ε inhibitor). Isoform selectivity and pharmacologic properties of the PI3K inhibitors contribute to the clinical activity and safety of individual agents. Ongoing investigations aim to improve the efficacy and long-term tolerability of PI3K inhibition through optimization of intermittent dosing strategies and development of novel agents.

Must Read References

Saxton, R.A., Sabatini, D. (2017). mTOR signaling in growth, metabolism, and disease. *Cell* 168 (6): 960–976.

A review on the mTOR signaling network and putative mechanisms of resistance to mTOR inhibition in cancer.

Song, M., Bode, A.M., Dong, Z. et al. (2019). AKT as a therapeutic target for cancer. *Cancer Res.* 79 (6): 1019–1031.

A comprehensive review of AKT inhibitors tested in animal models and clinical trials of various cancer types.

Vanhaesebroeck, B., Perry M.W.D., Brown, J.R. et al. (2021). PI3K inhibitors are finally coming of age. *Nat. Rev. Drug Discov.* 20 (10): 741–769.

A review of PI3K inhibitors that are clinically approved or in various stages of development. The article also outlines biological differences of the PI3K signaling pathway in solid tumors and lymphoma.

References

Abubaker, J., Bavi, P.P., Al-Harbi, S. et al. (2007). PIK3CA mutations are mutually exclusive with PTEN loss in diffuse large B-cell lymphoma. *Leukemia* 21 (11): 2368–2370. doi: 10.1038/sj.leu.2404873.

Aghajanian, C., Bell-mcguinn, K.M., Burris, H.A., 3rd. et al. (2018). A phase I, open-label, two-stage study to investigate the safety, tolerability, pharmacokinetics, and pharmacodynamics of the oral AKT inhibitor GSK2141795 in patients with solid tumors. *Invest. N. Drugs* 36 (6): 1016–1025. doi: 10.1007/s10637-018-0591-z.

Ahn, I.E. and Brown, J.R. (2021). Targeting Bruton's Tyrosine Kinase in CLL. *Front Immunol.* 12: 687458. doi: 10.3389/fimmu.2021.687458.

Alessi, D.R., Andjelkovic, M., Caudwell, B. et al. (1996). Mechanism of activation of protein kinase B by insulin and IGF-1. *EMBO J.* 15 (23): 6541–6551. https://www.ncbi.nlm.nih.gov/pubmed/8978681.

Algazi, A.P., Esteve-Puig, R., Nosrati, A. et al. (2018). Dual MEK/AKT inhibition with trametinib and GSK2141795 does not yield clinical benefit in metastatic NRAS-mutant and wild-type melanoma. *Pigment Cell Melanoma Res.* 31 (1): 110–114. doi: 10.1111/pcmr.12644.

Ali, K., Soond, D.R., Pineiro, R. et al. (2014). Inactivation of PI(3)K p110delta breaks regulatory T-cell-mediated immune tolerance to cancer. *Nature* 510 (7505): 407–411. doi: 10.1038/nature13444.

Ansell, S.M., Tang, H., Kurtin, P.J. et al. (2011). Temsirolimus and rituximab in patients with relapsed or refractory mantle cell lymphoma: a phase 2 study. *Lancet Oncol.* 12 (4): 361–368. doi: 10.1016/S1470-2045(11)70062-6.

Armand, P., Gannamaneni, S., Kim, H.T. et al. (2008). Improved survival in lymphoma patients receiving sirolimus for graft-versus-host disease prophylaxis after allogeneic hematopoietic stem-cell transplantation with reduced-intensity conditioning. *J. Clin. Oncol.: Off. J. Am. Soc. Clin. Oncol.* 26 (35): 5767–5774. doi: 10.1200/JCO.2008.17.7279.

Armand, P., Kim, H.T., Sainvil, M.M. et al. (2016). The addition of sirolimus to the graft-versus-host disease prophylaxis regimen in reduced intensity allogeneic stem cell transplantation for lymphoma: a multicentre randomized trial. *Br. J. Haematol.* 173 (1): 96–104. doi: 10.1111/bjh.13931.

Barr, P.M., Saylors, G.B., Spurgeon, S.E. et al. (2016). Phase 2 study of idelalisib and entospletinib: pneumonitis limits combination therapy in relapsed refractory CLL and NHL. *Blood* 127 (20): 2411–2415. doi: 10.1182/blood-2015-12-683516.

Blagden, S.P., Hamilton, A.L., Mileshkin, L. et al. (2019). Phase IB dose escalation and expansion study of AKT inhibitor afuresertib with carboplatin and paclitaxel in recurrent platinum-resistant ovarian cancer. *Clin. Cancer Res.* 25 (5): 1472–1478. doi: 10.1158/1078-0432.CCR-18-2277.

Brown, J.R., Byrd, J.C., Coutre, S.E. et al. (2014). Idelalisib, an inhibitor of phosphatidylinositol 3-kinase p110delta, for relapsed/refractory chronic lymphocytic leukemia. *Blood* 123 (22): 3390–3397. doi: 10.1182/blood-2013-11-535047.

Brown, J.R., Zelenetz, A., Furman, R. et al. (2020). Risk factors for grade 3/4 transaminase elevation in patients with chronic lymphocytic leukemia treated with idelalisib. *Leukemia* 34 (12): 3404–3407. doi: 10.1038/s41375-020-0974-y.

Burris, H.A., 3rd, Flinn, I.W., Patel, M.R. et al. (2018). Umbralisib, a novel PI3Kdelta and casein kinase-1epsilon inhibitor, in relapsed or refractory chronic lymphocytic leukaemia and lymphoma: an open-label, phase 1, dose-escalation, first-in-human study. *Lancet Oncol.* 19 (4): 486–496. doi: 10.1016/S1470-2045(18)30082-2.

Carpten, J.D., Faber, A.L., Horn, C. et al. (2007). A transforming mutation in the pleckstrin homology domain of AKT1 in cancer. *Nature* 448 (7152): 439–444. doi: 10.1038/nature05933.

Chapuy, B., Stewart, C., Dunford, A.J. et al. (2018). Molecular subtypes of diffuse large B cell lymphoma are associated with distinct pathogenic mechanisms and outcomes. *Nat. Med.* 24 (5): 679–690. doi: 10.1038/s41591-018-0016-8.

Chellappa, S., Kushekhar, K., Munthe, L.A. et al. (2019). The PI3K p110delta isoform inhibitor idelalisib preferentially inhibits human regulatory T cell function. *J. Immunol.* 202 (5): 1397–1405. doi: 10.4049/jimmunol.1701703.

Coleman, M., Belada, D., Casasnovas, R.O. et al. (2021). Phase 2 study of parsaclisib (INCB050465), a highly selective, next-generation PI3Kdelta inhibitor, in relapsed or refractory diffuse large B-cell lymphoma (CITADEL-202). *Leuk. Lymphoma* 62 (2): 368–376. doi: 10.1080/10428194.2020.1832660.

Dal Bo, M., Bomben, R., Hernandez, L. et al. (2015). The MYC/miR-17-92 axis in lymphoproliferative disorders: a common pathway with therapeutic potential. *Oncotarget* 6 (23): 19381–19392. doi: 10.18632/oncotarget.4574.

Dalle Pezze, P., Sonntag, A.G., Thien, A. et al. (2012). A dynamic network model of mTOR signaling reveals TSC-independent mTORC2 regulation. *Sci. Signal.* 5 (217): ra25. doi: 10.1126/scisignal.2002469.

Danilov, A.V., Herbaux, C., Walter, H.S. et al. (2020). Phase Ib study of tirabrutinib in combination with idelalisib or entospletinib in previously treated chronic lymphocytic leukemia. *Clin. Cancer Res.* 26 (12): 2810–2818. doi: 10.1158/1078-0432.CCR-19-3504.

Davids, M.S., Deng, J., Wiestner, A. et al. (2012). Decreased mitochondrial apoptotic priming underlies stroma-mediated treatment resistance in chronic lymphocytic leukemia. *Blood* 120 (17): 3501–3509. doi: 10.1182/blood-2012-02-414060.

Davids, M.S., Fisher, D.C., Tyekucheva, S. et al. (2021). A phase 1b/2 study of duvelisib in combination with FCR (DFCR) for frontline therapy for younger CLL patients. *Leukemia* 35 (4): 1064–1072. doi: 10.1038/s41375-020-01010-6.

Davids, M.S., O'Connor, O.A., Jurczak, W. et al. (2021). Integrated safety analysis of umbralisib, a dual PI3Kdelta/CK1epsilon inhibitor, in relapsed/refractory lymphoid malignancies. *Blood Adv.* doi: 10.1182/bloodadvances.2021005132.

Davis, R.J., Moore, E.C., Clavijo, P.E. et al. (2017). Anti-PD-L1 efficacy can be enhanced by inhibition of myeloid-derived suppressor cells with a selective inhibitor of PI3Kdelta/gamma. *Cancer Res.* 77 (10): 2607–2619. doi: 10.1158/0008-5472.CAN-16-2534.

Deng, C., Lipstein, M.R., Scotto, L. et al. (2017). Silencing c-Myc translation as a therapeutic strategy through targeting PI3Kdelta and CK1epsilon in hematological malignancies. *Blood* 129 (1): 88–99. doi: 10.1182/blood-2016-08-731240.

Doi, T., Tamura, K., Tanabe, Y. et al. (2015). Phase 1 pharmacokinetic study of the oral pan-AKT inhibitor MK-2206 in Japanese patients with advanced solid tumors. *Cancer Chemother. Pharmacol.* 76 (2): 409–416. doi: 10.1007/s00280-015-2810-z.

Dong, S., Harrington, B.K., Hu, E.Y. et al. (2019). PI3K p110delta inactivation antagonizes chronic lymphocytic leukemia and reverses T cell immune suppression. *J. Clin. Invest.* 129 (1): 122–136. doi: 10.1172/JCI99386.

Dreyling, M., Jurczak, W., Jerkeman, M. et al. (2016). Ibrutinib versus temsirolimus in patients with relapsed or refractory mantle-cell lymphoma: an international, randomised, open-label, phase 3 study. *Lancet* 387 (10020): 770–778. doi: 10.1016/S0140-6736(15)00667-4.

Dreyling, M., Santoro, A., Mollica, L. et al. (2017). Phosphatidylinositol 3-kinase inhibition by copanlisib in relapsed or refractory indolent lymphoma. *J. Clin. Oncol.: Off. J. Ame. Soc. Clin. Oncol.* 35 (35): 3898–3905. doi: 10.1200/JCO.2017.75.4648.

Dreyling, M., Santoro, A., Mollica, L. et al. (2020). Long-term safety and efficacy of the PI3K inhibitor copanlisib in patients with relapsed or refractory indolent lymphoma: 2-year follow-up of the CHRONOS-1 study. *Am. J. Hematol.* 95 (4): 362–371. doi: 10.1002/ajh.25711.

Dumble, M., Crouthamel, M.C., Zhang, S.Y. et al. (2014). Discovery of novel AKT inhibitors with enhanced anti-tumor effects in combination with the MEK inhibitor. *Plos One* 9 (6): e100880. doi: 10.1371/journal.pone.0100880.

Evans, C.A., Liu, T., Lescarbeau, A. et al. (2016). Discovery of a selective phosphoinositide-3-Kinase (PI3K)-gamma inhibitor (IPI-549) as an immuno-oncology clinical candidate. *ACS Med. Chem. Lett.* 7 (9): 862–867. doi: 10.1021/acsmedchemlett.6b00238.

Flinn, I.W., Cherry, M.A., Maris, M.B. et al. (2019). Combination trial of duvelisib (IPI-145) with rituximab or bendamustine/rituximab in patients with non-Hodgkin lymphoma or chronic lymphocytic leukemia. *Am. J. Hematol.* 94 (12): 1325–1334. doi: 10.1002/ajh.25634.

Flinn, I.W., Hillmen, P., Montillo, M. et al. (2018). The phase 3 DUO trial: duvelisib vs ofatumumab in relapsed and refractory CLL/SLL. *Blood* 132 (23): 2446–2455. doi: 10.1182/blood-2018-05-850461.

Flinn, I.W., Miller, C.B., Ardeshna, K.M. et al. (2019). DYNAMO: a phase II study of duvelisib (IPI-145) in patients with refractory indolent non-Hodgkin lymphoma. *J. Clin. Oncol.: Off. J. Am. Soc. Clin. Oncol.* 37 (11): 912–922. doi: 10.1200/JCO.18.00915.

Flinn, I.W., O'Brien, S., Kahl, B. et al. (2018a). Duvelisib, a novel oral dual inhibitor of PI3K-delta,gamma, is clinically active in advanced hematologic malignancies. *Blood* 131 (8): 877–887. doi: 10.1182/blood-2017-05-786566.

Flinn, I.W., Patel, M., Oki, Y. et al. (2018b). Duvelisib, an oral dual PI3K-delta, gamma inhibitor, shows clinical activity in indolent non-Hodgkin lymphoma in a phase 1 study. *Am. J. Hematol.* 93 (11): 1311–1317. doi: 10.1002/ajh.25228.

Forero-Torres, A., Ramchandren, R., Yacoub, A. et al. (2019). Parsaclisib, a potent and highly selective PI3Kdelta inhibitor, in patients with relapsed or refractory B-cell malignancies. *Blood* 133 (16): 1742–1752. doi: 10.1182/blood-2018-08-867499.

Fowler, N.H., Samaniego, F., Jurczak, W. et al. (2021). Umbralisib, a dual PI3Kdelta/CK1epsilon inhibitor in patients with relapsed or refractory indolent lymphoma. *J. Clin. Oncol.: Off. J. Am. Soc. Clin. Oncol.* 39 (15): 1609–1618. doi: 10.1200/JCO.20.03433.

Furman, R.R., Sharman, J.P., Coutre, S.E. et al. (2014). Idelalisib and rituximab in relapsed chronic lymphocytic leukemia. *N. Engl. J. Med.* 370 (11): 997–1007. doi: 10.1056/NEJMoa1315226.

Garcia, A., Kim, S., Bhavaraju, K. et al. (2010). Role of phosphoinositide 3-kinase beta in platelet aggregation and thromboxane A2 generation mediated by Gi signalling pathways. *Biochem. J.* 429 (2): 369–377. doi: 10.1042/BJ20100166.

Ghigo, A., Laffargue, M., Li, M. et al. (2017). PI3K and calcium signaling in cardiovascular disease. *Circ. Res.* 121 (3): 282–292. doi: 10.1161/CIRCRESAHA.117.310183.

Grabiner, B.C., Nardi, V., Birsoy, K. et al. (2014). A diverse array of cancer-associated MTOR mutations are hyperactivating and can predict rapamycin sensitivity. *Cancer Discov.* 4 (5): 554–563. doi: 10.1158/2159-8290.CD-13-0929.

Gribben, J.G., Jurczak, W., Jacobs, R.W. et al. (2020). Umbralisib plus ublituximab (U2) is superior to obinutuzumab plus chlorambucil (O+Chl) in patients with treatment naïve (TN) and relapsed/refractory (R/R) chronic lymphocytic leukemia (CLL): results from the phase 3 unity-CLL study. *Blood* 136: 37–39. (Conference Abstract) (In English). doi: 10.1182/blood-2020-134783.

Hanna, B.S., Roessner, P.M., Scheffold, A. et al. (2019). PI3Kdelta inhibition modulates regulatory and effector T-cell differentiation and function in chronic lymphocytic leukemia. *Leukemia* 33 (6): 1427–1438. doi: 10.1038/s41375-018-0318-3.

Harrington, L.S., Findlay, G.M., Gray, A. et al. (2004). The TSC1-2 tumor suppressor controls insulin-PI3K signaling via regulation of IRS proteins. *J. Cell Biol.* 166 (2): 213–223. doi: 10.1083/jcb.200403069.

Herman, S.E., Gordon, A.L., Wagner, A.J. et al. (2010). Phosphatidylinositol 3-kinase-delta inhibitor CAL-101 shows promising preclinical activity in chronic lymphocytic leukemia by antagonizing intrinsic and extrinsic cellular survival signals. *Blood* 116 (12): 2078–2088. doi: 10.1182/blood-2010-02-271171.

Hess, G., Herbrecht, R., Romaguera, J. et al. (2009). Phase III study to evaluate temsirolimus compared with investigator's choice therapy for the treatment of relapsed or refractory mantle cell lymphoma. *J. Clin. Oncol.: Off. J. Am. Soc. Clin. Oncol.* 27 (23): 3822–3829. doi: 10.1200/JCO.2008.20.7977.

Hess, G., Smith, S.M., Berkenblit, A. et al. (2009). Temsirolimus in mantle cell lymphoma and other non-Hodgkin lymphoma subtypes. *Semin. Oncol.* 36 (Suppl 3): S37–45. doi: 10.1053/j.seminoncol.2009.10.012.

Hillmen, P., Badoux, X., Delgado, J. et al. (2017). Safety results of terminated phase 2 study of idelalisib plus rituximab in treatment naive chronic lymphocytic leukemia (CLL) with del(17P). *Haematologica* 102: 172. (Conference Abstract) (In English). https://www.embase.com/search/results?subaction=viewrecord&id=L617379052&from=export.

Hirsch, E., Katanaev, V.L., Garlanda, C. et al. (2000). Central role for G protein-coupled phosphoinositide 3-kinase gamma in inflammation. *Science* 287 (5455): 1049–1053. doi: 10.1126/science.287.5455.1049.

Hoellenriegel, J., Meadows, S.A., Sivina, M. et al. (2011). The phosphoinositide 3′-kinase delta inhibitor, CAL-101, inhibits B-cell receptor signaling and chemokine networks in chronic lymphocytic leukemia. *Blood* 118 (13): 3603–3612. doi: 10.1182/blood-2011-05-352492.

Hopkins, B.D., Pauli, C., Du, X. et al. (2018). Suppression of insulin feedback enhances the efficacy of PI3K inhibitors. *Nature* 560 (7719): 499–503. doi: 10.1038/s41586-018-0343-4.

Horwitz, S.M., Koch, R., Porcu, P. et al. (2018). Activity of the PI3K-delta,gamma inhibitor duvelisib in a phase 1 trial and preclinical models of T-cell lymphoma. *Blood* 131 (8): 888–898. doi: 10.1182/blood-2017-08-802470.

Horwitz, S.M., Mehta-Shah, N., Pro, B. et al. (2019). Dose optimization of duvelisib in patients with relapsed or refractory peripheral T-cell lymphoma from the phase 2 primo trial: selection of regimen for the dose-expansion phase. *Blood* 134 (Supplement_1): 1567-1567. doi: 10.1182/blood-2019-121401.

Iacovelli, R., Palazzo, A., Mezi, S. et al. (2012). Incidence and risk of pulmonary toxicity in patients treated with mTOR inhibitors for malignancy. a meta-analysis of published trials. *Acta. Oncol.* 51 (7): 873–879. doi: 10.3109/0284186X.2012.705019.

Inoki, K., Corradetti, M.N., and Guan, K.L. (2005). Dysregulation of the TSC-mTOR pathway in human disease. *Nat. Genet.* 37 (1): 19–24. doi: 10.1038/ng1494.

Jakubowiak, A.J., Richardson, P.G., Zimmerman, T. et al. (2012). Perifosine plus lenalidomide and dexamethasone in relapsed and relapsed/refractory multiple myeloma: a phase I multiple myeloma research consortium study. *Br. J. Haematol.* 158 (4): 472–480. doi: 10.1111/j.1365-2141.2012.09173.x.

Janovska, P., Verner, J., Kohoutek, J. et al. (2018). Casein kinase 1 is a therapeutic target in chronic lymphocytic leukemia. *Blood* 131 (11): 1206–1218. doi: 10.1182/blood-2017-05-786947.

Jones, J.A., Robak, T., Brown, J.R. et al. (2017). Efficacy and safety of idelalisib in combination with ofatumumab for previously treated chronic lymphocytic leukaemia: an open-label, randomised phase 3 trial. *Lancet Haematol.* 4 (3): e114–e126. doi: 10.1016/S2352-3026(17)30019-4.

Kaneda, M.M., Messer, K.S., Ralainirina, N. et al. (2016). PI3Kgamma is a molecular switch that controls immune suppression. *Nature* 539 (7629): 437–442. doi: 10.1038/nature19834.

Knight, Z.A., Gonzalez, B., Feldman, M.E. et al. (2006). A pharmacological map of the PI3-K family defines a role for p110alpha in insulin signaling. *Cell* 125 (4): 733–747. doi: 10.1016/j.cell.2006.03.035.

Kohlhaas, V., Blakemore, S.J., Al-Maarri, M. et al. (2021). Active Akt signaling triggers CLL toward Richter transformation via overactivation of Notch1. *Blood* 137 (5): 646–660. doi: 10.1182/blood.2020005734.

Lampson, B.L. and Brown, J.R. (2021). The evolving use of phosphatidylinositol 3-kinase inhibitors for the treatment of chronic lymphocytic leukemia. *Hematol. Oncol. Clin. North Am.* 35 (4): 807–826. doi: 10.1016/j.hoc.2021.03.009.

Lampson, B.L., Kasar, S.N., Matos, T.R. et al. (2016). Idelalisib given front-line for treatment of chronic lymphocytic leukemia causes frequent immune-mediated hepatotoxicity. *Blood* 128 (2): 195–203. doi: 10.1182/blood-2016-03-707133.

Lampson, B.L., Kim, H.T., Davids, M.S. et al. (2019). Efficacy results of a phase 2 trial of first-line idelalisib plus ofatumumab in chronic lymphocytic leukemia. *Blood Adv.* 3 (7): 1167–1174. doi: 10.1182/bloodadvances.2018030221.

Larsen, J.T., Shanafelt, T.D., Leis, J.F. et al. (2017). Akt inhibitor MK-2206 in combination with bendamustine and rituximab in relapsed or refractory chronic lymphocytic leukemia: results from the N1087 alliance study. *Am. J. Hematol.* 92 (8): 759–763. doi: 10.1002/ajh.24762.

Lawrence, M.S., Stojanov, P., Mermel, C.H. et al. (2014). Discovery and saturation analysis of cancer genes across 21 tumour types. *Nature* 505 (7484): 495–501. doi: 10.1038/nature12912.

Liu, N., Rowley, B.R., Bull, C.O. et al. (2013). BAY 80-6946 is a highly selective intravenous PI3K inhibitor with potent p110alpha and p110delta activities in tumor cell lines and xenograft models. *Mol. Cancer Ther.* 12 (11): 2319–2330. doi: 10.1158/1535-7163.MCT-12-0993-T.

Louie, C.Y., DiMaio, M.A., Matsukuma, K.E. et al. (2015). Idelalisib-associated enterocolitis: clinicopathologic features and distinction from other enterocolitides. *Am. J. Surg. Pathol.* 39 (12): 1653–1660. doi: 10.1097/PAS.0000000000000525.

Maharaj, K., Powers, J.J., Achille, A. et al. (2020). The dual PI3Kdelta/CK1epsilon inhibitor umbralisib exhibits unique immunomodulatory effects on CLL T cells. *Blood Adv.* 4 (13): 3072–3084. doi: 10.1182/bloodadvances.2020001800.

Matasar, M.J., Capra, M., Ozcan, M. et al. (2021). Copanlisib plus rituximab versus placebo plus rituximab in patients with relapsed indolent non-Hodgkin lymphoma (CHRONOS-3): a double-blind, randomised, placebo-controlled, phase 3 trial. *Lancet Oncol.* 22 (5): 678–689. doi: 10.1016/S1470-2045(21)00145-5.

Mato, A.R., Ghosh, N., Schuster, S.J. et al. (2021). Phase 2 study of the safety and efficacy of umbralisib in patients with CLL who are intolerant to BTK or PI3Kdelta inhibitor therapy. *Blood* 137 (20): 2817–2826. doi: 10.1182/blood.2020007376.

Mehnert, J.M., Kaveney, A.D., Malhotra, J. et al. (2019). A phase I trial of MK-2206 and hydroxychloroquine in patients with advanced solid tumors. *Cancer Chemother. Pharmacol.* 84 (4): 899–907. doi: 10.1007/s00280-019-03919-x.

Moreno, O., Butler, T., Zann, V. et al. (2018). Safety, pharmacokinetics, and pharmacodynamics of ME-401, an oral, potent, and selective inhibitor of phosphatidylinositol 3-kinase P110delta, following single ascending dose administration to healthy volunteers. *Clin. Ther.* 40 (11): 1855–1867. doi: 10.1016/j.clinthera.2018.09.006.

Moreno, O. and Wood, J. (2019). Absorption, distribution, and binding profile of ME-401, a potent and selective oral small-molecule inhibitor of phosphatidylinositol 3-kinase delta (PI3Kdelta) in Animal and B-cell lymphoma models. *Target Oncol.* 14 (5): 603–611. doi: 10.1007/s11523-019-00668-y.

Morschhauser, F., Machiels, J.P., Salles, G. et al. (2020). On-target pharmacodynamic activity of the PI3K inhibitor copanlisib in paired biopsies from patients with malignant lymphoma and advanced solid tumors. *Mol. Cancer Ther.* 19 (2): 468–478. doi: 10.1158/1535-7163.MCT-19-0466.

O'Brien, S., Patel, M., Kahl, B.S. et al. (2018). Duvelisib, an oral dual PI3K-delta,gamma inhibitor, shows clinical and pharmacodynamic activity in chronic lymphocytic leukemia and small lymphocytic lymphoma in a phase 1 study. *Am. J. Hematol.* 93 (11): 1318–1326. doi: 10.1002/ajh.25243.

O'Brien, S.M., Lamanna, N., Kipps, T.J. et al. (2015). A phase 2 study of idelalisib plus rituximab in treatment-naive older patients with chronic lymphocytic leukemia. *Blood* 126 (25): 2686–2694. doi: 10.1182/blood-2015-03-630947.

O'Farrell, M., Ventura, R., Tai, A. et al. (2012). Preclinical characterization of PWT143, a novel selective and potent phosphatidylinositol 3-kinase delta (PI3K delta) inhibitor with ex-vivo activity in hematologic malignancies. *Blood* 120 (21). (Conference Abstract) (In English) (https://www.embase.com/search/results?subaction=viewrecord&id=L70962151&from=export) http://abstracts.hematologylibrary.org/cgi/content/abstract/120/21/2907?maxtoshow=&hits=80&RESULTFORMAT=&searchid=1&FIRSTINDEX=240&displaysectionid=Poster+Session&fdate=1/1/2012&tdate=12/31/2012&resourcetype=HWCIT.

Oki, Y., Fanale, M., Romaguera, J. et al. (2015). Phase II study of an AKT inhibitor MK2206 in patients with relapsed or refractory lymphoma. *Br. J. Haematol.* 171 (4): 463–470. doi: 10.1111/bjh.13603.

Okkenhaug, K., Bilancio, A., Farjot, G. et al. (2002). Impaired B and T cell antigen receptor signaling in p110delta PI 3-kinase mutant mice. *Science* 297 (5583): 1031–1034. doi: 10.1126/science.1073560.

Pachter, J.A. and Weaver, D.T. (2017). The dual PI3K-δ,γ inhibitor duvelisib stimulates anti-tumor immunity and enhances efficacy of immune checkpoint and co-stimulatory antibodies in a B cell lymphoma model. *Blood* 130: 1541. doi: 10.1182/blood.V130.Suppl_1.1541.1541.

Pagel, J.M., Reddy, N., Jagadeesh, D. et al. (2021). Efficacy and safety of the PI3Kδ inhibitor zandelisib (ME-401) on an intermittent schedule (IS) in patients with relapsed/refractory follicular lymphoma (FL) with progression of disease within 24 months of first-line chemoimmunotherapy (POD24). *J. Clin. Oncol.* 39 (15_suppl): 7550-7550. doi: 10.1200/JCO.2021.39.15_suppl.7550.

Patnaik, A., Appleman, L.J., Tolcher, A.W. et al. (2016). First-in-human phase I study of copanlisib (BAY 80-6946), an intravenous pan-class I phosphatidylinositol 3-kinase inhibitor, in patients with advanced solid tumors and non-Hodgkin's lymphomas. *Ann. Oncol.: Official Journal of the European Society for Medical Oncology / ESMO* 27 (10): 1928–1940. doi: 10.1093/annonc/mdw282.

Paul, J., Soujon, M., Wengner, A.M. et al. (2017). Simultaneous inhibition of PI3Kdelta and PI3Kalpha induces ABC-DLBCL regression by blocking BCR-dependent and -independent activation of NF-kappaB and AKT. *Cancer Cell* 31 (1): 64–78. doi: 10.1016/j.ccell.2016.12.003.

Pro, B., Brammer, J.E., Casulo, C. et al. (2020). Duvelisib in patients with relapsed/refractory peripheral T-cell lymphoma from the phase 2 primo trial: dose optimization efficacy update and expansion phase initial results. *Blood* 136: 38–39. doi: 10.1182/blood-2020-140412.

Psyrri, A., Papageorgiou, S., Liakata, E. et al. (2009). Phosphatidylinositol 3′-kinase catalytic subunit alpha gene amplification contributes to the pathogenesis of mantle cell lymphoma. *Clin. Cancer Res.* 15 (18): 5724–5732. doi: 10.1158/1078-0432.CCR-08-3215.

Ragon, B.K., Odenike, O., Baer, M.R. et al. (2019). Oral MEK 1/2 inhibitor trametinib in combination with AKT inhibitor GSK2141795 in patients with acute myeloid leukemia with RAS mutations: a phase II study. *Clin Lymphoma Myeloma Leuk* 19 (7): 431–440e13. doi: 10.1016/j.clml.2019.03.015.

Rhodes, N., Heerding, D.A., Duckett, D.R. et al. (2008). Characterization of an Akt kinase inhibitor with potent pharmacodynamic and antitumor activity. *Cancer Res.* 68 (7): 2366–2374. doi: 10.1158/0008-5472.CAN-07-5783.

Richardson, P.G., Nagler, A., Ben-Yehuda, D. et al. (2013). Randomized placebo-controlled phase III study of perifosine combined with bortezomib and dexamethasone in relapsed, refractory multiple myeloma patients previously treated with bortezomib. *Blood* 122 (21). (Conference Abstract) (In English). https://www.embase.com/search/results?subaction=viewrecord&id=L71266736&from=exporthttp://bloodjournal.hematologylibrary.org/content/122/21/3189.abstract?sid=e4ac49ee-db15-44bc-92f1-7212f0461b12.

Samuels, Y., Wang, Z., Bardelli, A. et al. (2004). High frequency of mutations of the PIK3CA gene in human cancers. *Science* 304 (5670): 554. doi: 10.1126/science.1096502.

Sarbassov, D.D., Guertin, D.A., Ali, S.M. et al. (2005). Phosphorylation and regulation of Akt/PKB by the rictor-mTOR complex. *Science* 307 (5712): 1098–1101. doi: 10.1126/science.1106148.

Sasaki, T., Irie-Sasaki, J., Jones, R.G. et al. (2000). Function of PI3Kgamma in thymocyte development, T cell activation, and neutrophil migration. *Science* 287 (5455): 1040–1046. doi: 10.1126/science.287.5455.1040.

Sato, A., Kayama, H., Shojima, K. et al. (2015). The Wnt5a-Ror2 axis promotes the signaling circuit between interleukin-12 and interferon-gamma in colitis. *Sci. Rep.* 5: 10536. doi: 10.1038/srep10536.

Schmitz, R., Young, R.M., Ceribelli, M. et al. (2012). Burkitt lymphoma pathogenesis and therapeutic targets from structural and functional genomics. *Nature* 490 (7418): 116–120. doi: 10.1038/nature11378.

Schneeweiss, A., Hess, D., Joerger, M. et al. (2019). Phase 1 dose escalation study of the allosteric AKT inhibitor BAY 1125976 in advanced solid cancer-lack of association between activating AKT mutation and AKT inhibition-derived efficacy. *Cancers (Basel)* 11 (12). doi: 10.3390/cancers11121987.

Schreiber, S., Hoellein, A., Decker, T. et al. (2015). Everolimus maintenance in patients with mantle cell lymphoma not eligible for intensive therapy: results of a prematurely closed phase 2 study. *Leuk. Lymphoma* 56 (11): 3227–3229. doi: 10.3109/10428194.2015.1028055.

Scott, W.J., Hentemann, M.F., Rowley, R.B. et al. (2016). Discovery and SAR of novel 2,3-dihydroimidazo[1,2-c] quinazoline PI3K inhibitors: identification of copanlisib (BAY 80-6946). *ChemMedChem* 11 (14): 1517–1530. doi: 10.1002/cmdc.201600148.

Sehn, L.H., Hallek, M., Jurczak, W. et al. (2016). A retrospective analysis of pneumocystis jirovecii pneumonia infection in patients receiving idelalisib in clinical trials. *Blood* 128 (22): 3705-3705. doi: 10.1182/blood.V128.22.3705.3705.

Sharman, J.P., Coutre, S.E., Furman, R.R. et al. (2019). Final results of a randomized, phase III study of rituximab with or without idelalisib followed by open-label idelalisib in patients with relapsed chronic lymphocytic leukemia. *J. Clin. Oncol.: Off. J. Am. Soc. Clin. Oncol.* 37 (16): 1391–1402. doi: 10.1200/JCO.18.01460.

Shin, N., Stubbs, M., Koblish, H. et al. (2020). Parsaclisib is a next-generation phosphoinositide 3-kinase delta inhibitor with reduced hepatotoxicity and potent antitumor and immunomodulatory activities in models of B-cell malignancy. *J. Pharmacol. Exp. Ther.* 374 (1): 211–222. doi: 10.1124/jpet.120.265538.

Smith, S.M., van Besien, K., Karrison, T. et al. (2010). Temsirolimus has activity in non-mantle cell non-Hodgkin's lymphoma subtypes: the University of Chicago phase II consortium. *J. Cli. Oncol.: Off. J. Am. Soc. Clin. Oncol.* 28 (31): 4740–4746. doi: 10.1200/JCO.2010.29.2813.

Somoza, J.R., Koditek, D., Villasenor, A.G. et al. (2015). Structural, biochemical, and biophysical characterization of idelalisib binding to phosphoinositide 3-kinase delta. *J. Biol. Chem.* 290 (13): 8439–8446. doi: 10.1074/jbc.M114.634683.

Song, M., Bode, A.M., Dong, Z. et al. (2019). AKT as a therapeutic target for cancer. *Cancer Res.* 79 (6): 1019–1031. doi: 10.1158/0008-5472.CAN-18-2738.

Spencer, A., Yoon, S.S., Harrison, S.J. et al. (2014). The novel AKT inhibitor afuresertib shows favorable safety, pharmacokinetics, and clinical activity in multiple myeloma. *Blood* 124 (14): 2190–2195. doi: 10.1182/blood-2014-03-559963.

Srinivasan, L., Sasaki, Y., Calado, D.P. et al. (2009). PI3 kinase signals BCR-dependent mature B cell survival. *Cell* 139 (3): 573–586. doi: 10.1016/j.cell.2009.08.041.

Stephens, L., Anderson, K., Stokoe, D. et al. (1998). Protein kinase B kinases that mediate phosphatidylinositol 3,4,5-trisphosphate-dependent activation of protein kinase B. *Science* 279 (5351): 710–714. doi: 10.1126/science.279.5351.710.

Sugimura, R., He, X.C., Venkatraman, A. et al. (2012). Noncanonical Wnt signaling maintains hematopoietic stem cells in the niche. *Cell* 150 (2): 351–365. doi: 10.1016/j.cell.2012.05.041.

Tam, C.S., Opat, S., Simpson, D. et al. (2021). Zanubrutinib for the treatment of relapsed or refractory mantle cell lymphoma. *Blood Adv.* 5 (12): 2577–2585. doi: 10.1182/bloodadvances.2020004074.

Vanhaesebroeck, B., Ali, K., Bilancio, A. et al. (2005). Signalling by PI3K isoforms: insights from gene-targeted mice. *Trends Biochem. Sci.* 30 (4): 194–204. doi: 10.1016/j.tibs.2005.02.008.

Vanhaesebroeck, B., Perry, M.W.D., Brown, J.R. et al. (2021). PI3K inhibitors are finally coming of age. *Nat. Rev. Drug. Discov.* 20 (10): 741–769. doi: 10.1038/s41573-021-00209-1.

Walker, E.H., Pacold, M.E., Perisic, O. et al. (2000). Structural determinants of phosphoinositide 3-kinase inhibition by wortmannin, LY294002, quercetin, myricetin, and staurosporine. *Mol. Cell* 6 (4): 909–919. doi: 10.1016/s1097-2765(05)00089-4.

Wang, J., Xu-Monette, Z.Y., Jabbar, K.J. et al. (2017). AKT Hyperactivation and the Potential of AKT-targeted therapy in diffuse large B-cell lymphoma. *Am. J. Pathol.* 187 (8): 1700–1716. doi: 10.1016/j.ajpath.2017.04.009.

Wang, M., Popplewell, L.L., Collins, R.H., Jr. et al. (2014). Everolimus for patients with mantle cell lymphoma refractory to or intolerant of bortezomib: multicentre, single-arm, phase 2 study. *Br. J. Haematol.* 165 (4): 510–518. doi: 10.1111/bjh.12780.

Wang, M., Rule, S., Zinzani, P.L. et al. (2018). Acalabrutinib in relapsed or refractory mantle cell lymphoma (ACE-LY-004): a single-arm, multicentre, phase 2 trial. *Lancet* 391 (10121): 659–667. doi: 10.1016/S0140-6736(17)33108-2.

Webb, L.M., Vigorito, E., Wymann, M.P. et al. (2005). Cutting edge: t cell development requires the combined activities of the p110gamma and p110delta catalytic isoforms of phosphatidylinositol 3-kinase. *J. Immunol.* 175 (5): 2783–2787. doi: 10.4049/jimmunol.175.5.2783.

Willemsen-Seegers, N., Uitdehaag, J.C.M., Prinsen, M.B.W. et al. (2017). Compound selectivity and target residence time of kinase inhibitors studied with surface plasmon resonance. *J. Mol. Biol.* 429 (4): 574–586. doi: 10.1016/j.jmb.2016.12.019.

Winkler, D.G., Faia, K.L., DiNitto, J.P. et al. (2013). PI3K-delta and PI3K-gamma inhibition by IPI-145 abrogates immune responses and suppresses activity in autoimmune and inflammatory disease models. *Chem. Biol.* 20 (11): 1364–1374. doi: 10.1016/j.chembiol.2013.09.017.

Witzig, T.E., Geyer, S.M., Ghobrial, I. et al. (2005). Phase II trial of single-agent temsirolimus (CCI-779) for relapsed mantle cell lymphoma. *J. Clin. Oncol.: Off. J. Am. Soc. Clin. Oncol.* 23 (23): 5347–5356. doi: 10.1200/JCO.2005.13.466.

Xing, Y., Lin, N.U., Maurer, M.A. et al. (2019). Phase II trial of AKT inhibitor MK-2206 in patients with advanced breast cancer who have tumors with PIK3CA or AKT mutations, and/or PTEN loss/PTEN mutation. *Breast Cancer Res.* 21 (1): 78. doi: 10.1186/s13058-019-1154-8.

Yap, T.A., Yan, L., Patnaik, A. et al. (2011). First-in-man clinical trial of the oral pan-AKT inhibitor MK-2206 in patients with advanced solid tumors. *J. Clin. Oncol.: Off. J. Am. Soc. Clin. Oncol.* 29 (35): 4688–4695. doi: 10.1200/JCO.2011.35.5263.

Yue, E.W., Li, Y.L., Douty, B. et al. (2019). INCB050465 (Parsaclisib), a novel next-generation inhibitor of phosphoinositide 3-kinase delta (PI3Kdelta). *ACS Med. Chem. Lett.* 10 (11): 1554–1560. doi: 10.1021/acsmedchemlett.9b00334.

Zelenetz, A.D., Barrientos, J.C., Brown, J.R. et al. (2017). Idelalisib or placebo in combination with bendamustine and rituximab in patients with relapsed or refractory chronic lymphocytic leukaemia: interim results from a phase 3, randomised, double-blind, placebo-controlled trial. *Lancet Oncol.* 18 (3): 297–311. doi: 10.1016/S1470-2045(16)30671-4.

Zelenetz, A.D., Reddy, N., Jagadeesh, D. et al. (2020). Tolerability and durable respones of the PI3Kδ inhibitor ME-401 administered on an intermittent schedule in relapsed/refractory (R/R) follicular lymphoma (FL) and other B-cell malignancies. *J. Clin. Oncol.* 38 (15_suppl): 8016-8016. doi: 10.1200/JCO.2020.38.15_suppl.8016.

7

Clinical Experience with Phosphatidylinositol 3-Kinase Inhibitors in Hematologic Malignancies

Alessandro Broccoli[1,2] *and Pier Luigi Zinzani*[1,2]

[1] *IRCCS Azienda Ospedaliero-Universitaria di Bologna, Bologna, Italy*
[2] *Istituto di Ematologia "Seràgnoli," Dipartimento di Medicina Specialistica, Diagnostica e Sperimentale, Università degli Studi, Bologna, Italy*

Take Home Messages

- The PI3K pathway is one of the most frequently dysregulated pathways across all of cancer biology.
- Drugs targeting the various isoform of PI3K are associated with promising activity, although many have distinct toxicity profiles depending on their selectivity.
- Despite the widespread occurrence of PI3K dysregulation in lymphoma, drugs targeting the pathway are only active as single agents in select forms of lymphoma (e.g. CLL, FL, and MZL).
- Combinations of PI3K inhibitors with other targeted drugs and anti-CD20 antibodies appear to improve their efficacy, though none of these combinations have received regulatory approval in lymphoma.

Introduction

Phosphatidyl-inositol 3-kinases (PI3K) are a family of heterodimeric lipid kinases that integrate signals from different cell surface receptors, such as the B-cell receptor, integrins, chemokine, and growth factors receptors, and in this way regulate most of the cellular pathways involved in proliferation, metabolism, protein synthesis, and survival. Three classes of PI3K have been described in humans, with class I being the most frequently implicated in cancer. The heterodimeric structure of each enzyme is composed of a regulatory subunit and a catalytic subunit. The former is activated by a cell surface receptor, which in turn recruits its catalytic subunit, catalyzing the phosphorylation of phosphatidylinositol 3,4,5-biphosphate (PIP_2) to phosphatidylinositol 3,4,5-triphosphate (PIP_3). PIP_3 may be dephosphorylated back to PIP_2 by phosphatase and tensin homolog (PTEN), and can interact with its downstream effectors, namely, the 3-phosphoinositide-dependent protein kinase 1 (PDK1) . PDK1 in turn can activate the serine–threonine kinase Akt, which ultimately leads to the transcription of genes involved in regulation of proliferative and apoptosis (Figure 7.1). When it is not interacting with cell surface receptors, the regulatory subunit is capable of inactivating the catalytic potential of the catalytic subunit.

Class IA PI3K are composed by three subclasses of enzymes (or isoforms), termed PI3Kα, β, and δ, composed of the regulatory subunits p85α, p85β, and p85δ, respectively. Class IB PI3K is composed by the catalytic subunit p110γ, with the regulatory subunits p101 and p84/87PIKAP. Among all the isoforms of class I PI3K, the PI3Kδ and PI3Kγ isoforms are those preferentially expressed in leukocytes and modulate both innate and adaptive immune functions (Cantley 2002; Katso et al. 2001; Liu et al. 2009; Vanhaesebroeck et al. 1997, 2012).

Given the complexity and importance of the PI3K-Akt signaling cascade, the pharmacological PI3K inhibition results in a series of scenarios (Lampson and Brown 2017; Seiler et al. 2016):

- Inhibition of cytokine signaling from the microenvironment through chemokine-mediated and adhesion molecules-mediated pro-survival signals, by means of mechanisms mostly relying on p110δ.
- Functional impairment of $CD8^+$ T-lymphocytes and reduction in the ability of $CD4^+$ T-lymphocytes to proliferate, expand, and differentiate into helper T-cell subsets, as a consequence of p110δ inhibition, on which converge signals from the T-cell receptor.
- Reduced chemotaxis of activated $CD4^+$ and $CD8^+$ T-cells via the stimulation of chemokine receptors, as a result of p110γ blockade.
- Decreased T-regulatory lymphocyte functions, which consequently counterbalance the impaired T-$CD4^+$ and $CD8^+$ function.
- Possible enhancement of direct anti-tumor activity.

These effects appear of particular importance in lymphoproliferative malignancies, as lack of p110δ and p110γ in knockout mice was shown to be associated with impaired

Precision Cancer Therapies: Targeting Oncogenic Drivers and Signaling Pathways in Lymphoid Malignancies: From Concept to Practice, Volume 1, First Edition. Edited by Owen A. O'Connor, Stephen M. Ansell, and John F. Seymour.

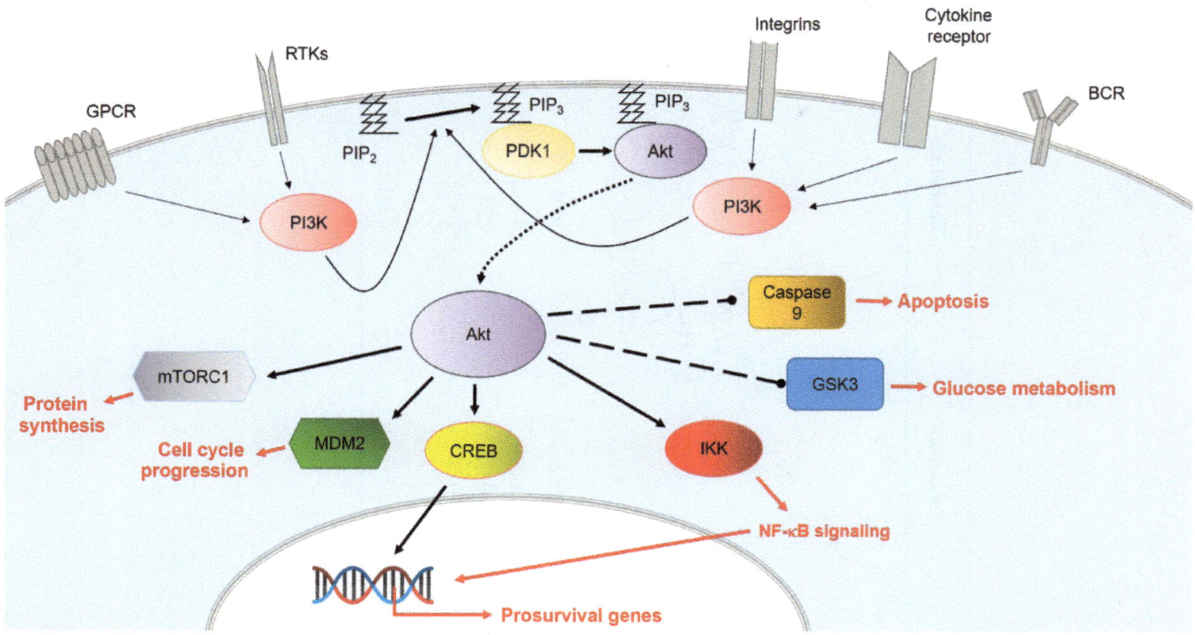

Figure 7.1 Simplified PI3K-dependent signaling, converging on Akt, which in turn activates downstream signaling pathways. PI3K activation is a consequence of signals from G protein-coupled receptors (GPCR), receptor tyrosine kinase (RTKs), integrins, cytokine receptor, B-cell receptor (BCR). PIP_2, phosphatidylinositol 3,4,5-biphosphate; PIP_3, phosphatidylinositol 3,4,5-triphosphate; PDK1, 3-phosphoinositide-dependent protein kinase 1; mTORC1, mammalian target of rapamycin complex 1; MDM2, mouse double minute 2 homolog; CREB, cyclic AMP response element-binding protein; IKK, IκB kinase; GSK3, glycogen synthase kinase-3. Arrows indicate activation pathways. Dashed lines indicate inhibitory pathways. Final effectors are labeled in red.

immune response and B-cell development. Similarly, mutations in the *PIK3CD* gene (encoding p110δ) have been associated with increased cancer susceptibility and occurrence of B-cell lymphomas (Crank et al. 2014; Kracker et al. 2014; Okkenhaug and Vanhaesebroeck 2003; Rommel et al. 2007). For this reason, there is a strong rationale to develop agents specifically designed to target PI3K (Sabbah et al. 2021).

This chapter will discuss in detail the commercially available PI3K inhibitors in terms of their mechanism of action and clinical application in lymphoproliferative malignancies, when applied either as single agents and/or combined with other lymphoma-directed drugs. Further, we will provide a glimpse of PI3K inhibitors in development within clinical trials (Table 7.1).

Idelalisib

Idelalisib (5-fluoro-3-phenyl-2-[(S)-1-(9H-purin-6-ylamino)-propyl]-3H-quinazolin-4-one) is a potent and highly selective inhibitor of the δ isoform of PI3K (Lannutti et al. 2011). The initial phase 1 studies with idelalisib have demonstrated its promising anti-tumor activity in patients with previously treated indolent non-Hodgkin's lymphomas (NHL) (Flinn et al. 2014) and chronic lymphocytic leukemia (CLL) (Brown et al. 2014).

Idelalisib as single agent in non-Hodgkin's lymphomas. The bulk of data regarding the efficacy and safety of idelalisib in patients with relapsed or refractory NHL comes from a phase 2 study involving 125 patients with disease refractory to rituximab and an alkylating agent or with relapse within six months after receiving these therapies, thus being considered double refractory to rituximab and alkylators, whether administered together or sequentially (Gopal et al. 2014).

The patients in this study received idelalisib orally, at the dose of 150 mg twice daily (b.i.d.), until disease progression, unacceptable toxicity, or withdrawal from the study for any cause. The median age of the patients was 64 years, most with advanced-stage (III-IV according to Ann Arbor) disease. Elevated lactate dehydrogenase was documented in one-third of the patients and 26% of them had lesions that were 7 cm or more in at least one dimension. A total of 58% of the patients enrolled had follicular lymphoma (FL): among those, 79% of whom displayed intermediate-risk or high-risk disease according to the FL International Prognostic Index (FLIPI). Among the remaining, 22% had small lymphocytic lymphoma (SLL), 12% marginal zone lymphoma (MZL), and 8% lymphoplasmocytic lymphoma (LPL), with or without Waldenström's macroglobulinemia (WM). Patients had received a median of 4 prior regimens, ranging from 2 to 12, with 79% having disease refractory to two or more previous treatment lines.

Table 7.1 Approved and experimental PI3K inhibitors.

	Idelalisib	Copanlisib	Duvelisib	Umbralisib	Parsaclisib	Zandelisib
Structure	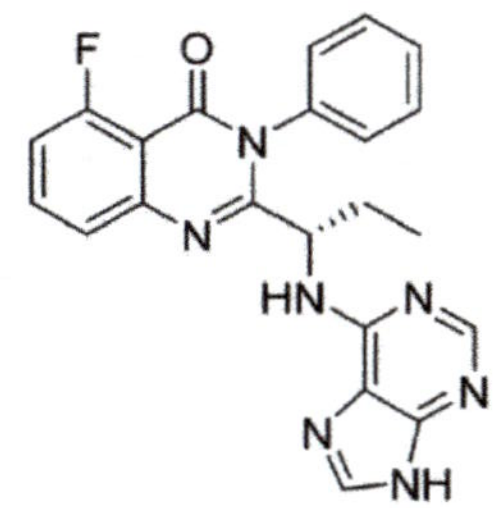	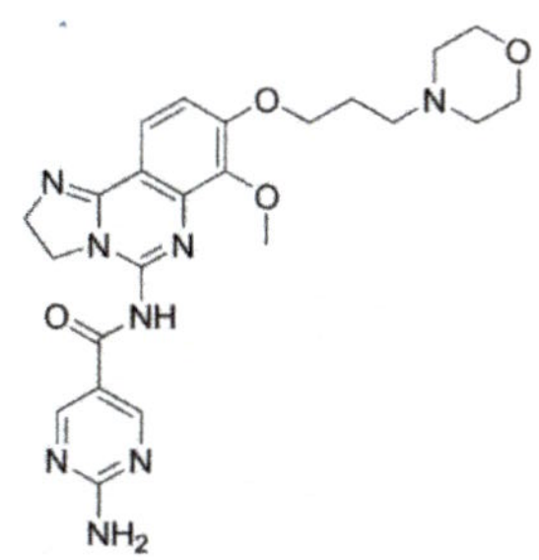	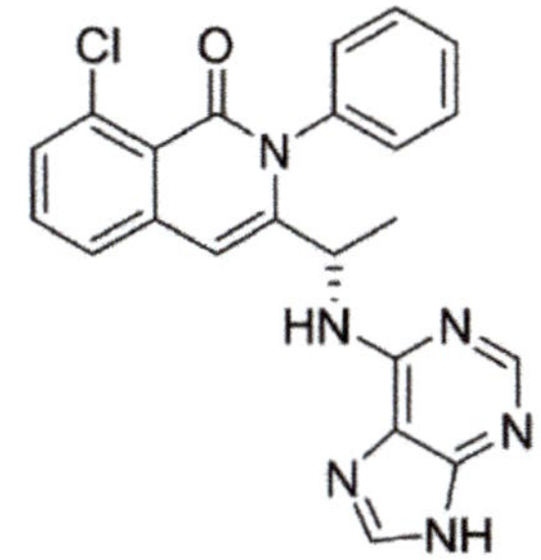	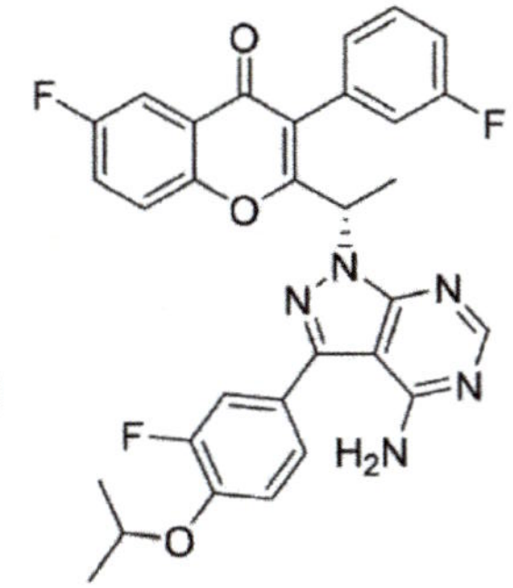	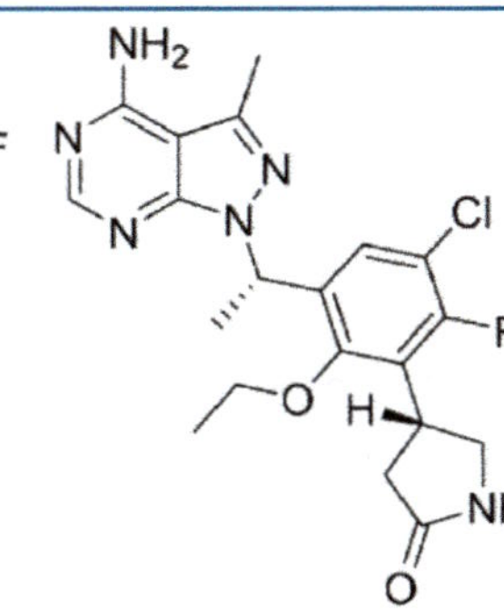	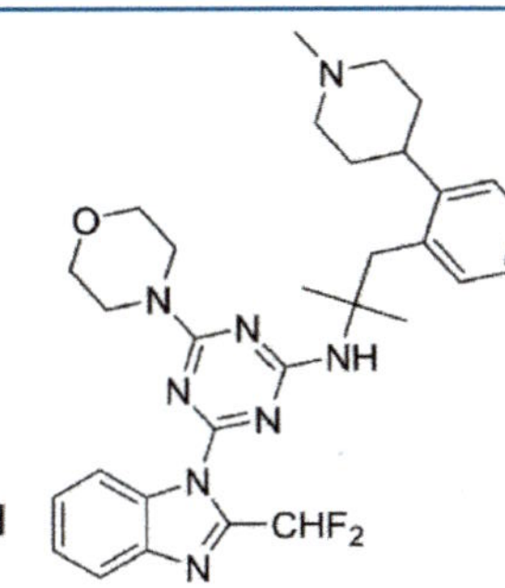
Target	PI3Kδ	PI3Kα + PI3Kδ	PI3Kγ + PI3Kδ	PI3Kδ + CK1ε	PI3Kδ	PI3Kδ
IC_{50} PI3Kα	820	0.5	1 602	>9 000	>20 000	5 022
IC_{50} PI3Kβ	565	3.7	85	>1 000	>20 000	208
IC_{50} PI3Kγ	89	6.4	27	>1 000	>10 000	2 137
IC_{50} PI3Kδ	2.5	0.7	2.5	22.23	1.1	5
Route	Oral	Intravenous	Oral	Oral	Oral	Oral

Abbreviations: CK1e = casein kinase-1ε; IC50 = half maximal inhibitory concentration (expressed as nM).

Single-agent idelalisib produced an objective response in 57% of the patients, and 90% of the evaluable population had some reduction in the size of the lymph nodes during treatment. A complete response (CR) was documented in 6%, and a partial response (PR) in 50%, on the basis of the assessment by an independent review committee. Responses were seen across all subgroups, and favorable outcomes were observed regardless clinical status, age, or sex of the patient, prior therapy, or refractoriness to the latest therapy. The observed median time to response (TTR) was 1.9 months, with a median duration of response (DOR) of 12.5 months. Importantly, this exceeded the median DOR obtained with the latest treatment before idelalisib, which was 5.9 months. A total of 34% of patients could continue treatment for at least 12 months (Wagner-Johnston et al. 2021). The median progression-free survival (PFS) and DOR were 11.0 and 11.8 months for patients with FL, 22.2 and 20.4 months for LPL/WM, and 6.6 and 18.4 months for MZL. Median overall survival (OS) after extended follow-up was 48.6 months (Wagner-Johnston et al. 2021).

Patients with FL have been analyzed separately in a subgroup analysis published later (Salles et al. 2017): the overall response rate (ORR) was 55.6%, with a CR in 13.9% of the cases and a PR in 41.7%. The median OS for this subgroup of patients had not been reached, with 69.8% alive at 24 months (100% for those achieving a CR, 71% for patients in PR, 64% for those who had a stable disease, 22% in case of disease progression as best response). Notably, a *post-hoc* analysis on 37 patients with FL who had shown early disease progression (i.e. ≤24 months; POD24) after initial chemoimmunotherapy showed that idelalisib displays anti-tumor activity in such a high-risk subset (Gopal et al. 2017). After a median duration of idelalisib treatment of 8.2 months, 21 out of 37 patients obtained a response (57%), with 5 CR (14%), and 16 PR (43%). The response rates were not significantly different between patients with very early initial disease progression (≤12 months after initial therapy) or between 12 and 24 months. The median DOR on idelalisib for all the 37 of these patients with prior POD24 was 12 months, with a median PFS of 11 months (8 and 14 months for the subgroups with progression within 12 months and between 12 and 24 months, respectively) (Gopal et al. 2017).

Idelalisib and rituximab in chronic lymphocytic leukemia. Furman and co-workers first presented the results of the combination of idelalisib and rituximab in patients with pre-treated CLL in a phase 3 placebo-controlled randomized study against single-agent rituximab (+ placebo). A total of 220 patients were enrolled in this trial, 110 per study arm, with a median age of 71 years and a median cumulative illness rating scale (CIRS) of 8. A deletion of the short arm of chromosome 17 (del17p) was found in 42%, and 45% of the patients enrolled in the idelalisib + rituximab and single-agent rituximab arms, respectively, while an unmutated immunoglobulin variable heavy chain (IGHV) status was found in 83% and 85% of the cases, respectively. Patients had received a median of three previous treatment lines, mainly fludarabine- or bendamustine-based chemotherapy regimens, together with rituximab in the vast majority of cases (Furman et al. 2014).

Rituximab was given at the standard initial dose of 375 mg/m^2, followed by 500 mg/m^2 every two weeks for four doses, then every four weeks for three doses, for a total of eight infusions. Patients randomized in the investigational arm also received idelalisib at the dose of 150 mg b.i.d., as established in the phase 1 trial (Brown et al. 2014). The ORR was 84% for patients receiving the combination therapy *versus* 16% of those receiving rituximab + placebo; no CR was seen in either arm. At 24 weeks, the rate of PFS was 93% in the combination arm compared with 46% in the rituximab arm, with a median OS not reached in either arm (Furman et al. 2014).

The study was terminated early due to the evident superiority of the combination of idelalisib + rituximab over single-agent rituximab. Upon study termination and unblinding, patients could be moved to an extension study to receive open label idelalisib monotherapy, regardless the treatment arm they were initially allocated. Overall, 161 patients transitioned from the primary study to the unblinded extension study, 75 from the idelalisib + rituximab arm, and 86 from the rituximab + placebo arm. Patients in the rituximab + placebo arm who experienced disease progression and then moved to the idelalisib extension study achieved an objective response in 48% of the cases; the ORR was 68% for patients in the extension arm if their disease had not manifest progression after rituximab + placebo (Sharman et al. 2019). The median PFS according to cytogenetic and IGHV mutational status for patients receiving idelalisib + rituximab then idelalisib in the extension study was 20.8 months *versus* 18.7 months (neither del17p nor *TP53* mutations *vs.* either del17p or *TP53* mutations) and 22.1 months *versus* 19.4 months (*IGHV* mutated *vs.* IGHV unmutated status). Conversely, patients receiving rituximab + placebo in the primary study displayed a PFS of 4.0 months *versus* 8.1 months (presence of del17p or *TP53* mutations *vs.* no del17p/*TP53* mutations) and 8.5 months versus 5.6 months (mutated *vs.* unmutated IGHV status). OS rates at 24 months were 69.8% and 51.5% for each treatment arm, respectively (Sharman et al. 2019).

A *post-hoc* analysis of the same study was aimed at evaluating the impact of complex karyotype – defined as the presence of at least three distinct chromosomal abnormalities in more than one metaphase – in the response to idelalisib + rituximab. The incidence of complex karyotype was comparable between treatment groups, being 41% in the idelalisib + rituximab arm and 42% in the rituximab + placebo arm. A higher percentage of patients with complex karyotype also harbored del(17p) or *TP53* mutations. Patients who received the combination of idelalisib + rituximab had an

ORR of 81% and 89% depending on the presence or not of a complex karyotype ($p = 0.35$) and displayed comparable PFS (median of 20.9 and 19.4 months, respectively). The deleterious impact of complex karyotype was confirmed in patients receiving rituximab + placebo: a median OS of 28.3 months was observed in patients receiving idelalisib + rituximab compared to 9.2 months in those receiving rituximab + placebo (Kreuzer et al. 2020).

The potential effectiveness of idelalisib as initial therapy was evaluated in 64 treatment-naïve older patients with CLL or SLL, with a median age of 71 years. Patients received eight rituximab infusions plus idelalisib, as previously described, for 48 weeks; if no disease progression was documented, idelalisib could be continued on an extension study. The median time on treatment was 22.4 months, the ORR was 97%, including 19% CR. Importantly, the ORR was 100% in patients with del(17p)/*TP53* mutations and 97% in those with unmutated IGHV. PFS was 83% at 36 months (O'Brien et al. 2015).

Results of the combination of idelalisib + rituximab in real-world settings outside clinical trials corroborate the findings of the prospective studies: longer PFS was associated with a lower median number of prior therapies, underscoring the potential effectiveness of this combination in patients with del(17p) or *TP53* disruptions in both frontline and relapsed/refractory settings. The significant toxic effects of the combination, especially when used as frontline treatment, still remain a key issue (Eyre et al. 2021).

Toxicity issues and their management. The median duration of treatment with idelalisib in the phase 2 registration trial involving patients with indolent lymphomas (Gopal et al. 2014) was 6.6 months. The most frequently reported adverse events, involving at least 20% of the patients, were: diarrhea (43%), fatigue (30%), nausea (30%), cough (29%), and pyrexia (28%). Among grade 3 or higher toxic effects, diarrhea (13% of the cases), pneumonia (7%), and dyspnea (3%) were the most relevant. The most common laboratory abnormalities of at least grade 3 occurring during treatment included neutropenia (27% of the patients) and elevations in level of serum alanine or aspartate aminotransferases (13%). Adverse events leading to the discontinuation of the drug were documented in 20% of the cases: importantly, colitis and pneumonia/pneumonitis were the cause of treatment withdrawal in 3% and 2% of the patients, respectively. Dose reductions to 100 mg b.i.d. or 75 mg b.i.d. were required in 34% of the treated patients, most frequently because of aminotransferase elevation, diarrhea, or neutropenia (Gopal et al. 2014).

More than 90% of the patients with relapsed or refractory CLL enrolled in the phase 3 trial had at least one adverse event. In the idelalisib + rituximab group, the five most common adverse events were pyrexia (29%), fatigue (24%), nausea (24%), chills (22%), and diarrhea (19%). In the rituximab + placebo group, the adverse events were similar to those in the idelalisib group, with the most common being infusion-related reactions (28%), fatigue (27%), cough (25%), nausea (21%), and dyspnea (19%). In the idelalisib + rituximab arm, grade 3 or higher diarrhea was reported in 4% of the cases and grade 3 or higher rash was reported in 2% of the cases, with no grade 3 or higher diarrhea or rash reported in the rituximab + placebo group. Aminotransferase elevation occurred more frequently in patients receiving idelalisib + rituximab (35% any grade, 5% grade ≥3 between 8 and 16 weeks from treatment start) than in those receiving rituximab + placebo (19%). No patients discontinued the study drug because of aminotransferase elevations. At least one serious adverse event occurred in 40% of patients in the idelalisib + rituximab group and in 35% of patients in the rituximab + placebo group. Pneumonia (6% and 8%) and febrile neutropenia (5% and 6%) were the most frequent serious adverse events in either group, respectively. Adverse events leading to study-drug discontinuation were reported in 8% of the cases in the idelalisib + rituximab group (mainly consisting of gastrointestinal and skin disorders) and in 10% of the cases in the rituximab + placebo group (predominantly infections and respiratory disorders) (Furman et al. 2014). Among patients treated frontline with idelalisib and rituximab, the incidence of adverse events was much more pronounced. Diarrhea, including colitis, was the most frequent adverse event (any grade), seen in 64% of patients; it was followed by rash (58%), pyrexia (42%), nausea (38%), chills (36%), cough (33%), and fatigue (31%). Elevation of alanine and aspartate aminotransferase was seen in 67% of patients, with grade ≥3 in 23% of the cases (Lampson et al. 2016; O'Brien et al. 2015).

In light of the toxic effects encountered during the registration trial leading to dose reductions or discontinuations, with immune-mediated effects and infection being the leading cause of treatment withdrawal, general recommendations on the management of side effects and on prophylaxis have been elaborated and published. These are aimed at reducing the risk of potentially life-threatening adverse events by offering a guidance to treating physicians in the management of laboratory abnormalities, diarrhea, and infectious complications, thus improving patients' adherence to treatment (Coutré et al. 2015; Cuneo et al. 2019; Zinzani et al. 2019).

- Management of diarrhea. Among idelalisib-treated patients who reported diarrhea or colitis, the median time to onset of any grade diarrhea or colitis was 1.9 months. Interestingly, the median time to onset of grades 1–2 diarrhea was 1.5 months, while for grades 3–4 it was 7.1 months, thus reflecting a bi-modal presentation of this symptom. Patients who experience new onset diarrhea while on treatment with idelalisib should be investigated to rule out an infectious cause. Treatment should be withdrawn in case of grade >3 diarrhea, or grade 2 persisting for more than two days. Non-absorbed steroids, like oral budesonide (3 mg three times a day [t.i.d]), should be applied if diarrhea persists beyond

48 hours after withdrawal of the drug and maintained until resolution, provided concomitant infections have been excluded. In case of grades 1–2 diarrhea, no drug discontinuation is required, and symptomatic or antibiotic therapy could be administered concomitantly. Dietary measures, with light and frequent meals, and adequate hydration are always recommended. Treatment rechallenge with idelalisib is feasible after the patient has recovered; dosage reductions should be considered.

- Management of aminotransferase elevation. Transaminitis (i.e. elevation of alanine and/or aspartate aminotransferase) is a frequent event during the treatment with idelalisib, as a consequence of hepatocellular injury secondary to an immune-mediated effect elicited by the PI3Kδ inhibition in regulatory T-cells. Grades 1–2 transaminase elevation does not require drug withdrawal, but careful monitoring is warranted. Discontinuation is mandatory in case of grade >3 transaminitis. Treatment may be resumed at a lower dose in patients experiencing grade 3 transaminitis with recovery to normal levels upon discontinuation, while idelalisib should be discontinued permanently if toxicity reached grade 4. Oral steroid treatment (1 mg/kg of prednisone or equivalent) is required in case of transaminitis ≥5 times above the upper normal level and persisting for at least seven days.
- Management of pneumonitis. Drug-mediated lung injury in patients receiving idelalisib resembles those of hypersensitivity pneumonitis or organizing pneumonia, without evidence of microbiological pathogens. Clinical suspicion is heightened in presence of cough, dyspnea, shortness of breath, inspiratory rales, or reduction in oxygen saturation. Bronchoalveolar lavage is needed to rule out an infectious cause. Thoracic computed tomography scan is a necessary highly informative diagnostic tool. Steroids and non-invasive ventilation to support oxygenation, when required, are mainstays of care. Idelalisib must be stopped and should not be resumed.
- Prophylaxis of infections. *Pneumocystis jiroveci* pneumonia and cytomegalovirus (CMV)-related disease have been prominent causes of adverse events and increased mortality in trials with idelalisib. Trimethoprim/sulfamethoxazole (TMP) is therefore required during treatment with idelalisib and continued for at least two to six months after discontinuation. Alternative treatments include atovaquone, pentamidine, or dapsone, if patients are intolerant to TMP. CMV viremia needs to be monitored regularly, at least on a monthly basis; pre-emptive therapy is recommended for CMV-DNA ≥100 000 copies/ml or rising values in two consecutive controls. Lamivudine HepB prophylaxis should be considered in patients with a positive titer of hepatitis B virus (HBV) anti-core antibodies (HBcAb), provided HBV-DNA is not detectable at baseline.

Combination therapy in non-Hodgkin's lymphomas. Idelalisib has been combined with lenalidomide and rituximab in two phase 1 trials involving respectively patients with relapsed and refractory lenalidomide-naïve mantle cell lymphoma (MCL, A051201 trial) and FL relapsing at least six months after a previous rituximab-containing regimen (A051202 trial) (Smith et al. 2017). Lenalidomide was given at the dose of 15 mg/day and 10 mg/day in patients with MCL and FL, respectively, for 21 consecutive days over a cycle of 28 days. MCL patients received standard-dose rituximab weekly during cycle 1, while in FL it was given on days 8–15–22 of cycle 1 and day 1 of cycle 2. Idelalisib was given at the dose of 150 mg b.i.d. in each trial. Safety and tolerability of the combination were the primary endpoints of each study.

The combination of idelalisib, lenalidomide, and rituximab in these settings proved to be excessively toxic. Among the first eight patients enrolled, four experienced a grade 4 sepsis, a grade 4 hypotension with grade 3 rash and fever, a grade 4 transaminitis with fever and a grade 3 pulmonary infection with grade 3 maculopapular rash. All toxic events developed within 9–20 days after treatment inception, coinciding with rituximab infusions. Grade 3 rashes and transaminitis have been observed after protocol amendment consisting of the removal of rituximab. Due to this unexpected serious toxic profile, both trials have been permanently closed.

Approved indications. Idelalisib as single agent is approved for the treatment of adult patients with FL refractory to at least two previous treatment lines, including an alkylator and rituximab. In combination with rituximab, it has received the approval for the treatment of adult patients with CLL after at least one previous treatment line. The combination of idelalisib and rituximab is also approved for treatment naïve CLL harboring the del(17p) and/or *TP53* mutations. Utilization for the latter indication is at present limited by the significant toxicity issues.

Copanlisib

Copanlisib intravenously administered PI3K inhibitor with preferential activity against the p110α and p110δ isoforms, relative to the p110β and p110γ isoforms. It has demonstrated anti-tumor and pro-apoptotic activity in various tumor cell lines and xenograft models. A first-in-human phase 1 study established the maximum tolerated dose of copanlisib as 0.8 mg/kg administered on days 1, 8, and 15 of a 28-day cycle (Patnaik et al. 2016). In an expansion cohort including patients with pre-treated NHL, the rate of severe toxicities was low and there were early signs of clinical efficacy, including some CR and PR in all six patients with relapsed or refractory FL and one of the three patients with diffuse large B-cell lymphoma (DLBCL).

Applications as single agent. An initial phase 2 study evaluated the efficacy and safety of intravenous copanlisib, administered intermittently at the dose of 0.8 mg/kg on days 1, 8, 15 every 28 days, in patients with heavily pre-treated relapsed or refractory, indolent, or aggressive NHL (Dreyling et al. 2017a). The study population comprised two cohorts of 30 patients each, with either indolent NHL or CLL, or aggressive NHL, relapsed or refractory to two or more prior lines of therapy. The indolent cohort consisted of histologically confirmed FL (grades 1–3a), MZL, LPL/WM, or CLL. Aggressive lymphomas included grade 3b FL, transformed indolent lymphoma, DLBCL, mediastinal large B-cell lymphoma, MCL, unspecified peripheral T-cell lymphoma (PTCL), anaplastic large-cell lymphoma primary (systemic type), or angioimmunoblastic T-cell lymphoma. A total of 84 patients received copanlisib: 33 in the indolent cohort and 34 in the aggressive cohort; 17 additional patients with aggressive lymphoma (4 MCL and 13 PTCL) were enrolled into an expansion cohort. The ORR was 44% in the indolent cohort and 29% in the aggressive cohort. CR was observed in 20% and PR in 20% of FL patients. A PR was also observed in 39% of CLL cases, in 67% of MZL, and in the only patient with SLL. The ORR for the aggressive lymphoma expansion cohort was 27%: objective responses were achieved in patients with DLBCL (ORR 7%), PTCL (21%), MCL (64%), and transformed FL (33%). Median TTR was 52 days in the indolent cohort and 51 days in the aggressive cohort. Median PFS was 294 days in the indolent cohort and 70 days in the aggressive cohort. At 12 months, PFS was 45% and 13% in the indolent and aggressive cohorts, respectively. The median DOR was 390 days and 166 days in the indolent and aggressive cohorts, respectively. Median OS was 657 days in the indolent cohort and 183 days in the aggressive cohort. At 12 months, OS was 69% and 42% in patients with indolent and aggressive lymphoma, respectively (Dreyling et al. 2017a).

In the single-arm, phase 2 CHRONOS-1 study, 142 patients with relapsed or refractory indolent NHL received copanlisib at the dose of 60 mg as a one-hour infusion on days 1, 8, and 15 of a 28-day cycle (Dreyling et al. 2017b). The treatment was given until disease progression or unacceptable toxicity. The majority of the enrolled patients had FL (73%), followed by MZL, SLL, and LPL/WM (16%, 6%, and 4%, respectively), with a median age of 63 years and a previous treatment history of at least two lines. An advanced Ann Arbor stage (III–IV) of disease was present in 81% of the cases, and the median number of previous regimes was 3 (range 2–9). An ORR of 61% was observed, with 17% of patients achieving a CR and 44% a PR. Median TTR was 53 days (range 41–296 days). Disease stability was obtained in 29% of the cases (Dreyling et al. 2017b, 2020). In the 104 patients with FL, the ORR was 59%, including 20% CR and 39% PR. In the subset of patients with MZL, the CR rate was 13% and the PR rate 65%, resulting in an ORR of 78% (Panayiotidis et al. 2021). Objective response rates of 60% and 57%, respectively, were found in patients whose disease was refractory or responsive to the last therapy. At the most recent update, the median DOR was 14.1 months and the median duration of CR was 26 months, at a median follow-up of 16 months. Patients with FL had a median DOR of 12 months. The median PFS was 13 months and the median OS was 43 months, at a median follow-up of 14 and 32 months, respectively.

Safety profile. The most common treatment-emergent adverse events of any grade were transient hyperglycemia (50%), diarrhea (35%), transient hypertension (29%), neutropenia (28%), pyrexia (26%), and fatigue (26%). The most common grade 3 adverse events were hyperglycemia (33%) and hypertension (24%), and the most common grade 4 adverse events were neutropenia (15%) and hyperglycemia (7%). Serious toxic events were reported in 79 patients (56%) and included pneumonia (11%), pyrexia (6%), hyperglycemia (5%), and pneumonitis (4%); overall, rates of incidence of pneumonitis (6%) and colitis (0.7%) remained low. In 27% of the cases, copanlisib was discontinued due to an adverse event not associated with disease progression, of which the majority (15%) occurred within the first six months of treatment and were highest in the first three cycles. The most common toxic events leading to permanent discontinuation included pneumonitis (4%), neutropenia (3%), diarrhea, hyperglycemia, and thrombocytopenia (2% each). Importantly, the highest incidence of adverse events was recorded early, within the first six months of treatment, with a reduced incidence and grade in the 6–12 months and >12 months treatment intervals. An exception was grade 3 diarrhea, which was reported in 11% of patients treated for more than 12 months compared with 5% of patients treated for less than six months (Dreyling et al. 2017b, 2020).

Copanlisib + rituximab in indolent non-Hodgkin's lymphomas. This combination was explored in CHRONOS-3, a multicenter, double-blind, randomized, placebo-controlled, phase 3 study. This trial involved patients with histologically confirmed CD20-positive indolent B-cell NHL relapsed after the last anti-CD20 monoclonal antibody-containing therapy, free of progression and treatment for at least 12 months, or at least six months if unwilling or unfit to receive chemotherapy. Randomization ratio was 2:1 to copanlisib (60 mg intravenously on an intermittent schedule on days 1, 8, and 15 every 28 days) + rituximab (375 mg/m^2 on a weekly basis during cycle 1 then on day 1 of cycles 3, 5, 7, and 9) or placebo + rituximab. A total of 307 patients were allocated to the copanlisib + rituximab arm and 151 to the placebo + rituximab arm. FL was the most frequent histology, accounting for 60% of patients in each arm; MZL was also well represented, with 21% and 19% of patients in the experimental and control arm, respectively. Other histologies were SLL and LPL/WM. Half of the patients had received at least two previous therapies. A total of 80% of patients were progression and treatment-free for at least 12 months since their previous rituximab-containing regimen, whereas all the others were judged unfit (or were unwilling) to receive chemotherapy (Matasar et al. 2021a).

At a median follow-up of 19.2 months, the combination copanlisib + rituximab demonstrated a statistically and clinically significant improvement in PFS *versus* placebo + rituximab, with a median PFS of 21.5 months *versus* 13.8 months ($p < 0.0001$). The ORR was 81% in the copanlisib + rituximab group and 34% in the placebo + rituximab arm, with CR observed in 34% and 15% of the cases, respectively, and a median DOR of 20.4 months and 17.3 months, respectively. Grades 3–4 hyperglycemia occurred in 56% of the patients in the copanlisib + rituximab group and in 8% of those in the placebo + rituximab group; similarly, grades 3–4 hypertension was more common in the experimental than in the control arm (40% *vs.* 9% of the cases). Serious treatment-emergent adverse events were reported in 47% of patients receiving copanlisib + rituximab and 18% of patients receiving placebo + rituximab. Treatment discontinuation because of an adverse event occurred in 34% of patients in the experimental arm; on the contrary, the most common cause of treatment discontinuation in the control arm was represented by disease progression (44% of the cases of discontinuation) (Matasar et al. 2021a).

Copanlisib + chemoimmunotherapy in indolent B-cell lymphomas. The phase 3 CHRONOS-4 study (NCT02626455) investigates the intermittent administration of copanlisib (45 mg, increasing to 60 mg in case of no dose-limiting toxicity) in combination with rituximab + bendamustine (BR) or rituximab + cyclophosphamide, doxorubicin, vincristine, and prednisone (R-CHOP) in patients with relapsed indolent B-cell lymphoma, including FL, MZL, SLL, LPL/WM, after one to three previous lines of therapy. So far, 10 patients have received the RB + copanlisib combination and 11 have been enrolled in the R-CHOP + copanlisib arm. Median age at enrollment was 62 and 64 years for either arm, respectively. The ORR was 90% for BR + copanlisib and 100% for R-CHOP + copanlisib, with a CR rate of 50% and 30%, respectively. Hyperglycemia and hypertension were the most common treatment-emergent adverse events, along with cytopenias likely attributable to the chemotherapy (Matasar et al. 2021b).

Copanlisib in relapsed and refractory DLBCL. A phase 2 study of single-agent copanlisib (at the dose of 60 mg on days 1, 8, 15 of a 28-day cycle until progression or unacceptable toxicity) was conducted in 67 patients with relapsed/refractory DLBCL, after a median of three previous therapies, at a median age of 69 years. More than three-quarters of patients had disease refractory to their last systemic therapy. Previous autologous stem cell transplant was performed in 3% of the patients enrolled, while 21% of the cases were transformed from a previous indolent lymphoma. The ORR was 19%, with a CR in 8% of the cases: patients with an activated B-cell (ABC) cell of origin had a higher ORR (32%) than patients with a germinal center B-cell (GCB) like cell of origin (13%). Likewise, patients with ABC-DLBCL had a longer median PFS than GCB-DLBCL, 2.4 months *versus* 1.7 months, respectively. The median PFS in the overall cohort was 1.8 months, while the median OS was 7.4 months. Hypertension (33%) and hyperglycemia (22%) were the most frequent grade 3 adverse events, while the most significant grade 4 toxicity was hyperglycemia (9%), as expected. Pneumonitis was documented in 5% of the patients, while infections were recorded in 8% (Lenz et al. 2020).

Gemcitabine and copanlisib in T-cell lymphomas. This combination was explored in the phase 1/2 COSMOS study, which enrolled 28 patients with relapsed or refractory PTCL. PTCL, not otherwise specified and angioimmunoblastic T-cell lymphoma were the most common disease entities (46% and 32% of the enrolled patients, respectively). Median age at enrollment was 63 years. Advanced-stage disease was documented in 82% of the patients, which was mostly refractory to the last treatment line. In the phase 1 part of the study, six patients received escalating doses of intravenous copanlisib (45 mg or 60 mg) on days 1, 8, and 15, concomitantly with fixed-dose gemcitabine (1000 mg/m^2 on days 1 and 8) in 28-day cycles. Dose-limiting toxicity was not observed in the dose-escalation phase and 60 mg copanlisib was selected for phase 2 evaluation. A total of 25 patients (including those enrolled in the phase 1 part) were enrolled in the phase 2 of the study (Yhim et al. 2021).

The ORR was 72%, with a CR rate of 32%. The median DOR was 8.2 months, the PFS was 6.9 months and the median OS was not reached. A higher, although not statistically significantly different, CR rate was observed in patients with angioimmunoblastic T-cell lymphoma than in those affected by PTCL, not otherwise specified (55.6% *vs.* 15.4%, $p = 0.074$); nevertheless, PFS was significantly longer (13.0 *vs.* 5.1 months, $p = 0.024$). The most frequent grade ≥3 adverse events were represented by transient hyperglycemia (57%), neutropenia (45%), thrombocytopenia, (37%), and transient hypertension (19%). All the adverse events were manageable with appropriate supportive care and none were fatal. Copanlisib dose reductions to 45 and 30 mg were required in four and one patients because of cytopenias (Yhim et al. 2021).

Approved indications. At present, copanlisib is approved for the treatment of adult patients with FL who have experienced disease relapse after receiving at least two prior systemic treatment lines.

Duvelisib

Duvelisib is an oral dual inhibitor of PI3Kδ and PI3Kγ. Its rationale of the use rests on the fact that the dual inhibition of both δ and γ isoforms may provide greater benefit than blocking the function of one isoform only. As said, the δ isoform is mainly involved in tumor growth and survival, whereas the γ isoform significantly contributes in sustaining leukemia and lymphoma cells in a protective microenvironment through the differentiation and migration of CD4$^+$ T-cells and M2 tumor-associated macrophages (Cantley 2002;

Katso et al. 2001; Liu et al. 2009; Seiler et al. 2016; Vanhaesebroeck et al. 1997, 2012).

In a phase 1, open-label, dose-escalation study in 210 patients with various hematologic malignancies, including indolent NHL, CLL/SLL, and T-cell NHL but also including some patients with aggressive NHL, acute leukemias, multiple myeloma, myelodysplastic syndrome, or myelofibrosis, duvelisib was given b.i.d. in an initial dose-finding phase (31 patients) at doses ranging from 8 to 100 mg. The expansion phase with 179 patients included indolent NHL, CLL, or T-cell lymphomas, using 25 mg or 75 mg b.i.d. Treated patients achieved a response at a median time of 1.8 months, with an ORR of 58% in patients affected by indolent lymphomas, 56% in pretreated CLL patients, 50% in PTCL, and 32% in cutaneous T-cell lymphomas (CTCL) (Flinn et al. 2018a, 2018b). A subgroup of 18 patients with treatment-naïve CLL was also enrolled, receiving duvelisib at the fixed dose of 25 mg b.i.d., with an ORR of 83% (all PR), regardless of their IGHV mutational status or del(17p)/*TP53* status (O'Brien et al. 2018).

The DOR was 16.9 months, with a median PFS of 14.7 months and a probability of being alive at 24 months of 71.7%. Severe (grade ≥3) adverse events included elevation of liver enzymes (39%), diarrhea (26%), and neutropenia (29%). Three patients, all receiving duvelisib at the dose of 75 mg b.i.d., died as a consequence of an adverse event (*Escherichia coli* sepsis, acute respiratory failure, and fungal pneumonia) (Flinn et al. 2018a).

Duvelisib as single agent in chronic lymphocytic leukemia. The phase 3 DUO trial was a randomized study of duvelisib *versus* ofatumumab monotherapy for patients with relapsed or refractory CLL and SLL. Patients were randomized 1:1 to oral duvelisib 25 mg b.i.d. (160 patients) or ofatumumab (159 patients). Patient characteristics were well balanced between treatment arms: 56% of patients in both arms had Rai stage III disease at the time of treatment inception, at a median time from initial diagnosis of 7.5 years in the duvelisib arm and 6.7 years in the ofatumumab arm. Approximately one-third of patients in each arm had del(17p) or *TP53* disruptions, whereas an unmutated IGHV status was present in 69% and 73% of the patients in each arm. The median number of prior therapies was 2 in each arm (Flinn et al. 2018c).

The study met its primary study endpoint by significantly improving PFS obtained with duvelisib compared with ofatumumab for all patients (median, 13.3 months *vs.* 9.9 months, $p < 0.0001$). This was true also for patients with del(17p) and/or *TP53* mutations. The ORR was significantly higher with duvelisib (74% *vs.* 45% in each arm, $p < 0.0001$) regardless of del(17p) status. The most common adverse events were diarrhea (51%), neutropenia (33%), pyrexia (29%), nausea (23%), anemia (23%), and cough (21%) in the duvelisib arm, whereas neutropenia (21%) and infusion reactions (19%) were the most common side effects in the ofatumumab arm, as expected (Flinn et al. 2018c).

Duvelisib as single agent in indolent non-Hodgkin's lymphomas. The phase 2, single-arm, open-label DYNAMO trial was designed to investigate the efficacy and safety of single-agent duvelisib in patients with indolent NHL refractory (i.e. with no response or with disease progression within six months after completion of therapy) to rituximab and to either chemotherapy (with an alkylator-containing or purine analog-containing regimen) or radioimmunotherapy. The trial enrolled 129 patients with histologically confirmed FL (83 patients), SLL (28 patients), and MZL (18 patients). Median age was 65 years, with 85% of patients presenting with stage III-IV disease according to the Ann Arbor staging system. The median number of previous treatment lines was 3, and 40% of the enrolled population received at least four previous therapies before duvelisib. Prior autologous stem cell transplantation was performed in 5% of the cases. Duvelisib was given at the fixed dose of 25 mg b.i.d., continuously in 28-day cycles, until disease progression, unacceptable toxicity, or patient's death (Flinn et al. 2019a).

The ORR was 47%, mainly consisting of PR (CR rate <2%). It was 42% in patients with FL, 68% for SLL, and 39% for MZL. Median TTR was 1.87 months and the median DOR was 10 months. Median PFS was 9.5 months and median OS 28.9 months.

The most frequent toxic effects were diarrhea (49%), nausea (30%), neutropenia (29%), fatigue (28%), and cough (27%). Colitis and pneumonitis were reported in 8% and 5% of the patients, respectively. Serious opportunistic infections have been reported in three cases, all recovered: bronchopulmonary aspergillosis, CMV pneumonia, and *P. jiroveci* pneumonia. Alanine and aspartate aminotransferase elevation was documented in 5% and 3% of the cases, respectively. Treatment discontinuation because of a treatment-emergent adverse event happened in 31% of the cases: pneumonia, pneumonitis, colitis, and diarrhea were the side effects that most frequently led to treatment discontinuation (Flinn et al. 2019a).

Duvelisib + rituximab or bendamustine/rituximab. The association of duvelisib with rituximab (arm 1) or rituximab + bendamustine (arm 2) was explored in a phase 1 study involving patients with relapsed or refractory NHL or CLL. Patients in arm 1 received rituximab (375 mg/m^2 weekly for two 4-week cycles) concomitantly with duvelisib until disease progression or intolerance. Patients in arm 2 received rituximab (375 mg/m^2 on day 1), bendamustine (90 mg/m^2 in NHL or 70 mg/m^2 in CLL on days 1–2 for six cycles), together with duvelisib until progression or intolerance (Flinn et al. 2019b). Duvelisib doses of 50 mg and 75 mg b.i.d. were tested during dose escalation. The maximum tolerated dose was not reached; however, a dose of 25 mg b.i.d. was chosen for the subsequent expansion phase, according to the results of previously reported phase 1 study (Flinn et al. 2018a, 2018b). Overall, 46 patients (27 with NHL and 19 with CLL) were treated. Among patients with NHL, 41% in arm 1 and 21% in arm 2 had FL, whereas 7% in arm 1 and 37% in arm 2 had DLBCL. The median number of previous treatments was 3 and 2 for each arm, respectively.

The ORR was 71.8%, with highest rates achieved in patients with CLL (89% and 75% in either arm, respectively). Patients with NHL obtained an objective response in 71% and 58% of the cases according to treatment arm (however, with a FL predominance in arm 1 and a DLBCL predominance in arm 2). Overall, the CR rate was 15%. Median PFS was 13.7 months. The median DOR was 15.1 months for CLL patients in arm 1, 16.9 for CLL patients in arm 2, 5.0 months for lymphoma patients in arm 1, and 6.2 for lymphoma patients in arm 2. The adverse events of the drug combinations were consistent with single-agent toxicities, mostly consisting of neutropenia (48%), fatigue (41%), and rash (41%) (Flinn et al. 2019b).

Single agent and combinations in T-cell lymphomas. Duvelisib was applied as single agent in a phase 1 trial involving 16 patients with PTCL and 19 with CTCL with relapsed and refractory disease. The drug was administered on a dose-escalation basis, starting from 25 mg b.i.d. up to 100 mg b.i.d. on a 28-day cycle; the maximum tolerated dose was set at 75 mg b.i.d., and 77% of the enrolled patients were treated at this dose. In the PTCL population, the ORR was 50%, with three CR and five PR, all occurring within the first two to four months of treatment. Median OS and PFS were 8.4 and 8.3 months, respectively. In the CTCL population, six patients obtained a PR, all within four months since treatment inception. Median PFS was 4.5 months, with one-year PFS and OS being 26.5% and 78.9%, respectively. The most relevant all-grade adverse events were transaminase elevation (57% of cases), diarrhea (31%), and neutropenia (20%); grades 3–4 transaminitis was described in 40% of patients. Severe adverse events were reported in 57% of patients, including pneumonia (20%), colitis (11%), and pyrexia (9%). Pharmacodynamic results showed that a reduction of serum cytokines and chemokines related to T-cell activation and migration and to the microenvironment (such as CCL22, CXCL13, tumor necrosis factor-α, matrix metallopeptidase-9, and interleukin-16) occurred within eight days of starting treatment (Horwitz et al. 2018a). The phase 2 PRIMO trial explored single-agent duvelisib in PTCL: the dose optimization phased compared the dose of 25 mg b.i.d. with 75 mg b.i.d. in 33 patients, while the subsequent expansion phase explored 75 mg b.i.d. In the dose optimization phase, the ORR was 35% (per investigator assessment) in the 25 mg b.i.d. dose cohort and 54% (per investigator assessment, up to 62% per independent review committee) in the 75 mg b.i.d. dose cohort, with a CR rate of 25% and 31%, respectively. Data from the initial 38 patients treated in the dose-expansion phase with duvelisib given at the dose of 75 mg b.i.d. confirms its activity in PTCL: 53% of patients have reached an objective response at a median time of 55 days, with a CR in 34% of the cases. The median DOR was 233 days. A total of 84% of patients discontinued treatment, mainly because of disease progression (50% of the cases) or an adverse event (18% of the cases). Survival data is not yet mature, as enrollment is ingoing (Pro et al. 2020).

Based on these results and on an *in vitro* documented synergism, a phase 1 trial of duvelisib + romidepsin (arm A) and duvelisib + bortezomib (arm B) was initiated in relapsed and refractory PTCL and CTCL patients. The study had a 3 + 3 design with expansion cohorts at maximum tolerated dose: duvelisib was given at 25 mg b.i.d., 50 mg b.i.d., or 75 mg b.i.d., romidepsin at 10 mg/m^2 on days 1, 8, and 15, and bortezomib at 1 mg/m^2 on days 1, 4, 8, and 11, on a 28-day cycle. The maximum tolerated dose of duvelisib was not reached in combination with romidepsin, thus the expansion cohort was treated with 75 mg b.i.d.; on the contrary, the dose established for the expansion cohort in arm B was 25 mg b.i.d. A total of 38 patients in arm A and 31 in arm B were evaluable for response. The combination duvelisib + romidepsin produced an ORR of 55% (59% in PTCL and 45% in CTCL patients), with a CR rate of 24% (33% in PTCL and 0 in CTCL patients). AITL and PTCL-NOS appeared as the most druggable entities with this combination, with 75% and 64% of ORR, and 63% and 36% of CR rate, respectively. The combination duvelisib + bortezomib yielded an ORR of 35% (44% in PTCL and 27% in CTCL patients), with a CR rate of 13% (25% in PTCL and 0 in CTCL patients). Again, AITL and PTCL-NOS showed 75% and 50% of ORR, and 50% and 25% of CR rate, respectively. Grades 3–4 transaminitis was the most important safety concern; however, its incidence and grade were much lower than with single-agent duvelisib (15% in arm A, no cases in arm B when duvelisib was given at 25 mg b.i.d.) (Horwitz et al. 2018b).

Approved indications. At present, duvelisib is approved for the treatment of adult patients with refractory FL after at least two prior systemic treatment lines. It is also approved in CLL patients who have failed at least two previous lines of therapy.

Umbralisib

Umbralisib is a novel, next-generation inhibitor of PI3Kδ and casein kinase-1ε (CK-1ε); it exhibits a chemical structure that is substantially different from that of idelalisib and duvelisib, yielding to a more selective PI3Kδ inhibition. Moreover, it displays limited inhibition of cytochrome P450 and reaches levels of plasma exposure that permit once-daily dosing. *In vitro* models have shown that umbralisib inhibits the downstream signaling of PI3Kδ with a cytotoxicity profile equivalent to idelalisib. Importantly, it has been shows that umbralisib, but not idelalisib, uniquely inhibits CK1ε. CK1ε regulates phosphorylation of 4E-binding protein 1 and thereby regulates the translation of oncoproteins such as c-Myc, bcl-2, and cyclin D1. CK1ε also activates the non-canonical Wnt5a signaling, being implicated in promoting interleukin-12-induced interferon-γ signaling in colitis (Bryja et al. 2007; Sato et al. 2015).

In a phase 1, dose-escalation study enrolling patients with histologically confirmed B-cell or T-cell NHL (including PTCL), CLL/SLL, and Hodgkin's lymphoma whose disease had relapsed after, or was refractory to, at least one previous treatment regimen, umbralisib was given once daily at doses ranging from 50 to 1800 mg. A total of 90 patients were enrolled and treated with umbralisib, including 27% with CLL, 54% with B-cell NHL, 12% with Hodgkin's lymphoma, and 7% with other hematologic malignancies. The most common treatment-emergent adverse events were diarrhea (43%), nausea (42%), and fatigue (31%). The most common grade 3 or 4 adverse events were neutropenia (13%), anemia (9%), and thrombocytopenia (7%). Serious adverse events were: pneumonia (3%), lung infection (1%), febrile neutropenia (1%), and colitis (2%). The maximum tolerated dose was 1200 mg, and 800 mg was selected as the recommended phase 2 dose. The ORR was 37%, with 33% of patients achieving a PR. Responses occurred at doses greater than 800 mg (Burris et al. 2018).

Umbralisib as single agent in non-Hodgkin's lymphomas. The UNITY-NHL trial was a phase 2, open-label study enrolling 208 patients with FL (56%), MZL (33%), and SLL (11%) who have failed at least one (for MZL) or two (for FL and SLL) previous systemic therapy including an anti-CD20-containing regimen (plus an alkylator for FL and SLL). Median age at enrollment was 66 years. Umbralisib was administered at the fixed dose of 800 mg once daily with food on a 28-day cycle. The ORR was 49% in patients with MZL, 45% in patients with FL, and 50% for SLL patients. A CR was recorded in 16%, 5%, and 5% of the patients, respectively. The median DOR was not reached for patients with MZL, and it was 11.1 months and 18.3 months for patients with FL and SLL, respectively. The median PFS was not reached in patients with MZL, whereas in FL and SLL patients it was 10.6 and 20.9 months, respectively. The incidence of treatment-emergent adverse events recapitulated that of the phase 1 study; grade 3 diarrhea was recorded in 10% of the cases, while non-infectious colitis was rare (2% overall, with grade ≥3 incidence less than 1%) (Davids et al. 2021; Fowler et al. 2021).

Umbralisib as single agent in chronic lymphocytic leukemia. Umbralisib was evaluated at the dose of 800 mg once daily in 51 CLL patients who proved to be intolerant to a previous Bruton's tyrosine kinase (BTK) or PI3K inhibitor. Patients' median age was 70 years, with a median of two prior lines of therapy. Del(17p) or *TP53* mutations were recorded in 24% of the patients, while an IGHV unmutated status was seen in 65% of the cases. The most common adverse events leading to prior BTK or PI3K inhibitor discontinuation were rash (27%), arthralgia (18%), and atrial fibrillation (16%). The median PFS obtained in this study was 23.5 months, with 58% of patients remaining on umbralisib for a longer duration than on prior BTK/PI3K inhibitor. The most common grade ≥3 toxicities on umbralisib were neutropenia (18%), leukocytosis (14%), thrombocytopenia (12%), and pneumonia (12%) (Mato et al. 2021).

Umbralisib + ublituximab. The safety of the combination of umbralisib and the anti-CD20 antibody ublituximab (U2 regimen) was evaluated in a phase 1/1b study in 22 patients with CLL and 53 with aggressive and indolent NHL. In the dose-escalation portion, ublituximab was given at the dose of 900 mg (lymphomas) and 600 or 900 mg (CLL) for 12 cycles. Umbralisib was given orally once daily at 800 or 1200 mg (initial formulation) or 400–1200 mg (micronized formulation) in the phase 1 dose-escalation portion, and at 800–1200 mg in the phase 1b portion until progression or toxicity. The maximum tolerated dose was not reached in either the CLL or NHL cohort, and only one dose-limiting toxicity was observed. The incidence of grade ≥3 adverse events was low, including diarrhea (8%), pneumonia (8%), or hepatic toxicity (4%). The ORR for all patients was 46%, with 17% CR. More precisely, CLL patients responded in 62% of the cases, with a CR in 10% of the cases; patients with aggressive lymphoma achieved an ORR of 24%, with a CR in 12% of the cases; the ORR in indolent lymphomas reached 57%, with a CR in 30% of the instances. The median DOR reached 20 months (Lunning et al. 2019). Data on 72 patients with MZL receiving the U2 combination within the phase 2 UNITY-NHL trial has been recently disclosed (Chavez et al. 2021). U2 produced an ORR of 68% in patients treated with a median of two prior regimens, with 19% of the patients achieving a CR. At a median follow-up of 16 months, the median DOR was not reached, and 90% of the enrolled patients displayed a reduction in disease burden from baseline.

Combinations with ibrutinib ± ublituximab. The combination of umbralisib + ibrutinib was evaluated in a phase 1/1b study with 21 CLL and 21 MCL patients, previously treated with a median number of 2 systemic therapies. No dose-limiting toxicities were observed and the maximum-tolerated dose of umbralisib was not reached, thus the recommended phase 2 dose was 800 mg once daily. Toxic effects recapitulated those observed with any of the drugs (Davids et al. 2019).

The combination of ublituximab + umbralisib + ibrutinib was explored in a phase 1 study with dose-escalation and dose-expansion phases involving patients with relapsed or refractory CLL/SLL (23 patients) and NHL (23 patients). In the dose-escalation portion, patients were treated in cycles of 28 days with escalating doses of umbralisib (400, 600, or 800 mg) and fixed doses of ublituximab (900 mg) and ibrutinib (420 mg in CLL and 560 mg in non-Hodgkin's lymphomas). The maximum tolerated dose of umbralisib was not reached, thus the recommended dose for the dose-expansion phase was 800 mg once daily. The ORR was 84%. The toxicity profile was consistent with that of each drug, without any new warnings. The incidence of atrial fibrillation, in particular, did not exceed 4% (Nastoupil et al. 2019).

Approved indications. Umbralisib is currently indicated for the treatment of adult patients with relapsed or refractory MZL who have received at least one prior anti-CD20-based regimen and with relapsed or refractory FL who have received at least three prior lines of systemic therapy.

Parsaclisib

Parsaclisib is a potent and highly selective next-generation PI3Kδ inhibitor displaying more than 19 000-fold selectivity for PI3Kδ over other PI3K class I isoforms. Preclinical experience with parsaclisib demonstrated no hepatotoxicity, along with the capacity of potently inhibiting the proliferation of malignant human B-cells at very low concentrations.

In the phase 1/2 CITADEL-101 study, parsaclisib was evaluated in patients with relapsed or refractory B-cell malignancies, alone or in combination with a Janus kinase 1 inhibitor (itacitinib) or chemotherapy (rituximab, ifosfamide, carboplatin, and etoposide, R-ICE). Parsaclisib monotherapy (5–45 mg once daily) was administered to 72 patients testing expansion doses of 20 and 30 mg once daily. An intermittent dosing at 20 mg once daily for nine weeks, then once weekly, was also explored after initial protocol amendment. No dose-limiting toxicities were identified, and the maximum tolerated dose was not reached. In NHL, the ORR to monotherapy was 71% in FL, 78% in MZL, 67% in MCL, and 30% in DLBCL. The majority (93%) of responses occurred at approximately nine weeks since treatment inception. The most common treatment-emergent adverse events were diarrhea/colitis (36%), nausea (36%), fatigue (31%), and rash (31%). Serious adverse events were diarrhea/colitis (nine cases), pyrexia (four cases), hypotension (three cases), and sepsis (three cases). Results on the combination of parsaclisib with either itacitinib or R-ICE are still preliminary, as just a few patients have been enrolled in each arm (Forero-Torres et al. 2019).

Single-agent parsaclisib in specific lymphoma subtypes. The phase 2 CITADEL-202 trial explored single-agent parsaclisib, at the dose of 20 mg daily for eight weeks followed by 20 mg once weekly, in patients with relapsed or refractory DLBCL, according to their previous exposure to a BTK inhibitor (five patients) or not (55 patients). The median age at enrollment was 70 years, and most patients had received three to five prior systemic treatments. In 16 cases, the diagnosis of DLBCL followed a previous diagnosis of indolent lymphoma. The ORR was 26% in BTK inhibitor-naïve patients and 20% (one patient out of five) in patients previously exposed to BTK inhibitors. The median DOR in BTK inhibitor-naïve patients was 6.2 months, with a median PFS of 2.2 months. The futility boundary was crossed at the *interim* analysis of BTK inhibitor-naïve patients, thus resulting in a negative study (Coleman et al. 2021).

In the phase 2 CITADEL-203 trial (NCT03126019), parsaclisib was applied as a single agent in patients with relapsed and refractory FL at two dosing groups (20 mg daily for eight weeks followed by either 20 mg once weekly or 2.5 mg daily). Data is available for the first 106 patients, with a median age of 67 years and a median number of previous therapies of 2. The ORR was 70%, with a CR in 14% of the cases, with a median TTR of eight weeks and a median PFS of 15.8 months, at a median follow-up of 10.2 months (Lynch et al. 2020).

The phase 2 CITADEL-204 study (NCT03144674) is exploring parsaclisib monotherapy (same scheduled as in CITADEL-203) in relapsed and refractory MZL, regardless their presentation as nodal (31% of the cases), extranodal (33%), or splenic (35%). So far, data for 94 BTK inhibitor-naïve patients evaluable for response has been disclosed. Median number of systemic therapies was 2, with a median age at enrollment of 71 years. The ORR was 54%, being 48%, 50%, and 64% for patients with nodal, extranodal, or splenic MZL, respectively. The median TTR was eight months, the median DOR was 9.3 months, and the median PFS was 13.8 months, at a median follow-up of 11.1 months (Phillips et al. 2020).

CITADEL-205 (NCT03235544) is now enrolling MCL patients previously treated with ibrutinib in order to receive single-agent parsaclisib (see above for treatment schedule). Data is available for the first 47 patients enrolled (median age was 70 years, with a median number of previous therapies of 3). The ORR and CR rate were 28% and 2%, respectively. At a median follow-up of 10.2 months, the median DOR was 7.3 months, with a TTR of 7.6 weeks, and the median PFS was 3.7 months (Zinzani et al. 2020).

Zandelisib

Zandelisib is a highly selective potent inhibitor of PI3Kδ, at present under investigation. Compared to idelalisib, it binds to its target 37-fold more tightly and remains bound 138 times longer, resulting in profound PI3Kδ inhibition (Moreno and Wood 2019). The administration schedule for zandelisib is unique among all the other PI3K inhibitors: treatment cycles 1 and 2 (i.e. response induction therapy) consist of a daily administration at the fixed dose of 60 mg, for 28 consecutive days each cycle. Starting from cycle 3, the drug is administered at the same dose for the first seven days of the cycle, with no administration between days 8 and 28 (intermittent dosing therapy). This allows for regulatory T-cell recovery, with the possible reduction of the onset of immune-related toxic effects commonly associated with this class of agents. In a phase 1b study, zandelisib (± rituximab) was administered in a cohort of 37 patients with relapsed or refractory FL, 41% of them with disease refractory to previous rituximab. The ORR was 87%, regardless of early (≤24 months) or late disease progression after frontline therapy, with a CR rate of 27%. A low incidence of grade ≥3 adverse events was observed, with neutropenia in 16% of the cases, transaminitis in 8% of the cases, diarrhea and colitis in 5% of the cases each. The median DOR was not reached at a median follow-up of 13 months (Pagel et al. 2021).

The phase 2 TIDAL trial (NCT03768505) is now enrolling patients with FL and MZL relapsed or refractory to at least two prior systemic therapies, with a planned target population of 120 FL and 60 MZL cases. Zandelisib is administered continuously as a single agent for the first two cycles, then on a 7 days "on" 21 days "off" schedule, as previously outlined. The randomized phase 3 COASTAL trial (NCT04745832) is instead aimed at evaluating the efficacy of zandelisib combined with rituximab (6 cycles + 20 cycles of single-agent zandelisib as maintenance) in comparison to standard chemoimmunotherapy (rituximab + bendamustine or rituximab + cyclophosphamide, doxorubicin, vincristine, and prednisone) in patients with relapsed or refractory FL or MZL who have received at least one prior systemic therapy.

Amdizalisib (HMPL-689)

HMPL-689 is a potent and highly selective PI3Kδ inhibitor given orally once daily. Phase 1 dose finding trials are now enrolling patients in China, the United States, and Europe, with doses ranging from 5 to 50 mg, involving patients affected by FL, MZL, MCL, cutaneous B-cell lymphomas, LPL/WM, CLL and SLL, and PTCL. A phase 2 registration trial is enrolling patients with relapsed and refractory FL (about 100 patients expected) and MZL (about 80 patients expected) who have failed at least one previous anti-CD20-containing treatment.

Conclusion

PI3K inhibitors have been widely approved in the treatment of indolent NHL, mainly FL, in case of disease relapse or refractoriness to anti-CD20 agents, alkylators, or purine analogs. Their efficacy has been confirmed in phases 2 and 3 clinical trials and potential combinations with monoclonal antibodies, chemotherapy, or targeted agents are under investigation (Table 7.2). Treatment-emergent toxicities are still an issue, given that a significant proportion of patients experience extra-hematologic – and prevalently immune-mediated – adverse effects and display enhanced infectious morbidity. Newer PI3K inhibitors, with higher selectivity toward the PI3Kδ isoform or with a mechanism of action that combines the inhibition of multiple substrates, may display enhanced on-target effect with a concomitant reduction in adverse events.

The choice of the most suitable PI3K inhibitor is of crucial importance in clinical practice (Figure 7.2): treatment decisions should be a consequence of the balance between expected results and potential side effects in light of the peculiar patient's disease history and comorbidities.

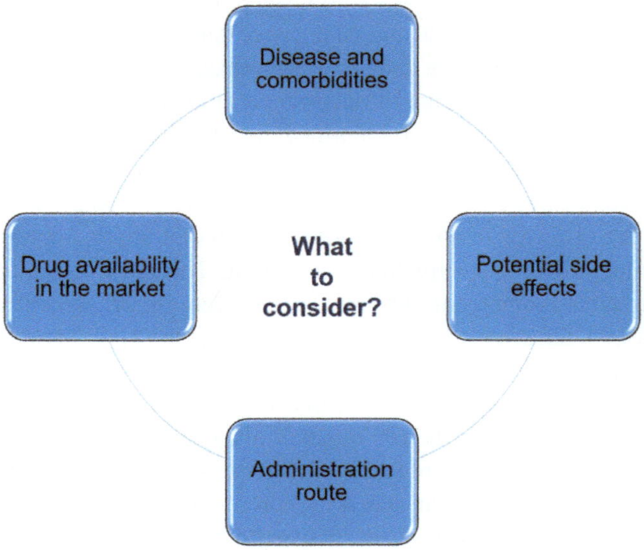

Figure 7.2 Factors implicating in the choice of the most suitable PI3K inhibitor.

Table 7.2 Summary of the efficacy of each PI3K inhibitor in different histologic subtypes. The data present the overall response rate as a percentage, and the complete response rate also as a percentage in the brackets alongside.

	FL	MZL	SLL	CLL (*)	References
Idelalisib	**56% (14%)**	—	—	**84% (10%)**	(Furman et al. 2014; Gopal et al. 2014)
Copanlisib	**59% (20%)**	78% (13%)	—	—	(Dreyling et al. 2017b)
Duvelisib	**42% (1%)**	39% (6%)	68% (0)	**74% (0.6%)**	(Flinn et al. 2018c, 2019a)
Umbralisib	**45% (15%)**	**49% (16%)**	50% (5%)	—	(Fowler et al. 2021)
Parsaclisib	71% (21%)	78% (33%)	—	33% (0)	(Forero-Torres et al. 2019)

(*) Data refers to pretreated patients only and not to those treated frontline.
Abbreviations: CLL = chronic lymphocytic leukemia; FL = follicular lymphoma; MZL = marginal zone lymphoma; SLL = small lymphocytic lymphoma
Data written in bold refers to the specific subset(s) in which the molecule has approval.

Must Read References

Furman, R.R., Sharman, J.R., Coutre, S.E. et al. (2014). Idelalisib and rituximab in relapsed chronic lymphocytic leukemia. *N. Engl. J. Med.* 370 (11): 997–1007.

Burris, H.A., 3rd, Flinn, I.W., Patel, M.R. et al. (2018). Umbralisib, a novel PI3Kδ and casein kinase-1ε inhibitor, in relapsed or refractory chronic lymphocytic leukaemia and lymphoma: an open-label, phase 1, dose-escalation, first-in-human study. *Lancet Oncol.* 19 (4): 486–496.

Matasar, M.J., Capra, M., Özcan, M. et al. (2021a). Copanlisib plus rituximab versus placebo plus rituximab in patients with relapsed indolent non-Hodgkin lymphoma (CHRONOS-3): a double-blind, randomised, placebo-controlled, phase 3 trial. *Lancet Oncol.* 22 (5): 678–689.

Sharman, J.P., Coutre, S.E., Furman, R.R. et al. (2019). Final results of a randomized, phase III study of rituximab with or without idelalisib followed by open-label idelalisib in patients with relapsed chronic lymphocytic leukemia. *J. Clin. Oncol.* 37 (16): 1391–1402.

References

Brown, J.R., Byrd, J.C., Coutre, S.E. et al. (2014). Idelalisib, an inhibitor of phosphatidylinositol 3-kinase p110δ, for relapsed/refractory chronic lymphocytic leukemia. *Blood* 123 (22): 3390–3397.

Bryja, V., Schulte, G., Rawal, N. et al. (2007). Wnt-5a induces Dishevelled phosphorylation and dopaminergic differentiation via a CK1-dependent mechanism. *J. Cell Sci.* 120 (Pt 4): 586–595.

Burris, H.A., 3rd, Flinn, I.W., Patel, M.R. et al. (2018). Umbralisib, a novel PI3Kδ and casein kinase-1ε inhibitor, in relapsed or refractory chronic lymphocytic leukaemia and lymphoma: an open-label, phase 1, dose-escalation, first-in-human study. *Lancet Oncol.* 19 (4): 486–496.

Cantley, L.C. (2002). The phosphoinositide 3-kinase pathway. *Science* 296 (5573): 1655–1657.

Chavez, J.C., Goldschmidt, N., Samaniego, F. et al. (2021). The combination of umbralisib plus ublituximab is active in patients with relapsed or refractory marginal zone lymphoma (MZL): results from the phase 2 global Unity-NHL trial. *Blood (ASH Annual Meeting Abstracts)* 138 (suppl 1): 45.

Coleman, M., Belada, D., Casasnovas, R.O. et al. (2021). Phase 2 study of parsaclisib (INCB050465), a highly selective, next-generation PI3Kδ inhibitor, in relapsed or refractory diffuse large B-cell lymphoma (CITADEL-202). *Leuk Lymphoma* 62 (2): 368–376.

Coutré, S.E., Barrientos, J.C., Brown, J.R. et al. (2015). Management of adverse events associated with idelalisib treatment: expert panel opinion. *Leuk. Lymphoma* 56 (10): 2779–2786.

Crank, M.C., Grossman, J.K., Moir, S. et al. (2014). Mutations in PIK3CD can cause hyper IgM syndrome (HIGM) associated with increased cancer susceptibility. *J. Clin. Immunol.* 34 (3): 272–276.

Cuneo, A., Barosi, G., Danesi, R. et al. (2019). Management of adverse events associated with idelalisib treatment in chronic lymphocytic leukemia and follicular lymphoma: a multidisciplinary position paper. *Hematol. Oncol.* 37 (1): 3–14.

Davids, M.S., Kim, H.T., Nicotra, A. et al. (2019). Umbralisib in combination with ibrutinib in patients with relapsed or refractory chronic lymphocytic leukaemia or mantle cell lymphoma: a multicentre phase 1–1b study. *Lancet. Haematol.* 6 (1): e38–e47.

Davids, M.S., O'Connor, O.A., Jurczak, W. et al. (2021). Integrated safety analysis of umbralisib, a dual PI3Kδ/CK1ε inhibitor, in relapsed/refractory lymphoid malignancies. *Blood Adv.* 5 (23): 5332–5343.

Dreyling, M., Morschhauser, F., Bouabdallah, K. et al. (2017a). Phase II study of copanlisib, a PI3K inhibitor, in relapsed or refractory, indolent or aggressive lymphoma. *Ann. Oncol.* 28 (9): 2169–2178.

Dreyling, M., Santoro, A., Mollica, L. et al. (2017b). Phosphatidylinositol 3-kinase inhibition by copanlisib in relapsed or refractory indolent lymphoma. *J. Clin. Oncol.* 35 (35): 3898–3905.

Dreyling, M., Santoro, M.L. et al. (2020). Long-term safety and efficacy of the PI3K inhibitor copanlisib in patients with relapsed or refractory indolent lymphoma: 2-year follow-up of the CHRONOS-1 study. *Am. J. Hematol.* 95 (4): 362–371.

Eyre, T.A., Preston, G., Kagdi, H. et al. (2021). A retrospective observational study to evaluate the clinical outcomes and routine management of patients with chronic lymphocytic leukaemia treated with idelalisib and rituximab in the UK and Ireland (RETRO-idel). *Br. J. Haematol.* 194 (1): 69–77.

Flinn, I.W., Cherry, M.A., Maris, M.B. et al. (2019b). Combination trial of duvelisib (IPI-145) with rituximab or bendamustine/rituximab in patients with non-Hodgkin lymphoma or chronic lymphocytic leukemia. *Am. J. Hematol.* 94 (12): 1325–1334.

Flinn, I.W., Hillmen, P., Montillo, M. et al. (2018c). The phase 3 DUO trial: duvelisib vs ofatumumab in relapsed and refractory CLL/SLL. *Blood* 132 (23): 2446–2455.

Flinn, I.W., Kahl, B.S., Leonard, J.P. et al. (2014). Idelalisib, a selective inhibitor of phosphatidylinositol 3-kinase-δ, as therapy for previously treated indolent non-Hodgkin lymphoma. *Blood* 123 (22): 3406–3413.

Flinn, I.W., Miller, C.B., Ardeshna, K.M. et al. (2019a). DYNAMO: a phase II study of Duvelisib (IPI-145) in patients with refractory indolent Non-Hodgkin Lymphoma. *J. Clin. Oncol.* 37 (11): 912–922.

Flinn, I.W., O'Brien, S., Kahl, B. et al. (2018a). Duvelisib, a novel oral dual inhibitor of PI3K-δ,γ, is clinically active in advanced hematologic malignancies. *Blood* 131 (8): 877–887.

Flinn, I.W., Patel, M., Oki, Y. et al. (2018b). Duvelisib, an oral dual PI3K-δ, γ inhibitor, shows clinical activity in indolent non-Hodgkin lymphoma in a phase 1 study. *Am. J. Hematol.* 93 (11): 1311–1317.

Forero-Torres, A., Ramchandren, R., Yacoub, A. et al. (2019). Parsaclisib, a potent and highly selective PI3Kδ inhibitor, in patients with relapsed or refractory B-cell malignancies. *Blood* 133 (16): 1742–1752.

Fowler, N.H., Samaniego, F., Jurczak, W. et al. (2021). Umbralisib, a dual PI3Kδ/CK1ε inhibitor in patients with relapsed or refractory indolent lymphoma. *J. Clin. Oncol.* 39 (15): 1609–1618.

Furman, R.R., Sharman, J.R., Coutre, S.E. et al. (2014). Idelalisib and rituximab in relapsed chronic lymphocytic leukemia. *N. Engl. J. Med.* 370 (11): 997–1007.

Gopal, A.K., Kahl, B.S., de Vos, S. et al. (2014). PI3Kδ inhibition by idelalisib in patients with relapsed indolent lymphoma. *N. Engl. J. Med.* 370 (11): 1008–1018.

Gopal, A.K., Kahl, B.S., Flowers, C.R. et al. (2017). Idelalisib is effective in patients with high-risk follicular lymphoma and early relapse after initial chemoimmunotherapy. *Blood* 129 (22): 3037–3039.

Horwitz, S.M., Koch, R., Porcu, P. et al. (2018a). Activity of the PI3K-δ,γ inhibitor duvelisib in a phase 1 trial and preclinical models of T-cell lymphoma. *Blood* 131 (8): 888–898.

Horwitz, S.M., Moskowitz, A.J., Jacobsen, E.D. et al. (2018b). The combination of duvelisib, a PI3K-δ,γ inhibitor, and romidepsin is highly active in relapsed/refractory peripheral T-cell lymphoma with low rates of transaminits: results of parallel multicentre, phase 1 combination studies with expansion cohorts. *Blood (ASH Annual Meeting Abstracts)* 132 (suppl. 1): abstr 683.

Katso, R., Okkenhaug, K., Ahmadi, K. et al. (2001). Cellular function of phosphoinositide 3-kinases: implications for development, homeostasis, and cancer. *Annu. Rev. Cell Dev. Biol.* 17: 615–675.

Kracker, S., Curtis, J., Ibrahim, M.A. et al. (2014). Occurrence of B-cell lymphomas in patients with activated phosphoinositide 3-kinase delta syndrome. *J. Allergy Clin. Immunol.* 134 (1): 233–236.

Kreuzer, K.A., Furman, R.R., Stilgenbauer, S. et al. (2020). The impact of complex karyotype on the overall survival of patients with relapsed chronic lymphocytic leukemia treated with idelalisib plus rituximab. *Leukemia* 34 (1): 296–300.

Lampson, B.L. and Brown, J.R. (2017). PI3Kδ-selective and PI3Kα/δ-combinatorial inhibitors in clinical development for B-cell non-Hodgkin lymphoma. *Expert Opin Investig Drugs* 26: 1267–1279.

Lampson, B.L., Kasar, S.N., Matos, T.R. et al. (2016). Idelalisib given front-line for treatment of chronic lymphocytic leukemia causes frequent immune-mediated hepatotoxicity. *Blood* 128 (2): 195–203.

Lannutti, B.J., Meadows, S.A., Herman, S.E.M. et al. (2011). CAL-101, a p110δ selective phosphatidylinositol-3-kinase inhibitor for the treatment of B-cell malignancies, inhibits PI3K signaling and cellular viability. *Blood* 117 (2): 591–594.

Lenz, G., Hawkes, E., Verhoef, G. et al. (2020). Single-agent activity of phosphatidylinositol 3-kinase inhibition with copanlisib in patients with molecularly defined relapsed or refractory diffuse large B-cell lymphoma. *Leukemia* 34 (8): 2184–2197.

Liu, P., Cheng, H., Roberts, T.M. et al. (2009). Targeting the phosphoinositide 3-kinase pathway in cancer. *Nat. Rev. Drug. Discov.* 8 (8): 627–644.

Lunning, M., Vose, J., Nastoupil, L. et al. (2019). Ublituximab and umbralisib in relapsed/refractory B-cell non-Hodgkin lymphoma and chronic lymphocytic leukemia. *Blood* 134 (21): 1811–1820.

Lynch, R.C., Paneesha, S., Avigdor, A. et al. (2020). Phase 2 study evaluating the efficacy and safety of parsaclisib in patients with relapsed or refractory follicular lymphoma (CITADEL-203). *Blood (ASH Annual Meeting Abstracts)* 136 (supp 1): 36–37.

Matasar, M.J., Capra, M., Özcan, M. et al. (2021a). Copanlisib plus rituximab versus placebo plus rituximab in patients with relapsed indolent non-Hodgkin lymphoma (CHRONOS-3): a double-blind, randomised, placebo-controlled, phase 3 trial. *Lancet Oncol.* 22 (5): 678–689.

Matasar, M.J., Dreyling, M., Leppä, S. et al. (2021b). Feasibility of combining the phosphatidylinositol 3-Kinase inhibitor copanlisib with rituximab-based immunochemotherapy in patients with relapsed indolent B-cell lymphoma. *Clin. Lymphoma Myeloma Leuk.* 21 (11): e886–e894.

Mato, A.R., Ghosh, N., Schuster, S.J. et al. (2021). Phase 2 study of the safety and efficacy of umbralisib in patients with CLL who are intolerant to BTK or PI3Kδ inhibitor therapy. *Blood* 137 (20): 2817–2826.

Moreno, O. and Wood, J. (2019). Absorption, distribution, and binding profile of ME-401, a potent and selective oral small-molecule inhibitor of phosphatidylinositol 3-kinase δ (PI3Kδ) in animal and B-cell lymphoma models. *Target Oncol.* 14 (5): 603–611.

Nastoupil, L.J., Lunning, M.A., Vose, J.M. et al. (2019). Tolerability and activity of ublituximab, umbralisib, and ibrutinib in patients with chronic lymphocytic leukaemia and non-Hodgkin lymphoma: a phase 1 dose escalation and expansion trial. *Lancet Haematol.* 6 (2): e100–e109.

O'Brien, S., Patel, M., Kahl, B.S. et al. (2018). Duvelisib, an oral dual PI3K-δ,γ inhibitor, shows clinical and pharmacodynamic activity in chronic lymphocytic leukemia and small lymphocytic lymphoma in a phase 1 study. *Am. J. Hematol.* 93 (11): 1318–1326.

O'Brien, S.M., Lamanna, N., Kipps, T.J. et al. (2015). A phase 2 study of idelalisib plus rituximab in treatment-naïve older patients with chronic lymphocytic leukemia. *Blood* 126 (25): 2686–2694.

Okkenhaug, K. and Vanhaesebroeck, B. (2003). PI3K-signalling in B- and T-cells: insights from gene-targeted mice. *Biochem. Soc. Trans.* 31 (Pt 1): 270–274.

Pagel, J.M., Reddy, N., Jagadeesh, D. et al. (2021). Efficacy and safety of the PI3Kδ inhibitor zandelisib (ME-401) on an intermittent schedule (IS) in patients with relapsed/refractory follicular lymphoma (FL) with progression of disease within 24 months of first-line chemoimmunotherapy (POD24). *J. Clin. Oncol. (ASCO Annual Meeting Abstracts)* 39 (15,suppl): abstr7550.

Panayiotidis, P., Follows, G.A., Mollica, L. et al. (2021). Efficacy and safety of copanlisib in patients with relapsed or refractory marginal zone lymphoma. *Blood Adv.* 5 (3): 823–828.

Patnaik, A., Appleman, L.J., Tolcher, A.W. et al. (2016). First-in-human phase I study of copanlisib (BAY 80-6946), an intravenous pan-class I phosphatidylinositol 3-kinase inhibitor, in patients with advanced solid tumors and non-Hodgkin's lymphomas. *Ann. Oncol.* 27 (10): 1928–1940.

Phillips, T.J., Corradini, P., Gurion, R. et al. (2020). Phase 2 study evaluating the efficacy and safety of parsaclisib in patients with relapsed or refractory marginal zone lymphoma (CITADEL-204). *Blood (ASH Annual Meeting Abstracts)* 136 (supp 1): 27–28.

Pro, B., Brammer, J.E., Casulo, C. et al. (2020). Duvelisib in patients with relapsed/refractory peripheral T-cell lymphoma from the phase 2 primo trial: dose optimization efficacy update and expansion phase initial results. *Blood (ASH Annual Meeting Abstracts)* 136: abstr 44.

Rommel, C., Camps, M., and Ji, H. (2007). PI3K delta and PI3K gamma: partners in crime in inflammation in rheumatoid arthritis and beyond? *Nat. Rev. Immunol.* 7 (3): 191–201.

Sabbah, D.A., Hajjo, R., Bardaweel, S.K. et al. (2021). Phosphatidylinositol 3-kinase (PI3K) inhibitors: a recent update on inhibitor design and clinical trials (2016–2020). *Expert. Opin. Ther. Pat.* 31 (10): 877–892.

Salles, G., Schuster, S.J., de Vos, S. et al. (2017). Efficacy and safety of idelalisib in patients with relapsed, rituximab- and alkylating agent-refractory follicular lymphoma: a subgroup analysis of a phase 2 study. *Haematol.* 102 (4): e156–e159.

Sato, A., Kayama, H., Shojima, K. et al. (2015). The Wnt5a-Ror2 axis promotes the signaling circuit between interleukin-12 and interferon-γ in colitis. *Sci. Rep.* 5: 10536.

Seiler, T., Hutter, G., and Dreyling, M. (2016). The emerging role of PI3K inhibitors in the treatment of hematological malignancies: preclinical data and clinical progress to date. *Drugs* 76: 639–646.

Sharman, J.P., Coutre, S.E., Furman, R.R. et al. (2019). Final results of a randomized, phase III study of rituximab with or without idelalisib followed by open-label idelalisib in patients with relapsed chronic lymphocytic leukemia. *J. Clin. Oncol.* 37 (16): 1391–1402.

Smith, S.M., Pitcher, B.N., Jung, S.H. et al. (2017). Safety and tolerability of idelalisib, lenalidomide, and rituximab in relapsed and refractory lymphoma: the alliance for clinical trials in oncology A051201 and A051202 phase 1 trials. *Lancet Haematol.* 4 (4): e176–e182.

Vanhaesebroeck, B., Leevers, S.J., Panayotou, G. et al. (1997). Phosphoinositide 3-kinases: a conserved family of signal transducers. *Trends Biochem. Sci.* 22 (7): 267–272.

Vanhaesebroeck, B., Stephens, L., and Hawkins, P. (2012). PI3K signalling: the path to discovery and understanding. *Nat. Rev. Mol. Cell Biol.* 13 (3): 195–203.

Wagner-Johnston, N.D., Schuster, S.J., de Vos, S. et al. (2021). Outcomes of patients with up to 6 years of follow-up from a phase 2 study of idelalisib for relapsed indolent lymphomas. *Leuk. Lymphoma* 62 (5): 1077–1087.

Yhim, H.Y., Kim, T., Kim, S.J. et al. (2021). Combination treatment of copanlisib and gemcitabine in relapsed/refractory PTCL (COSMOS): an open-label phase I/II trial. *Ann. Oncol.* 32 (4): 552–559.

Zinzani, P.L., Delwail, V., Paneesha, S. et al. (2020). Phase 2 study evaluating the efficacy and safety of parsaclisib in patients with relapsed or refractory mantle cell lymphoma previously treated with ibrutinib (CITADEL-205). *Blood (ASH Annual Meeting Abstracts)* 136 (supp 1): 43–44.

Zinzani, P.L., Rambaldi, A., Gaidano, G. et al. (2019). Infection control in patients treated for chronic lymphocytic leukemia with ibrutinib or idelalisib: recommendations from Italian society of hematology. *Leuk. Res.* 81: 88–94.

8

Clinical Experiences with Drugs Targeting mTOR

Thomas E. Witzig

Division of Hmeatology, Mayo Clinic, Rochester, MN, USA

Take Home Messages

- There are three mTORC1 inhibitors that have been widely tested in lymphoma – sirolimus (parent compound) and two derivatives referred to as rapalogs – temsirolimus and everolimus.
- There is clear single-agent activity in both relapsed Hodgkin's and non-Hodgkin's lymphoma – both indolent and aggressive and both B-cell and T-cell types.
- Combinations with chemoimmunotherapy such as bendamustine/rituximab, RCHOP, CHOP, and DHAP have been conducted and found safe and efficacious.
- The mTORC1/chemoimmunotherapy combinations have not been subjected to phase 3 trials.
- The mTORC1/mTORC2 dual inhibitors were developed with strong rationale but have not been tested in lymphoma to date.

Introduction

The PI3K/mTOR pathway has been under investigation as a therapeutic target for over 25 years. The biology of this pathway is nicely described in Chapter 5 "Principles of PI3K Biology and its Role in Cancer." The agents targeting the pathway at the PI3K enzyme level are comprehensively discussed in Chapter 7 "Clinical Experiences with Phosphatidylinositol 3-Kinase Inhibitors in Hematologic Malignancies." In this chapter, the discussion will focus on targeting the end of the signaling pathway at the level of the mammalian target of rapamycin (mTOR) complex. The discovery of rapamycin (sirolimus) preceded the discovery of its target – the mTOR. Rapamycin is a macrocyclic lactone produced by a strain of *Streptomyces hygroscopicus* found in the soil of the Vai Atore region of Easter Island (Rapa Nui). Its first described action was as an antifungal agent (Sehgal et al. 1975; Vezina et al. 1975). It was named rapamycin based on the discovery site (Rapa) and its antifungal activity (mycin). The target of rapamycin was not described until 1991 (Heitman et al. 1991) with further descriptions (Abraham 1998; Brunn et al. 1996; Sabers et al. 1995; Sehgal 1998) of the importance of this pathway and the methods to target it quickly following. These are more recently succinctly reviewed by Manning (2017). The mTOR is present in two distinct complexes (Chiang and Abraham 2007; Dann et al. 2007; Sabatini 2006), mTORC1 and mTORC2, and they have different substrate specificities and rapamycin sensitivities (Chiang and Abraham 2007; Dann et al. 2007; Inoki and Guan 2006; Sabatini 2006). This has become important to understand as the approved drugs discussed below are all mTORC1 selective agents. The result of signaling through the PI3K/mTOR signal pathway is the phosphorylation of 4E-BP1 resulting in a release of its binding to eIF4E. The liberated eIF4E then binds to eIF4G and the RNA helicase eIF4A, forming an active helicase that facilitates translation of mRNAs containing long, highly folded 5′ untranslated regions. This is important for lymphoma therapy because it results in messages encoding cyclin D1 and c-Myc, proteins important to the proliferation of aggressive lymphomas such as diffuse large B-cell lymphoma (DLBCL), Burkitt's lymphoma, and mantle cell lymphoma (MCL) (Easton and Houghton 2006; Faivre et al. 2006; Mamane et al. 2006). Finally, immunohistochemical staining of lymphoma tumors and cell lines documents the upregulation of the proteins in this pathway (Gupta et al. 2009).

Precision Cancer Therapies: Targeting Oncogenic Drivers and Signaling Pathways in Lymphoid Malignancies: From Concept to Practice, Volume 1, First Edition. Edited by Owen A. O'Connor, Stephen M. Ansell, and John F. Seymour.

Rapamycin (Sirolimus) Rapamune® (Pfizer) and Generic Sirolimus

The parent drug in this class is sirolimus. Sirolimus binds to the immunophilin FK Binding Protein-12 (FKBP-12) to generate the sirolimus:FKBP-12 immunosuppressive complex. In turn, this complex binds to mTORC1 and inhibits the antigenic and cytokine (IL2, IL4, and IL15) stimulation of the pathway thus inhibiting T-cell activation. Sirolimus also inhibits antibody production. Sirolimus is metabolized in the liver and gut wall with most metabolites excreted in the feces; only 2% is excreted in the urine. Therefore, sirolimus blood levels are monitored in those patients with liver dysfunction. Sirolimus is known to be a substrate for both cytochrome CYP3A4 and P-glycoprotein and thus dose modifications are necessary when used with other drugs that are metabolized through a similar mechanism such as cyclosporin, a substrate and inhibitor of CYP3A4 and P-glycoprotein and the azole antifungals which are also strong inhibitors of CYP3A4. Its approved uses are for prevention of rejection after a renal transplant and as treatment of pulmonary lymphangioleiomyomatosis.

Sirolimus has also been used to treat patients with congenital orbital lymphatic malformations. These cases are quite rare but a recent review (Shoji et al. 2020) found that 9 of 10 total patients who received sirolimus had disease response. These patients were all young (aged 1 week to 23 years). The dose ranged from 0.05 mg/kg twice a day (b.i.d.) to 1 mg b.i.d., and duration ranged from 6 to 53 months. All three patients who achieved a complete remission (CR) with sirolimus had lesions with a microcystic malformation component (Shoji et al. 2020).

There have been very few studies of sirolimus in lymphoma and no single-agent studies. A phase 1 study of sirolimus in combination with the histone deacetylase inhibitor vorinostat (Park et al. 2016) found that a dose of 4 mg PO sirolimus in combination with 300 mg of vorinostat was safe and recommended for further study. Two patients with relapsed Hodgkin's lymphoma (HL) were treated and one achieved disease response with an impressive partial remission (PR). (Armand et al. 2008) retrospectively analyzed the outcome of lymphoma patients treated with allogeneic transplantation by type of graft versus host prophylaxis. Patients who received sirolimus as part of the GVH preventive regimen had a statistically significant better outcome. The improvement was observed to be a reduced risk of lymphoma relapse rather than non-relapse mortality. This study provides an important clue that sirolimus had intrinsic anti-lymphoma efficacy.

The Rapamycin Analogs (Rapalogs)

Modifications to the structure of rapamycin were undertaken to deal with its solubility issues. The early development of these is reviewed by Dancy (2010). Although there are only a few studies in lymphoma patients with the parent compound sirolimus, there are many studies with the rapalogs. The results of these studies are first described for temsirolimus, given that they were initiated first followed by everolimus. These are summarized in Table 8.1.

Temsirolimus (CCI-779; Torisel)

Temsirolimus (Tem) is a dihydroester of rapamycin that was developed as an intravenous preparation by Wyeth Pharmaceuticals which then merged with Pfizer in 2009. Its original name in the literature was CCI-779. It is currently marketed by Pfizer for treatment of advanced renal cell carcinoma in the United States and for relapsed MCL in Europe. As of 2021, a generic version is now available in the United States from Fresenius Kabi.

- **Single-agent temsirolimus studies in relapsed mantle cell lymphoma:** The development of temsirolimus for lymphoma began with MCL because of the known overexpression of the cell cycle protein cyclin-D1 in MCL cells, and the recognition that cyclin-D1 mRNA is regulated by the mTOR pathway. In the first phase 2 trial conducted in 2002–2003 (Witzig et al. 2005), a flat dose of 250 mg/weekly was tested based on studies in solid tumors (Raymond et al. 2004). A total of 35 patients were enrolled with a median age of 70 years (range, 38–89) with most (91%) in advanced stages of disease. Patients had received a median of three prior therapies (range, 1–11), and 54% had disease refractory to the last treatment. The overall response rate (ORR) was 38% (13/34: 90% confidence interval [CI], 24–54%) with one (3%) CR and 12 (35%) PR. The median time-to-progression (TTP) in all patients was 6.5 months (95% CI, 2.9–8.3 months), and the duration of response (DOR) was 6.9 months (95% CI, 5.2–12.4 months). The main toxicity of the 250 mg weekly schedule was hematologic with 71% (25/35) having grade 3 and 11% (4/35) having grade 4 toxicities.

To reduce this myelosuppression the trial was amended by reducing the dose to 25 mg weekly IV (Ansell et al. 2008), and 29 additional patients were enrolled; 28 were evaluable for toxicity and 27 for efficacy. The patient characteristics were otherwise similar with a median of four prior therapies (range, 1–9), and 50% with disease refractory to the last treatment. With this new scheduled the ORR was 41% (11/27: 90% CI, 22–61%) with 1 (3%) CR and 10 (37%) PR; the median TTP was six months (95% CI, 3–11 months), and the median DOR was six months (range, 1–26 months). Hematologic toxicities were lower with the 25 mg weekly dose but remained the most common toxicity with 50% (14/28) grade 3 and 4% (1/28) grade 4 toxicities observed. The conclusion of the trial was to go forward with the flat dose of 25 mg weekly schedule in future trials.

Table 8.1 Summary of key studies of the mTORC1 inhibitors in lymphoma.

Agent	Year/References	Tumor type	Dose	# Patients	ORR	CR	PFS (median)
Tem	2005 (Witzig et al. 2005)	R/R MCL	250 mg	35	38%	3%	6.5 mo
Tem	2008 (Ansell et al. 2008)	R/R MCL	25 mg	29	41	4%	6 mo
Tem	2009 (Hess et al. 2009)	R/R MCL	175/75 or 25 mg	162	22%	2%	4.8 mo
Evero	2010 (Johnston et al. 2010)	R/R Hodgkin	10 mg	19	47	5%	6.2 mo
Tem	2010 (Smith et al. 2010)	R/R DLBCL	25 mg	32	28	13%	2.6
Tem	2010 (Smith et al. 2010)	R/R FL	25 mg	39	54	26%	12.7
Tem	2010 (Smith et al. 2010)	CLL/WM	25 mg	18	11	0%	4.6
Evero	2010 (Ghobrial et al. 2010)	R/R WM	10 mg	50	70	0	Not reached
Evero	2010 (Tobinai et al. 2010)	R/RNHL	5 or 10 mg	13	31%	15%	not reported
Tem/Rit	2011 (Ansell et al. 2011)	R/R MCL	25 mg	71	59	19%	10.9
Evero	2011 (Witzig et al. 2011)	R/R DLBCL/ MCL	10 mg	77	30%	4	3.4 mo
Evero	2014 (Ghobrial et al. 2014)	R/R WM	10 mg	60	73	0	21 mo
Tem/ Cladribine/R	2014 (Inwards et al. 2014)	R/R MCL	25 mg	17	94%	53%	18.7 mo
Evero	2014 (Wang et al. 2014)	R/R MCL failed Bort	10 mg	58	9%	0	4.4 mo
Evero	2015 (Witzig et al. 2015)	R/R T-cell	10 mg	16	44%	6%	4.1 mo
Tem/BR	2015 (Hess et al. 2015)	R/R MCL/FL	Tem d1, 8, 15 with BR	15	93%	33%	Not reached
Evero/RCHOP	2016 (Johnston et al. 2016; Witzig et al. 2017)	New DLBCL	10 mg d1–10 or 1–14	24	100	100	Not reached
Tem/BR	2020 (Hess et al. 2020)	R/R MCL/FL	50 mg with BR	39	89%	38%	1.55 yr
Tem/RDHAP	2020 (Witzens-Harig et al. 2021)	R/R DLBCL	25 mg or 50 mg with RDHAP	53	66%	24%	2 yr

Abbreviations: Bort = bortezomib; BR = bendamustine/rituximab; CR = complete response; DLBCL = diffuse large B-cell lymphoma; Evero = everolimus; FL = follicular lymphoma; MCL = mantle cell lymphoma; mo = months; NHL = non-Hodgkin's lymphoma; NR = not reported; ORR = overall response rate; PFS = progression-free survival; RCHOP = rituximab, cyclophosphamide, adriamycin, vincristine, prednisone; RDHAP = rituximab, dexamethasone, cytarabine, cisplatin; Tem = temsirolimus; WM = Waldenstrom's macroglobulinemia; yr = years.

Temsirolimus was moved into a large Phase 3 trial which employed a loading dose of 175 mg weekly × three weeks followed by either 75 or 25 mg weekly thereafter. The control arm was a regimen selected by the physician (Hess et al. 2009). The trial enrolled 162 patients between 2005 and 2007 and the result was an ORR of 22% (2% CR) in the Tem 175/25 mg arm versus 2% in investigator's choice ($p = 0.0019$). The median progression-free survival (PFS) for the three arms was 4.8, 3.4, and 1.9 months, respectively, with a hazard ratio of 0.44 for the Tem 175/75 versus investigator's choice arm. There was an overall survival (OS) benefit (median 12.8 vs. 9.7 months) of Tem 175/75 over investigator's choice. The most frequent grade 3 or 4 adverse events in the Tem groups were again hematologic. This established that inhibition of the PI3K/mTOR pathway was indeed effective in MCL and superior to chemotherapy available in that treatment era which was prior to the availability of Bruton's tyrosine kinase (BTK) inhibitors (Wang et al. 2013) or CAR-T cell therapy (Wang et al. 2020).

- **Single-agent temsirolimus for lymphomas other than mantle cell**: Smith et al. (2010) applied the Tem 25 mg IV weekly to other types of relapsed non-Hodgkin's lymphoma (NHL). The patients were stratified into three groups – Group A (DLBCL, transformed follicular lymphoma), Group B (follicular lymphoma [FL]), and Group C (chronic lymphocytic leukemia [CLL]/small lymphocytic lymphoma, and other indolent lymphomas). The median number of prior regimens for all patients was 2 and over 80% of all patients had failed rituximab or rituximab-containing regimens. The ORR was quite different between the three groups. Interestingly, the highest ORR (54%) was in the FL patients (Group B) with 28% ORR in aggressive NHL (Group A) and only 11% in relapsed CLL (Group C). Despite the excellent responses in FL this was never pursued with Tem; rather, the emergence of new drugs in FL shifted to the PI3K inhibitors (idelalisib, copanlisib, duvelisib, and umbralisib) which all eventually have become FDA-approved.

- **Combinations of temsirolimus with rituximab:** The above studies were the last single-agent temsirolimus studies, as the focus turned to combinations. Given the hematologic toxicity with temsirolimus, the logical next step was in combination with rituximab (Ansell et al. 2011). The study enrolled 71 patients with relapsed MCL (69 assessable) and utilized the 25 mg weekly IV temsirolimus with rituximab 375 mg/m^2 per week for four weeks during the first cycle and a single dose of rituximab every other 28-day cycle thereafter. Patients with responding disease after six cycles could continue treatment for a total of 12 cycles and were then observed without additional maintenance treatment (Ansell et al. 2011). The ORR was 59% (41/69 patients) with 19% achieving a CR. As expected, the ORR was higher for patients with rituximab-sensitive disease compared to those that were rituximab-refractory (63% vs. 52%, respectively). The median DOR for all responders was 10.6 months (11 months for the rituximab-sensitive; 6.6 months for rituximab refractory). Immunohistochemistry for tumor expression of phosphor-4EBP1 showed that the median TTP for patients with low phospho-4EBP1 expression was 10.0 months compared with 5.2 months for patients with high phospho-4EBP1 expression ($p = 0.02$). These encouraging results led to the next step to combine Tem/rituximab with a chemotherapy backbone.
- **Studies of temsirolimus with chemoimmunotherapy:** The Tem/rituximab regimen reviewed above (Ansell et al. 2011) was taken forward and combined with cladribine a purine nucleoside analog in a phase 1 study led by Inwards et al. (2014). There were 17 patients with relapsed MCL, and the dose determined to be safe was temsirolimus 25 mg IV weekly added to rituximab and cladribine at 375 mg/m^2 IV day 1 and 5 mg/m^2/day IV days 1–5 of a 28-day cycle, respectively. The ORR was 94% with 53% CR and the median PFS was 18.7 months.

Bendamustine is a commonly used chemotherapy agent for MCL in combination with rituximab (Rummel et al. 2005). However, since bendamustine/rituximab (BR) is not curative it has been combined with Tem (BeRT) in this initial study by Hess et al. (2015) and a case report by Zoellner et al. (2016). The phase 1 study included patients with relapsed disease (one to three prior therapies) and used bendamustine (90 mg/m^2, days 1, 2) and rituximab (375 mg/m^2, day 1) with temsirolimus in doses from 25 to 75 mg added on days 1, 8, 15 of a 28-day cycle. The phase 1 study included 15 (11 MCL, 4 FL) patients and reported an ORR and CR of 93% and 33%, respectively. Patients received a median of four cycles with 73% completing all planned cycles. The above schedule was confirmed without dose-limiting toxicity (DLT) criteria being met; therefore, the doses selected to move forward were the standard BR plus Tem 50 mg IV days 1, 8, and 15. The phase 2 portion of the BeRT study added 27 additional patients with either relapsed MCL or FL (Hess et al. 2020). In the entire 39 patient phase 1/2 study, 30 patients received the recommended BeRT dose with patients receiving a median of four cycles with dose intensities of all three drugs being over 95%. The regimen was well tolerated; 12 patients (31%) required growth factor support, 7 (18%) received a RBC transfusion, and 3 (8%) had a platelet transfusion. The ORR for all 37 evaluable patients was 89%, with rates of 89% and 90% for MCL and FL, respectively. The responses were durable with a median PFS of 1.6 years for all patients, 1.5 years for patients with MCL, and 1.82 years for patients with FL. The median OS has not yet been reached; however, the PFS and OS curves have not plateaued indicating the regimen is not curative.

The most recent strategy of adding Tem to standard chemoimmunotherapy was the STORM trial (Witzens-Harig et al. 2021) that enrolled patients with relapsed DLBCL who were considered candidates for salvage, platinum-based chemotherapy. In STORM, the investigators tested the standard RDHAP salvage chemoimmunotherapy regimen with rituximab 375 mg/m^2 (day 2) and DHAP (dexamethasone 40 mg days 3–6, cisplatin 100 mg/m^2 day 3, cytarabine 2×2 g/m^2 day 4). The Tem was delivered IV on days 1 and 8 of the 21-day cycle and Tem dose levels of 25, 50, 75, and 100 mg were tested. The phase 1 trial results recommended Tem 25 mg as the recommended dose for the extension cohort. A total of 53 patients were treated, and the ORR was 66% with 24% CR; 53% (28/53) of patients proceeded to high-dose therapy with stem cell rescue. The median DOR has not yet been reached and the PFS at 24 months was 53% in all patients and 78% in those who proceeded to stem cell transplantation (SCT). The OS at two years was 59% for all patients and 82% for patients who proceeded to SCT.

- **Summary of lymphoma studies with temsirolimus:** It has now been nearly 20 years since the initial testing of Tem for lymphoma. The mTORC1 targeted IV agent has clear single-agent activity against MCL, DLBCL, and FL with minimal activity in CLL. Tem has now been safely combined with rituximab, bendamustine (BeRT) and RDHAP (STORM). The Tem dose when given in combination can be 25–50 mg. However, if the 50 mg dose is used, one can expect a need for growth factors or dose reduction to 25 mg after repeated cycles. The results of BeRT and STORM offer opportunities for more widespread use in MCL and DLBCL and even relapsed FL. However, phase 3 trials will be necessary to definitively prove superiority over BR or RDHAP alone. Whether there is interest in these trials is unknown given the generic status of Tem and the newer treatments such as CAR-T (Wang et al. 2020).

Everolimus (RAD-001; Afinitor, Zortrees, Evertor)

Everolimus is an oral mTORC1 inhibitor developed by Novartis (Lebwohl et al. 2013) and first approved in Europe in 2003 and by the US FDA in 2009. It is a structural analog of rapamycin that contains a 2-hydroxethyl substitution at position 40. Its current approvals are for tuberous sclerosis complex, renal cell carcinoma, renal and hepatic transplant rejection, breast cancer, and neuroendocrine tumors. It is now available generically as Evertor (Biocon Pharma). The potential advantage of everolimus over sirolimus was its improved oral bioavailability due to its greater polarity (Kirchner et al. 2004). After oral administration it is rapidly absorbed within 1.3–1.8 hours and reaches a steady state within seven days. Flat dosing is used in adults since weight, age, and sex do not affect the levels; in children, weight-based dosing is necessary. The variation in metabolism of the drug between patients results in myelosuppression, and thus dose adjustments are frequently required (Kirchner et al. 2004). This variation cannot currently be predicted with standard assays. Its use in prevention of organ rejection is based on its acting downstream of the calcineurin inhibitors cyclosporin and tacrolimus, and thus these combinations are synergistic.

- **Single-agent trials of everolimus for relapsed lymphoma:** Yee et al. (2006) performed the first phase 1 trial of single-agent everolimus in patients with blood cancers. Two dose levels were studied – 5 and 10 mg daily PO with continuous dosing. Of the 27 patients enrolled only four had NHL (all relapsed MCL). The maximum tolerated dose (MTD) was determined to be 10 mg daily. No lymphoma patients responded, and the median number of cycles received was 1 indicating the refractory nature of this patient population. The study was useful at establishing the 5–10 mg/day dosing schedule and the toxicity profile in blood cancer patients. These reversible toxicities included grade 1 or 2 hyperlipidemia in 44%; anorexia in 37%, mucositis (oral aphthous ulcers) in 37%, diarrhea in 29%, hyperglycemia in 26% (six patients required insulin), and hypomagnesemia in 22%.

The recommended dose of 10 mg daily in 28-day cycles was used in a phase 2 trial (MC048G; NCT00436618) in relapsed lymphomas of multiple types that were stratified into three groups – aggressive, indolent, and uncommon (Johnston et al. 2010; Witzig et al. 2011; Zent et al. 2010). In this trial, the tumor response was assessed after two and six cycles, and then every three cycles until progression. The relapsed aggressive NHL group (Witzig et al. 2011) accrued 77 patients with the DLBCL subset the most common at 61% (41/77). The patient population had relapsed disease with a median of three previous therapies, while 32% of patients had undergone previous autologous stem cell transplant. The ORR in all 77 patients was 30% with all but one of the responses being a PR. The ORR varied slightly between types of NHL – 30% for DLBCL, 32% for MCL, and 38% for FL-III. The median DOR was 5.7 months. Grade 3 or 4 anemia, neutropenia, and thrombocytopenia occurred in 14%, 18%, and 38% of patients, respectively.

In the CLL arm (Zent et al. 2010), 18% (4/22) of patients experienced a PR. The most interesting aspect of this study was the first description of redistribution of malignant cells from the nodes to the blood with a signal transduction inhibitor. The absolute lymphocyte count (ALC) increased a median of 4.8-fold (range, 1.9- to 25.1-fold), and the clinically measurable lymphadenopathy decreased a median of 75.5% (range, 38–93%) compared with baseline measurements. This phenomenon occurred in eight (36%) patients. This redistribution from the nodes to blood was subsequently shown to be commonly observed with the BTK inhibitors. There was a second small (n = 7) study of everolimus for CLL (Decker et al. 2009) that found one responder.

The results of the 19 patients with R/R HL that were accrued to MC048G were reported separately (Johnston et al. 2010). They were heavily pretreated with a median of six prior therapies and 82% had failed stem cell transplant. The ORR (all PR) was a respectful 47% (9/19) with a median PFS of 6.2 months. The median DOR for the responders (CR/PR) was 7.1 months and four remained progression-free at 12 months.

Ghobrial et al. (2010) reported the results of single-agent everolimus in 50 patients with relapsed Waldenstrom's macroglobulinemia (WM) treated on MC048G. The ORR (complete response [CR] plus PR plus minimal response [MR]) was 70% with a PR of 42% and 28% MR. There was no CR. The estimated PFS rates at 6 and 12 months were 75% and 62%, respectively. Grade 3 or higher related toxicities were observed in 56% of patients with hematologic toxicities being the most common. Lung toxicity occurred in 10% of patients. Because of this success, the study was amended to accrue 10 additional patients (total of 60) and the follow-up was extended (Ghobrial et al. 2014). The ORR of all 60 patients remained similar at 73% with 50% PR. The median DOR had not been reached and median PFS was 21 months.

Members of the PI3K/mTOR pathway are also upregulated in malignant T-cells (Witzig et al. 2015). This provided a rationale to evaluate everolimus in 16 patients with relapsed T-cell NHL. The ORR in all patients was 44% (7/16) with one patient achieving a CR (PTCL-NOS) and six patients a PR (three MF, two PTCL-NOS, and one ALCL). The response rates within the different types of TCL were: 43% (3/7) in patients with CTCL; 75% (3/4) in patients with PTCL-NOS; and 20% (1/5) in other patients with TCL. The median DOR was 8.5 months with median OS of 10.2 months. Blood biomarker studies performed pre- and post-everolimus demonstrated a decrease in biologically active cytokines, namely, IL-8 and sIL2R (Witzig et al. 2015). There have been other case reports of everolimus activity in cutaneous anaplastic large cell NHL (Chumsri et al. 2008).

Tobinai et al. (2010) used the same schedule of everolimus in a phase 1 trial of 13 Japanese patients with relapsed NHL. Seven patients received 5 mg daily and six received 10 mg daily and none of the patients experienced DLT. There was one case of grade 1 non-infectious pneumonitis. The ORR was 31% (4/13). The pharmacokinetic studies revealed results similar to other studies.

Wang et al. (2014) published the results of a 58-patient multicenter trial of everolimus 10 mg daily in patients with relapsed MCL who had failed bortezomib. The study accrued patients between 2008 and 2011. The ORR was quite low at 9% when compared to the usual 30% ORR for relapsed MCL in other mTORC1 inhibitor studies which did not enroll patients who had received bortezomib (Witzig et al. 2005, 2011). In the phase 3 trial of Tem versus clinician's choice (Hess et al. 2009), the ORR was lower at 22% and 23% of enrolled patients had previously received bortezomib. Based on these results, it appears that failing bortezomib predicts for a lower ORR to mTORC1 targeted single agents.

- **Trials of adjuvant everolimus for prevention of relapse:** There have been two studies using everolimus as maintenance therapy after induction chemotherapy (Schoch et al. 2018; Witzig et al. 2018). The first approach used everolimus as maintenance after SCT. The dose of everolimus was adjusted to achieve a serum trough level between 3 and 15 ng/ml. In addition, rituximab maintenance was given every three months. A total of 49 patients were enrolled with 26 (53%) having MCL. The dose of everolimus needed to achieve the target serum level was 2.5 mg daily or qod. At the time of publication at a timepoint of 30 months post-enrollment, 58% of patients remained progression free and 93% were alive. This targeted concentration-level strategy uses a smaller dose of everolimus. What exactly it is contributing to the disease outcome beyond the maintenance rituximab awaits a phase 3 trial.

The second trial of maintenance everolimus was the PILLAR-2 trial (Witzig et al. 2018). This trial enrolled high-risk patients with DLBCL who were in their first CR based on a negative PET scan at the end of treatment. A total of 742 patients were randomized to one year of everolimus (n = 372) versus placebo (n = 370). Only 48% of everolimus patients completed the one year of treatment compared with 67% of placebo patients. The main reason was a higher adverse event rate between everolimus and placebo (30% vs. 12%), but a lower relapse rate (6% vs. 13%). Everolimus did not significantly improve DFS compared with placebo (hazard ratio 0.92).

- **Combination of everolimus with RCHOP for new, untreated DLBCL:** Given the single activity in relapsed DLBCL (Witzig et al. 2011), the importance of the PI3K/mTOR pathway in DLBCL cells (Roschewski et al. 2014), and the unmet need to improve RCHOP in upfront disease, a phase 1 and feasibility study in the NCTN Alliance group (study N1085) explored everolimus plus standard RCHOP for upfront treatment of DLBCL. The trial accrued 26 patients between 2012 and 2014 and used standard RCHOP with pegfilgrastim plus everolimus 10 mg days 1–10 (level 1) or 1–14 (level 2) every 21 days for six cycles. The median time from diagnosis to treatment (DtT) was 14 days which according to previous publications (Maurer et al. 2018) would predict an EFS24 of 56% in this patient population. The trial results demonstrated that the 10 mg dose days 1–14 was acceptable and the one to be taken forward. The ORR was 96% (23/24) as determined by PET imaging (Johnston et al. 2016). All patients have been assessed for EFS24 and there were no DLBCL relapses (Witzig et al. 2017).
- **Combination of everolimus with CHOP for T-cell lymphoma:** A 15-patient phase 1 trial of everolimus with CHOP (without pegfilgrastim) for new, untreated T-cell NHL was conducted (Kim et al. 2013). It determined that 5 mg of everolimus on days 1–14 was the MTD and should be used for further trials, although the combination was noted to be relatively toxic. There has been no further testing of everolimus/CHOP for T-cell NHL.

Summary of Lymphoma Studies of Everolimus

Everolimus has definite single-agent activity in many subtypes of B-cell and T-cell lymphoma. Given what we now know about the mTORC1/mTORC2 pathway it is not surprising that there is activity in lymphoma, and that it appears modest at best. The only combinations that have been tested are with RCHOP in DLBCL where the results have been encouraging and durable. To date, the authors have been unsuccessful in obtaining industry approval to evaluate everolimus plus RCHOP in a randomized phase 3 clinical trial. One reasonable question to pose at this juncture is, "why did the clinical development of everolimus in lymphoma stall?" While the combination of everolimus with RCHOP was impressive it was a small trial, and it came after the PILLAR-2 everolimus maintenance trial failed to meet its statistical goals. A phase 3 concept to evaluate everolimus/RCHOP versus RCHOP was developed in the NCTN but drug company interest waned as the drug became generic. At the same time as these events were occurring there was substantial interest and indeed FDA-approval of both oral and IV PI3K inhibitors that also showed activity in lymphoma. Investigators have now shifted attention to using PI3K inhibitors with RCHOP such as the ongoing trial parsaclisib/RCHOP (NCT04323956).

Despite these setbacks, these results remain important since they highlight the importance of targeting the PI3K/mTOR pathway. Recent data from experiments on DLBCL tumors has demonstrated that a multiprotein supercomplex formed by MYD88, TLR9, and the B-cell receptor (My-T-BCR) signals through mTOR (Phelan et al. 2018). Indeed, mTOR is an essential component of this My-T-BCR supercomplex. Thus, future studies may find increased benefit in patients with tumors that harbor this supercomplex. Despite the new agents that have impacted the treatment of HL, FL, and WM, patients will still fail and having an oral agent such as everolimus can be useful. In addition, the generic Tem and everolimus may make these treatments more cost-effective.

Ridaforolimus

Ridaforolimus is another rapalog that has been tested primarily in solid tumors and is currently not approved for any cancer. It is approved for use in drug-eluting stents (Saito et al. 2021).

Dual Inhibitors of mTORC1 and mTORC2

Mechanistic studies in lymphoma have demonstrated that DLBCL and MCL tumors have upregulated expression of both mTORC1 (pS6, 4EBP1) and mTORC2 (Akt) (Gupta et al. 2009; Hsieh and Ruggero 2010). Inhibition of only mTORC1 allows the pathway activation to continue through mTORC2. Indeed, treatment with rapamycin or rapalogs can upregulate mTORC2 through Akt and this can be blunted with combinations of HDAC inhibitors such as panobinostat (Gupta et al. 2009). It must also be recalled that the rapalogs are cytostatic drugs not cytotoxic as demonstrated in Figure 2 (Witzig et al. 2011). The promising results with rapalogs and a better understanding of these resistance mechanisms led to substantial efforts to develop dual mTORC1/2 inhibitors. The field is reviewed in the excellent report by Chen and Zhou (Chen and Zhou 2020). Here we review OSI-027 which has been investigated in lymphoma *in vitro* and in other cancers *in vivo*.

- **OSI-027**: OS-027 is an oral mTOR kinase inhibitor that binds to and inhibits both mTORC1 and mTORC2 complexes in lymphoma cells (Gupta et al. 2012). When tested *in vitro* on human lymphoma cell lines OSI-027 can inhibit the p70S6kinase (mTORC1) and pAkt (mTORC2) with anti-lymphoma activity in cell line and mouse models. The drug was tested in a large 128 patient broad phase 1 trial with no responses (5% stable disease) and was nephrotoxic (Mateo et al. 2016). Since no patients with lymphoma were included in the trial, the *in vitro/in vivo* results (Gupta et al. 2012) remain untested and unconfirmed. OSI Pharmaceuticals was acquired by Astellas Pharmaceuticals with no published plans to pursue additional studies with OSI-027.

Side Effects of mTORC1 Inhibitors

- **Myelosuppression**: The most important DLT for these drugs is myelosuppression. The initial studies of Tem used a 250 mg IV weekly schedule and 71% of patients experienced grade 3 and 11% grade 4 hematologic toxicity. Subsequent studies have found the 25 mg flat dose weekly to be better tolerated. Even so, in heavily pretreated patients or those with marrow involvement dose delays or the use of growth factors may be necessary to maintain the schedule. When Tem was combined with BR (BeRT) for patients with relapsed MCL or FL (Hess et al. 2020) 56% experienced grade 3/4 leukopenia and 36% grade 3/4 thrombocytopenia. In the STORM trial where Tem was combined with RDHAP (Witzens-Harig et al. 2021), the hematological toxicity was substantial as expected given the RDHAP. However, the incidence of febrile neutropenia was only 13%. For everolimus, again myelosuppression is commonly encountered. In the MC048G study of relapsed aggressive patients (Witzig et al. 2011), grade 3 or 4 anemia, neutropenia, and thrombocytopenia occurred in 14%, 18%, and 38% of patients, respectively. Although dosing was initiated at 10 mg PO qd, dose adjustments to 5 mg qd or qod were allowed. The combination of everolimus with CHOP-based chemotherapy has only been tested in two studies (Johnston et al. 2016; Kim et al. 2013; Witzig et al. 2017). In the everolimus/RCHOP study, the patients were newly diagnosed, untreated, and thus had better marrow function (Johnston et al. 2016; Witzig et al. 2017). Grade 3/4 neutropenia occurred in 75% of patients but febrile neutropenia in only 21%. In summary, the doses of Tem are recommended to be 25 mg IV weekly and everolimus at 10 mg daily with options of reducing to 5 mg qd or qod. Growth factor support is helpful and was mandated in the everolimus/RCHOP study (Johnston et al. 2016).
- **Pneumonitis**: The mTOR inhibitors as a class can cause a non-infectious pneumonitis. This can be asymptomatic or symptomatic with cough and shortness of breath. The asymptomatic cases are usually detected at the time of a restaging CT or PET/CT. In the large PILLAR-2 trial of adjuvant single-agent everolimus, the incidence of non-infectious pneumonitis that led to treatment discontinuation was 2% (Witzig et al. 2018). In patients with active lymphoma enrolled in MC048G, the incidence was 1% (Witzig et al. 2011). In the everolimus/RCHOP trial (Johnston et al. 2016), pneumonitis was not observed likely because prednisone was given at high dose for five days of each cycle as part of the RCHOP component of the regimen. Patients with asymptomatic pneumonitis by imaging can be observed and continued on drug. If they become symptomatic, then depending on severity, treatment with oral corticosteroids and/or interruption/dose reduction of the mTOR inhibitors is advised. Actual infection must always be kept in mind since these patients are immunosuppressed.
- **Aphthous ulcers/mucositis:** This is a unique side effect that occurs in patients treated with mTOR inhibitors usually within the first two months of therapy (Rugo et al. 2016). It is somewhat unusual and unpredictable and was documented as grade 3/4 in 3% of the patients in MC048G (Witzig et al. 2011). These can be very irritating for patients and often lead to interruption in dosing and/or dose reductions. There is much more experience in dealing with this

complication-n in women with breast cancer who are being treated with everolimus. Rugo et al. (2017) performed a phase 2 prevention trial where women starting everolimus 10 mg daily were given 10 ml of alcohol-free dexamethasone 0.5 mg per 5 ml oral solution (swish for two minutes and spit, four times daily [q.i.d.] for eight weeks). The incidence of grade ≥2 stomatitis was 3% compared to the historical control of 33% in the BOLERO-2 trial (Rugo et al. 2017). Although this prevention strategy has not been tried in the lymphoma setting, it appears to be an excellent preventive strategy.

- **Metabolic effects:** Given the key role of mTOR in metabolism it is not surprising that inhibition of mTOR could induce metabolic side effects. Both hyperglycemia and hyperlipidemia are commonly observed in patients on mTOR inhibitors. Patients with pre-existing diabetes or hyperlipidemia can expect to note worsening of those conditions requiring careful follow-up. The pathophysiology of these effects and recommended management has been reported by Busaidy et al. (2012). In lymphoma, as in other diseases where mTOR agents are used the incidence of grade 3/4 toxicity is low. For example, 8% of patients developed grade 3/4 hyperglycemia in MC058G (Witzig et al. 2011). The risk of grade 3/4 hyperlipidemia was even lower at 1% (Witzig et al. 2011). Thus, these metabolic side effects are important to note but are manageable. For patients with baseline diabetes and hyperlipidemia it is important to include the physician team managing those aspects of the patient's care at the start of mTORC inhibitor therapy.

Future Directions for mTOR Inhibitors in Lymphoma

In 2022, where do the mTOR inhibitors stand in the field of lymphoma? The biological rationale of targeting mTOR is strong and, as presented in this chapter, there is solid evidence for activity of both Tem and everolimus as single agents in both HL and NHL and both T-cell and B-cell subtypes. Both agents are available for use and are now generic. The studies of combinations with Tem have been with commonly used regimens such as BR (Hess et al. 2020) and RDHAP (Witzens-Harig et al. 2021) but in both these studies the patients had relapsed disease. There have not been any lymphoma trials that incorporated Tem upfront. In the study of everolimus with RCHOP (Johnston et al. 2016; Witzig et al. 2017) for newly diagnosed DLBCL patients, the results were very impressive and worthy of further study. Despite the above, neither Tem nor everolimus is widely used for the treatment of lymphoma as single agents, and although the combination trials that were conducted were encouraging they never proceeded to definitive phase 3 trials. Despite substantial efforts to develop mTORC1/mTORC2 inhibitors, none have been adequately tested in lymphoma. None of these studies in Table 8.1 used current mutation/pathway analysis to select for patients. Given our improved understanding of biology selecting lymphoma patients for mTORC1 inhibitor regimens holds real potential for enriching responses. Finally, to be successful a drug needs the full support and financial backing of pharmaceutical companies. This was present early on but as the lymphoma field moved into the eras of BTK inhibitors, PI3K inhibitors, CAR-T, and now bispecific antibodies the mTOR inhibitors were left behind.

Given these current realities, what are the opportunities? Despite all the new agents from the last decade, there remain major challenges for lymphoma patients. What could be or should be tested? The goal of any new trials should be to combine the mTORC1 inhibitor with chemoimmunotherapy. The advantage of this strategy is that it takes advantage of the targeted approach of the mTOR inhibitor with the established efficacy of chemoimmunotherapy. The goals would be improved ORR and CR rate and a lower relapse rate while largely avoiding any of the toxicities associated with chronic use of mTORC1 inhibitors. This is exactly what was accomplished with everolimus/RCHOP DLBCL × six cycles pilot (Witzig et al. 2017) but has yet to be confirmed in a phase 3. There remains unmet need to improve upfront therapy of basically all the NHL – FL, DLBCL, MCL, marginal cell, and peripheral T-cell. Since mTORC1 inhibitors have activity in all these diseases, there still remains opportunity for phase 3 trials. Since BeRT has been tested in relapsed (Hess et al. 2020) FL and given that ECOG2408 did not change the upfront treatment of FL from the current BR and rituximab maintenance standard (Evens et al. 2020), it would be plausible (and interesting) to test BR versus BeRT in new, untreated FL. For DLBCL testing the everolimus/RCHOP regimen in a trial where genomic testing to randomize patients by genomic signatures and pathway analysis (Chapuy et al. 2018; Phelan et al. 2018; Schmitz et al. 2018) would be the optimal strategy since the field has moved beyond randomization by gene expression profiling. Indeed, the National Clinical Trials Network is discussing a such a strategy where genomic testing would be a part of the randomization at cycle 2 to learn if the standard RCHOP can be improved upon. Upfront therapy of peripheral T-cell NHL (PTCL) was improved by brentuximab in the ECHELON-2 trial (Horwitz et al. 2019) but there is much room for improvement and the activity of everolimus in T-cell lymphoma (Witzig et al. 2015) could be explored in combination with the brentuximab-CHP regimen. The protocol situation in upfront MCL is saturated at this time with the three-arm NCTN trial (EA4181; NCT04115631) that is using the BR/cytarabine backbone with or without the BTK inhibitor acalabrutinib. Depending on the results there will be opportunity to add further with a BeRT-type regimen. The situation in salvage therapy for aggressive NHL remains stagnant with platinum-based regimens still the norm (Crump et al. 2014). This provides opportunities for combinations with mTOR inhibitors as recently described (Witzens-Harig et al. 2021). If any of these trials are conducted, they should include state-of-the art genomic studies to learn if specific signatures can guide therapy.

Whether any of these trials will ever be performed is uncertain at this time. The generic nature of these drugs can be an advantage in settings where cost is important; however, the pharmaceutical support is likely to be lacking in these settings. The heightened focus on targeting at the level of PI3K may also continue to dominate the field as it has over the last 10 years and thus the combination trials discussed above may occur with a PI3K inhibitor rather than an mTOR inhibitor. In the end, the rationale is strong for targeting the PI3K/mTOR pathway and these investigations will continue and should continue. Which drug class and specific drug wins will need to be driven by novel ideas, a specific genomically driven pathway signature that predicts response to mTOR inhibitor-containing regimens as well as pharmaceutical and NCTN support.

Must Read References

Hess, G., Wagner, K., Keller, U. et al. (2020). Final results of a phase l/ll trial of the combination bendamustine and rituximab with temsirolimus (BeRT) in relapsed mantle cell lymphoma and follicular lymphoma. *Hemasphere* 4 (3): e398. Epub 2020/07/11. doi: 10.1097/HS9.0000000000000398. PubMed PMID: 32647802; PMCID: PMC7306311.

Johnston, P.B., Laplant, B., McPhail, E. et al. (2016). Everolimus combined with R-CHOP-21 for new, untreated, diffuse large B-cell lymphoma (NCCTG 1085[Alliance]): safety and efficacy results of a phase 1 and feasibility trial. *Lancet Haemato.* 3 (7): e309-16. Epub 2016/07/05. doi: 10.1016/S2352-3026(16)30040-0. PubMed PMID: 27374464; PMCID: PMC4958393.

Witzens-Harig M., Viardot A., Keller U. et al. (2021). The mTOR inhibitor temsirolimus added to rituximab combined with dexamethasone, cytarabine, and cisplatinum (R-DHAP) for the Treatment of Patients With Relapsed or Refractory DLBCL - Results From the Phase-ll STORM Trial. *Hemasphere* 5 (10): e636. Epub 2021/10/01. doi: 10.1097/HS9.0000000000000636. PubMed PMID: 34589671; PMCID: PMC8476051.

References

Abraham, R.T. (1998). Mammalian target of rapamycin: immunosuppressive drugs uncover a novel pathway of cytokine receptor signaling. *Curr. Opin. Immunol.* 10 (3): 330–336.

Ansell, S.M., Inwards, D.J., Rowland, K.M., Jr. et al. (2008). Low-dose, single-agent temsirolimus for relapsed mantle cell lymphoma: a phase 2 trial in the North Central Cancer Treatment Group. *Cancer* 113 (3): 508–514.

Ansell, S.M., Tang, H., Kurtin, P.J. et al. (2011). Temsirolimus and rituximab in patients with relapsed or refractory mantle cell lymphoma: a phase 2 study. *Lancet Oncol.* 12 (4): 361–368.

Armand, P., Gannamaneni, S., Kim, H.T. et al. (2008). Improved survival in lymphoma patients receiving sirolimus for graft-versus-host disease prophylaxis after allogeneic hematopoietic stem-cell transplantation with reduced-intensity conditioning. *J. Clin. Oncol.* 26 (35): 5767–5774.

Brunn, G.J., Williams, J., Sabers, C. et al. (1996). Direct inhibition of the signaling functions of the mammalian target of rapamycin by the phosphoinositide 3-kinase inhibitors, wortmannin and LY294002. *EMBO J.* 15 (19): 5256–5267.

Busaidy, N.L., Farooki, A., Dowlati, A. et al. (2012). Management of metabolic effects associated with anticancer agents targeting the PI3K-Akt-mTOR pathway. *J. Clin. Oncol.* 30 (23): 2919–2928.

Chapuy, B., Stewart, C., Dunford, A.J. et al. (2018). Molecular subtypes of diffuse large B cell lymphoma are associated with distinct pathogenic mechanisms and outcomes. *Nat. Med.* 24 (5): 679–690.

Chen, Y. and Zhou, X. (2020). Research progress of mTOR inhibitors. *Eur. J. Med. Chem.* 208: 112820.

Chiang, G.G. and Abraham, R.T. (2007). Targeting the mTOR signaling network in cancer. *Trends. Mol. Med.* 13 (10): 433–442.

Chumsri, S., Zhao, M., Garofalo, M. et al. (2008). Inhibition of the mammalian target of rapamycin (mTOR) in a case of refractory primary cutaneous anaplastic large cell lymphoma. *Leuk. Lymphoma.* 49 (2): 359–361.

Crump, M., Kuruvilla, J., Couban, S. et al. (2014). Randomized comparison of gemcitabine, dexamethasone, and cisplatin versus dexamethasone, cytarabine, and cisplatin chemotherapy before autologous stem-cell transplantation for relapsed and refractory aggressive lymphomas: NCIC-CTG LY.12. *J. Clin. Oncol.* 32 (31): 3490–3496.

Dancey, J. (2010). mTOR signaling and drug development in cancer. *Nat. Rev. Clin. Oncol.* 7 (4): 209–219.

Dann, S.G., Selvaraj, A., and Thomas, G. (2007). mTOR complex1-S6K1 signaling: at the crossroads of obesity, diabetes and cancer. *Trends. Mol. Med.* 13 (6): 252–259.

Decker, T., Sandherr, M., Goetze, K. et al. (2009). A pilot trial of the mTOR (mammalian target of rapamycin) inhibitor RAD001 in patients with advanced B-CLL. *Ann. Hematol.* 88 (3): 221–227.

Easton, J.B. and Houghton, P.J. (2006). mTOR and cancer therapy. *Oncogene* 25 (48): 6436–6446.

Evens, A.M., Hong, F., Habermann, T.M. et al. (2020). A three-arm randomized phase II study of bendamustine/rituximab with bortezomib induction or lenalidomide continuation in untreated follicular lymphoma: ECOG-ACRIN E2408. *Clin. Cancer Res.* 26 (17): 4468–4477.

Faivre, S., Kroemer, G., and Raymond, E. (2006). Current development of mTOR inhibitors as anticancer agents. *Nat. Rev. Drug Discov.* 5 (8): 671–688.

Ghobrial, I.M., Gertz, M., Laplant, B. et al. (2010). Phase II trial of the oral mammalian target of rapamycin inhibitor everolimus in relapsed or refractory Waldenstrom macroglobulinemia. *J. Clin. Oncol.* 28 (8): 1408–1414.

Ghobrial, I.M., Witzig, T.E., Gertz, M. et al. (2014). Long-term results of the phase II trial of the oral mTOR inhibitor everolimus (RAD001) in relapsed or refractory Waldenstrom Macroglobulinemia. *Am. J. Hematol.* 89 (3): 237–242.

Gupta, M., Ansell, S.M., Novak, A.J. et al. (2009). Inhibition of histone deacetylase overcomes rapamycin-mediated resistance in diffuse large B-cell lymphoma by inhibiting Akt signaling through mTORC2. *Blood* 114 (14): 2926–2935.

Gupta, M., Hendrickson, A.E., Yun, S.S. et al. (2012). Dual mTORC1/mTORC2 inhibition diminishes Akt activation and induces Puma-dependent apoptosis in lymphoid malignancies. *Blood* 119 (2): 476–487.

Heitman, J., Movva, N.R., and Hall, M.N. (1991). Targets for cell cycle arrest by the immunosuppressant rapamycin in yeast. *Science* 253 (5022): 905–909.

Hess, G., Herbrecht, R., Romaguera, J. et al. (2009). Phase III study to evaluate temsirolimus compared with investigator's choice therapy for the treatment of relapsed or refractory mantle cell lymphoma. *J. Clin. Oncol.* 27 (23): 3822–3829.

Hess, G., Keller, U., Scholz, C.W. et al. (2015). Safety and efficacy of Temsirolimus in combination with Bendamustine and Rituximab in relapsed mantle cell and follicular lymphoma. *Leukemia* 29 (8): 1695–1701.

Hess, G., Wagner, K., Keller, U. et al. (2020). Final results of a phase I/II trial of the combination bendamustine and Rituximab with Temsirolimus (BeRT) in relapsed mantle cell lymphoma and follicular lymphoma. *Hemasphere* 4 (3): e398.

Horwitz, S., O'Connor, O.A., Pro, B. et al. (2019). Brentuximab vedotin with chemotherapy for CD30-positive peripheral T-cell lymphoma (ECHELON-2): a global, double-blind, randomised, phase 3 trial. *Lancet* 393 (10168): 229–240.

Hsieh, A.C. and Ruggero, D. (2010). Targeting eukaryotic translation initiation factor 4E (eIF4E) in cancer. *Clin. Cancer Res.* 16 (20): 4914–4920.

Inoki, K. and Guan, K.L. (2006). Complexity of the TOR signaling network. *Trends Cell Biol.* 16 (4): 206–212.

Inwards, D.J., Fishkin, P.A., LaPlant, B.R. et al. (2014). Phase I trial of rituximab, cladribine, and temsirolimus (RCT) for initial therapy of mantle cell lymphoma. *Ann. Oncol.* 25 (10): 2020–2024.

Johnston, P.B., Inwards, D.J., Colgan, J.P. et al. (2010). A phase II trial of the oral mTOR inhibitor everolimus in relapsed Hodgkin lymphoma. *Am. J. Hematol.* 85 (5): 320–324.

Johnston, P.B., LaPlant, B., McPhail, E. et al. (2016). Everolimus combined with R-CHOP-21 for new, untreated, diffuse large B-cell lymphoma (NCCTG 1085 [Alliance]): safety and efficacy results of a phase 1 and feasibility trial. *Lancet Haematol* 3 (7): e309–316.

Kim, S.J., Kang, H.J., Kim, J.S. et al. (2013). A phase I study of everolimus and CHOP in newly diagnosed peripheral T-cell lymphomas. *Invest. New Drugs* 31 (6): 1514–1521.

Kirchner, G.I., Meier-Wiedenbach, I., and Manns, M.P. (2004). Clinical pharmacokinetics of everolimus. *Clin. Pharmacokinet* 43 (2): 83–95.

Lebwohl, D., Anak, O., Sahmoud, T. et al. (2013). Development of everolimus, a novel oral mTOR inhibitor, across a spectrum of diseases. *Ann. N. Y. Acad. Sci.* 1291: 14–32.

Mamane, Y., Petroulakis, E., LeBacquer, O. et al. (2006). mTOR, translation initiation and cancer. *Oncogene* 25 (48): 6416–6422.

Manning, B.D. (2017). Game of TOR - The target of rapamycin rules four kingdoms. *N. Engl. J. Med.* 377 (13): 1297–1299.

Mateo, J., Olmos, D., Dumez, H. et al. (2016). A first in man, dose-finding study of the mTORC1/mTORC2 inhibitor OSI-027 in patients with advanced solid malignancies. *Br. J. Cancer* 114 (8): 889–896.

Maurer, M.J., Ghesquieres, H., Link, B.K. et al. (2018). Diagnosis-to-treatment interval is an important clinical factor in newly diagnosed diffuse large B-cell lymphoma and has implication for bias in clinical trials. *J. Clin. Oncol.* 36 (16): 1603–1610.

Park, H., Garrido-Laguna, I., Naing, A. et al. (2016). Phase I dose-escalation study of the mTOR inhibitor sirolimus and the HDAC inhibitor vorinostat in patients with advanced malignancy. *Oncotarget* 7 (41).

Phelan, J.D., Young, R.M., Webster, D.E. et al. (2018). A multiprotein supercomplex controlling oncogenic signalling in lymphoma. *Nature* 560 (7718): 387–391.

Raymond, E., Alexandre, J., Faivre, S. et al. (2004). Safety and pharmacokinetics of escalated doses of weekly intravenous infusion of CCI-779, a novel mTOR inhibitor, in patients with cancer. *J. Clin. Oncol.* 22 (12): 2336–2347.

Roschewski, M., Staudt, L.M., and Wilson, W.H. (2014). Diffuse large B-cell lymphoma-treatment approaches in the molecular era. *Nat Rev. Clin. Oncol.* 11 (1): 12–23.

Rugo, H.S., Hortobagyi, G.N., Yao, J. et al. (2016). Meta-analysis of stomatitis in clinical studies of everolimus: incidence and relationship with efficacy. *Ann. Oncol.* 27 (3): 519–525.

Rugo, H.S., Seneviratne, L., Beck, J.T. et al. (2017). Prevention of everolimus-related stomatitis in women with hormone receptor-positive, HER2-negative metastatic breast cancer using dexamethasone mouthwash (SWISH): a single-arm, phase 2 trial. *Lancet Oncol.* 18 (5): 654–662.

Rummel, M.J., Al-Batran, S.E., Kim, S.Z. et al. (2005). Bendamustine plus rituximab is effective and has a favorable toxicity profile in the treatment of mantle cell and low-grade non-Hodgkin's lymphoma. *J. Clin. Oncol.* 23 (15): 3383–3389.

Sabatini, D.M. (2006). mTOR and cancer: insights into a complex relationship. *Nat. Rev. Cancer* 6 (9): 729–734.

Sabers, C.J., Martin, M.M., Brunn, G.J. et al. (1995). Isolation of a protein target of the FKBP12-rapamycin complex in mammalian cells. *J. Biol. Chem.* 270 (2): 815–822.

Saito, S., Yamazaki, S., Otsuji, S. et al. (2021). Ridaforolimus eluting stent for the treatment of Japanese patients with coronary disease: 1 year outcomes of the JNIR study. *Cardiovasc Interv. Ther.* 36 (3): 273–280.

Schmitz, R., Wright, G.W., Huang, D.W. et al. (2018). Genetics and pathogenesis of diffuse large B-cell lymphoma. *N. Engl. J. Med.* 378 (15): 1396–1407.

Schoch, L., Asiama, A., Zahurak, M. et al. (2018). Pharmacokinetically-targeted dosed everolimus maintenance therapy in lymphoma patients. *Cancer Chemother. Pharmacol.* 81.

Sehgal, S.N. (1998). Rapamune (RAPA, rapamycin, sirolimus): mechanism of action immunosuppressive effect results from blockade of signal transduction and inhibition of cell cycle progression. *Clin. Biochem.* 31 (5): 335–340.

Sehgal, S.N., Baker, H., and Vezina, C. (1975). Rapamycin (AY-22,989), a new antifungal antibiotic. II. Fermentation, isolation and characterization. *J. Antibiot.* 28 (10): 727–732.

Shoji, M.K., Shishido, S., and Freitag, S.K. (2020). The use of sirolimus for treatment of orbital lymphatic malformations: a systematic review. *Ophthalmic Plast. Reconstr. Surg.* 36 (3): 215–221.

Smith, S.M., van Besien, K., Karrison, T. et al. (2010). Temsirolimus has activity in non-mantle cell non-Hodgkin's lymphoma subtypes: the University of Chicago phase II consortium. *J. Clin. Oncol.* 28 (31): 4740–4746.

Tobinai, K., Ogura, M., Maruyama, D. et al. (2010). Phase I study of the oral mammalian target of rapamycin inhibitor everolimus (RAD001) in Japanese patients with relapsed or refractory non-Hodgkin lymphoma. *Int. J. Hematol.* 92 (4): 563–570.

Vezina, C., Kudelski, A., and Sehgal, S.N. (1975). Rapamycin (AY-22,989), a new antifungal antibiotic. I. Taxonomy of the producing streptomycete and isolation of the active principle. *J. Antibiot.* 28 (10): 721–726.

Wang, M., Munoz, J., Goy, A. et al. (2020). KTE-X19 CAR T-cell therapy in relapsed or refractory mantle-cell lymphoma. *N. Engl. J. Med.* 382 (14): 1331–1342.

Wang, M., Popplewell, L.L., Collins, R.H., Jr. et al. (2014). Everolimus for patients with mantle cell lymphoma refractory to or intolerant of bortezomib: multicentre, single-arm, phase 2 study. *Br. J. Haematol.* 165 (4): 510–518.

Wang, M.L., Rule, S., Martin, P. et al. (2013). Targeting BTK with ibrutinib in relapsed or refractory mantle-cell lymphoma. *N. Engl. J. Med.* 369 (6): 507–516.

Witzens-Harig, M., Viardot, A., Keller, U. et al. (2021). The mTOR inhibitor temsirolimus added to rituximab combined with dexamethasone, cytarabine, and cisplatinum (R-DHAP) for the treatment of patients with relapsed or refractory DLBCL - results from the phase-II STORM trial. *Hemasphere* 5 (10): e636.

Witzig, T.E., Geyer, S.M., Ghobrial, I. et al. (2005). Phase II trial of single-agent temsirolimus (CCI-779) for relapsed mantle cell lymphoma. *J. Clin. Oncol.* 23 (23): 5347–5356.

Witzig, T.E., LaPlant, B., Habermann, T.M. et al. (2017). High rate of event-free survival at 24 months with everolimus/RCHOP for untreated diffuse large B-cell lymphoma: updated results from NCCTG N1085 (Alliance). *Blood Cancer J.* 7 (6): e576.

Witzig, T.E., Reeder, C., Han, J.J. et al. (2015). The mTORC1 inhibitor everolimus has antitumor activity in vitro and produces tumor responses in patients with relapsed T-cell lymphoma. *Blood* 126 (3): 328–335.

Witzig, T.E., Reeder, C.B., LaPlant, B.R. et al. (2011). A phase II trial of the oral mTOR inhibitor everolimus in relapsed aggressive lymphoma. *Leukemia* 25 (2): 341–347.

Witzig, T.E., Tobinai, K., Rigacci, L. et al. (2018). Adjuvant everolimus in high-risk diffuse large B-cell lymphoma: final results from the PILLAR-2 randomized phase III trial. *Ann. Oncol.* 29 (3): 707–714.

Yee, K.W., Zeng, Z., Konopleva, M. et al. (2006). Phase I/II study of the mammalian target of rapamycin inhibitor everolimus (RAD001) in patients with relapsed or refractory hematologic malignancies. *Clin. Cancer Res.* 12 (17): 5165–5173.

Zent, C.S., LaPlant, B.R., Johnston, P.B. et al. (2010). The treatment of recurrent/refractory chronic lymphocytic leukemia/small lymphocytic lymphoma (CLL) with everolimus results in clinical responses and mobilization of CLL cells into the circulation. *Cancer* 116 (9): 2201–2207.

Zoellner, A.K., Weiglein, T., Hutter, G. et al. (2016). Temsirolimus acts as additive with bendamustine in aggressive lymphoma. *Ann. Hematol.* 95 (3): 403–407.

9

PI3 Kinase, AKT, and mTOR Inhibitors

Joel McCay and John G. Gribben

Centre for Haemato-Oncology, Barts Cancer Institute, Queen Mary University of London, London, UK

Take Home Messages

- Phosphatidylinositol 3-kinase (PI3K) inhibitors are effective treatments for B-cell malignancies, but many have unique toxicities based on the differential expression of the four different PI3K isoforms in different body tissues and organs.
- Unique toxicities include autoimmune effects (colitis, hepatitis, pneumonitis, rash), opportunistic infections (cytomegalovirus [CMV], *Pneumocystis jirovecii* pneumonia [PJP]), hypertension, hyperglycemia, and neuropsychiatric changes. Inhibition of different PI3K isoforms is associated with different toxicities.
- Many toxicities associated with PI3K inhibitors can be effectively managed while continuing treatment, while others require drug discontinuation. Prompt attention to reported toxicities and adherence to prescribing information and expert guidelines are essential for optimal outcomes of patients receiving these therapies.

Introduction

Phosphatidylinositol-3-kinase (PI3K)/AKT signaling constitutes an important intracellular pathway that consists of two parts: PI3K and its downstream molecule AKT (also known as serine/threonine protein kinase B [PKB]) (Bilanges et al. 2019). AKT and the mammalian target of rapamycin (mTOR) signaling pathways are crucial to many aspects of signal transduction and biological processes including cell proliferation, apoptosis, metabolism, and angiogenesis, in physiological as well as in many pathological conditions including cancer. These pathways are so interconnected that they are usually regarded as a single pathway. Here we address the present status of the development of specific PI3K, AKT, and mTOR inhibitors, their clinical utility, and toxicities.

The PI3K/AKT/mTOR pathway is stimulated by receptor tyrosine kinase (RTK) and cytokine receptor activation (Figure 9.1). Tyrosine residues are then phosphorylated and provide anchor sites for PI3K translocation to the cell membrane, thereby participating in the transduction of various extracellular matrix molecules and cytokines. This signaling pathway also has important biological effects on cells, such as enhancing viability and inhibiting senescence, aging, and death and is associated with a range of physiological and pathological activities. Dysfunction of this pathway is related not only to the development of cancers but also many other human diseases. The structure and function of the PI3K/AKT/mTOR signaling pathway and its relationship with upstream and downstream molecules are complex, and further research is clearly needed for a complete understanding of the impacts of inhibiting this pathway. This review aims to summarize the recent research and clinical progress on the PI3K/AKT/mTOR signaling pathway in cancer.

The PI3K/AKT pathway is a key regulator of survival during cellular stress and the role of this pathway in cancer appears crucial (Datta et al. 1999). mTOR is a serine/threonine kinase ubiquitously expressed in mammalian cells (Hennessy et al. 2005). mTOR integrates signals initiated by a number of cellular stimuli to regulate downstream signaling and protein synthesis. It is involved in the initiation of ribosomal translation of mRNA into proteins necessary for cell growth, cell cycle progression, and cell metabolism through its downstream effectors, 4EBP1 and P70S6 kinase (S6K).

Somatic mutations and/or gains and losses of key genes are among a number of genetic alterations affecting these pathways in a number of different solid and hematological cancers. The activation of the PI3K/AKT/mTOR pathway results in a profound disturbance of control of cell growth and survival, leading to a competitive growth advantage, metastatic competence, angiogenesis, and therapy resistance. Therefore, although complex, this pathway is considered one

Precision Cancer Therapies: Targeting Oncogenic Drivers and Signaling Pathways in Lymphoid Malignancies: From Concept to Practice, Volume 1, First Edition. Edited by Owen A. O'Connor, Stephen M. Ansell, and John F. Seymour.

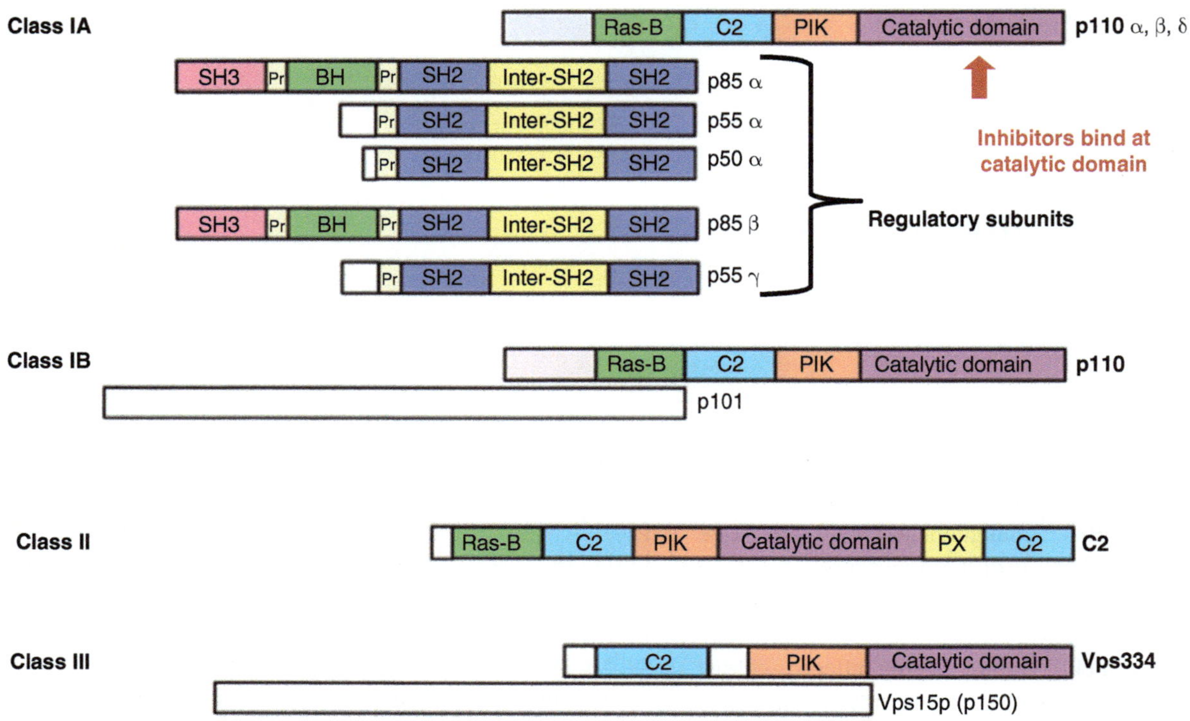

Figure 9.1 PI3K structure.

of the most attractive targets for the development of anti-cancer agents (Hennessy et al. 2005).

PI3K Structure and Functions

The PI3Ks constitute a lipid kinase family that has the capacity to phosphorylate inositol ring 3′-OH group in inositol phospholipids. The PI3K family is divided into three different classes (I, II, and III) in mammals (Figure 9.1). Class I PI3Ks are complex heterodimers composed of a catalytic (CAT) subunit (p110) and an adaptor/regulatory subunit (p85). This class is further divided into two subclasses: subclass IA (PI3Kα, β, and δ), which is activated by receptors with protein tyrosine kinase activity, and subclass IB (PI3Kγ), which is activated by receptors coupled with G proteins.

Activation of receptor protein tyrosine kinases results in tyrosine autophosphorylation (Figure 9.2). PI3K is then recruited to the cell membrane by directly binding to phosphotyrosine consensus residues of growth factor receptors or adaptors through one of the two SH2 domains in the adaptor subunit, leading to allosteric activation of the CAT subunit. PI3K activation rapidly leads to production of the second messenger phosphatidylinositol-3,4,5-triphosphate ($PI3,4,5\text{-}P_3$) which then recruits to the membrane a subset of signaling proteins with pleckstrin homology (PH) domains, including protein serine/threonine kinase-3′-phosphoinositide-dependent kinase 1 (PDK1) and AKT.

AKT Structure and Functions

AKT kinases belong to the AGC kinase family, related to AMP/GMP kinases and protein kinase C. They consist of three conserved domains, an N-terminal PH domain, a central kinase CAT domain, and a C-terminal extension (EXT) containing a regulatory hydrophobic motif (HM). Among the AKT isoforms, the PH domains are ~80% identical and ~30% identical to PH domains in pleckstrin and other proteins. The linker (LINK) region connecting the PH domain to the CAT domain is poorly conserved among the AKT isoforms (17–46% identical) and has no significant homology to any other human protein. The consensus CAT domain is ~90% identical among the AKT isoforms and is closely related to the PKC, PKA, SGK, and S6 subfamilies of the AGC kinase family. The C-terminal EXT is ~70% identical among the AKT isoforms and is most closely related to the PKC family.

AKT regulates several cell processes involved in cell survival and cell cycle progression and can inactivate pro-apoptotic factors including Bad and Procaspase-9, as well as the Forkhead family of transcription factors that induce the expression of other pro-apoptotic factors, such as Fas-ligand (FasL). AKT activation has been related to increased resistance of cancer cells to apoptosis mediated by tumor necrosis factor-related apoptosis inducing ligand (TRAIL)/APO-2L. AKT also activates IκB kinase (IKK), a positive regulator of NF-κB. Several targets of AKT are involved in protein synthesis, glycogen metabolism, and cell cycle regulation (Fresno-Vara et al. 2004) including mTOR, glycogen synthase

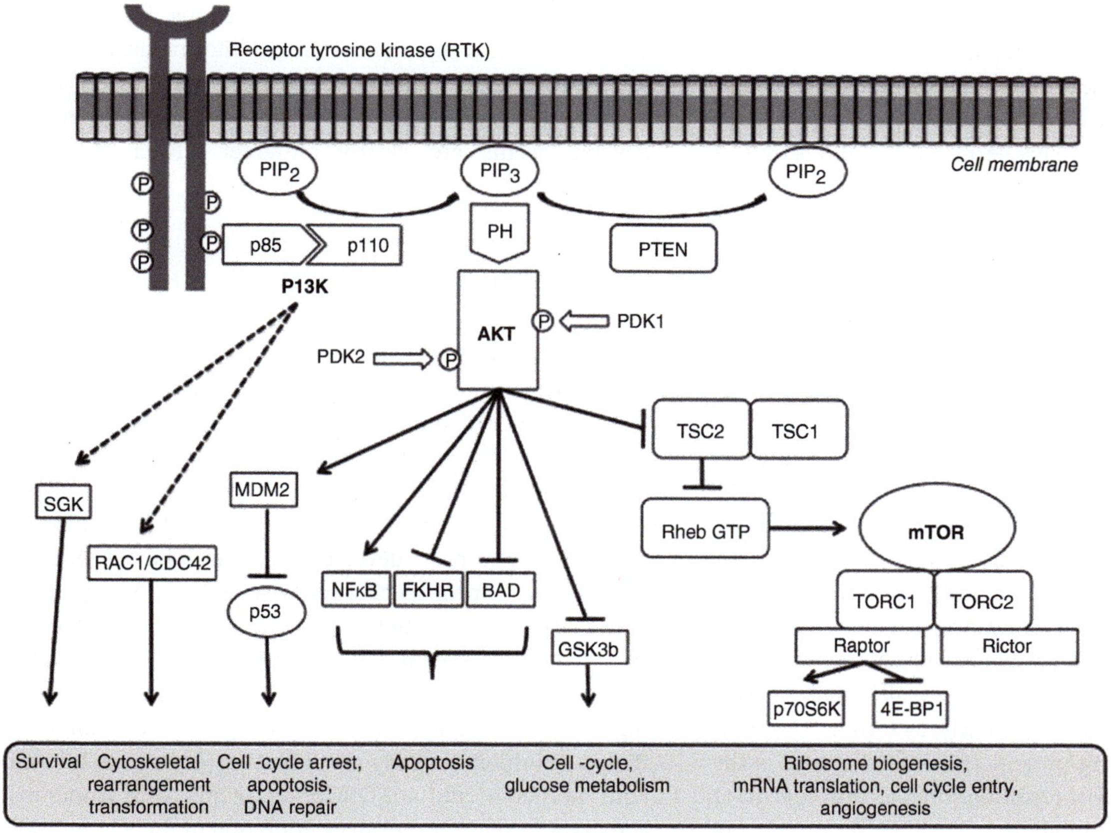

Figure 9.2 Schematic representation of the PI3K/AKT/mTOR pathway.

kinase-3 (GSK3), insulin receptor substrate-1 (IRS-1), the cyclin-dependent kinase inhibitors $p21^{CIP1/WAF1}$, and $p27^{KIP1}$. AKT triggers a network that positively regulates G1/S cell cycle progression through inactivation of GSK3-β, leading to increased cyclin D1, and inhibition of the Forkhead family transcription factors and the tumor suppressor tuberin (TSC2), ultimately resulting in the reduction in p27Kip1.

mTOR Structure and Functions

mTOR is a key highly evolutionarily conserved protein that is essential for life, and embryonic mTOR mutations are lethal. mTOR activity is controlled by positive and negative upstream regulators which transmit signals to mTOR through PI3K/AKT (Hay and Sonenberg 2004) Positive regulators include growth factors and receptors, including insulin-like growth factor-1 (IGF-1) and its receptor IFGR-1, members of the human epidermal growth factor receptor (HER) family and associated ligands, and vascular endothelial growth factor receptors (VEGFRs) and their ligands. Negative regulators of mTOR activity include phosphatase and tensin homolog (PTEN) that inhibits signaling through the PI3K/AKT pathway, and tuberous sclerosis complex (TSC) 1 (hamartin) and TSC2 (tuberin). Phosphorylation of TSC2 by AKT releases its inhibitory effect on mTOR and upregulates mTOR activity. mTOR activity is carried out by two distinct complexes: mTORC1 and mTORC2. The mTORC1 complex is made up of mTOR, Raptor, mLST8, and PRAS40 and activates S6K and inactivates 4EBP1, leading to protein translation and cell growth (Burris et al. 2018). It is extremely sensitive to rapamycin and represents the target of first-generation mTOR inhibitors. The mTORC2 complex is composed of mTOR, Rictor, Sin 1, and mLST8. mTORC2 is less sensitive to rapamycin and its role in normal cell function and oncogenesis has not been as well clarified as mTORC1, but it is known to promote cell proliferation and survival by AKT activation. The canonical pathway of mTOR activation depends on mitogen-driven signaling through PI3K/AKT, although alternative non-AKT-dependent activation through the Ras/MEK/ERK pathway is also recognized (Memmott and Dennis 2009). mTOR activation leads to increased protein synthesis, several of which have been implicated in the pathogenesis of multiple tumors, such as cyclin D1, and hypoxia-Inducible Factor (HIF).

PTEN as a Regulator of the PI3K/AKT/mTOR Pathway

Phosphatase and tensin homolog (PTEN) is a phosphatase with dual activity on proteins and lipids and is a key molecule downstream of the PI3K/AKT pathway. The main lipid substrate of PTEN is PI3,4,5-P_3. PTEN acts as a negative regulator of PI3K/AKT signaling and loss of PTEN activity leads to PI3K/AKT pathway activation. PTEN acts as a tumor suppressor by inhibiting cell growth and enhancing cellular sensitivity to apoptosis. PTEN is frequently mutated in several human cancers and PTEN germ cell mutations result in the rare hereditary syndrome known as Cowden's disease, associated with a higher risk of several different cancers, including breast, thyroid, and endometrial cancers (Simpson and Parson 2001).

mTOR Inhibitors

Rapamycin has long been known to have broad anti-cancer activity, but its use as an anti-cancer agent was hampered by its unfavorable pharmacokinetic properties. The rapamycin analogs, temsirolimus, everolimus, and ridaforolimus, have a more favorable pharmacokinetic profile, and opened up the era of mTOR inhibitors as anti-cancer agents. These agents have similar structure and mechanism of action, but different pharmacokinetic properties. They are all small molecule inhibitors that function intracellularly, by forming a complex with the FK506 binding protein-12 (FKBP-12) that is then recognized by mTOR. The resulting complex prevents mTOR activity, leading to inhibition of cell cycle progression, survival, and angiogenesis. All of these inhibitors affect only mTORC1, and not mTORC2 (Faivre et al. 2006).

Temsirolimus: Phase 3 Trials

Temsirolimus is a pro-drug whose primary active metabolite is rapamycin. Temsirolimus is administered intravenously on a once-weekly schedule. It has been approved for the treatment of patients with advanced renal cell carcinoma (RCC) and mantle cell lymphoma (MCL). The pivotal registration trial in MCL was a phase 3 trial where 62 patients with relapsed or refractory MCL were randomly assigned to receive one of two temsirolimus regimens: 175 mg weekly for three weeks followed by either 75 mg (175/75 mg) or 25 mg (175/25 mg) weekly, or investigator's choice therapy (Hess et al. 2009). Patients treated with temsirolimus 175/75 mg had significantly longer progression-free survival (PFS) than those treated with investigator's choice therapy [$p = 0.0009$; hazard ratio (HR) = 0.44]. Furthermore, objective response rate (ORR) was significantly higher in the 175/75 mg group (22%) compared with the investigator's choice group (2%; $p = 0.0019$), while there was no statistical difference in overall survival (OS).

Adverse events (AE) observed in patients treated with mTOR inhibitors are fairly constant, irrespective of each specific indication, and include stomatitis and skin rash, non-infectious pneumonitis, elevated blood levels of glucose, cholesterol, and triglycerides, as well as immune-related events including increased incidence of infections. We should of course remember that the mTOR inhibitor rapamycin is still widely used as an immunosuppressant agent in the transplantation setting. These metabolic and immune-related adverse events are clearly on-target effects of mTOR inhibition.

PI3K and Dual PI3K/mTOR Inhibitors

First-generation PI3K inhibitors, such as wortmannin and LY294002, bind all class I PI3Ks and are termed "pan-inhibitors." These compounds can be considered as pre-clinical tools to characterize this complex pathway and they were never fully developed as anti-cancer drugs for clinical use. Second-generation inhibitors with better pharmacokinetic properties have been developed and are characterized by greater and isoform-specific selective activity (Martini et al. 2013). Third generation of compounds comprises the so-called "dual PI3K/mTOR inhibitors" were developed after recognition that the CAT sites of PI3K and mTOR share a high degree of sequence homology. A potential advantage is that they inhibit not only all PI3K class I isoforms but also both mTORC1 and mTORC2. In theory, this combined activity would lead to stronger inhibition of the whole PI3K/AKT/mTOR pathway.

The first in class PI3K inhibitor idelalisib was approved by the US Food and Drug Administration (FDA) and is used in the treatment of relapsed/refractory chronic lymphocytic leukemia (CLL)/small lymphocytic lymphoma (SLL) and follicular lymphoma (FL) (US Food and Drug Administration 2014). Duvelisib was approved for the treatment of adult patients with relapsed or refractory CLL/SLL after at least two prior therapies. Copanlisib has subsequently been approved for relapsed FL in patients who have received at least two prior systemic therapies. Umbralisib received accelerated approval in February 2021 as a treatment for patients with marginal zone lymphoma who previously received at least one anti-CD20 regimen or FL previously treated with three or more lines of therapy. There are multiple other PI3K agents currently in development and these target various combinations of PI3K isoforms (Figure 9.3). Despite the therapeutic benefit, there have been concerns about the severe and sometimes fatal adverse effects of this class of drug. Several side effects are unusual and have poorly understood mechanisms including autoimmune dysfunction, opportunistic infections, skin toxicity, hypertension, and hyperglycemia. An understanding of these unusual toxicities, as well as a good grasp of management principles, will be important as more PI3K inhibitors are approved and become incorporated into routine practice.

Idelalisib is the first in class PI3K inhibitor licensed (US Food and Drug Administration 2014). The pivotal study in

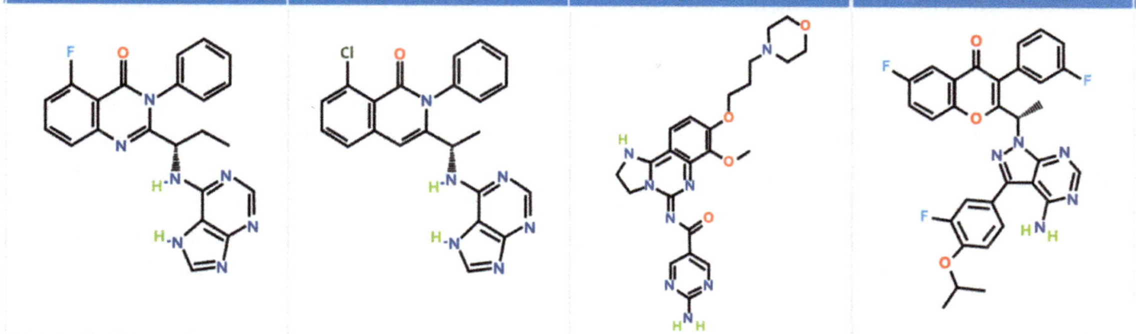

Isoform	Idelalisib	Duvelisib	Copanlisib	Umbralisib
	K_d (nM)			
PI3Kα	600	40	0.04	>10,000
PI3Kβ	19	0.89	1.5	>10,000
PI3Kγ	9.1	0.21	0.31	1,400
PI3Kδ	1.2	0.047	0.068	6.2
CK1ε	>30,000	>30,000	>6,000	180

Figure 9.3 Approved PI3K inhibitors and their specificity for isoforms.

CLL showed that idelalisib combined with the anti-CD20 monoclonal antibody rituximab (IdR) led to a significant improvement in PFS and OS compared to rituximab monotherapy alone (Furman et al. 2014). A total of 220 patients with relapsed CLL were randomized to idelalisib at a dose of 150 mg twice daily (b.i.d.) with rituximab infusion given every two weeks for four doses followed by four weekly for a total of eight doses versus rituximab given in combination with placebo. Rituximab was given at a dose of 375 mg initially before escalation to 500 mg/m^2 in both treatment arms. The median time since CLL diagnosis was 9 years and patients had received a median of three prior lines of therapy, including chemoimmunotherapy (CI). Most patients had advanced stage disease with *TP53* mutation 40% and more than 80% had immunoglobulin heavy chain variation (IGHV) unmutated status and these factors were balanced in both arms. The PFS in the idelalisib treatment arms was not reached versus 5.5 months in the rituximab arm alone. The 12-month OS in the idelalisib and rituximab/placebo group was 92% and 80%, respectively ($p = 0.02$).

In an open-label, phase 2 study, 125 patients with indolent non-Hodgkin's lymphomas with disease refractory to rituximab and an alkylating agent or relapsed within six months after receipt of those therapies were administered idelalisib, 150 mg b.i.d., until the disease progressed or the patient withdrew from the study. The primary endpoint was the overall rate of response and was 54% in FL and 61% in SLL (Gopal et al. 2014).

Until recently, PI3K inhibitors had not been compared with other novel agents, but recent data presented at The American Society of Hematology from the ASCEND trial (NCT02970318) assessed the PFS of CLL patients in three treatment arms to compare the effects of CI versus targeted agents (Jurczak et al. 2021). Patients were randomized to either the Bruton's tyrosine kinase inhibitor (BTKi) acalabrutinib, IdR, or a conventional chemoimmunotherapy bendamustine–rituximab (BR). A total of 310 patients were randomized across the three groups and reviewed over a period of 36 months. A clear benefit of acalabrutinib was shown where at a median of 36-month follow-up with the median PFS not reached, whereas the median PFS was 16.2 months for IdR and 18.2 months for BR. Tolerability and the ability to remain on therapy was a major problem for IdR with severe adverse effects (SAE) reported in 63% of patients, significantly higher than those in the BR or BTKi arms.

Since the initial approval of idelalisib by the FDA further inroads into the successful use of PI3K inhibitors have been made with the approval of duvelisib, copanlisib, and umbralisib (FDA 2020). Although like idelalisib they inhibit class I PI3K, umbralisib is more than 1000-fold more selective for the δ isoform of PI3K compared to α and β forms and 200-fold more selective relative to the γ isoform (Burris et al. 2018). Its dual activity of inhibiting casein kinase-1ε, often associated with downstream activation of eukaryotic initiation factor 4F (eIF4F) which in turn leads to C-MYC translation, is also likely to have significant anti-tumor effects (Bhat et al. 2015). The CHRONOS-1 study was a multicenter trial that examined the use of copanlisib in 142 patients with histologically confirmed indolent B-cell lymphoma who had relapsed after or were refractory to ≥2 prior treatments and who received copanlisib 60 mg on days 1, 8, and 15 (28-day cycle) (Dreyling et al. 2020). The primary efficacy endpoint was ORR after ≥4 cycles (independent assessment). The predominant histology was FL (n = 104). The ORR was 60.6%.

Despite these promising results in a heavily pre-treated cohort, safety surrounding the use of PI3K inhibitors remains a major issue. Autoimmune complications, increased risk of bowel perforations, and life-threatening infections are part of the well-documented side effect profile. Other side effects depending on class inhibition have been reported such as hypertension, hepatotoxicity, and hyperglycemia (www.medicines.org.uk n.d.). Concerning side effects were reported following initial data in the phase 3 trial comparing idelalisib–rituximab versus rituximab-placebo (Furman et al. 2014). The P13K inhibitor arm showed increased grade 3 adverse events across the cohort compared to the rituximab-placebo arm (56% vs. 48%) more commonly diarrhea, pyrexia, and rigors, though each arm had a >10% chance of any adverse effect, suggesting that PI3K inhibitors alone are not the sole reason contributing to adverse events (AE) in this disease cohort.

To date, six trials have been halted due to several safety concerns in both CLL and non-Hodgkin's lymphoma (NHL) and this has largely hindered the introduction and development of PI3K inhibitors in a population in which traditional CI is neither appropriate nor effective (Gilead Sciences 2018a, 2018b, 2018c, 2018d, 2019a, 2019b). When used in combination with lenalidomide and rituximab severe life-threatening transaminitis, hypertension, and septic shock were encountered shortly after idelalisib treatment (Cheah et al. 2015). Intensive care unit admission was required for three of the patients and as a result of this the use of idelalisib outside of a clinical trial or approved setting is not recommended (Coutré et al. 2015). The use of idelalisib now carries with it a "black box" warning for the risk of life-threatening infection, including opportunistic infections including CMV and PJP, bowel perforation, severe transaminitis, and autoimmune-mediated toxicity.

The UNITY-CLL phase 3 trial assessed the pan-class I P13K inhibitor umbralisib in combination with ublituximab (U2) versus the CI regimen of obinutuzumab–chlorambucil (OC) (Gribben et al. 2020). A total of 421 patients who had either treatment naive or relapsed/refractory disease requiring treatment per iwCLL criteria were randomized accordingly. Groups were stratified based on the presence or absence of *TP53* deletion as well as being treatment naive versus previously treated. The primary endpoint was PFS in the two groups with the secondary endpoints including OR and safety. The two years PFS in the PI3K inhibit arm was significantly greater than the CI arm (61% vs. 40%; $p < 0.0001$) with the median PS in each group 32 months and 18 months, respectively. Two-year PFS was significantly better in the previously untreated group versus previously treated in the PI3K arm (77% vs. 41%) though each significantly outperformed the CI group (2-year PFS 52% and 25% in untreated vs. treated, respectively). Although increased rates of grade 3 side effects were seen in the PI3K arm for transaminitis (8% vs. 1%), colitis (2% vs. 1%), and opportunistic infection (6% vs. 2%), these appear less common with U2 than with other PI3Ki, especially in the treatment naïve cohort. The treatment naive population had higher rates of diarrhea and urticarial reactions whereas the previously treated cohort had significantly higher rates of neutropenia.

Further research is needed to better understand the mechanisms underlying the cause for and prevention of toxicity profiles associated with PI3K inhibitors. Their potential as a targeted therapy in treatment refractory CLL offers promising results. Further development of next-generation drugs and better understanding of dosing regimens should lead to improved outcomes and side effect profiles for patients.

Multiple trials are looking at newer PI3K inhibitors such as duvelisib and umbralisib and their effect on CLL and NHL (Burris et al. 2016; Davids and Brown 2013; Gopal et al. 2014; Infinity Pharmaceuticals, Inc n.d.). Interestingly, they seem to have comparable activity across CLL and NHL with duvelisib and umbralisib having better ORR than idelalisib.

Umbralisib may have improved ORR when used in diffuse large B-cell lymphoma (DLBCL) when compared with idelalisib or duvelisib as well as lower rates of grades 3 and 4 hepatotoxicity, diarrhea, colitis, and lower rates of discontinuation of treatment (Burris et al. 2016; Coutré et al. 2015; Davids and Brown 2013; Flinn et al. 2018; Gopal et al. 2014; Gribben et al. 2020; Infinity Pharmaceuticals, Inc n.d.; O'Connor et al. 2015). Though promising, many of these studies have small numbers of patients and more research is needed. At present, there are 14 active clinical trials running using newer agents such as buparlisib and umbralisib with other agents, such as immune checkpoint inhibitors to further understand their potential use in CLL and NHL (clinicaltrials.gov n.d.).

PI3K Isoforms and Expression Throughout the Body

Though often demonstrating upregulated activity in lymphoid malignancies as well as many other solid organ cancers, PI3K is crucial in normal cell signaling pathways. Variable expression levels throughout the body as well as variable isoform expression of PI3K are important in understanding the ways in which toxicities manifest with these agents (Fruman et al. 2017). The three different classes of PI3K are further subcategorized into eight different isoforms with particular isoforms implicated more so than others in the underlying mechanisms of toxicity development. The class I δ and γ isoforms are particularly important in T-cell activation and differentiation into various T helper subsets as well as maintaining homeostatic mechanisms involved in blood pressure regulation (Denley et al. 2007). Below we describe the various mechanisms and how understanding of isoform expression can lead to a fuller understating of management and prevention of AEs.

Immune Toxicity and Management

The immune mediated effects of PI3K inhibition can be better understood by knowledge of the expression of PI3K isoforms on various cell types. The PI3Kδ isoform is upregulated in T-regulatory cells which allow for tumor survival and growth within the tumor microenvironment (TME) in many malignancies, such as CLL. Inversely, their role in autoimmune disease is characterized by absent or altered T-regulatory cell populations (Dubovsky et al. 2013). This absence of T-regulatory cells leads to impaired immune tolerance as well as other mechanisms preventing autoimmune disease development (Roessner and Seiffert 2020). T-regulatory cells, as characterized by cell surface expression of CD4+ and CD25+, were reduced in patients receiving PI3K inhibitors compared to healthy controls (Maharaj et al. 2020). Although both umbralisib and duvelisib reduced T-regulatory cell numbers, they did not fall below the range of healthy controls, whereas a greater reduction was seen with idelalisib, potentially offering some of the explanation to the immune-related toxicity profile. Another mechanism may be related the effects of idelalisib on interleukin (IL) production. Patients treated with idelalisib were found to have lower levels of the anti-inflammatory IL-10 and higher levels of the pro-inflammatory IL-12. These results were not observed with umbralisib. Given this abnormal pattern of cytokine profile variation, it is likely that this is also a contributor to many of the unwanted autoimmune effects experienced with idelalisib.

Colitis

Colitis is a well-documented complication of treatment with PI3K inhibitors, especially idelalisib. Rates of all grades of colitis vary across studies from 29% to 64% with rates of grade 3 or worse reported as 5–42% (Hanlon and Brander 2020). One study found that patients with grade 3 or greater side effects had evidence of an abnormal T-lymphocyte infiltrate on biopsy following colonoscopy (O'Brien et al. 2015).

One study has shown the effects of IL-10 signaling defects on the T-cell repertoire and the development of inflammatory bowel disease (IBD) in infants (Werner et al. 2020). Loss of the IL-10 receptor on T-cells skewed the differentiation and promotion of T helper 17 cells in IBD, contributing to the autoimmune development of the condition (Immunology.org 2016). This loss of IL-10 highlights the importance that suppression of IL-10 seen in idelalisib therapy may have on rates of colitis. Although rates of colitis are much lower with umbralisib, case reports of grade 3 colitis do exist (Bajaj et al. 2021).

Initial steps to prevent severe colitis development can be implemented prior to drug initiation to reduce the chances of severe colitis ensuing. Selection of the right patient to avoid on-target off-tumor effects, for example those with IBD patients, previous abdominal surgery, or those at high risk of perforation or ulcers. In those who go on to develop colitis while on treatment, the appropriate first-line investigations include stool culture to rule out infective pathology, daily abdominal examination, and adequate nutrition and supportive care. Early liaison with gastrointestinal specialty teams and accurate stool chart measurement to aid in the grading of colitis is important. Studies describe both infective and non-infective colitis and suggest those with infective focus should have appropriate anti-microbial therapy (Gribben et al. 2020). Patients with grade 3 or worse colitis should be referred for endoscopy as well as discussion around the use of steroids, usually oral budesonide 9 mg in milder cases (www.medicines.org.uk n.d.). In extreme cases, or when tablets are not suitable, intravenous prednisolone at a dose of 1 mg/kg should be considered with tapering doses once the colitis has resolved (Coutré et al. 2015). Early dietetic involvement should be sought with severe cases referred for parenteral nutrition until colitis has resolved. Less severe cases should adhere to dietary advice from specialists such as low fiber and low residue (NHS Choices 2019). Cessation of the PI3K inhibitor is advised, though it can be considered to restart, at typically a lower dose, once colitis has subsided following patient and specialist discussion. Those with grades 1–2 colitis are often able to carry on with the medication provided they feel they are able to do so. Once oral nutrition has been established routine monitoring of electrolytes to prevent refeeding syndrome as well as B-vitamin supplementation should be initiated if not already in place (National Institute for Health and Care Excellence 2018).

Hepatitis

The hepatotoxic complications of PI3K inhibition are one of the most common reasons for treatment cessation or dose reduction across numerous trials. The rates of grade 3 hepatotoxicity or greater have been reported in as many as 40% of individuals. The typical picture is that of elevation of the transaminases aspartate transaminase (AST) and alanine transaminase (ALT) with rates significantly higher in treatment naive CLL patients and those with pre-existing liver conditions (O'Brien et al. 2015). A case of fatality was reported in idelalisib in combination with the CD20 inhibitor ofatumumab causing severe liver failure as well as profound sepsis (Furman et al. 2014). Mouse models have shown that the inhibition of PI3K in mice with parietal hepatectomy leads to reduced hepatocyte regeneration and abnormal liver architecture formation, compared to those which did not receive inhibition (Jackson et al. 2008). This mechanism was shown to reduce macrophage infiltration and ultimately the production of cytokines, such as IL-6, for hepatocyte priming and proliferation.

The elevation of either AST or ALT to a limit of five times the upper limit of normal (ULN) is considered a grade 3 AE and at this point treatment cessation should occur. Only when toxicity has returned to grade 1 or below treatment should be restarted and often at a lower dose (www.medicines.org.uk n.d.). Even when introduced at a lower dose over a quarter of patients may experience recurrence of significant hepatotoxicity (Coutré et al. 2015). Compared to colitis or pneumonitis the pathophysiological time frame of hepatotoxicity onset is usually in the first three months. As a result, twice monthly monitoring of liver function tests is advised during this period before being extended. Elevation to greater than 20× the ULN should lead to complete cessation and no retrial of the drug as well as considering the use of steroids. Imaging of the abdomen and liver can be useful to rule out any thrombogenic etiology as well as full viral and autoimmune screen. Though bilirubin is not usually affected it should be monitored closely. Regular coagulopathy screens should be performed, and patients counseled on the risk of excessive alcohol use during this time as well as review of other hepatotoxic drugs they may be taking. Vitamin K is of unknown significance in severe hepatotoxicity though should be considered when concurrent bleeding is present.

Pneumonitis

Pneumonitis as a result of PI3K inhibitors has been reported and usually presents with similar symptoms to that of acute respiratory distress syndromes (ARDS). Symptoms of dry cough, oxygen desaturation, fever, and shortness of breath were commonly reported with an oxygen saturation reduction of 5% or more considered significant to investigate for pneumonitis (www.medicines.org.uk n.d.). As many as 14% of patients have reported pneumonitis across PI3K inhibitor studies, though cases of severe grade 3 or worse pneumonitis are not as common as other immune-mediated toxicities (Coutré et al. 2015).

The immune mechanism behind pneumonitis development is still not fully understood, though some hypotheses suggest the upregulation of the innate immune system (Fruman et al. 2017). Levels of PD-1 and CTLA4 expression on T-regulatory cells were also found to be reduced in patients on duvelisib compared to healthy controls which may offer an explanation as to the mechanism of pneumonitis development as well as other autoimmune toxicities (Maharaj et al. 2020). Changes to dendritic cell function and tumor-associated macrophage populations following reduced IL-10 and increased IL-12 production following the use of PI3K inhibitors have also been shown in mouse models (Bhattacharyya et al. 2004).

Avoiding a PI3K inhibitor in those with pre-existing lung conditions such as chronic obstructive pulmonary disease or asthma is good practice as well as those with significant smoking history. Regular observation and pulse oximetry in clinic is suggested and those with signs of clinical or objective hypoxia should have an arterial blood gas, chest X-ray, and receive oxygen supplementation. A full respiratory viral screen should be performed to rule out infective causes as well as a COVID-19 swab and treated accordingly with antivirals ± steroids in positive cases (Centers for Disease Control and Prevention 2020). The chest X-ray appearance characteristically shows bilateral pulmonary infiltrates but in severe cases an ARDS picture may be seen with or without pleural effusions. Empirical antibiotics should be used in the case of suspected concomitant bacterial infection and if suitable neutropenic protocols implemented for treatment of atypical organisms as well as antifungal and antiviral prophylaxis (Nice.org.uk 2012). Holding the PI3K should occur in those with grade 2 or worse AE and a high-resolution CT performed with consideration of high-dose steroids (O'Brien et al. 2015). In those who continue to deteriorate high-flow oxygen, early ITU involvement, non-invasive ventilation, and mechanical ventilation should be discussed early. In these cases, PI3K inhibitors should not be initiated again (www.medicines.org.uk n.d.).

Skin Rash

Infusion-related reactions or cutaneous skin rashes have been widely reported in idelalisib use. Though more commonly reactions are grade 1 or 2 requiring only anti-histamine treatment and paracetamol for fever, severe cases such as Stevens–Johnson syndrome have occurred. Earlier recognition, drug cessation, and liaison with dermatology are crucial in these often fatal manifestations. In this scenario, idelalisib and other PI3K inhibitors should be discontinued permanently (www.medicines.org.uk n.d.).

Homeostatic Toxicity

The PI3Kγ isoform has been shown to be expressed on cardiovascular myocytes and endothelial vascular cells which impact on myogenic vascular tone (Carnevale and Lembo 2012). Further research in the PI3K/AKT axis in vascular endothelial cells leads to downstream signaling pathways which lead to vasodilation of smooth muscle cells via vascular endothelial growth factor (VEGF) and therefore an important factor in blood pressure homeostasis. Depending on whether the signaling from PI3K is mediated via PTEN or AKT largely impacts on the homeostatic mechanism deployed (i.e. vasoconstriction or vasodilation) (Perrotta et al. 2016). Single nucleotide polymorphisms in the *PIK3R5* gene have also been shown to have an association with drug-induced hypertension from other novel agents such as the Fms related receptor tyrosine kinase 3 (FLT-3) inhibitor sorafenib (Quintanilha et al. 2022).

PI3K is also expressed on muscle and adipose tissue. Following insulin treatment in mouse models, PI3K activated and adipocytes from diabetic patients had reduced expression of PI3K (Nelson et al. 2014). Evidence of insulin resistance in hepatocytes and adipocytes has been shown as well as abnormal lipid and glucose metabolism due to PI3K inhibition and subsequent loss of the AKT pathway, crucial in these homeostatic mechanisms (Huang et al. 2018). Activated AKT is upregulated in insulin sensitive tissues, and murine models with knockout AKT or PI3K protein expression have been shown to have increased insulin resistance, leptin resistance, and increased adipose tissue (Matasar et al. 2021).

Hypertension and Hyperglycemia

The CHRONOS studies showed significant activity with copanlisib with ORR in heavily treated NHL patients of around 60% as single agent and over 80% when used in combination with rituximab (Matasar et al. 2021). The action of copanlisib is predominantly focused on the α and γ isoforms and the side effect profile differs from that of other licensed PI3K inhibitors. In the CHRONOS 3 trial, the AE profile was significantly different compared to idelalisib with no immune-related toxicities reported. Previous history of hypertension and diabetes was equal in the PI3K and rituximab arm in comparison to the control group of placebo and rituximab. Despite this the rates of grade 2/3 hypertension were significantly higher in the PI3K arm versus the control (40% vs. 9%) as well as grade 3 hyperglycemia (48% and 8%). There was also a proportion of patients developing grade 4 hyperglycemia (8%) indicating the need for regular monitoring of blood sugars in those at high risk as well as routinely in clinic. In the product literature for copanlisib, the manufacturers express concerns around hyperglycemia and hypertension whereas these side effects are not routinely expected in other PI3K such as idelalisib or umbralisib (Aliqopa US HCP n.d.). A recent phase 2 trial using the pan-class I inhibitor buparlisib in metastatic hormone receptor triple negative breast cancer showed incidences of grade 3 hyperglycemia also (6%), though to less of a degree than that in the CHRONOS 3 trial notwithstanding the smaller patient number studied.

Management of hypertension should include careful selection of patients with a history of hypertension, though this adverse event varies in incidence across the individual PI3K inhibitors. Regular monitoring of blood pressure and signs of end organ damage such as fundoscopy and urinalysis for proteinuria during treatment cycles in clinic is vital. The guidelines around treatment cessation suggest that if blood pressure is greater than 150/90 mm/Hg (grade 3), copanlisib should be held and continue to monitor blood pressure until less than this reading on two consecutive occasions before re-administration. As copanlisib is given in weekly infusions, delaying of infusion until hypertension is under control can be a challenge logistically and should be discussed with the patient and multidisciplinary team. As blood pressure is likely to remain elevated six to eight hours after infusion, empowering patients to check their blood pressure at home is a good safety netting strategy. If hypertension remains greater than 150/90 mm/Hg initiation of anti-hypertensive treatment should be administered based on local or national guidance (NICE 2019). Should there be signs of malignant hypertension or hypertensive crisis (>180/120 mm/Hg) patients should be admitted to hospital for observation as well as treatment to reduce blood pressure gradually (NICE 2019).

Hyperglycemia was more commonly encountered in those taking copanlisib with some patients reporting serious hyperglycemic events. Again, appropriate selection of patients at risk of hyperglycemic episodes or those with poorly controlled diabetes remains important in serious AE prevention. Glucose levels tend to peak around five to eight hours after infusion, so establishing blood glucose levels at this time is a sensible option, especially for those with a history of diabetes. Early involvement of diabetic specialist nurses and doctors in those receiving insulin or other hypoglycemic medication is important. Avoiding concomitant use of other medications, such as steroids, reduces the risk of significant glycemic events and dietician input around low GI index foods can also be a helpful adjunct in prevention. Copanlisib should not be administered if fasting glucose is >8.9/mmol/l or random >11.1mmol/l. In those with persistent hyperglycemia, dose reduction should be considered and in those with life-threatening hyperglycemic episodes or complications, such as diabetic ketoacidosis, treatment cessation or alternative options should be considered (Aliqopa US HCP n.d.).

Myelosuppression and Opportunistic Infection

Myelosuppression exists as a risk in PI3K inhibitors. Regardless of the isoform inhibition targeted, neutropenia, lymphopenia, and susceptibility to atypical opportunistic infections have been documented extensively in PI3K inhibitors (Aliqopa US HCP n.d.; Hanlon and Brander 2020; Perrotta et al. 2016). The rates of neutropenia of any grade are documented as higher in idelalisib (>50%) versus the pan-class I inhibitor copanlisib (33%), though monitoring should occur irrespective of the PI3K inhibitor (CLL Society 2016).

CMV and Pneumocystis pneumonia (PCP) have been reported in the use of idelalisib and have been shown to alter T-cell and dendritic cell populations, in turn affecting CD8+ naive T-cells. Even those with no evidence of neutropenia or lymphopenia should commence PJP prophylaxis to mitigate this risk (Braun et al. 2021). Recent data showed the inability of CLL patients untreated, on immunochemotherapy or targeted drugs such as Bruton's tyrosine kinase (BTK) inhibitors to produce an antibody response following

COVID-19 vaccination compared to healthy control patients. Patients on treatment such as BTKi were found to have significantly lower rates of detectable antibody titers (16%) to COVID-19 vaccinations compared to treatment naive patients (55%), emphasizing the deep effects malignancies and immunotherapies have on humoral immunity (Herishanu et al. 2021).

Myelosuppression

Though the thresholds for holding treatment vary, a neutrophil count of $<0.5 \times 10^3$ cells/mm^3 is considered standard across product literature for different PI3K inhibitors (www.medicines.org.uk n.d.). Counts should be monitored every two weeks and every week should the neutrophil count drop below 1×10^3 cells/mm^3. In those with neutropenic fever, appropriate anti-microbial therapy should be taken as well as prophylactic antibiotics and antiviral medication in those $<0.5 \times 10^3$ cells/mm^3 without fever. The use of granulocyte colony stimulating factor (GCSF) has not been studied but should be considered. Dose cessation or reduction should occur when neutrophil levels are $<0.5 \times 10^3$ cells/mm^3 and not restarted until above this level. A platelet count $>25 \times 10^9$ /l is considered safe for the administration of most PI3K inhibitors.

Atypical Infection

The use of PJP prophylaxis using low-dose co-trimoxazole, or if contraindicated dapsone, atovaquone, or pentamidine nebulizers, is recommended due to the rates of PJP infection in those not receiving prophylaxis and the significance of infection in heavily immunocompromised patients. PJP prophylaxis should be started at the time of treatment and continued for two to six months after cessation. Patients with signs of hypoxia on exertion, dry cough, or fever should have a chest X-ray to identify pulmonary infiltrates. Those with any features suggestive of PJP should be discussed for consideration of bronchoalveolar lavage and treatment dose cotrimoxazole initiated.

CMV screening with CMV DNA should occur monthly and those with a previous history of CMV pneumonitis or infection should be discussed with virologists for prophylaxis consideration. Letermovir is not yet licensed for primary prophylaxis outside of a hematopoietic stem cell transplant setting (www.nice.org.uk n.d.). Those with rising CMV DNA levels or signs of CMV infection should be initiated on ganciclovir or valganciclovir and in severe or resistant infections foscarnet or cidofovir (Cytomegalovirus (CMV) Treatment & Management: Medical Care, Consultations, Activity 2021). In both CMV and PJP infection, PI3K inhibitors should be held and a decision to re-commence them should be made with the multidisciplinary team and often at a lower dose.

Vaccination

Despite evidence that vaccination response in CLL patients is often impaired, seasonal vaccinations against pneumococcal and influenza are recommended (Schuh et al. 2018). COVID-19 data suggests that three primary doses of the vaccine should be given as well as a fourth booster dose three months after in immunocompromised individuals. Hypogammaglobulinemia remains both a complication of CLL itself and the treatment of the disease and regular monitoring of immunoglobulin levels in those with recurrent infections should be performed. Those with IgG <5g/L and recurrent infection should be considered for regular intravenous immunoglobulin infusion.

Neuropsychiatric Problems

Though rare, symptoms of altered mood, anxiety, confusion, and, in severe cases, suicidal ideation have been reported with PI3K inhibitors. These effects occur most commonly with the pan-class I inhibitor buparlisib. In one study, the rate of moderate depressive or anxiety symptoms was seen in 22% and 16% of patients, respectively (Garrido-Castro et al. 2020). The expression of PI3K in neuronal signaling and in chronic neurodegenerative disorders has been demonstrated in some studies; however, the exact mechanisms and role it plays are still not understood (Sánchez-Alegría et al. 2018; Xu et al. 2020). Evidence of upregulation of the p110δ isoform was seen leading to altered signaling in schizophrenic patients, hence why some of the side effects described with buparlisib are low mood or depression (Gross and Bassell 2014). Treatment involves regular psychiatric assessment using recognized tools to categorize the severity of mood disorder in patients. Early assessment by psychiatric specialists and cessation of PI3K treatment in those high risk or with concerning symptoms. Initiation of anti-depressant medications should be discussed with pharmacists and psychiatrists to ensure no interactions with other concomitant medications (www.medicines.org.uk n.d.). Regular screening in clinic should be performed in all patients on PI3K inhibitors, especially those known to cross the blood brain barrier, such as buparlisib (de Gooijer et al. 2018).

PI3K Treatment in NHL

PI3K inhibitors and their use in often heavily treated relapse NHL patients remain an important and useful option in the ongoing goal of cure in many diseases such as CLL. Though issues around their safety previously have hindered the large-scale uptake and use of them compared to other novel agents, such as BTKi, they still have an important role to play. Better understanding around the various isoforms of PI3K, their expression throughout different tissues, and their role in disease will help better plan treatment regimens and understand toxicity profiles in greater details. For example, early-phase studies of idelalisib reported inferior responses in MCL compared with other NHLs. Our group therefore studied expression of isoforms and assessed their contribution to PI3K signaling in MCL (Martorana et al. 2021). We found that although p110δ was highly expressed in MCL, p110α showed wide variation and expression which increased significantly with relapse. Loss of PTEN expression was found in 16% of cases, whereas PIK3CA and PIK3R1 mutations were absent. Although p110δ inhibition was sufficient to block B-cell receptor-mediated PI3K activation, combined p110α and p110δ inhibition was necessary to abolish constitutive PI3K activation (Iyengar et al. 2013). In addition, pictilisib (GDC-0941), a predominantly p110α/δ inhibitor, was significantly more active compared with idelalisib against MCL cell lines and primary samples. We found that a high PIK3CA/PIK3CD ratio identified a subset of primary MCLs resistant to idelalisib and this ratio increased significantly with relapse. These findings support the use of dual p110α/p110δ inhibitors in MCL and suggest a role for p110α in disease progression.

In general, fewer pan-inhibitor classes such as umbralisib, copanlisib, or buparlisib have better response rates and PFS as well as more tolerable immune-mediated toxicity profiles. Given the large number of trials ongoing with these agents and further development of others, it is likely that their use will become more frequent and safer as we understand them more. Despite these improvements, precautions and guidelines should still be followed to maximize on-tumor on-target desired effects and minimize off-tumor on-target unwanted effects.

AKT Inhibitors

Despite the important role in cell signaling, the widespread use and development of AKT inhibitors is substantially less than that of PI3K or MTOR inhibitors. Despite the lack of licensed agents, there have been promising phase 2 trials with capivasertib and ipatasertib which are now entering phase 3 in triple negative breast cancer (Faes and Dormond 2015) (Table 9.1). Their use in combination therapies with checkpoint inhibitors or CDK4/6 inhibitors has also been studied in this field with ongoing trials. They predominantly act by competitively inhibiting ATP on either class of AKT1, 2, or 3 with multiple agents having pan-class effect. Other mechanisms of action include inhibition of DNA synthase and inhibition of the sodium-potassium ATPase pump activity in cells (Hirai et al. 2010).

MK-2206 is an allosteric pan-AKT inhibitor shown to be effective in enhancing anti-tumor activity in breast cancer patients when combined with chemotherapy but of more relevance in CLL patients (Larsen et al. 2017). A phase 2 trial has shown that when used in combination with bendamustine and rituximab for six cycles, ORR were excellent at 92% with PFS 16–24 months in a relapsed/refractory cohort of CLL patients (Oki et al. 2015). The most commonly experienced grade 3 or above side effects were neutropenia, rash, diarrhea, and thrombocytopenia. Overall, the regime was relatively well tolerated. Another phase 2 demonstrating the safety profile of MK-2206 in relapsed/refractory lymphoma patients showed that as a single agent it is well tolerated and safe (Larsen et al. 2017). In this trial, 25 classical Hodgkin's lymphoma patients were given the oral agent once weekly for one year, with the most common side effect being rash, though few had grade 3 or more (15%). Despite the ORR only being 20%, this demonstrates the safe use of AKT inhibitors and the potential for their use as another regime compared to checkpoint inhibitors (CI).

Conclusion

While most PI3K inhibitors are generally selective, there are subtle differences in the relative selectivity of these agents which could explain in part some of the variations in toxicity profiles seen. However, the severity of these toxicity profiles is highly variable and often poorly explained by differences in specificity and potency. Given that all PI3K inhibitors are highly selective potent low nanomolar inhibitors of PI3K, other mechanisms appear to be at work which determine a patient's risk of severe toxicity Is it possible that other off-target effects, such as those seen in BTKi on the TEC family of kinases, could be responsible for some of the immune-mediated toxicities which are similar in appearance to graft versus host disease. It is reasonable to hypothesize that complementary, synergistic inhibition of other kinases within the cytoplasm may enhance toxicity or efficacy of PI3K inhibitors, though more research is needed in this area. Clinically it is apparent that differences in drug toxicities exist but this is also apparent at a biochemical level with the marked differences in cytokine profile expression, T-regulatory cell numbers, and T-cell repertoire phenotype. These differences at a scientific level need to be better understood to hone in on the advantages of the available target agents now at our disposal.

Table 9.1 A list of AKT inhibitors under pre-clinical and clinical development.

Number	Trial title	Malignancy	Drug
1	AZD5363 in Patients With Advanced Solid Tumors Harboring AKT Mutations	Breast Prostate Advance solid organ	Drug: AZD5363 Drug: Enzalutamide Drug: Fulvestrant
2	Testing AZD5363 as a Potential Targeted Treatment in Cancers With AKT Genetic Changes (MATCH-Subprotocol Y)	Advanced lymphoma Advanced malignant solid neoplasm Hematopoietic and lymphoid cell neoplasm	Drug: Capivasertib
3	AKT Inhibitor, Ipatasertib, With Endocrine and CDK 4/6 Inhibitor for Patients with Metastatic Breast Cancer (TAKTIC)	Breast	Drug: Ipatasertib Drug: Fulvestrant Drug: Aromatase inhibitor Drug: Palbociclib
4	mTORC1/2 Inhibitor AZD2014 or the Oral AKT Inhibitor AZD5363 for Recurrent Endometrial and Ovarian	BRCA1 mutation carrier BRCA2 mutation carrier Endometrial adenocarcinoma (and 13 more ...)	Drug: Capivasertib Other: Laboratory Biomarker Analysis Drug: Olaparib (and 2 more ...)
5	A Study of Ipatasertib in Combination With Paclitaxel as a Treatment for Participants With PIK3CA/AKT1/PTEN-Altered, Locally Advanced or Metastatic, Triple-Negative Breast Cancer or Hormone Receptor-Positive, HER2-Negative Breast Cancer	Breast cancer	Drug: Ipatasertib Drug: Paclitaxel Drug: Placebo
6	Everolimus in Castrated Resistant Prostate Cancer(CRPC)Patients With PI3K-AKT-mTOR Signaling Pathway Deficiency	Prostate cancer	Drug: Everolimus Drug: Placebo
7	Testing the Addition of Ipatasertib to Usual Chemotherapy and Radiation for Stage III-IVB Head and Neck Cancer	Head and neck carcinoma of unknown primary Locally advanced head and neck squamous cell carcinoma Locally advanced hypopharyngeal squamous cell carcinoma (and 22 more ...)	Drug: Cisplatin Drug: Ipatasertib Radiation: Radiation therapy
8	Vismodegib, FAK Inhibitor GSK2256098, Capivasertib, and Abemaciclib in Treating Patients With Progressive Meningiomas	Intracranial meningioma Recurrent meningioma NF2 gene mutation	Drug: Vismodegib Drug: FAK inhibitor GSK2256098 Drug: Capivasertib Drug: Abemaciclib
9	Ipatasertib + Pertuzumab + Trastuzumab in Advanced HER2+ PI3KCA-mutant Breast Cancer Patients	Metastatic breast cancer	Drug: Ipatasertib Drug: Trastuzumab Drug: Pertuzumab
10	Uprosertib, Dabrafenib, and Trametinib in Treating Patients With Stage IIIC-IV Cancer	Hematopoietic and lymphoid cell neoplasm Locally advanced malignant solid neoplasm Locally advanced melanoma (and 6 more ...)	Drug: Dabrafenib mesylate Drug: Trametinib dimethyl sulfoxide Drug: Uprosertib

11	A Study to Assess the Effect of Capivasertib on Midazolam in Patients With Advanced Solid Tumors	Solid tumor	Drug: Capivasertib Drug: Midazolam
12	Inetetamab Plus Rapamycin and Chemotherapy for HER2+ Metastatic Breast Cancer With Abnormal Activation of PAM Pathway	Breast cancer	Drug: Inetetamab Drug: Rapamycin Drug: Pyrotinib Drug: Chemotherapy
13	AKT Inhibitor MK2206 and Hydroxychloroquine in Treating Patients With Advanced Solid Tumors, Melanoma, Prostate or Kidney Cancer	Advanced malignant solid neoplasm Stage III cutaneous melanoma AJCC v7 Stage III prostate cancer AJCC v7 (and 7 more ...)	Drug: AKT inhibitor MK2206 Drug: Hydroxychloroquine
14	Fulvestrant ± AKT Inhibition in Advanced Aromatase Inhibitor Resistant Breast Cancer	Estrogen receptor positive breast cancer	Drug: AZD5363 Drug: Placebo Drug: Fulvestrant
15	Bicalutamide With or Without AKT Inhibitor MK2206 in Treating Patients With Previously Treated Prostate Cancer	Recurrent prostate carcinoma Stage I prostate cancer AJCC v7 Stage IIA prostate cancer AJCC v7 (and 2 more ...)	Drug: AKT inhibitor MK2206 Drug: Bicalutamide Other: Clinical observation Other: Laboratory biomarker analysis
16	Safety, Tolerability & Potential Anti-cancer Activity of Increasing Doses of AZD5363 in Different Treatment Schedules	Advanced solid malignancy Safety and tolerability Pharmacokinetics (and 11 more ...)	Drug: AZD5363
17	Rapamycin Treatment for Activated Phosphoinositide 3-Kinase δ Syndrome	Activated PI3K-delta syndrome Immunodeficiency primary	Drug: Rapamycin
18	Investigating Safety, Tolerability and Efficacy of AZD5363 When Combined With Paclitaxel in Breast Cancer Patients	Advanced or metastatic breast cancer ER+ve advanced or metastatic breast cancer	Drug: AZD5363 when combined with weekly paclitaxel Drug: AZD5363when combined with weekly paclitaxel Drug: A placebo in combination with weekly paclitaxel
19	A Study of the Safety and Tolerability in Participants With PIK3CA-related Overgrowth Spectrum or Proteus Syndrome Who Are Being Treated With Miransertib (MK-7075) in Other Studies (MK-7075–006)	PIK3CA-related overgrowth spectrum (PROS)/ Proteus syndrome (PS)	Drug: Miransertib
20	Study of Miransertib (MK-7075) in Participants With PIK3CA-related Overgrowth Spectrum and Proteus Syndrome (MOSAIC) (MK-7075–002)	PIK3CA-related overgrowth spectrum (PROS)/ Proteus syndrome	Drug: Miransertib
21	TAS-117 in Patients With Advanced Solid Tumors Harboring Germline PTEN Mutations	Advanced or metastatic solid tumors irrespective of gene alterations Advanced or metastatic solid tumors with germline PTEN inactivating mutations	Drug: TAS-117
22	A Study of TAS0612 in Participants With Advanced or Metastatic Solid Tumor Cancer	Advanced or metastatic solid tumors	Drug: TAS0612
23	Perifosine and Torisel (Temsirolimus) for Recurrent/Progressive Malignant Gliomas	Brain tumor, recurrent Glioblastoma Anaplastic astrocytoma (and 2 more ...)	Procedure: Cytoreductive surgery Drug: Perifosine Drug: Temsirolimus

Must Read References

Bilanges, B., Posor, Y., and Vanhaesebroeck, B. (2019). PI3K isoforms in cell signaling and vesicle trafficking. *Nat. Rev. Mol. Cell Biol.* 20: 515–534.

Burris, H.A., Flinn, I.W., Patel, M.R. et al. (2018). Umbralisib, a novel PI3Kδ and casein kinase-1ε inhibitor, in relapsed or refractory chronic lymphocytic leukaemia and lymphoma: an open-label, phase 1, dose-escalation, first-in-human study. *Lancet Oncol.* 19 (4): 486–496.

Dreyling, M., Santoro, A., Mollica, L. et al. (2020 April). Long-term safety and efficacy of the PI3K inhibitor copanlisib in patients with relapsed or refractory indolent lymphoma: 2-year follow-up of the CHRONOS-1 study. *Am. J. Hematol.* 95 (4): 362–371.

Faivre, S., Kroemer, G., and Raymond, E. (2006). Current development of mTOR inhibitors as anticancer agents. *Nat. Rev. Drug Discov.* 5: 671–688.

Flinn, I.W., O'Brien, S., Kahl, B. et al. (2018). Duvelisib, a novel oral dual inhibitor of PI3K-δ,γ, is clinically active in advanced hematologic malignancies. *Blood* [online] 131 (8): 877–887.

Furman, R.R., Sharman, J.P., Coutre, S.E. et al. (2014). Idelalisib and rituximab in relapsed chronic lymphocytic leukemia. *N. Engl. J. Med.* 370: 997–1007.

Gopal, A.K., Kahl, B.S., de Vos, S. et al. (2014). PI3KÎ′ inhibition by idelalisib in patients with relapsed indolent lymphoma. *N. Engl. J. Med.* 370: 1008–1018.

Martorana, F., Motta, G., Pavone, G. et al. (2021). AKT inhibitors: new weapons in the fight against breast cancer? *Front. Pharmacol.* 12.

References

Aliqopa US HCP. (n.d.). *Dosing & administration - dose modification & toxicity management.* [online] Available at https://www.hcp.aliqopa-us.com/dosing-administration/dose-modifications. (accessed 2 March, 2022).

Bajaj, S., Barrett, S.M., Nakhleh, R.E. et al. (2021). Umbralisib-induced immune-mediated colitis: a concerning adverse effect of the novel PI3Kδ/CK1ε inhibitor. *ACG Case Rep. J.* [online] 8 (11): e00701. Available at https://www.ncbi.nlm.nih.gov/pmc/articles/PMC8613332 (accessed 2 March 2022).

Bhat, M., Robichaud, N., Hulea, L. et al. (2015). Targeting the translation machinery in cancer. *Nat. Rev. Drug Discov.* [online] 14 (4): 261–278. Available at https://www.nature.com/articles/nrd4505 (accessed 22 January 2022).

Bhattacharyya, S., Sen, P., Wallet, M. et al. (2004). Immunoregulation of dendritic cells by IL-10 is mediated through suppression of the PI3K/Akt pathway and of IκB kinase activity. *Blood*, [online] 104 (4): 1100–1109. Available at https://ashpublications.org/blood/article/104/4/1100/18483/Immunoregulation-of-dendritic-cells-by-IL-10-is (accessed 6 March 2022).

Bilanges, B., Posor, Y., and Vanhaesebroeck, B. (2019). PI3K isoforms in cell signaling and vesicle trafficking. *Nat. Rev. Mol. Cell Biol.* 20: 515–534.

Braun, C., Schlaweck, S., Daecke, S.N. et al. (2021). The PI3Kδ inhibitor idelalisib impairs the function of human dendritic cells. *Cancer Immunol. Immunother.* 70 (12): 3693–3700.

Burris, H.A., Flinn, I., Lunning, M.A. et al. (2016). Long-term follow-up of the PI3Kδ inhibitor TGR-1202 to demonstrate a differentiated safety profile and high response rates in CLL and NHL: integrated-analysis of TGR-1202 monotherapy and combined with ublituximab. *J. Clin. Oncol.* 34 (15_suppl): 7512–7512.

Burris, H.A., Flinn, I.W., Patel, M.R. et al. (2018). Umbralisib, a novel PI3Kδ and casein kinase-1ε inhibitor, in relapsed or refractory chronic lymphocytic leukaemia and lymphoma: an open-label, phase 1, dose-escalation, first-in-human study. *Lancet Oncol.* 19 (4): 486–496. Available at https://pubmed.ncbi.nlm.nih.gov/29475723 (accessed 2 March 2022).

Carnevale, D. and Lembo, G. (2012). PI3K in hypertension: a novel therapeutic target controlling vascular myogenic tone and target organ damage. *Cardiovasc. Res.* 95 (4): 403–408.

Centers for Disease Control and Prevention (2020). *Interim clinical guidance for management of patients with confirmed 2019 novel coronavirus (2019-nCoV) infection.* [online] Centers for Disease Control and Prevention. Available at https://www.cdc.gov/coronavirus/2019-ncov/hcp/clinical-guidance-management-patients.html. (accessed 2 March, 2022).

Cheah, C.Y., Nastoupil, L.J., Neelapu, S.S. et al. (2015). Lenalidomide, idelalisib, and rituximab are unacceptably toxic in patients with relapsed/refractory indolent lymphoma. *Blood* [online] 125 (21): 3357–3359. Available at https://www.ncbi.nlm.nih.gov/pmc/articles/PMC5161005 (accessed 2 March 2022).

clinicaltrials.gov. (n.d.). *Search of: PI3K | recruiting, not yet recruiting, active, not recruiting, enrolling by invitation studies | CLL - list results - ClinicalTrials.gov.* [online] Available at https://clinicaltrials.gov/ct2/results?term=PI3K&cond=CLL&Search=Apply&recrs=b&recrs=a&recrs=f&recrs=d&age_v=&gndr=&type=&rslt= (accessed 2 March 2022).

CLL Society. (2016). *Commentary on Idelalisib by Dr. Richard Furman.* [online] Available at https://cllsociety.org/2016/03/commentary-idelalisib-dr-richard-furman/ (accessed 6 March 2022).

Coutré, S.E., Barrientos, J.C., Brown, J.R. et al. (2015). Management of adverse events associated with idelalisib treatment: expert panel opinion. *Leuk. Lymphoma* 56 (10): 2779–2786.

Cytomegalovirus (CMV) Treatment & Management: Medical Care, Consultations, Activity. (2021). eMedicine. [online] Available at https://emedicine.medscape.com/article/215702t

reatment#:~:text=The%20drug%20of%20choice%20for (accessed 2 March, 2022).

Datta, S.R., Brunet, A., and Greenberg, M.E. (1999). Cellular survival: a play in three AKTs. *Genes Dev.* 13: 2905–2927.

Davids, M.S. and Brown, J.R. (2013). Phosphoinositide 3′-Kinase inhibition in chronic lymphocytic leukemia. *Hematol. Oncol. Clin. North Am.* 27 (2): 329–339.

de Gooijer, M.C., Zhang, P., Buil, L.C.M. et al. (2018). Buparlisib is a brain penetrable pan-PI3K inhibitor. *Sci. Rep.* [online] 8 (1): 10784. Available at https://www.nature.com/articles/s41598-018-29062-w (accessed 6 March 2022).

Denley, A., Kang, S., Karst, U. et al. (2007). Oncogenic signaling of class I PI3K isoforms. *Oncogene* 27 (18): 2561–2574.

Dreyling, M., Santoro, A., Mollica, L. et al. (2020 April). Long-term safety and efficacy of the PI3K inhibitor copanlisib in patients with relapsed or refractory indolent lymphoma: 2-year follow-up of the CHRONOS-1 study. *Am. J. Hematol.* 95 (4): 362–371.

Dubovsky, J.A., Beckwith, K.A., Natarajan, G. et al. (2013). Ibrutinib is an irreversible molecular inhibitor of ITK driving a Th1-selective pressure in T lymphocytes. *Blood* 122 (15): 2539–2549.

Faes, S. and Dormond, O. (2015). PI3K and AKT: unfaithful partners in cancer. *Int. J. Mol. Sci.* 16 (9): 21138–21152.

Faivre, S., Kroemer, G., and Raymond, E. (2006). Current development of mTOR inhibitors as anticancer agents. *Nat. Rev. Drug Discov.* 5: 671–88.

(2020). *FDA approves new treatment for adults with relapsed follicular lymphoma.* [online] FDA. Available at https://www.fda.gov/news-events/press-announcements/fda-approves-new-treatment-adults-relapsed-follicular-lymphoma (accessed 2 March 2022).

Flinn, I.W., O'Brien, S., Kahl, B. et al. (2018). Duvelisib, a novel oral dual inhibitor of PI3K-δ,γ, is clinically active in advanced hematologic malignancies. *Blood* [online] 131 (8): 877–887. Available at https://pubmed.ncbi.nlm.nih.gov/29191916 (accessed 2 March 2022).

Fresno-Vara, J.A., Casado, E., De Castro, J. et al. (2004). PI3K/AKT signaling pathway and cancer. *Cancer Treat. Rev.* 30: 193–204.

Fruman, D.A., Chiu, H., Hopkins, B.D. et al. (2017). The PI3K pathway in human disease. *Cell* [online] 170 (4): 605–635. Available at https://www.cell.com/cell/pdf/S0092-8674(17)30865-6.pdf.

Furman, R.R., Sharman, J.P., Coutre, S.E. et al. (2014). Idelalisib and rituximab in relapsed chronic lymphocytic leukemia. *N. Engl. J. Med.* 370: 997–1007.

Garrido-Castro, A.C., Saura, C., Barroso-Sousa, R. et al. (2020). Phase 2 study of buparlisib (BKM120), a pan-class I PI3K inhibitor, in patients with metastatic triple-negative breast cancer. *Breast Cancer Res.* 22 (1).

Gilead Sciences (2018a). *A phase 3, randomized, double-blind, placebo-controlled study evaluating the efficacy and safety of idelalisib (GS-1101) in combination with rituximab for previously treated indolent non-Hodgkin lymphomas.* [online] clinicaltrials.gov. Available at https://clinicaltrials.gov/ct2/show/NCT01732913 (accessed 2 March 2022).

Gilead Sciences (2018b). *A phase 3, randomized, double-blind, placebo-controlled study evaluating the efficacy and safety of idelalisib (GS-1101) in combination with bendamustine and rituximab for previously treated indolent non-Hodgkin lymphomas.* [online] clinicaltrials.gov. Available at https://clinicaltrials.gov/ct2/show/NCT01732926 (accessed 2 March 2022).

Gilead Sciences (2018c). *A phase 3, randomized, open-label study evaluating the efficacy and safety of idelalisib in combination with obinutuzumab compared to chlorambucil in combination with obinutuzumab for previously untreated chronic lymphocytic leukemia.* [online] clinicaltrials.gov. Available at https://clinicaltrials.gov/ct2/show/NCT01980875 (accessed 2 March 2022).

Gilead Sciences (2018d). *A phase 2, single arm study evaluating the efficacy and safety of idelalisib in combination with rituximab in patients with previously untreated chronic lymphocytic leukemia with 17p deletion.* [online] clinicaltrials.gov. Available at https://clinicaltrials.gov/ct2/show/NCT02044822 (accessed 2 March 2022).

Gilead Sciences (2019a). *A phase 3, double-blind extension study evaluating the efficacy and safety of two different dose levels of single-agent idelalisib (GS-1101) for previously treated chronic lymphocytic leukemia a companion trial to study GS-US-312-0116: a phase 3, randomized, double-blind, placebo-controlled study evaluating the efficacy and safety of idelalisib (GS-1101) in combination with rituximab for previously treated chronic lymphocytic leukemia.* [online] clinicaltrials.gov. Available at https://clinicaltrials.gov/ct2/show/NCT01539291 (accessed 2 March 2022).

Gilead Sciences (2019b). *A phase 2, single arm study evaluating the safety and efficacy of idelalisib in combination with rituximab for previously untreated follicular lymphoma and small lymphocytic lymphoma.* [online] clinicaltrials.gov. Available at https://clinicaltrials.gov/ct2/show/NCT02258529 (accessed 2 March 2022).

Gopal, A.K., Kahl, B.S., de Vos, S. et al. (2014). PI3KÎ´ inhibition by idelalisib in patients with relapsed indolent lymphoma. *N. Engl. J. Med.* 370: 1008–1018.

Gribben, J., Jurczak, W., Jacobs, R. et al. (2020). *Umbralisib plus ublituximab (U2) is superior to obinutuzumab plus chlorambucil (O+Chl) in patients with treatment naïve (TN) and relapsed/refractory (R/R) chronic lymphocytic leukemia (CLL): results from the phase 3 unity-CLL study.* [online] ash.confex.com. Available at https://ash.confex.com/ash/2020/webprogram/Paper134783.html (accessed 2 March 2022).

Gross, C. and Bassell, G.J. (2014). Neuron-specific regulation of class I PI3K catalytic subunits and their dysfunction in brain disorders. *Front. Mol. Neurosci.* 7.

Hanlon, A. and Brander, D.M. (2020). Managing toxicities of phosphatidylinositol-3-kinase (PI3K) inhibitors. *Hematology* 2020 (1): 346–356.

Hay, N. and Sonenberg, N. (2004). Upstream and downstream of mTOR. *Genes Dev.* 18: 1926–1945.

Hennessy, B.T., Smith, D.L., Ram, P.T. et al. (2005). Exploiting the PI3K/AKT pathway for cancer drug discovery. *Nat. Rev. Drug Discov.* 4: 988–1004.

Herishanu, Y., Avivi, I., Aharon, A. et al. (2021). Efficacy of the BNT162b2 mRNA COVID-19 vaccine in patients with chronic lymphocytic leukemia. *Blood* Jun 10 137 (23): 3165–3173.

Hess, G., Herbrecht, R., Romaguera, J. et al. (2009). Phase III study to evaluate temsirolimus compared with investigator's choice therapy for the treatment of relapsed or refractory mantle cell lymphoma. *J. Clin. Oncol.* 27: 3822–3829.

Hirai, H., Sootome, H., Nakatsuru, Y. et al. (2010). MK-2206, an allosteric Akt inhibitor, enhances antitumor efficacy by standard chemotherapeutic agents or molecular targeted drugs in vitro and in vivo. *Mol. Cancer Ther.* 9 (7): 1956–1967.

Huang, X., Liu, G., Guo, J. et al. (2018). The PI3K/AKT pathway in obesity and type 2 diabetes. *Int. J. Biol. Sci.* [online] 14 (11): 1483–1496. Available at https://www.ncbi.nlm.nih.gov/pmc/articles/PMC6158718. (Accessed 2 March 2022).

Immunology.org. (2016). *Th17 cells | British society for immunology*. [online] Available at https://www.immunology.org/public-information/bitesized-immunology/cells/th17-cells.

Infinity Pharmaceuticals, Inc. (n.d.). *PI3K-Gamma*. [online] Available at https://www.infi.com/home/our-development-program/pi3k-gamma (accessed 2 March 2022).

Iyengar, S., Clear, A., Bödör, C. et al. (2013). P110α-mediated constitutive PI3K signaling limits the efficacy of p110δ-selective inhibition in mantle cell lymphoma, particularly with multiple relapse. *Blood* 2013 (121): 2274–2284.

Jackson, L.N., Larson, S.D., Silva, S.R. et al. (2008). PI3K/Akt activation is critical for early hepatic regeneration after partial hepatectomy. *Am. J. Physiol.-Gastroint. Liver Physiol.* 294 (6): G1401–G1410.

Jurczak, W. et al. (2021). *Three-Year Follow-up of the Ascend Trial: acalabrutinib Vs Rituximab Plus Idelalisib or Bendamustine in Relapsed/Refractory Chronic Lymphocytic Leukemia*. [online] ash.confex.com. Available at https://ash.confex.com/ash/2021/webprogram/Paper146570.html (accessed 2 March 2022).

Larsen, J.T., Shanafelt, T.D., Leis, J.F. et al. (2017). Akt inhibitor MK-2206 in combination with bendamustine and rituximab in relapsed or refractory chronic lymphocytic leukemia: results from the N1087 alliance study. *Am. J. Hematol.* 92: 759–763.

Maharaj, K., Powers, J.J., Achille, A. et al. (2020). The dual PI3Kδ/CK1ε inhibitor umbralisib exhibits unique immunomodulatory effects on CLL T cells. *Blood Adv.* [online] 4 (13): 3072–3084. Available at https://www.ncbi.nlm.nih.gov/pmc/articles/PMC7362385 (accessed 2 March 2022).

Martini, M., Ciraolo, E., Gulluni, F. et al. (2013). PI3K in cancer: any good news? *Front. Oncol.* 3: 108.

Martorana, F., Motta, G., Pavone, G. et al. (2021). AKT inhibitors: new weapons in the fight against breast cancer? *Front. Pharmacol.* 12.

Matasar, M.J., Capra, M., Özcan, M. et al. (2021). Copanlisib plus rituximab versus placebo plus rituximab in patients with relapsed indolent non-Hodgkin lymphoma (CHRONOS-3): a double-blind, randomised, placebo-controlled, phase 3 trial. *Lancet Oncol.* 22 (5): 678–689.

Memmott, R.M. and Dennis, P.A. (2009). AKT-dependent and -independent mechanisms of mTOR regulation in cancer. *Cell. Signal.* 21: 656–664.

National Institute for Health and Care Excellence (2018). *NICE CG32 refeeding guidelines: retrospective audit comparing dietetic and medical practice of vitamin prescriptions, blood checks and K+, PO43- & Mg2+ replacement including discharge medications | NICE*. [online] NICE. Available at https://www.nice.org.uk/sharedlearning/nice-cg32-refeeding-guidelines-retrospective-audit-comparing-dietetic-and-medical-practice-of-vitamin-prescriptions-blood-checks-and-k-po43-mg2-replacement-including-discharge-medications-at-st-george-s-hospital-london.

Nelson, V.L.B., Jiang, Y.-P., Dickman, K.G. et al. (2014). Adipose tissue insulin resistance due to loss of PI3K p110α leads to decreased energy expenditure and obesity. *Am. J. Physiol. Endocrinol. Metabolism* [online] 306 (10): E1205–E1216. Available at https://www.ncbi.nlm.nih.gov/pmc/articles/PMC4025064 (accessed 6 March 2022).

Nelson, V.L.B., Jiang, Y.-P., Dickman, K.G. et al. (2014). Adipose tissue insulin resistance due to loss of PI3K p110α leads to decreased energy expenditure and obesity. *Am. J. Physiol. Endocrinol. Metabolism* [online] 306 (10): E1205–E1216. Available at https://www.ncbi.nlm.nih.gov/pmc/articles/PMC4025064.

NHS Choices (2019). *Living with - Ulcerative colitis*. [online] Available at https://www.nhs.uk/conditions/ulcerative-colitis/living-with.

NICE (2019). Overview | hypertension in adults: diagnosis and management | guidance | NICE. [online] Nice.org.uk. Available at https://www.nice.org.uk/guidance/ng136.

Nice.org.uk. (2012). *Overview | neutropenic sepsis: prevention and management in people with cancer | guidance | NICE*. [online] Available at https://www.nice.org.uk/Guidance/CG151.

O'Brien, S.M., Lamanna, N., Kipps, T.J. et al. (2015). A phase 2 study of idelalisib plus rituximab in treatment-naïve older patients with chronic lymphocytic leukemia. *Blood* 126 (25): 2686–2694.

O'Connor, O.A., Flinn, I.W., Patel, M.R. et al. (2015). TGR-1202, a novel once daily PI3K-delta inhibitor, demonstrates clinical activity with a favorable safety profile in patients with CLL and B-Cell Lymphoma. *Blood* [online] 126 (23): 4154. Available at https://www.sciencedirect.com/science/article/pii/S0006497118511447 (accessed 2 March 2022).

Oki, Y., Fanale, M., Romaguera, J. et al. (2015). Phase II study of an AKT inhibitor MK2206 in patients with relapsed or refractory lymphoma. *Br. J. Haematol.* [online] 171 (4): 463–470.

Perrotta, M., Lembo, G., and Carnevale, D. (2016). The multifaceted roles of PI3Kγ in hypertension, vascular biology, and inflammation. *Int. J. Mol. Sci.* 17 (11): 1858.

Quintanilha, J.C.F., Racioppi, A., Wang, J. et al. (2022). PIK3R5 genetic predictors of hypertension induced by VEGF-pathway inhibitors. *Pharmacogenomics J.* [online] 22 (1): 82–88. Available at https://www.nature.com/articles/s41397-021-00261-5?proof=t%3B+see+alsowww.sussex.ac.uk%2Fbroadcast%2Fread%2F53376 (accessed 6 March 2022).

Roessner, P.M. and Seiffert, M. (2020). T-cells in chronic lymphocytic leukemia: guardians or drivers of disease? *Leukemia* 3: 2012–2024.

Sánchez-Alegría, K., Flores-León, M., Avila-Muñoz, E. et al. (2018). PI3K signaling in neurons: a central node for the control of multiple functions. *Int. J. Mol. Sci.* [online] 19 (12): 3725. Available at https://www.ncbi.nlm.nih.gov/pmc/articles/PMC6321294/pdf/ijms-19-03725.pdf (accessed 29 October 2022).

Schuh, A.H., Parry-Jones, N., Appleby, N. et al. (2018). Guideline for the treatment of chronic lymphocytic leukaemia. *Br. J. Haematol.* 182 (3): 344–359.

Simpson, L. and Parson, R. (2001). PTEN: life as a tumor suppressor. *Exp. Cell Res.* 264: 29–41.

US Food and Drug Administration. Prescribing information: zydelig (idelalisib). 2014. https://www.accessdata.fda.gov/drugsatfda_docs/label/2014/206545lbl.pdf (accessed February 2022).

Werner, L., Lee, Y.N., Rechavi, E. et al. (2020). Alterations in T and B cell receptor repertoires patterns in patients with IL10 signaling defects and history of infantile-onset IBD. *Front. Immunol.* 11.

www.medicines.org.uk. (n.d.). *Zydelig 100mg film-coated tablets - Summary of product characteristics (SmPC) - (emc).* [online] Available at https://www.medicines.org.uk/emc/medicine/29202#gref (accessed 2 March 2022).

www.nice.org.uk. (n.d.). *Overview | letermovir for preventing cytomegalovirus disease after a stem cell transplant | guidance | NICE.* [online] Available at https://www.nice.org.uk/guidance/ta591 (accessed 2 March, 2022).

Xu, F., Na, L., Li, Y. et al. (2020). Roles of the PI3K/AKT/mTOR signaling pathways in neurodegenerative diseases and tumours. *Cell Biosci.* 10 (1).

Section III

Targeting Programmed Cell Death

10

Principles for Understanding Mechanisms of Cell Death and Their Role in Cancer Biology

Sarah T. Diepstraten[1,2], *John E. La Marca*[1,2], *David C.S. Huang*[1,2], *and Gemma L. Kelly*[1,2]

[1] *The Walter and Eliza Hall Institute of Medical Research, Melbourne, Victoria, Australia*
[2] *The Department of Medical Biology, The University of Melbourne, Melbourne, Victoria, Australia*

Take Home Messages

- Apoptosis is controlled by two distinct but ultimately convergent pathways.
- Upon a death stimuli, the relative expression and physical interaction between the pro-survival family proteins and pro-apoptotic family proteins determine whether a cell lives or dies.
- Different healthy cells and cancerous cells rely on diverse one or more pro-survival proteins for their survival and growth.
- The intrinsic apoptosis pathway is frequently deregulated in cancer.

Introduction

Cell death is a critical physiological process needed to remove damaged, infected, or superfluous cells. It is estimated that in an average human up to 330 billion cells die and are replaced with new cells each day (Sender and Milo 2021). This, alongside other tumor suppressive processes, ensures that unwanted or damaged cells that could form tumors are safely and efficiently destroyed. As such, evasion from cell death is a key hallmark of malignant diseases (Hanahan and Weinberg 2011) and can arise through many different mechanisms (Kelly and Strasser 2011), resulting in reduced sensitivity to developmental cues and permitting the expansion of cancerous cells. Understanding the pathways to cell death and the different ways cancer cells can disable the cell death machinery can inform the most effective ways to treat a particular cancer. Many anti-cancer therapies act to induce cell death preferentially in cancer cells, often through induction of DNA damage which activates the critical tumor suppressor protein, TP53. Activated TP53 then serves to block tumor growth by upregulation of hundreds of target genes involved in diverse cellular pathways, including DNA repair, cell cycle arrest, cellular senescence, and a form of programmed cell death termed apoptosis (Aubrey et al. 2018; Lieschke et al. 2018; Yonish-Rouach et al. 1991). In recent years, anti-cancer therapeutics that aims to induce cell death through direct manipulation of key components of the apoptosis pathway downstream of TP53 has been developed. These drugs are termed BH3-mimetics, because they mimic the function of the natural pro-apoptotic BH3-only proteins (e.g. BIM and PUMA) that are critical for the induction of apoptosis signaling. BH3 mimetic drugs work by directly inhibiting key apoptosis inhibitory proteins (called pro-survival B-cell lymphoma 2 [BCL2] proteins), such as BCL2 or mantle cell lymphoma 1 (MCL-1), to trigger cancerous cells to undergo apoptosis (Diepstraten et al. 2022; Merino et al. 2018). Knowledge about which pro-survival BCL2 protein is essential for the growth of a particular cancer is therefore critical for the application of BH3-mimetic drugs in cancer patients. Subsequent chapter will focus on the pre-clinical and clinical application of BH3 mimetic drugs for cancer therapy. Here, we endeavor to provide a basic explanation of the cellular apoptotic cell death pathway that these drugs target and provide a historical perspective of where the field started, the critical discoveries that led to the expansion of this field of research, and ultimately led to these new anti-cancer drugs for patients.

A Historical Perspective

The concept of cellular death was first observed and reported in 1842 by the German scientist and philosopher, Carl Vogt,

Precision Cancer Therapies: Targeting Oncogenic Drivers and Signaling Pathways in Lymphoid Malignancies: From Concept to Practice, Volume 1, First Edition. Edited by Owen A. O'Connor, Stephen M. Ansell, and John F. Seymour.

who was studying the midwife toad using a crude microscope and observed that cells in the cartilage would die and be replaced (Vogt 1842). It was later in 1885 that the German anatomist Walther Flemming used early cellular staining dyes alongside light microscopy to observe epithelial cells in the lining of regressive mammalian ovarian follicles that displayed nuclei breaking up into smaller parts and then disappearing, a phenomenon he termed chromatolysis and which is now a well-recognized feature of apoptotic cells (Clarke and Clarke 1996). It was much later in 1965 that the Australian pathologist John Kerr used an electron microscope to observe the distinct nature of this cell death pathway compared to cell death that arose from acute injury in rat liver cells and he termed this type of death "shrinkage necrosis" (Kerr 1965). The programmed nature of this pathway during embryogenesis was also reported by Richard Lockshin (1969) and John Saunders (1966). It was during a sabbatical at the University of Aberdeen, when Kerr worked with pathologists Alastair Currie and Andrew Wyllie, that the importance of this programmed cell death process in many cell types and settings was realized, including embryogenesis but also in therapy-induced tissue remodeling and in cancerous cells where the rate of proliferation outweighed the propensity to undergo cell death (Kerr et al. 1972). With input from their colleague James Cormack, a professor of Greek studies at the University of Aberdeen, they coined the term "apoptosis" which in Greek means "dropping off" or "falling off" to describe the natural process of leaves falling from a tree in autumn. Their seminal paper described the morphological changes and stages associated with cells undergoing apoptosis, such as nuclear condensation, and the formation of apoptotic bodies that were ultimately engulfed by phagosomes (Kerr et al. 1972).

While the impact of these discoveries is widely recognized now, the field of apoptosis research was slow to grow initially and only really expanded in the late 1970s/early 1980s, with the discovery of the first genes involved in apoptosis and the role of dysregulated expression of these genes in cancer. With the development of the nematode *Caenorhabditis elegans* as a model for genetic studies by Sydney Brenner, John Sulston, and H. Robert Horvitz (Sulston and Horvitz 1977), it was recognized that this cell death pathway was evolutionarily conserved (Hedgecock et al. 1983). *Ced3* was discovered as a mutation that causes abnormal accumulation of cells in *C. elegans* in Horvitz's laboratory by Hilary Ellis (Ellis and Horvitz 1986). In humans, the first apoptosis pathway gene to be identified was the one encoding the pro-survival protein BCL2 that was found through sequencing the abnormal chromosomal t14;18 translocation present in a large fraction of patients with follicular lymphoma (Bakhshi et al. 1985; Cleary and Sklar 1985; Fukuhara and Rowley 1978; Tsujimoto and Croce 1986; Tsujimoto et al. 1984). To understand the role of BCL2, David Vaux, then working in the laboratories of Suzanne Cory and Jerry Adams, cloned the *BCL2* gene into an expression construct and introduced it into the mouse interleukin 3 (IL-3) dependent myeloid cell line FDC-P1. This led to the exciting discovery that, in contrast to the parental cells that stopped proliferating and rapidly died when IL-3 was withdrawn, such BCL2 expressing FDC-P1 cells still stopped proliferating but remained viable following cytokine withdrawal (Vaux et al. 1988). In this way, Vaux and colleagues were able to uncouple the proliferative capacity of immortalized cells from their survival and identified BCL2 as the first cell survival protein in any species. Mice were generated that overexpressed BCL2 and shown not to be tumor-prone but the cells derived from these mice were highly resistant to death stimuli (Mcdonnell et al. 1989). Subsequently, Andreas Strasser, using the lymphoma prone *Eμ-Myc* transgenic mouse model of aggressive B-cell lymphomas developed by Jerry Adams (Adams et al. 1985), was able to show the powerful role of blocking cell death in tumorigenesis. Strasser generated *Eμ-BCL2* transgenic mice and noted that these mice that had enforced overexpression of BCL2 in the B-lineage cells did not develop lymphomas at a young age but when these mice were crossed with *Eμ-Myc* transgenic mice, a rapid acceleration in lymphoma onset was observed (Strasser et al. 1990). It is now recognized that overexpression of each pro-survival BCL2 family protein can elicit the same acceleration in tumorigenesis (Campbell et al. 2010; Swanson et al. 2004).

Apoptotic Pathways

Consistent with the early reports describing cells undergoing apoptosis (Kerr et al. 1972), there are characteristic morphological cellular changes associated with apoptosis, including cell shrinkage, membrane blebbing, and DNA fragmentation that reflect the orderly, and immunologically silent, manner in which the dying cell is dismantled (as demonstrated by live cell imaging in Mcarthur et al. (2018)). The apoptotic cell death pathway is evolutionally conserved at a basic level back to *C. elegans* (Ellis and Horvitz 1986; Vaux et al. 1992b) and much is already known about the cellular pathways that are activated in cells undergoing apoptosis.

There are two distinct albeit ultimately converging cellular apoptotic pathways, the intrinsic (also called the BCL2 regulated) and the extrinsic (also called death receptor induced) pathways, as first demonstrated by the observations that BCL2 overexpression could not inhibit FAS/APO-1/CD95 death receptor induced apoptosis in lymphoid cells and that overexpression of BCL2 synergized with loss of FAS in driving severe lymphadenopathy in mice (Strasser et al. 1995) (Figure 10.1). These two pathways ultimately converge on the activation of a group of proteins called cysteine aspartic proteases (caspases) that are responsible for the orderly demolition of the dying cells (Van Opdenbosch and Lamkanfi

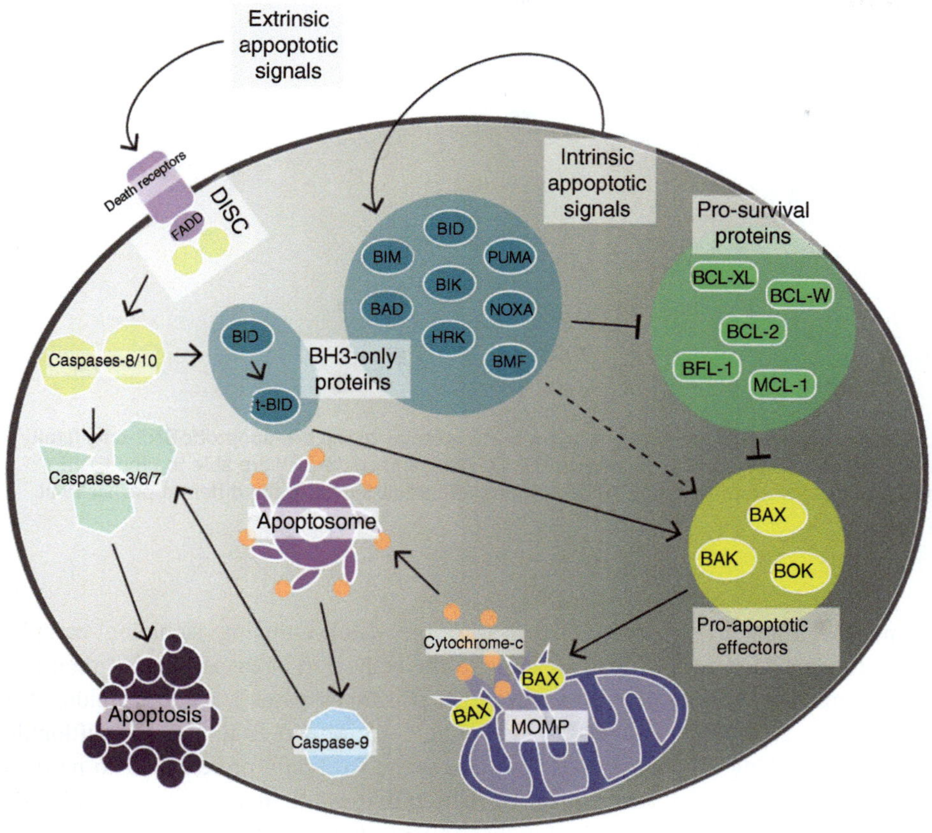

Figure 10.1 **Apoptotic pathways:** Apoptosis can be elicited by the intrinsic (BCL2 regulated) pathway and by the extrinsic (death receptor) pathway. These two pathways are distinct but ultimately converge on the activation of caspases that serve to demolish the cell. The intrinsic pathway is triggered by developmental cues, cytokine withdrawal, or DNA damage which is initially sensed by the BH3-only proteins that can inhibit the pro-survival proteins, leading to activation of the pro-apoptotic effectors BAX and BAK that oligomerize and cause breaches in the inner mitochondrial membrane. Consequently, the apoptosome forms that activate the initiator caspase, caspase 9, can then activate the effector caspases, caspases 3, 6, 7. By contrast the extrinsic pathway is activated through death receptor binding that leads to formation of the DISC that can activate the initiator caspase, caspase 8 (and caspase 10 in humans) that can subsequently activate the effectors caspase 3, 6, 7. Caspase 8 can also cleave the BH3-only protein BID to form t-BID that can then proceed to amplify the apoptotic signal through BAX/BAK-mediated apoptosis involving the mitochondria.

2019). Caspases are expressed as inactive zymogens consisting of small and large pro-domains that require activation and cleavage of the small domain for them to function (Lamkanfi et al. 2002). They can be broadly categorized based on their functions into initiator caspases that have N-terminal domains for the recruitment of adaptor proteins, either a caspase activation and recruitment domain (CARD) or a death effector domain (DED), and effector caspases that are activated by the initiator caspases and proceed to degrade hundreds of cellular protein substrates. The large family of caspases means that some caspases play a fundamental role in the two distinct apoptotic pathways that will be discussed below, and others function in inflammatory responses that will not be the focus of this chapter.

The intrinsic or BCL2 regulated pathway is activated in response to diverse stimuli, such as cytokine deprivation, DNA damage, and developmental cues. The pathway is regulated by the relative expression and interactions of pro-apoptotic and pro-survival proteins of the wider BCL2 protein family (Czabotar et al. 2014; Moldoveanu et al. 2014; Singh et al. 2019). The binding interactions of the different pro-apoptotic and pro-survival proteins are summarized in Figure 10.2. The first group of proteins to respond to stimuli are the pro-apoptotic BH3-only proteins (BIM, BAD, BID, NOXA, PUMA, HRK, BMF, BIK) that become upregulated and/or stabilized in stressed cells. The BH3-only proteins bind via their BH3-domain into the hydrophobic groove of the pro-survival BCL2 family proteins (BCL2, BCL-XL, MCL-1, BCL-W, A1/BFL-1, BCL-W), preventing the pro-survival proteins from binding and thus restraining the pro-apoptotic BAX and BAK apoptosis effector proteins (Chen et al. 2005; Willis et al. 2005, 2007). While some BH3-only proteins (BIM, PUMA, t-BID) can bind to all of the pro-survival proteins, others display selectivity in their binding (e.g. NOXA binds only to MCL-1 and A1/BFL-1, BAD binds only to BCL2, BCL-XL, and BCL-W) (Chen et al. 2005; Kuwana et al. 2005).

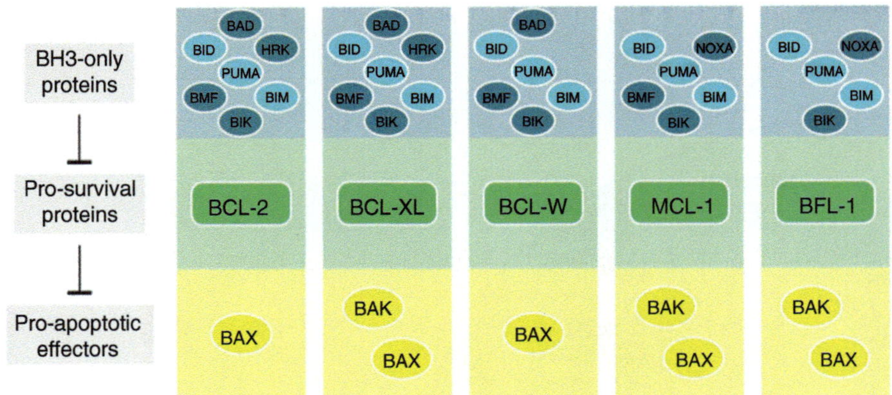

Figure 10.2 Schematic summarizing the binding interactions of the different pro-survival proteins to the pro-apoptotic BH3-only family proteins and the pro-apoptotic effector proteins BAX and BAK. Some BH3-only proteins (PUMA, BIM, and t-BID) are able to bind to all pro-survival proteins, whereas other BH3-only proteins are more selective in their binding affinities. Similarly, the different pro-survival proteins bind preferentially to BAX or BAK.

Additionally, there is evidence that BAX and BAK might also be activated directly by certain BH3-only proteins, such as PUMA, BIM, and activated BID (t-BID) (Certo et al. 2006; Kim et al. 2006a; Kuwana et al. 2005; Letai et al. 2002; Oh et al. 2006; Walensky et al. 2006). Of note, cells lacking all BH3-only proteins can still be induced to undergo BAX/BAK-dependent apoptosis by genetic removal or drug-mediated inhibition of the pro-survival BCL2 proteins (O'Neill et al. 2016). This reveals that unleashing of BAX and/or BAK from their restraint by the pro-survival BCL2 proteins is sufficient for induction of apoptotic cell death. Activated BAX and BAK oligomerize and form holes in the mitochondrial outer membrane, allowing release of cytochrome c into the cytosol (Cosentino and Garcia-Saez 2017; Moldoveanu and Czabotar 2020). Cytochrome c together with seven molecules of the apoptotic protease activating factor-1 (APAF-1) and deoxy adenosine tri-phosphate (dATP) form the apoptosome that recruits pro-caspase 9 via CARD–CARD interactions leading to auto-proteolytic activation caspase-9 (Salvesen and Dixit 1999). Caspase 9 then activates the effector caspases-3, 6, and 7 that can then proceed to degrade their specific protein substrates and thereby dismantle the dying cell (Hakem et al. 1998; Timmer and Salvesen 2007).

The extrinsic or death receptor-induced apoptotic pathway is activated in response to death ligands binding to their cognate death receptors, as indicated by the name (Strasser et al. 2009). Binding of ligands to the death receptors (members of the tumor necrosis factor receptor [TNFR] family containing an intracellular death domain) stimulates these receptors to bind via death domains in their intracellular domain to the death domains in adaptors proteins *FAS*-associated death domain (FADD) and TNFR associated death domain (TRADD) (Ashkenazi and Dixit 1998). FADD binds via its death effector domain (DED to the DED of the initiator caspase, pro-caspase 8 (and also pro-caspase-10 in humans), recruiting it into the death-inducing signaling complex (DISC) leading to the activation of caspase 8 that then proceeds to activate the effector caspases 3, 6, and 7 (Boldin et al. 1996; Kischkel et al. 1995; Muzio et al. 1996). Additionally caspase 8 can cleave the BH3-only protein BID to produce truncated BID (t-BID) that can then activate BAX and BAX-mediated induced apoptosis, thereby connecting the two apoptotic pathways (Billen et al. 2008; Li et al. 1998; Luo et al. 1998). For some cell types, such as hepatocytes, amplification of the extrinsic apoptotic signal via t-BID and stimulation of intrinsic apoptosis are required for efficient cell killing and these cells are termed "type 2" cells (Jost et al. 2009; Yin et al. 1999). For some other cell types, mostly lymphoid ones, caspase 8-mediated activation of effector caspases is sufficient to kill the cells and these cells are termed "type 1" cells (Lamhamedi-Cherradi et al. 2003; Wilson et al. 2009). The precise reasons for these cell type differences in susceptibility to extrinsic apoptotic signaling are still not fully known but may relate to expression levels of the X-linked inhibitor of apoptosis protein (XIAP) that can block the caspase cascade. Specifically, there is evidence that XIAP is degraded in thymocytes but induced in hepatocytes upon FAS signaling and therefore greater caspase activity is required to demolish type II cells. This is backed by evidence from mice with genetically deleted XIAP that shows loss of XIAP does not affect killing of thymocytes but does increase the killing of hepatocytes in response to FAS signaling (Jost et al. 2009).

The importance of the extrinsic pathway to apoptosis came from the analysis of mice that had acquired a spontaneous mutation in FAS, termed *lpr* mice (Watanabe-Fukunaga et al. 1992). Such mice display lymphadenopathy and splenomegaly due to the accumulation of lymphoid cells that were not dying via the extrinsic apoptotic pathway in response to normal developmental cues. These mice also develop systemic autoimmune disease with anti-nuclear antibodies

(ANA) and on analysis were found to have an accumulation of non-malignant TCR-α/β^+, $CD3^+$, $B220^+$, $CD4^-$, $CD8^-$ lymphocytes which are thought to represent previously activated T-cells that did not die after repeated T-cell receptor (TCR) stimulation (Watanabe-Fukunaga et al. 1992). Cells taken from the *lpr* mutant mice could not be killed *in vitro* using agonistic FAS antibodies (Watanabe-Fukunaga et al. 1992). In humans, a similar disease called autoimmune lymphoproliferative syndrome (ALPS) has been identified which is also due to mutations in FAS and is also characterized by lymphadenopathy, hepato-splenomegaly, and autoimmune phenomena (e.g. autoimmune anemia and thrombocytopenia, urticarial rash, and glomerulo-nephritis) (Rieux-Laucat et al. 1995; Sneller et al. 1997).

The distinct nature of the two apoptotic pathways was most elegantly demonstrated by crossing BIM-deficient mice that also display lymphoadenopathy due to reduced intrinsic apoptotic signaling ([Bouillet et al. 1999] and described in later sections), with *lpr* mutant mice leading to compound mutant mice that had much more severe disease relative to the single pathway defective mice (Hughes et al. 2008).

Other Cell Death Pathways

There are now a large number of additional cell death pathways identified. These include well-defined lytic forms of programmed cell death, such as pyroptosis, that function to protect cells from invading pathogens, and necroptosis which appears important in inflammatory disorders and neurodegenerative disorders (Bedoui et al. 2020; Green 2019; Vandenabeele et al. 2010). Additional cell death pathways include ferroptosis which is an iron-dependent form of cell death characterized by extensive lipid peroxidation (Dixon et al. 2012; Jiang et al. 2021). While these programmed lytic cell death pathways provide critical functions to eliminate cells under specific circumstances, their reported importance in cancer therapy is still emerging and not yet as well established as for the apoptotic pathways. Therefore, we refer readers to comprehensive reviews on these cell death pathways (Bedoui et al. 2020; Bergsbaken et al. 2009; Green 2019; Jiang et al. 2021; Weinlich et al. 2017) and will focus here on the apoptotic pathways.

The Role of Intrinsic Apoptosis in Normal Cells – Lessons from Gene Knockout Mice

The first discoveries about cell death were made in the context of development. Cell death is required to balance cell proliferation in order to maintain the size and morphology of organs and tissues. Excessive cell death can lead to tissue degeneration such as in Parkinson's disease and motor neurone disease, while aberrant survival of cells can give rise to cancer. Therefore, cell death pathways are increasingly important targets for the therapy of diverse diseases. The intrinsic apoptosis pathway, regulated by the BCL2 family proteins, has been intensely studied in both normal and disease states in order to facilitate therapeutic targeting of cell death, for example with BH3-mimetic drugs in cancer patients. Elucidating the role of the BCL2 family proteins in mediating the death and survival of diverse healthy cell types, thereby determining how well tolerated these drugs will be by cancer patients, has been uncovered primarily through studies of gene knockout mice.

BCL2 Family Pro-survival Proteins

While the BCL2 family pro-survival proteins are often considered to have redundant roles in inhibiting apoptosis, especially *in vitro*, they exhibit marked tissue and temporal specificity which results in a complex web of interactions governing apoptosis within the whole organism. Notably, the protein expression of a particular BCL2 family member within a particular tissue or cell type is not necessarily indicative of the importance of that particular family member in driving or preventing cell death (Diepstraten et al. 2022). Therefore, studies on gene knockout mice are necessary to determine the true dependencies of particular cell types on BCL2 pro-survival family members for ongoing survival. As mentioned earlier, this allows for the prediction of potential side effects from therapies targeting these pro-survival proteins, but importantly it also provides insight into the potential dependencies of cancer cells which arise from diverse cell types. While much knowledge can be gained from the analysis of gene knockout mice, potential dependencies can still be missed, particularly if the genes also have important roles at early developmental stages (e.g. for BCL-X [Motoyama et al. 1995]) and then targeted cell type specific gene knockouts are required.

BCL2

Expression of BCL2 can be detected in many embryonic and adult tissues. However, studies of *Bcl2* gene knockout mice revealed that BCL2 is largely dispensable for prenatal development. BCL2-deficient mice are viable with no obvious defects at birth (Kamada et al. 1995; Nakayama et al. 1993; Veis et al. 1993b). However, by one to two weeks of age they are noticeably smaller than wild-type littermates and most die at three to five weeks, with only 10% surviving to adulthood (Kamada et al. 1995). The early mortality of BCL2-deficient mice is attributed to renal failure due to polycystic kidney disease (Kamada et al. 1995; Nakayama et al. 1993; Veis et al. 1993b). Examination of the developing kidneys of the embryo showed increased apoptosis of epithelial cells (Sorenson et al. 1995), while postnatal analysis of

BCL2-deficient mice revealed hyperproliferation of kidney epithelium and interstitium and increased blood urea and serum creatinine levels (Veis et al. 1993b).

Interestingly, given the high levels of BCL2 expression in the hematopoietic system, hematopoiesis in these mice is initially normal, including the differentiation and maturation of lymphoid cells in the spleen and thymus (Nakayama et al. 1993; Veis et al. 1993b). However, by four weeks of age, the spleen and thymus begin to atrophy due to catastrophic apoptosis of mature BCL2-deficient lymphoid cells (Kamada et al. 1995; Nakayama et al. 1993; Veis et al. 1993b). Upon isolation and culture *ex vivo*, BCL2-deficient lymphoid cells showed abnormally reduced lifespan and increased sensitivity to apoptotic signals (Kamada et al. 1995; Nakayama et al. 1993; Veis et al. 1993b), while neutrophils appeared unaffected by loss of BCL2 (Veis et al. 1993a).

BCL2-deficient mice also show loss of hair pigmentation during the second hair follicle cycle, as BCL2 is required for the survival of melanocyte progenitors (Kamada et al. 1995; Mak et al. 2006; Nishimura et al. 2005; Veis et al. 1993b). Finally, BCL2 has been found to be required for the postnatal maintenance of specific subsets of neurons, including motoneurons, sensory neurons, and sympathetic neurons (Michaelidis et al. 1996), and for the survival of epithelial progenitors responsible for colonizing the villi in the small intestine (Kamada et al. 1995).

BCL-XL

BCL-XL deficiency (the gene that encodes BCL-XL is termed *Bcl2l1*) is embryonic lethal, with mice dying around embryonic day 13 (Motoyama et al. 1995). Analysis of BCL-XL-deficient embryos revealed prolific and aberrant apoptosis of immature neurons in the brain, spinal cord, and dorsal root ganglia. Loss of BCL-XL also caused increased apoptosis of hematopoietic cells in the fetal liver (Motoyama et al. 1995). Examination of the lymphatic system in chimeric BCL-XL knockout mice revealed significantly increased apoptosis of immature T- and B-cells upon loss of BCL-XL, though the surviving progenitor cells were still capable of maturation (Ma et al. 1995; Motoyama et al. 1995). From these studies it was established that BCL-XL is essential for the survival of the developing neurological and hematopoietic systems. Due to its embryonic lethality, targeted conditional knockout of BCL-XL has been undertaken in various tissue types to further dissect the cell types dependent on this protein for survival.

Mice generated with conditional knockout of BCL-XL in erythroid cells showed massive splenomegaly by three to five months of age and increased mortality (Wagner et al. 2000). Analysis of peripheral blood at three months revealed that BCL-XL-deficient mice were severely anemic and also had greatly reduced (<10% of control mice) numbers of platelets (Wagner et al. 2000). Enlarged spleens in these mice accumulated excessive numbers of immature erythroid cells with a marked decrease in the number of T and B lymphocytes compared to control mice. Subsequent studies established that BCL-XL-deficient mice exhibit ineffective erythropoiesis and that BCL-XL is required to prevent apoptosis of erythroblasts at the final stages of maturation (Rhodes et al. 2005). Outside of the hematopoietic system, conditional loss of BCL-XL in postmitotic neurons (but not in immature neural progenitor cells) in the brains of adult mice resulted in increased apoptosis and numerous behavioral defects, including self-injurious behaviors and hyperactivity (Nakamura et al. 2016). More recently, BCL-XL was shown to be critical for the survival of certain renal epithelial cells in the adult (Brinkmann et al. 2020).

MCL-1

Of all the BCL2 family protein knockout mice, the phenotype of MCL-1-deficient mice is most severe. MCL-1-deficient embryos fail to implant and die at E3.5 (Rinkenberger et al. 2000). *In vitro* analysis of these blastocysts revealed no evidence of excessive apoptosis in the inner cell mass, suggesting that a defect in the outer trophoblast layer could explain the implantation failure. This lack of apparent apoptosis led to the hypothesis that MCL-1 may have essential non-apoptotic roles in development.

Much of the work to elucidate the survival dependencies of tissues on MCL-1 has been achieved using conditional knockout models where MCL-1 is depleted only in the tissue of interest. These experiments have revealed essential roles for MCL-1 in both progenitor and mature cells of the hematopoietic system, including T- and B-cells (Opferman et al. 2003), hematopoietic stem cells (Opferman et al. 2005), mast cells, and basophils (Lilla et al. 2011), neutrophils, but not macrophages (Dzhagalov et al. 2007). MCL-1 is also required for survival of early erythroid progenitors (Turnis et al. 2021), hepatocytes in the liver (Vick et al. 2009), antigen-activated B lymphocytes in the germinal center (Vikstrom et al. 2010), antibody secreting plasma cells (Peperzak et al. 2013), and intestinal epithelial cells (Healy et al. 2020). In addition, MCL-1 is essential for the survival of cardiomyocytes; loss of MCL-1 in these cells caused rapid cardiomyopathy and death (Thomas et al. 2013). Altogether, these studies suggest that MCL-1 is the predominant pro-survival factor in a highly diverse set of cell types.

A1/BFL-1

A1 (BFL-1 in humans) is a poorly studied pro-survival protein which is predominantly expressed in hematopoietic cells. A1 has three functional isoforms in the murine genome. Mice deficient for A1 isoform a (A1-a) showed enhanced apoptosis of activated mast cells (Xiang et al. 2001) and peripheral neutrophils (Hamasaki et al. 1998). Complete knockout of all A1 isoforms in mice has only recently become possible by sequential gene targeting in ES cells (Schenk et al. 2017). Despite its widespread expression in hematopoietic cells, mice deficient for all three functional A1 isoforms appear phenotypically normal and show only minor defects in the hematopoietic compartment, with small reductions in specific subsets of T-cells and in conventional dendritic cells (Schenk et al. 2017).

BCL-W

BCL-W is expressed in diverse tissues including the colon, brain, and testes (O'Reilly et al. 2001). BCL-W-deficient mice appear normal; however, males are sterile due to excessive apoptosis of cells in the seminiferous tubules, including Sertoli cells and spermatocytes (Print et al. 1998). BCL-W has also been found to contribute to the survival of gut epithelial cells (O'Reilly et al. 2001).

Combined Knockout of Pro-survival Proteins

Loss of single alleles of the genes for MCL-1 and BCL-XL results in severe and developmentally lethal craniofacial defects (Grabow et al. 2018), while conditional loss of single alleles of the genes for MCL-1 and BCL-XL in hepatocytes caused spontaneous apoptosis of these cells, indicating that both MCL-1 and BCL-XL play crucial roles in hepatocyte survival (Hikita et al. 2009). In contrast, mice with combined loss of a single alleles of the genes for MCL-1 and BCL2 or BCL-XL and BCL2 showed no obvious defects (Grabow et al. 2018). In many instances, targeting of more than one pro-survival protein may be required to effectively initiate apoptosis. These studies shed light onto the potential BH3 mimetic drug combination therapies that may be tolerated and those which may be too toxic to healthy tissues to progress into the clinic, such as combining MCL-1 inhibitors with BCL-XL inhibitors.

BCL2 Family Pro-apoptotic Effector Proteins

The question of whether apoptosis is truly essential for development has been explored using mice deficient in the critical pro-apoptotic effector proteins BAK and BAX. BAK-deficient mice show no overt defects besides a slight increase in platelet numbers (Mason et al. 2007), while BAX-deficient mice exhibit mild lymphoid hyperplasia (Knudson et al. 1995). BAX was also found to be required for proper formation of the retina (Pequignot et al. 2003). BAX has also an important role in development of the reproductive system, with BAX-deficient female mice showing ovarian abnormalities, while BAX-deficient male mice accumulated premeiotic germ cells and were infertile (Knudson et al. 1995). BAX and BAK are thought to have largely redundant roles, which may explain the lack of serious defects in BAX-deficient and BAK-deficient mice. In contrast, only 10% of BAK/BAX double knockout mice survive to adulthood and these display severe developmental defects including webbed feet, imperforate vaginal canals, and accumulation of hematopoietic and neuronal cells (Lindsten et al. 2000).

The fact that some BAK/BAX double knockout mice survive to adulthood led to the hypothesis that other pro-apoptotic proteins may be compensating for their absence. The poorly studied pro-apoptotic protein BOK was examined as a possibility for this role due to its structural similarities to BAK and BAX. While BOK-deficient mice are viable with no abnormalities (Ke et al. 2012), BAK/BAX/BOK-deficient mice show more severe abnormalities than BAK/BAX-deficient mice, with increases in the proportion of mice with facial clefting, omphalocele, and exencephaly (Ke et al. 2018). However, a small number of BAK/BAX/BOK mice still survive to adulthood suggesting that viable, albeit abnormal, development can occur in the absence of the intrinsic apoptosis pathway (Table 10.1) (Ke et al. 2018).

BH3-only Proteins

Due to the complex interactions between the pro-apoptotic BH3-only proteins and pro-survival proteins, the expression of BH3-only proteins can help to determine the dependency of a particular cell type on a particular pro-survival protein.

Table 10.1 Intrinsic apoptosis pathway gene knockout mice and their phenotypes.

Genotype	Description	Overt phenotype	Cell types affected	References
Bcl2$^{-/-}$	BCL2 deficient in all tissues	Early mortality Polycystic kidney disease Involution of spleen and thymus Loss of hair pigmentation	Apoptosis of mature lymphoid cells, subsets of neurons, intestinal epithelial cells, melanocytes	(Kamada et al. 1995; Michaelidis et al. 1996; Nakayama et al. 1993; Veis et al. 1993b)
Bcl-x$^{-/-}$	BCL-XL deficient in all tissues	Embryonic lethality at E13	Apoptosis of immature neurons, immature lymphoid cells	(Motoyama et al. 1995; Ma et al. 1995)
Bcl-x$^{MMTV\text{-}Cre}$	BCL-XL deficient in erythroid cells	Splenomegaly Early mortality	Apoptosis of erythroblasts, platelets	(Rhodes et al. 2005; Wagner et al. 2000)
Bcl-x$^{Emx1\text{-}Cre}$, ***Bcl-x***$^{Nex\text{-}Cre}$	BCL-XL deficient in neurons	Behavioral defects	Apoptosis of postmitotic neurons	(Nakamura et al. 2016)

(Continued)

Table 10.1 (Continued)

Genotype	Description	Overt phenotype	Cell types affected	References
Mcl1 $^{-/-}$	MCL-1 deficient in all tissues	Embryonic lethality at E3.5, implantation failure		(Rinkenberger et al. 2000)
Mcl1 $^{Lck\text{-}Cre}$, ***Mcl1*** $^{CD19\text{-}Cre}$	MCL-1 deficient in T-cells, B-cells or		Apoptosis of lymphocytes	(Opferman et al. 2003)
Mcl1 $^{Mx1\text{-}Cre}$	MCL-1 deficient in hematopoietic stem cells		Apoptosis of hematopoietic stem and progenitor cells	(Opferman et al. 2005)
Mcl1 ^{LysMcre}	MCL-1 deficient in myeloid cells		Apoptosis of neutrophils	(Dzhagalov et al. 2007)
Mcl1 $^{Cpa3\text{-}Cre}$	MCL-1 deficient in mast cells, basophils, subsets of T-cells, and subsets of hematopoietic progenitors		Apoptosis of mast cells and basophils	(Lilla et al. 2011)
Mcl1 ^{AlbCre}	MCL-1 deficient in hepatocytes		Apoptosis of hepatocytes	(Vick et al. 2009)
Mcl1 $^{EpoR\text{-}Cre}$	MCL-1		Apoptosis of early erythroid progenitors	(Turnis et al. 2021)
Mcl1 ^{MerCreMer}	MCL-1 deficient in cardiomyocytes		Apoptosis of cardiomyocytes	(Thomas et al. 2013)
Mcl1 $^{Aicda\text{-}Cre}$	MCL-1 deficient in B-cells after antigen activation		Apoptosis of activated B-cells in germinal center	(Vikstrom et al. 2010)
MCL1 $^{Villin\text{-}Cre}$	MCL-1 deficient in intestinal epithelial cells	Chronic inflammation, hyperproliferative crypts, development of intestinal tumors	Apoptosis of intestinal epithelial cells	(Healy et al. 2020)
A1-a $^{-/-}$	A1 isoform a deficient in all tissues	No overt defects	Apoptosis of activated mast cells, peripheral neutrophils	(Hamasaki et al. 1998; Xiang et al. 2001)
A1 $^{-/-}$	A1 deficient (all functional isoforms) in all tissues	No overt defects	Apoptosis of conventional dendritic cells	(Schenk et al. 2017)
Bcl-w $^{-/-}$	BCL-W deficient in all tissues	Male sterility	Apoptosis of Sertoli cells, spermatocytes, gut epithelial cells	(Print et al. 1998; O'Reilly et al. 2001)
Mcl1 $^{+/-}$ ***Bcl-x*** $^{+/-}$	Heterozygous for MCL-1 and BCL-XL expression in all tissues	Developmentally lethal craniofacial defects	Apoptosis of hepatocytes	(Grabow et al. 2018; Hikita et al. 2009)
Mcl1 $^{+/-}$ ***Bcl2*** $^{+/-}$	Heterozygous for MCL-1 and BCL-XL expression in all tissues	No overt defects	—	(Grabow et al. 2018)
Bcl2 $^{+/-}$ ***Bcl-x*** $^{+/-}$	Heterozygous for MCL-1 and BCL-XL expression in all tissues	No overt defects	—	(Grabow et al. 2018)
Bak $^{-/-}$	BAK deficient in all tissues	No overt defects	Slight accumulation of platelets	(Mason et al. 2007)
Bax $^{-/-}$	BAX deficient in all tissues	Defects in retina Reproductive defects in females Male infertility	Progressive accumulation of lymphoid cells Accumulation of premeiotic germ cells	(Knudson et al. 1995; Pequignot et al. 2003)
Bax $^{-/-}$ ***Bak*** $^{-/-}$	Deficient for both BAX and BAK in all tissues	Early mortality Webbed feet Imperforate vaginal canals Omphaloceles Exencephaly	Accumulation of hematopoietic and neuronal cells Lymphocytes resistant apoptosis induced by diverse stressors	(Ke et al. 2018; Lindsten et al. 2000)

(Continued)

Table 10.1 (Continued)

Genotype	Description	Overt phenotype	Cell types affected	References
Bok$^{-/-}$	BOK deficient in all tissues	No overt defects	—	(Ke et al. 2012)
Bax$^{-/-}$*Bak*$^{-/-}$*Bok*$^{-/-}$	Deficient for BAX, BAK, and BOK in all tissues	Early mortality Webbed feet Facial clefting Omphaloceles Exencephaly	—	(Ke et al. 2018)
Bim$^{-/-}$	BIM deficient in all tissues	Autoimmune kidney disease	Accumulation of lymphoid and myeloid cells Accumulation of autoreactive thymocytes and B-cells Lymphocytes resistant to apoptosis induced by DNA damage, cytokine deprivation, and ER stress	(Bouillet et al. 1999; Enders et al. 2003; Puthalakath et al. 2007)
Puma$^{-/-}$	PUMA deficient in all tissues	No overt defects	Lymphocytes and fibroblasts resistant to DNA damage and y-irradiation	(Jeffers et al. 2003; Villunger et al. 2003)
Noxa$^{-/-}$	NOXA deficient in all tissues	No overt defects	Fibroblasts resistant to DNA damage	(Villunger et al. 2003; Shibue et al. 2003)
Bid$^{-/-}$	BID deficient in all tissues	No overt defects	Hepatocytes resistant to Fas-induced apoptosis	(Yin et al. 1999)
Bik$^{-/-}$	BIK deficient in all tissues	No overt defects	—	(Coultas et al. 2004)
Bmf$^{-/-}$	BMF deficient in all tissues	No overt defects	Accumulation of lymphoid cells Lymphocytes resistant to apoptosis induced by glucocorticoids or histone deacetylase inhibition	(Labi et al. 2008)
Bad$^{-/-}$	BAD deficient in all tissues	No overt defects Progress to diffuse large B-cell lymphoma with aging	Mild accumulation of platelets	(Kelly et al. 2010; Ranger et al. 2003)
Hrk$^{-/-}$	HRK deficient in all tissues	No overt defects	Motoneurons resistant to cell death following resection, superior cervical ganglia resistant to cell death triggered by nerve growth factor removal	(Imaizumi et al. 2004)
Bim$^{-/-}$*Puma*$^{-/-}$	Deficient for both BIM and PUMA in all tissues	Splenomegaly Lymphadenopathy Prone to lymphoma development	Accumulation of lymphocytes and thymocytes Lymphocytes resistant to apoptosis induced by diverse stressors	(Erlacher et al. 2006)
Bim$^{-/-}$*Puma*$^{-/-}$*Bid*$^{-/-}$	Deficient for BIM, PUMA, and BID in all tissues	Early mortality Webbed feet Imperforate vaginal canals Enlarged thymi Splenomegaly lymphadenopathy	Accumulation of hematopoietic cells Lymphocytes resistant to apoptosis induced by diverse stressors	(Ren et al. 2010)

For example, cells may express high levels of MCL-1, but if this MCL-1 is sequestered by high levels of one or more BH3-only proteins binding to MCL-1, the contribution of MCL-1 protein to the survival of a cell may be nullified.

BIM-deficient mice (the gene that encodes BIM is called *Bcl2l11*) have excessive accumulation of lymphoid and myeloid cells in peripheral blood, spleen, and lymph nodes (Bouillet et al. 1999). BIM is also required for the deletion of autoreactive thymocytes (Bouillet et al. 1999) and B-cells (Enders et al. 2003), with most older BIM-deficient mice (on a mixed C57BL/6x129SV background) dying from autoimmune kidney disease (Bouillet et al. 1999). Loss of BIM protects diverse hematopoietic cell types from DNA-damaging agents, including chemotherapeutic drugs (Bouillet et al. 1999; Erlacher et al. 2005) and also from cytokine deprivation (Bouillet et al. 1999) as well as ER stress (Puthalakath et al. 2007). Interestingly, all defects caused by the absence of pro-survival BCL2, detailed earlier, can be prevented by the concomitant loss of pro-apoptotic BIM, demonstrating the importance of the balance between pro-apoptotic and pro-survival proteins (Bouillet et al. 2001).

PUMA-deficient (the gene that encodes PUMA is called *Bbc3*) mice show no obvious developmental defects. PUMA-deficient lymphocytes show resistance to DNA-damaging agents and y-irradiation (Jeffers et al. 2003; Villunger et al. 2003). NOXA-deficient (the gene that encodes NOXA is termed *Pmaip1*) mice (Shibue et al. 2003; Villunger et al. 2003), BID-deficient mice (Yin et al. 1999), and BIK-deficient mice (Coultas et al. 2004) show no marked developmental defects. BMF-deficient mice exhibit progressive lymphoid hyperplasia (Labi et al. 2008). BAD-deficient mice show a mild increase in platelets (Kelly et al. 2010; Ranger et al. 2003), while HRK-deficient mice showed normal development and HRK loss was found to be neuroprotective (Imaizumi et al. 2004). The relatively mild phenotypes of several of the BH3-only protein-deficient mice are likely due to their redundant and overlapping roles in promoting apoptosis. Indeed, more substantial defects, such as lymphadenopathy and webbed feet, were observed in BIM/PUMA double knockout and BIM/PUMA/BID triple knockout mice (Erlacher et al. 2006; Ren et al. 2010).

The Dysregulation of Apoptosis in Cancer

While the idea that evasion of cell death could contribute to tumorigenesis was first illustrated by studies which showed that overexpression of the pro-survival protein BCL2 in mice could accelerate oncogene-driven tumor development (Strasser et al. 1990; Vaux et al. 1992a, 1988), we now know that escape from apoptosis, a hallmark of cancer, can be achieved by alterations at multiple levels of the intrinsic apoptosis pathway. In all cases, these molecular changes result in an environment which strongly favors cell survival even in the face of increased pro-apoptotic signals.

The two main ways that cancer cells overcome apoptosis are by upregulating one or more pro-survival BCL2 proteins which protect the cells from pro-apoptotic signals, or by losing expression of one or more pro-apoptotic proteins, thereby diminishing the pro-apoptotic signal itself.

Overexpression of pro-survival BCL2 family members has long been established as a mechanism which facilitates tumorigenesis. The first studies showing BCL2 overexpression could accelerate MYC-driven lymphomagenesis in mice (Strasser et al. 1990; Vaux et al. 1992a, 1988) have since been replicated with overexpression of other pro-survival proteins, showing that this is a class effect. Overexpression of MCL-1 in the hematopoietic system of mice resulted in lymphoid cells with profound resistance to cytotoxic agents (Campbell et al. 2010). Moreover, MCL-1 overexpression could accelerate MYC-driven lymphomagenesis resulting in death of mice around birth from stem/progenitor cell tumors. Similarly, overexpression of BCL-XL specifically in the B-cell compartment resulted in aggressive acute leukemias representing an early stage of B-cell development (Swanson et al. 2004).

Notably, a diversity of human cancers has been shown to overexpress pro-survival proteins. This is commonly achieved by amplification of the locus encoding pro-survival proteins, for example MCL-1 and BCL-XL in diverse human cancers (Beroukhim et al. 2010), or by translocations of pro-survival proteins into the proximity of transcriptional enhancers, for example translocation of BCL2 into the immunoglobulin heavy chain locus in follicular lymphoma (Yunis et al. 1987). An alternative mechanism which can cause upregulation of pro-survival proteins is the loss of repressive microRNAs, small non-coding RNAs which can regulate diverse cellular signaling pathways. For example, loss of miR-15a and miR-16–1, which normally represses expression of BCL-2, occurs frequently in chronic lymphocytic leukemia (Cimmino et al. 2005). Increased expression of pro-survival proteins can also be induced in cancer cells by factors provided by the tumor microenvironment. Activation of the NF-κB pathway by signaling by cytokines or other factors from the lymph node niche has been shown to upregulate BCL2, BCL-XL, and BFL-1 thereby contributing to the survival of resident chronic lymphocytic leukemia cells (Haselager et al. 2021; Jayappa et al. 2017; Thijssen et al. 2015). While high expression levels of particular pro-survival proteins do not necessarily indicate dependency on said protein for ongoing survival, cancer types which may be sensitive to therapies targeting pro-survival overexpression can be identified using shRNA knockdown, CRISPR/Cas9-mediated gene deletion, or application of BH3-mimetic drugs that inhibit certain pro-survival proteins. Much research focus has been applied to identify the pro-survival proteins which are not only highly expressed but also essential to protect the survival of particular malignant cells, in the hopes of identifying vulnerabilities which can be exploited for cancer therapy.

Over 10% of human cancers have amplification of the *MCL1* locus (Beroukhim et al. 2010) and increased MCL-1 protein expression has been observed in diverse malignancies, including in lymphoma and leukemia (Aichberger et al. 2005; Cho-Vega et al. 2004). An essential role for MCL-1 in the survival has been established for numerous malignancies, including diverse blood cancers, such as Burkitt's lymphoma (Kelly et al. 2014), acute myeloid leukemia (Glaser et al. 2012), acute lymphoblastic leukemia (Koss et al. 2013), T-cell lymphoma (Grabow et al. 2014; Spinner et al. 2016), and multiple myeloma (Gong et al. 2016), as well as certain solid cancers, such as non-small cell lung cancer (Zhang et al. 2011), breast cancer (Xiao et al. 2015), and melanoma (Boisvert-Adamo et al. 2009).

Amplification of *BCL2L1*, which encodes BCL-XL, is also a common somatic copy-number change detected among human cancers (Beroukhim et al. 2010), and BCL-XL is known to be highly expressed particularly in solid tumors, including colorectal cancer (Scherr et al. 2016), gastric cancer (Kondo et al. 1996), bladder cancer (Kirsh et al. 1998), and breast cancer (Olopade et al. 1997). Cancers with established dependencies on BCL-XL for survival include natural killer/T-cell lymphomas (Sejic et al. 2020) and malignant pleural mesothelioma (Arulananda et al. 2020). In addition, high expression levels of BCL-XL were found to correlate with general resistance to anti-cancer drugs in a panel of 60 human cancer cell lines, highlighting its important role in securing the survival of diverse malignancies (Amundson et al. 2000). Furthermore, BCL-XL, along with BCL-W, has been found to safeguard the survival of senescent cells (Yosef et al. 2016). This finding suggests that the use of drugs targeting BCL-XL (and possibly BCL-W) in combination with anti-cancer therapies which promote senescence of malignant cells could be a promising therapeutic strategy (Gayle et al. 2019).

Overexpression of BCL2 was first identified in blood cancers (Pegoraro et al. 1984; Tsujimoto et al. 1987) and is particularly prevalent in follicular lymphomas, most of which have characteristic IgH:BCL2 t(14;18) chromosomal translocations, as well as in MCL, Waldenstrom's macroglobulinemia, and chronic lymphocytic leukemia (Roberts and Huang 2017). High BCL2 expression has also been reported in subsets of lung (Pezzella et al. 1993), breast (Monaghan et al. 1992), and prostate (McDonnell et al. 1992) cancers. BCL2 is known to be critical for the survival of chronic lymphocytic leukemia (Souers et al. 2013), multiple myeloma with t(11;14) translocations (Touzeau et al. 2014) and acute myeloid leukemia (Pan et al. 2014), along with small-cell lung cancers (Lochmann et al. 2018) and estrogen receptor-positive breast cancers (Vaillant et al. 2013), which express high levels of BCL2.

High expression of BCL-W has been identified in subsets of non-Hodgkin's lymphoma, though its role in the survival of these malignant cells is disputed (Adams et al. 2017, 2020; Diepstraten et al. 2020). BFL-1 is highly expressed in hematological malignancies, such as B chronic lymphocytic leukemia (Morales et al. 2005), MCL (Nagy et al. 2003), and diffuse large B-cell lymphoma (Feuerhake et al. 2005). Interestingly, higher BFL-1 expression is associated with more severe disease in breast cancer (Yoon et al. 2003) and melanoma (Riker et al. 2008). BFL-1 also has an increasingly recognized role in promoting resistance to a variety of anti-cancer therapies, including chemotherapies and drugs targeting the apoptosis pathway (Vogler 2012).

It is important to note that the dependency of cancer cells on a particular pro-survival BCL2 protein for sustained survival is not always due to the aberrant expression of this protein and instead can reflect the cell of origin of the tumor. For example, multiple myeloma cells are sensitive to MCL-1 inhibitors (Kotschy et al. 2016), and while it is known MCL-1 can be overexpressed in multiple myeloma (Wuilleme-Toumi et al. 2005), the cells of origin for this tumor are plasma cells that are themselves highly MCL-1 dependent (Peperzak et al. 2013).

Aside from increased expression of pro-survival proteins, the second mechanism by which cancer cells can evade apoptosis is by loss of pro-apoptotic protein expression. Epigenetic silencing of the genes for pro-apoptotic BH3-only proteins BIM, PUMA, and NOXA frequently occurs in Burkitt's lymphoma (Garrison et al. 2008; Mestre-Escorihuela et al. 2007; Richter-Larrea et al. 2010), while hypermethylation of the promoters of the *HRK*, *BIK*, and *BAD* genes has been observed in diverse cancers, including colorectal cancer (Obata et al. 2003), glioma (Kim et al. 2006b), and myeloma (Pompeia et al. 2004), respectively. Silencing of the pro-apoptotic effector proteins BAX and BAK has been reported in multiple myeloma (Pompeia et al. 2004). Deletion of the genes for certain pro-apoptotic proteins has also been identified. Deletion of *BIM* is common in MCL (Mestre-Escorihuela et al. 2007), while inactivating mutations in BAX and/or BAK have been reported in colorectal cancer (Miquel et al. 2005) and gastrointestinal cancers (Ionov et al. 2000).

Due to the critical role that caspases play in executing apoptosis, it may be anticipated that they would be commonly lost or deactivated in cancer cells to aid in evasion of cell death. However, compared with BCL2 family members, the genes for caspases are rarely mutated in human cancers and more research is required to elucidate their exact functions in the development and ongoing survival of malignant cells (Jäger and Zwacka 2010; Olsson and Zhivotovsky 2011). The reason why caspases are not frequently lost in human cancer could be that activation of pro-apoptotic BAX and BAK can still kill cells effectively even when caspases are disabled (Marsden et al. 2002).

Taken together, these studies highlight the complexities of the apoptosis pathway and the changes that can occur at the many levels of regulation to give cancer cells a survival advantage. A thorough understanding of the fundamental roles of apoptosis pathway members in both normal and cancer cells is essential to drive the development of pharmacological interventions targeting cell death pathways. With the advent of BH3-mimetic drugs which directly inhibit pro-survival BCL2 family proteins to trigger apoptosis, and the current progression of these new anti-cancer drugs into the clinic, the knowledge gained from these fundamental studies into cell death has become more vital than ever.

Must Read References

Bedoui, S., Herold, M.J., and Strasser, A. (2020). Emerging connectivity of programmed cell death pathways and its physiological implications. *Nat. Rev. Mol. Cell Biol.* 21: 678–695.

Bouillet, P., Metcalf, D., Huang, D.C.S. et al. (1999). Proapoptotic Bcl-2 relative Bim required for certain apoptotic responses, leukocyte homeostasis, and to preclude autoimmunity. *Science* 286: 1735–1738.

Chen, L., Willis, S.N., Wei, A. et al. (2005). Differential targeting of pro-survival Bcl-2 proteins by their BH3-only ligands allows complementary apoptotic function. *Mol. Cell* 17: 393–403.

Clarke, P.G. and Clarke, S. (1996). Nineteenth century research on naturally occurring cell death and related phenomena. *Anat. Embryol.* 193: 81–99.

Diepstraten, S.T., Anderson, M.A., Czabotar, P.E. et al. (2022). The manipulation of apoptosis for cancer therapy using BH3-mimetic drugs. *Nat. Rev. Cancer.* 22: 45–64.

Jost, P.J., Grabow, S., Gray, D. et al. (2009). XIAP discriminates between type I and type II FAS-induced apoptosis. *Nature* 460: 1035–1039.

Kamada, S., Shimono, A., Shinto, Y. et al. (1995). *bcl-2* deficiency in mice leads to pleiotropic abnormalities: accelerated lymphoid cell death in thymus andspleen, polycystic kidney, hair hypopigmentation, and distorted small intestine. *Cancer Res.* 55: 354–359.

Kerr, J.F., Wyllie, A.H., and Currie, A.R. (1972). Apoptosis: a basic biological phenomenon with wide-ranging implications in tissue kinetics. *Br. J. Cancer* 26: 239–257.

Vaux, D.L., Cory, S., and Adams, J.M. (1988). *Bcl*-2 gene promotes haemopoietic cell survival and cooperates with c-*myc* to immortalize pre-B cells. *Nature* 335: 440–442.

Watanabe-Fukunaga, R., Brannan, C.I., Copeland, N.G. et al. (1992). Lymphoproliferation disorder in mice explained by defects in Fas antigen that mediates apoptosis. *Nature* 356: 314–317.

References

Adams, C.M., Kim, A.S., Mitra, R. et al. (2017). BCL-W has a fundamental role in B cell survival and lymphomagenesis. *J. Clin. Invest.* 127: 635–650.

Adams, C.M., Mitra, R., Vogel, A.N. et al. (2020). Targeting BCL-W and BCL-XL as a therapeutic strategy for Hodgkin lymphoma. *Leukemia* 34: 947–952.

Adams, J.M., Harris, A.W., Pinkert, C.A. et al. (1985). The c-myc oncogene driven by immunoglobulin enhancers induces lymphoid malignancy in transgenic mice. *Nature* 318: 533–538.

Aichberger, K.J., Mayerhofer, M., Krauth, M.T. et al. (2005). Identification of mcl-1 as a BCR/ABL-dependent target in chronic myeloid leukemia (CML): evidence for cooperative antileukemic effects of imatinib and mcl-1 antisense oligonucleotides. *Blood* 105: 3303–3311.

Amundson, S.A., Myers, T.G., Scudiero, D. et al. (2000). An informatics approach identifying markers of chemosensitivity in human cancer cell lines. *Cancer Res.* 60: 6101–6110.

Arulananda, S., O'brien, M., Evangelista, M. et al. (2020). BCL-XL is an actionable target for treatment of malignant pleural mesothelioma. *Cell Death Discov.* 6: 114.

Ashkenazi, A. and Dixit, V.M. (1998). Death receptors: signaling and modulation. *Science* 281: 1305–1308.

Aubrey, B.J., Kelly, G.L., Janic, A. et al. (2018). How does p53 induce apoptosis and how does this relate to p53-mediated tumour suppression? *Cell Death Differ.* 25: 104–113.

Bakhshi, A., Jensen, J.P., Goldman, P. et al. (1985). Cloning the chromosomal breakpoint of t(14;18) human lymphomas: clustering around J_H on chromosome 14 and near a transcriptional unit on 18. *Cell* 41: 899–906.

Bedoui, S., Herold, M.J., and Strasser, A. (2020). Emerging connectivity of programmed cell death pathways and its physiological implications. *Nat. Rev. Mol. Cell Biol.* 21: 678–695.

Bergsbaken, T., Fink, S.L., and Cookson, B.T. (2009). Pyroptosis: host cell death and inflammation. *Nat. Rev. Microbiol.* 7: 99–109.

Beroukhim, R., Mermel, C., Porter, D. et al. (2010). The landscape of somatic copy-number alteration across human cancers. *Nature* 463: 899–905.

Billen, L.P., Shamas-din, A., and Andrews, D.W. (2008). Bid: a Bax-like BH3 protein. *Oncogene* 27 (Suppl 1): S93–104.

Boisvert-Adamo, K., Longmate, W., Abel, E.V. et al. (2009). Mcl-1 is required for melanoma cell resistance to anoikis. *Mol. Cancer Res.* 7: 549–556.

Boldin, M.P., Goncharov, T.M., Goltsev, Y.V. et al. (1996). Involvement of MACH, a novel MORT1/FADD-interacting protease, in Fas/APO-1- and TNF receptor-induced cell death. *Cell* 85: 803–815.

Bouillet, P., Cory, S., Zhang, L.-C. et al. (2001). Degenerative disorders caused by Bcl-2 deficiency are prevented by loss of its BH3-only antagonist Bim. *Dev. Cell* 1: 645–653.

Bouillet, P., Metcalf, D., Huang, D.C.S. et al. (1999). Proapoptotic Bcl-2 relative Bim required for certain apoptotic responses, leukocyte homeostasis, and to preclude autoimmunity. *Science* 286: 1735–1738.

Brinkmann, K., Waring, P., Glaser, S.P. et al. (2020). BCL-XL exerts a protective role against anemia caused by radiation-induced kidney damage. *Embo J.* e105561.

Campbell, K.J., Bath, M.L., Turner, M.L. et al. (2010). Elevated Mcl-1 perturbs lymphopoiesis, promotes transformation of hematopoietic stem/progenitor cells, and enhances drug resistance. *Blood* 116: 3197–3207.

Certo, M., Del Gaizo Moore, V., Nishino, M. et al. (2006). Mitochondria primed by death signals determine cellular addiction to antiapoptotic BCL-2 family members. *Cancer Cell* 9: 351–365.

Chen, L., Willis, S.N., Wei, A. et al. (2005). Differential targeting of pro-survival Bcl-2 proteins by their BH3-only ligands allows complementary apoptotic function. *Mol. Cell* 17: 393–403.

Cho-Vega, J.H., Rassidakis, G.Z., Admirand, J.H. et al. (2004). MCL-1 expression in B-cell non-Hodgkin's lymphomas. *Hum. Pathol.* 35: 1095–1100.

Cimmino, A., Calin, G.A., Fabbri, M. et al. (2005). miR-15 and miR-16 induce apoptosis by targeting BCL2. *Proc. Natl. Acad. Sci. U.S.A.* 102: 13944–13949.

Clarke, P.G. and Clarke, S. (1996). Nineteenth century research on naturally occurring cell death and related phenomena. *Anat. Embryol.* 193: 81–99.

Cleary, M.L. and Sklar, J. (1985). Nucleotide sequence of a t(14;18) chromosomal breakpoint in follicular lymphoma and demonstration of a breakpoint-cluster region near a transcriptionally active locus on chromosome 18. *Proc. Natl. Acad. Sci. U.S.A.* 82: 7439–7443.

Cosentino, K. and Garcia-Saez, A.J. (2017). Bax and bak pores: are we closing the circle? *Trends Cell Biol.* 27: 266–275.

Coultas, L., Bouillet, P., Stanley, E.G. et al. (2004). Proapoptotic BH3-only Bcl-2 family member Bik/Blk/Nbk is expressed in hemopoietic and endothelial cells but is redundant for their programmed death. *Mol. Cell Biol.* 24: 1570–1581.

Czabotar, P.E., Lessene, G., Strasser, A. et al. (2014). Control of apoptosis by the BCL-2 protein family: implications for physiology and therapy. *Nat. Rev. Mol. Cell Biol.* 15: 49–63.

Diepstraten, S.T., Anderson, M.A., Czabotar, P.E. et al. (2022). The manipulation of apoptosis for cancer therapy using BH3-mimetic drugs. *Nat. Rev. Cancer. 22: 45–64.*

Diepstraten, S.T., Chang, C., Tai, L. et al. (2020). BCL-W is dispensable for the sustained survival of select Burkitt lymphoma and diffuse large B-cell lymphoma cell lines. *Blood Adv.* 4: 356–366.

Dixon, S.J., Lemberg, K.M., Lamprecht, M.R. et al. (2012). Ferroptosis: an iron-dependent form of nonapoptotic cell death. *Cell* 149: 1060–1072.

Dzhagalov, I., St John, A., and He, Y.W. (2007). The antiapoptotic protein Mcl-1 is essential for the survival of neutrophils but not macrophages. *Blood* 109: 1620–1626.

Ellis, H.M. and Horvitz, H.R. (1986). Genetic control of programmed cell death in the nematode C. elegans. *Cell* 44: 817–829.

Enders, A., Bouillet, P., Puthalakath, H. et al. (2003). Loss of the pro-apoptotic BH3-only Bcl-2 family member Bim inhibits BCR stimulation-induced apoptosis and deletion of autoreative B cells. *J. Exp. Med.* 198: 1119–1126.

Erlacher, M., Laabi, V., Manzl, C. et al. (2006). Puma cooperates with Bim, the rate-limiting BH3-only protein in cell death during lymphocyte development, in apoptosis induction. *J. Exp. Med.* 203: 2939–2951.

Erlacher, M., Michalak, E.M., Kelly, P.N. et al. (2005). BH3-only proteins Puma and Bim are rate-limiting for {gamma} -radiation and glucocorticoid-induced apoptosis of lymphoid cells in vivo. *Blood* 106: 4131–4138.

Feuerhake, F., Kutok, J.L., Monti, S. et al. (2005). NFkappaB activity, function, and target-gene signatures in primary mediastinal large B-cell lymphoma and diffuse large B-cell lymphoma subtypes. *Blood* 106: 1392–1399.

Fukuhara, S. and Rowley, J.D. (1978). Chromosome 14 translocations in non-Burkitt lymphomas. *Int. J. Cancer* 22: 14–21.

Garrison, S.P., Jeffers, J.R., Yang, C. et al. (2008). Selection against PUMA gene expression in Myc-driven B-cell lymphomagenesis. *Mol. Cell Biol.* 28: 5391–5402.

Gayle, S.S., Sahni, J.M., Webb, B.M. et al. (2019). Targeting BCL-xL improves the efficacy of bromodomain and extra-terminal protein inhibitors in triple-negative breast cancer by eliciting the death of senescent cells. *J. Biol. Chem.* 294: 875–886.

Glaser, S., Lee, E.F., Trounson, E. et al. (2012). Anti-apoptotic Mcl-1 is essential for the development and sustained growth of acute myeloid leukemia. *Genes Dev.* 26: 120–125.

Gong, J.N., Khong, T., Segal, D. et al. (2016). Hierarchy for targeting prosurvival BCL2 family proteins in multiple myeloma: pivotal role of MCL1. *Blood* 128: 1834–1844.

Grabow, S., Delbridge, A.R., Valente, L.J. et al. (2014). MCL-1 but not BCL-XL is critical for the development and sustained expansion of thymic lymphoma in p53-deficient mice. *Blood* 124: 3939–3946.

Grabow, S., Kueh, A.J., Ke, F. et al. (2018). Subtle changes in the levels of BCL-2 proteins cause severe craniofacial abnormalities. *Cell Rep.* 24: 3285–3295 e4.

Green, D.R. (2019). The coming decade of cell death research: five riddles. *Cell* 177: 1094–1107.

Hakem, R., Hakem, A., Duncan, G.S. et al. (1998). Differential requirement for caspase 9 in apoptotic pathways in vivo. *Cell* 94: 339–352.

Hamasaki, A., Sendo, F., Nakayama, K. et al. (1998). Accelerated neutrophil apoptosis in mice lacking A1-a, a subtype of the *bcl-2*-related A1 gene. *J. Exp. Med.* 188: 1985–1992.

Hanahan, D. and Weinberg, R.A. (2011). Hallmarks of cancer: the next generation. *Cell* 144: 646–674.

Haselager, M., Thijssen, R., West, C. et al. (2021). Regulation of Bcl-XL by non-canonical NF-κB in the context of CD40-induced drug resistance in CLL. *Cell Death & Differentiation* 28: 1658–1668.

Healy, M.E., Boege, Y., Hodder, M.C. et al. (2020). MCL1 is required for maintenance of intestinal homeostasis and prevention of carcinogenesis in mice. *Gastroenterol.* 159: 183–199.

Hedgecock, E.M., Sulston, J.E., and Thomson, J.N. (1983). Mutations affecting programmed cell deaths in the nematode. *Caenorhabditis elegans. Science* 220: 1277–1279.

Hikita, H., Takehara, T., Shimizu, S. et al. (2009). Mcl-1 and Bcl-xL cooperatively maintain integrity of hepatocytes in developing and adult murine liver. *Hepatol.* 50: 1217–1226.

Hughes, P.D., Belz, G.T., Fortner, K. et al. (2008). Apoptosis regulators Fas and Bim cooperate in shutdown of chronic immune responses and prevention of autoimmunity. *Immunity* 28: 197–205.

Imaizumi, K., Benito, A., Kiryu-seo, S. et al. (2004). Critical role for DP5/Harakiri, a Bcl-2 homology domain 3-only Bcl-2 family member, in axotomy-induced neuronal cell death. *J. Neurosci.* 24: 3721–3725.

Ionov, Y., Yamamoto, H., Krajewski, S. et al. (2000). Mutational inactivation of the proapoptotic gene BAX confers selective advantage during tumor clonal evolution. *Proc. Natl. Acad. Sci. U.S.A.* 97: 10872–10877.

Jäger, R. and Zwacka, R.M. (2010). The enigmatic roles of caspases in tumor development. *Cancers (Basel)* 2: 1952–1979.

Jayappa, K.D., Portell, C.A., Gordon, V.L. et al. (2017). Microenvironmental agonists generate de novo phenotypic resistance to combined ibrutinib plus venetoclax in CLL and MCL. *Blood Adv.* 1: 933–946.

Jeffers, J.R., Parganas, E., Lee, Y. et al. (2003). Puma is an essential mediator of p53-dependent and -independent apoptotic pathways. *Cancer Cell* 4: 321–328.

Jiang, X., Stockwell, B.R., and Conrad, M. (2021). Ferroptosis: mechanisms, biology and role in disease. *Nat. Rev. Mol. Cell Biol.* 22: 266–282.

Jost, P.J., Grabow, S., Gray, D. et al. (2009). XIAP discriminates between type I and type II FAS-induced apoptosis. *Nature* 460: 1035–1039.

Kamada, S., Shimono, A., Shinto, Y. et al. (1995). *bcl-2* deficiency in mice leads to pleiotropic abnormalities: accelerated lymphoid cell death in thymus andspleen, polycystic kidney, hair hypopigmentation, and distorted small intestine. *Cancer Res.* 55: 354–359.

Ke, F., Voss, A., Kerr, J.B. et al. (2012). BCL-2 family member BOK is widely expressed but its loss has only minimal impact in mice. *Cell Death Differ.* 19: 915–925.

Ke, F.F.S., Vanyai, H.K., Cowan, A.D. et al. (2018). Embryogenesis and adult life in the absence of intrinsic apoptosis effectors BAX, BAK, and BOK. *Cell* 173: 1217–1230 e17.

Kelly, G.L., Grabow, S., Glaser, S.P. et al. (2014). Targeting of MCL-1 kills MYC-driven mouse and human lymphomas even when they bear mutations in p53. *Genes Dev.* 28: 58–70.

Kelly, G.L. and Strasser, A. (2011). The essential role of evasion from cell death in cancer. *Adv. Cancer Res.* 111: 39–96.

Kelly, P.N., White, M.J., Goschnick, M.W. et al. (2010). Individual and overlapping roles of BH3-only proteins Bim and Bad in apoptosis of lymphocytes and platelets and in suppression of thymic lymphoma development. *Cell Death Differ.* 17: 1655–1664.

Kerr, J.F. (1965). A histochemical study of hypertrophy and ischaemic injury of rat liver with special reference to changes in lysosomes. *J. Pathol. Bacteriol.* 90: 419–435.

Kerr, J.F., Wyllie, A.H., and Currie, A.R. (1972). Apoptosis: a basic biological phenomenon with wide-ranging implications in tissue kinetics. *Br. J. Cancer* 26: 239–257.

Kim, H., Rafiuddin-shah, M., Tu, H.C. et al. (2006a). Hierarchical regulation of mitochondrion-dependent apoptosis by BCL-2 subfamilies. *Nat. Cell Biol.* 8: 1348–1358.

Kim, T.Y., Zhong, S., Fields, C.R. et al. (2006b). Epigenomic profiling reveals novel and frequent targets of aberrant DNA methylation-mediated silencing in malignant glioma. *Cancer Res.* 66: 7490–7501.

Kirsh, E.J., Baunoch, D.A., and Stadler, W.M. (1998). Expression of bcl-2 and bcl-X in bladder cancer. *J. Urol.* 159: 1348–1353.

Kischkel, F.C., Hellbardt, S., Behrmann, I. et al. (1995). Cytotoxicity-dependent APO-1 (Fas/CD95) - associated proteins form a death-inducing signaling complex (DISC) with the receptor. *EMBO J.* 14: 5579–5588.

Knudson, C.M., Tung, K.S.K., Tourtellotte, W.G. et al. (1995). Bax-deficient mice with lymphoid hyperplasia and male germ cell death. *Science* 270: 96–99.

Kondo, S., Shinomura, Y., Kanayama, S. et al. (1996). Over-expression of bcl-xL gene in human gastric adenomas and carcinomas. *Int. J. Cancer* 68: 727–730.

Koss, B., Morrison, J., Perciavalle, R.M. et al. (2013). Requirement for antiapoptotic MCL-1 in the survival of BCR-ABL B-lineage acute lymphoblastic leukemia. *Blood* 122: 1587–1598.

Kotschy, A., Szlavik, Z., Murray, J. et al. (2016). The MCL1 inhibitor S63845 is tolerable and effective in diverse cancer models. *Nature* 538: 477–482.

Kuwana, T., Bouchier-hayes, L., Chipuk, J.E. et al. (2005). BH3 domains of BH3-only proteins differentially regulate bax-mediated mitochondrial membrane permeabilization both directly and indirectly. *Mol. Cell* 17: 525–535.

Labi, V., Erlacher, M., Kiessling, S. et al. (2008). Loss of the BH3-only protein Bmf impairs B cell homeostasis and accelerates gamma irradiation-induced thymic lymphoma development. *J. Exp. Med.* 205: 641–655.

Lamhamedi-Cherradi, S.E., Zheng, S.J., Maguschak, K.A. et al. (2003). Defective thymocyte apoptosis and accelerated autoimmune diseases in TRAIL-/- mice. *Nat. Immunol.* 4: 255–260.

Lamkanfi, M., Declercq, W., Kalai, M. et al. (2002). Alice in caspase land. A phylogenetic analysis of caspases from worm to man. *Cell Death Differ.* 9: 358–361.

Letai, A., Bassik, M., Walensky, L. et al. (2002). Distinct BH3 domains either sensitize or activate mitochondrial apoptosis, serving as prototype cancer therapeutics. *Cancer Cell* 2: 183–192.

Li, H., Zhu, H., Xu, C.-J. et al. (1998). Cleavage of BID by caspase 8 mediates the mitochondrial damage in the Fas pathway of apoptosis. *Cell* 94: 491–501.

Lieschke, E., Wang, Z., Kelly, G.L. et al. (2018). Discussion of some "knowns" and some "unknowns" about the tumour suppressor. *J. Mol. Cell Biol.* 53.

Lilla, J.N., Chen, C.C., Mukai, K. et al. (2011). Reduced mast cell and basophil numbers and function in Cpa3-Cre; Mcl-1fl/fl mice. *Blood* 118: 6930–6938.

Lindsten, T., Ross, A.J., King, A. et al. (2000). The combined functions of proapoptotic Bcl-2 family members Bak and Bax are essential for normal development of multiple tissues. *Mol. Cell* 6: 1389–1399.

Lochmann, T.L., Floros, K.V., Naseri, M. et al. (2018). Venetoclax is effective in small-cell lung cancers with high BCL-2 expression. *Clin. Cancer Res.* 24: 360–369.

Lockshin, R.A. (1969). Programmed cell death. Activation of lysis by a mechanism involving the synthesis of protein. *J. Insect Physiol.* 15: 1505–1516.

Luo, X., Budlhardjo, I., Zou, H. et al. (1998). Bid, a Bcl-2 interacting protein, mediates cytochrome *c* release from mitochondria in response to activation of cell surface death receptors. *Cell* 94: 481–490.

Ma, A., Pena, J.C., Chang, B. et al. (1995). Bclx regulates the survival of double-positive thymocytes. *Proc. Natl. Acad. Sci. U.S.A.* 92: 4763–4767.

Mak, -S.-S., Moriyama, M., Nishioka, E. et al. (2006). Indispensable role of Bcl2 in the development of the melanocyte stem cell. *Develop. Biol.* 291: 144–153.

Marsden, V., O'connor, L., O'REILLY, L.A. et al. (2002). Apoptosis initiated by Bcl–2-regulated caspase activation independently of the cytochrome *c*/Apaf–1/caspase–9 apoptosome. *Nature* 419: 634–637.

Mason, K.D., Carpinelli, M.R., Fletcher, J.I. et al. (2007). Programmed anuclear cell death delimits platelet life span. *Cell* 128: 1173–1186.

Mcarthur, K., Whitehead, L.W., Heddleston, J.M. et al. (2018). BAK/BAX macropores facilitate inner mitochondrial membrane herniation and mtDNA efflux. *Science* 359: eaao6047.

Mcdonnell, T.J., Deane, N., Platt, F.M. et al. (1989). *bcl-2*-immunoglobulin transgenic mice demonstrate extended B cell survival and follicular lymphoproliferation. *Cell* 57: 79–88.

McDonnell, T.J., Troncoso, P., Brisbay, S.M. et al. (1992). Expression of the proto-oncogene Bcl-2 in the prostate and its association with emergence of androgen-independent prostate cancer. *Cancer Res* 52: 6940–6944.

Merino, D., Kelly, G.L., Lessene, G. et al. (2018). BH3-mimetic drugs: blazing the trail for new cancer medicines. *Cancer Cell* 34: 879–891.

Mestre-Escorihuela, C., Rubio-moscardo, F., Richter, J.A. et al. (2007). Homozygous deletions localize novel tumor suppressor genes in B-cell lymphomas. *Blood* 109: 271–280.

Michaelidis, T.M., Sendtner, M., Cooper, J.D. et al. (1996). Inactivation of *bcl-2* results in progressive degeneration of motoneurons, sympathetic and sensory neurons during early postnatal development. *Neuron* 17: 75–89.

Miquel, C., Borrini, F., Grandjouan, S. et al. (2005). Role of bax mutations in apoptosis in colorectal cancers with microsatellite instability. *Am. J. Clin. Pathol.* 123: 562–570.

Moldoveanu, T. and Czabotar, P.E. (2020). BAX, BAK, and BOK: a coming of age for the BCL-2 family effector proteins. *Cold Spring Harb. Perspect. Biol.* 12.

Moldoveanu, T., Follis, A.V., Kriwacki, R.W. et al. (2014). Many players in BCL-2 family affairs. *Trends Biochem Sci.* 39: 101–111.

Monaghan, P., Robertson, D., Amos, T.A.S. et al. (1992). Ultrastructural localization of BCL-2 protein. *J. Histochem. Cytochem.* 40: 1819–1825.

Morales, A.A., Olsson, A., Celsing, F. et al. (2005). High expression of bfl-1 contributes to the apoptosis resistant phenotype in B-cell chronic lymphocytic leukemia. *Int. J. Cancer* 113: 730–737.

Motoyama, N., Wang, F.P., Roth, K.A. et al. (1995). Massive cell death of immature hematopoietic cells and neurons in Bcl-x deficient mice. *Science* 267: 1506–1510.

Muzio, M., Chinnaiyan, A.M., Kischkel, F.C. et al. (1996). FLICE, a novel FADD homologous ICE/CED-3-like protease, is recruited to the CD95 (Fas/Apo-1) death-inducing signaling complex. *Cell* 85: 817–827.

Nagy, B., Lundan, T., Larramendy, M.L. et al. (2003). Abnormal expression of apoptosis-related genes in hematological malignancies: overexpression of MYC is poor prognostic sign in mantle cell lymphoma. *Br. J. Haematol.* 120: 434–441.

Nakamura, A., Swahari, V., Plestant, C. et al. (2016). Bcl-xL is essential for the survival and function of differentiated neurons in the cortex that control complex behaviors. *J. Neurosci.: The Off. J. Soc. Neurosci.* 36: 5448–5461.

Nakayama, K.-I., Nakayama, K., Izumi, N. et al. (1993). Disappearance of the lymphoid system in Bcl-2 homozygous mutant chimeric mice. *Science* 261: 1584–1588.

Nishimura, E.K., Granter, S.R., and Fisher, D.E. (2005). Mechanisms of hair graying: incomplete melanocyte stem cell maintenance in the niche. *Science* 307: 720–724.

O'Neill, K.L., Huang, K., Zhang, J. et al. (2016). Inactivation of prosurvival Bcl-2 proteins activates Bax/Bak through the outer mitochondrial membrane. *Genes Dev.* 30: 973–988.

O'Reilly, L.A., Print, C., Hausmann, G. et al. (2001). Tissue expression and subcellular localization of the pro-survival molecule Bcl-w. *Cell Death Differ.* 8: 486–494.

Obata, T., Toyota, M., Satoh, A. et al. (2003). Identification of HRK as a target of epigenetic inactivation in colorectal and gastric cancer. *Clin. Cancer Res.* 9: 6410–6418.

Oh, K.J., Barbuto, S., Pitter, K. et al. (2006). A membrane-targeted BID BCL-2 homology 3 peptide is sufficient for high potency activation of BAX in vitro. *J. Biol. Chem.* 281: 36999–37008.

Olopade, O.I., Adeyanju, M.O., Safa, A.R. et al. (1997). Overexpression of BCL-x protein in primary breast cancer is associated with high tumor grade and nodal metastases. *Cancer J. Sci. Am.* 3: 230–237.

Olsson, M. and Zhivotovsky, B. (2011). Caspases and cancer. *Cell Death Differ.* 18: 1441–1449.

Opferman, J., Iwasaki, H., Ong, C.C. et al. (2005). Obligate role of anti-apoptotic MCL-1 in the survival of hematopoietic stem cells. *Science* 307: 1101–1104.

Opferman, J.T., Letai, A., Beard, C. et al. (2003). Development and maintenance of B and T lymphocytes requires antiapoptotic MCL-1. *Nature* 426: 671–676.

Pan, R., Hogdal, L.J., Benito, J.M. et al. (2014). Selective BCL-2 inhibition by ABT-199 causes on-target cell death in acute myeloid leukemia. *Cancer Discov.* 4: 362–375.

Pegoraro, L., Palumbo, A., Erikson, J. et al. (1984). A 14;18 and an 8;14 chromosome translocation in a cell line derived from an acute B-cell leukemia. *Proc. Natl. Acad. Sci. U.S.A.* 81: 7166–7170.

Peperzak, V., Vikstrom, I., Walker, J. et al. (2013). Mcl-1 is essential for the survival of plasma cells. *Nat. Immunol.* 14: 290–297.

Pequignot, M.O., Provost, A.C., Salle, S. et al. (2003). Major role of BAX in apoptosis during retinal development and in establishment of a functional postnatal retina. *Dev. Dyn.* 228: 231–238.

Pezzella, F., Turley, H., Kuzu, I. et al. (1993). *bcl*-2 protein in non-small-cell lung carcinoma. *N. Engl. J. Med.* 329: 690–694.

Pompeia, C., Hodge, D.R., Plass, C. et al. (2004). Microarray analysis of epigenetic silencing of gene expression in the KAS-6/1 multiple myeloma cell line. *Cancer Res.* 64: 3465–3473.

Print, C.G., Loveland, K.L., Gibson, L. et al. (1998). Apoptosis regulator Bcl-w is essential for spermatogenesis but appears otherwise redundant. *Proc. Natl. Acad. Sci. U.S.A.* 95: 12424–12431.

Puthalakath, H., O'Reilly, L.A., Gunn, P. et al. (2007). ER stress triggers apoptosis by activating BH3-only protein Bim. *Cell* 129: 1337–1349.

Ranger, A.M., Zha, J., Harada, H. et al. (2003). *Bad*-deficient mice develop diffuse large B cell lymphoma. *Proc. Natl. Acad. Sci. U.S.A.* 100: 9324–9329.

Ren, D., Tu, H.C., Kim, H. et al. (2010). BID, BIM, and PUMA are essential for activation of the BAX- and BAK-dependent cell death program. *Science* 330: 1390–1393.

Rhodes, M.M., Kopsombut, P., Bondurant, M.C. et al. (2005). Bcl-x(L) prevents apoptosis of late-stage erythroblasts but does not mediate the antiapoptotic effect of erythropoietin. *Blood* 106: 1857–1863.

Richter-Larrea, J.A., Robles, E.F., Fresquet, V. et al. (2010). Reversion of epigenetically mediated BIM silencing overcomes chemoresistance in Burkitt lymphoma. *Blood* 116: 2531–2542.

Rieux-Laucat, F., Le Deist, F., Hivroz, C. et al. (1995). Mutations in Fas associated with human lymphoproliferative syndrome and autoimmunity. *Science* 268: 1347–1349.

Riker, A.I., Enkemann, S.A., Fodstad, O. et al. (2008). The gene expression profiles of primary and metastatic melanoma yields a transition point of tumor progression and metastasis. *BMC Med. Genomics* 1: 13.

Rinkenberger, J.L., Horning, S., Klocke, B. et al. (2000). Mcl-1 deficiency results in peri-implantation embryonic lethality. *Genes Dev.* 14: 23–27.

Roberts, A.W. and Huang, D. (2017). Targeting BCL2 with BH3 mimetics: basic science and clinical application of venetoclax in chronic lymphocytic leukemia and related B cell malignancies. *Clin. Pharmacol. Ther.* 101: 89–98.

Salvesen, G.S. and Dixit, V.M. (1999). Caspase activation: the induced-proximity model. *Proc. Natl. Acad. Sci. U.S.A.* 96: 10964–10967.

Saunders, J.W., JR. (1966). Death in embryonic systems. *Science* 154: 604–612.

Schenk, R.L., Tuzlak, S., Carrington, E.M. et al. (2017). Characterisation of mice lacking all functional isoforms of the pro-survival BCL-2 family member A1 reveals minor defects in the haematopoietic compartment. *Cell Death Differ* 24: 534–545.

Scherr, A.L., Gdynia, G., Salou, M. et al. (2016). Bcl-xL is an oncogenic driver in colorectal cancer. *Cell Death Dis.* 7: e2342.

Sejic, N., George, L.C., Tierney, R.J. et al. (2020). BCL-XL inhibition by BH3-mimetic drugs induces apoptosis in models of Epstein-Barr virus-associated T/NK-cell lymphoma. *Blood Adv.* 4: 4775–4787.

Sender, R. and Milo, R. (2021). The distribution of cellular turnover in the human body. *Nat. Med.* 27: 45–48.

Shibue, T., Takeda, K., Oda, E. et al. (2003). Integral role of Noxa in p53-mediated apoptotic response. *Genes Dev.* 17: 2233–2238.

Singh, R., Letai, A., and Sarosiek, K. (2019). Regulation of apoptosis in health and disease: the balancing act of BCL-2 family proteins. *Nat. Rev. Mol. Cell Biol.* 20: 175–193.

Sneller, M.C., Wang, J., Dale, J.K. et al. (1997). Clinical, immunologic and genetic features of an autoimmune lymphoproliferative syndrome associated with abnormal lymphocyte apoptosis. *Blood* 89: 1341–1348.

Sorenson, C.M., Rogers, S.A., Korsmeyer, S.J. et al. (1995). Fulminant metanephric apoptosis and abnormal kidney development in bcl-2-deficient mice. *Am. J. Physiol.* 268: F73–F81.

Souers, A.J., Leverson, J.D., Boghaert, E.R. et al. (2013). ABT-199, a potent and selective BCL-2 inhibitor, achieves antitumor activity while sparing platelets. *Nat. Med.* 19: 202–208.

Spinner, S., Crispatzu, G., Yi, J.H. et al. (2016). Re-activation of mitochondrial apoptosis inhibits T-cell lymphoma survival and treatment resistance. *Leukemia* 30: 1520–1530.

Strasser, A., Harris, A.W., Bath, M.L. et al. (1990). Novel primitive lymphoid tumours induced in transgenic mice by cooperation between *myc* and *bcl-2*. *Nature* 348: 331–333.

Strasser, A., Harris, A.W., Huang, D.C.S. et al. (1995). Bcl-2 and Fas/APO-1 regulate distinct pathways to lymphocyte apoptosis. *EMBO J.* 14: 6136–6147.

Strasser, A., Jost, P.J., and Nagata, S. (2009). The many roles of FAS receptor signaling in the immune system. *Immunity* 30: 180–192.

Sulston, J.E. and Horvitz, H.R. (1977). Postembryonic cell lineages of the nematode. *Caenorhabditis Elegans. Dev. Biol.* 56: 110–156.

Swanson, P.J., Kuslak, S.L., Fang, W. et al. (2004). Fatal acute lymphoblastic leukemia in mice transgenic for B cell-restricted bcl-xL and c-myc. *J. Immunol.* 172: 6684–6691.

Thijssen, R., Slinger, E., Weller, K. et al. (2015). Resistance to ABT-199 induced by microenvironmental signals in chronic lymphocytic leukemia can be counteracted by CD20 antibodies or kinase inhibitors. *Haematol.* 100: e302–e306.

Thomas, R.L., Roberts, D.J., Kubli, D.A. et al. (2013). Loss of MCL-1 leads to impaired autophagy and rapid development of heart failure. *Genes Dev.* 27: 1365–1377.

Timmer, J.C. and Salvesen, G.S. (2007). Caspase substrates. *Cell Death Differ* 14: 66–72.

Touzeau, C., Dousset, C., Le Gouill, S. et al. (2014). The Bcl-2 specific BH3 mimetic ABT-199: a promising targeted therapy for t(11;14) multiple myeloma. *Leukemia* 28: 210–212.

Tsujimoto, Y. and Croce, C.M. (1986). Analysis of the structure, transcripts, and protein products of *bcl-2*, the gene involved in human follicular lymphoma. *Proc. Natl. Acad. Sci. U.S.A.* 83: 5214–5218.

Tsujimoto, Y., Finger, L.R., Yunis, J. et al. (1984). Cloning of the chromosome breakpoint of neoplastic B cells with the t(14;18) chromosome translocation. *Science* 226: 1097–1099.

Tsujimoto, Y., Ikegaki, N., and Croce, C.M. (1987). Characterization of the protein product of *bcl-2*, the gene involved in human follicular lymphoma. *Oncogene* 2: 3–7.

Turnis, M.E., Kaminska, E., Smith, K.H. et al. (2021). Requirement for antiapoptotic MCL-1 during early erythropoiesis. *Blood* 137: 1945–1958.

Vaillant, F., Merino, D., Lee, L. et al. (2013). Targeting BCL-2 with the BH3 mimetic ABT-199 in estrogen receptor-positive breast cancer. *Cancer Cell* 24: 120–129.

Van Opdenbosch, N. and Lamkanfi, M. (2019). Caspases in cell death, inflammation, and disease. *Immunity* 50: 1352–1364.

Vandenabeele, P., Galluzzi, L., Vanden Berghe, T. et al. (2010). Molecular mechanisms of necroptosis: an ordered cellular explosion. *Nat. Rev. Mol. Cell Biol.* 11: 700–714.

Vaux, D.L., Aguila, H.L., and Weissman, I.L. (1992a). *Bcl-2* prevents death of factor-deprived cells but fails to prevent apoptosis in targets of cell mediated killing. *Int. Immunol.* 4: 821–824.

Vaux, D.L., Cory, S., and Adams, J.M. (1988). *Bcl-2* gene promotes haemopoietic cell survival and cooperates with c-*myc* to immortalize pre-B cells. *Nature* 335: 440–442.

Vaux, D.L., Weissman, I.L., and Kim, S.K. (1992b). Prevention of programmed cell death in *Caenorhabditis elegans* by human *bcl-2*. *Science* 258: 1955–1957.

Veis, D.J., Sentman, C.L., Bach, E.A. et al. (1993a). Expression of the Bcl-2 protein in murine and human thymocytes and in peripheral T lymphocytes. *J. Immunol.* 151: 2546–2554.

Veis, D.J., Sorenson, C.M., Shutter, J.R. et al. (1993b). Bcl-2-deficient mice demonstrate fulminant lymphoid apoptosis, polycystic kidneys, and hypopigmented hair. *Cell* 75: 229–240.

Vick, B., Weber, A., Urbanik, T. et al. (2009). Knockout of myeloid cell leukemia-1 induces liver damage and increases apoptosis susceptibility of murine hepatocytes. *Hepatol.* 49: 627–636.

Vikstrom, I., Carotta, S., Luethje, K. et al. (2010). Mcl-1 is essential for germinal center formation and B cell memory. *Science* 330: 1095–1099.

Villunger, A., Michalak, E.M., Coultas, L. et al. (2003). p53- and drug-induced apoptotic responses mediated by BH3-only proteins puma and noxa. *Science* 302: 1036–1038.

Vogler, M. (2012). BCL2A1: the underdog in the BCL2 family. *Cell Death Differ* 19: 67–74.

Vogt, C. (1842). Untersuchungen uber die Entwicklungsgeschichte der Geburtshelferkrote (*Alytes obstertricians*). In: (ed. J.U. Gassman). Solothurn.

Wagner, K.U., Claudio, E., Rucker, E.B., 3rd et al. (2000). Conditional deletion of the Bcl-x gene from erythroid cells results in hemolytic anemia and profound splenomegaly. *Development* 127: 4949–4958.

Walensky, L.D., Pitter, K., Morash, J. et al. (2006). A stapled BID BH3 helix directly binds and activates BAX. *Mol. Cell* 24: 199–210.

Watanabe-Fukunaga, R., Brannan, C.I., Copeland, N.G. et al. (1992). Lymphoproliferation disorder in mice explained by defects in Fas antigen that mediates apoptosis. *Nature* 356: 314–317.

Weinlich, R., Oberst, A., Beere, H.M. et al. (2017). Necroptosis in development, inflammation and disease. *Nat. Rev. Mol. Cell Biol.* 18: 127–136.

Willis, S.N., Chen, L., Dewson, G. et al. (2005). Proapoptotic Bak is sequestered by Mcl-1 and Bcl-xL, but not Bcl-2, until displaced by BH3-only proteins. *Genes Dev.* 19: 1294–1305.

Willis, S.N., Fletcher, J.I., Kaufmann, T. et al. (2007). Apoptosis initiated when BH3 ligands engage multiple Bcl-2 homologs, not Bax or Bak. *Science* 315: 856–859.

Wilson, N.S., Dixit, V., and Ashkenazi, A. (2009). Death receptor signal transducers: nodes of coordination in immune signaling networks. *Nat. Immunol.* 10: 348–355.

Wuilleme-Toumi, S., Robillard, N., Gomez, P. et al. (2005). Mcl-1 is overexpressed in multiple myeloma and associated with relapse and shorter survival. *Leukemia* 19: 1248–1252.

Xiang, Z., Ahmed, A.A., Moller, C. et al. (2001). Essential role of the prosurvival bcl-2 homologue A1 in mast cell survival after allergic activation. *J. Exp. Med.* 194: 1561–1569.

Xiao, Y., Nimmer, P., Sheppard, G.S. et al. (2015). MCL-1 is a key determinant of breast cancer cell survival: validation of MCL-1 dependency utilizing a highly selective small molecule inhibitor. *Mol. Cancer Ther.* 14: 1837–1847.

Yin, X.-M., Wang, K., Gross, A. et al. (1999). Bid-deficient mice are resistant to Fas-induced hepatocellular apoptosis. *Nature* 400: 886–891.

Yonish-Rouach, E., Resnitzky, D., Lotem, J. et al. (1991). Wild-type p53 induces apoptosis of myeloid leukaemic cells that is inhibited by interleukin-6. *Nature* 352: 345–347.

Yoon, H.-S., Hong, S.-H., Kang, H.-J. et al. (2003). Bfl-1 gene expression in breast cancer: its relationship with other prognostic factors. *J. Korean Med. Sci.* 18: 225–230.

Yosef, R., Pilpel, N., Tokarsky-Amiel, R. et al. (2016). Directed elimination of senescent cells by inhibition of BCL-W and BCL-XL. *Nat. Commun.* 7: 11190.

Yunis, J.J., Frizzera, G., Oken, M.M. et al. (1987). Multiple recurrent genomic defects in follicular lymphoma. A possible model for cancer. *N. Engl. J. Med.* 316: 79–84.

Zhang, H., Guttikonda, S., Roberts, L. et al. (2011). Mcl-1 is critical for survival in a subgroup of non-small-cell lung cancer cell lines. *Oncogene* 30: 1963–1968.

11

Pharmacologic Features of Drugs Targeting BCL2 Family Members

Jennifer K. Lue[1] *and Owen A. O'Connor*[2]

[1] *Memorial Sloan Kettering Cancer Center Lymphoma Service, New York, NY, USA*
[2] *Department of Medicine, Division of Hematology and Medical Oncology, T-Cell Malignancies Program University of Virginia Comprehensive Cancer Center Department of Microbiology, Immunology and Cancer Biology University of Virginia, Charlottesville, VA, USA*

Take Home Messages

- The balance of pro- and anti-apoptotic proteins dictates a cell's fate with regard to its survival or programmed cell death.
- Cancer cells tend to be "upregulated" with regard to the anti-apoptotic pathways and "repressed" with regard to the pro-apoptotic pathways, favoring survival.
- A tendency toward "upregulation" of anti-apoptotic pathways renders cells more resistant to traditional chemotherapy.
- Numerous small molecule strategies have been shown to intervene in this biology, readjusting the balance between pro-survival and pro-death signaling, with at least one agent already approved for the treatment of chronic lymphocytic leukemia (CLL).

Introduction

Apoptosis, or programmed cell death, is an essential process in development and tissue homeostasis. The biology is regulated by complex interactions between pro-apoptotic (i.e. pro-death) and anti-apoptotic (i.e. pro-survival) proteins. The delicate balance between these opposing forces dictates a cell's fate and plays a critical role in tumorigenesis. Alterations that lead to the deregulation of this balance in favor of cell survival can lead to the development of various human ailments, including cancer. Despite the frequent dysregulation of these pathways across all malignant diseases, the lymphomas stand out as the disease group where both biology and pharmacology blend, albeit not perfectly, to establish important proof-of-principal concepts. In this fascinating disease context, not only do alterations in these cell death pathways contribute directly to lymphomagenesis, but they can also render malignant cells resistant to conventional chemotherapeutic agents, serving as an escape mechanism over time.

Over the past several decades, attempts to leverage our understanding of the dysregulation of cell death pathways have led to many novel cancer therapeutics, starting from the introduction of traditional non-specific chemotherapy agents to more recent agents that target very specific interactions among the cast of members governing the balance between pro-death and pro-survival. Members of the BCL2 family are the key components of the intrinsic mitochondrial apoptotic pathway and share sequence homology, known as BCL2 homology (BH) domains, which influence structure and function (Cory et al. 2003). As outlined in greater detail in the preceding chapter, BCL2 family members can be divided into two distinct groups: (i) anti-apoptotic proteins which include BCL2, BCL-X_L, BCL-$_W$, MCL-1, and A1/BFL-1; and (ii) pro-apoptotic proteins such as BAX, BAK, BOK, BIM, PUMA, BID, BIK, BAD, and NOXA. These two groups share certain BH domains, with pro-survival proteins sharing all four BH domains (BH1, BH2, BH3, and BH4), while pro-apoptotic proteins share only BH3 homology, specifically with BAX, BAK, and BOK sharing BH1-3, and BIK, BID, BAD, BIM, PUMA, and NOXA harboring only the BH3 domain, which is the basis for referring to these specific proteins as "BH3-only proteins" (Huang and Strasser 2000; Youle and Strasser 2008). Again, the balance between the two distinct functional groups influences the survival of a cell. While the biological mechanisms

Precision Cancer Therapies: Targeting Oncogenic Drivers and Signaling Pathways in Lymphoid Malignancies: From Concept to Practice, Volume 1,
First Edition. Edited by Owen A. O'Connor, Stephen M. Ansell, and John F. Seymour.

of the apoptotic pathway have been discussed in detail in preceding chapters, herein we will review the history and pharmacological features of drugs that induce apoptosis and possible biomarkers that can predict response to these agents.

Historical Perspective: From the Discovery of BCL2 to Therapeutic Applications

It has been over three decades since the initial discovery of BCL2 (Reed et al. 1988) and its role in tumorigenesis. This fundamental observation has laid the foundation for our understanding of the critical role BCL2 plays in controlling cell fate and provided insights on how we might leverage that understanding to develop pro-apoptotic pharmacological agents (Figure 11.1). In 1984, Tsujimoto and colleagues were the first to identify BCL2 (Tsujimoto et al. 1985), specifically cloning portions of the *BCL2* gene and associated t(14;18) translocation, which was identified in 1978 (Fukuhara and Rowley 1978), as a characteristic genetic feature of human follicular lymphoma (FL) (Tsujimoto et al. 1984, 1985). Shortly thereafter, Reed et al. (1988) were the first to describe *BCL2* as an oncogene, demonstrating that *BCL2* constructs could enhance the tumorigenicity of transfected cells. Subsequently, further insights on how BCL2 functions as an oncogene was described through elegant experiments in which retroviral constructs of *BCL2* were introduced into two cell lines: the pro-B cell line LyHy7 and the myeloid line, FDC-P1, both of which had obligatory requirements for interleukin 3 (IL-3) supplementation (Vaux et al. 1988). Upon introduction of the retroviral construct, both cell lines were able to survive in the absence of IL-3 supplementation and

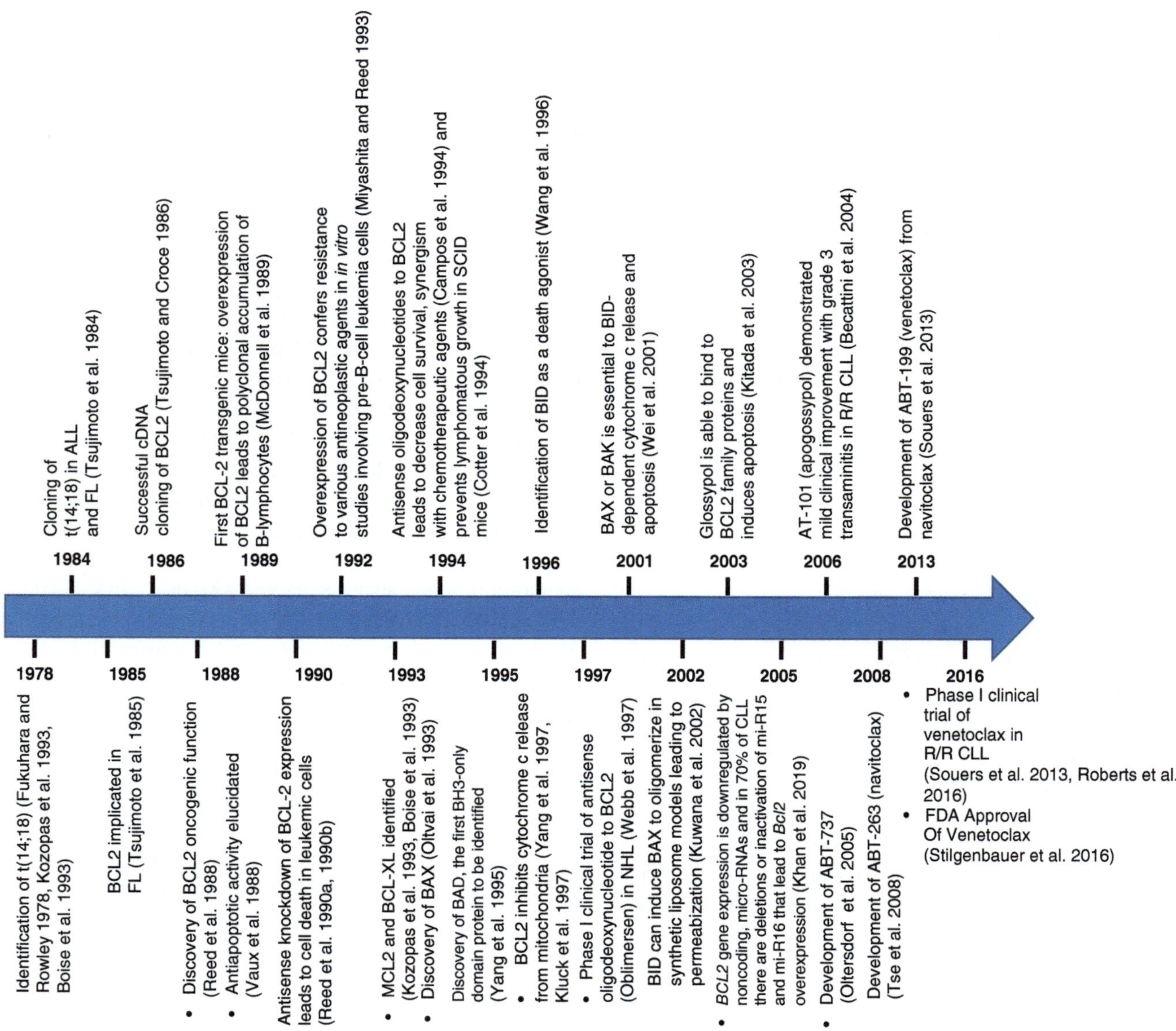

Figure 11.1 Binding relationships between the BH3-only proteins and BCL2 protein family members. Note: The darkened BH3-only proteins bind to the specific anti-apoptotic protein shown below.

were noted to be arrested in G0 phase of cell cycle. With the re-introduction of the IL-3 stimulus, even after several weeks of deprivation, the BCL2 overexpressing cells began to proliferate once again. The first BCL2 transgenic mice were developed in 1989 and revealed that the overexpression of BCL2 resulted in polyclonal accumulation of B lymphocytes (McDonnell et al. 1989). Taken together, it was thought that BCL2 functions as an escape mechanism to avoid cell death, permitting a cell to acquire additional oncogenic hits eventually leading to enhanced proliferation. In fact, activation of BCL2 alone is not sufficient to drive lymphomagenesis in the Eμ-*BCL2* mouse model, where mice initially developed polyclonal follicular hyperplasia, followed by a latency period prior to the development of high-grade lymphoma, with 50% of the mice acquiring a secondary *c-myc* rearrangement (McDonnell and Korsmeyer 1991). Additional insight which supported BCL2 as an anti-apoptotic protein was provided by the antisense oligonucleotide knockdown of BCL2 expression in leukemic cells (Reed et al. 1990a, Reed et al. 1990b) followed by the revelation that BCL2 sequesters cytochrome c release from the mitochondria (Kluck et al. 1997; Yang et al. 1997). In sum, the aforementioned history unequivocally established *BCL2* as a *bona fide* oncogene, and the first known inhibitor of programmed cell death.

The discovery of other essential members of the BCL2 family such as the pro-survival MCL1 and BCL-X_L occurred in 1993, expanding our knowledge of the many intricately interacting layers of anti-apoptotic mechanisms in mammalian cells. Other notable events in the evolution of our understanding of this biology include the identification of pro-apoptotic proteins such as BAX (Oltvai et al. 1993) and BID (Wang et al. 1996). BAX, or its close relative BAK, homodimerizes and heterodimerizes with BCL2, subsequently forming mitochondrial apoptotic channels, permeabilizing the mitochondrial membrane, allowing for cytochrome c release into the cytosol, and activation of caspase proteins (Kuwana et al. 2002; Wei et al. 2001). In 1995, Yang and colleagues were the first to describe the BH3-only protein identified as BAD, which was discovered using the yeast two-hybrid screening system and lambda expression cloning. BAD was found to dimerize with BCL2 and BCL-X_L, stimulating cell death, mitigating the influence of a strong pro-apoptotic influence (Yang et al. 1995). Afterward, additional members of the BCL2 family were discovered in the mid-1990s as well as the delineation of BCL2 family protein structures, in turn allowing for a more comprehensive understanding of how pro- and anti-apoptotic members of the BCL2 family interact. It is likely because of this very complex, nuanced, and redundant biology that it took so long to successfully translate this understanding of apoptosis signaling to the clinic. This fertile history has now led to a host of potential therapeutic strategies which are now having a major impact on our ability to treat lymphoid malignancies with these highly targeted drugs.

BCL2 as a Biomarker

It may appear obvious that markers of pro-death and pro-survival signaling should be able to identify prognostic or predictive biomarkers. However, the complexity of this biology, manifests in part through the innumerable interaction of its members, makes understanding the precise equipoise that any cell might exhibit with regard to its life and death balance challenging to quantify.

Overexpression and upregulation of BCL2 anti-apoptotic family members are hallmark of lymphomagenesis and acquired drug resistance. In particular, BCL2 anti-apoptotic family members induce programmed cell death by binding and neutralizing pro-apoptotic proteins, preventing mitochondrial membrane permeabilization (Brunelle and Letai 2009; Llambi et al. 2011). As noted above, translocation of BCL2 to the immunoglobulin heavy chain locus [t(14;18) (q32;a21)] is observed in nearly 90% all of FL leading to constitutive expression of BCL2 (Weiss et al. 1987). However, although an early driving event, BCL2 overexpression alone is insufficient to drive lymphomagenesis. For example, mouse models, such as the Eμ-*BCL2* model in which mice developed follicular hyperplasia, followed by a long latency, can develop high-grade lymphomas with several tumors acquiring a secondary *c-myc* rearrangement (McDonnell and Korsmeyer 1991). Despite this, somatic mutations in *BCL2* correlate with a decrease in overall survival (OS) and an increased risk for transformation in FL patients, partially due to the increased binding affinity of BCL2 to pro-apoptotic proteins such as BIM and PUMA, leading to their sequestration (Correia et al. 2015). The observation that BCL2 is perhaps not the most potent sole driver of lymphomagenesis is underscored in studies that have demonstrated modest activity of drugs targeting this biology in FL (Davids et al. 2017). In another example, approximately 20% of diffuse large B-cell lymphomas (DLBCL) harbor *Bcl2* translocations (Schuetz et al. 2012) which also have been shown to translate into an inferior OS (Iqbal et al. 2006). The presence of a *BCL2* translocation along with an *MYC* translocation is characteristic of "double hit" lymphomas, an aggressive lymphoma with notoriously poor outcomes after treatment with R-CHOP (Landsburg et al. 2017; Petrich et al. 2014), a pattern also observed in double-expressor lymphomas which are defined by the co-overexpression of BCL2 and MYC without the presence of cytogenetic translocations (Swerdlow et al. 2016). Despite the presence of BCL2 overexpression in FL and DLBCL, single-agent activity of venetoclax has demonstrated an overall response rate (ORR) of only 38% and 18%, respectively (Davids et al. 2017), further emphasizing the complexity of multiple pathways involved in their lymphomagenesis, and lending itself to the rationale of combinational therapy with BCL2 inhibitors in these lymphoma subtypes. As such, BCL2 overexpression alone has proven to be a suboptimal biomarker to predict clinical benefit from single-agent BCL2 inhibitors.

Targeting BCL2 Family Members

One of the first reports establishing an association between BCL2 and chemoresistance arose from the observation that overexpression of BCL2 in leukemic and lymphoid cells leads to resistance to cell death from a host of anti-neoplastic agents such dexamethasone, and traditional cytotoxic drugs including methotrexate, cytarabine, etoposide, vincristine, and cisplatin (Miyashita and Reed 1992, 1993). In fact, BCL2 was associated with chemotherapy resistance in patients with acute myeloid leukemia (AML), an observation supported by the finding that the antisense oligodeoxynucleotides to BCL2 mRNA led to improved sensitivity of AML cells to cytarabine *in vitro* (Campos et al. 1994). Given its complex role in cancer biology, as both an early precursor event in certain tumors as well as a means of acquired chemoresistance, most attention to drug discovery in this space has been dedicated to development of BCL2 antagonists. Clinical summary of BCL-2 targeting approaches are summarized in Table 11.1.

Antisense Approaches for Targeting BCL2

Early attempts to target BCL2 family proteins included antisense-based therapy followed by BH3 mimetics or small molecule inhibitors that interfere with the sequestering of pro-apoptotic proteins by anti-apoptotic proteins, with subsequent stimulation of BAX/BAK-dependent apoptosis. Genasense (oblimersen) was one of the first approaches employing antisense-based technology to target a specific disease-associated biology. Oblimersen is an 18-mer antisense oligonucleotide to BCL2 mRNA which targeted the reading frame of BCL2, therefore preventing translation. Our group originally demonstrated that oblimersen in combination with bortezomib, which modulated many BH3-only proteins in a manner that would favor apoptosis, could sensitize B-cell lymphoma cells to cytotoxic chemotherapy such as cyclophosphamide, providing further evidence that targeting the BCL2 axis can overcome inherent chemotherapeutic resistance and function synergistically with other novel agents (O'Connor et al. 2006). While oblimersen was studied in other malignant therapeutic areas such as melanoma, studies were also conducted in patients with relapsed/refractory (R/R) non-Hodgkin's lymphoma (NHL). A phase 1 clinical trial of oblimersen in R/R NHL demonstrated an overall favorable toxicity profile with minor clinical responses. Notably, six of eight patients treated on this trial achieved a complete response (CR) on subsequent therapy, potentially suggesting that BCL2 antisense therapy was able to overcome intrinsic or acquired drug resistance (Webb et al. 1997). Several studies explored the merits of various combination therapies, including one with rituximab (Pro et al. 2008). Although pre-clinical and early clinical studies were promising, phase 3 clinical trials in AML (Marcucci et al. 2007), melanoma (Kirkwood et al. 2005), and chronic lymphocytic leukemia (CLL) (O'Brien et al. 2009) did not lead to an FDA approval in any indication despite achieving their primary endpoint of improved CRs in CLL as well as an improved progression-free survival (PFS) (a secondary end point) in melanoma.

Natural Anti-apoptotic Compounds

While antisense therapy was leading the field of apoptosis-based drug development, the development of small molecule BCL2 antagonists was not far behind. BH3 mimetics are peptides that resemble the BH3 domains of BCL2 family proteins and aim to disrupt pro-apoptotic/anti-apoptotic protein complexes, such as BCL2:BAX, which consequentially render BAX free to form mitochondrial apoptosis channels, facilitating the release of cytochrome c into the cytosol, initiating cell destruction. Gossypol, a derivative of the cotton plant [*Gossypium sp.*], was originally developed as a male contraceptive (Coutinho 2002). Gossypol was shown to bind and antagonize BCL2 family proteins, particularly BCL-X_L (Kitada et al. 2003), leading to the notion it could be used as a possible anti-cancer therapeutic. Ironically, it was precisely these pro-apoptotic effects that led to its initial use as a male contraceptive, leading to increased death of sperm cells (Coutinho 2002). Two clinical trials in patients with R/R B-cell lymphoma (NCT00275431, NCT00440388) were launched; however, these studies did not provide sufficient support to advance the development of glossypol for oncology, likely due to the unfavorable pharmacologic features of the natural product which contained two highly reactive aldehyde moieties. Based on these experiences, subsequent analogs of gossypol were developed, including apogossypol (AT-101) (Becattini et al. 2004), in which the two reactive aldehyde groups were strategically removed. Paoluzzi et al. (2008) illustrated that AT-101 was synergistic with carfilzomib, etoposide, doxorubicin, and 4-hydroxycyclophosphamide (4-HC) in mantle cell lymphoma (MCL) cell lines, but, interestingly, was only synergistic in a transformed DLBCL cell line when sequentially administered with 4-HC, again highlighting the potential of BCL2 inhibition as a sensitizing agent. Given promising *in vitro* and *in vivo* results, a phase 1 trial of AT-101 in R/R CLL with high-risk features was conducted demonstrating limited efficacy and untoward toxicity (grade 3 transaminitis) (James et al. 2006). In combination with rituximab in R/R CLL, AT-101 demonstrated an underwhelming ORR of 42% with no CRs (Castro et al. 2007), which stifled further clinical development.

Small Molecule Inhibitors of BCL2 Family Members

Validated strategies have established the merits of targeting of BCL2 family members. By definition, pure BH3 mimetics directly bind to the BH3-domain pocket of anti-apoptotic

Table 11.1 BCL2 antagonists.

Drug	Mechanism of action	Pre-clinical studies	Clinical trial	Results	Chemical structure
Oblimersen	Antisense oligonucleotide	Combinations with bortezomib sensitize B-cell lymphoma to cytotoxic therapy (O'Connor et al. 2006)	Phase 1 non-Hodgkin's lymphoma (Webb et al. 1997) Phase 2 R/RNHL (in combination with rituximab) (Pro et al. 2008)	1 CR, 3 SD, 5 PD ORR:42% CR: 10 PR: 8 Median DOR: 12 months	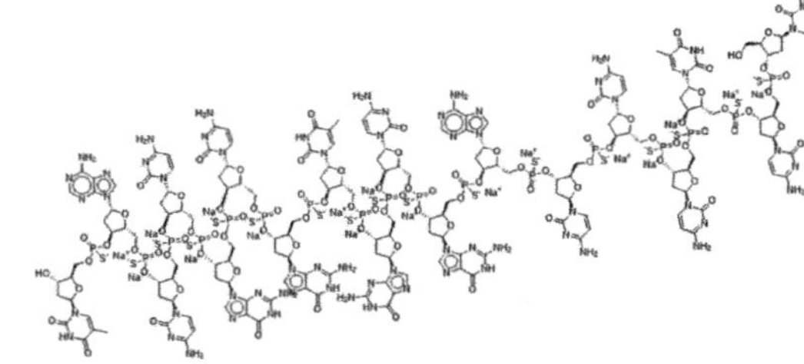
Gossypol	Inhibitor of BCL2 family members, including BCL-X_L	Developed a male contraceptive (Coutinho 2002)	Relapsed/refractory B-cell lymphoma (NCT00275431 NCT00440388)	–	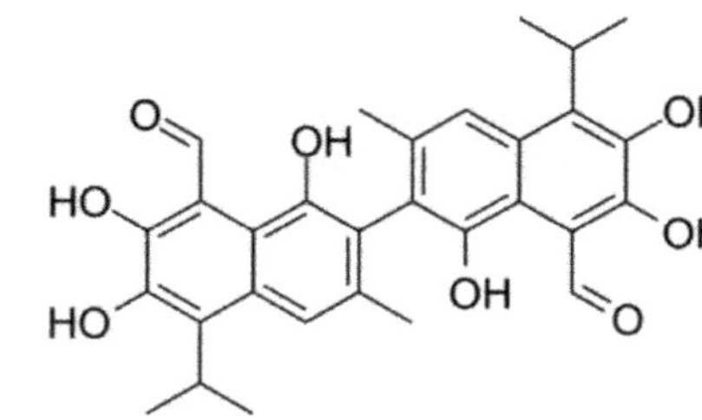
Apogossypol (AT-101)	Inhibitor of BCL2 family members, including BCL-X_L	Synergistic with proteasome inhibitors and cytotoxic chemotherapy (Paoluzzi et al. 2008)	Phase 1 R/R CLL (James et al. 2006) Phase 2 in combination with rituximab in R/R CLL (Castro et al. 2007)	5/6 patients with decrease lymphocyte count 6/6 reduction in lymphadenopathy 5/5 reduction in palpable spleen ORR: 42% (5/12)	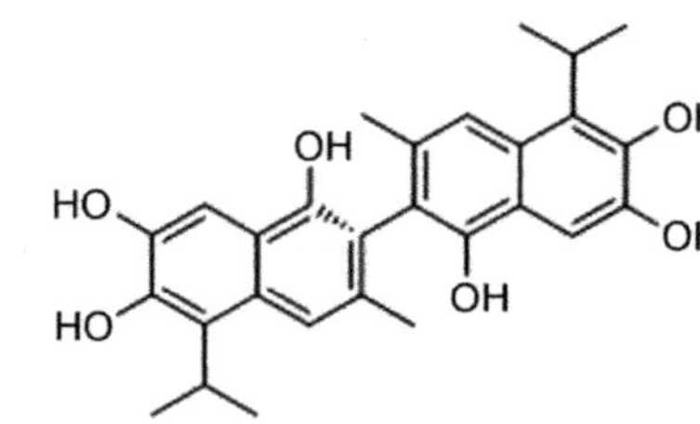
Obatoclax	Inhibitor of BCL2, MCL-1, BCL-X_L, and BCL-$_W$	First BCL2 inhibitor, binds to BH3 binding groove of BCL2 and related proteins (Nguyen et al. 2007; Pérez-Galán et al. 2008)	Phase 1 R/R CLL (O'Brien et al. 2009) Phase 2 in combination with FR in R/R CLL (Brown et al. 2015)	1/26 PR ORR: 85% (11/13) CR: 54% (7/13)	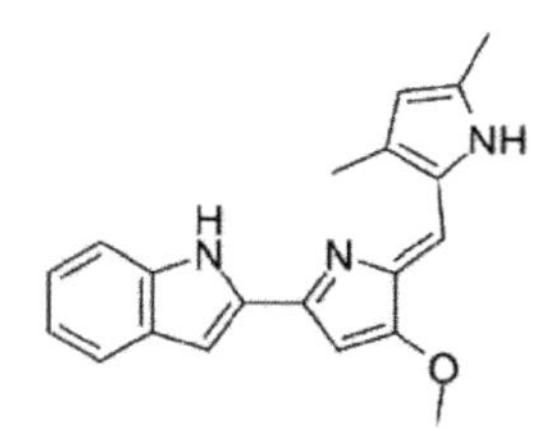
Navitoclax	Inhibitor BCL2, BCL-X_L, BCL-$_W$	Synergistic with bortezomib with preferential sensitivity to B-cell lymphomas (Paoluzzi et al. 2008)	Phase 1 in NHL (Wilson et al. 2010) Phase 1 R/R CLL (Roberts et al. 2012)	ORR: 22% (10/46, all PRs) mPFS: 455 d ORR: 31% (9/29) mPFS: 25 mo	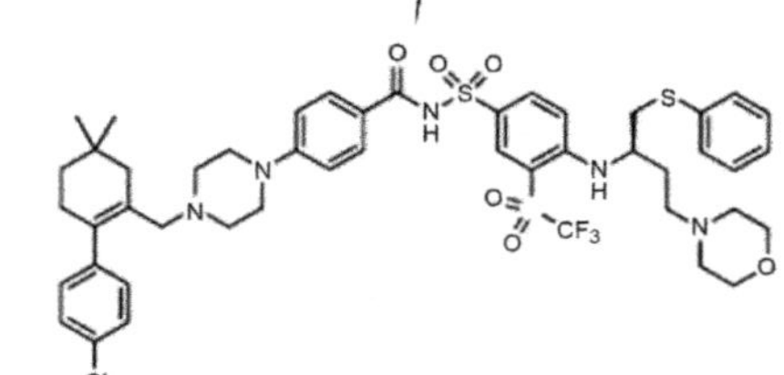

(Continued)

Table 11.1 (Continued)

Drug	Mechanism of action	Pre-clinical studies	Clinical trial	Results	Chemical structure
Venetoclax*	Antagonist of BCL2	Developed through reverse engineering of navitoclax (Souers et al. 2013)	Phase 1 R/R CLL (Roberts et al. 2016) Phase 2 R/R CLL with del(17p) (Stilgenbauer et al. 2016)	ORR: 79% (92/116) CR: 20% (23/116) ORR 79% (85/107) CR: 8% (8/107)	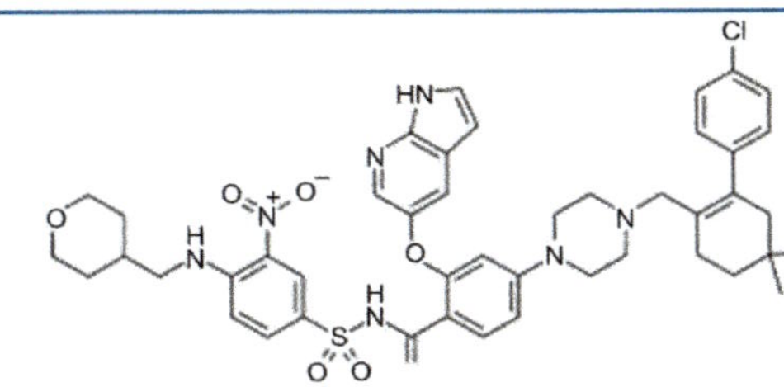
Lisaftoclax (APG-2575)	Antagonist of BCL2	Synergistic with lenalidomide in MM models (Xie et al. 2020)	Phase 1 in CLL and NHL (Ailawadhi et al. 2021)	ORR: 85.7% (12/14)**	-
BGB-11417	Antagonist of BCL2 (including BCL2 G101V)	Binds more potently to WT and Mutant BCL2 compared to venetoclax (Hu et al. 2020)	Phase 1R/R B-cell lymphoma (Cheah et al. 2021)	-	-

Abbreviations: CLL = chronic lymphocytic leukemia; CR = complete response; d = days; DOR = duration of response; mPFS = improved progression-free survival; mo = months; NHL = Non-Hodgkin's lymphoma; ORR = = overall response rate; PD = progression of disease; PR = partial response; R/R = relapse/refractory; SD = stable disease; WT = wild-type; MM = multiple myeloma

*FDA approved

**CLL patients only

proteins, thereby preventing the inhibition of pro-apoptotic proteins by anti-apoptotic proteins. During the course of the development BH3-mimetics, cellular tools have been proposed in order to validate the function of these small molecules given the observation of indirect mechanisms, such as upregulation of NOXA a pro-apoptotic protein, drive apoptosis rather than direct binding of anti-apoptotic proteins by the BH3 mimetics (Soderquist and Eastman 2016). These cell-based validation models include: (i) screening of BH3 mimetics that target BCL2 in human CLL cells *ex vivo* as these cells will rapidly undergo apoptosis (<6 hours) (Del Gaizo Moore et al. 2007); (ii) evaluation of inhibitors of BCL-X_L in platelets, given their critical dependence on BCL-X_L (Zhang et al. 2007); and (iii) BH3-mimetics targeting MCL-1 should trigger the accumulation of MCL-1 in cells dependent on MCL-1 such as in the $p185^+$ B-ALL model described by Koss et al. (2016). The $p185^+$ B-ALL model is derived from a B-ALL cell line that is dependent on MCL-1 in which *Mcl-1* is deleted by drug selection, and cDNAs encoding BCL2, BCL-X_L, BCL-$_W$, MCL-1, or BFL-1 are transduced. Subsequently, these models can be used to evaluate BH3-mimetics targeting each respective BCL2 family member.

Another strategy to determine the sensitivity of cells to anti-apoptotic drugs was conceptualized by Letai et al. in an assay commonly referred to as "*BH3 profiling*." BH3 profiling is based on measuring the permeabilization of the outer mitochondrial membrane, and thus cytochrome c release, in well-controlled experimental conditions where the exact concentrations of specific BH3 peptides are applied (Del Gaizo Moore and Letai 2013). In this setting, by utilizing sensitizing peptides, the level of mitochondrial apoptotic priming (relative threshold at which a cell commits to apoptosis) and dependence on specific BCL2 family proteins can be quantified (Certo et al. 2006). This strategy has been used to identify a cell's dependency on BCL2 family members and has been employed to identify potentially synergistic drug combinations with BCL2-targeted molecules. Similarly, other methods such as the measurement of mitochondrial membrane potential, as shown by Paoluzzi et al. (2008), can also identify synergistic drug combinations with BCL2 antagonists, and can be a useful approach to quantitate synergistic drug combinations.

Obatoclax, a non-specific inhibitor of BCL2 family proteins, binds not only to BCL2 but also to MCL-1, BCL-X_L, and BCL-$_W$, was one of the first inhibitors of BCL2 to be developed (Nguyen et al. 2007; Pérez-Galán et al. 2008). Specifically, obatoclax is a hydrophobic indole bipyrrole compound that binds to the BH3 binding groove of BCL2 and related proteins. Clinical applications of obatoclax were limited by unusual neurological symptoms including somnolence, euphoria, and ataxia with one observed partial response (PR) (1/26) in a single-agent study in R/R CLL (O'Brien et al. 2009). When obatoclax was combined with fludarabine and rituximab in patients with R/R CLL, the ORR and CR rates were 85% and 54%, respectively. While promising, no randomized study was ever conducted to definitively establish the contribution of obatoclax (Brown et al. 2015).

In an effort to develop more selective inhibitors, Oltersdorf et al. (2005) utilized a nuclear magnetic resonance-based drug screening approach focusing on the hydrophobic BH3 binding pocket of BCL-X_L which led to the development of the laboratory tool compound ABT-737, which binds to BCL-X_L, BCL2, and BCL-$_W$. ABT-737 demonstrated *in vitro* and *in vivo* activity in a variety of solid tumor models, including small cell lung carcinoma (Hann et al. 2008), as well as synergy with other chemotherapeutic agents such as paclitaxel (Oltersdorf et al. 2005). In lymphoma models including primary patient samples, Paoluzzi et al. demonstrated selective sensitivity of ABT-737 in B-cell malignancies, including MCL and DLBCL (0.025–0.42 μM), with T-cell lymphoma models displaying less sensitivity with IC50s in the micromolar range (2.92–5.65 μM). Moreover, the group also demonstrated that the combination of ABT-737 with bortezomib leads to enhanced apoptosis in *in vitro* and *in vivo* B-cell lymphoma models (Paoluzzi et al. 2008).

Navitoclax (ABT-263), a first-in-class orally bioavailable BCL2 family antagonist and derivative of ABT-737 (Tse et al. 2008), demonstrated an identical protein binding profile and similar *in vivo* and *in vitro* activity. Notably, pre-clinical experiences with ABT-737 and navitoclax demonstrated rapid thrombocytopenia due to apoptosis of circulating platelets, revealing their dependence on BCL-X_L (Mason et al. 2007). Despite this early finding, navitoclax was advanced into the clinic given the compelling preclinical data and its oral administration. As one might have predicted, in the first-in-human phase 1 clinical trial of navitoclax, the dose-limiting toxicity was thrombocytopenia, with 29% of patients experiencing grade 3/4 thrombocytopenia (Wilson et al. 2010). Navitoclax would then go on to be evaluated in a dedicated phase 1 trial in patients with R/R CLL, where it produced an ORR of 31%, all of which were PRs (Roberts et al. 2012). Once again, the dose-limiting toxicity was thrombocytopenia. Extensive research regarding the mechanism of thrombocytopenia revealed that BH3-mimetics that target BCL-X_L induce dose-related thrombocytopenia that not only affects the number of circulating platelets but also the hemostatic functionality of the remaining platelets as BCL-X_L is critical in platelet function (Schoenwaelder et al. 2011). Furthermore, exposure to BCL-X_L inhibition preferentially leads to apoptosis of aged/senescence platelets due to the fact that BCL-X_L levels decrease over time in order to prime an older platelet for cell death (Mason et al. 2007).

Despite encouraging results from early clinical trials, there was substantial concern regarding the thrombocytopenia observed in the clinic, which ultimately limited dose escalation and compromised efficacy of navitoclax. As such, venetoclax, a more specific small molecule inhibitor of BCL2 was developed (Souers et al. 2013). Derived from navitoclax using reverse engineering methods leading to the replacement of an indole moiety with an azaindole in the binding pocket of BCL2, venetoclax binds to BCL2 with higher affinity (Ki < 0.010 nM), and, more importantly, has a significantly lower binding affinity toward BCL-X_L (Ki = 48 nM) and BCL-w (Ki = 245 nM), with the former potentially circumventing the thrombocytopenia issues observed in the navitoclax clinical trials (Gandhi et al. 2011; Wilson et al. 2010). The fact that BCL2 family members share BH domains makes it extremely challenging to develop selective BCL2 antagonists; however, Souers et al. (2013) modeled venetoclax to bind to Asp103 of BCL2, which is one of the few amino acid differences within the BH3-binding domain between BCL2 and BCL-X_L (Glu96 is corresponding amino acid in the later), leading to preferential binding to BCL2 thus avoiding the undesirable thrombocytopenia observed when antagonizing BCL-X_L. In fact, venetoclax was significantly less potent against human platelets *ex vivo* than navitoclax [EC50 5.5 μM vs. 0.083 μM], which was confirmed in dog models as well. Given this rationale, venetoclax was advanced into the clinic. A phase 1, first-in-human study of venetoclax in patients with R/R CLL and NHL led to significant and rapid tumor shrinkage and concomitant tumor lysis syndrome (TLS) in the first three subjects within the dose-escalation cohort (Roberts et al. 2016; Souers et al. 2013). Ultimately, TLS occurred in 10 of 56 patients, with three clinical cases of TLS and eight cases of laboratory TLS. One patient experienced sudden death during an episode of TLS, another required hemodialysis, and an additional patient had transient acute kidney injury. The majority of patients (9 of 10) with TLS resumed treatment with venetoclax and only one patient experienced a recurrence of TLS (Roberts et al. 2016).

As a direct result of this unusual TLS experience, an extended dose ramp-up schema along with TLS prophylaxis and monitoring strategies, including stepwise dose escalation while hospitalized, were implemented in a subsequent protocol amendment (Roberts et al. 2016). Remarkably, the thrombocytopenia seen with navitoclax was largely mitigated, making the development of venetoclax one of the truly remarkable examples of translational medicine, bridging sophisticated chemical structure–function relationships to produce an improved therapeutic with the desired drug features. Of the 116 patients evaluated (including dose escalation n = 56, and expansion n = 60) in the phase 1 trial, the majority of patients responded with an ORR of 79% and a CR rate of 20%. Notably, responses were observed in high-risk disease sub-sets such as those with del(17p). To elucidate the potential benefit observed in CLL patients with 17p deletion, a dedicated phase 2 clinical trial was conducted which demonstrated an ORR of 79% (85/107) with 8% CRs (8/107) (Stilgenbauer et al. 2016). Nearly 38 years since the t(14;18) translocation was identified, and nearly 25 years since the first phase 1 of a clinical trial exploring the merits of targeting this biology, venetoclax became the first BH3 mimetic to receive FDA approval for the treatment of CLL with 17p deletion in 2016. Since then, venetoclax has achieved FDA approval for a number of indications including AML and CLL and is presently being evaluated in a host of clinical trials.

Novel BCL2 Inhibitors on the Horizon

Given the success of venetoclax, additional BCL2 antagonists have entered early development. Lisaftoclax (APG-2575, Ascentage) has entered clinical evaluation for CLL, NHL, AML, multiple myeloma, and T-cell prolymphocytic leukemia. A phase 1 trial focusing on lisaftoclax in CLL and other hematological malignancies was initiated using a daily ramp-up, which interestingly produced no observed TLS events (Ailawadhi et al. 2021). Of the 14 evaluable CLL/SLL patients, 12 achieved a PR (ORR 85.7%), with a median time to response of three cycles (range: two to seven cycles). As such, given the fact that venetoclax requires a five-week ramp-up, lisaftoclax appears to be an attractive alternative with daily dose ramp-up schedule and shorter time to optimal therapeutic dosing, with little to no risk of TLS.

With chronic exposure to venetoclax mutations such as G101V in *BCL2* have been reported and implicated in drug resistance (Blombery et al. 2019). In order to develop agents that would overcome common mutations leading to drug resistance, BeiGene developed BGB-11417, a selective inhibitor of BCL2 that binds more potently to both wild-type (0.035 nM vs. 1.3 nM) and mutant BCL2 (G101V-mutated) (0.28 nM vs. 34 nM) compared to venetoclax. This also translated to lower IC50s in various hematological cell lines and xenograft models, including DLBCL when comparing BGB-11417 to venetoclax (Hu et al. 2020). BGB-11417 is actively being studied in a phase 1 trial in patients with R/R B-cell malignancies with a reported tolerable safety profile using a weekly or daily dose ramp-up (Cheah et al. 2021).

Mechanisms of Resistance to BCL2 Inhibitors

The differential activity observed across lymphoma subtypes when exposed to venetoclax or BCL2 inhibitors can be partially explained by innate differences in the biological networks that lead to primary resistance. These intrinsic mechanisms of resistance are driven by compensatory upregulation of other anti-apoptotic proteins through a variety of pathways. The limited activity observed in FL and DLBCL to single-agent venetoclax may be due to the upregulation of other pro-survival proteins such as BCL-X_L and MCL1. In fact, Adams et al. described that along with *BCL-2*, *BCL-X_L* is overexpressed in both germinal center and activated B-cell DLBCL (Adams et al. 2017), suggesting that DLBCL cells may drive the anti-apoptotic escape message through the activity of *BCL-X_L* when pressured with venetoclax. This observation was also found in FL patient samples, suggesting that the redundancy in anti-apoptotic BCL2 members works cooperatively to promote a pro-survival state.

The tumor microenvironment has also been implicated in promoting resistance to BCL2 inhibition. In particular, several lines of evidence have demonstrated that drugs affecting the microenvironment, including the ILs and CD40L, can stimulate the enhanced expression of MCL-1, BCL-X_L, and survivin (Chiron et al. 2016; Jayappa et al. 2017) in both CLL and MCL patient samples. Given the potential activity in CLL and evidence of pre-clinical synergy, as well as the impact of BTK inhibitors on the tumor microenvironment, the combination of ibrutinib and venetoclax has been studied. Primary patient MCL and CLL samples demonstrated sensitivity to dual inhibition of BCL2 and BTK (Cervantes-Gomez et al. 2015; Chiron et al. 2015). However, other data suggests that primary patient CLL and MCL samples have impaired sensitivity to this combination. This intrinsic resistance was attributed to the generation of stimuli including IL-10, CD40L, and cytosine guanine dinucleotide-oligodeoxynucleotide (a TLR9 pathway agonist) in the microenvironment, leading to NF-κB activation and in turn the enhanced expression of MCL-1, BCL-X_L, and survivin (Jayappa et al. 2017). The addition of antagonists to MCL-1, BCL-XL, or survivin was synergistic with the ibrutinib and venetoclax, overcoming anti-apoptotic drug resistance. Similarly, co-culture of CD40L positive cells with IL-6, IL-10, IGF-1, and BAFF induced *ex vivo* expression of NF-κB in primary MCL cells, leading to the upregulation of BCL-X_L and downregulation of BIM, BAX, and BAK (Chiron et al. 2016), thus creating an anti-apoptotic environment. The finding of upregulation of BCL-X_L is further supported by the dynamic profiling of circulating tumor DNA undertaken in the AIM study, which investigated the merits of the combination of ibrutinib and venetoclax in R/R MCL (Agarwal et al. 2019; Tam et al. 2018). Baseline genomic mutations in SWI-SNF chromatin modeling complex and/or loss of chromosome 9p were present in patients whose disease did not respond to this combination, leading to upregulation of *BCL-X_L*, providing a selective survival advantage (Agarwal et al. 2019). Taken together, it is clear that drugs that influence the microenvironment can modulate the apoptotic threshold by changing the expression of BCL-X_L and MCL-1, contributing to resistance to BCL2 inhibition, reinforcing further the complexity of this biology across a spectrum of lymphoma subtypes. These dynamic interactions further underscore the need to deconvolute the interactions and the importance of combinational therapy.

Despite CR rates of approximately 20–50% as a single agent or in combination with rituximab (Roberts et al. 2016; Seymour et al. 2018), acquired or secondary resistance to venetoclax or BCL2 inhibitor exposure is linked to treatment failure (Roberts et al. 2019). This acquired resistance is thought to be secondary to two mechanisms: (i) as shown in cells with intrinsic drug resistance, an increased dependence on compensatory anti-apoptotic proteins, BCL-X_L and MCL-1; and (ii) the acquisition of mutations within the BCL2 protein that impairs the binding of venetoclax. Robust data regarding dependency on alternative anti-apoptotic proteins has been reported given the long-term follow-up with CLL and MCL patients treated with venetoclax. A genome-wide screen of OCI-LY1, a venetoclax-resistant lymphoid cell line, revealed overexpression of MCL-1 and dysregulation in AMKP signaling, which were associated with metabolic reprogramming of the mitochondria, specifically with resistant cell lines demonstrating a higher rate of basal and maximal oxygen consumption (Guièze et al. 2019). Upon exposure to the MCL-1 inhibitor S63845, the resistant OCI-LY1 cell line was re-sensitized to venetoclax and demonstrated synergy when exposed to both drugs simultaneously. The overexpression of both MCL-1 and AMPK was also confirmed in primary CLL patient samples who progressed on venetoclax therapy. Further studies have shown that increased phosphorylation of MCL-1 secondary to the upregulation of cyclin E (Cdk2) competes with the ubiquitination of MCL-1, preventing MCL-1 degradation, thus promoting sequestration of pro-apoptotic proteins (Choudhary et al. 2015). Additionally, Choudhary et al. (2015) described that acquired resistance to venetoclax was driven by the activation of PI3K/AKT/mTOR pathway in turn leading to the upregulation of MCL-1 and BCL-X_L. This resistance was reversed upon treatment with inhibitors of PI3K/AKT/mTOR signaling such as idelalisib (Choudhary et al. 2015). The role of AKT in venetoclax resistance was further supported by the fact that in venetoclax-exposed FL models, phosphorylated AKT and FOXO3a (a transcription factor of BIM expression) were both present in elevated levels, leading to the sequestration of BIM (Bodo et al. 2016).

As alluded to earlier, and as shown with the use of many other small molecule inhibitors in malignant disease, the accumulation of mutations in BCL2 leading to reduced affinity of venetoclax to BCL2 has been, and in all likelihood, will continue to be described (Birkinshaw et al. 2019; Blombery et al. 2020). The finding that patients who experience intrinsic or acquired drug resistance may harbor a host of mutations in differing subclones suggests the emergence of a polyclonal mechanism of resistance (Blombery et al. 2020), which will likely be mitigated to some extent with the earlier use of combinatorial platforms.

Novel Mechanisms to Overcome BCL2 Resistance

Targeting MCL1

The compensatory or even redundant expression of anti-apoptotic proteins following BCL2 inhibitor exposure has led to the development of MCL-1 inhibitors and, more recently, novel mechanisms to target BCL-X_L. A-1210477 was the first selective MCL-1 inhibitor ($K_i = 0.000\,454\ \mu M$), preventing the interaction between MCL-1 and BIM (Bruncko et al. 2015; Leverson et al. 2015), which interestingly synergizes with navitoclax in multiple myeloma cell lines. S63845, another selective inhibitor of MCL-1 ($K_d = 0.19$ nM), potently induced apoptosis in venetoclax resistant multiple myeloma cells, and more notably, was approximately 1000-fold more cytotoxic than A-1210477 (Kotschy et al. 2016). S63845 binds to the conserved Arg26, while an aromatic scaffold interacts with the hydrophobic pocket P2, and a trifluoromethyl moiety spans across into P4, effectively allowing the drug to displace pro-apoptotic proteins from the hydrophobic pocket of MCL-1. A related compound, S64315/MIK665 (Ki = 0.048 nM for MCL-1), has demonstrated synergy with select BCL2 inhibitors in *in vivo* models (Halilovic et al. 2019), and has transitioned into clinical evaluation for lymphoma and multiple myeloma (NCT02992483) and AML and myelodysplastic syndrome (NCT02979366). The development of oral MCL-1 inhibitors, AMG176 (Ki = 0.06 nM for MCL-1) and its derivative AMG397 demonstrated potent activity in a range of hematological malignancies including lymphoma (Caenepeel et al. 2018, 2020). The lead compound, AMG397, was subsequently evaluated in a phase 1 clinical trial (NCT03465540); however, due to the possibility of cardiac toxicity in light that MCL-1 is essential for normal cardiac myocyte function (Wang et al. 2013), the trial was placed on an FDA hold and eventually terminated due to strategic decision to advance another MCL-1 inhibitor, AMG176 (Caenepeel et al. 2018) (NCT02675452). Other MCL-2 inhibitors including AZD5991 (NCT03218683) and ABBV-467 (NCT04178902) have also entered phase 1 clinical trial evaluation, with the later also terminated for strategic considerations.

PROTAC Strategies for Targeting Apoptotic Family Members

Although much of the focus over the past decades has centered on small molecule inhibitors, a novel technology that represents a promising approach to specifically and selectively target anti-apoptotic proteins is proteolysis-targeting chimeras (PROTACs). PROTACs are heterobifunctional molecules that simultaneously bind a target protein (i.e. oncogene) and an E3 ubiquitin ligase to drive the degradation of a target protein by the proteasome (refer to chapter on PROTACs for more detail). Using this technology, various oncogenic proteins have been targeted including MCL-1 and BCL-X_L. What is unique to this drug technology is that using specific E3 ligases that are differentially expressed in malignant/target cells versus normal cells, it becomes possible to circumvent unwanted side effects observed with tissue non-selective approaches. In particular, IMiD compounds such as lenalidomide are able to recruit cereblon (CRBN), which in turn forms an E3 ubiquitin ligase complex. Wang et al. (2019) developed two series of PROTACs against MCL-1, utilizing a CRBN-binding E3 ligase. The authors linked CRBN-binding pomalidomide to a dual inhibitor of MCL-1/BCL2 (S1-6 and NAP1) and demonstrated that their PROTAC led to superior cytotoxic death in H23 cells compared to A-1210477 (Wang et al. 2019). Another protein degrader, dMCL1-2 modeled after the MCL-1 inhibitor A-1210477 and thalidomide, induced degradation of MCL-1 at nanomolar concentrations as early as three hours in multiple myeloma cell lines (Papatzimas et al. 2019). An MCL-1 PROTAC has yet to enter the clinic; however, it theoretically may be safer than MCL-1 inhibition where cardiotoxicity is a concern, if a selective E3 ligase is incorporated.

Given the undesirable effects of inhibition of BCL-X_L in platelets observed with navitoclax, the application of PROTAC technology to degrade BCL-X_L has been gradually emerging. This concept is thought to be a superior method as targeted degradation of an oncogenic protein by a PROTAC can be achieved by selecting an E3 ligase that is differentially expressed in a malignant cell compared to normal tissues/platelets, thus preventing degradation of the protein in off-target cells. As a result, Khan et al. (2019) devised a PROTAC (DT2216) against BCL-X_L that bypassed the thrombocytopenia observed with small molecule inhibition of BCL-X_L by utilizing von Hippel–Lindau as the target E3 ligase, which is poorly expressed in platelets. In fact, DT2216 was shown to selectively degrade BCL-X_L in malignant hematological cell lines but not in platelets. Taken together, PROTACs targeting the resistance mechanism of BCL2 inhibition is a potential therapeutic platform that warrants further attention and development in lymphoid and other hematological malignancies.

Conclusions

The evasion of apoptosis is a key hallmark of cancer biology, with BCL2 being one of the first anti-apoptotic protein discovered. As our understanding of the complex biology that drives B-cell lymphoma continues to become increasingly more sophisticated, a host of new targeted therapies will gradually become more and more apparent. However, we must learn from the history of BCL2 inhibition as well as other small molecule inhibitors and think about strategies to avoid potential resistance mechanisms earlier in a treatment course. The generation of cell lines resistant to a particular drug in the laboratory can provide insight into the potential mechanisms of acquired drug resistance. Such information could be used to configure multi-agent combinations that simultaneously target the protein of interest as well as pathways leading to resistance. And perhaps, more novel technologies, such as PROTAC therapy, can be applied to completely degrade an oncogene, thus potentially avoiding the acquisition of mutations that arise from small molecule exposure. However, it is likely that even PROTACs will need to be applied in combinations as it likely does not address primary resistant apoptosis mechanisms (i.e. upregulation of BCL-X_L or MCL-1) and the complex biological nature of tumors. The potential of targeting and manipulation of the various components of this complex biology has proven their value and is likely only in the earliest phases of their evolution.

Must Read References

Khan, S., Zhang, X., Lv, D. et al. (2019). A selective BCL-X(L) PROTAC degrader achieves safe and potent antitumor activity. *Nature Med.* 25 (12): 1938–1947.

Reed, J.C., Cuddy, M., Slabiak, T. et al. (1988). Oncogenic potential of bcl-2 demonstrated by gene transfer. *Nature* 336 (6196): 259–261.

Souers, A.J., Leverson, J.D., Boghaert, E.R. et al. (2013). ABT-199, a potent and selective BCL-2 inhibitor, achieves antitumor activity while sparing platelets. *Nature Med.* 19 (2): 202–208.

Tsujimoto, Y., Cossman, J., Jaffe, E. et al. (1985). Involvement of the bcl-2 gene in human follicular lymphoma. *Science* 228 (4706): 1440–1443.

References

Adams, C.M., Mitra, R., Gong, J.Z. et al. (2017). Non-Hodgkin and Hodgkin lymphomas select for overexpression of BCLW. *Clin. Cancer Res.* 23 (22): 7119–7129.

Agarwal, R., Chan, Y.-C., Tam, C.S. et al. (2019). Dynamic molecular monitoring reveals that SWI–SNF mutations mediate resistance to ibrutinib plus venetoclax in mantle cell lymphoma. *Nature Med.* 25 (1): 119–129.

Ailawadhi, S., Chanan-Khan, A.A.A., Chen, Z. et al. (2021). First-in-human study of lisaftoclax (APG-2575), a novel BCL-2 inhibitor (BCL-2i), in patients (pts) with relapsed/refractory (R/R) CLL and other hematologic malignancies (HMs). *J. Clini. Oncol.* 39 (15_suppl): 7502-.

Becattini, B., Kitada, S., Leone, M. et al. (2004). Rational design and real time, in-cell detection of the proapoptotic activity of a novel compound targeting Bcl-X(L). *Chem. Biol.* 11 (3): 389–395.

Birkinshaw, R.W., Gong, J.N., Luo, C.S. et al. (2019). Structures of BCL-2 in complex with venetoclax reveal the molecular basis of resistance mutations. *Nat. Comm.* 10 (1): 2385.

Blombery, P., Anderson, M.A., Gong, J.N. et al. (2019). Acquisition of the recurrent Gly101Val mutation in BCL2 confers resistance to venetoclax in patients with progressive chronic lymphocytic leukemia. *Cancer Discov.* 9 (3): 342–353.

Blombery, P., Thompson, E.R., Nguyen, T. et al. (2020). Multiple BCL2 mutations cooccurring with Gly101Val emerge in chronic lymphocytic leukemia progression on venetoclax. *Blood* 135 (10): 773–777.

Bodo, J., Zhao, X., Durkin, L. et al. (2016). Acquired resistance to venetoclax (ABT-199) in t(14;18) positive lymphoma cells. *Oncotarget* 7 (43): 70000–70010.

Boise, L.H., González-García, M., Postema, C.E. et al. (1993). bcl-x, a bcl-2-related gene that functions as a dominant regulator of apoptotic cell death. *Cell* 74 (4): 597–608.

Brown, J.R., Tesar, B., Yu, L. et al. (2015). Obatoclax in combination with fludarabine and rituximab is well-tolerated and shows promising clinical activity in relapsed chronic lymphocytic leukemia. *Leuk. Lymphoma* 56 (12): 3336–3342.

Bruncko, M., Wang, L., Sheppard, G.S. et al. (2015). Structure-guided design of a series of MCL-1 inhibitors with high affinity and selectivity. *J. Med. Chem.* 58 (5): 2180–2194.

Brunelle, J.K. and Letai, A. (2009). Control of mitochondrial apoptosis by the Bcl-2 family. *J. Cell Sci.* 122 (Pt 4): 437–441.

Caenepeel, S., Brown, S.P., Belmontes, B. et al. (2018). AMG 176, a selective MCL1 inhibitor, is effective in hematologic cancer models alone and in combination with established therapies. *Cancer Dis.* 8 (12): 1582–1597.

Caenepeel, S., Karen, R., Belmontes, B. et al. (2020). Abstract 6218: discovery and preclinical evaluation of AMG 397, a potent, selective and orally bioavailable MCL1 inhibitor. *Cancer Res.* 80 (16 Supplement): 6218-.

Campos, L., Sabido, O., Rouault, J.P. et al. (1994). Effects of BCL-2 antisense oligodeoxynucleotides on in vitro proliferation and survival of normal marrow progenitors and leukemic cells. *Blood* 84 (2): 595–600.

Castro, J.E., Loria, O.J., Aguillon, R.A. et al. (2007). A phase II, open label study of AT-101 in combination with rituximab in patients with relapsed or refractory chronic lymphocytic leukemia. Evaluation of two dose regimens. *Blood* 110 (11): 3119-.

Certo, M., Del Gaizo Moore, V., Nishino, M. et al. (2006). Mitochondria primed by death signals determine cellular addiction to antiapoptotic BCL-2 family members. *Cancer Cell* 9 (5): 351–365.

Cervantes-Gomez, F., Lamothe, B., Woyach, J.A. et al. (2015). Pharmacological and protein profiling suggests venetoclax (ABT-199) as optimal partner with ibrutinib in chronic lymphocytic leukemia. *Clin. Cancer Res.: An Official J. Am. Ass. Cancer Res.* 21 (16): 3705–3715.

Cheah, C.Y., Verner, E., Tam, C.S. et al. (2021). Preliminary safety data from patients (PTS) with relapsed/refractory (R/R) B-cell malignancies treated with the novel B-cell Lymphoma 2 (BCL2) inhibitor BGB-11417. *Hematol. Oncol.* 39 (S2).

Chiron, D., Bellanger, C., Papin, A. et al. (2016). Rational targeted therapies to overcome microenvironment-dependent expansion of mantle cell lymphoma. *Blood* 128 (24): 2808–2818.

Chiron, D., Dousset, C., Brosseau, C. et al. (2015). Biological rational for sequential targeting of Bruton tyrosine kinase and Bcl-2 to overcome CD40-induced ABT-199 resistance in mantle cell lymphoma. *Oncotarget* 6 (11): 8750–8759.

Choudhary, G.S., Al-Harbi, S., Mazumder, S. et al. (2015). MCL-1 and BCL-xL-dependent resistance to the BCL-2 inhibitor ABT-199 can be overcome by preventing PI3K/AKT/mTOR activation in lymphoid malignancies. *Cell Death Dis.* 6 (1): e1593.

Choudhary, G.S., Tat, T.T., Misra, S. et al. (2015). Cyclin E/Cdk2-dependent phosphorylation of Mcl-1 determines its stability and cellular sensitivity to BH3 mimetics. *Oncotarget* 6 (19): 16912–16925.

Cimmino, A., Calin, G.A., Fabbri, M. et al. (2005). <em>miR-15</em> and <em>miR-16</em> induce apoptosis by targeting BCL2. *Proc. Natl. Acad. Sci. U.S.A.* 102 (39): 13944–13949.

Correia, C., Schneider, P.A., Dai, H. et al. (2015). BCL2 mutations are associated with increased risk of transformation and shortened survival in follicular lymphoma. *Blood* 125 (4): 658–667.

Cory, S., Huang, D.C., and Adams, J.M. (2003). The Bcl-2 family: roles in cell survival and oncogenesis. *Oncogene* 22 (53): 8590–8607.

Cotter, F.E., Johnson, P., Hall, P. et al. (1994). Antisense oligonucleotides suppress B-cell lymphoma growth in a SCID-hu mouse model. *Oncogene* 9 (10): 3049–3055.

Coutinho, E.M. (2002). Gossypol: a contraceptive for men. *Contraception* 65 (4): 259–263.

Davids, M.S., Roberts, A.W., Seymour, J.F. et al. (2017). Phase I first-in-human study of venetoclax in patients with relapsed or refractory non-Hodgkin lymphoma. *J. Clin. Oncol.: Official J. Am. Soc. Clin. Oncol.* 35 (8): 826–833.

Del Gaizo Moore, V., Brown, J.R., Certo, M. et al. (2007). Chronic lymphocytic leukemia requires BCL2 to sequester prodeath BIM, explaining sensitivity to BCL2 antagonist ABT-737. *J. Clin. Invest.* 117 (1): 112–121.

Del Gaizo Moore, V. and Letai, A. (2013). BH3 profiling–measuring integrated function of the mitochondrial apoptotic pathway to predict cell fate decisions. *Cancer Lett.* 332 (2): 202–205.

Fukuhara, S. and Rowley, J.D. (1978). Chromosome 14 translocations in non-Burkitt lymphomas. *International Journal of Cancer* 22 (1): 14–21.

Gandhi, L., Camidge, D.R., Ribeiro de Oliveira, M. et al. (2011). Phase I study of Navitoclax (ABT-263), a novel Bcl-2 family inhibitor, in patients with small-cell lung cancer and other solid tumors. *J. Clin. Oncol.: Official J. Am. Soc. Clin. Oncol.* 29 (7): 909–916.

Guièze, R., Liu, V.M., Rosebrock, D. et al. (2019). Mitochondrial reprogramming underlies resistance to BCL-2 inhibition in lymphoid malignancies. *Cancer Cell* 36 (4): 369–84.e13.

Halilovic, E., Chanrion, M., Mistry, P. et al. (2019). Abstract 4477: MIK665/S64315, a novel Mcl-1 inhibitor, in combination with Bcl-2 inhibitors exhibits strong synergistic antitumor activity in a range of hematologic malignancies. *Cancer Res.* 79 (13 Supplement): 4477-.

Hann, C.L., Daniel, V.C., Sugar, E.A. et al. (2008). Therapeutic efficacy of ABT-737, a selective inhibitor of BCL-2, in small cell lung cancer. *Cancer Res.* 68 (7): 2321–2328.

Hu, N., Guo, Y., Xue, H. et al. (2020). Abstract 3077: preclinical characterization of BGB-11417, a potent and selective Bcl-2 inhibitor with superior antitumor activities in haematological tumor models. *Cancer Res.* 80 (16 Supplement): 3077-.

Huang, D.C. and Strasser, A. (2000). BH3-Only proteins-essential initiators of apoptotic cell death. *Cell* 103 (6): 839–842.

Iqbal, J., Neppalli, V.T., Wright, G. et al. (2006). BCL2 expression is a prognostic marker for the activated B-cell-like type of diffuse large B-cell lymphoma. *J. Clin. Oncol.: Official J. Am. Soc. Clin. Oncol.* 24 (6): 961–968.

James, D.F., Castro, J.E., Loria, O. et al. (2006). AT-101, a small molecule Bcl-2 antagonist, in treatment naïve CLL patients (pts) with high risk features; Preliminary results from an ongoing phase I trial. *J. Clin. Oncol.* 24 (18_suppl): 6605-.

Jayappa, K.D., Portell, C.A., Gordon, V.L. et al. (2017). Microenvironmental agonists generate de novo phenotypic resistance to combined ibrutinib plus venetoclax in CLL and MCL. *Blood Adv.* 1 (14): 933–946.

Khan, S., Zhang, X., Lv, D. et al. (2019). A selective BCL-X(L) PROTAC degrader achieves safe and potent antitumor activity. *Nature Med.* 25 (12): 1938–1947.

Kirkwood, J.M., Bedikian, A.Y., Millward, M.J. et al. (2005). Long-term survival results of a randomized multinational phase 3 trial of dacarbazine (DTIC) with or without Bcl-2 antisense (oblimersen sodium) in patients (pts) with advanced malignant melanoma (MM). *J. Clin. Oncol.* 23 (16_suppl): 7506-.

Kitada, S., Leone, M., Sareth, S. et al. (2003). Discovery, characterization, and structure-activity relationships studies of proapoptotic polyphenols targeting B-cell lymphocyte/leukemia-2 proteins. *J. Med. Chem.* 46 (20): 4259–4264.

Kluck, R.M., Bossy-Wetzel, E., Green, D.R. et al. (1997). The release of cytochrome c from mitochondria: a primary site for Bcl-2 regulation of apoptosis. *Science* 275 (5303): 1132–1136.

Koss, B., Ryan, J., Budhraja, A. et al. (2016). Defining specificity and on-target activity of BH3-mimetics using engineered B-ALL cell lines. *Oncotarget* 7 (10): 11500–11511.

Kotschy, A., Szlavik, Z., Murray, J. et al. (2016). The MCL1 inhibitor S63845 is tolerable and effective in diverse cancer models. *Nature* 538 (7626): 477–482.

Kozopas, K.M., Yang, T., Buchan, H.L. et al. (1993). MCL1, a gene expressed in programmed myeloid cell differentiation, has sequence similarity to BCL2. *Proc. Natl. Acad. Sci. U.S.A.* 90 (8): 3516–3520.

Kuwana, T., Mackey, M.R., Perkins, G. et al. (2002). Bid, Bax, and lipids cooperate to form supramolecular openings in the outer mitochondrial membrane. *Cell* 111 (3): 331–342.

Landsburg, D.J., Falkiewicz, M.K., Maly, J. et al. (2017). Outcomes of patients with double-hit lymphoma who achieve first complete remission. *J. Clin. Oncol.: Official J. Am. Soc. Clin. Oncol.* 35 (20): 2260–2267.

Leverson, J.D., Zhang, H., Chen, J. et al. (2015). Potent and selective small-molecule MCL-1 inhibitors demonstrate on-target cancer cell killing activity as single agents and in combination with ABT-263 (navitoclax). *Cell Death Dis.* 6 (1): e1590.

Llambi, F., Moldoveanu, T., Tait, S.W. et al. (2011). A unified model of mammalian BCL-2 protein family interactions at the mitochondria. *Molecular Cell* 44 (4): 517–531.

Marcucci, G., Moser, B., Blum, W. et al. (2007). A phase III randomized trial of intensive induction and consolidation chemotherapy ± oblimersen, a pro-apoptotic Bcl-2 antisense oligonucleotide in untreated acute myeloid leukemia patients >60 years old. *J. Clin. Oncol.* 25 (18_suppl): 7012-.

Mason, K.D., Carpinelli, M.R., Fletcher, J.I. et al. (2007). Programmed anuclear cell death delimits platelet life span. *Cell* 128 (6): 1173–1186.

McDonnell, T.J., Deane, N., Platt, F.M. et al. (1989). bcl-2-immunoglobulin transgenic mice demonstrate extended B cell survival and follicular lymphoproliferation. *Cell* 57 (1): 79–88.

McDonnell, T.J. and Korsmeyer, S.J. (1991). Progression from lymphoid hyperplasia to high-grade malignant lymphoma in mice transgenic for the t(14; 18). *Nature* 349 (6306): 254–256.

Miyashita, T. and Reed, J.C. (1992). bcl-2 gene transfer increases relative resistance of S49.1 and WEHI7.2 lymphoid cells to cell death and DNA fragmentation induced by glucocorticoids and multiple chemotherapeutic drugs. *Cancer Res.* 52 (19): 5407–5411.

Miyashita, T. and Reed, J.C. (1993). Bcl-2 oncoprotein blocks chemotherapy-induced apoptosis in a human leukemia cell line. *Blood* 81 (1): 151–157.

Nguyen, M., Marcellus, R.C., Roulston, A. et al. (2007). Small molecule obatoclax (GX15-070) antagonizes MCL-1 and overcomes MCL-1-mediated resistance to apoptosis. *Proc. Natl. Acad. Sci. U.S.A.* 104 (49): 19512–19517.

O'Brien, S., Moore, J.O., Boyd, T.E. et al. (2009). 5-year survival in patients with relapsed or refractory chronic lymphocytic leukemia in a randomized, phase III trial of fludarabine plus cyclophosphamide with or without oblimersen. *J. Clin. Oncol.: Official J. Am. Soc. Clin. Oncol.* 27 (31): 5208–5212.

O'Brien, S.M., Claxton, D.F., Crump, M. et al. (2009). Phase I study of obatoclax mesylate (GX15-070), a small molecule pan-Bcl-2 family antagonist, in patients with advanced chronic lymphocytic leukemia. *Blood* 113 (2): 299–305.

O'Connor, O.A., Smith, E.A., Toner, L.E. et al. (2006). The combination of the proteasome inhibitor bortezomib and the bcl-2 antisense molecule oblimersen sensitizes human B-cell lymphomas to cyclophosphamide. *Clin. Cancer Res.: An Official J. Am. Assoc. Cancer Res.* 12 (9): 2902–2911.

Oltersdorf, T., Elmore, S.W., Shoemaker, A.R. et al. (2005). An inhibitor of Bcl-2 family proteins induces regression of solid tumours. *Nature* 435 (7042): 677–681.

Oltvai, Z.N., Milliman, C.L., and Korsmeyer, S.J. (1993). Bcl-2 heterodimerizes in vivo with a conserved homolog, Bax, that accelerates programmed cell death. *Cell* 74 (4): 609–619.

Paoluzzi, L., Gonen, M., Bhagat, G. et al. (2008). The BH3-only mimetic ABT-737 synergizes the antineoplastic activity of proteasome inhibitors in lymphoid malignancies. *Blood* 112 (7): 2906–2916.

Paoluzzi, L., Gonen, M., Gardner, J.R. et al. (2008). Targeting Bcl-2 family members with the BH3 mimetic AT-101 markedly enhances the therapeutic effects of chemotherapeutic agents in in vitro and in vivo models of B-cell lymphoma. *Blood* 111 (11): 5350–5358.

Papatzimas, J.W., Gorobets, E., Maity, R. et al. (2019). From inhibition to degradation: targeting the antiapoptotic protein myeloid cell leukemia 1 (MCL1). *J. Med. Chem.* 62 (11): 5522–5540.

Pérez-Galán, P., Roué, G., López-Guerra, M. et al. (2008). BCL-2 phosphorylation modulates sensitivity to the BH3 mimetic GX15-070 (Obatoclax) and reduces its synergistic interaction with bortezomib in chronic lymphocytic leukemia cells. *Leukemia* 22 (9): 1712–1720.

Petrich, A.M., Gandhi, M., Jovanovic, B. et al. (2014). Impact of induction regimen and stem cell transplantation on outcomes in double-hit lymphoma: a multicenter retrospective analysis. *Blood* 124 (15): 2354–2361.

Pro, B., Leber, B., Smith, M. et al. (2008). Phase II multicenter study of oblimersen sodium, a Bcl-2 antisense oligonucleotide, in combination with rituximab in patients with recurrent B-cell non-Hodgkin lymphoma. *Br. J. Haematol.* 143 (3): 355–360.

Reed, J.C., Cuddy, M., Haldar, S. et al. (1990a). BCL2-mediated tumorigenicity of a human T-lymphoid cell line: synergy with MYC and inhibition by BCL2 antisense. *Proc. Natl. Acad. Sci. U.S.A.* 87 (10): 3660–3664.

Reed, J.C., Cuddy, M., Slabiak, T. et al. (1988). Oncogenic potential of bcl-2 demonstrated by gene transfer. *Nature* 336 (6196): 259–261.

Reed, J.C., Stein, C., Subasinghe, C. et al. (1990b). Antisense-mediated inhibition of BCL2 protooncogene expression and leukemic cell growth and survival: comparisons of phosphodiester and phosphorothioate oligodeoxynucleotides. *Cancer Res.* 50 (20): 6565–6570.

Roberts, A.W., Davids, M.S., Pagel, J.M. et al. (2016). Targeting BCL2 with Venetoclax in Relapsed Chronic Lymphocytic Leukemia. *N. Engl. J. Med.* 374 (4): 311–322.

Roberts, A.W., Ma, S., Kipps, T.J. et al. (2019). Efficacy of venetoclax in relapsed chronic lymphocytic leukemia is influenced by disease and response variables. *Blood* 134 (2): 111–122.

Roberts, A.W., Seymour, J.F., Brown, J.R. et al. (2012). Substantial susceptibility of chronic lymphocytic leukemia to BCL2 inhibition: results of a phase I study of navitoclax in patients with relapsed or refractory disease. *J. Clin. Oncol.: Official J. Am. Soc. Clin. Oncol.* 30 (5): 488–496.

Schoenwaelder, S.M., Jarman, K.E., Gardiner, E.E. et al. (2011). Bcl-xL-inhibitory BH3 mimetics can induce a transient thrombocytopathy that undermines the hemostatic function of platelets. *Blood* 118 (6): 1663–1674.

Schuetz, J.M., Johnson, N.A., Morin, R.D. et al. (2012). BCL2 mutations in diffuse large B-cell lymphoma. *Leukemia* 26 (6): 1383–1390.

Seymour, J.F., Kipps, T.J., Eichhorst, B. et al. (2018). Venetoclax-rituximab in relapsed or refractory chronic lymphocytic leukemia. *N. Engl. J. Med.* 378 (12): 1107–1120.

Soderquist, S. and Eastman, A.R. (2016). BCL2 inhibitors as anticancer drugs: a plethora of misleading BH3 mimetics. *Mol. Cancer Ther.* 15 (9): 2011–2017.

Souers, A.J., Leverson, J.D., Boghaert, E.R. et al. (2013). ABT-199, a potent and selective BCL-2 inhibitor, achieves antitumor activity while sparing platelets. *Nature Med.* 19 (2): 202–208.

Stilgenbauer, S., Eichhorst, B., Schetelig, J. et al. (2016). Venetoclax in relapsed or refractory chronic lymphocytic leukaemia with 17p deletion: a multicentre, open-label, phase 2 study. *Lancet Oncol.* 17 (6): 768–778.

Swerdlow, S.H., Campo, E., Pileri, S.A. et al. (2016). The 2016 revision of the World Health Organization classification of lymphoid neoplasms. *Blood* 127 (20): 2375–2390.

Tam, C.S., Anderson, M.A., Pott, C. et al. (2018). Ibrutinib plus venetoclax for the treatment of mantle-cell lymphoma. *N. Engl. J. Med.* 378 (13): 1211–1223.

Tse, C., Shoemaker, A.R., Adickes, J. et al. (2008). ABT-263: a potent and orally bioavailable Bcl-2 family inhibitor. *Cancer Res.* 68 (9): 3421–3428.

Tsujimoto, Y., Cossman, J., Jaffe, E. et al. (1985). Involvement of the bcl-2 gene in human follicular lymphoma. *Science* 228 (4706): 1440–1443.

Tsujimoto, Y. and Croce, C.M. (1986). Analysis of the structure, transcripts, and protein products of bcl-2, the gene involved in human follicular lymphoma. *Proc. Natl Acad. Sci. U.S.A.* 83 (14): 5214–5218.

Tsujimoto, Y., Finger, L.R., Yunis, J. et al. (1984). Cloning of the chromosome breakpoint of neoplastic B cells with the t(14;18) chromosome translocation. *Science* 226 (4678): 1097–1099.

Vaux, D.L., Cory, S., and Adams, J.M. (1988). Bcl-2 gene promotes haemopoietic cell survival and cooperates with c-myc to immortalize pre-B cells. *Nature* 335 (6189): 440–442.

Wang, K., Yin, X.M., Chao, D.T. et al. (1996). BID: a novel BH3 domain-only death agonist. *Genes & Development* 10 (22): 2859–2869.

Wang, X., Bathina, M., Lynch, J. et al. (2013). Deletion of MCL-1 causes lethal cardiac failure and mitochondrial dysfunction. *Genes & Development* 27 (12): 1351–1364.

Wang, Z., He, N., Guo, Z. et al. (2019). Proteolysis targeting chimeras for the selective degradation of Mcl-1/Bcl-2 derived from nonselective target binding ligands. *J. Med. Chem.* 62 (17): 8152–8163.

Webb, A., Cunningham, D., Cotter, F. et al. (1997). BCL-2 antisense therapy in patients with non-Hodgkin lymphoma. *Lancet* 349 (9059): 1137–1141.

Wei, M.C., Zong, W.X., Cheng, E.H. et al. (2001). Proapoptotic BAX and BAK: a requisite gateway to mitochondrial dysfunction and death. *Science* 292 (5517): 727–730.

Weiss, L.M., Warnke, R.A., Sklar, J. et al. (1987). Molecular analysis of the t(14;18) chromosomal translocation in malignant lymphomas. *N. Engl. J. Med.* 317 (19): 1185–1189.

Wilson, W.H., O'Connor, O.A., Czuczman, M.S. et al. (2010). Navitoclax, a targeted high-affinity inhibitor of BCL-2, in lymphoid malignancies: a phase 1 dose-escalation study of safety, pharmacokinetics, pharmacodynamics, and antitumour activity. *Lancet Oncol.* 11 (12): 1149–1159.

Xie, Y., FU, C., Yan, L. et al. (2020). Targeting 1q21 amplification with APG2575 and lenalidomide to sensitize BCL-2 inhibition with the decrease of MCL-1 protein in high risk MM models. *Blood* 136 (Supplement 1): 46–47.

Yang, E., Zha, J., Jockel, J. et al. (1995). Bad, a heterodimeric partner for Bcl-XL and Bcl-2, displaces Bax and promotes cell death. *Cell* 80 (2): 285–291.

Yang, J., Liu, X., Bhalla, K. et al. (1997). Prevention of apoptosis by Bcl-2: release of cytochrome c from mitochondria blocked. *Science* 275 (5303): 1129–1132.

Youle, R.J. and Strasser, A. (2008). The BCL-2 protein family: opposing activities that mediate cell death. *Nat. Rev. Mol. Cell Biol.* 9 (1): 47–59.

Zhang, H., Nimmer, P.M., Tahir, S.K. et al. (2007). Bcl-2 family proteins are essential for platelet survival. *Cell Death Differ.* 14 (5): 943–951.

12

Clinical Experience with Pro-Apoptotic Agents

Thomas E. Lew[1,2] *and John F. Seymour*[1,3]

[1] *Department of Haematology, The Royal Melbourne Hospital and Peter MacCallum Cancer Centre, Melbourne, Victoria, Australia*
[2] *Blood Cells and Blood Cancer Division, Walter and Eliza Hall Institute of Medical Research, Parkville, Victoria, Australia*
[3] *Faculty of Medicine, Dentistry and Health Sciences, The University of Melbourne, Parkville, Victoria, Australia*

Take Home Messages

- BH3-mimetics are a novel class of small molecule inhibitors of BCL2 family proteins, which restore apoptosis in malignant cells that depend on these proteins for survival.
- The orally bioavailable selective BCL2 inhibitor, venetoclax, is the most clinically advanced and only currently approved BH3-mimetic.
- The major toxicities of venetoclax include tumor lysis syndrome and neutropenia, although these are readily preventable/manageable with established protocols.
- Venetoclax achieves frequent and deep remissions in CLL/SLL, and is now a standard of care regimen in relapsed and frontline disease as fixed-duration combination therapy with anti-CD20 monoclonal antibodies.
- Venetoclax is also active against other B-NHLs, especially MCL and Waldenstrom's macroglobulinemia, and may improve outcomes when added to conventional chemoimmunotherapy in aggressive B-cell neoplasms, likely at the expense of increased myelosuppression, although confirmatory randomized data is awaited.
- Venetoclax resistance can be mediated through *BCL2* mutations, upregulation of alternative BCL2 family members, p53 aberrations, and genomic instability or defects in other components of the intrinsic cellular death pathway.
- Future research will focus on therapeutics targeting other BCL2 family members, clinically validated biomarkers for BH3-mimetic sensitivity and novel combinations to improve efficacy.

Introduction

BCL2 and the intrinsic cell death pathway are critical regulators of cell survival, frequently perturbed by cancer cells resulting in evasion of programmed cell death (Cory and Adams 2002). Initially identified as the fusion partner of the immunoglobulin heavy chain gene locus in the classic t(14;18) translocation of follicular lymphoma (FL), BCL2 overexpression was recognized to confer resistance to apoptosis (Vaux et al. 1988). This seminal observation instigated the ensuing decades of research that characterized the complex mechanisms of intrinsic cell death and laid the foundations for the development of therapeutics capable of restoring apoptosis in malignant cells (Delbridge et al. 2016). The biology of intrinsic cell death is outlined in further detail in an earlier chapter of this volume.

The first attempt to target BCL2 using the antisense oligonucleotide oblimersen (G3139) demonstrated limited clinical efficacy in chronic lymphocytic leukemia/small cell lymphoma (CLL/SLL), and B-cell non-Hodgkin's lymphoma (B-NHL) was limited (O'Brien et al. 2005, 2009a; Pro et al. 2008) and subsequent pre-clinical studies cast doubt over its capacity to effectively target BCL2 in tumor cells (Kang and Reynolds 2009). In contrast with oblimersen, BH3-mimetics are specific, potent, and selective small molecule inhibitors of BCL2 family proteins, which disable their capacity to sequester "pro-death" BH3-only molecules. Released from the inhibitory action of BCL2 and related proteins, these pro-apoptotic BH3-only proteins are then able to activate the downstream effector molecules BAX and BAK, which dimerize on the mitochondrial outer membrane surface and permeabilize it, triggering the release of cytochrome C, caspase activation and committing the cell to apoptosis (Figure 12.1). BH3-mimetics are distinguished by their various selectivity for members of the BCL2 family (BCL2, BCL-X_L, MCL-1, etc.), and healthy and malignant cell types exhibit variable dependencies on these proteins to maintain survival (Merino et al. 2018). The pharmacology of BH3-mimetics is discussed in further detail in a previous chapter in this volume.

The most clinically advanced and only licensed BH3-mimetic is venetoclax (ABT-199/GDC-0199), an orally bioavailable selective inhibitor of BCL2 (Souers et al. 2013). In CLL/SLL, BCL2 is universally overexpressed and crucial to

Precision Cancer Therapies: Targeting Oncogenic Drivers and Signaling Pathways in Lymphoid Malignancies: From Concept to Practice, Volume 1, First Edition. Edited by Owen A. O'Connor, Stephen M. Ansell, and John F. Seymour.

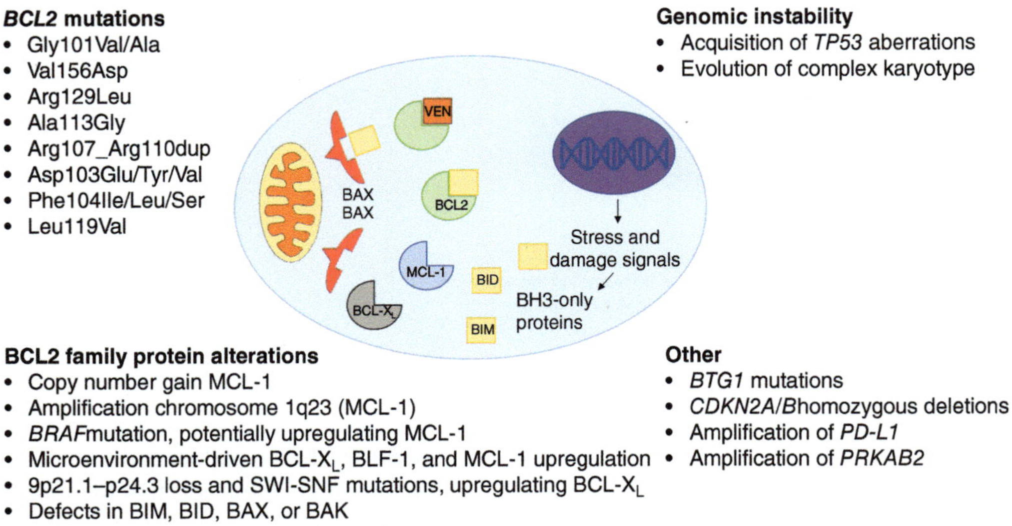

Figure 12.1 Mechanisms of venetoclax resistance in B-cell malignancies.

the evasion of cellular apoptosis (Robertson et al. 1996), underpinning the potent clinical efficacy of venetoclax in patients with this disease and the first regulatory approval for a BH3-mimetic drug for this indication (Roberts et al. 2016). In contrast to inhibitors of B-cell receptor signaling (BCRis), venetoclax frequently induces deep remissions and undetectable measurable residual disease (uMRD) status in patients with CLL/SLL, facilitating time-limited combination therapies (Lew et al. 2020). To date, venetoclax has regulatory approval in the United States, Europe, and many other countries for the management of relapsed and frontline CLL/SLL and acute myeloid leukemia (AML), with promising data in myeloma and many B-NHLs. Another clinically advanced but currently unregistered BH3-mimetic is the predecessor molecule to venetoclax, the BCL2/BCL-X_L/BCL-w inhibitor navitoclax (ABT-263), whose clinical efficacy in CLL/SLL was compromised by dose-limiting thrombocytopenia due to the reliance of platelets on BCL-X_L for survival (Mason et al. 2007; Roberts et al. 2012). Other BH3-mimetics with reported clinical data include the pan-BCL2 family inhibitor obatoclax, which demonstrated limited selectivity for BCL2, minimal clinical efficacy, and troublesome off-target neuropsychiatric toxicities in phase 1 trials (Hwang et al. 2010; O'Brien et al., 2009b), and the MCL-1 inhibitor AMG-176, which achieved infrequent responses (12%) in relapsed/refractory (R/R) multiple myeloma (Spencer et al. 2019). More recently, preliminary safety and efficacy data have been presented in abstract form from the first-in-human studies of two selective BCL2-inhibitors, BGB-11417 and lisaftoclax (APG2575), in patients with CLL/SLL and B-NHLs (Ailawadhi et al. 2021; Cheah et al. 2021). Many other BH3-mimetic compounds are in the early phases of clinical development (Roberts et al. 2021).

BH3-mimetics represent an exciting novel class of rationally designed and highly targeted therapeutics, capable of inducing rapid and deep remissions in CLL, AML, and B-NHL. This chapter will principally focus on clinical data regarding the safety and efficacy of venetoclax and navitoclax in lymphoid neoplasms, and their combination with anti-CD20 monoclonal antibodies and conventional chemotherapy. The role of BH3-mimetics in combination with other targeted agents will be discussed in the following sections.

Safety and Toxicities of Pro-apoptotic Agents

The most significant adverse effects (AEs) of venetoclax and navitoclax are cytopenias and tumor lysis syndrome (TLS), although both can be readily prevented or treated in the majority of cases without significant clinical sequela. Because the earliest clinical use and approvals for venetoclax were in patients with CLL/SLL, the majority of the safety data available are derived from patients with this condition.

Tumor Lysis Syndrome

Consistent with its mechanism of action of direct activation of apoptosis, clinically significant TLS is a well-described toxicity of venetoclax, most commonly seen in the context of CLL/SLL, and rarely in mantle cell lymphoma (MCL). During the dose ramp-up of the earliest phase 1/1b studies of venetoclax in patients with CLL/SLL, there were two fatalities due to clinical TLS and one instance of acute renal failure requiring dialysis (Roberts et al. 2016; Seymour et al. 2017). In response, the protocol was adapted for the expansion cohort of the phase 1 study, with an initial dose of 20 mg daily, weekly step-wise dose escalation and an aggressive TLS risk-adapted prophylaxis and monitoring program. Patients with any lymph node ≥10 cm or ≥ 5cm with an absolute lymphocyte count (ALC) $\geq 25 \times 10^9/l$ are considered at high-risk for TLS, and inpatient monitoring, IV hydration, and consideration of prophylactic rasburicase are recommended. Utilizing this strategy, there was only one case of laboratory TLS and no clinical TLS among the 60 patient expansion cohort of the phase 1 study (Roberts et al. 2016). The safety of this approach was further validated in a cohort of 350 patients receiving venetoclax for CLL, in which no patients met formal Howard criteria for laboratory or clinical TLS, although investigator assessed TLS and brief dose interruptions were required in a minority of patients, with all ultimately escalating to the recommended dose of 400 mg daily (Davids et al. 2018a). In addition to CLL/SLL disease burden, patients with impaired renal function are also at increased risk of TLS and warrant close attention. Drug–drug interactions that increase venetoclax levels, such as concomitant administration of potent CYP3A4 inhibitors, also potentiate TLS risk and should be avoided during dose ramp-up. Typically, TLS occurs within 6–24 hours of venetoclax initiation or dose escalation (Fischer et al. 2020). As venetoclax is increasingly used in combination, many regimens are designed with a lead-in using anti-CD20 monoclonal antibodies or Bruton's tyrosine kinase inhibitors (BTKis) which may reduce tumor bulk, reclassify the patient's TLS risk, and facilitate less intensive monitoring procedures (Al-sawaf et al. 2020; Jain et al. 2019). Despite this theoretical benefit, in a phase 1b study of venetoclax–obinutuzumab, laboratory TLS was uncommon, clinical TLS did not occur, and TLS rates did not differ between cohorts treated with venetoclax or obinutuzumab first, likely reflecting the effectiveness of the dose ramp-up strategy to mitigate the majority of TLS risk irrespective of sequencing (Flinn et al. 2019). In the phase 3 CLL14 study which defined the standard of care use of venetoclax in patients with previously untreated CLL/SLL and comorbidities or renal impairment, patients were randomized to one year of venetoclax plus obinutuzumab or chlorambucil plus obinutuzumab. In the trial design, patients received three to four doses of obinutuzumab prior to venetoclax, with three instances of laboratory TLS during the obinutuzumab run-in and no cases after commencement of venetoclax (Fischer et al. 2019a). The phase 3 MURANO study defined the standard approach in patients with R/R CLL by randomizing patients to two years of venetoclax plus rituximab or bendamustine–rituximab (BR). In this study, rituximab commenced after the venetoclax dose ramp-up and grade 3/4 TLS occurred in 3.1% of patients, with only one instance of clinical TLS (elevated creatinine) (Seymour et al. 2018). Overall, clinicians should be vigilant of the risk of TLS, but note that clinically significant sequela is rare with the careful application of the established ramp-up and risk-adapted prophylaxis strategy recommended in the product information (Abbvie 2016). When used in the frontline setting, clinicians should be cognizant that TLS can also occur during the obinutuzumab run-in prior to the initiation of venetoclax.

Outside the context of CLL/SLL, clinical TLS has been reported in patients receiving venetoclax for MCL, including one fatality. For this disease, an initial dose of 20 mg daily, weekly dose ramp-up and vigilant TLS prophylaxis and monitoring is strongly recommended (Davids et al. 2018b). For patients with less intrinsically sensitive disease such as FL and diffuse large B-cell lymphoma (DLBCL), patients have been safely commenced at doses of 400 mg daily and up-titrated to 800–1200 mg daily with rare, manageable laboratory TLS and no instances of clinical TLS (Davids et al. 2017).

Myeloid Compartment Toxicities and Infections

Cytopenias are commonly observed in patients receiving venetoclax, particularly neutropenia, as BCL2 supports survival of granulocyte-macrophage precursor cells (Leverson et al. 2015). In a pooled analysis of 350 patients receiving venetoclax 400 mg daily as monotherapy for CLL, the most common grade 3/4 toxicities were neutropenia (37%), anemia (17%), and thrombocytopenia (14%), although these most frequently emerged during dose ramp-up and the first three months of therapy, with a low rate of new onset severe cytopenias subsequently. Neutropenia was the most common reason for dose reductions or interruptions (required in 9% of patients), whereas this was rarely required for anemia or thrombocytopenia (<2%). Granulocyte colony stimulating factor (G-CSF) support or brief dose pauses led to resolution of neutropenia in the majority of cases, and permanent discontinuation due to cytopenias was very rare (<1%). Serious infections occurred in 15% of patients with grade 3/4 neutropenia and death due to infectious complications was rare (~1%). Opportunistic infections such as *Pneumocystis jiroveci* pneumonia, invasive fungal diseases, or herpetic eruptions are very uncommon, even in among heavily pre-treated patients (3.1%), and no specific prophylaxis is generally warranted (Davids et al. 2018a).

Consistent with these observations in the monotherapy setting, grade 3/4 neutropenia was commonly observed in the MURANO trial. Although grade 3/4 neutropenia occurred more frequently in the venetoclax–rituximab arm than with BR (58% vs. 39%), febrile neutropenia was uncommon (4% vs. 10%) and rates of infections and infestations were comparable (18% vs. 22%) (Seymour et al. 2018). Similarly in the CLL14 study, grade 3/4 neutropenia occurred in 53% of the venetoclax–obinutuzumab and 48% in the chlorambucil–obinutuzumab arm and grade 3/4 infections occurred in 18% and 15%, respectively (Fischer et al. 2019a). In summary, clinicians should be conscious that neutropenia is a frequent toxicity of venetoclax; however, the use of G-CSF and/or a treatment pause in persistent cases is typically effective, such that premature discontinuation of therapy due to cytopenias is rarely if ever appropriate and can adversely impact therapeutic benefit (Mato et al. 2020). Although infectious sequela can occur, these are comparable to rates seen with chemo-immunotherapy regimens. Outside of

CLL/SLL, cytopenias were less frequently reported among similarly heavily pre-treated cohorts of patients with MCL, FL, and DLBCL (grade 3/4 anemia 15%, neutropenia 11%) (Davids et al. 2017, 2021a).

A recent report of patients treated with longer term continuous venetoclax for heavily pre-treated CLL/SLL found that 28% of patients experienced persistent cytopenias (≥4 months), with 80% of such patients demonstrating clonal myeloid abnormalities. Although treatment-related myeloid neoplasms (tMNs) were described, these exclusively occurred in the setting of prior fludarabine exposure at rates comparable to historical cohorts. Interestingly, mutations of the intrinsic death pathway effector *BAX* were identified in the myeloid compartment in 32% of evaluable patients with a low burden of bone marrow (BM) CLL. Although these mutations conferred resistance to venetoclax, there were not clearly associated with the emergence of myeloid neoplasms (Blombery et al. 2021). These findings are of uncertain relevance to patients receiving time-limited venetoclax, but nevertheless demonstrate that chronic BH3-mimetic therapy can exert on-target survival pressures and clonal selection within the non-malignant myeloid compartment. In patients with persistent cytopenias on venetoclax, especially those with prior fludarabine exposure, BM evaluation, cytogenetics, and molecular studies are recommended to exclude tMN.

Gastrointestinal Toxicities

Most patients (75%) will experience transient gastrointestinal AEs on venetoclax, typically mild diarrhea or nausea. Grade 3/4 gastrointestinal symptoms are rare and typically transient (median duration five days) at 400 mg, but become more troublesome at higher doses. Most incidences emerge during dose ramp-up and resolve over time, although a small subset of patients will have persistent mild symptoms (Davids et al. 2018a). After infectious or other clinically suspected etiologies are excluded, supportive care measures such as anti-emetics and/or anti-motility agents are generally effective and facilitate ongoing treatment in the majority of cases (Fischer et al. 2020). Alternative drug formulations are being explored that may improve gastrointestinal tolerance (Kala and Chinni 2021; Salem et al. 2021).

Thrombocytopenia and Navitoclax

The precursor to venetoclax, navitoclax, is a small molecule BCL2 inhibitor that exhibits a concomitant 200-fold inhibitory action on BCL-X_L and BCL-w. The toxicity profile to navitoclax is similar to venetoclax, with frequent neutropenia, uncommon infectious complications, and transient, typically low-grade, gastrointestinal symptoms. However, navitoclax additionally causes dose-related acute thrombocytopenia due to the reliance of platelets on BCL-X_L for survival (Mason et al. 2007), with nadirs two to five days after dose initiation, partial recovery during ongoing dosing and full resolution with drug cessation. Grade 3/4 thrombocytopenia occurred in 30–50% of patients receiving navitoclax in early phase trials, although clinically significant bleeding has only been rarely reported XXX (De Vos et al. 2021; Kipps et al. 2015; Roberts et al. 2015, 2019; Wilson et al. 2010), perhaps due to the greater susceptibility of older platelets to apoptosis and persistence of younger, more hemostatically effective platelets. Due to this dose-limiting toxicity, the clinical development of navitoclax was de-prioritized in favor of venetoclax, whose selectivity of BCL2 preserved platelets (Kipps et al. 2015; Roberts et al. 2012). Therefore, the anti-neoplastic efficacy of navitoclax has not been studied at doses likely required to optimally inhibit BCL2 or to determine the potential anti-tumor effect of potent BCL-X_L inhibition. Partially due to this, TLS with navitoclax has also been observed in only a small proportion of patients (Kipps et al. 2015; Roberts et al. 2012). Nevertheless, the clinical potential of targeting BCL-X_L remains an area of significant interest, as BCL-X_L upregulation has been implicated in venetoclax resistance and responses to navitoclax have been observed in a range of lymphoid malignancies (summarized in Table 12.1) (Agarwal et al. 2019; Blombery et al. 2019a). Alternative scheduling or novel drug formulations may enable safe delivery of BCL-X_L inhibitors and reveal their true therapeutic potential (Balachander et al. 2020; Pullarkat et al. 2021).

Efficacy of Venetoclax in Chronic Lymphocytic Leukemia/Small Cell Lymphoma

Phase 1/2 Studies

Published clinical trial data for venetoclax in CLL is summarized in Table 12.2. In the first-in-human and expansion cohorts of the phase 1 study, venetoclax achieved an overall response rate (ORR) of 79%, including complete responses in 20%to be and undetectable BM disease by flow cytometry in 5%. These results were particularly encouraging given the study cohort was enriched for high-risk features including multiple prior therapies, *TP53* aberrations, fludarabine-refractoriness, and immunoglobulin heavy chain variable region (IGHV) unmutated status. Indeed, venetoclax achieved consistent response rates and deep remission across these high-risk subsets (Roberts et al. 2016). The efficacy of venetoclax in high-risk disease was formally evaluated in a subsequent phase 2 study of 158 patients with CLL/SLL harboring del(17p), where high response rates (ORR 86%) and frequent deep remissions (complete response rate [CRR] 53%) were again demonstrated. Furthermore, uMRD by flow cytometry (defined as <1 CLL cell per 10 000 leucocytes, when

Table 12.1 Clinical trials of navitoclax in hematological malignancies.

Study	Cohort	Design	ORR/CRRMRD	PFS/OS	III/IV toxicity (>10%)	Note
Phase 1						
(Wilson et al. 2010) NCT00406809	$n = 55$ RR lymphoid malignancies	Dose escalation of navitoclax given 14 or 21 days out of 21-day cycle	ORR 22%	Median PFS 16 mo (among responders)	Neutropenia 31% Thrombocytopenia 53%	Continuous dosing appeared to reduce platelet nadir
(Roberts et al. 2012) NCT00481091	$n = 29$ RR CLL	Dose escalation of navitoclax given 14 or 21 days out of 21-day cycle	ORR 35% among patients receiving ≥110 mg daily	Median PFS 25 mo	Neutropenia 28% Thrombocytopenia 28%	Navitoclax MTD: 250 mg daily
(Roberts et al. 2015) NCT00788684	$n = 29$ Previously treated B-cell malignancies FL ($n = 12$) Aggressive lymphoma ($n = 9$) CLL/SLL ($n = 5$)	3 + 3 dose escalation of navitoclax 200–325 mg daily + rituximab × 4	FL: ORR 75%; CRR 42% Aggressive lymphoma: ORR 11%; CRR 11% CLL: ORR 100%; CRR 0%	Median PFS 11 mo	Neutropenia 28% Thrombocytopenia 17%	Navitoclax MTD: 250 mg daily
(Pullarkat et al. 2021) NCT03181126	$n = 47$ Pediatric and adult RR ALL	Dose escalation of low-dose navitoclax with venetoclax 400 mg daily, plus chemotherapy	ORR 66%; CRR 60%; uMRD 34%	Median DOR 4.2 mo Median OS 7.8 mo 28% proceeded to CAR-T or alloSCT	Febrile neutropenia 47% Neutropenia 38% Thrombocytopenia 26%	Recommended phase 2 dose of navitoclax 50 mg daily for adult, 25mg if <45 kg, with venetoclax 400 mg daily and chemotherapy
Phase 2						
(Kipps et al. 2015) NCT01087151	$n = 118$ Previously untreated CLL/SLL	Randomized 1:1:1 A: Rituximab × 8 B: Rituximab × 8 + navitoclax 12 wk C: Rituximab × 8 + indefinite venetoclax Navitoclax 100 mg daily for 1st week, then 250 mg daily	A: ORR 35%; CRR 0% B: ORR 55%; CRR 0% C: ORR 75%; CRR 5%	A: Median PFS 9.1 mo B: Median PFS 15.6 mo C: Not reached	Arm C Neutropenia 45% Thrombocytopenia 33% Liver enzyme increase 25%	Study closed prematurely due to sponsor decision to develop ABT-199 (venetoclax)
(De Vos et al. 2021) NCT00406809	$N = 26$ Previously treated B-cell malignancies A: FL ($n = 11$) B: Other ($n = 15$)	Navitoclax 150 mg daily for 1st week, then 250 mg daily. Optional escalation to 325 mg daily if well tolerated. Continuous dosing	A: ORR 9%; CRR 9% B: ORR 33%; CRR 0%	Median PFS 4.9 mo Median OS 24.8 mo	Thrombocytopenia 39% Neutropenia 31%	

Abbreviations: ALL = acute lymphoblastic leukemia; AlloSCT = allogeneic stem cell transplant; CAR-T = chimeric antigen-receptor T-cell; CLL/SLL = chronic lymphocytic leukemia/small lymphocytic lymphoma; CRR = complete response rate; DOR = duration of response; FL = follicular lymphoma; mo = months; MTD = maximum tolerated dose; ORR = overall response rate; OS = overall survival; PFS = progression-free survival; uMRD = unmeasurable minimal residual disease.

≥200 000 leukocytes are analyzed) was observed in the peripheral blood (PB) and BM of 30% and 13%, respectively (Stilgenbauer et al. 2016, 2018). These observations were in distinct contrast to the other highly effective targeted agents in CLL, namely, BCRis such as ibrutinib and idelalisib, where durable remissions can be achieved for patients with high-risk disease but deep remissions are rare and indefinite therapy is required (Byrd et al. 2013; Furman et al. 2014). Venetoclax monotherapy has also demonstrated efficacy in the context of BCRi resistance or intolerance (Coutre et al. 2018; Jones et al. 2018), although refractoriness to BCRis is associated with inferior response rates and disease control after venetoclax on multivariate analyses (Roberts et al. 2019). Venetoclax monotherapy was also associated significantly improved

Table 12.2 Clinical trials of venetoclax with or without anti-CD20 antibodies or chemotherapy in CLL/SLL.

Study	Cohort	Design	ORR/CRRMRD	PFS/OS	III/IV toxicity (>10%)	Note
Phase 1/2						
(Roberts et al. 2016) **NCT01328626**	R/R Dose finding: $n = 56$ Expansion: $n = 60$	Phase 1 150–1 200 mg venetoclax daily* 400 mg venetoclax daily*	ORR 79%; CRR 20% BM flow cytometry-neg 5%	15 mo PFS 66% 24 mo OS 84%	Three cases clinical TLS, one fatal Neutropenia 41% Anemia 12% Thrombocytopenia 12%	
(Stilgenbauer et al. 2016; Stilgenbauer et al. 2018) **NCT01889186**	del(17p) R/R: $n = 158$ TN: $n = 5$	Phase 2 400 mg venetoclax daily*	ORR 77%; CRR 20% PB uMRD 30% BM uMRD 13%	24 mo PFS 54% 24 mo OS 73%	No clinical TLS Neutropenia 40% Anemia 15% Thrombocytopenia 15% Pneumonia 10%	
(Seymour et al. 2017; Ma et al. 2021) **NCT01682616**	R/R $n = 49$	Phase 1b 200–400 mg venetoclax daily^ + rituximab × 6	ORR 86%; CRR 53% BM uMRD 61%	5 yr PFS 56% 5 year OS 86%	Two cases clinical TLS, one fatal Neutropenia 53% Anemia 14% Thrombocytopenia 16% Febrile neutropenia 12% Infections and infestations 16%	Among 33 patients with deep remission (CR or uMRD), 14 continued venetoclax and 19 ceased with similar PFS
(Coutre et al. 2018) **NCT02141282**	Idelalisib exposed $n = 36$	Phase 2 400 mg venetoclax daily*	ORR 67%; CRR 8% PB uMRD 22% BM uMRD 6%	12 mo PFS 79% 12 mo OS 94%	No clinical TLS Neutropenia 50% Thrombocytopenia 25% Anemia 17%	
(Jones et al. 2018) **NCT02141282**	Ibrutinib exposed $n = 91$	Phase 2 400 mg venetoclax daily*	ORR 65%; CRR 9% PM uMRD 26% BM uMRD 5%	Median PFS 25 mo 12 mo OS 92%	Two cases laboratory TLS Neutropenia 51% Anemia 29% Thrombocytopenia 29% Lymphopenia 1% Febrile neutropenia 11%	
(Flinn et al. 2019) **NCT01685892**	R/R: $n = 50$ TN: $n = 32$	Phase 1b 100–400 mg venetoclax daily$^{\&}$ + obinutuzumab × 6	R/R ORR 95%; CRR 37% PM uMRD 64% BM uMRD 62% TN ORR 100%; CRR 78% PM uMRD 91% BM uMRD 78%	R/R 24 mo PFS 85% OS NA TN 24 mo PFS 91% OS NA	Neutropenia 53–58% Thrombocytopenia 22% Infection 13–29%	

(Cochrane et al. 2021) NCT02980731	RR $n = 210$	Phase 3b 400 mg venetoclax daily#	ORR 77%; CRR 19% QoL + 9.3 points by EORTC QLQ-C30	12 mo PFS 83% 12 mo OS 88%	Neutropenia 32% Thrombocytopenia 17% Anemia 11%
Phase 3					
MURANO (Seymour et al. 2018; Kater et al. 2020a; Kater et al. 2019; Kater et al. 2020b) NCT02005471	R/R Venetoclax + rituximab $n = 194$	400 mg venetoclax daily 24 mo + rituximab × 6+	ORR 93%; CRR 27% PB uMRD 62% BM uMRD 27%	Median PFS 54 mo 5 yr OS 82%	TLS 3%, one case clinical TLS Neutropenia 58% Infection 18%
	Bendamustine + rituximab $n = 195$	70 mg/m^2 bendamustine D1 + D2 Q28D × 6 + rituximab × 6	ORR 68%; CRR 8% PB uMRD 13% BM uMRD 2%	Median PFS 17 mo 5 yr OS 62%	TLS 1%, one case clinical TLS Neutropenia 39% Infection 22%
CLL14 (Fischer et al. 2019a; Al-sawaf et al. 2020; Fischer et al. 2019b) NCT02242942	TN CIRS > 6 or CrCl < 70 Venetoclax + obinutuzumab $n = 216$	400 mg venetoclax daily 12 mo + obinutuzumab × 6	ORR 85%; CRR 50% PB uMRD 76% BM uMRD 57%	3 yr PFS 82% 24 mo OS 92%	Three cases lab TLS Neutropenia 53% Infection 18%
	Chlorambucil + obinutuzumab $n = 216$	0.5 mg/kg chlorambucil D1 + D15 Q28D × 12 + obinutuzumabx6	ORR 71%; CRR 23% PB uMRD 35% BM uMRD 17%	3 yr PFS 50% 24 mo OS 93%	Five cases lab TLS Neutropenia 48% Infection 15%
Venetoclax plus chemotherapy					
CLL2-BAG (Cramer et al. 2018) NCT02401503	$n = 63$ TN: $n = 34$ RR: $n = 29$	Debulking *if tumor bulk* (ALC > 25 000/ul or adenopathy ≥ 5 cm): 70 mg/m^2 bendamustine D1 + D2 Q28D × 2 Induction: Venetoclax + obinutuzumab (two cycles) Maintenance: Venetoclax up to 24 mo s + obinutuzumab	TN: ORR 100%; CRR 50% PB uMRD 91% RR: ORR 90%; CRR 28% PB uMRD 83%	TN: 15 mo PFS 100% 15 mo OS 100% RR: 15 mo PFS 92% 15 mo OS 95%	Neutropenia 44% Infections 14% Thrombocytopenia 13% Anemia 11%

Abbreviations: CIRS = Cumulative Illness Rating Scale; CrCl = creatinine clearance; EORTC QLQ-C30 = European Organization for Research and Treatment of Cancer Quality of Life Questionnaire Core 30; mo = months; QoL = quality of life; yr = year.

*Continuous therapy until progression, death, or other reason to withdraw from trial.

^Continuous venetoclax therapy, cessation permitted in good response at clinician discretion.

&Continuous venetoclax for patients with relapse and refractory disease, fixed-duration therapy for 12 months in treatment naive patients with optional additional 12 months of therapy if not in CR or BM MRD-neg response.

#Continuous therapy until progression, unacceptable toxicity or two years total therapy. Patients in countries without commercial access to venetoclax could continue for a further two years if ongoing clinical benefit.

quality-of-life among patients with R/R CLL in the single-arm VENICE II study (Cochrane et al. 2021).

Supported by *in vitro* and clinical evidence of synergy between anti-CD20 monoclonal antibodies and BH3-mimetics (Kipps et al. 2015; Roberts et al. 2015; Souers et al. 2013), 49 patients were enrolled in a phase 1b study of venetoclax plus rituximab, achieving frequent and deep responses (ORR 86%; CRR 53%), with a remarkable frequency of BM uMRD in a R/R cohort (61%). Hematological toxicities predominated, with no unexpected AEs observed with the combination regimen (Seymour et al. 2017). At the latest follow-up, the five-year estimated progression-free survival (PFS) and overall survival (OS) rates were 56% and 86%, respectively. Among 33 patients who attained complete remission (CR) or uMRD, 14 elected to continue venetoclax monotherapy and 19 ceased, with comparable PFS between the two groups (ongoing response at five years in 71% for ongoing therapy and 79% for fixed-duration) (Ma et al. 2021). Although non-randomized, these results suggest that venetoclax can be ceased among patients in deep response without compromising durability of disease control, with the potential advantages of minimizing toxicity, cost, and the selection pressure for venetoclax-resistant subclones. A phase 1b study of venetoclax–obinutuzumab has also demonstrated responses in 95–100% of patients, with rates of BM uMRD ranging from 62% to 78% across treatment-naive and R/R cohorts (Flinn et al. 2019). Although a formal randomized comparison of venetoclax with or without anti-CD20 antibodies has not been performed and cohort characteristics differ significantly between monotherapy and combination studies, these datasets and other non-randomized comparisons suggest that depth of remission is substantially increased through combination, without increase in clinically serious AEs (Lew et al. 2020). Overall, early phase clinical trials demonstrated frequent, deep and durable remissions were achievable with venetoclax, including patients with biologically adverse disease. Furthermore, observation that uMRD could be attained in the majority of patients with durable treatment-free remissions led to the preferential development of the fixed-duration regimens that were evaluated in phase 3 trials and defined current standard of care approaches.

Combining Venetoclax with Conventional Chemotherapy in CLL/SLL

The potent single-agent efficacy of venetoclax in CLL/SLL and frequent neutropenia somewhat dissuade combination with chemotherapy, which may add little additional efficacy and likely synergistic myelosuppression. Nevertheless, the phase 2 CLL2-BAG study investigated the use of bendamustine for two cycles to debulk disease in patients with high tumor volume, followed by obinutuzumab and venetoclax for up to two years. Of the patients who received debulking chemotherapy (31 treatment-naive; 14 R/R), 53% had responsive disease, approximately one-third of patients experienced grade 3/4 AEs and the majority of patients with high TLS risk due to ALC or bulky adenopathy had resolution of these high-risk features prior to venetoclax. Response rates, survival outcomes, and toxicities were comparable to other anti-CD20 combination regimens (Cramer et al. 2018). Given the low incidence of clinical TLS with venetoclax using standard protocols, the utility of debulking chemotherapy is unclear and may increase short and longer term toxicities. The availability of other potent targeted agents with evidence of synergistic efficacy and non-overlapping toxicities has focused research efforts on these "chemotherapy-free" combination regimens (Hillmen et al. 2019; Jain et al. 2019).

Phase 3 Studies

For patients with R/R disease, the MURANO study randomized subjects to receive venetoclax for two years after completion of the five-week dose ramp-up combined with six doses of rituximab or BR for six cycles. Patients receiving venetoclax–rituximab demonstrated superior response rates, response depth, PFS, and OS. At most recent follow-up, the median PFS after venetoclax–rituximab was 54 months, with an estimated OS of 82% at five years. PB uMRD was achieved in 62% of patents, and ~40% of patients with PB uMRD at the end of fixed-duration venetoclax treatment maintained ongoing uMRD after three years off therapy, demonstrating deep treatment-free remissions can be sustained after time-limited combination therapy (Kater et al. 2019, 2020a, 2020b; Seymour et al. 2018).

The CLL14 trial randomized treatment-naive patients with co-morbidities (Cumulative illness rating score >6) or renal impairment (creatinine clearance <70 ml/min) to 12 months of venetoclax or chlorambucil, each combined with six cycles of obinutuzumab. The venetoclax regimen demonstrated superior response depth and PFS with comparable toxicity and OS (Fischer et al. 2019a). In the venetoclax–obinutuzumab cohort, 76% of patients attained PB uMRD and the estimated three-year PFS was 82% (Al-sawaf et al. 2020; Fischer et al. 2019b). In both MURANO and CLL14, superiority of the venetoclax-based regimen was observed across subgroups, with greatest benefit among patients with del(17p), *TP53* mutations, and IGHV unmutated status, for whom outcomes after conventional chemo-immunotherapy are inferior (Strati et al. 2014). Whether a subset of patients may benefit from more prolonged venetoclax treatment remains controversial, although deepening of response beyond two years of therapy is rare (Lew et al. 2020). To date, randomized data is lacking to support the use of venetoclax-based regimens for treatment-naive fit patients, in distinction to ibrutinib which has demonstrated superiority to the standard chemo-immunotherapy regimen FCR (fludarabine, cyclophosphamide, rituximab)

(Shanafelt et al. 2019). Recruitment has completed for the CLL13 study (FCR/BR vs. venetoclax–rituximab vs. venetoclax–obinutuzumab vs. obinutuzumab–ibrutinib–venetoclax; NCT02950051) and the results are awaited. In the absence of these data, venetoclax- or BTKi-based regimens are recommended over chemo-immunotherapy for fit patients with disease harboring *TP53* aberrations, for whom durable remissions are not achieved with FCR. For fit patients with p53 wild-type, IGHV mutated disease, FCR achieves very durable remissions and likely cures in ~50–60%, and best frontline management for this subgroup will likely remain controversial for some time (Thompson et al. 2016).

Venetoclax Re-treatment

Emerging evidence suggests that many patients who cease venetoclax in deep response may retain sensitivity to BCL2 inhibition at disease relapse. This is congruent with the observation that resistance mutations are typically observed only after prolonged exposure, and have not been detected among patients treated with time-limited venetoclax-based regimens to date (Blombery et al. 2019a). After a median time off therapy of 3.2 years, six patients (32%) who ceased in deep response in the 1b study of venetoclax–rituximab have had progressive disease (PD), and four have been re-treated with venetoclax–rituximab. All had ceased drug for >24 months and all had responsive disease, with second remissions ranging from 19 to 43 months (three ongoing) (Ma et al. 2021). In two separate preliminary reports each with 18 response-evaluable patients with similar results, venetoclax-based re-treatment achieved responses in 72% of patients, including CRs and remissions beyond one year (Harrup et al. 2020; Thompson et al. 2020b). Although longer term follow-up of larger cohorts is required, these data suggest that re-treatment is effective for some patients with PD after time-limited therapy. Further study of clinico-pathological predictors of successful re-treatment is warranted to maximize the therapeutic benefit of this strategy (Wu et al. 2021).

Efficacy of Venetoclax in Other B-cell Neoplasms

Mantle Cell Lymphoma

BCL2 is frequently upregulated in MCL, driven by defective degradation by the E3 ubiquitin ligase FBXO10 and increased transcription through BTK signaling driven activation of the nuclear factor-kappa B pathway (Li et al. 2016). BCL2 inhibition potently induces apoptosis in cell lines and primary MCL cells, especially in cells with a high BCL2 to MCL-1 ratio (Touzeau et al. 2011). These preclinical observations made BCL2 inhibition an attractive strategy warranting clinical trials in patients with MCL (summarized in Table 12.3).

In the phase 1 first-in-human study of venetoclax in B-NHL, venetoclax achieved an ORR of 75% and CRR of 21% in a cohort of 28 patients with R/R MCL. These patients were heavily pre-treated (median three prior lines), but naive to BTKis (Davids et al. 2017). The median PFS and duration of response (DOR) were 11 and 16 months, respectively, with prolonged DOR among the six patients attaining a CR (median 32 months) (Davids et al. 2021a). Since this formal prospective evaluation, published data on single-agent venetoclax is derived predominantly from retrospective cohorts, as prospective studies have focused on combinations with other targeted therapies, especially BTKis (see following chapter) (Tam et al. 2018).

In a retrospective analysis of 20 patients who received venetoclax for high-risk, BTKi-exposed MCL, response rates were modest (ORR/CRR: 53%/18%) and the median PFS was poor at three months (Eyre et al. 2019). In another retrospective study of 24 patients with high-risk MCL (median five prior lines of therapy; 67% BTKi-resistant), venetoclax-based regimens (83% monotherapy ± anti-CD20 antibody) similarly achieved an ORR of 50% and CRR of 21%, with a median PFS of eight months (Zhao et al. 2020). A multicenter retrospective analysis of 81 patients with RR MCL (median three prior lines of therapy; 91% BTKi-exposed), venetoclax-based regimens (75% monotherapy ± anti-CD20 antibody) achieved an ORR of 42% and CRR of 18%, with a median time on venetoclax of three months (Sawalha et al. 2020). Overall, these data suggest that although venetoclax achieves responses in MCL, including some deep remissions, the duration of benefit is short-lived in heavily pre-treated patients, especially those with BTKi-resistant disease. The greatest benefit of venetoclax in MCL is therefore likely to be derived in earlier lines of therapy, or in combination with other targeted agents.

Follicular Lymphoma

BCL2 is overexpressed in FL via the canonical chromosomal translocation, t(14;18), establishing a central role in disease biology and an attractive therapeutic target (Galteland et al. 2005). Clinical trials investigating venetoclax monotherapy or combined with anti-CD20 monoclonal antibodies or chemotherapy are summarized in Table 12.3. Venetoclax monotherapy achieved modest responses among 29 patients with heavily pre-treated FL in the first-in-human phase 1 study (ORR 38%; CR 17%), with a median PFS and DOR of 11 and 27 months, respectively. As seen in CLL and MCL, greater response depth was associated with prolonged DOR (PR: median DOR 10 months; CR: median DOR 38 months) (Davids et al. 2017, 2021a). Higher response rates were observed in cohorts assigned doses ≥900 mg daily, with an ORR of 44% among those assigned 1200 mg daily compared to

Table 12.3 Studies of venetoclax with or without anti-CD20 antibodies or chemotherapy in B-NHL.

Study	Cohort	Design	ORR/ CRRMRD	PFS/OS	III/IV toxicity (>10%)	Note
Mantle cell lymphoma						
(Davids et al. 2021a; Davids et al. 2017) NCT01328626	$n = 28$ RR MCL (median 3 prior lines of therapy) Lenalidomide and ibrutinib naive 18% bortezomib exposed	Phase 1 dose escalation venetoclax monotherapy 200–1 200 mg daily	ORR 75%; CRR 21%	Median PFS 11 mo Median DOR 16 mo 12 mo OS: 82%	Overall cohort Anemia 15% Neutropenia 11%	RP2D 800 mg
(Eyre et al. 2019)	$n = 20$ RR MCL (median 3 prior lines of therapy) BTKi exposed (90% resistant)	Retrospective analysis of venetoclax at doses of 200–1 200 mg daily	ORR 53%; CRR 18%	Median PFS 3 mo Median OS 9 mo	Pneumonia 15%	
(Zhao et al. 2020)	$n = 24$ RR MCL (median 5 prior lines of therapy) BTKi resistant: 67%	Retrospective analysis of venetoclax-based regimens: Monotherapy: $n = 12$ + anti-CD20 antibody: $n = 8$ + BTKi: $n = 3$ + chemotherapy: $n = 1$	ORR 50%; CRR 21%	Median PFS 8 mo Median OS 13.5 mo	NA	
(Sawalha et al. 2020)	$n = 81$ RR MCL (median 3 prior lines of therapy)	Retrospective analysis of venetoclax-based regimens: Monotherapy: $n = 50$ + anti-CD20 antibody: $n = 11$ + BTKi: $n = 16$ + other: $n = 4$	ORR 42%; CRR 18%	Median duration of venetoclax treatment 3 mo Median OS 13 mo	NA	
Follicular lymphoma						
(Davids et al. 2021a; Davids et al. 2017) NCT01328626	$n = 29$ RR FL	Phase 1 dose escalation venetoclax monotherapy 200–1 200 mg daily	ORR 38%; CRR 17%	Median PFS 11 mo Median DOR 27 mo 12 mo OS: 100%	Overall cohort Anemia 15% Neutropenia 11%	RP2D 1 200 mg
(De Vos et al. 2018) NCT01594229	$n = 32$ RR FL	Phase 1b dose escalation of venetoclax 50-1200mg daily plus bendamustine-rutiximabx6	ORR 75% CR 38%	Median PFS and OS not reached	Overall cohort Neutropenia 60% Lymphopenia 38%	RP2D 800 mg in combination with bendamustine–rituximab

CAVALLI Ib **(Zelenetz et al. 2019)** **NCT02055820**	$n = 24$ RR FL: $n = 4$ TN FL: $n = 20$	Phase 1b dose escalation of venetoclax 200–800 mg in combination with R/G-CHOP	ORR 83%; CRR 75%	12 mo PFS 100% Ven-R-CHOP and 90% Ven-G-CHOP	Overall cohort Neutropenia 54% Febrile neutropenia 33% Thrombocytopenia 17% Anemia 13%	RP2D 800 mg C1D4-10 and D1-10 for subsequent cycles
(Stathis et al. 2019) **NCT02877550**	$n = 25$ TN FL	Phase 1 trial of venetoclax 600–800 mg daily plus obinutuzumab for six cycles, followed by obinutuzumab maintenance (two years)	ORR 88%; CRR 68%	12 mo PFS 77%	Neutropenia 28%	RP2D 800 mg in combination with obinutuzumab
(Zinzani et al. 2020) **NCT02187861**	$n = 163$ RR FL Arm A: $n = 52$ Arm B: $n = 51$ Arm C: $n = 51$ Safety run-in: $n = 9$	Phase 2 study of: Arm A: Venetoclax 800 mg daily for one year plus rituximab C1D1, 8, 15, 22 & D1 of C4, C6, C8, C12 Arm B: Venetoclax 800 mg daily for one year plus bendamustine–rituximab × 6 Arm C: Bendamustine–rituximab × 6	Arm A: ORR 35%; CRR 17% Arm B: ORR 84%; CRR 75% Arm C: ORR 84%; CRR 69%	18- mo PFS Arm A: 27% Arm B: 62% Arm C:59%	Arm A: Neutropenia 25% Arm B: Neutropenia 59% Thrombocytopenia 45% Anemia 14% Febrile neutropenia 12% Arm C: Neutropenia 28%	
Diffuse large B-cell lymphoma and aggressive B-cell lymphomas						
(Davids et al. 2021a; Davids et al. 2017) **NCT01328626**	$n = 34$ RR DLBCL and PMBCL (two patients)	Phase 1 dose escalation venetoclax monotherapy 200–1 200 mg daily	ORR 18%; CRR 12%	Median PFS 1 mo 12 mo OS: 32%	Overall cohort Anemia 15% Neutropenia 11%	RP2D 1 200 mg
(De Vos et al. 2018) **NCT01594229**	$n = 22$ RR DLBCL	Phase 1b dose escalation of venetoclax 50–1 200 mg daily plus bendamustine–rituximab × 6	ORR 41%; CR 14%	Median PFS 4 mo Median OS 15 mo	Overall cohort Neutropenia 60% Lymphopenia 38% Thrombocytopenia 28% Anemia 17%	RP2D 800 mg in combination with bendamustine–rituximab
CAVALLI 1b **(Zelenetz et al. 2019)** **NCT02055820**	$n = 18$ TN DLBCL	Phase 1b dose escalation of venetoclax 200–800 mg in combination with R/G-CHOP	ORR 89%; CRR 89%	12 mo PFS 70% Ven-R-CHOP and 100% Ven-G-CHOP	Overall cohort Neutropenia 54% Febrile neutropenia 33% Thrombocytopenia 17% Anemia 13%	RP2D 800 mg C1D4-10 and D1-10 for subsequent cycles

(*Continued*)

Table 12.3 (Continued)

Study	Cohort	Design	ORR/ CRRMRD	PFS/OS	III/IV toxicity (>10%)	Note
(Rutherford et al. 2021) **NCT03036904**	$n = 30$ TN aggressive B-NHL DHL: $n = 15$ DLBCL: $n = 9$ Transformed NHL: $n = 2$ HGBCL-NOS: $n = 2$ PMBCL: $n = 2$	Phase 1 dose escalation of venetoclax 400–800 mg in combination with dose-adjusted-R-EPOCH	ORR 97%; CRR 93%	24 mo PFS: 83% 24 mo OS: 90%	Neutropenia 83% Thrombocytopenia 70% Febrile neutropenia 63% Anemia 60% Serious gastrointestinal AEs 27%	RP2D 600 mg for five days per cycle
CAVALLI phase 2 **(Morschhauser et al. 2021)** **NCT02055820**	$n = 206$ TN DLBCL IPI 2–5	Phase 2 study of venetoclax-Rx8 plus CHOPx6-8	ORR 83%; CRR 69%	24 mo PFS: 80% 24 mo OS: 86%	Neutropenia 68% Febrile neutropenia 31% Infections 23% Anemia 24% Thrombocytopenia 22% Leucopenia 10%	Improved PFS compared to historical R-CHOP control (GOYA), esp if BCL2 + by IHC
(Davids et al. 2021b) **NCT03054896**	$n = 27$ DLBCL-RT	Phase 2 of C1 DA-R-EPOCH, followed by venetoclax ramp-up, then venetoclax 400 mg D1-10 of C2-6 of DA-R-EPOCH followed by alloSCT/ CAR-T or venetoclax 400 mg daily maintenance	ORR 62%; CRR 50%	Median PFS 10 mo Median OS 20 mo	Neutropenia 58% Anemia 62% Thrombocytopenia 50% Febrile neutropenia 38% Hypophosphatemia 23% Hyponatremia 15% Hyperglycemia 15%	

Abbreviations: alloSCT = allogeneic stem cell transplant; BTKi = Bruton's tyrosine kinase inhibitor; CAR-T = chimeric antigen-receptor T-cell; CHOP = cyclophosphamide, adriamycin, vincristine & prednisolone; CRR = complete response rate; D = day; DA = dose adjusted; DHL = double-hit lymphoma; DLBCL = diffuse large B-cell lymphoma; EPOCH = etoposide, prednisolone, vincristine, cyclophosphamide, adriamycin; FL = follicular lymphoma; G = obinutuzumab; IHC = immunohistochemistry; IPI = international prognostic indexR; MCL = mantle cell lymphoma; mo = months; ORR = overall response rate; PFS = progression-free survival; PMBCL = primary mediastinal B-cell lymphoma; R = rituximab; RP2D = recommended phase 2 dose; RR= relapsed/refractory; TN = treatment naïve.

13% among those receiving ≤600 mg daily, suggesting a dose–response relationship. Although promising, the modest single-agent efficacy suggested that combination with chemotherapy or other novel agents would be required to improve outcomes. A phase 1 study of 25 treatment-naive patients investigated doses of venetoclax 600–800 mg daily combined with obinutuzumab for six cycles, followed by two years of obinutuzumab maintenance among patients with disease response. Among the 11 response-evaluable patients, the ORR/CRR was 82%/45% with two instances of PD. Grade 3/4 toxicities to date have been predominantly hematological (neutropenia 28%, febrile neutropenia 8%), with one discontinuation due to thrombocytopenia, hepatic enzyme rise, and pneumonitis (Stathis et al. 2019). Although preliminary, these response rates appear comparable to those after obinutuzumab-chemotherapy for frontline management of FL in the GALLIUM study (ORR/CRR: 89%/20%) (Marcus et al. 2017).

Based on pre-clinical evidence of synergy (Souers et al. 2013), a phase 1b study investigated venetoclax combined with BR in patients with B-NHL, including 32 patients with R/R FL. In the FL cohort, the regimen achieved an ORR of 75% and CRR of 38%, and the median PFS had not been reached at the time of the reporting, although follow-up was short. Across the overall cohort, grade 3/4 neutropenia occurred in 60%, although febrile neutropenia was rare (8%). A maximum tolerated dose of venetoclax in combination with BR was not reached, and the investigators concluded that 800 mg daily was recommended for phase 2 trials (De Vos et al. 2018). The similarly designed phase 1b CAVALLI study examined the combination of venetoclax with CHOP (cyclophosphamide, doxorubicin, vincristine, and prednisolone) with rituximab or obinutuzumab. Grade 3/4 neutropenia and febrile neutropenia were common (54% and 33%, respectively), requiring protocol adjustments to deliver venetoclax over a fixed period (C1D4-10 and D1-10 for subsequent cycles) rather than continuously. Nevertheless, disease responses among the 24 patients with FL (20 treatment-naive; 4 R/R) were robust, with an ORR of 83%, CRR of 75%, and a 12-month PFS between 90% and 100% across the rituximab- and obinutuzumab-treated cohorts (Zelenetz et al. 2019). These results compared favorably to the R-CHOP arm of the contemporaneous phase 3 REVELANCE study (R-CHOP vs. R-lenalidomide in patients with treatment-naive FL), which reported an ORR of 65%, CRR of 53%, and an estimated three-year PFS rate of 78% (Morschhauser et al. 2018). Within the limitations of cross-trial comparisons, these data suggest that the addition of venetoclax to standard chemotherapy regimens may improve response rates, although likely at the expense of increased rates of severe neutropenia and its complications.

The best data currently available to inform the potential utility of adding venetoclax to conventional chemotherapy in FL comes from the randomized phase 2 CONTRALTO study, in which patients with R/R FL were assigned at investigator discretion to receive either one year of venetoclax plus rituximab (arm A, $n = 52$) or a chemotherapy-containing regimen. Patients in the chemotherapy-containing cohort were randomized 1:1 to receive six cycles BR with one year of venetoclax (arm B, $n = 51$) or without (arm C, $n = 51$). While the response rates in the BR cohorts were similar with or without venetoclax (ORR 84%; CRR 69–75%), responses were less frequent in the venetoclax–rituximab cohort (ORR 35%; CRR 17%). These response data correlated to PFS outcomes, with no difference in the BR cohorts with or without venetoclax (estimated 18-month PFS 62% vs. 59%), but significantly inferior outcomes in the venetoclax–rituximab arm (estimated 18-month PFS 27%). Furthermore, toxicity was increased with the addition of venetoclax to BR (grade 3/4 neutropenia: 59% vs. 28%; febrile neutropenia 12% vs. 6%) and dose reductions and treatment discontinuations were more common. In somewhat disappointing contrast to CLL/SLL, this non-randomized study demonstrated inferior efficacy with venetoclax-rituximab compared to conventional chemotherapy in R/R FL, and increased toxicity without improved efficacy when venetoclax was added to BR (Zinzani et al. 2020).

Overall, venetoclax is active in FL and can achieve CRs in a subset of patients. Despite the high prevalence of t(14;18) and the associated overexpression of BCL2 seen in FL, clinical data has demonstrated inferior efficacy with BCL2 inhibition compared to CLL/SLL or MCL. Although an abbreviated dosing schedule may reduce toxicities and dose interruptions when venetoclax is added to chemo-immunotherapy, the lack of evidence for increased efficacy over conventional approaches casts doubt over this strategy. Future success with venetoclax for patients with this disease will require better selection of patients with BCL2-dependent biology or more efficacious combinations with reduced likelihood of synergistic myelosuppression, preferentially with targeted agents.

Diffuse Large B-cell Lymphoma and Other Aggressive B-cell Lymphomas

Venetoclax monotherapy has limited efficacy in R/R DLBCL, achieving an ORR of 18% (CRR 12%) and median PFS of one month among 34 patients in the phase 1 study (Davids et al. 2017). These results suggested that venetoclax is active in some patients with DLBCL, but combination therapy or biomarker identification of likely responders would be required to improve clinical utility. For example, BH3 profiling of primary aggressive B-NHL cells demonstrates that approximately one-third harbor defects in pro-apoptotic proteins such as BAX, BAK, BIM, or BID that confer venetoclax resistance (Rys et al. 2021). Although further validation is required, these assays may ultimately prove useful clinical tools to predict response to BH3-mimetic drugs. In the phase

1b study of venetoclax plus BR, the ORR among 22 patients with R/R DLBCL was 41% (CRR 14%), with poor PFS (median four months) (De Vos et al. 2018). In the phase 1b CAVALLI study, outcomes among 18 patients with treatment-naive DLBCL were more promising when venetoclax was added to rituximab/obinutuzumab-CHOP, with a CRR of 89% and an estimated 12-month PFS rate between 70% and 100%. Interestingly, CRs were achieved among seven out of eight patients with double-expressor status, and three out of four patients with MYC rearrangements by fluorescent *in situ* hybridization (FISH), suggesting that the addition of venetoclax may improve efficacy within these higher risk subsets (Zelenetz et al. 2019).

These results led to the larger phase 2 CAVALLI study of 206 patients with treatment-naive DLBCL and an international prognostic index (IPI) of 2–5. The R-CHOP arm of the contemporaneous GOYA study (rituximab vs. obinutuzumab plus CHOP in frontline DLBCL) was used as a pre-specified covariate-adjusted historical control (Sehn et al. 2020). Patients received CHOP for six cycles, with the option for a further two cycles at investigator discretion (utilized in <10% of patients), with venetoclax 800 mg on C1 D4-10 and D1-10 for cycles 2–8 and standard rituximab. The patients were similar to the IPI 2–5 R-CHOP cohort of GOYA across baseline characteristics, although elevated BCL2 expression by immunohistochemistry was more prevalent in the CAVALLI cohort (58% vs. 49%). Six or more cycles of R-CHOP were completed in 74% of patients, and 70% completed the planned venetoclax treatment. Relative dose intensity for CHOP was similar across the cohorts, although rituximab intensity was reduced among venetoclax-treated patients due to dose delays. Although response rates were comparable between groups, the CAVALLI cohort demonstrated significantly superior PFS compared to historical controls in the overall population (hazard ratio [HR] 0.61; 95% CI [0.43–0.87]) and particularly among patients with high BCL2 expression by immunohistochemistry (HR 0.55; 95% CI [0.34–0.89]). The two-year OS was 86% in the overall CAVALLI cohort and 81% in the covariate-adjusted GOYA R-CHOP control, without a statistically significant difference (HR 0.72; 95% CI [0.48–1.10]). Toxicities were more common among venetoclax-treated patients, with higher rates of grade 3/4 AEs (86% vs. 66%) and serious AEs (56% vs. 41%), which were predominantly related to myelosuppression and febrile neutropenia. There was no increase in fatal AEs (2% in CAVALLI vs. 5% in GOYA controls) (Morschhauser et al. 2021). Overall, these data suggest that venetoclax can be added to R-CHOP without compromising dose intensity, although hematologic and infectious complications are likely increased. The suggestion of improved efficacy, particularly among patients with BCL2 overexpression by immunohistochemistry, is promising and requires formal study in randomized trials, which are currently active (NCT03984448).

A recently published phase 1 study reported the safety and preliminary efficacy of venetoclax added to six cycles of dose-adjusted-R-EPOCH (etoposide, prednisolone, vincristine, cyclophosphamide, and doxorubicin) in 30 patients with treatment-naive aggressive B-cell lymphoid neoplasms (50% with BCL2 and MYC rearrangements by FISH, "double-hit lymphoma" [DHL]). Although unacceptable dose-limiting toxicities were not observed at the maximum dose level (800 mg for 10 days per cycle), the investigators selected 600 mg for five days as the recommended phase 2 dose in combination with R-EPOCH due to improved overall tolerability and reduced duration of cytopenias to facilitate maintenance of chemotherapy dose intensity. Venetoclax dose reductions and discontinuations were required in five patients (17%), and 30% of patients discontinued treatment due to toxicity. Grade 3/4 hematologic complications were common (neutropenia, 83%; thrombocytopenia, 70%; anemia, 60%) and 63% of patients experienced febrile neutropenia. There was one septic death, one instance of intracranial hemorrhage and eight instances of serious gastrointestinal complications including ileus, colonic perforation, and bowel obstruction. Although toxicities were common, 93% of patients achieved a CR and the estimated 24-month PFS was 83%, representing impressive efficacy in this high-risk cohort. Among patients with DHL, 87% attained a CR and the estimated 24-month PFS was 65%. Overall, this study suggests that the addition of venetoclax to R-EPOCH is associated with a high rate of toxicities and likely compromises chemotherapy dose intensification, although this may be offset by potentially improved outcomes among high-risk populations for whom current standard regimens are associated with poor outcomes (Oki et al. 2014). Alliance 051701, a randomized study of venetoclax plus R-CHOP/EPOCH for patients with double-hit or double-expressor DLBCL is currently active (NCT03984448), and will hopefully provide clarity on the trade-off of toxicity and efficacy. Critically, preliminary analysis showed an excess of deaths (six vs. one) in the R-EPOCH arm with the addition of venetoclax, leading to the closure of this arm. The randomization in the R-CHOP backbone cohort for double-expressor cases continues (Abramson et al. 2021). Titration of venetoclax dose and exposure will require close attention in future trials to optimize efficacy without inducing unacceptable toxicity or compromised chemotherapy delivery.

Overall, current data suggests that the addition of venetoclax to standard chemo-immunotherapy regimens in aggressive B-cell lymphomas has the potential to improve outcomes for some patients, but likely at the expense of increased neutropenia and infectious complications (summarized Table 12.3). Evaluation of this strategy in randomized trials is clearly needed, as are biomarkers of BCL2 dependence, which will ideally enable identification of patients most likely to benefit (Punnoose et al. 2021). Progress in the biological subtyping of

DLBCL by molecular profiling may also identify patients whose disease is most vulnerable to BCL2 inhibition, and warrants dedicated study in future clinical trials (Schmitz et al. 2018).

Richter Transformation

In contrast to CLL/SLL, evidence to inform use of venetoclax to treat Richter transformation (RT) is scarce. Seven patients with DLBCL-type RT received venetoclax monotherapy in the first-in-human phase 1 study, three of whom achieved a partial response (PR) (Davids et al. 2017). Preliminary data is available from a phase 2 study in which 26 patients received a cycle of dose-adjusted-R-EPOCH, followed by accelerated inpatient venetoclax ramp-up and subsequently venetoclax 400 mg daily on D1-10 of the remaining five R-EPOCH cycles. Patients achieving objective disease response were planned to proceed to alloSCT, chimeric antigen receptor T-cell (CAR-T) therapy, or venetoclax 400 mg daily maintenance. The ORR was 62% and CRR was 50%, with a median PFS and OS of 10 and 20 months, respectively. Of the 18 candidates for cellular therapy, nine (50%) have proceeded to alloSCT or CAR-T (Davids et al. 2021b). Consistent with other trials combining venetoclax with intensive chemotherapy, hematologic toxicity and frequent febrile neutropenia (38%) were reported, with no instances of TLS. Given the dismal historical outcomes of patients with RT (Langerbeins et al. 2014; Rogers et al. 2018), these results are highly promising. Although longer term follow-up and evaluation in randomized studies are awaited, this preliminary evidence of efficacy may offset the increase toxicity profile in this high-risk patient population for whom improved therapies are desperately needed.

Waldenstrom's Macroglobulinemia

Gene expression analyses have identified that BCL2 is frequently upregulated in Waldenstrom's macroglobulinemia, with a transcriptional profile more closely resembling CLL than multiple myeloma (Chng et al. 2006; Hunter et al. 2016). Consistent with this preclinical evidence of a pathobiological role of BCL2, all four patients with Waldenstrom's macroglobulinemia who received venetoclax in the phase 1 study in patients with B-NHL attained a PR, with a median PFS and DOR 30 and 25 months, respectively (Davids et al. 2021a, 2017). In a phase 2 study of venetoclax monotherapy 800 mg daily for two years in 32 patients with RR Waldenstrom's macroglobulinemia (median two prior lines of therapy; 50% BTKi-exposed; *CXCR4* mutations 53%), the ORR was 84% with a major response rate of 81% and median PFS of 30 months. The major toxicity was neutropenia (44% grade 3/4) (Castillo et al. 2021). These results suggest significant clinical activity in Waldenstrom's macroglobulinemia, and trials investigating venetoclax combination with other targeted agents are currently active (NCT04840602).

Marginal Zone Lymphoma

Data specifically pertaining to patients with marginal zone lymphoma (MZL) is limited. Among the three patients who received venetoclax in the phase 1 study in B-NHL, two PRs were observed, with a median PFS and DOR of 21 and 20 months, respectively (Davids et al. 2017, 2021a). Six patients with RR MZL received venetoclax–BR in the phase 1b study, achieving an ORR of 100% and CRR of 50%. The median PFS and DOR were 12 and 10 months, respectively (De Vos et al. 2018). As seen with other therapeutic advances, dedicated analyses of this indolent subtype are made difficult by their relatively rarity and insights are largely extrapolated from broader cohorts of B-cell malignancies (Broccoli and Zinzani 2020).

Acute Lymphoblastic Leukemia/Lymphoma

Based on preclinical evidence of dependence on BCL2 and BCL-X_L (Alford et al. 2015; Del Gaizo Moore et al. 2008; Khaw et al. 2016), several small series have investigated the use of BH3-mimetics in acute lymphoblastic leukemia/lymphoma (ALL). In an early report of a phase 1 study of 18 predominantly older adults with Philadelphia chromosome negative ALL (56% treatment naive), escalating doses of venetoclax (400–600 mg daily) were added to mini-hyper-CVD/MA (cyclophosphamide, vincristine, dexamethasone, alternating with cycles of methotrexate and cytarabine) followed by alloSCT or venetoclax plus POMP (6-mercaptopurine, vincristine, methotrexate, and prednisolone) maintenance. The most common grade 3/4 AE was febrile neutropenia (39%). Among the 10 patients with treatment-naive ALL, the ORR/CRR was 100%/90%, with uMRD by flow cytometry in all instances of CR. Six patients proceed to alloSCT with no disease relapse over a median follow-up of 11 months. Among the eight patients with R/R disease, 38% achieved a CR and 25% attained uMRD, with two ongoing responses up to ~4 months. In a retrospective analysis of patients with R/R T-ALL, 13 patients received venetoclax with chemotherapy and 60% of evaluable patients achieved a morphological CR, although the median OS was short (eight months) (Richard-Carpentier et al. 2020). In the largest published study to date, 47 pediatric and adult patients with R/R ALL (40% T-cell ALL) received escalating doses of navitoclax (25–100 mg daily) in combination with venetoclax 400 mg daily and chemotherapy/asparaginase. Complete responses were achieved in 60% of patients, with comparable results across B-cell, T-cell, adult and pediatric subgroups. BM uMRD was attained in 34% of patients, and 28% of subjects proceeded to alloSCT or CAR-T therapy. Grade 3/4 toxicities were predominantly hematological, including febrile neutropenia in 47% of patients. Correlative BH3 profiling confirmed frequent BCL2 and BCL-X_L dependency in ALL cells, and the capacity for dependency switching during treatment as a potential mechanism of resistance to BCL2 inhibition (Pullarkat et al. 2021).

Overall, these data suggest that BH3-mimetics have activity in ALL and achieve deep responses that facilitate progression to cellular therapies in the R/R setting. These are particularly important in the context of T-ALL, where effective therapeutic options are limited for patients with R/R disease (McMahon and Luger 2019), and for older patients, for whom currently modalities are frequently unacceptably toxic or do not achieve durable control (Sawalha and Advani 2018).

Lessons from Venetoclax in Lymphoid Neoplasms Other than CLL/SLL

Venetoclax has single-agent activity in a broad range of lymphoid neoplasms, with MCL and Waldenstrom's macroglobulinemia demonstrating the greatest intrinsic sensitivity to BCL2 inhibition. In these two diseases, combination regimens with anti-CD20 monoclonal antibodies or other targeted agents are likely to be potent, and may challenge current standard of care regimens in the near future (e.g. NCT03112174, NCT04273139, and NCT03523975). In FL and DLBCL, responses are less consistent; however, subsets of patients can achieve deep and durable remissions. Further research to prospectively identify patients with sensitive disease may improve the clinical utility of BH3-mimetics in these diseases. The addition of venetoclax to conventional chemotherapy results in synergistic myelosuppression, which may be attenuated through abbreviated courses of venetoclax instead of continuous dosing. Despite added toxicity, preliminary data suggests that the addition of venetoclax to conventional chemotherapy may improve response rates among high-risk neoplasms with historically poor outcomes, such as RT, DHL, and high-risk ALL. However, this may also be associated with increased toxicity, and potentially even increased early deaths as shown with the intensive R-EPOCH backbone (Abramson et al. 2021). Randomized data in DLBCL is required to confirm the preliminary evidence of improved outcomes with venetoclax-R-CHOP observed in the CAVALLI study.

Associations and Mechanisms of Resistance to Pro-apoptotic Agents

Our current understanding of the mechanisms of resistance to BH3-mimetics is predominantly derived from cohorts of patients with heavily pre-treated R/R CLL receiving continuous venetoclax monotherapy. While critical insights have been made, their relevance to patients receiving frontline fixed-duration combination regimens is uncertain, as are their implications for other disease types. In the context of indefinite venetoclax monotherapy for R/R CLL, the clinico-pathological factors associated with inferior PFS on multivariate analysis include disease bulk (≥5 cm), BCRi or fludarabine refractoriness, *TP53* aberrations, and *NOTCH1* mutations (Roberts et al. 2019). Among patients who received venetoclax–rituximab for R/R CLL in the MURANO study, high genomic complexity was associated with inferior PFS, and lower uMRD rates were observed among patients with disease harboring *TP53*, *NOTCH1*, *BRAF*, and *BIRC3* mutations (Kater et al. 2020b). Furthermore, among patients who attained uMRD, del(17p), genomic complexity or IGHV unmutated status was associated accelerated MRD recrudescence and shorter time to PD (Kater et al. 2020a). On multivariate analysis of the venetoclax–obinutuzumab cohort of CLL14, only del(17p) was associated with inferior PFS (Tausch et al. 2020). Overall, although patients with traditional risk factors benefit most from the use of venetoclax-based regimens instead of chemo-immunotherapy, they nevertheless retain an adverse prognosis, especially those with *TP53* aberrant disease. Consistent with these clinical observations, *in vitro* experiments suggest that although venetoclax is active against p53 perturbed CLL (Anderson et al. 2016), these lesions facilitate survival and the evolution of resistance with prolonged sublethal exposure to BCL2 inhibitors (Thijssen et al. 2021).

The best characterized biological mechanisms of venetoclax resistance in CLL/SLL are acquisition of *BCL2* resistance mutations and upregulation of alternative pro-survival proteins such as BCL-X_L and MCL-1. Expansion of clones with genomic instability and other genetic mutations have been described among patients with early progression and RT on venetoclax, although their precise role in resistant disease biology requires further study (Guieze et al. 2019; Herling et al. 2018). The first described *BCL2* mutation, Gly101Val, was detected among patients with prolonged venetoclax exposure (median 36 months) and impairs venetoclax binding to the alpha-helical groove of BCL2 without compromising its affinity for BH3-only proteins (Blombery et al. 2019a). Several *BCL2* resistance mutations have now been identified, including in patients with FL and MCL, and have not been detected in pre-treatment samples (Blombery et al. 2019b, 2020; Lucas et al. 2020; Tausch et al. 2019; Thompson et al. 2020a). Interestingly, distinct mutations frequently co-occur within individuals and are present in a highly variable proportion of any single patient's CLL cell population (<1 to 83%), implying that multiple resistance mechanisms likely co-exist within the leukemic population (Blombery et al. 2020). Supporting this hypothesis, distinct subclones with wild-type *BCL2* but overexpression of BCL-X_L and MCL-1 have been found to co-exist separately alongside *BCL2*-mutated populations within individual patients (Blombery et al. 2019a, 2020). Alternative pro-survival proteins may also be upregulated by the lymph node microenvironment to confer resistance, and *in vitro* evidence suggests BCRis may disrupt this mechanism (Thijssen et al. 2015). Upregulation of BCL-X_L has also been implicated in resistance to venetoclax–ibrutinib therapy for MCL, where chromosome 9p21.1–p24.3 loss and/or mutations in components of the SWI–SNF chromatin-remodeling complex were identified in all patients with primary resistance and two-thirds of patients with relapsed disease. The consequence of these abnormalities was upregulation of BCL-X_L transcription, and concomitant BCL-X_L inhibition restored cytotoxicity (Agarwal et al. 2019). Other described resistance mechanisms in patients with CLL/SLL include chromosome 1q23 amplification and overexpression of MCL-1, with associated changes to mitochondrial metabolism (Guieze et al. 2019). Among eight patients with early PD and frequent RT, whole-exome sequencing of identified recurrent mutations in *BTG1* and homozygous deletions of *CDKN2A/B*, *PD-L1* amplification in one case, and a *BRAF* mutation postulated to augment MCL-1 expression (Herling et al. 2018). Emergence of *TP53* aberrations or cytogenetically complex disease has been frequently observed in patients with PD on venetoclax, further implicating genomic instability in the development of resistance (Anderson et al. 2017; Lin et al. 2020). As previously discussed, primary venetoclax resistance due to defects in other components of the intrinsic death pathway is frequently detectable in primary DLBCL cells, and upregulation of MCL-1 is associated with *in vitro* resistance in primary indolent B-NHL cells (Rys et al. 2021).

Overall, among patients receiving indefinite venetoclax monotherapy for CLL/SLL, resistant disease is typically oligoclonal, with multiple co-existing mechanisms including *BCL2* mutations and upregulation of alternative BCL2-family proteins. Mechanisms may differ among patients with early PD, where expansion of clones with genomic instability is frequently observed. Although resistance mechanisms outside of CLL are less well understood, parallel observations in FL and MCL have been reported (Figure 12.1). These observations support the use of time-limited combination regimens which may remove the sustained selection pressure for *BCL2*-mutated subclones, and indeed, no *BCL2* mutations have been detected among patients treated with time-limited therapy to date. Concomitant BTK inhibition may subvert the upregulation of alternative BCL2-family proteins by the tumor microenvironment, and combination trials have demonstrated frequent deep remission in CLL and MCL (Jain et al. 2019; Portell et al. 2021; Tam et al. 2018; Wierda et al. 2020). Further investigation is ongoing into the clinical development of BCL-X_L and MCL-1 inhibitors to eradicate venetoclax-resistant subpopulations and hopefully enhance the curative potential of BH3-mimetic-based regimens (Roberts et al. 2021).

Must Read References

Roberts, A.W., Wei, A.H., and Huang D.C.S. (2021 September 30). BCL2 and MCL1 inhibitors for hematologic malignancies. *Blood* 138 (13): 1120–1136.

Lew, T.E., Anderson, M.A., and Seymour, J.F. (2020 May 23). Promises and pitfalls of targeted agents in chronic lymphocytic leukemia. *Cancer Drug Resist.* 3 (3): 415–444.

Davids, M.S., Roberts, A.W., Kenkre, V.P. et al. (2021). Long-term follow-up of patients with relapsed or refractory non-Hodgkin lymphoma treated with venetoclax in a phase I, first-in-human study. *Clin. Cancer Res.* 27 (17): 4690–5.

Roberts, A.W., Davids, M.S., Pagel, J.M. et al. (2016). Targeting BCL2 with venetoclax in relapsed chronic lymphocytic leukemia. *N. Engl. J. Med.* 374 (4): 311–322.

Fischer, K., Al-Sawaf, O., Bahlo, J. et al. (2019). Venetoclax and obinutuzumab in patients with CLL and coexisting conditions. *N. Engl. J. Med* 380 (23): 2225–2236.

Seymour, J.F., Kipps, T.J., Eichhorst, B. et al. (2018). Venetoclax-rituximab in relapsed or refractory chronic lymphocytic leukemia. *N. Engl. J. Med.* 378 (12): 1107–20.

References

Abbvie. (2016). Venclexta (Venetoclax) tablets full prescribing information.

Abramson, J.S., Ruppert, A.S., Giri, S. et al. (2021). Randomized phase II/III study of DA-EPOCH-R ± venetoclax in previously untreated double hit lymphoma: initial results from Alliance A051701. *Blood* 138 (Suppl1): 523 (Abstract).

Agarwal, R., Chan, Y.C., Tam, C.S. et al. (2019). Dynamic molecular monitoring reveals that SWI-SNF mutations mediate resistance to ibrutinib plus venetoclax in mantle cell lymphoma. *Nat. Med.* 25: 119–129.

Ailawadhi, S., Chanan-khan, A.A.A., Chen, Z. et al. (2021). First-in-human study of lisaftoclax (APG-2575), a novel BCL-2 inhibitor (BCL-2i), in patients (pts) with relapsed/refractory (R/R) CLL and other hematologic malignancies (HMs). *J. Clin. Oncol.* 39: 7502-7502.

Alford, S.E., Kothari, A., Loeff, F.C. et al. (2015). BH3 inhibitor sensitivity and Bcl-2 dependence in primary acute lymphoblastic leukemia cells. *Cancer Res.* 75: 1366–1375.

Al-sawaf, O., Zhang, C., Tandon, M. et al. (2020). Venetoclax plus obinutuzumab versus chlorambucil plus obinutuzumab for previously untreated chronic lymphocytic leukaemia (CLL14): follow-up results from a multicentre, open-label, randomised, phase 3 trial. *Lancet Oncol.* 21: 1188–1200.

Anderson, M.A., Deng, J., Seymour, J.F. et al. (2016). The BCL2 selective inhibitor venetoclax induces rapid onset apoptosis of CLL cells in patients via a TP53-independent mechanism. *Blood* 127: 3215–3224.

Anderson, M.A., Tam, C., Lew, T.E. et al. (2017). Clinicopathological features and outcomes of progression of CLL on the BCL2 inhibitor venetoclax. *Blood* 129: 3362–3370.

Balachander, S.B., Criscione, S.W., Byth, K.F. et al. (2020). AZD4320, A dual inhibitor of Bcl-2 and Bcl-x(L), induces tumor regression in hematologic cancer models without dose-limiting thrombocytopenia. *Clin. Cancer Res.* 26: 6535–6549.

Blombery, P., Anderson, M.A., Gong, J.N. et al. (2019a). Acquisition of the recurrent Gly101Val mutation in BCL2 confers resistance to venetoclax in patients with progressive chronic lymphocytic leukemia. *Cancer Discov.* 9: 342–353.

Blombery, P., Birkinshaw, R.W., Nguyen, T. et al. (2019b). Characterization of a novel venetoclax resistance mutation

(BCL2 Phe104Ile) observed in follicular lymphoma. *Br. J. Haematol.* 186: e188–e191.

Blombery, P., Lew, T.E., Dengler, M.A. et al. (2021). Clonal hematopoiesis, myeloid disorders and BAX-mutated myelopoiesis in patients receiving venetoclax for CLL. *Blood.* epub ahead of print.

Blombery, P., Thompson, E.R., Nguyen, T. et al. (2020). Multiple BCL2 mutations cooccurring with Gly101Val emerge in chronic lymphocytic leukemia progression on venetoclax. *Blood* 135: 773–777.

Broccoli, A. and Zinzani, P.L. (2020). How do we sequence therapy for marginal zone lymphomas? *Hematology* 2020: 295–305.

Byrd, J.C., Furman, R.R., Coutre, S.E. et al. (2013). Targeting BTK with ibrutinib in relapsed chronic lymphocytic leukemia. *N. Engl. J. Med.* 369: 32–42.

Castillo, J.J., Allan, J.N., Siddiqi, T. et al. (2021). Venetoclax in previously treated waldenström macroglobulinemia. *J. Clin. Oncol.* epub ahead of print.

Cheah, C., Verner, E., Tam, C. et al. (2021). Preliminary safety data from patients with relapsed/refractory B-cell malignancies treated with the novel B-cell lymphoma (BCL2) inhibitor BGB-11417. *Hematol. Oncol.* 39.

Chng, W.J., Schop, R.F., Price-Troska, T. et al. (2006). Gene-expression profiling of Waldenstrom macroglobulinemia reveals a phenotype more similar to chronic lymphocytic leukemia than multiple myeloma. *Blood* 108: 2755–2763.

Cochrane, T., Enrico, A., Gomez-Almaguer, D. et al. (2021). Impact of venetoclax monotherapy on the quality of life of patients with relapsed or refractory chronic lymphocytic leukemia: results from the phase 3b VENICE II trial. *Leuk. Lymphoma* epub ahead of print.

Cory, S. and Adams, J.M. (2002). The Bcl2 family: regulators of the cellular life-or-death switch. *Nat. Rev. Cancer* 2: 647–656.

Coutre, S., Choi, M., Furman, R.R. et al. (2018). Venetoclax for patients with chronic lymphocytic leukemia who progressed during or after idelalisib therapy. *Blood* 131: 1704–1711.

Cramer, P., Von Tresckow, J., Bahlo, J. et al. (2018). Bendamustine followed by obinutuzumab and venetoclax in chronic lymphocytic leukaemia (CLL2-BAG): primary endpoint analysis of a multicentre, open-label, phase 2 trial. *Lancet Oncol.* 19: 1215–1228.

Davids, M.S., Hallek, M., Wierda, W. et al. (2018a). Comprehensive safety analysis of venetoclax monotherapy for patients with relapsed/refractory chronic lymphocytic leukemia. *Clin. Cancer Res.* 24: 4371–4379.

Davids, M.S., Roberts, A.W., Kenkre, V.P. et al. (2021a). Long-term follow-up of patients with relapsed or refractory non-Hodgkin lymphoma treated with venetoclax in a phase I, first-in-human study. *Clin. Cancer Res.* 27: 4690–4695.

Davids, M.S., Roberts, A.W., Seymour, J.F. et al. (2017). Phase I first-in-human study of venetoclax in patients with relapsed or refractory non-Hodgkin lymphoma. *J. Clin. Oncol.* 35: 826–833.

Davids, M.S., Rogers, K.A., Tyekucheva, S., PH.D. et al. (2021b). Venetoclax plus dose-adjusted R-EPOCH (VR-EPOCH) for Richter's syndrome. *Blood.* Epub ahead of print.

Davids, M.S., Von Keudell, G., Portell, C.A. et al. (2018b). Revised dose ramp-up to mitigate the risk of tumor lysis syndrome when initiating venetoclax in patients with mantle cell lymphoma. *J. Clin. Oncol.* 36 (35): 3525–3527.

De Vos, S., Leonard, J.P., Friedberg, J.W. et al. (2021). Safety and efficacy of navitoclax, a BCL-2 and BCL-X(L) inhibitor, in patients with relapsed or refractory lymphoid malignancies: results from a phase 2a study. *Leuk. Lymphoma* 62: 810–818.

De Vos, S., Swinnen, L.J., Wang, D. et al. (2018). Venetoclax, bendamustine, and rituximab in patients with relapsed or refractory NHL: a phase Ib dose-finding study. *Ann. Oncol.* 29: 1932–1938.

Del Gaizo Moore, V., Schlis, K.D., Sallan, S.E. et al. (2008). BCL-2 dependence and ABT-737 sensitivity in acute lymphoblastic leukemia. *Blood* 111: 2300–2309.

Delbridge, A.R., Grabow, S., Strasser, A. et al. (2016). Thirty years of BCL-2: translating cell death discoveries into novel cancer therapies. *Nat. Rev. Cancer* 16: 99–109.

Eyre, T.A., Walter, H.S., Iyengar, S. et al. (2019). Efficacy of venetoclax monotherapy in patients with relapsed, refractory mantle cell lymphoma after Bruton tyrosine kinase inhibitor therapy. *Haematologica* 104: e68–e71.

Fischer, K., Al-Sawaf, O., Bahlo, J. et al. (2019a). Venetoclax and obinutuzumab in patients with CLL and coexisting conditions. *N. Engl. J. Med.* 380: 2225–2236.

Fischer, K., Al-Sawaf, O., and Hallek, M. (2020). Preventing and monitoring for tumor lysis syndrome and other toxicities of venetoclax during treatment of chronic lymphocytic leukemia. *Hematol. Am. Soc. Hematol. Educ. Program.* 2020: 357–362.

Fischer, K., Ritgen, M., Al-Sawaf, O. et al. (2019b). Quantitative analysis of minimal residual disease (MRD) shows high rates of undetectable MRD after fixed-duration chemotherapy-free treatment and serves as surrogate marker for progression-free survival: a prospective analysis of the randomized CLL14 trial. *Blood* 134: 36-36.

Flinn, I.W., Gribben, J.G., Dyer, M.J.S. et al. (2019). Phase 1b study of venetoclax-obinutuzumab in previously untreated and relapsed/refractory chronic lymphocytic leukemia. *Blood* 133: 2765–2775.

Furman, R.R., Sharman, J.P., Coutre, S.E. et al. (2014). Idelalisib and rituximab in relapsed chronic lymphocytic leukemia. *N. Engl. J. Med.* 370: 997–1007.

Galteland, E., Sivertsen, E.A., Svendsrud, D.H. et al. (2005). Translocation t(14;18) and gain of chromosome 18/BCL2: effects on BCL2 expression and apoptosis in B-cell non-Hodgkin's lymphomas. *Leukemia* 19: 2313–2323.

Guieze, R., Liu, V.M., Rosebrock, D. et al. (2019). Mitochondrial reprogramming underlies resistance to BCL-2 inhibition in lymphoid malignancies. *Cancer Cell* 36: 369–384 e13.

Harrup, R.A., Owen, C., D'Rozario, J. et al. (2020). Efficacy of subsequent novel targeted therapies, including repeated venetoclax-rituximab (VenR), in patients (Pts) with relapsed/refractory chronic lymphocytic leukemia (R/R CLL) previously treated with fixed-duration venr in the murano study. *Blood* 136: 44–45.

Herling, C.D., Abedpour, N., Weiss, J. et al. (2018). Clonal dynamics towards the development of venetoclax resistance in chronic lymphocytic leukemia. *Nat. Commun.* 9: 727.

Hillmen, P., Rawstron, A.C., Brock, K. et al. (2019). Ibrutinib plus venetoclax in relapsed/refractory chronic lymphocytic leukemia: the CLARITY study. *J. Clin. Oncol.* 37: 2722–2729.

Hunter, Z.R., Xu, L., Yang, G. et al. (2016). Transcriptome sequencing reveals a profile that corresponds to genomic variants in Waldenström macroglobulinemia. *Blood* 128: 827–838.

Hwang, J.J., Kuruvilla, J., Mendelson, D. et al. (2010). Phase I dose finding studies of obatoclax (GX15-070), a small molecule pan-BCL-2 family antagonist, in patients with advanced solid tumors or lymphoma. *Clin. Cancer Res.* 16: 4038–4045.

Jain, N., Keating, M., Thompson, P. et al. (2019). Ibrutinib and venetoclax for first-line treatment of CLL. *N. Engl. J. Med.* 380: 2095–2103.

Jones, J.A., Mato, A.R., Wierda, W.G. et al. (2018). Venetoclax for chronic lymphocytic leukaemia progressing after ibrutinib: an interim analysis of a multicentre, open-label, phase 2 trial. *Lancet Oncol.* 19: 65–75.

Kala, S.G. and Chinni, S. (2021). Development and characterization of venetoclax nanocrystals for oral bioavailability enhancement. *AAPS PharmSciTech* 22: 92.

Kang, M.H. and Reynolds, C.P. (2009). Bcl-2 inhibitors: targeting mitochondrial apoptotic pathways in cancer therapy. *Clin. Cancer Res.* 15: 1126–1132.

Kater, A.P., Kipps, T.J., Eichhorst, B. et al. (2020a). Five-year analysis of murano study demonstrates enduring undetectable minimal residual disease (uMRD) in a subset of relapsed/refractory chronic lymphocytic leukemia (R/R CLL) patients (Pts) following fixed-duration venetoclax-rituximab (VenR) therapy (Tx). *Blood* 136: 19–21.

Kater, A.P., Seymour, J.F., Hillmen, P. et al. (2019). Fixed duration of venetoclax-rituximab in relapsed/refractory chronic lymphocytic leukemia eradicates minimal residual disease and prolongs survival: post-treatment follow-up of the MURANO phase III study. *J. Clin. Oncol.* 37: 269–277.

Kater, A.P., Wu, J.Q., Kipps, T. et al. (2020b). Venetoclax plus rituximab in relapsed chronic lymphocytic leukemia: 4-year results and evaluation of impact of genomic complexity and gene mutations from the MURANO phase III study. *J. Clin. Oncol.* 38 (34): 4042–4054.

Khaw, S.L., Suryani, S., Evans, K. et al. (2016). Venetoclax responses of pediatric ALL xenografts reveal sensitivity of MLL-rearranged leukemia. *Blood* 128: 1382–1395.

Kipps, T.J., Eradat, H., Grosicki, S. et al. (2015). A phase 2 study of the BH3 mimetic BCL2 inhibitor navitoclax (ABT-263) with or without rituximab, in previously untreated B-cell chronic lymphocytic leukemia. *Leuk. Lymphoma* 56: 2826–2833.

Langerbeins, P., Busch, R., Anheier, N. et al. (2014). Poor efficacy and tolerability of R-CHOP in relapsed/refractory chronic lymphocytic leukemia and Richter transformation. *Am. J. Hematol.* 89: E239–43.

Leverson, J.D., Phillips, D.C., Mitten, M.J. et al. (2015). Exploiting selective BCL-2 family inhibitors to dissect cell survival dependencies and define improved strategies for cancer therapy. *Sci. Transl. Med.* 7: 279ra40.

Lew, T.E., Anderson, M.A., Lin, V.S. et al. (2020). Undetectable peripheral blood MRD should be the goal of venetoclax in CLL, but attainment plateaus after 24 months. *Blood Adv.* 4: 165–173.

Li, Y., Bouchlaka, M.N., Wolff, J. et al. (2016). FBXO10 deficiency and BTK activation upregulate BCL2 expression in mantle cell lymphoma. *Oncogene* 35: 6223–6234.

Lin, V.S., Lew, T.E., Handunnetti, S.M. et al. (2020). BTK inhibitor therapy is effective in patients with CLL resistant to venetoclax. *Blood* 135 (25): 2266–2270.

Lucas, F., Larkin, K., Gregory, C.T. et al. (2020). Novel BCL2 mutations in venetoclax-resistant, ibrutinib-resistant CLL patients with BTK/PLCG2 mutations. *Blood* 135: 2192–2195.

Ma, S., Seymour, J.F., Brander, D.M. et al. (2021). Efficacy of venetoclax plus rituximab for relapsed CLL: 5-year follow-up of continuous or limited- duration therapy. *Blood* 138: 836–846.

Marcus, R., Davies, A., Ando, K. et al. (2017). Obinutuzumab for the first-line treatment of follicular lymphoma. *N. Engl. J. Med.* 377: 1331–1344.

Mason, K.D., Carpinelli, M.R., Fletcher, J.I. et al. (2007). Programmed anuclear cell death delimits platelet life span. *Cell* 128: 1173–1186.

Mato, A.R., Sharman, J.P., Biondo, J.M.L. et al. (2020). The impact of early discontinuation/dose modification of venetoclax on outcomes in patients with relapsed/refractory chronic lymphocytic leukemia: post-hoc analyses from the phase III MURANO study. *Haematologica*. Online ahead of print.

McMahon, C.M. and Luger, S.M. (2019). Relapsed T cell ALL: current approaches and new directions. *Curr. Hematol. Malig. Rep.* 14: 83–93.

Merino, D., Kelly, G.L., Lessene, G. et al. (2018). BH3-mimetic drugs: blazing the trail for new cancer medicines. *Cancer Cell* 34: 879–891.

Morschhauser, F., Feugier, P., Flinn, I.W. et al. (2021). A phase 2 study of venetoclax plus R-CHOP as first-line treatment for patients with diffuse large B-cell lymphoma. *Blood* 137: 600–609.

Morschhauser, F., Fowler, N.H., Feugier, P. et al. (2018). Rituximab plus lenalidomide in advanced untreated follicular lymphoma. *N. Engl. J. Med.* 379: 934–947.

O'Brien, S., Moore, J.O., Boyd, T.E. et al. (2009a). 5-year survival in patients with relapsed or refractory chronic lymphocytic leukemia in a randomized, phase III trial of fludarabine plus cyclophosphamide with or without oblimersen. *J. Clin. Oncol.* 27: 5208–5212.

O'Brien, S.M., Claxton, D.F., Crump, M. et al. (2009b). Phase I study of obatoclax mesylate (GX15-070), a small molecule pan-Bcl-2 family antagonist, in patients with advanced chronic lymphocytic leukemia. *Blood* 113: 299–305.

O'Brien, S.M., Cunningham, C.C., Golenkov, A.K. et al. (2005). Phase I to II multicenter study of oblimersen sodium, a Bcl-2 antisense oligonucleotide, in patients with advanced chronic lymphocytic leukemia. *J. Clin. Oncol.* 23: 7697–7702.

Oki, Y., Noorani, M., Lin, P. et al. (2014). Double hit lymphoma: the MD Anderson Cancer Center clinical experience. *Br. J. Haematol.* 166: 891–901.

Portell, C.A., Wages, N.A., Kahl, B.S. et al. (2021). Dose finding study of ibrutinib and venetoclax in relapsed or refractory mantle cell lymphoma. *Blood Adv.*epub ahead of print.

Pro, B., Leber, B., Smith, M. et al. (2008). Phase II multicenter study of oblimersen sodium, a Bcl-2 antisense oligonucleotide, in combination with rituximab in patients with recurrent B-cell non-Hodgkin lymphoma. *Br. J. Haematol.* 143: 355–360.

Pullarkat, V.A., Lacayo, N.J., Jabbour, E. et al. (2021). Venetoclax and navitoclax in combination with chemotherapy in patients with relapsed or refractory acute lymphoblastic leukemia and lymphoblastic lymphoma. *Cancer Discov.* 11: 1440–1453.

Punnoose, E., Peale, F.V., Szafer-Glusman, E. et al. (2021). BCL2 expression in first-line diffuse large B-cell lymphoma identifies a patient population with poor prognosis. *Clin. Lymphoma Myeloma Leuk.* 21: 267–278.e10.

Richard-Carpentier, G., Jabbour, E., Short, N.J. et al. (2020). Clinical experience with venetoclax combined with chemotherapy for relapsed or refractory T-cell acute lymphoblastic leukemia. *Clin. Lymphoma Myeloma Leuk.* 20: 212–218.

Roberts, A.W., Advani, R.H., Kahl, B.S. et al. (2015). Phase 1 study of the safety, pharmacokinetics, and antitumour activity of the BCL2 inhibitor navitoclax in combination with rituximab in patients with relapsed or refractory CD20+ lymphoid malignancies. *Br. J. Haematol.* 170: 669–678.

Roberts, A.W., Davids, M.S., Pagel, J.M. et al. (2016). Targeting BCL2 with venetoclax in relapsed chronic lymphocytic leukemia. *N. Engl. J. Med.* 374: 311–322.

Roberts, A.W., MA, S., Kipps, T.J. et al. (2019). Efficacy of venetoclax in relapsed chronic lymphocytic leukemia is influenced by disease and response variables. *Blood* 134: 111–122.

Roberts, A.W., Seymour, J.F., Brown, J.R. et al. (2012). Substantial susceptibility of chronic lymphocytic leukemia to BCL2 inhibition: results of a phase I study of navitoclax in patients with relapsed or refractory disease. *J. Clin. Oncol.* 30: 488–496.

Roberts, A.W., Wei, A.H., and Huang, D.C.S. (2021). BCL2 and MCL1 inhibitors for hematologic malignancies. *Blood* 138: 1120–1136.

Robertson, L.E., Plunkett, W., Mcconnell, K. et al. (1996). Bcl-2 expression in chronic lymphocytic leukemia and its correlation with the induction of apoptosis and clinical outcome. *Leukemia* 10: 456–459.

Rogers, K.A., Huang, Y., Ruppert, A.S. et al. (2018). A single-institution retrospective cohort study of first-line R-EPOCH chemoimmunotherapy for Richter syndrome demonstrating complex chronic lymphocytic leukaemia karyotype as an adverse prognostic factor. *Br. J. Haematol.* 180: 259–266.

Rutherford, S.C., Abramson, J.S., Bartlett, N.L. et al. (2021). Venetoclax with dose-adjusted EPOCH-R as initial therapy for patients with aggressive B-cell lymphoma: a single-arm, multicentre, phase 1 study. *Lancet Haematol.* 8 (11): e818–e827.

Rys, R.N., Wever, C.M., Geoffrion, D. et al. (2021). Apoptotic blocks in primary non-Hodgkin B cell lymphomas identified by BH3 profiling. *Cancers (Basel)* 13: 1002.

Salem, A.H., Tao, Z.F., Bueno, O.F. et al. (2021). Expanding the repertoire for "large small molecules": prodrug ABBV-167 efficiently converts to venetoclax with reduced food effect in healthy volunteers. *Mol. Cancer Ther.* 20: 999–1008.

Sawalha, Y. and Advani, A.S. (2018). Management of older adults with acute lymphoblastic leukemia: challenges & current approaches. *Int. J. Hematol. Oncol.* 7: Ijh02.

Sawalha, Y., Goyal, S., Switchenko, J.M. et al. (2020). Outcomes of patients with relapsed mantle cell lymphoma treated with venetoclax: a multicenter retrospective analysis. *Blood* 136: 4–6.

Schmitz, R., Wright, G.W., Huang, D.W. et al. (2018). Genetics and pathogenesis of diffuse large B-cell lymphoma. *N. Engl. J. Med.* 378: 1396–1407.

Sehn, L.H., Martelli, M., Trněný, M. et al. (2020). A randomized, open-label, Phase III study of obinutuzumab or rituximab plus CHOP in patients with previously untreated diffuse large B-Cell lymphoma: final analysis of GOYA. *J. Hematol. Oncol.* 13: 71.

Seymour, J.F., Kipps, T.J., Eichhorst, B. et al. (2018). Venetoclax-rituximab in relapsed or refractory chronic lymphocytic leukemia. *N. Engl. J. Med.* 378: 1107–1120.

Seymour, J.F., Ma, S., Brander, D.M. et al. (2017). Venetoclax plus rituximab in relapsed or refractory chronic lymphocytic leukaemia: a phase 1b study. *Lancet Oncol.* 18: 230–240.

Shanafelt, T.D., Wang, X.V., Kay, N.E. et al. (2019). Ibrutinib-rituximab or chemoimmunotherapy for chronic lymphocytic leukemia. *N. Engl. J. Med.* 381: 432–443.

Souers, A.J., Leverson, J.D., Boghaert, E.R. et al. (2013). ABT-199, a potent and selective BCL-2 inhibitor, achieves antitumor activity while sparing platelets. *Nat. Med.* 19: 202–208.

Spencer, A., Rosenberg, A.S., Jakubowiak, A. et al. (2019). A phase 1, first-in-human study of AMG 176, a selective MCL-1 inhibitor, in patients with relapsed or refractory multiple myeloma. *Clin. Lymphoma Myeloma Leuk.* 19: e53–e54.

Stathis, A., Mey, U., Schär, S. et al. (2019). SAKK 35/15: a phase I trial of obinutuzumab in combination with venetoclax in previously untreated follicular lymphoma patients. *Hematol. Oncol.* 37: 118–119.

Stilgenbauer, S., Eichhorst, B., Schetelig, J. et al. (2016). Venetoclax in relapsed or refractory chronic lymphocytic leukaemia with 17p deletion: a multicentre, open-label, phase 2 study. *Lancet Oncol.* 17: 768–778.

Stilgenbauer, S., Eichhorst, B., Schetelig, J. et al. (2018). Venetoclax for patients with chronic lymphocytic leukemia with 17p deletion: results from the full population of a phase II pivotal trial. *J. Clin. Oncol.* 36: 1973–1980.

Strati, P., Keating, M.J., O'Brien, S.M. et al. (2014). Outcomes of first-line treatment for chronic lymphocytic leukemia with 17p deletion. *Haematologica* 99: 1350–1355.

Tam, C.S., Anderson, M.A., Pott, C. et al. (2018). Ibrutinib plus venetoclax for the treatment of mantle-cell lymphoma. *N. Engl. J. Med.* 378: 1211–1223.

Tausch, E., Close, W., Dolnik, A. et al. (2019). Venetoclax resistance and acquired BCL2 mutations in chronic lymphocytic leukemia. *Haematologica* 104: e434–e437.

Tausch, E., Schneider, C., Robrecht, S. et al. (2020). Prognostic and predictive impact of genetic markers in patients with CLL treated with obinutuzumab and venetoclax. *Blood* 135: 2402–2412.

Thijssen, R., Diepstraten, S.T., Moujalled, D. et al. (2021). Intact TP-53 function is essential for sustaining durable responses to BH3-mimetic drugs in leukemias. *Blood* 137: 2721–2735.

Thijssen, R., Slinger, E., Weller, K. et al. (2015). Resistance to ABT-199 induced by microenvironmental signals in chronic lymphocytic leukemia can be counteracted by CD20 antibodies or kinase inhibitors. *Haematologica* 100: e302.

Thompson, E.R., Nguyen, T., Kankanige, Y. et al. (2020a). High clonal complexity of resistance mechanisms occurring at progression after single-agent targeted therapy strategies in chronic lymphocytic leukemia. *Blood* 136: 15–16.

Thompson, M.C., Allan, J.N., Sail, K. et al. (2020b). Venetoclax re-treatment of chronic lymphocytic leukemia (CLL) patients after a previous venetoclax-based regimen. *Blood* 136: 39–41.

Thompson, P.A., Tam, C.S., O'Brien, S.M. et al. (2016). Fludarabine, cyclophosphamide, and rituximab treatment achieves long-term disease-free survival in IGHV-mutated chronic lymphocytic leukemia. *Blood* 127: 303–309.

Touzeau, C., Dousset, C., Bodet, L. et al. (2011). ABT-737 induces apoptosis in mantle cell lymphoma cells with a Bcl-2high/Mcl-1low profile and synergizes with other antineoplastic agents. *Clin. Cancer Res.* 17: 5973–5981.

Vaux, D.L., Cory, S., and Adams, J.M. (1988). Bcl-2 gene promotes haemopoietic cell survival and cooperates with c-myc to immortalize pre-B cells. *Nature* 335: 440–442.

Wierda, W.G., TAM, C.S., Allan, J.N. et al. (2020). Ibrutinib (Ibr) plus venetoclax (Ven) for first-line treatment of chronic lymphocytic leukemia (CLL)/small lymphocytic lymphoma (SLL): 1-year disease-free survival (DFS) results from the MRD cohort of the phase 2 CAPTIVATE study. *Blood* 136: 16–17.

Wilson, W.H., O'Connor, O.A., Czuczman, M.S. et al. (2010). Navitoclax, a targeted high-affinity inhibitor of BCL-2, in lymphoid malignancies: a phase 1 dose-escalation study of safety, pharmacokinetics, pharmacodynamics, and antitumour activity. *Lancet Oncol.* 11: 1149–1159.

Wu, J.Q., Seymour, J.F., Eichhorst, B. et al. (2021). Unfavourable genetics impact MRD response to venetoclax+rituximab retreatment in relapsed or refractory chronic lymphocytic leukemia: phase 3 MURANO substudy. *Haematol. Oncol.* 39.

Zelenetz, A.D., Salles, G., Mason, K.D. et al. (2019). Venetoclax plus R- or G-CHOP in non-Hodgkin lymphoma: results from the CAVALLI phase 1b trial. *Blood* 133: 1964–1976.

Zhao, S., Kanagal-Shamanna, R., Navsaria, L. et al. (2020). Efficacy of venetoclax in high risk relapsed mantle cell lymphoma (MCL) - outcomes and mutation profile from venetoclax resistant MCL patients. *Am. J. Hematol.* 95: 623–629.

Zinzani, P.L., Flinn, I.W., Yuen, S.L.S. et al. (2020). Venetoclax-rituximab with or without bendamustine vs bendamustine-rituximab in relapsed/refractory follicular lymphoma. *Blood* 136: 2628–2637.

13

Promising Combinations of Drugs Targeting Apoptosis

William G. Wierda

D.B. Lane Cancer Research Distinguished Professor of Medicine Section Head, CLL Department of Leukemia Division of Cancer Medicine Holcombe Blvd, Unit 428, Houston, TX, USA

Take Home Messages

- Dysregulation of apoptosis is fundamental to almost every type of malignant disease.
- Tumor cells have evolved elaborate mechanisms to circumnavigate cell death.
- Combinations of drugs that target both the direct mechanisms of apoptosis, as well as those redundant pathways favoring survival, offer the prospect of improving efficacy and deepening the complete response rate.

Introduction: Background and Disease Perspective

The monoclonal leukemic B-cells of patients with chronic lymphocytic leukemia (CLL) circulate in blood and lymphatics between microenvironments, including lymph nodes, liver and spleen, bone marrow, and secondary lymphoid tissue. These long-lived cells are in a dynamic interplay of proliferation and apoptosis, with the microenvironments providing critical support and signaling for CLL cell growth and survival. CLL cell turnover and longevity ultimately lead to accumulation of the cells and the typical pattern of progressive disease is rising lymphocyte count, enlarging lymph nodes liver and spleen and progressive cytopenias, secondary to crowding out of normal hematopoietic elements in the bone marrow.

Many critical surface and intracellular molecules participate in, and are responsible for, microenvironment interactions, proliferation, and resistance to physiological senescence-related apoptosis observed in this disease. The B-cell receptor (BCR) signaling pathway is one critical pathway for CLL pathophysiology, and protein members of this pathway have been targeted with small molecule inhibitors successfully for therapeutic intervention, particularly Bruton's tyrosine kinase (BTK) and phosphoinositide 3-kinase (PI3K). One mechanism of action for the inhibitors of BCR signaling is to disrupt and block the ability of CLL cells to interact with their microenvironment, resulting in release of CLL cells from these protective and stimulating niches. The era of targeted therapy for CLL was ushered in with development of the orally administered irreversible small molecule BTK inhibitor (BTKi), ibrutinib. Multiple phase 3 trials reported improved progression-free survival (PFS) with irreversible BTKi-based treatment comparing across the spectrum of patient age, comorbidities, and chemoimmunotherapy (CIT) intensity (Burger et al. 2020; Moreno et al. 2019; Shanafelt et al. 2019; Sharman et al. 2020; Woyach et al. 2018). BTKi-based treatment is highly effective at reducing the bulk of disease, especially in lymph nodes, and achieving disease control; deep remissions are uncommon, but can rarely occur with prolonged treatment, and treatment is typically continuous, until progression, which can be many years (Byrd et al. 2015; Coutre et al. 2017; O'Brien et al. 2014, 2018). Finally, BTKi-based treatments work by a p53-independent mechanism and are effective for biologically high-risk CLL, particularly del(17p) and mutated *TP53* CLL, where CIT is not recommended (Ahn et al. 2020; O'Brien et al. 2014; Stilgenbauer et al. 2018).

The malignant CLL cells commonly harbor characteristic chromosome aberrations; chromosome deletions are hallmark of the disease. The majority of patients have leukemia cells harboring deletion of a portion of the long arm of chromosome 13 [del(13q)]. Two important microRNA (miR) genes, miR15 and miR16, were identified in the critical minimal deleted region of del(13q) and were noted to be deleted or downregulated in more than two-thirds of all CLL

Precision Cancer Therapies: Targeting Oncogenic Drivers and Signaling Pathways in Lymphoid Malignancies: From Concept to Practice, Volume 1, First Edition. Edited by Owen A. O'Connor, Stephen M. Ansell, and John F. Seymour.

cases (Calin et al. 2002). MicroRNAs are non-translated small RNAs that function to regulate gene expression. Both miR15 and miR16 bind and downregulate *BCL2* transcript levels. The absence of miR15 and miR16 in cases with del(13q) leads to increased BCL2 expression (Cimmino et al. 2005) and resultant resistance to apoptosis. BCL2 is universally overexpressed by leukemia cells of patients with CLL.

Small molecule inhibitor blockade of BCL2 protein favors the stoichiometry of BCL2 family members toward pro-apoptosis, thus exposure of CLL cells to a small molecule inhibitor potently induces apoptosis, but not in normal hematopoietic cells. Lowering of the apoptotic threshold in CLL cells through inhibition of BCL2 also establishes an opportunity to synergize other therapeutic agents. Additionally, this mechanism of action is independent of p53, making it particularly appealing for patients with high-risk disease which lacks normal *TP53*, such as those with del(17p) and patients who have mutated *TP53*.

CLL is a chronic disease with heterogeneous clinical course and timeline between patients. No clinical trial has shown survival benefit with early treatment for CLL, including with targeted therapy, therefore, treatment is only initiated when patients develop active disease requiring treatment according to the standard International Working Group on CLL (iwCLL) criteria. Active CLL requiring treatment is manifest by progressive disease-related symptoms, such as fatigue, drenching night sweats, or unintentional weight loss; massively enlarged lymph nodes, liver or spleen; or progressive anemia or thrombocytopenia (Hallek et al. 2018). Patients who do not display active CLL can be monitored and observed, some for many years.

Historically, standard treatment for CLL consisted of CIT, with the intent of achieving disease remission, followed by a period of time off treatment for the duration of the remission. Deeper response, such as with complete remission (CR), was correlated with longer remission duration and PFS. Disease relapse ultimately was expected and retreatment initiated with evidence of active, progressive disease. Depth of response, further reflected by level of measurable residual disease (MRD) status in blood and bone marrow, is an important endpoint for CIT-based treatment and fixed-duration targeted therapy. Undetectable MRD (uMRD) measured at a level of 10^{-4} sensitivity (uMRD4) has been used as a treatment endpoint correlated with longer PFS, time-to-next treatment, and overall survival (OS) and certainly curative treatment could not be demonstrated without achieving uMRD status.

Clinical Development of BCL2 Inhibitors

BCL2 is a fundamental protein in the biochemistry and survival of CLL cells. Overexpression of BCL2 by CLL cells favors the biochemical stoichiometry toward survival and resistance to apoptosis. When BCL2 function is blocked in CLL cells, the cells undergo apoptosis and are eliminated by a p53-independent mechanism. *In vitro* treatment of CLL cells with navitoclax (ABT-263), the small molecule inhibitor of BCL2, BCL-w, and BCL-xL, potently induced cell death. A phase 1/2 trial of orally administered navitoclax was conducted and generated promising results. The majority of patients treated in the study had greater than 50% reduction in leukemia counts and some patients experienced reduction in lymph node size (Roberts et al. 2012). The dose-limiting toxicity was thrombocytopenia secondary to accelerated platelet senescence from inhibition of BCL-xL in platelets. Given this activity and observed toxicity, venetoclax (ABT-199) was designed as a molecule with greater affinity for BCL2 and reduced affinity for BCL-xL (Souers et al. 2013). Venetoclax is a once daily, orally available small molecule inhibitor of BCL2 (BCL2i) that is now broadly approved for treatment of patients with CLL.

Venetoclax Monotherapy for CLL

Venetoclax is approved for treatment of patients with CLL, both as monotherapy and combined with a CD20 antibody, which came about through several clinical trials demonstrating efficacy, safety, and tolerability, including trials in first-line and relapsed or refractory (R/R) CLL and with monotherapy and combinations with continuous and fixed-duration treatment (Tables 13.1 and 13.2). Venetoclax was initially studied in a phase 1 clinical trial (M12-175) that included patients with CLL as well as other lymphoid malignancies (Davids et al. 2017; Roberts et al. 2016). In early trials, tumor lysis syndrome (TLS) was identified as a significant risk but the phase 1 trial did not identify a maximum tolerated dose or dose-limiting toxicity. The occurrence of clinical TLS was mitigated by assessing pretreatment TLS risk determined by absolute lymphocyte count and maximal diameter of lymph node disease by CT scan imaging and initiating risk-directed monitoring and interventions through a weekly ramp-up schedule over five weeks. The effective dose identified for CLL in this trial was 400 mg daily and an overall response rate (ORR) of 79% and CR rate of 20% were reported in 116 patients with R/R CLL with a median PFS of 25 months.

The pivotal trial that led to initial approval for venetoclax as continuous monotherapy was a phase 2 trial for R/R del(17p) CLL (M13-982, Table 13.1) (Stilgenbauer et al. 2016). This trial demonstrated a CR rate of 20%, ORR of 77%, and median PFS of 27 months with continuous venetoclax monotherapy in a population of heavily previously treated patients with del(17p) CLL. In addition, uMRD4 responses were demonstrated in this very high-risk population of patients (Table 13.1). Continuous monotherapy was also investigated in patients intolerant of, or with disease refractory to, BCR signaling pathway inhibitors

Table 13.1 Venetoclax-based treatment for relapsed/refractory CLL.

Study	Phase	Treatment	Population	N	ORR	CR/CRi	uMRD4	mPFS (mo)	24-mo PFS	OS	NCT#
M12-175 (Roberts et al. 2016)	1/2	VEN-cont'	R/R	116	79%	20%	NP	25	49%	84% (24 mo)	01328626
M13-982 (Stilgenbauer et al. 2016, 2018)	2	VEN-cont'	R/R (TN = 5) Del(17p)	158	77%	20%	30% (PB)	27	54%	73% (24 mo)	01889186
M14-032 (Coutre et al. 2018; Jones et al. 2018)	2	VEN-cont'	R/R BTKi Ref/Intol PI3Ki Ref/Intol	91 36	65% 67%	9% 8%	26% (PB) 20% (PB)	25 NR	75% (12 mo) 79% (12 mo)	91% (12 mo) 94% (12 mo)	02141282
UK Real World (Eyre et al. 2019)	2	VEN-cont'	R/R	105	88%	30%	ITT NP	NR	65% (12 mo)	75% (12 mo)	NA
VENICE II (Cochrane et al. 2022)	3b	VEN-24 cycles	R/R	210	77%	19%	NP	NR	83% (12 mo)	88% (12 mo)	02980731
M13-365 (Ma et al. 2021, Seymour et al. 2018)	1b	VEN-cont' + RIT-6 cycles	R/R	49	86%	53%	61% (BM)	67	46% (72 mo)	79% (72 mo)	01682616
GNE-VO (Flinn et al. 2019)	1b	VEN-12 cycles + OBIN-6 cycles	R/R	43	95%	37%	64% (PB) 62% (BM)	NR	85%	NP	01685892
MURANO (Kater et al. 2019; Kater et al. 2020; Seymour et al. 2018)	3	VEN-24 cycles + RIT-6 cycles vs. BEN-6 cycles + RIT-6 cycle	R/R	194 195	92.3% 72.3%	8% 4%	62% (PB) 27% (BM) 13% (PB) 2% (BM)	54 17	57% (48 mo) 5% (48 mo)	85% (48 mo) 67% (48 mo)	02005471
CLARITY (Hillmen et al. 2019)	2	IBR-14–26 cycles + VEN-12–24 cycles	R/R	53	89% (1-yr combo)	51% (1-yr combo)	53% (PB) 36% (BM) (1-yr combo)	NR	NP	100%	NP
OSU-IVO (Rogers et al. 2018)	1b	IBR-13 cycles + VEN-12 cycles + OBIN-8 cycles	R/R	12	92%	42%	92% (PB) 58% (BM)	NR	92%	100%	02427451
CLL2-BAG (Cramer et al. 2018)	2	BEN-2 cycles + OBIN-6 cycles; M VEN-cont'	R/R	29	90%	28%	83% (PB) 14% (BM)	NR	83% (15 mo)	90% (15 mo)	02401503
GNE-VBR (Stilgenbauer et al. 2021)	1b	BEN-6 cycles + RIT-6 cycles + VEN-cont' (R/R)	R/R	33	91%	44%	58% (PB) 27% (BM)	NR	87%	NP	01671904

Abbreviations: ACA = acalabrutinib; BEN = bendamustine; BM = bone marrow; BTKi = Bruton's tyrosine kinase inhibitor; cont' = continuous; CR/CRi = complete remission/CR with incomplete count recovery; DFCI = Dana Farber Cancer Institute; GNE = Genentech sponsored study; IBR = ibrutinib; ITT = intent to treat; M = maintenance; MDACC = MD Anderson Cancer Center; mo = months; mPFS = median PFS; N = number; NP = not provided; NR = not reached; ORR = overall response rate; OS = overall survival; OSU = Ohio State University; PB = peripheral blood; PFS = progression-free survival; R/R = relapsed/refractory; Ref/Intol = refractory and/or intolerant; RIT = rituximab; TN = treatment naive; uMRD4 = undetectable measurable residual disease (10^{-4} sensitivity); VEN = venetoclax; vs. = versus; ZAN = zanubrutinib.

Table 13.2 Venetoclax-based treatment for treatment-naive CLL.

Study	Phase	Treatment	Population	N	ORR	CR/CRi	uMRD4	mPFS (mo)	24-mo PFS	OS	NCT#
GNE-VO (Flinn et al. 2019)	1b	VEN-12 cycles + OBIN-6 cycles	TN	32	100%	78%	72% (PB) 78% (BM)	NR	91%	NP	01685892
CLL14 (Al-Sawaf et al. 2020; Fischer et al. 2019)	3	VEN-12 cycles + OBIN-6 cycles vs. CHLOR-12 cycles + OBIN-6 cycles	TN CIRS >6; CrCl <70 ml/min	216 216	85% 71%	50% 23%	76% (PB) 57% (BM) 35% (PB) 17% (BM)	NR 36	74% (48 mo) 35% (48 mo)	85% (48 mo) 83% (48 mo)	02242942
MDACC (Jain et al. 2019, 2021)	2	IBR-27+ cycles + VEN-24 cycles	TN	80	100% (1 yr)	88% (1 yr)	56% (12 cycles combo) (BM) 66% (24 cycles combo) (BM)	NR	93% (36 mo)	96% (36 mo)	02756897
CAPTIVATE (MRD Cohort) (Wierda et al. 2021)	2	IBR-15 cycles + VEN-12 cycles	TN	164	97%	46%	75% (PB) 68% (BM)	NR	95% (30 mo)	NP	02910583
CAPTIVATE (FD Cohort) (Tam et al. 2022)	2	IBR-15 cycles + VEN-12 cycles	TN	159	96%	55%	77% (PB) 60% (BM)	NR	95% (24 mo)	98% (24 mo)	02910583
GLOW (Kater et al. 2022)	3	IBR-15 cycles + VEN-12 cycles vs. CHLOR-6 cycles + OBIN-6 cycles	TN Age≥ 65 yr or younger with CIRS score >6; CrCl <70 ml/min	106 105	87% 85%	39% 11%	55% (PB) 56% (BM) 39% (PB) 21% (BM)	NR 21 mo	84% 44%	NP	03462719
HOVON 139/ GiVe (Kater et al. 2018; Kersting et al. 2022)	2	OBIN-2 cycles then VEN-12 cycles + OBIN-6 cycles then 1:1 VEN-12 cycles (FD) vs. VEN to uMRD4 (MRD)	TN FD MRD	67 32 30	94% 78% 97%	31% 41% 60%	88% (PB) 79% (BM) 72% (PB) 59% (BM) 57% (PB) 57% (BM)	NP	85% (36 mo)	94% (36 mo)	NP
DFCI-AVO (Davids et al. 2021)	2	ACA-15+ cycles + VEN-12+ cycles + OBIN-6 cycles	TN	37	97% (@ cycle 16)	43% (@ cycle 16)	86% (PB) 86% (BM) (@ cycle 16)	NR	100% (24 mo)	NP	03580928
BOVen (Soumerai et al. 2021)	2	OBIN-8 cycles + VEN-8–24 cycles + ZAN-8–24 cycles	TN	37	100%	57%	95% (PB) 89% (BM)	NR	NP	NP	03824483
GIVe (Huber et al. 2022)	2	OBIN-6 cycles + IBR-12 cycles + VEN-12 cycles – then IBR-1–24 cycles (uMRD)	TN Del(17p)/m-TP53	41	100%	59% (@ cycle15)	78% (PB) 66% (BM) overall	NR	95%	95%	02758665
CLL2-BAG (Cramer et al. 2018)	2	BEN-2 cycles + OBIN-6 cycles; M VEN-cont'	TN	34	100%	50%	91% (PB) 12%(BM)	NR	100% (15 mo)	100% (15 mo)	02401503

(Continued)

Table 13.2 (Continued)

Study	Phase	Treatment	Population	N	ORR	CR/CRi	uMRD4	mPFS (mo)	24-mo PFS	OS	NCT#
GNE-VBO/R (Stilgenbauer et al. 2021)	1b	BEN-6 cycles + OBIN-6 or RIT-6 cycles VEN-12 cycles	TN (VBO) TN (VBR)	22 27	100% 100%	68% 44%	89% (PB) 50% (BM) 71% (PB) 41% (BM)	NR NR	100% 96%	NP	01671904

Abbreviations: ACA = acalabrutinib; BEN = bendamustine; BM = bone marrow; BTKi = Bruton's tyrosine kinase inhibitor; cont' = continuous; CR/CRi = complete remission/CR with incomplete count recovery; DFCI = Dana Farber Cancer Institute; FD = fixed duration; GNE = Genentech sponsored study; IBR, ibrutinib; ITT = intent to treat; M = maintenance; MDACC = MD Anderson Cancer Center; mo = months; mPFS = median PFS; MRD = measurable residual disease; N = number; NP = not provided; NR = not reached; ORR = overall response rate; OS = overall survival; OSU = Ohio State University; PB = peripheral blood; PFS = progression-free survival; R/R = relapsed/refractory; Ref/Intol = refractory and/or intolerant; RIT = rituximab; TN = treatment naive; uMRD4 = undetectable measurable residual disease (10^{-4} sensitivity); VEN = venetoclax; vs. = versus; ZAN = zanubrutinib.

(M14-032), including ibrutinib (n = 91) and idelalisib (n = 36) (Coutre et al. 2018; Jones et al. 2018). The ORR of 65% and 67% and CR rates of 9% and 8% were notable and durable with one-year PFS of 75% and 79% for patients who were BTKi- or PI3Ki-refractory or intolerant, respectively.

The VENICE II trial evaluated 24 cycles fixed-duration venetoclax in previously treated patients with CLL (Table 13.1) (Cochrane et al. 2022). This trial reported an ORR of 77%, CR rate of 19%, and one-year PFS of 83%. Longer follow-up is needed to understand the relevance of fixed-duration venetoclax monotherapy for R/R CLL and to potentially provide insights into importance of the addition of CD20 monoclonal antibody (mAb) in this setting.

Venetoclax Plus CD20 Monoclonal Antibody for CLL

Venetoclax was initially combined with the CD20 mAb, rituximab, in a phase 1b trial exploring tolerability of this combination for R/R patients with CLL (M13-365, Table 13.1) which also established the possibility of time-limited therapy after attainment of a deep remission (Seymour et al. 2017). In addition, venetoclax was studied with obinutuzumab in another phase 1b trial that enrolled both first-line and relapsed CLL (GNE-VO, Tables 13.1 and 13.2) (Flinn et al. 2019). This trial evaluated schedules of treatment initiated first with obinutuzumab then venetoclax ramp-up and *vice versa*. Both schedules were shown to be similarly safe; initiation of obinutuzumab for cycle 1, with initiation of venetoclax ramp-up starting on day 22 of cycle 1, was selected as the preferred schedule.

Large, randomized phase 3 clinical trials demonstrated improved PFS with fixed-duration venetoclax-based therapy over CIT (Tables 13.1 and 13.2) (Al-Sawaf et al. 2020; Fischer et al. 2019; Kater et al. 2019; Seymour et al. 2018). The MURANO trial evaluated venetoclax plus rituximab for patients with previously treated CLL (Kater et al. 2019; Seymour et al. 2018). Patients in the control arm received the standard six cycles bendamustine plus rituximab (BR). Venetoclax was given for 24 cycles total with the first six cycles including rituximab was given to patients in the experimental arm. The ORR of 92% versus 72%, CR rate of 8% versus 4%, blood uMRD4 status of 62% versus 13%, and four-year PFS of 57% versus 5% were all superior for the venetoclax–rituximab treated patients versus standard BR, respectively. Furthermore, the four-year OS was 85% versus 67% and statistically significantly higher for the venetoclax-treated patients (Table 13.1).

The CLL14 trial evaluated venetoclax plus obinutuzumab in treatment naive CLL and compared to treatment with chlorambucil plus obinutuzumab (Fischer et al. 2019). Venetoclax was given for 12 cycles as was chlorambucil, the first six cycles included obinutuzumab for both arms. In CLL14 trial, cycle 1 was treatment with obinutuzumab initiated alone; venetoclax ramp-up was initiated on day 22 of cycle 1. Cycle 1 obinutuzumab single agent was highly effective at reducing lymphocytosis prior to initiating venetoclax. There was no age restriction for enrollment on CLL14, inclusion required cumulative illness rating scale score (CIRS) of >6, but patients treated on this trial tended to be older, with median age of 72 years. This trial showed remarkably improved outcomes and depth of remission associated with venetoclax-based therapy over CIT. The ORR of 85% versus 71%, CR rate of 50% versus 23%, blood uMRD4 status of 76% versus 35%, and four-year PFS of 74% versus 35% were markedly superior for the venetoclax–obinutuzumab treated patients versus chlorambucil plus obinutuzumab, respectively. No difference in OS has been observed with current trial follow-up.

Venetoclax Plus BTK Inhibitor for CLL

The rationale for combining BTKi with BCL2i was built on clinically complimentary activity; BTKi is highly active in treating and shrinking nodal disease and BCL2i is highly effective at eliminating cell from blood and bone marrow. Interference with and release of CLL cells from the microenvironment induced by BTKi, potentially making the CLL cells more susceptible to venetoclax-induced apoptosis, also forms a basis for therapeutic synergy between these agents. Furthermore, *in vitro* studies demonstrated reduced MCL1 levels with BTKi treatment potentially making cells more vulnerable to BCL2i-induced apoptosis (Cervantes-Gomez et al. 2015). These targeted agents have non-overlapping toxicities. Combined targeted therapy with BTKi and BCL2i was evaluated in three early, phase 1/2 clinical trials (Tables 13.1 and 13.2) (Hillmen et al. 2019; Jain et al. 2019; Wierda et al. 2021). Ibrutinib monotherapy was initiated to debulk disease and potentially reduce risk of TLS in all three trials, then venetoclax was added for 12–24 total cycles of combined therapy. Data was initially available for the MD Anderson (Jain et al. 2019) and UK CLARITY (Hillmen et al. 2019) studies, which clearly demonstrated high uMRD4 rate in both first-line and relapsed CLL. The CAPTIVATE study investigated 12 cycles of combined ibrutinib and venetoclax followed by randomization based on confirmed uMRD4 status (Wierda et al. 2021). Patients who were confirmed MRD undetectable were randomized to continued ibrutinib single agent versus placebo and those unconfirmed for uMRD4 were randomized to continued ibrutinib single agent versus continued combined therapy. The post-randomization, one-year disease-free survival rate was similar between patients assigned to placebo versus continued ibrutinib. Therefore, this trial provides support for fixed-duration combined targeted therapy, with the expectation for durable remission following treatment discontinuation, particularly for patients who achieve uMRD4 status by end of combined treatment. None of the three trials identified major safety or tolerability concerns with this combination. Remaining questions with this strategy include whether there is any role for the addition of a CD20 mAb, predictive markers for response and outcomes, optimal duration of combined treatment, how to manage relapsed disease after exposure to such combinations and clinical characteristics of CLL refractory to targeted therapy. A randomized comparison of venetoclax plus obinutuzumab versus venetoclax plus BTKi is ongoing in CLL17 of the German CLL Study Group.

The phase 3 GLOW trial demonstrated superior PFS with first-line, all oral, fixed-duration ibrutinib plus venetoclax compared with that seen with a standard CIT regimen (chlorambucil plus obinutuzumab) (Table 13.2) (Kater et al. 2022). The trial population included patients over 65 years and younger patients with comorbidities. Superior efficacy was demonstrated by longer PFS, a higher uMRD4 rate at three months after the end of treatment, higher CR rate, and longer time to next treatment. Ibrutinib plus venetoclax was highly effective at achieving bone marrow uMRD4 status versus that seen with CIT (52% vs. 17%); uMRD4 status was maintained after the first year of treatment in 84% versus 29% of patients, respectively. There was a higher observed rate of toxicities with ibrutinib plus venetoclax on GLOW than reported for CAPTIVATE. Advanced age is associated with an increased proportion of patients with comorbidities and preexisting conditions and increased potential for side effects and toxicities. The median age for patients enrolled in GLOW was 71 years, 10 years greater than for patients enrolled in CAPTIVATE and more consistent with the age of patients treated in community practice.

There was no difference in OS between the treatment arms in GLOW. There was similar overall mortality rate with available follow-up; however, there were more early deaths (first three months and on treatment) for the ibrutinib plus venetoclax-treated patients and more deaths in follow-up after end of treatment for the CIT-treated patients. The number of cardiac deaths and adverse events was greater for the ibrutinib plus venetoclax-treated patients, raising concern for the potential role of ibrutinib in these infrequent but significant events. Other trials have raised similar concerns for cardiac-related events associated with ibrutinib, particularly in older patients with pre-existing cardiac conditions.

Venetoclax Plus BTK Inhibitor and CD20 Monoclonal Antibody for CLL

Venetoclax was also combined with BTKi (ibrutinib (Huber et al. 2022; Rogers et al. 2018) or acalabrutinib (Davids et al. 2021) or zanubrutinib (Soumerai et al. 2021)) and obinutuzumab for a triplet regimen (Tables 13.1 and 13.2). These trials showed similar tolerability and safety with each of these combinations. Response rates, including uMRD4, were consistently high; however, with limited number of enrolled patients and considering they are early phase trials, it is difficult to compare and understand whether these combinations were superior to venetoclax plus obinutuzumab or venetoclax plus BTKi. Nevertheless, these trials show tolerability and safety for these triplet combinations and data from phase 3 trials will be needed to assess benefits from triplet versus doublet therapies in clinical trials (Table 13.3).

Venetoclax Plus Chemoimmunotherapy

Chemoimmunotherapy is highly effective at reducing the bulk of CLL but comes with the burden of poor tolerability in older individuals, immuno- and myelosuppression, and risk for long-term marrow damage leading to myelodysplastic syndrome and acute myeloid leukemia associated with genotoxic chemotherapy. Clinical trials evaluated the potential benefit of initiating treatment with CIT, followed by consolidation with venetoclax-based therapy, including CD20 mAb

Table 13.3 Select ongoing phase 3 clinical trials including venetoclax in first-line CLL.

Trial	Subgroup	N	Status*	MRD status	Treatment arms			
GAIA/CLL13 (NCT02950051)	Fit pts	920	Enrolled	Primary objective	Ibr**Ven**Ob	**Ven**Ob	**Ven**R	CIT FCR/BR
EA9161 (NCT03701282)	Fit, 18–69 yo	720	Enrolled	Secondary objective	Ibr**Ven**Ob	IbrOb		
ACE-CL-311 (NCT03836261)	All pts	780	Enrolling	Secondary objective	Aca**Ven**Ob	Aca**Ven**		CIT FCR/BR
CRISTALLO (NCT04285567)	Fit pts	165	Enrolling	Primary objective	**Ven**Ob			CIT FCR/BR
A041702 (NCT03737981)	≥70 yo	454	Enrolling	Secondary objective	Ibr**Ven**Ob	IbrOb		
CLL17 (NCT04608318)	All pts	897	Enrolling	Secondary objective	Ibr	**Ven**Ob	Ibr**Ven**	
MAJIC (NCT05057494)	All pts	600	Pending	Primary objective	Aca**Ven**	**Ven**Ob		

*Status as of May 2022.
Abbreviations: Aca = acalabrutinib; BR = bendamustine plus rituximab; CIT = chemoimmunotherapy; FCR = fludarabine, cyclophosphamide, rituximab; Ibr = ibrutinib; MRD = measurable residual disease; N = number; Ob = obinutuzumab; Pts = patients; R = rituximab; Ven = venetoclax; yo = years old; Zanub = zanubrutinib.

(Tables 13.1 and 13.2) (Cramer et al. 2018; Stilgenbauer et al. 2021). These trials demonstrated tolerability of this treatment and effective debulking prior to venetoclax ramp-up; however, targeted therapy, particularly venetoclax, has enabled non-chemotherapy-based treatment which is well tolerated and does not have the risks described with CIT. Therefore, there is discussion and debate of any long-term benefit for the inclusion of chemotherapy in these combination regimens.

Venetoclax Toxicities and Side Effects in CLL

TLS Risk Mitigation and Management in CLL

Clinical and laboratory TLS were mitigated through stratification by risk for tumor lysis based on bulk of nodal disease and risk-based monitoring and management with a gradual venetoclax ramp-up over five weeks. With this strategy, laboratory TLS risk is extremely low and risk for clinical TLS is even lower. Standard of care first-line treatment with venetoclax-based therapy should be according to the CLL14 regimen (Fischer et al. 2019). Allopurinol or other urate-reducing agent should be initiated before treatment and cycle 1 treatment is with obinutuzumab monotherapy, which typically results in rapid resolution of lymphocytosis. Indeed, treatment for cycle 1 with obinutuzumab monotherapy can effectively decrease TLS-risk category, notably bringing most high- and medium-risk patients down to medium- and low-risk TLS category, respectively (Fischer et al. 2019; Kater et al. 2018). Prior to initiating venetoclax on day 22 of cycle 1, patients should have a staging CT of chest, abdomen, and pelvis to fully evaluate risk for TLS upon starting the venetoclax ramp-up. Similarly, effective debulking and significant reduction in patients high-risk for TLS was reported with BTKi treatment for two to three months prior to initiating venetoclax therapy (Hillmen et al. 2019; Jain et al. 2019; Kater et al. 2022; Wierda et al. 2021).

Venetoclax-associated Neutropenia

Neutropenia is a direct on-target drug effect and can be exacerbated in patients who have extensive marrow involvement with CLL or when venetoclax is combined with other myelosuppressive agents such as chemotherapy. The use of hematopoietic growth factor in early treatment cycles to support dosing until bone marrow can be cleared of disease is favored over early treatment interruption and dose reduction. The rationale for achieving the venetoclax target dose, not interrupting venetoclax dosing and maintaining target dose with use of neutrophil growth factor support to maintain absolute neutrophil count greater than 1000 neutrophils/μl, is that the CLL bone marrow burden is initially high and maintaining venetoclax dose intensity early will clear the marrow and allow for better recovery of counts. Among patients treated with venetoclax and obinutuzumab in CLL14, 53% experienced grade ≥3 neutropenia and 14% experienced grade ≥3 thrombocytopenia (Fischer et al. 2019). Once the marrow has been effectively cleared, which usually takes three to six cycles of treatment, then dose reduction is favored over continued growth factor if recurrent neutropenia is encountered. Infection grade ≥3 occurred in 18% of patients treated with venetoclax-based therapy in this study.

Venetoclax is a cytochrome P450 3A (CYP3A) substrate, and when taken concurrently with CYP3A inhibitors, such as "azole" antifungal agents, the pharmacokinetics are altered leading to increased venetoclax exposure. Venetoclax dose reduction by 50% and 75% is recommended when combined with moderate and strong inhibitors of CYP3A, respectively (Freise et al. 2017).

Risk for Progression and Resistance Mechanisms

CLL cells generally have an increased intrinsic sensitivity to venetoclax-induced apoptosis compared to other B-cell malignancies, such as DLBCL, likely related to increased BCL2 expression and other mechanisms in CLL cells and microenvironment. This is reflected in the increased risk for TLS with initiation and the impressive response rates and depth of remission that are achieved even with monotherapy. In the first-line setting with venetoclax plus obinutuzumab, shorter PFS was associated with presence of del(17p); additional predictive factors may be identified with longer follow-up (Tausch et al. 2020). An early analysis or R/R patients on continuous venetoclax revealed that fludarabine-refractory disease and complex karyotype were predictive of early progression on venetoclax therapy (Anderson et al. 2017). Characteristics associated with lower CR rate and shorter duration of response with venetoclax-based treatment in R/R CLL include presence of bulky lymph nodes (≥5 cm) and refractoriness to BTKi (Roberts et al. 2019). Shorter response duration among responders was associated with abnormalities in *TP53* and mutated *NOTCH1* (Roberts et al. 2019). These might be patients for whom active allo-SCT planning is initiated or cellular therapy on clinical trial. Longer duration of response was clearly associated with achieving uMRD4 status. Consideration for continued venetoclax monotherapy after combination with rituximab for R/R CLL should be given to patients with persistent MRD4 at the end of 24 cycles of venetoclax and for those with *TP53* abnormality (deletion or mutation), since these patients are more likely to progress sooner upon discontinuing venetoclax (Kater et al. 2019, 2020).

Several mechanisms of acquired clinical resistance to venetoclax-based treatment have been described. These have been explored and some confirmed in clinical samples from patients who develop resistance. Mutations that block venetoclax binding of BCL2 have been described in samples from patients who develop clinical resistance, including: G101V (Blombery et al. 2019), D103Y (Tausch et al. 2019), and F104I (Tausch et al. 2019). Additionally, resistance mechanisms may include increased expression of other anti-apoptotic BCL2 family proteins, such as MCL-1 and BCL-xL, which raise the threshold of apoptosis and decrease cell dependence on BCL2 (Haselager et al. 2020). One potential mechanism for increasing BCL-xL levels is through reduction in miR-377 (Al-Harbi et al. 2015). Resistance is likely multifactorial and currently is an area of active investigation.

Current Knowledge Gaps and Opportunities for Future Work with Venetoclax

Venetoclax was evaluated in phase 3 clinical trials with fixed-duration treatment for 12 cycles venetoclax with the first six cycles combined with obinutuzumab in first-line (CLL14) and for 24 cycles with the first six cycles combined with rituximab in the R/R setting (MURANO). Although the rate of uMRD4 in blood is high at end of therapy with venetoclax-based treatment in both of these settings, there are opportunities for optimizing this strategy. Certainly, not all patients require same duration of treatment to achieve uMRD4 status, therefore, with fixed-duration treatment it is likely that some patients will be overtreated and others undertreated. Identifying the optimal duration of treatment therefore is needed and is likely to be individualized. Trials with MRD4 as treatment endpoint are needed to further clarify this issue.

While approximately half of patients with mutated-IGHV who receive six cycles of FCR (fludarabine, cyclophosphamide, rituximab) in the first-line setting remain progression-free beyond 10 years, many of whom remain in an uMRD4 state, it is unclear if similar results can be achieved with venetoclax-based therapy. Clarification of this will come with longer follow-up from trials. Additionally, early indication of this may come from monitoring for MRD4 relapse on current clinical trials.

Progress in therapy will likely be reflected in a higher proportion of treated patients achieving uMRD4 status with shorter treatment duration. Now that next-generation sequencing (NGS) methodology is commercially available for MRD evaluation, uMRD6 (10^{-6} sensitivity) may become goal of treatment. Curative strategies will need to strive for uMRD6 as treatment goal in future trials. Optimizing combinations of targeted therapies to achieve this end is the basis for many current phase 2 clinical trials. Optimal sequencing of targeted therapy has yet to be clarified as well as optimized combined therapy.

While a high proportion of patients achieve uMRD4 status as best response, it is unclear if this is associated with correction of immune dysfunction and restoration of immune function in patients with CLL. This is currently under investigation. Immune dysfunction resulting in increased risk for infection and second cancers continues to be a major challenge with this disease.

With fixed-duration venetoclax-based treatment, the majority of patients complete treatment and achieve uMRD4 remission. Several studies demonstrated that response is expected with retreatment, with better anticipated results expected for patient to have longer remission duration with initial treatment. Limited data gives confirmation to this expectation. Additionally, no studies have been conducted to clarify optimal targeted therapeutic sequencing. Table 13.4 summarizes strategies for next treatment based on available data and clinical experience.

Table 13.4 Therapeutic sequencing strategy for relapsed/refractory CLL.

Prior treatment				
CIT	**Venetoclax**	**BTKi**	**Recommendation for next treatment**	**Allo-SCT planning**
Yes	No **OR** completed prior BCL2i with remission	No	Ven + CD20 mAb (fixed duration) **OR** BTKi (continuous)	No
		Yes (intolerant)	Alternative BTKi (continuous) **OR** Ven + CD20 mAb (fixed duration) **OR** PI3Ki (continuous) + R	No
		Yes (refractory)	VEN + CD20 mAb **OR** PI3Ki (continuous) + R	Short-term
	Yes (refractory)	No	BTKi (continuous)	Long-term
		Yes (intolerant)	Alternative BTKi (continuous) **OR** PI3Ki (continuous) + R	Long-term
		Yes (refractory)	Clinical trial CIT if no *TP53* abnormality to debulk	Immediate
No	No **OR** completed prior BCL2i with remission	No	Ven + CD20 mAb (fixed duration) **OR** BTKi (continuous)	No
		Yes (intolerant)	Alternative BTKi (continuous) **OR** Ven + CD20 mAb (fixed duration) **OR** PI3Ki (continuous) + R	No
		Yes (refractory)	Ven + CD20 mAb (fixed duration)	Long-term
	Yes (refractory)	No	BTKi (continuous)	No
		Yes (intolerant)	Alternative BTKi (continuous) **OR** PI3Ki (continuous) + R	No
		Yes (refractory)	Clinical trial CIT if no *TP53* abnormality to debulk	Immediate

Abbreviations: Allo-SCT = allogeneic stem cell transplant; BCL2i = B-cell lymphoma 2 inhibitor; BTKi = Bruton's tyrosine kinase inhibitor; CIT = chemoimmunotherapy; PI3Ki = PI3 kinase inhibitor; R = rituximab; Ven = venetoclax.

Must Read References

Roberts, A.W., Seymour, J.F., Brown, J.R. et al. (2012). Substantial susceptibility of chronic lymphocytic leukemia to BCL2 inhibition: results of a phase I study of navitoclax in patients with relapsed or refractory disease. *J. Clin. Oncol.* 30: 488–496.

Roberts, A.W., Davids, M.S., Pagel, J.M. et al. (2016). Targeting BCL2 with venetoclax in relapsed chronic lymphocytic leukemia. *N. Engl. J. Med.* 374: 311–322.

Al-Sawaf O., Zhang, C., Tandon, M. et al. (2020). Venetoclax plus obinutuzumab versus chlorambucil plus obinutuzumab for previously untreated chronic lymphocytic leukaemia (CLL14): follow-up results from a multicentre, open-label, randomised, phase 3 trial. *Lancet. Oncol.* 21: 1188–1200.

Cervantes-Gomez, F., Lamothe, B., Woyach, J.A. et al. (2015). Pharmacological and protein profiling suggests venetoclax (ABT-199) as optimal partner with ibrutinib in chronic lymphocytic leukemia. *Clin. Cancer Res.* 21: 3705–3715.

References

Ahn, I.E., Tian, X., and Wiestner, A. (2020). Ibrutinib for chronic lymphocytic leukemia with TP53 alterations. *N. Engl. J. Med.* 383: 498–500.

Al-Harbi, S., Choudhary, G.S., Ebron, J.S. et al. (2015). miR-377-dependent BCL-xL regulation drives chemotherapeutic resistance in B-cell lymphoid malignancies. *Mol. Cancer* 14: 185.

Al-Sawaf, O., Zhang, C., Lu, T. et al. (2021). Minimal residual disease dynamics after venetoclax-obinutuzumab treatment: extended off-treatment follow-up from the randomized CLL14 study. *J. Clin. Oncol.* 39: 4049–4060.

Al-Sawaf, O., Zhang, C., Robrecht, S. et al. (2020). Clonal dynamics after venetoclax-obinutuzumab therapy: novel insights from the randomized, phase 3 CLL14 trial. *Blood* 136: 22–23.

Al-Sawaf, O., Zhang, C., Tandon, M. et al. (2020). Venetoclax plus obinutuzumab versus chlorambucil plus obinutuzumab for previously untreated chronic lymphocytic leukaemia (CLL14): follow-up results from a multicentre, open-label, randomised, phase 3 trial. *Lancet Oncol.* 21: 1188–1200.

Anderson, M.A., Tam, C., Lew, T.E. et al. (2017). Clinicopathological features and outcomes of progression of CLL on the BCL2 inhibitor venetoclax. *Blood* 129: 3362–3370.

Blombery, P., Anderson, M.A., Gong, J.N. et al. (2019). Acquisition of the recurrent gly101Val mutation in BCL2 confers resistance to venetoclax in patients with progressive chronic lymphocytic leukemia. *Cancer Discov.* 9: 342–353.

Burger, J.A., Barr, P.M., Robak, T. et al. (2020). Long-term efficacy and safety of first-line ibrutinib treatment for patients with CLL/SLL: 5 years of follow-up from the phase 3 RESONATE-2 study. *Leukemia*. 34: 787–798.

Byrd, J.C., Furman, R.R., Coutre, S.E. et al. (2015). Three-year follow-up of treatment-naive and previously treated patients with CLL and SLL receiving single-agent ibrutinib. *Blood* 125: 2497–2506.

Calin, G.A., Dumitru, C.D., Shimizu, M. et al. (2002). Frequent deletions and down-regulation of micro- RNA genes miR15 and miR16 at 13q14 in chronic lymphocytic leukemia. *Proc. Natl. Acad. Sci. U.S.A.* 99: 15524–15529.

Cervantes-Gomez, F., Lamothe, B., Woyach, J.A. et al. (2015). Pharmacological and protein profiling suggests venetoclax (ABT-199) as optimal partner with ibrutinib in chronic lymphocytic leukemia. *Clin. Cancer Res.* 21: 3705–3715.

Cimmino, A., Calin, G.A., Fabbri, M. et al. (2005). miR-15 and miR-16 induce apoptosis by targeting BCL2. *Proc. Natl. Acad. Sci. U.S.A.* 102: 13944–13949.

Cochrane, T., Enrico, A., Gomez-Almaguer, D. et al. (2022). Impact of venetoclax monotherapy on the quality of life of patients with relapsed or refractory chronic lymphocytic leukemia: results from the phase 3b VENICE II trial. *Leuk. Lymphoma* 63: 304–314.

Coutre, S., Choi, M., Furman, R.R. et al. (2018). Venetoclax for patients with chronic lymphocytic leukemia who progressed during or after idelalisib therapy. *Blood* 131: 1704–1711.

Coutre, S.E., Furman, R.R., Flinn, I.W. et al. (2017). Extended treatment with single-agent ibrutinib at the 420 mg dose leads to durable responses in chronic lymphocytic leukemia/small lymphocytic lymphoma. *Clin. Cancer Res.* 23: 1149–1155.

Cramer, P., von Tresckow, J., Bahlo, J. et al. (2018). Bendamustine followed by obinutuzumab and venetoclax in chronic lymphocytic leukaemia (CLL2-BAG): primary endpoint analysis of a multicentre, open-label, phase 2 trial. *Lancet Oncol.* 19: 1215–1228.

Davids, M.S., Lampson, B.L., Tyekucheva, S. et al. (2021). Acalabrutinib, venetoclax, and obinutuzumab as frontline treatment for chronic lymphocytic leukaemia: a single-arm, open-label, phase 2 study. *Lancet Oncol.* 22: 1391–1402.

Davids, M.S., Roberts, A.W., Seymour, J.F. et al. (2017). Phase I first-in-human study of venetoclax in patients with relapsed or refractory non-Hodgkin lymphoma. *J. Clin. Oncol.* 35: 826–833.

Eyre, T.A., Kirkwood, A.A., Gohill, S. et al. (2019). Efficacy of venetoclax monotherapy in patients with relapsed chronic lymphocytic leukaemia in the post-BCR inhibitor setting: a UK wide analysis. *Br. J. Haematol.* 185: 656–669.

Fischer, K., Al-Sawaf, O., Bahlo, J. et al. (2019). Venetoclax and obinutuzumab in patients with CLL and coexisting conditions. *N. Engl. J. Med.* 380: 2225–2236.

Flinn, I.W., Gribben, J.G., Dyer, M.J.S. et al. (2019). Phase 1b study of venetoclax-obinutuzumab in previously untreated and relapsed/refractory chronic lymphocytic leukemia. *Blood* 133: 2765–2775.

Freise, K.J., Shebley, M., and Salem, A.H. (2017). Quantitative prediction of the effect of CYP3A inhibitors and inducers on venetoclax pharmacokinetics using a physiologically based pharmacokinetic model. *J. Clin. Pharmacol.* 57: 796–804.

Hallek, M., Cheson, B.D., Catovsky, D. et al. (2018). iwCLL guidelines for diagnosis, indications for treatment, response assessment, and supportive management of CLL. *Blood* 131: 2745–2760.

Haselager, M.V., Kielbassa, K., Ter Burg, J. et al. (2020). Changes in Bcl-2 members after ibrutinib or venetoclax uncover functional hierarchy in determining resistance to venetoclax in CLL. *Blood* 136: 2918–2926.

Hillmen, P., Rawstron, A.C., Brock, K. et al. (2019). Ibrutinib plus venetoclax in relapsed/refractory chronic lymphocytic leukemia: the CLARITY study. *J. Clin. Oncol.* 37: 2722–2729.

Huber, H., Edenhofer, S., von Tresckow, J. et al. (2022). Obinutuzumab (GA-101), ibrutinib, and venetoclax (GIVe) frontline treatment for high-risk chronic lymphocytic leukemia. *Blood* 139: 1318–1329.

Jain, N., Keating, M., Thompson, P. et al. (2019). Ibrutinib and venetoclax for first-line treatment of CLL. *N. Engl. J. Med.* 380: 2095–2103.

Jain, N., Keating, M., Thompson, P. et al. (2021). Ibrutinib plus venetoclax for first-line treatment of chronic lymphocytic leukemia: a nonrandomized phase 2 trial. *JAMA Oncol.* 7: 1213–1219.

Jones, J.A., Mato, A.R., Wierda, W.G. et al. (2018). Venetoclax for chronic lymphocytic leukaemia progressing after ibrutinib: an interim analysis of a multicentre, open-label, phase 2 trial. *Lancet Oncol.* 19: 65–75.

Kater, A., Owen, C., Moreno, C. et al. (2022). Fixed-duration ibrutinib-venetoclax in patients with chronic lymphocytic leukemia and comorbidities. NEJM Evidence 0:Epub ahead of print.

Kater, A.P., Kersting, S., van Norden, Y. et al. (2018). Obinutuzumab pretreatment abrogates tumor lysis risk while maintaining undetectable MRD for venetoclax + obinutuzumab in CLL. *Blood Adv.* 2: 3566–3571.

Kater, A.P., Kipps, T.J., Eichhorst, B. et al. (2020). Five-year analysis of murano study demonstrates enduring undetectable minimal residual disease (uMRD) in a subset of relapsed/refractory chronic lymphocytic leukemia (R/R CLL) patients (Pts) following fixed-duration venetoclax-rituximab (VenR) therapy (Tx). *Blood* 136: 19–21.

Kater, A.P., Seymour, J.F., Hillmen, P. et al. (2019). Fixed duration of venetoclax-rituximab in relapsed/refractory chronic lymphocytic leukemia eradicates minimal residual disease and prolongs survival: post-treatment follow-up of the MURANO phase III study. *J. Clin. Oncol.* 37: 269–277.

Kater, A.P., Wu, J.Q., Kipps, T. et al. (2020). Venetoclax plus rituximab in relapsed chronic lymphocytic leukemia: 4-year results and evaluation of impact of genomic complexity and gene mutations from the MURANO phase III study. *J. Clin. Oncol.* 38: 4042–4054.

Kersting, S., Dubois, J., Nasserinejad, K. et al. (2022). Venetoclax consolidation after fixed-duration venetoclax plus obinutuzumab for previously untreated chronic lymphocytic leukaemia (HOVON 139/GiVe): primary endpoint analysis of a multicentre, open-label, randomised, parallel-group, phase 2 trial. *Lancet Haematol.* 9: e190–e199.

Ma, S., Seymour, J.F., Brander, D.M. et al. (2021). Efficacy of venetoclax plus rituximab for relapsed CLL: 5-year follow-up of continuous or limited- duration therapy. *Blood* 138: 836–846.

Moreno, C., Greil, R., Demirkan, F. et al. (2019). Ibrutinib plus obinutuzumab versus chlorambucil plus obinutuzumab in first-line treatment of chronic lymphocytic leukaemia (iLLUMINATE): a multicentre, randomised, open-label, phase 3 trial. *Lancet Oncol.* 20: 43–56.

O'Brien, S., Furman, R.R., Coutre, S. et al. (2018). Single-agent ibrutinib in treatment-naive and relapsed/refractory chronic lymphocytic leukemia: a 5-year experience. *Blood* 131: 1910–1919.

O'Brien, S., Furman, R.R., Coutre, S.E. et al. (2014). Ibrutinib as initial therapy for elderly patients with chronic lymphocytic leukaemia or small lymphocytic lymphoma: an open-label, multicentre, phase 1b/2 trial. *Lancet Oncol.* 15: 48–58.

Roberts, A.W., Davids, M.S., Pagel, J.M. et al. (2016). Targeting BCL2 with venetoclax in relapsed chronic lymphocytic leukemia. *N. Engl. J. Med.* 374: 311–322.

Roberts, A.W., Ma, S., Kipps, T.J. et al. (2019). Efficacy of venetoclax in relapsed chronic lymphocytic leukemia is influenced by disease and response variables. *Blood* 134: 111–122.

Roberts, A.W., Seymour, J.F., Brown, J.R. et al. (2012). Substantial susceptibility of chronic lymphocytic leukemia to BCL2 inhibition: results of a phase I study of navitoclax in patients with relapsed or refractory disease. *J. Clin. Oncol.* 30: 488–496.

Rogers, K.A., Huang, Y., Ruppert, A.S. et al. (2018). Phase 1b study of obinutuzumab, ibrutinib, and venetoclax in relapsed and refractory chronic lymphocytic leukemia. *Blood* 132: 1568–1572.

Seymour, J.F., Kipps, T.J., Eichhorst, B. et al. (2018). Venetoclax-rituximab in relapsed or refractory chronic lymphocytic leukemia. *N. Engl. J. Med.* 378: 1107–1120.

Seymour, J.F., Ma, S., Brander, D.M. et al. (2017). Venetoclax plus rituximab in relapsed or refractory chronic lymphocytic leukaemia: a phase 1b study. *Lancet Oncol.* 18: 230–240.

Shanafelt, T.D., Wang, X.V., Kay, N.E. et al. (2019). Ibrutinib-rituximab or chemoimmunotherapy for chronic lymphocytic leukemia. *N. Engl. J. Med.* 381: 432–443.

Sharman, J.P., Egyed, M., Jurczak, W. et al. (2020). Acalabrutinib with or without obinutuzumab versus chlorambucil and obinutuzmab for treatment-naive chronic lymphocytic leukaemia (ELEVATE TN): a randomised, controlled, phase 3 trial. *Lancet* 395: 1278–1291.

Souers, A.J., Leverson, J.D., Boghaert, E.R. et al. (2013). ABT-199, a potent and selective BCL-2 inhibitor, achieves antitumor activity while sparing platelets. *Nat. Med.* 19: 202–208.

Soumerai, J.D., Mato, A.R., Dogan, A. et al. (2021). Zanubrutinib, obinutuzumab, and venetoclax with minimal residual disease-driven discontinuation in previously untreated patients with chronic lymphocytic leukaemia or small lymphocytic lymphoma: a multicentre, single-arm, phase 2 trial. *Lancet Haematol* 8: e879–e890.

Stilgenbauer, S., Eichhorst, B., Schetelig, J. et al. (2016). Venetoclax in relapsed or refractory chronic lymphocytic leukaemia with 17p deletion: a multicentre, open-label, phase 2 study. *Lancet Oncol.* 17: 768–778.

Stilgenbauer, S., Eichhorst, B., Schetelig, J. et al. (2018). Venetoclax for patients with chronic lymphocytic leukemia with 17p deletion: results from the full population of a phase II pivotal trial. *J. Clin. Oncol.* 36: 1973–1980.

Stilgenbauer, S., Morschhauser, F., Wendtner, C.M. et al. (2021). Venetoclax plus bendamustine-rituximab or bendamustine-obinutuzumab in chronic lymphocytic leukemia: final results of a phase 1b study (GO28440). *Haematologica* 106: 2834–2844.

Tam, C.S., Allan, J.N., Siddiqi, T. et al. (2022). Fixed-duration ibrutinib plus venetoclax for first-line treatment of CLL: primary analysis of the CAPTIVATE FD cohort. *Blood.* 139: 3278–3289.

Tausch, E., Close, W., Dolnik, A. et al. (2019). Venetoclax resistance and acquired BCL2 mutations in chronic lymphocytic leukemia. *Haematologica* 104: e434–e437.

Tausch, E., Schneider, C., Robrecht, S. et al. (2020). Prognostic and predictive impact of genetic markers in patients with CLL treated with obinutuzumab and venetoclax. *Blood* 135: 2402–2412.

Wierda, W.G., Allan, J.N., Siddiqi, T. et al. (2021). Ibrutinib plus venetoclax for first-line treatment of chronic lymphocytic leukemia: primary analysis results from the minimal residual disease cohort of the randomized phase II CAPTIVATE study. *J. Clin. Oncol.* 39: 3853–3865.

Woyach, J.A., Ruppert, A.S., Heerema, N.A. et al. (2018). Ibrutinib regimens versus chemoimmunotherapy in older patients with untreated CLL. *N. Engl. J. Med.* 379: 2517–2528.

Section IV

Targeting the Cancer Epigenome

14

The Role of Epigenetic Dysregulation in Lymphoma Biology

Qing Deng[1] *and Michael R. Green*[1,2]

[1] *Department of Lymphoma & Myeloma, University of Texas MD Anderson Cancer Center, Houston, TX, USA*
[2] *Department of Genomic Medicine, University of Texas MD Anderson Cancer Center, Houston, TX, USA*

Take Home Messages

- Germinal center B-cell development and terminal differentiation are controlled by large epigenetically regulated shifts in transcriptional states.
- Somatic mutations of chromatin modifiers are highly prevalent in germinal center B-cell derived malignancies.
- Mutations of histone "writer" proteins such as KMT2D, CREBBP, and EZH2 deregulate the normal activation of gene regulatory elements that control germinal center B-cell development.
- Mutations in HIST1 and BAF complex genes deregulate the epigenome of B-cell lymphoma by perturbing chromatin structure.

Introduction: Germinal Center B (GCB)-cells and GCB-derived Lymphomas

B-cell development is a complex multi-step process that has evolved to allow for the generation of high-affinity immunoglobulins against pathogens and humoral recall responses upon re-challenge (Nutt et al. 2015). For T-cell-dependent antigens, the differentiation from mature naive B-cells to terminally differentiated plasma cells or memory B-cells occurs via the germinal center (GC) reaction. Entry into the GC upon antigen encounter is regulated by transient expression of MYC and IRF4, which promote the expression of BCL6 and POU2AF1 (Obf1) (Dominguez-Sola et al. 2012; Ochiai et al. 2013). In the dark zone (DZ) of the GC, centroblasts undergo rounds of proliferation and edit their immunoglobulin genes through somatic hypermutation (SHM). This program is regulated by BCL6, which recruits co-repressor complexes to suppress the expression of genes involved in cell cycle and DNA repair checkpoints, B-cell receptor (BCR) signaling, and antigen presentation. After multiple rounds of division and SHM, GCB cells stop proliferating and enter the light zone (LZ) of the GC as centrocytes where they interact with follicular dendritic cells (FDCs) and T follicular helper (TFH) cells. FDCs inhibit apoptosis of GCB cells through Notch:Notch ligand interactions and provide antigen that is taken up and presented on major histocompatibility complex (MHC) class II. Based upon the amount of antigen that is captured by their immunoglobulin and presented on MHC class II, GCB cells compete for limiting interactions with TFH cells that provide survival signals through CD40:CD40 ligand interactions. Those that fail to compete for these survival signals die by neglect, whereas GCB cells with the higher affinity for their antigen form the immune synapses with TFH cells, where their fate is determined by the amount of CD40 signal that they receive from this interaction. Lower levels of signaling result in activation of MYC and re-entry to the DZ for addition rounds of proliferation and SHM (Dominguez-Sola et al. 2012; Gitlin et al. 2014), or differentiation into memory B-cells through a pre-memory B-cell state regulated by BACH2 (Shinnakasu et al. 2016). GCB cells with the highest affinity for their antigens form the most stable contacts with TFH cells and receive the strongest CD40 signaling (Ise et al. 2018), leading to plasma cell differentiation through a plasmablast state regulated by IRF4, PRDM1, and XBP1. Thus, B-cell development consists of complex and dynamic shifts in transcriptional programs at multiple cell fate transitions that are linked to extrinsic signals and are regulated by transcription factors (Figure 14.1). These transcription factors recruit co-repressor or co-activator complexes that epigenetically control gene expression by post-translationally modifying histones and/or remodeling chromatin structure, thereby driving large,

Precision Cancer Therapies: Targeting Oncogenic Drivers and Signaling Pathways in Lymphoid Malignancies: From Concept to Practice, Volume 1, First Edition. Edited by Owen A. O'Connor, Stephen M. Ansell, and John F. Seymour.

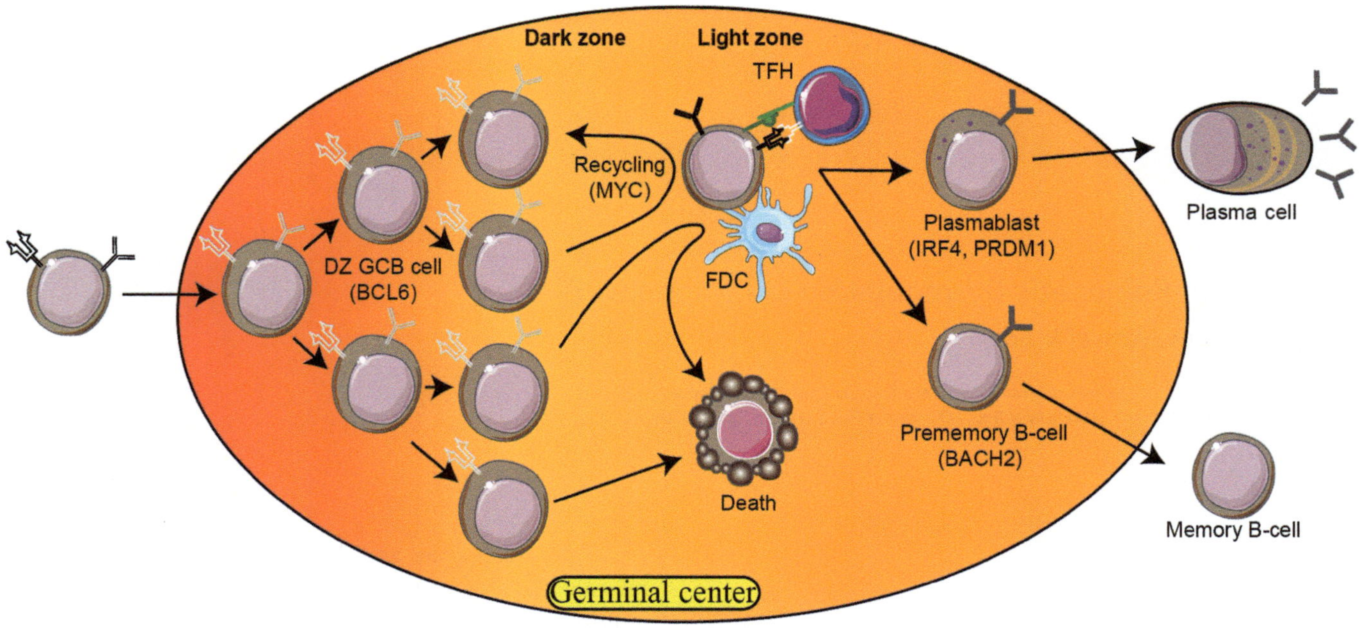

Figure 14.1 Transcriptional control of the germinal center reaction. Affinity maturation and terminal differentiation through the germinal center reaction require broad epigenetic and transcriptional changes that are regulated by transcription factors and their associated co-activator/co-repressor proteins. Normal epigenetic control of B-cell development is dysregulated in B-cell lymphoma via a variety of genetic mechanisms.

dynamic and highly coordinated shifts in the epigenome and transcriptome during cell fate transitions.

As GCB cells possess many of the hallmarks of cancer (e.g. high proliferative rate, suppressed DNA damage response), it is perhaps not surprising that the majority of non-Hodgkin's lymphomas arise from GCB cells. In GCB-derived lymphomas such as diffuse large B-cell lymphoma (DLBCL), follicular lymphoma (FL), and Burkitt's lymphoma (BL), the epigenetic and transcriptional programs that naturally occur during B-cell development are hijacked by genetic alterations that directly or indirectly change the function of transcription factors and/or chromatin modifying genes. This leads to the aberrant perpetuation of the GCB cell state, including the suppression of epigenetic and transcriptional programs that drive immune interactions and terminal differentiation. Here, we review the role of mutations in chromatin-modifying genes and their impact on the biology of GCB-derived lymphomas.

Mutations Altering DNA Modifications and Structure

Methylation of cytosine nucleotides is a well-established mechanism of gene silencing, and aberrant DNA methylation can drive cancer through the silencing of tumor suppressor genes. DNA is methylated by DNA methyltransferase enzymes that either act *de novo* (DNMT3A/B) or maintain methylation during replication (DNMT1). DNA methylation can either be passively lost or actively removed by TET enzymes (TET1, TET2, TET3) that catalyze the sequential oxidation of 5-methylcytosine (5mC) to 5-hydroxymethylcytosine (5hmC) and other oxidized derivatives that are repaired to cytosine (Ko et al. 2015). Higher 5mC is associated with gene silencing and can contribute to tumorigenesis through silencing of tumor suppressor genes, while 5hmC functions as an epigenetic mark that is associated with enhancer activation. DLBCLs have a high degree of inter-tumor and intra-tumor heterogeneity in DNA methylation (De et al. 2013) and the degree to which the DNA methylome differs from normal B-cells is associated with patient survival (Chambwe et al. 2014). Mutations of the *TET2* gene lead to an increase of 5mC and a loss of 5hmC but are only observed in a subset of patients. The remaining degree of heterogeneity in DNA methylation and hydroxymethylation may therefore either be stochastic or acquired through mechanisms that remain to be defined.

TET2

TET2 loss-of-function mutations are observed in ~10% of DLBCL, are a core feature of the ST2 subtype (Wright et al. 2020), and are associated with genome-wide DNA methylation profiles in primary tumors (Asmar et al. 2013). Conditional deletion of *Tet2* either within hematopoietic stem cells or B-cells leads to a significant increase in GCB cells following immunization, but this effect is not observed when *Tet2* is selectively deleted within GCB cells (Dominguez et al. 2018). Plasma cells are also reduced in *Tet2* knock-out mice, suggesting a defect in GC exit and terminal differentiation. Molecular analysis of *Tet2* deficient GCB cells identified downregulation of genes that are normally induced in centrocytes within the LZ, with a significant enrichment of BCL6 target genes and pathways that are also deregulated by CREBBP mutation. Mechanistically, *Tet2* deletion results in the accumulation of 5mC at promoters (Rosikiewicz et al. 2020) and the loss of 5hmC at enhancers (Dominguez et al. 2018), resulting in the reduced expression of genes that are induced within the LZ and involved in GC exit. Demethylation by *Tet2* may occur in cooperation with activation-induced cytidine deaminase (AID), and regions of hypermethylation were highly similar in Tet2 knock-out and AID knock-out GCB cells, suggestive of disrupted AID-mediated demethylation (Rosikiewicz et al. 2020) (Figure 14.2).

A recent study employing conditional knock-out of both *Tet2* and *Tet3* in B-cells (*Tet2/3*^{dKO}) (Shukla et al. 2022) observed a high penetrance lymphoma phenotype, with downregulated genes resembling those observed previously (Dominguez et al. 2018). However, they also noted a significant upregulation of genes involved DNA repair pathways associated with the resolution of secondary DNA structure. Upon close inspection, they noted that Tet2/3^{dKO} cells had a significant accumulation of G-quadruplexes (a planar structure formed by a stranded DNA molecule when four guanines within a G-rich region interact via hydrogen bonds)

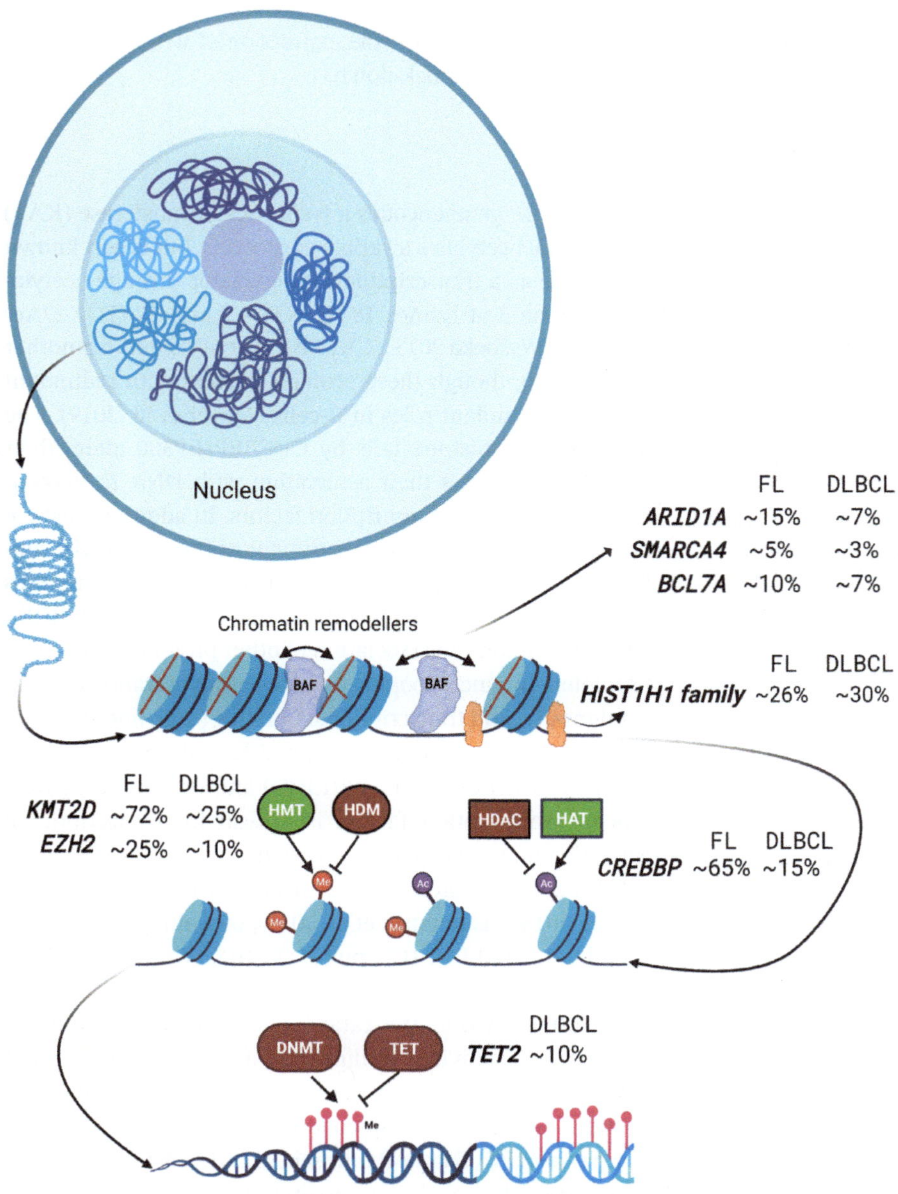

Figure 14.2 Schematic of frequently mutated epigenetic modifiers in B-cell lymphoma. Genetic alterations in B-cell lymphoma target genes with a role in chromatin remodeling, histone post-translational modification (acetylation and methylation), and DNA methylation and hydroxymethylation.

and R-loops (a DNA/RNA hybrid formed when transcribed RNA binds to single-stranded DNA) within a few days of knock-out. These G-quadruplexes and R-loops were enriched at highly transcribed regions and were also associated with increased genomic instability and genetic translocations at AID targets such as the immunoglobulin switch region. TET loss-of-function may therefore also contribute to lymphomagenesis by promoting genetic instability (Shukla et al. 2022).

Mutations Altering Writers of Histone Post-translational Modifications

The reversible post-translational modification of histone tails is a fundamental mechanism transcriptional control. Depending on their positional context relative to the transcriptional start site of a gene, histones will be decorated by "writer" proteins that add various post-translational modifications that are capable of activating or suppressing transcription by acting as docking sites for "reader" proteins that control DNA accessibility, chromatin conformation, and the recruitment of transcriptional machinery. Mutations of genes that encode "writers" of histone post-translational modifying enzymes, including histone methyltransferases (*KMT2D*, EZH2) and histone acetyltransferases (*CREBBP*), are characteristics of FL and the newly characterized EZB/C3 subset of DLBCL (Chapuy et al. 2018; Wright et al. 2020) (Figure 14.2). Mutations in these genes often co-occur within a given tumor, and likely have cooperating roles that are yet to be defined (Green 2018; Ma et al. 2021). However, the function of individual gene mutations has been characterized using genetically engineered mouse models (GEMMs) and cell line models, providing insight into epigenetic mechanisms of B-cell development that is deregulated in lymphoma.

KMT2D

The *KMT2D* gene (aka *MLL2*) encodes a SET domain-containing lysine methyltransferase that catalyzes enhancer H3K4 mono-methylation, either independently or as part of multi-protein COMPASS-like complexes that are preferentially associated with developmentally regulated genes (Ford and Dingwall 2015). Enhancer H3K4me1 leads to the recruitment of transcriptional co-activators that drive enhancer–promoter looping and transcriptional activation. The *KMT2D* gene is mutated ~72% of FL and ~25% of DLBCL (~54% of the EZB/C3 subtype), primarily consisting of premature stop codons or frameshifts that result in a truncation or loss of KMT2D protein (Zhang et al. 2015). Missense mutations of *KMT2D* predominantly affect the SET domain in the C-terminal portion of the gene and reduce methyltransferase activity (Zhang et al. 2015), though it is unclear whether the protein retains some activity as a scaffold. The effect of Kmt2d loss on GCB cell development and lymphomagenesis has been investigated in murine models using shRNA-mediated knock-down (Ortega-Molina et al. 2015) or conditional knock-out (Zhang et al. 2015). Knock-down/knock-out of *Kmt2d* in murine B-cells did not lead to a significant change in early stages of B-cell development. However, following immunization mice with Kmt2d knock-out/knock-down showed a marked increase in GCB cell frequency and perturbed class-switch recombination, indicative of a defect in normal B-cell maturation following *Kmt2d* loss. At a functional level, loss of *Kmt2d* was associated with the upregulation of pathways involved in proliferation and DNA repair, which led to a proliferative advantage of *Kmt2d*-null cells within the GC reaction (Zhang et al. 2015). This may occur as a downstream consequence of direct targets of *Kmt2d*, such as *Tnfaip3*, the expression of which is reduced following *Kmt2d* knock-down.

CREBBP

The *CREBBP* gene encodes a lysine acetyltransferase (KAT) protein that acetylates a variety of proteins, but is best known for its role as a transcriptional co-activator through acetylation histone 3 at lysines 18 (H3K18Ac) and 27 (H3K27Ac) (Calo and Wysocka 2013). CREBBP is homologous to another KAT, EP300, though these proteins possess both redundant and non-redundant roles in B-cells (Meyer et al. 2019). The acetylation of histone tails by CREBBP/EP300 alters their charge and loosens their association with DNA to make it more accessible to transcription factors. In addition, histone acetylation results in the recruitment of bromodomain-containing proteins such as chromatin remodeling complexes that drive nucleosome shuffling and eviction, and BRD4 which facilitates the association of other proteins that lead to promoter–enhancer looping, the formation of transcriptional condensates, and transcriptional bursting (Calo and Wysocka 2013; Filippakopoulos and Knapp 2012; Gibson et al. 2019). The recruitment of CREBBP/EP300 and/or other co-activators by transcription factors is critical for transcriptional activation and target gene expression.

CREBBP is mutated in ~65% of FL and 10–15% of DLBCL (Green 2018; Pasqualucci et al. 2011), including 53% of EZB/C3 subtype of DLBCL (Chapuy et al. 2018; Wright et al. 2020). The majority of these mutations result in single amino acid substitutions within the catalytic KAT domain leading to reduced KAT activity (Mullighan et al. 2011; Pasqualucci et al. 2011), though DLBCLs possess a significantly higher frequency of premature stop codon and frameshift mutations compared to FL (Garcia-Ramirez et al. 2017). Multiple studies evaluating the evolutionary hierarchy of FL through sequencing of paired biopsies or tumor cell subpopulations have shown that *CREBBP* mutations are acquired as early events during the genetic evolution of FL (Green et al. 2013,

2015; Kridel et al. 2016; Okosun et al. 2014; Pasqualucci et al. 2014). Analysis of primary human FL tumors has identified an association between the presence of *CREBBP* mutations and loss of MHC class II expression, as well as changes in the frequency and phenotype of tumor-infiltrating T-cells (Green et al. 2015; Han et al. 2022). Reducing tumor cell MHC class II expression has been found to enhance lymphomagenesis (Hashwah et al. 2017), suggesting that *CREBBP* mutations may in part drive lymphoma through immune evasion of FL progenitors via reduced antigen presentation.

Knock-out/knock-down of *Crebbp* in murine B-cells is not alone sufficient to drive lymphomagenesis but increases the penetrance and decreases the latency of lymphoma driven by *Bcl2* overexpression (Garcia-Ramirez et al. 2017; Jiang et al. 2017; Zhang et al. 2017). Regions of reduced H3K27Ac in these tumors were significantly enriched for enhancer elements that were previously found to be bound by the BCL6 transcription factor, and were accompanied by reduced expression of genes and pathways that are suppressed by BCL6 including antigen presentation on MHC class II, BCR signaling, and interferon signaling (Jiang et al. 2017; Meyer et al. 2019). At the pathway level, these results were consistent with observations from primary human FLs, but key differences were noted with respect to the magnitude of change observed in association with knock-out/knock-down of *Crebbp* in murine B-cells compared to those observed in association with *CREBBP* point mutations in primary tumors. The use of CRISPR/Cas9 gene editing to introduce the *CREBBP* R1446C KAT domain hotspot mutation into a lymphoma cell line later revealed that the *CREBBP* R1446C mutation causes a more severe reduction H3K27Ac and gene expression compared to isogenic cells bearing biallelic frameshift mutations (KO) (Mondello et al. 2020). This was associated with a more profound suppression of BCL6 target genes, including those with a role in antigen presentation on MHC class II and interferon signaling, in cells bearing the *CREBBP R1446C* mutation compared to isogenic KOs. The BCL6 transcription factor acts as a transcriptional repressor through the recruitment of multi-protein co-repressor complexes such as the SMRT/HDAC3 complex that leads to histone deacetylation. These data therefore suggested that CREBBP mutation may lead to a loss antagonism between CREBBP and BCL6-HDAC3, which may be potentially targetable with an HDAC3-selective inhibitor. In line with this, treatment of *CREBBP* mutant cells with HDAC3 inhibitor restored histone acetylation and expression of genes that were reduced in association with *CREBBP* mutation, including genes with a role in antigen presentation and interferon signaling. However, this effect was not restricted to *CREBBP* mutant cells, due to the normal antagonism between CREBBP and BCL6-HDAC3 that exists independently of mutation. That is, *CREBBP* mutation drove a reduced baseline expression of genes that are antagonistically regulated by CREBBP and BCL6-HDAC3 (Figure 14.2), but HDAC3 inhibition was able to promote the expression of these genes in both wild-type (WT) and mutant cells.

CREBBP mutations have also been observed to be associated with reduced acetylation of non-histone proteins such as p53 and BCL6 (Pasqualucci et al. 2011). Consistent with this, conditional knock-out of *Crebbp* in murine B-cells leads to a significant attenuation of p53 acetylation in response to DNA damage, and reduced DNA damage response (Horton et al. 2017). It is therefore likely that perturbed acetylation of non-histone proteins play an important role in the pathobiology of *CREBBP* mutant tumors, but the relative importance of these changes and their interplay with histone acetylation remains to be defined. Loss of Crebbp function in conditional knock-out mice and via inducible Cas9-KO has also been found to result in compensation by Ep300, highlighting a potentially targetable paralogous-lethality associated with *CREBBP* nonsense/frameshift mutations that could be exploited using EP300 inhibition (Meyer et al. 2019). However, it is unclear to what degree EP300 is able to compensate for CREBBP in the setting of KAT domain point mutations. It will therefore be important to determine whether all recurrent *CREBBP* KAT domain point mutations have similar functional consequences, and how these proteins affect the function EP300 and/or the alternate wild-type CREBBP allele.

EZH2

The EZH2 gene encodes the catalytic subunit of the polycomb repressor 2 (PRC2) complex, which catalyzes the trimethylation methylation H3K27 (H3K27me3). This transcriptionally repressive mark has an important role in controlling the expression of developmentally regulated genes via the formation of "bivalent" promoters that possess both activating H3K4 trimethylation (H3K4me3) and repressive H3K27me3. Following developmental cues, these genes can be stably repressed or rapidly activated via the removal of either H3K4me3 or H3K27me3, respectively. Within the context of B-cells, the normal function of EZH2 is to epigenetically repress a subset of genes that are highly expressed in naive B-cells by creating bivalency at genes with H3K4me3-marked promoters, or by catalyzing the addition of H3K27me3 at gene promoters which do not carry the H3K4me3 mark. Some prominent examples of bivalent promoters in GCB cells include transcription factors that are involved in GC exit and terminal differentiation, such as *PRDM1*, *IRF4*, and *XBP1* (Beguelin et al. 2013; Souroullas et al. 2016), and the cell cycle regulators *CDKN1A* and *CDKN1B* (Beguelin et al. 2013). These genes are targets of the BCL6 transcription factor, master regulator of the GC reaction, which recruits EZH2 through a multi-protein complex including CBX8 and BCOR (Beguelin et al. 2016). Components of the PRC2 complex, including EZH2, are highly expressed in GCB cells (Raaphorst et al. 2000; Van Galen et al. 2004; Velichutina et al. 2010), and GCB-specific deletion of EZH2 in conditional knock-out mice significantly attenuates GC development (Beguelin et al. 2013), highlighting its critical role in GCB cell development that is independent of its somatic mutation. Silencing of the BCL6 target gene, *Cdkn1a*, by EZH2 is particularly important for promoting B-cell proliferation and GC formation, and deletion of *Cdkn1a* is sufficient to rescue GC formation in EZH2 conditional knock-out mice (Beguelin et al. 2017).

Mutations of EZH2 occur in 15–25% of FL and 5–10% of DLBCL (Green 2018) (25–45% of the EZB/C3 subtype of DLBCL (Chapuy et al. 2018; Wright et al. 2020); EZH2 mutation is a seed feature for the EZB subtype). These are predominantly missense mutations at Y641 (Morin et al. 2010), or less frequently A677 (Mccabe et al. 2012a), within the catalytic SET domain that creates a neomorphic change in activity. Specifically, the mutant allele possesses higher activity compared to the wild-type allele when using H3K27me2 as a substrate, but lower activity when using H3K27me0 or H3K27me1 as a substrate (Mccabe et al. 2012a; Yap et al. 2011). EZH2 mutations are always acquired as heterozygous events, and thus the mutant allele acts in concert with the wild-type allele to increase H3K27me3 (Yap et al. 2011).

Viral overexpression or conditional knock-in of the $EZH2^{Y641}$ allele within murine GCB cells leads to GC hyperplasia following immunization, though alone is insufficient to promote lymphomagenesis (Beguelin et al. 2013; Souroullas et al. 2016). Early studies showed that this may result from deepening repression of canonical EZH2 target genes within GCB cells, such as *Prdm1* and *Irf4*, as well as spreading of the H3K27me3 mark to a large number of neighboring promoters (Beguelin et al. 2020) (*de novo* targets). The spreading of H3K27me3 may be restricted within topologically associated domains (TADs), leading to the coordinated repression of neighboring tumor suppressor genes (Donaldson-Collier et al. 2019). A number of these genes are involved in GC exit and terminal differentiation, first suggesting that their stable repression may contribute to lymphomagenesis in part by maintaining a GCB-specific epigenetic and transcriptional program and preventing GC exit (Beguelin et al. 2013; Souroullas et al. 2016). However, Beguelin *et al.* recently showed that GCB cells from $EZH2^{Y641}$ conditional knock-in mice accumulate within the LZ of the GC and have no significant block in terminal differentiation (Beguelin et al. 2020). The LZ polarization of EZH2-mutant B-cells is in part driven by the aberrant repression of genes that mediate interaction with TFH cells, leading to a loss of immune synapse formation, reduced CD40:CD40LG signaling, attenuated MYC expression, and reduced recycling to the DZ of the GC. However, EZH2-mutant GCB cells increased their association with FDCs and showed increased rates of proliferation within the LZ that was sensitive to FDC blockade. They were thereby able to maintain GC reactions in the absence of CD40 signaling. EZH2 mutations may therefore serve to deregulate normal programs of GCB-cell development that orchestrate clonal selection within the LZ, allowing GCB cells to survive and proliferate within the LZ in a manner that is independent of their affinity for antigen, but dependent upon FDCs.

Consistent with a perturbation of T-cell interactions associated with EZH2 mutations, analysis of DLBCL tumors with loss of MHC class I and MHC class II expression identified an association with EZH2 mutations (Ennishi et al. 2019). However, it is unclear if this association may have been driven by the co-association with other mutations that are highly frequent in the EZB/C3 subtype of DLBCL, such as CREBBP mutation, because these mutations were not evaluated. Furthermore, although loss of MHC expression tended to be associated with reduced frequencies of tumor-infiltrating CD4 and CD8 T-cells (Ennishi et al. 2019), comparison of DLBCL tumors by EZH2 mutation status alone did not identify any significant differences between EZH2 wild-type and mutant cases (Beguelin et al. 2020). The consequences of EZH2 mutations on immune interactions and the lymphoma microenvironment therefore require further investigation.

EZH2 mutant DLBCL is sensitive to catalytic inhibitors of EZH2, providing a rationale for targeting EZH2 in FL and DLBCL (Mccabe et al. 2012b). Indeed, results of the phase 2 study of tazemetostat in relapsed/refractory FL (Morschhauser et al. 2019) showed a high response rate in EZH2 mutant tumors. However, responses were also observed in EZH2 wild-type cases. As EZH2 mutations occur in only 15–25% of FLs, treatment of an unselected patient population with tazemetostat would be expected to result in a relatively equal proportion of EZH2 mutant and EZH2 wild-type patients among responders. Thus, while EZH2 mutation is indicative of a targetable biology, this biology may also exist in the absence of mutation and be related to the critical role for EZH2 in normal GCB development (Beguelin et al. 2013).

Mutations Altering Higher Order Chromatin Structure

Chromatin is assembled into higher order topological structures that can be broadly categorized into "compartment B," consisting of closed chromatin with less interactions that is inactive, or "compartment A," consisting of more open chromatin with more interactions that is active and demarcated as TADs. The transition from naive to GCB cells following activation is associated with the opening of chromatin at thousands of sites, which is accompanied by increased promoter and enhancer interactivity (Bunting et al. 2016). This requires the remodeling of chromatin through the shuffling and eviction of nucleosomes, and changes in chromatin topology supervised by architectural proteins. Although it is clear that these processes can be deregulated by genetic alterations in GCB-derived lymphomas, their precise mechanistic contribution to disease etiology remains a subject of active investigation.

BAF Chromatin Remodeling Complex

BAF complexes drive the ATP-dependent mobilization and eviction of nucleosomes to convert chromatin from inactive to active states (Centore et al. 2020), and its continuous activity is required to maintain local accessibility and activity of enhancers (Iurlaro et al. 2021; Schick et al. 2021). BAF assembly occurs in a modular fashion to yield stoichiometrically distinct complexes: canonical BAF (cBAF), polybromo-associated BAF (PBAF), or non-canonical BAF (ncBAF). All three complexes contain one of the two mutually exclusive ATPases, SMARCA4 (aka Brg1) or SMARCA2 (aka Brm), which form the ATPase module with other proteins (Mashtalir et al. 2018). The core module containing SMARCB, SMARCC, SMARCD, and SMARCE proteins is assembled first. Binding of ARID1A or ARID1B to the BAF core facilitates binding of the ATPase module and yields the cBAF complex. Alternatively, binding of ARID2 to the BAF core can facilitate binding of a PBRM1-associated ATPase module and yields the PBAF complex. ARID-independent assembly can yield the ncBAF complex containing BRD9. These complexes assemble in a competitive fashion, dependent upon the relative abundance of complex-defining subunits and modules (Mashtalir et al. 2018). BAF complexes have both common and non-overlapping functions (Centore et al. 2020); for example, BRD9 can specifically tether ncBAF to a subset of *MYC* regulatory elements (Centore et al. 2020), and PBAF has been shown to regulate accessibility at IFNγ-responsive genes (Pan et al. 2018). These complex-specific roles are likely driven by differences in transcription factor interactomes.

GCB-derived lymphomas feature highly recurrent somatic mutations in genes encoding subunits of BAF complexes (Bouska et al. 2017; Ma et al. 2021; Wright et al. 2020). The most commonly affected BAF complex genes in lymphoma are *SMARCA4* (in 34% of pediatric BL, 17% of adult BL, 3.4% of DLBCL, and 4.5% of FL), *ARID1A* (~20% of pediatric/adult BL, 7.4% of DLBCL, and 14.6% of FL), and *BCL7A* (7.5% of pediatric/adult BL, 7.4% of DLBCL, and 10.6% of FL) (Ma et al. 2021) (Figure 14.2). Among DLBCLs, BAF mutations are particularly enriched in the newly defined EZB/C3 DLBCL subtype (Chapuy et al. 2018; Wright et al. 2020). *SMARCA4* is primarily targeted by inactivating mutations within the SNF2 or helicase domains, which inactivate the protein (Stanton et al. 2017), while most *ARID1A* mutations yield truncated proteins (frameshift and premature stop codon) and likely lead to loss of protein expression. Coding mutations of *BCL7A* are primarily missense mutations within the N-terminal conserved region of the protein (Ma et al. 2021) that may alter its association with the BAF complex (Balinas-Gavira et al. 2020). However, the mutation frequency of *BCL7A* in many studies may be underestimated due to the failure to account for splice site mutations (Balinas-Gavira et al. 2020) and mutations of its *cis*-regulatory element (Mathelier et al. 2015). Loss-of-function mutations in different BAF genes have the clear potential to alter distinct BAF complexes and transcription factor programs, but the degree to which alternative subunits (e.g. SMARCA2, ARID1B, BCL7B/C) may compensate for their loss is unclear. Knock-out of BCL7A in lymphoma cell lines leads to a proliferative advantage and increased expression of genes involved in B-cell activation (Balinas-Gavira et al. 2020). However, the functional consequence of *ARID1A* and *SMARCA4* mutations has not yet been investigated in the setting of B-cell lymphoma.

Linker Histones

The highly conserved HIST1H1 family of linker histones is encoded by eight genes that are functionally redundant but show differing patterns of expression during development (Izzo et al. 2008). *HIST1H1B*, *HIST1H1C*, *HIST1H1D*, and *HIST1H1E* are collectively mutated in ~30% of FL (Green et al. 2015; Li et al. 2014; Okosun et al. 2014) and ~26% of DLBCL (Yusufova et al. 2021), with the highest frequency within the MCD/C5 subtype of DLBCL (Chapuy et al. 2018; Wright et al. 2020), and primarily affect the globular domains of the protein. Linker histones reside outside of the core nucleosome particle and drive chromatin compaction by binding "linker DNA" between nucleosomes and "stiffening" the chromatin fiber, thereby reducing interactions. In addition, oligonucleosomes assembled in complex with HIST1H1 provide better substrates for PRC2 (Martin et al. 2006), providing a further platform for epigenetic repression. Mutations in the globular domain of HIST1H1 prevent their association with chromatin and lead to a gain of chromatin interactivity (Li et al. 2014; Yusufova et al. 2021). Mice with knock-out of *Hist1h1c* and *Hist1h1e* ($H1c^{-/-}H1e^{-/-}$) feature enlarged GCs with a selective expansion of centrocytes and an increased competitive advantage within the LZ compared to WT B-cells, associated with increased proliferation (Yusufova et al. 2021). Mechanistically, $H1c^{-/-}H1e^{-/-}$ featured focal decompaction of chromatin demarcated by TAD boundaries, with a subset of regions undergoing B-to-A (inactive to active) compartment switch with increased interactivity and expression. Decompacted regions showed increased H3K27me2 and reduced H3K27me3, and were highly enriched for developmentally regulated PRC2 target genes with roles in self-renewal. $H1c^{-/-}H1e^{-/-}$ cooperated with the VavP-Bcl2 allele to reduce the latency of lymphoma development, and endowed the lymphomas with the ability to be serially passaged in immunodeficient mice, possibly related to the enhanced stem-like properties associated with

H1c$^{-/-}$*H1e*$^{-/-}$ (Yusufova et al. 2021). Mutations of HIST1H1 genes may therefore drive lymphoma by derepressing genes that endowing GCB cells with increased capacity for self-renewal and enhanced competitive advantage within the GC reaction (Figure 14.2).

Must Read References

Beguelin, W., Teater, M., Meydan, C., Hoehn, K.B., Phillip, J.M. et al. (2020). Mutant EZH2 induces a pre-malignant lymphoma niche by reprogramming the immune response. *Cancer Cell* 37: 655–673 e11.

Chapuy, B., Stewart, C., Dunford, A.J., Kim, J., Kamburov, A. et al. (2018). Molecular subtypes of diffuse large B cell lymphoma are associated with distinct pathogenic mechanisms and outcomes. *Nat. Med.* 24: 679–690.

De, S., Shaknovich, R., Riester, M., Elemento, O., Geng, H. et al. (2013). Aberration in DNA methylation in B-cell lymphomas has a complex origin and increases with disease severity. *PLoS Genet.* 9: e1003137.

Mondello, P., Tadros, S., Teater, M., Fontan, L., Chang, A.Y. et al. (2020). Selective inhibition of HDAC3 targets synthetic vulnerabilities and activates immune surveillance in lymphoma. *Cancer Discov.* 10: 440–459.

Pasqualucci, L., Dominguez-Sola, D., Chiarenza, A., Fabbri, G., Grunn, A. et al. (2011). Inactivating mutations of acetyltransferase genes in B-cell lymphoma. *Nature* 471: 189–195.

Zhang, J., Dominguez-Sola, D., Hussein, S., Lee, J.E., Holmes, A.B. et al. (2015). Disruption of KMT2D perturbs germinal center B cell development and promotes lymphomagenesis. *Nat. Med.* 21: 1190–1198.

References

Asmar, F., Punj, V., Christensen, J., Pedersen, M.T., Pedersen, A. et al. (2013). Genome-wide profiling identifies a DNA methylation signature that associates with TET2 mutations in diffuse large B-cell lymphoma. *Haematologica* 98: 1912–1920.

Balinas-Gavira, C., Rodriguez, M.I., Andrades, A., Cuadros, M., Alvarez-Perez, J.C. et al. (2020). Frequent mutations in the amino-terminal domain of BCL7A impair its tumor suppressor role in DLBCL. *Leukemia* 34: 2722–2735.

Beguelin, W., Popovic, R., Teater, M., Jiang, Y., Bunting, K.L. et al. (2013). EZH2 is required for germinal center formation and somatic EZH2 mutations promote lymphoid transformation. *Cancer Cell* 23: 677–692.

Beguelin, W., Rivas, M.A., Calvo Fernandez, M.T., Teater, M., Purwada, A. et al. (2017). EZH2 enables germinal centre formation through epigenetic silencing of CDKN1A and an Rb-E2F1 feedback loop. *Nat. Commun.* 8: 877.

Beguelin, W., Teater, M., Gearhart, M.D., Calvo Fernandez, M.T., Goldstein, R.L. et al. (2016). EZH2 and BCL6 cooperate to assemble CBX8-BCOR complex to repress bivalent promoters, mediate germinal center formation and lymphomagenesis. *Cancer Cell* 30: 197–213.

Beguelin, W., Teater, M., Meydan, C., Hoehn, K.B., Phillip, J.M. et al. (2020). Mutant EZH2 induces a pre-malignant lymphoma niche by reprogramming the immune response. *Cancer Cell* 37: 655–673 e11.

Bouska, A., BI, C., Lone, W., Zhang, W., Kedwaii, A. et al. (2017). Adult high-grade B-cell lymphoma with Burkitt lymphoma signature: genomic features and potential therapeutic targets. *Blood* 130: 1819–1831.

Bunting, K.L., Soong, T.D., Singh, R., Jiang, Y., Beguelin, W. et al. (2016). Multi-tiered reorganization of the genome during B cell affinity maturation anchored by a germinal center-specific locus control region. *Immunity* 45: 497–512.

Calo, E. and Wysocka, J. (2013). Modification of enhancer chromatin: what, how, and why? *Mol. Cell* 49: 825–837.

Centore, R.C., Sandoval, G.J., Soares, L.M.M., Kadoch, C., and Chan, H.M. (2020). Mammalian SWI/SNF chromatin remodeling complexes: emerging mechanisms and therapeutic strategies. *Trends Genet.* 36: 936–950.

Chambwe, N., Kormaksson, M., Geng, H., De, S., Michor, F. et al. (2014). Variability in DNA methylation defines novel epigenetic subgroups of DLBCL associated with different clinical outcomes. *Blood* 123: 1699–1708.

Chapuy, B., Stewart, C., Dunford, A.J., Kim, J., Kamburov, A. et al. (2018). Molecular subtypes of diffuse large B cell lymphoma are associated with distinct pathogenic mechanisms and outcomes. *Nat. Med.* 24: 679–690.

De, S., Shaknovich, R., Riester, M., Elemento, O., Geng, H. et al. (2013). Aberration in DNA methylation in B-cell lymphomas has a complex origin and increases with disease severity. *PLoS Genet.* 9: e1003137.

Dominguez, P.M., Ghamlouch, H., Rosikiewicz, W., Kumar, P., Beguelin, W. et al. (2018). TET2 deficiency causes germinal center hyperplasia, impairs plasma cell differentiation, and promotes B-cell lymphomagenesis. *Cancer Discov.* 8: 1632–1653.

Dominguez-Sola, D., Victora, G.D., Ying, C.Y., Phan, R.T., Saito, M. et al. (2012). The proto-oncogene MYC is required for selection in the germinal center and cyclic reentry. *Nat. Immunol.* 13: 1083–1091.

Donaldson-Collier, M.C., Sungalee, S., Zufferey, M., Tavernari, D., Katanayeva, N. et al. (2019). EZH2 oncogenic mutations drive epigenetic, transcriptional, and structural changes within chromatin domains. *Nat. Genet.* 51: 517–528.

Ennishi, D., Takata, K., Beguelin, W., Duns, G., Mottok, A. et al. (2019). Molecular and genetic characterization of MHC deficiency identifies EZH2 as therapeutic target for enhancing immune recognition. *Cancer Discov.* 9: 546–563.

Filippakopoulos, P. and Knapp, S. (2012). The bromodomain interaction module. *FEBS Lett.* 586: 2692–2704.

Ford, D.J. and Dingwall, A.K. (2015). The cancer COMPASS: navigating the functions of MLL complexes in cancer. *Cancer Genet.* 208: 178–191.

Garcia-Ramirez, I., Tadros, S., Gonzalez-Herrero, I., Martin-Lorenzo, A., Rodriguez-Hernandez, G. et al. (2017). Crebbp loss cooperates with Bcl2 over-expression to promote lymphoma in mice. *Blood* 129: 2645–2656.

Gibson, B.A., Doolittle, L.K., Schneider, M.W.G., Jensen, L.E., Gamarra, N. et al. (2019). Organization of chromatin by intrinsic and regulated phase separation. *Cell* 179: 470–484 e21.

Gitlin, A.D., Shulman, Z., and Nussenzweig, M.C. (2014). Clonal selection in the germinal centre by regulated proliferation and hypermutation. *Nature* 509: 637–640.

Green, M.R. (2018). Chromatin modifying gene mutations in follicular lymphoma. *Blood* 131: 595–604.

Green, M.R., Gentles, A.J., Nair, R.V., Irish, J.M., Kihira, S. et al. (2013). Hierarchy in somatic mutations arising during genomic evolution and progression of follicular lymphoma. *Blood* 121: 1604–1611.

Green, M.R., Kihira, S., Liu, C.L., Nair, R.V., Salari, R. et al. (2015). Mutations in early follicular lymphoma progenitors are associated with suppressed antigen presentation. *Proc. Natl. Acad. Sci. U.S.A.* 112: E1116–25.

Han, G., Deng, Q., Dai, E., Dang, M., Ma, J. et al. (2022). Follicular lymphoma microenvironment characteristics associated with tumor cell mutations and MHC class II expression. *Blood Cancer Disc* 3 (5): 428–443.

Hashwah, H., Schmid, C.A., Kasser, S., Bertram, K., Stelling, A. et al. (2017). Inactivation of CREBBP expands the germinal center B cell compartment, down-regulates MHCII expression and promotes DLBCL growth. *Proc. Natl. Acad. Sci. U.S.A.* 114 (36): 9701–9706.

Horton, S.J., Giotopoulos, G., Yun, H., Vohra, S., Sheppard, O. et al. (2017). Early loss of Crebbp confers malignant stem cell properties on lymphoid progenitors. *Nat. Cell Biol.* 19: 11093–11104.

Ise, W., Fujii, K., Shiroguchi, K., Ito, A., Kometani, K. et al. (2018). T follicular helper cell-germinal center B cell interaction strength regulates entry into plasma cell or recycling germinal center cell fate. *Immunity* 48: 702–715 e4.

Iurlaro, M., Stadler, M.B., Masoni, F., Jagani, Z., Galli, G.G. et al. (2021). Mammalian SWI/SNF continuously restores local accessibility to chromatin. *Nat. Genet.* 53: 279–287.

Izzo, A., Kamieniarz, K., and Schneider, R. (2008). The histone H1 family: specific members, specific functions? *Biol. Chem.* 389: 333–343.

Jiang, Y., Ortega-Molina, A., Geng, H., Ying, H.Y., Hatzi, K. et al. (2017). CREBBP inactivation promotes the development of HDAC3-dependent lymphomas. *Cancer Discov.* 7: 38–53.

Ko, M., An, J., and Rao, A. (2015). DNA methylation and hydroxymethylation in hematologic differentiation and transformation. *Curr. Opin. Cell Biol.* 37: 91–101.

Kridel, R., Chan, F.C., Mottok, A., Boyle, M., Farinha, P. et al. (2016). Histological transformation and progression in follicular lymphoma: a clonal evolution study. *PLoS Med.* 13: e1002197.

Li, H., Kaminski, M.S., Li, Y., Yildiz, M., Ouillette, P. et al. (2014). Mutations in linker histone genes HIST1H1 B, C, D, and E; OCT2 (POU2F2); IRF8; and ARID1A underlying the pathogenesis of follicular lymphoma. *Blood* 123: 1487–1498.

Ma, M.C.J., Tadros, S., Bouska, A., Heavican, T., Yang, H. et al. (2021). Subtype-specific and co-occurring genetic alterations in B-cell non-Hodgkin lymphoma. *Haematologica* 107 (3): 690–701.

Martin, C., Cao, R., and Zhang, Y. (2006). Substrate preferences of the EZH2 histone methyltransferase complex. *J. Biol. Chem.* 281: 8365–8370.

Mashtalir, N., D'Avino, A.R., Michel, B.C., Luo, J., Pan, J. et al. (2018). Modular organization and assembly of SWI/SNF family chromatin remodeling complexes. *Cell* 175: 1272–1288 e20.

Mathelier, A., Lefebvre, C., Zhang, A.W., Arenillas, D.J., Ding, J. et al. (2015). Cis-regulatory somatic mutations and gene-expression alteration in B-cell lymphomas. *Genome Biol.* 16: 84.

Mccabe, M.T., Graves, A.P., Ganji, G., Diaz, E., Halsey, W.S. et al. (2012a). Mutation of A677 in histone methyltransferase EZH2 in human B-cell lymphoma promotes hypertrimethylation of histone H3 on lysine 27 (H3K27). *Proc. Natl. Acad. Sci. U.S.A.* 109: 2989–2994.

Mccabe, M.T., Ott, H.M., Ganji, G., Korenchuk, S., Thompson, C. et al. (2012b). EZH2 inhibition as a therapeutic strategy for lymphoma with EZH2-activating mutations. *Nature* 492: 108–112.

Meyer, S.N., Scuoppo, C., Vlasevska, S., Bal, E., Holmes, A.B. et al. (2019). Unique and shared epigenetic programs of the CREBBP and EP300 acetyltransferases in germinal center B cells reveal targetable dependencies in lymphoma. *Immunity* 51: 535–547.

Mondello, P., Tadros, S., Teater, M., Fontan, L., Chang, A.Y. et al. (2020). Selective inhibition of HDAC3 targets synthetic vulnerabilities and activates immune surveillance in lymphoma. *Cancer Discov.* 10: 440–459.

Morin, R.D., Johnson, N.A., Severson, T.M., Mungall, A.J., An, J. et al. (2010). Somatic mutations altering EZH2 (Tyr641) in follicular and diffuse large B-cell lymphomas of germinal-center origin. *Nat. Genet.* 42: 181–185.

Morschhauser, F., Tilly, H., Chaidos, A., Phillips, T., Ribrag, V. et al. (2019). Phase 2 multicenter study of tazemetostat, an EZH2 inhibitor, in patients with relapsed or refractory follicular lymphoma. *Blood* 134: 123.

Mullighan, C.G., Zhang, J., Kasper, L.H., Lerach, S., Payne-Turner, D. et al. (2011). CREBBP mutations in relapsed acute lymphoblastic leukaemia. *Nature* 471: 235–239.

Nutt, S.L., Hodgkin, P.D., Tarlinton, D.M., and Corcoran, L.M. (2015). The generation of antibody-secreting plasma cells. *Nat. Rev. Immunol.* 15: 160–171.

Ochiai, K., Maienschein-Cline, M., Simonetti, G., Chen, J., Rosenthal, R. et al. (2013). Transcriptional regulation of germinal center B and plasma cell fates by dynamical control of IRF4. *Immunity* 38: 918–929.

Okosun, J., Bodor, C., Wang, J., Araf, S., Yang, C.Y. et al. (2014). Integrated genomic analysis identifies recurrent mutations and evolution patterns driving the initiation and progression of follicular lymphoma. *Nat. Genet.* 46: 176–181.

Ortega-Molina, A., Boss, I.W., Canela, A., Pan, H., Jiang, Y. et al. (2015). The histone lysine methyltransferase KMT2D sustains a gene expression program that represses B cell lymphoma development. *Nat. Med.* 21: 1199–1208.

Pan, D., Kobayashi, A., Jiang, P., Ferrari De Andrade, L., Tay, R.E. et al. (2018). A major chromatin regulator determines resistance of tumor cells to T cell-mediated killing. *Science* 359: 770–775.

Pasqualucci, L., Dominguez-Sola, D., Chiarenza, A., Fabbri, G., Grunn, A. et al. (2011). Inactivating mutations of acetyltransferase genes in B-cell lymphoma. *Nature* 471: 189–195.

Pasqualucci, L., Khiabanian, H., Fangazio, M., Vasishtha, M., Messina, M. et al. (2014). Genetics of follicular lymphoma transformation. *Cell Rep.* 6: 130–140.

Raaphorst, F.M., Van Kemenade, F.J., Fieret, E., Hamer, K.M., Satijn, D.P. et al. (2000). Cutting edge: polycomb gene expression patterns reflect distinct B cell differentiation stages in human germinal centers. *J. Immunol.* 164: 1–4.

Rosikiewicz, W., Chen, X., Dominguez, P.M., Ghamlouch, H., Aoufouchi, S. et al. (2020). TET2 deficiency reprograms the germinal center B cell epigenome and silences genes linked to lymphomagenesis. *Sci. Adv.* 6: eaay5872.

Schick, S., Grosche, S., Kohl, K.E., Drpic, D., Jaeger, M.G. et al. (2021). Acute BAF perturbation causes immediate changes in chromatin accessibility. *Nat. Genet.* 53: 269–278.

Shinnakasu, R., Inoue, T., Kometani, K., Moriyama, S., Adachi, Y. et al. (2016). Regulated selection of germinal-center cells into the memory B cell compartment. *Nat. Immunol.* 17: 861–869.

Shukla, V., Samaniego-Castruita, D., Dong, Z., Gonzalez-Avalos, E., Yan, Q. et al. (2022). TET deficiency perturbs mature B cell homeostasis and promotes oncogenesis associated with accumulation of G-quadruplex and R-loop structures. *Nat. Immunol.* 23: 99–108.

Souroullas, G.P., Jeck, W.R., Parker, J.S., Simon, J.M., Liu, J.Y. et al. (2016). An oncogenic Ezh2 mutation induces tumors through global redistribution of histone 3 lysine 27 trimethylation. *Nat. Med.* 22: 632–640.

Stanton, B.Z., Hodges, C., Calarco, J.P., Braun, S.M., Ku, W.L. et al. (2017). Smarca4 ATPase mutations disrupt direct eviction of PRC1 from chromatin. *Nat. Genet.* 49: 282–288.

Van Galen, J.C., Dukers, D.F., Giroth, C., Sewalt, R.G., Otte, A.P. et al. (2004). Distinct expression patterns of polycomb oncoproteins and their binding partners during the germinal center reaction. *Eur. J. Immunol.* 34: 1870–1881.

Velichutina, I., Shaknovich, R., Geng, H., Johnson, N.A., Gascoyne, R.D. et al. (2010). EZH2-mediated epigenetic silencing in germinal center B cells contributes to proliferation and lymphomagenesis. *Blood* 116: 5247–5255.

Wright, G.W., Huang, D.W., Phelan, J.D., Coulibaly, Z.A., Roulland, S. et al. (2020). A probabilistic classification tool for genetic subtypes of diffuse large B cell lymphoma with therapeutic implications. *Cancer Cell* 37: 551–568 e14.

Yap, D.B., Chu, J., Berg, T., Schapira, M., Cheng, S.W. et al. (2011). Somatic mutations at EZH2 Y641 act dominantly through a mechanism of selectively altered PRC2 catalytic activity, to increase H3K27 trimethylation. *Blood* 117: 2451–2459.

Yusufova, N., Kloetgen, A., Teater, M., Osunsade, A., Camarillo, J.M. et al. (2021). Histone H1 loss drives lymphoma by disrupting 3D chromatin architecture. *Nature 589: 299–305.*

Zhang, J., Dominguez-Sola, D., Hussein, S., Lee, J.E., Holmes, A.B. et al. (2015). Disruption of KMT2D perturbs germinal center B cell development and promotes lymphomagenesis. *Nat. Med.* 21: 1190–1198.

Zhang, J., Vlasevska, S., Wells, V.A., Nataraj, S., Holmes, A.B. et al. (2017). The crebbp acetyltransferase is a haploinsufficient tumor suppressor in B cell lymphoma. *Cancer Discov.* 7: 322–337.

15

Quantitating and Characterizing the Effects of Epigenetic Targeted Drugs

Emily Gruber[1], Alexander C. Lewis[1], and Lev M. Kats[1,2]

[1] The Peter MacCallum Cancer Centre, Melbourne, Victoria, Australia
[2] The Sir Peter MacCallum Department of Oncology, University of Melbourne, Parkville, Victoria, Australia

Take Home Messages

- Technological advancements now enable precise analysis of various aspects of chromatin, with some methods capable of interrogating changes in individual cells.
- The effect of an epigenetic drug on chromatin and transcriptional output is complex and highly context dependent.
- Maximizing the efficacy of epigenetic drugs ultimately depends on a detailed understanding of their impact not only on malignant cells but also on non-malignant cells and in particular immune cells.

Introduction

Although mutational processes undoubtedly underpin oncogenic transformation, it has now become apparent that alterations that are not caused by changes in DNA sequence play an equally fundamental role in every aspect of cancer biology. So-called "epigenetic" changes, that is modifications to chromatin that affect its accessibility to or interaction with various protein factors, regulate not only transcription but also DNA replication and repair (Dawson 2017). The epigenetic state of a cell is stable but potentially reversible and is propagated during mitosis, passing information to daughter cells. As such, the epigenome controls both the phenotype of a particular cell (i.e. what a cell is doing at a given moment) as well as its capabilities (i.e. the ability of a cell to respond to a stimulus) and that of its progeny. In the context of cancer, these features enable malignant cells to rapidly adapt to changing environments during disease progression and withstand insults imposed by the immune system and anti-cancer therapies (Ushijima et al. 2021).

Chromatin structure and function is regulated at multiple levels by proteins that deposit, detect, or remove covalent modifications on DNA and histones and facilitate the complex three-dimensional folding of the genome (Allis and Jenuwein 2016). As discussed elsewhere in this book, genes encoding epigenetic regulators are among the most frequently mutated functional class in cancer, including in lymphoid malignancies (Cancer Genome Atlas Research 2013). Drugs that target many and varied epigenetic regulators are in development and are increasingly entering clinical use (Bates 2020; Cheng et al. 2019b; Dawson 2017; Marzluff et al. 2008; Ribeiro et al. 2019). Beyond their cell autonomous effects on cancer cells, an emerging theme is that epigenetic-focused drugs affect anti-cancer immunity by altering antigen presentation and differentiation of immune cells (Hogg et al. 2020). It is also important to note that biological processes such as kinase signaling cascades and metabolic pathways impinge on the epigenome (Lu and Thompson 2012). For that reason, many drugs that do not directly bind to or inhibit epigenetic regulators nonetheless have profound effects on chromatin that ultimately underpins the cellular response.

To understand how the epigenetic state of a cell has been altered by oncogenic processes or perturbed by drug treatment, it has been necessary to develop methodologies that enable the different aspects of chromatin to be analyzed. Epigenetic changes can occur uniformly across the entire genome, but more commonly they are confined to specific genomic regions. The dramatic drop in the cost of DNA sequencing over the past decade coupled with faster and more powerful computing has fueled a rapid increase in the number of techniques that can precisely map epigenetic features on a genome-wide level. Multiplexed analyses that simultaneously quantify several parameters and technological advancements that reduce the amount of input material that is required have now made it possible to study chromatin with incredible granularity.

In this chapter, we begin by summarizing widely used methods for mapping the epigenetic state. Our aim is not to present an exhaustive catalog of experimental protocols, but rather to outline general principles. We then discuss emerging single-cell techniques that are beginning to revolutionize

Precision Cancer Therapies: Targeting Oncogenic Drivers and Signaling Pathways in Lymphoid Malignancies: From Concept to Practice, Volume 1, First Edition. Edited by Owen A. O'Connor, Stephen M. Ansell, and John F. Seymour.

out understanding of non-genetic heterogeneity and plasticity. In the final section, we consider the complex molecular and cellular phenotypes induced by epigenetic drugs. We hope that this will aid readers in interpreting the vast number of publications that analyze the epigenome of cancer at baseline and in response to therapy and provide would-be-investigators with considerations for optimal experimental design.

Experimental Analysis of the Epigenome

DNA Methylation

Covalently linked DNA modifications affect gene expression and DNA repair and are frequently dysregulated in many cancers (Schübeler 2015; Stirzaker et al. 2014). Methylation of the 5′ position of cytosine (5mC) is the most common such alteration in mammals and is catalyzed by the DNA methyltransferase (DNMT) family of enzymes. Related, but far less abundant modifications are 5-hydroxymethylcytosine (5hmC), 5-formylcytosine (5fC), and 5-carboxylcytosine (5caC) that are derived from 5mC via sequential oxidation by the ten-eleven translocation (TET) hydroxymethylases. Although previously thought to be transient intermediates in the process of DNA demethylation, 5hmC is now recognized as a bona-fide epigenetic mark in its own right and analysis of the function of 5fC and 5caC is ongoing (Lio and Rao 2019).

In most tissues, DNA methylation occurs almost exclusively in the context of the sequence 5′-CG-3′, also referred to as a CpG dinucleotide. The exceptions are embryonic stem cells and neuronal tissues, where non-CpG methylation is more common, and accounts for ~20% of all methylation (Lister et al. 2009). There are ~28 million CpG sites in the human genome dispersed in a non-uniform pattern. The highest density of CpGs occurs in clusters termed CpG islands (CGIs) that often overlap with proximal promoters of house-keeping genes, followed by regions of intermediate CpG frequency usually found in gene bodies. The bulk of the rest of the genome is largely depleted of CpGs, although they are also found at lower frequency in CGI "shores," non-CGI promoters, and distal regulatory elements. Broadly, CGI promoter methylation is associated with gene silencing whereas gene body methylation is associated with active transcription. It is important to note, however, that these relationships are correlative and frequently break down especially in the context of acute perturbation (Spainhour et al. 2019). The extent to which altered DNA methylation is sufficient or necessary to influence gene expression remains under investigation (Schübeler 2015). Both *hyper*- and *hypo*-methylation states have been identified in different cancers, including seemingly opposing patterns in the same tumor type (Glass et al. 2017).

Numerous methods have been developed to analyze the methylome of cells that differs significantly with respect to the amount and quality of input DNA that is required, the regions of the genome that are covered, whether or not methylation is measured at single base-pair resolution, the complexity of the analysis, and the cost. These considerations are critical when selecting a particular approach. For example, if the loss of DNA methylation is expected to be "global," such as following treatment with hypomethylating agents (HMAs) (e.g. azacitidine), then measurement of a subset of representative highly methylated regions may be sufficient. In most other cases, however, methylation needs to be specifically measured at regions of interest and cannot be inferred from what may be occurring elsewhere in the genome. Broadly, methods can be divided into two types: conversion based and affinity based. Below we outline the principles, advantages, and limitations of some of the most commonly applied experimental workflows.

Bisulfite Conversion Methods

Methods for differential chemical conversion of unmethylated and methylated cytosines in DNA by sodium bisulfite were first developed in the mid-1990s and revolutionized methylome analysis (Clark et al. 1994; Frommer et al. 1992). Under specific conditions, bisulfite treatment of DNA deaminates unmethylated cytosines, but not 5mC or 5hmC, to uracil. When bisulfite-treated DNA is subsequently utilized as a polymerase chain reaction (PCR) template, cytosines that were unmethylated in the original sample are amplified as thymines, whereas 5mC and 5hmC residues remain as cytosines. Using this approach, it is possible to determine the methylation status of individual cytosines on either strand of a DNA template.

A simple protocol that takes advantage of this process and can be applied to estimate global DNA methylation levels in a sample is LINE-PCR (Yang et al. 2004). The human genome contains >15 000 long interspersed nucleotide elements (LINE), a subtype of retrotransposon that is widespread in all eukaryotic genomes. LINE regions are usually maintained in a heavily methylated state by the maintenance DNA methyltransferase DNMT1. If DNMT1 is pharmacologically inhibited or genetically depleted, methylation of LINE is lost following rounds of cell division (Yang et al. 2004). Using universal primers, it is possible to simultaneously amplify thousands of LINE regions from bisulfite converted DNA and their methylation status can then be measured using various approaches such as direct sequencing, pyrosequencing, or selective restriction digestion.

At the other end of the spectrum is whole-genome bisulfite sequencing (WGBS), theoretically capable of quantifying the percentage of methylation for every cytosine in the genome (Olova et al. 2018; Stirzaker et al. 2014). In early protocols, WGBS involved shearing genomic DNA, ligation of methylated adapters, followed by bisulfite conversion, PCR amplification, and next-generation sequencing (NGS) (Lister et al. 2009). Upward of 200 million paired-end reads are required to achieve sufficient sequencing coverage across the genome for a single sample, until recently making the cost prohibitive for most applications. However, with the cost of NGS continuing to fall, WGBS has become much more widely utilized. This in turn has driven the development of various modifications to all aspects of the original protocol, including amplification-free library preparation that reduces the amount of input DNA by several orders of magnitude (micrograms to nanograms) (Miura et al. 2012). It should be noted that each protocol has the potential to introduce unique biases and artifacts in the final sequencing output, and caution is required when comparing between datasets generated by different WGBS methods (Olova et al. 2018).

Intermediate alternatives that assess a subset of residues of interest have also been developed. Reduced representation bisulfite sequencing (RRBS) preferentially "selects" CpG-rich regions during library preparation by incorporating a restriction digestion step using a methylation-insensitive restriction enzyme such as MspI (Gu et al. 2010; Meissner et al. 2005). In a typical RRBS experiment, ~20 million reads are sufficient to provide coverage of ~1 million CpGs. Along similar lines but based on hybridization of bisulfite-converted DNA to arrays that contain predesigned probes, the Illumina Infinium Human Methylation 450 K BeadChip provides quantitative information on the methylation status of ~480 000 individual cytosines (Bibikova et al. 2011). BeadChip technology requires a little material, is compatible with DNA extracted from formalin-fixed, paraffin-embedded (FFPE) samples, and has been extensively used by The Cancer Genome Atlas consortium to map DNA methylation levels in thousands of tumors (Cancer Genome Atlas Research 2013). Common to both RRBS and BeadChip protocols is the fact that although only a relatively small fraction (<5%) of all CpGs are covered, the analysis is highly enriched for sites with a putative regulatory role such as those in promoters and enhancers (Akalin et al. 2012; Bibikova et al. 2011). Although this significantly reduces cost and complexity of analysis, an important caveat is that epigenetic events occurring in CpG poor areas that may be functionally significant are not visible.

Affinity-based Methods

Affinity-based methods utilize reagents that selectively bind to and capture methylated DNA fragments that can subsequently be quantified by hybridization or sequencing. Methylated DNA immunoprecipitation (MeDIP) and capture of methylated DNA by methyl-CpG binding domain-base proteins (MBDCap) are two variations on a theme that utilize antibodies specific for 5mC and a methyl-CpG binding domain protein, respectively (Serre et al. 2010; Weber et al. 2005). Neither protocol provides single base-pair resolution, but rather enrichment of methylated DNA fragments that contain multiple CpGs. In MeDIP, immunoprecipitation of single-stranded DNA favors coverage of regions of comparatively low CpG density. In contrast, MBDCap utilizes double-stranded DNA fragments and can capture regions of both high and low CpG density (Nair et al. 2011). Notably, however, because in both cases the efficiency of capture is dependent on the number and frequency of CpGs within a particular fragment, DNA methylation can be compared for the same genomic region between different samples, but not for different regions within the same sample (Stirzaker et al. 2014).

A major advantage of MeDIP and MBDCap is their capacity to provide comparatively broad coverage of the genome at low sequencing cost. For this reason, investigators have recently optimized these methods for analysis of circulating tumor DNA (ctDNA) (Aberg et al. 2017; Shen and Laird 2013). In comparison with recurrent mutations that are limited in number and often require a priori knowledge to enable sensitive detection, cancer-associated DNA methylation changes affect large parts of the genome, are reflective of cancer type, and are therefore well suited to monitor disease recurrence and treatment response in liquid biopsies (Keller et al. 2021).

Detection of 5hmC

Standard bisulfite conversion methods cannot discriminate between 5mC and its oxidized derivatives. OxBS-seq and TAB-seq are two protocols that incorporate additional steps into bisulfite sequencing to enable mapping of 5hmC in genomic DNA at single nucleotide resolution (Booth et al. 2012; Yu et al. 2012). In OxBS-Seq, 5hmC is chemically converted to uracil in a two-step process under conditions that leave 5mC unchanged (Booth et al. 2012). TAB-seq utilizes a combination of b-glucosyltransferase and TET1 treatment to convert cytosine and 5mC to uracil, while maintaining 5hmC (Booth et al. 2012; Yu et al. 2012). Affinity-based methods that specifically detect anti-5hmC such as anti-CMS have also been developed but have not been as widely used (Huang et al. 2012).

Histone Modifications, Histone Variants, and Chromatin-associated Proteins

The basic unit of chromatin is the nucleosome consisting of ~147 bp of DNA wrapped around a histone octamer comprising two copies of each of the four core histones – H2A, H2B, H3, and H4. H2A, H2B, H3 (and the linker histone H1) are encoded by multiple genetic isoforms that vary by a small number of amino acids and have non-identical functions (Marzluff et al. 2008). Histones are also decorated by a myriad of post-translational modifications (PTMs) including acetylation, methylation, phosphorylation, ubiquitination, and sumoylation (Zhao and Garcia 2015). The modifications occur on specific amino acids on the N-terminal tails of histones that protrude from the nucleosome core particle, and both the residues that are modified, as well as the specific PTM, ultimately influence chromatin function and transcription. Thus, the same PTM on different residues (e.g. histone 3 lysine 4 trimethylation [H3K4me3] or H3K27me3) or different PTMs on the same residue (e.g. H3K27me3 or H3K27ac) can have opposing effects on transcriptional output (Bannister and Kouzarides 2011).

As with DNA methylation, histone variants and PTMs are not uniformly distributed across the genome but are specifically associated with particular genomic features. Some modifications are enriched at transcription start sites or active enhancers, whereas others are predominantly present in gene bodies. A specific PTM can also play multiple roles in different regions of the genome, or indeed at different times during the cell cycle. A case in point is H2AT120Ph, that is enriched at centromeres and transcription start sites, where it has been implicated in chromosomal segregation and transcriptional activation, respectively (Aihara et al. 2016; Kawashima et al. 2010). During epigenetic reprogramming, alterations in chromatin patterns can be local or global depending on the nature of the stimulus. Detection of regional perturbations is reliant on the availability of highly specific affinity reagents (usually antibodies), whereas global changes in variant expression or PTM abundance can be accurately quantified by mass spectrometry-based proteomics. As outlined below, the two approaches have unique advantages.

Antibody-based Techniques for Mapping the Chromatin State

Among the most extensively used methods for analyzing the epigenome is chromatin immunoprecipitation with sequencing (ChIP-seq). In addition to genome-wide identification of histone variants and PTMs, ChIP-seq can also be applied to map chromatin-associated proteins including epigenetic readers, writers, and erasers as well as DNA binding transcription factors. A typical ChIP-seq protocol begins with chemical cross-linking of DNA and associated proteins followed by fragmentation. Antibodies that specifically recognize a particular histone PTM (or other factor in question) are then used to immunoprecipitate DNA fragments bound to them from the chromatin pool. The covalent links between DNA and protein are then reversed and NGS libraries prepared and sequenced (Robertson et al. 2007). Sequencing reads are mapped back to the genome enabling regions that are enriched for a particular modification compared with background to be identified (Nakato and Sakata 2021). Although early methods required tens of millions of cells for the procedure, progressive NGS improvements over the past decade now mean that analysis of many PTMs can be performed from thousands or even hundreds of cells (Lara-Astiaso et al. 2014).

One significant drawback of standard ChIP-seq methods is the need for chemical cross-linking that can alter antigen–antibody reactivity and generate false positive interactions between proteins and DNA. To overcome the need for cross-linking, cleavage under targets and release using nuclease (CUT&RUN) and cleavage under targets and tagmentation (CUT&Tag) were developed (Kaya-Okur et al. 2019; Skene and Henikoff 2017). These approaches tether DNA modifying enzymes to antibodies that bind to chromatin proteins or PTMs in their native conformation in permeabilized cells, thereby directing the enzymatic activity to specific genome regions. In CUT&RUN, an antibody targeting a protein of interest is used to direct protein A-MNase to excise DNA fragments from surrounding chromatin that are subsequently isolated and sequenced (Skene and Henikoff 2017). In CUT&Tag, regions of DNA surrounding the protein bound by the specific antibody are "tagmented" using a protein A-Tn5 fusion loaded with sequencing adapters (Kaya-Okur et al. 2019). Both methods can be used on very few cells, and in the case of CUT&Tag, individual cells can be analyzed.

Proteomic Analysis of Histones

Although mass spectrometry cannot map histone variants or PTMs to specific regions of the genome, it is a powerful alternative for the study of chromatin biology, especially in situations where antibody-based methods cannot be applied. Over 500 different histone PTMs have been detected, of which only a small subset (<15%) have validated antibodies (Zhao and Garcia 2015). Antibody assays analyze a single modification at a time, whereas proteomics can simultaneously measure many PTMs and variants, providing valuable insights into histone "cross-talk." Proteomics can also quantify variant specific PTMs and distinguish variants that are too homologous to be differentially detected by antibodies (El Kennani et al. 2018).

Numerous histone extraction methods and mass spectrometry protocols have been described. The most common "bottom-up" approach involves proteolysis of histone extracts using trypsin, separation of peptides by high-performance liquid chromatography (HPLC), and identification by tandem mass spectrometry (MS-MS) (Huang et al. 2015). However, because histones are rich in arginine and lysine, some regions get digested into peptides that are too small for HPLC-coupled MS-MS analysis. Detection of PTMs in these regions requires alterative techniques, such as "top-down" analyses that quantify large peptides or intact proteins.

Chromatin Accessibility

The physical compaction of DNA in the nucleus plays a fundamental role in the regulation of gene expression. Chromatin exists in two broad states of condensation – highly condensed or "closed" heterochromatin and relatively unwound or "open" euchromatin. Regulatory regions of actively transcribed genes, including gene-bodies, promoters, enhancers, and insulators, occur at open regions of chromatin and are thus accessible to transcriptional regulatory machinery (Klemm et al. 2019). On the other hand, regions where nucleosomes are compactly organized are closed and inaccessible to DNA binding factors and broadly associated with transcriptional silencing.

Although leukemias and lymphoid malignancies have a relatively low mutational burden, they often harbor malignant driver mutations in epigenetic regulators, including chromatin remodeling proteins such as *ARID1A* and *CHD2* (Jiang et al. 2013). Patterns in chromatin accessibility have been used to characterize cell-type-specific signatures, differentiate normal from leukemic cells, define sub-types of lymphoid leukemias and lymphomas, distinguish between malignant and non-malignant T-cells from individuals with lymphoid malignancies, and provide prognostic indication of response to epigenetic drugs in patients (Corces et al. 2016; Lara-Astiaso et al. 2014; Mehrmohamadi et al. 2018; Qu et al. 2017; Rendeiro et al. 2016).

Experimentally, chromatin accessibility is primarily quantitated by NGS of enzymatically cleaved DNA (DNase-seq, ATAC-seq, MNase-seq) or methylated DNA (NOME-seq) that is accessible to various molecular probes (Klemm et al. 2019). DNase I-hypersensitive site sequencing (DNase-seq) and assay for transposase-accessible chromatin using sequencing (ATAC-seq) are assays that profile open chromatin by sequencing cleaved DNA fragments that are accessible to DNase I and transposase, respectively. Nucleosome occupancy and methylome sequencing (NOME-seq) utilizes a CpG methyltransferase to demarcate accessible chromatin. Unlike DNase-seq, ATAC-seq, and NOME-seq, which sequence accessible chromatin, micrococcal nuclease digestion with sequencing (MNase-seq) uses MNase to cleave and digest accessible chromatin, enabling nucleosome occupancy profiling through sequencing DNA fragments that are associated with single nucleosomes. Despite the wide range of molecular probes and experimental protocols for assessing the accessible chromatin landscape, high correlation has been observed across methods (Klemm et al. 2019).

For DNase-seq, two main experimental methods have been developed: end-capture and double-cut. Both protocols begin with the partial DNase I-mediated DNA digest, using DNase I concentrations and incubation times that enable the preferential cleavage of open chromatin over DNA spanning nucleosomes (Klemm et al. 2019; Liu et al. 2019). The subsequent library preparations differ between the two methods. In theory, all DNase I cut sites are sequenced with the end-capture method, whereas the double-cut method only sequences fragments arising from two proximal cleavage events within accessible chromatin (Klemm et al. 2019; Liu et al. 2019). Following DNase I digest, the end-capture method proceeds with the ligation of adaptors to each DNase cut site, digestion with a type II restriction enzyme and enrichment of ~20 bp fragments (Klemm et al. 2019; Liu et al. 2019). On the other hand, the double-cut method utilizes a gel-electrophoresis size-selection step, to enrich for digested DNA fragments that lie within DNase hypersensitivity sites (Klemm et al. 2019; Liu et al. 2019). Although the end-capture method identifies more DNase I cut sites, the double-cut method is more widely utilized due to the simplified procedure and results in a higher specificity and signal-to-noise ratio (Klemm et al. 2019; Liu et al. 2019).

ATAC-seq utilizes a hyperactive Tn5 transposase to simultaneously cleave and ligate sequencing adaptors into genomic regions of accessible chromatin. Subsequent PCR amplification enriches for proximal double-cleavage events within accessible genomic regions. ATAC-seq is widely used to profile the population-average chromatin landscape as the experimental method is relatively simple and rapid, requires scarce material (as few as 500 cells and even single-cell resolution), and shows high concordance with DNase-seq protocols (Buenrostro et al. 2013; Klemm et al. 2019; Satpathy et al. 2019). In comparison, DNase-seq is time-consuming and requires more starting material. In addition to defining open and closed genomic regions, ATAC-seq can identify transcription factor binding sites, or "footprints," within accessible chromatin and provide nucleosome positioning information given sufficient depth of paired-end sequencing.

Genome Organization

Higher order chromatin structures, including chromosomal territories, A/B compartments corresponding to permissive/repressed chromatin, respectively, topologically associating domains (TADs), and chromosomal looping, can regulate transcription by bringing linearly distal genomic regions into close proximity. Three-dimensional (3D) chromatin architecture is important for transcriptional regulation, DNA replication, X chromosome inactivation, cell identity and cell fate decisions, VDJ recombination, and immune response modulation (Kempfer and Pombo 2020; Schmitt et al. 2016; Scourzic et al. 2021). Given the interplay between the 3D chromatin landscape and regulation of cellular processes, it is not surprising to find it dysregulated in human diseases. Aberrant chromatin organization has been linked to several immune disorders, including lymphoid malignancies. Compartment A/B switching, disruption of TAD boundaries, modulation in TAD activity, and dysregulated enhancer–promoter loop formations have been reported to contribute to aberrant gene expression that drives malignant transformation and proliferation in B-cell acute lymphoblastic leukemia (B-ALL), diffuse large B-cell lymphoma (DLBCL), T-cell acute lymphoblastic leukemia (T-ALL), mantle cell lymphoma (MCL), and multiple myeloma (MM) (Scourzic et al. 2021).

Chromosome conformation capture (3C)-based assays have become the primary protocols for examining the relationship between distal genomic loci and gene expression, by measuring long-range chromatin interactions through proximity ligation of fragmented cross-linked DNA (Kempfer and Pombo 2020). The original method, 3C, first described by Dekker et al. (2002), measures physical chromatin interactions between two genomic loci of interest (one vs. one). Following formaldehyde cross-linking of DNA/RNA/protein interactions, chromatin is enzymatically fragmented and the proximal cross-linked fragment ends ligated and purified. The resulting 3C library contains chimeric DNA fragments of all physically interacting, but linearly distal, DNA loci across the genome. PCR, using primers against regions of interest, is subsequently performed to quantify the interaction frequency between two long-range genomic loci. As such, 3C is low-throughput and requires prior knowledge of interacting distal genomic regions (Dekker et al. 2002; Kempfer and Pombo 2020).

The advent of NGS enabled 3C to be adapted for high-throughput quantification of genome-wide chromatin interactions at increasing resolution (Kempfer and Pombo 2020; Schmitt et al. 2016). Circular chromosome conformation capture (4C) quantifies all interactions made with a genomic locus of interest (one vs. all). Chromosome conformation capture carbon copy (5C) measures all genomic interactions made within a large region (many vs. many). Unlike 3C, 4C, and 5C, which require prior knowledge of the interacting genomic locus or region of interest, Hi-C provides an unbiased and genome-wide map of all intra- (*cis*) and inter- (*trans*) chromosomal interactions (all vs. all). Hi-C demarcates ligation junctions with biotin through DNA cross-linking and fragmentation, followed by biotinylation then ligation of fragment ends, and sonication to further shear the DNA fragments. Biotin is then cleaved from the ends of unligated fragments and biotin-labeled ligated-junctions enriched with streptavidin-coated magnetic beads. The Hi-C library is subsequently sequenced. Hi-C is currently the most widely used method for assessing long-range chromatin interactions (Kempfer and Pombo 2020; Schmitt et al. 2016). Although Hi-C provides an unbiased and genome-wide method for assessing physical chromatin interactions, Hi-C typically requires millions of cells, millions to billions of paired-end reads, and thus incurs high sequencing costs, and is lower in resolution when compared to other 3C-based methods with the same sequencing depth. The resolution of 3C-based methods refers to the size of the genomic windows which is permissible for the detection of chromatin interactions. Thus, a smaller genomic bin size corresponds with an increase in resolution. Due to high sequencing costs, Hi-C is typically conducted at a relatively low resolution (50 kb–1 Mb), which is capable of detecting A/B compartments and TADs, but unable to identify fine-scale chromatin loops and enhancer–promoter interactions which require <10 kb resolutions.

In recent years, computational and experimental advances have increased the mapping resolution of genome-wide chromatin interactions, while improving cost-effectiveness. Computational approaches, including HiCPlus, HiCNN, hicGAN, Deephic, HiCSR, and EnHiC, utilize mathematical modeling and machine learning to predict increasing resolutions from low-resolution Hi-C data (Chang et al. 2018; Hu and Ma 2021). Furthermore, the Hi-C methodology has been adapted to provide high resolution of all chromatin interactions associated with a specific protein probe (ChIA-PET, HiChIP, PLAC-seq) or genomic sequence probe (Capture-HiC) (Kempfer and Pombo 2020; Schmitt et al. 2016). Capture-HiC utilizes DNA and RNA oligonucleotide probes to hybridize to and enrich for specific regulatory loci fragments (e.g. promoter and enhancer regions) in a Hi-C library (Kempfer and Pombo 2020; Schmitt et al. 2016). The targeted enrichment of specific genome-wide interactions enables deep sequencing and high resolution at a significantly reduced cost. Chromatin interaction analysis by paired-end tag sequencing (ChIA-PET), Hi-C with ChIP sequencing (HiChIP), and proximity ligation-assisted ChIP sequencing (PLAC-Seq) combine Hi-C and ChIP to incorporate information about the association of DNA-binding proteins with physically interacting genomic loci (Kempfer and Pombo 2020; Schmitt et al. 2016). The major difference between ChIA-PET and HiChIP/PLAC-seq is when chromatin immunoprecipitation occurs; ChIA-PET performs protein pull-down prior to proximity ligation, whereas immunoprecipitation occurs downstream of *in situ* Hi-C and proximity ligation in the HiChIP/PLAC-seq methods. Since chromatin interactions are captured on intact nuclei in HiChIP/PLAC-seq, these methods require significantly fewer cells and provide increased sensitivity.

Emerging Technologies for Epigenomic Analysis of Single Cells

Intratumoral heterogeneity at the level of genetics, epigenetics, transcriptomics, proteomics, and spatial organization within a microenvironment is hallmark of cancer which underpin tumor evolution, metastasis, clinical response, and therapeutic resistance. Genetic diversity within tumors has been widely studied, with specific mutations associated with poor clinical and therapeutic outcomes. However, underlying genetic events cannot explain a large proportion of therapeutic response and resistance in cancers, especially in hematopoietic malignancies that have a low mutational burden, yet display inconsistent responses to therapeutic pressures (Bell et al. 2019). Thus, recent years have seen a greater appreciation for the role of non-genetic heterogeneity in cancer evolution and therapy resistance.

Epigenetic heterogeneity refers to the diversity of epigenetic states across a genetically clonal population of cells. Quantitating the epigenome and transcriptome using population-average ("bulk") methodologies is limited in their ability to measure non-genetic heterogeneity (Figure 15.1). Furthermore, experiments using cancer cell lines may not accurately recapitulate the epigenetic diversity seen in patients. Bulk sequencing methodologies have since been adapted in order to delineate non-genetic heterogeneity within a malignant population at single-cell resolution (Lim et al. 2020). Understanding intratumor heterogeneity will provide greater insight into the mechanisms that underpin tumorigenesis and therapeutic resistance, which will aid in the identification of prognostic markers and development of novel effective therapeutic strategies, ultimately improving clinical outcomes.

Early single-cell DNA and RNA sequencing methods were restricted in the total number of cells that could be analyzed in a single experiment (up to 100 single cells) (Navin et al. 2011; Tang et al. 2009). Although they provided important insights, they were limited in their ability to capture low-frequency cell populations and hence accurately measure the full heterogeneity of complex tumors. Recent advances, such as the improvements to library amplification and development of unique molecular identifiers (UMIs), barcoding strategies, high-throughput platforms, and computational methods, have greatly increased the number of cells that can be sequenced, improved the quality and reproducibility of the

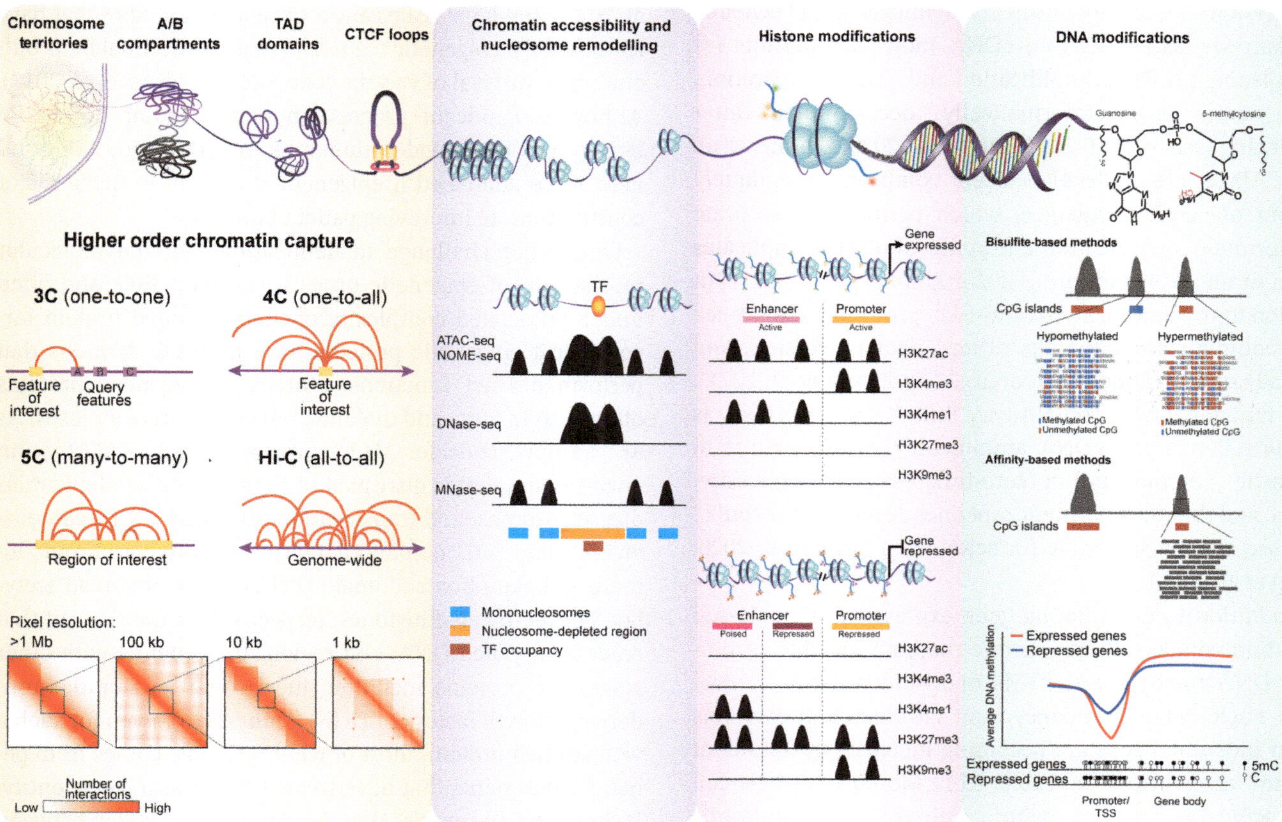

Figure 15.1 Methods for quantitating the epigenome. Epigenetic regulation of gene expression is depicted at the top at increasing resolution (left to right) from chromosome territories to DNA modifications. 1st panel: Chromosome territories, A/B compartments, TAD domains, and DNA looping can be measures using higher order chromatin capture methods including 3C, 4C, 5C, and Hi-C. 3C in a low-throughput method requires prior knowledge of both the locus of interest and query features. 4C, 5C, and Hi-C utilize next-generation sequencing to measure all DNA interactions with a specific locus, all interacting loci within a given region, or all interactions genome-wide, respectively. Chromatin interactions identified with high-throughput higher order chromatin capture methods are visualized as a heatmap of a matrix (n × n), where the genome (Hi-C) or regions of interest (4C and 5C) are divided into n bins of equal size and each element of the matrix contains the population-average probability of bin-i and bin-j interacting. 2nd panel: Chromatin accessibility is primarily quantitated by next-generation sequencing of enzymatically cleaved DNA (ATAC-seq, DNase-seq, MNase-seq) or methylated DNA (NOME-seq) that is accessible to various molecular probes. Collectively, these methods can identify "open" regions of chromatin, transcription factor binding sites, or "footprints," within accessible chromatin, and nucleosome positioning. 3rd panel: Methods that measure post-translational modifications (PTMs) of histone tails include ChIP-seq, CUT&RUN, and CUT&TAG. The co-localization of PTMs and their proximity to genes can define gene features (e.g. promoters and enhancers) and their state of function. 4th panel: The methylation status of cytosines across the genome can be measured using bisulfite-based methods (WGBS, RRBS) and affinity-based methods (MeDIP, MBDCap). Bisulfite-based methods are able to determine the methylation status of individual cytosines on either strand of a DNA template. Affinity-based methods utilize antibodies to enrich for methylated DNA fragments.

data, and significantly improved cost-effectiveness (Lim et al. 2020). Droplet microfluidics is the most widely used high-throughput platform to isolate single cells for high-throughput single-cell sequencing (Islam et al. 2014; Lim et al. 2020; Zilionis et al. 2017). This method encapsulates an individual cell within a single droplet where cell lysis and DNA/RNA barcoding occur. Single-cell RNA-sequencing (scRNA-seq) methods using droplet microfluidics occur in four stages: (i) single-cell isolation, (ii) reverse transcription and barcoding, (iii) cDNA amplification, and (iv) library preparation and sequencing (Islam et al. 2014; Lim et al. 2020; Zilionis et al. 2017). Reverse transcription occurs with oligonucleotides comprised four components: an oligo-dT primer, a cell-specific barcode sequence, a molecule-specific barcode (UMI), and a PCR or sequencing primer. The integration of cell-specific barcode sequences into cDNA molecules permits for multiplexing of cDNA amplification and library preparation, which can be bioinformatically deconvoluted after sequencing (Islam et al. 2014; Lim et al. 2020; Zilionis et al. 2017). UMIs are molecular labels comprised a uniquely random nucleotide sequence, which permits the accurate bioinformatic identification and removal of PCR duplicates (Islam et al. 2014; Lim et al. 2020; Zilionis et al. 2017). In addition to the optimization of wet-lab protocols, scRNA-seq also requires specialized algorithms, data processing, and normalization methods (Fan et al. 2020; Zhang et al. 2021). Since individual cells contain very little RNA, scRNA-seq is heavily reliant upon cDNA amplification which results in stochastic dropout and a zero-inflated gene expression matrix, and thus bioinformatic pipelines developed for "bulk" RNA-seq are inappropriate for scRNA-seq (Fan et al. 2020; Zhang et al. 2021).

In addition to quantitating gene expression at single-cell resolution, single-cell epigenomic methods capable of profiling DNA methylation, PTMs of histones, DNA accessibility, nucleosome occupancy, and chromatin interactions within individual cells are becoming increasingly abundant and are summarized in Table 15.1. Moreover, single-cell sequencing methods are being combined into multi-omic assays, enabling simultaneous examination of the transcriptome and multiple levels of the epigenome (Table 15.1). Given that the epigenome is multifaceted with highly complex relationships across epigenomic levels, cells are equipped with an arsenal of mechanisms to ensure a gene is activated or repressed. Therefore, perturbations within one layer of the epigenome may not uniformly impact gene expression at all affected loci. For example, not all genes are upregulated when their promoters become hypomethylated following DNMT1 inhibition. Such instances are discussed in greater detail in the next section. Single-cell multi-omic methods provide the ability to study the interplay between the different layers of the epigenome and gene expression. However, single-cell multi-omic protocols are still under active investigation to overcome the limitations that exist in current methods including low-throughput, low coverage, poor mapping efficiencies, and high costs.

Molecular and Cellular Effects of Epigenetic Drugs

The past decade has seen a rapid rise in the number of small molecules targeting epigenetic regulators (Table 15.2). Although many remain in pre-clinical or early clinical assessment, a number have entered clinical use (Bates 2020). Two notable developments have fueled this trend; the discovery through genome sequencing that genes encoding epigenetic regulators are frequently mutated in cancer (Kandoth et al. 2013), and large-scale cancer dependency studies that have identified the epigenetic regulators that are essential for proliferation or survival of various cancer cells (Meyers et al. 2017). Although significant progress in understanding chromatin biology has been made, numerous important questions still need to be addressed if epigenetic drugs are to make major contributions to improving patient outcomes.

One major challenge in delineating the true molecular mechanism of epigenetic drugs is the incredible and often underappreciated complexity of their intended protein targets. Most epigenetic proteins have multiple domains that perform distinct functions. Moreover, epigenetic proteins often exist in large and dynamic multi-protein complexes. As an example, consider MLL1 (also known as KMT2A), an onco-protein that is disrupted in a subset of acute leukemias due to chromosomal translocations at 11q23. MLL1 contains an enzymatic SET domain that writes H3K4me3; a bromodomain and plant homeodomain (PHD) fingers that read acetylated or methylated histones, respectively; a CxxC motif that reads methylated DNA; and regions that interact with other epigenetic proteins including menin and lens epithelium-derived growth factor (LEDGF) (Slany 2016). Even for such a well-studied protein, most of what we know comes from genetic experiments that have treated MLL1 as a single entity. It should be no surprise that there is limited overlap between the phenotypes caused by loss of the entire protein and pharmacological interference with a particular domain.

The recruitment and activity of epigenetic proteins at chromatin is also highly context dependent and can vary in different genomic regions (Figure 15.2). MLL1 fusion proteins physically interact with the scaffold protein Menin and are co-localized widely across the genome in MLL1-rearranged leukemic cells. However, disruption of the MLL1 fusion–Menin interaction by small molecule inhibitors causes displacement of the MLL1 fusion protein at *MEIS1* and *MEF2C* loci, but not at *HOXA* loci (Krivtsov et al. 2019). Similarly, the bromodomain inhibitor JQ1 has been posited to induce preferential displacement of its target BRD4 at so-called super-enhancer regions that control genes which maintain cell identity (Lovén et al. 2013). Interestingly, BRD4 contains two bromodomains

Table 15.1 Epigenetic and multi-omic single-cell methods.

DNA methylation		
scRRBS-seq	Genomic DNA is fragmented with restriction enzymes, followed by bisulfite treatment to convert unmethylated cytosines to thymines, amplification, and sequencing. Provides high coverage over dense CpG regions including CpG islands and promoters.	(Guo et al. 2015)
scPBAT	Bisulfite treatment of genomic DNA simultaneously fragments DNA and converts unmethylated cytosines to thymines. Next, multiple rounds of random priming and extension occur, followed by PCR amplification and sequencing. Provides genome-wide coverage of CpGs.	(Smallwood et al. 2014)
scCGI-seq	Genomic DNA is fragmented using a cocktail of methylation sensitive restriction enzymes followed by multiple displacement amplification, which selectively enriches for densely methylated CpG regions.	(Han et al. 2017)
sci-MET	Utilizes a single-cell combinatorial indexing strategy whereby: (1) thousands of intact nuclei are sorted into each well and indexed with well-specific barcodes during transposase tagmentation, (ii) nuclei are pooled and redistributed such that there is a low probability of two nuclei harboring the same well-specific indexes residing in the same new well, (iii) DNA is bisulfite treated, and (iv) PCR amplification incorporates a second index. The combinatorial indexes provide a cell-specific barcode. High-throughput method with high alignment efficiency.	(Mulqueen et al. 2018)
Histone modifications		
scChIP-seq	Utilizes droplet microfluidics to encapsulate individual cells within a single drop where cell lysis, chromatin fragmentation with MNase, and cell-specific DNA barcoding occur. DNA is subsequently pooled and chromatin immunoprecipitation performed. This is a high-throughput method, however, provides low coverage per cell.	(Rotem et al. 2015)
scChIC-seq	The single-cell chromatin immunocleavage sequencing (scChIC-seq) method uses a MNase conjugated to a specific antibody to target MNase to specific histone marks. Cleaved target sites are subsequently selectively PCR amplified. This method provides a high number of unique reads per cell, however, is low-throughput as single-cell libraries are not multiplexed.	(Ku et al. 2019)
scCUT&TAG	Pooled nuclei are incubated with an antibody of interest and chromatin tagmented at target loci with a Tn5 transposase-protein A fusion. Individual tagmented nuclei are subsequently encapsulated within single droplets and processed as per scATAC-seq methods. This is a cost-effective and high-throughput method, however, provides a low number of unique reads per cell.	(Bartosovic et al. 2021)
CoBATCH	Combinatorial barcoding and targeted chromatin release (CoBATCH) incorporates a combinatorial indexing strategy with barcoded Tn5 transposase-protein A fusions (PAT). Pooled nuclei are incubated with an antibody of interest, sorted into wells (~2 000 nuclei/well) then tagmented and indexed with well-specific barcoded PATs. Tagmented nuclei are redistributed to ensure a low probability of two same-indexed nuclei being present in the same well, and PCR amplification subsequently performed with well-specific primers. This is a high-throughput method that provides a high number of unique reads per cell.	(Wang et al. 2019)
iACT-seq	Index multiplexing strategy of antibody-guided chromatin tagmentation (iACT-seq) utilizes a similar and slightly simplified method to CoBATCH; however, rather than incubating the nuclei with the target antibody, the barcoded PATs are initially incubated with the antibody of interest to form antibody-bound-PATs prior to nuclei tagmentation and barcoding.	(Carter et al. 2019)
scChIL-seq	The single-cell chromatin integration labeling (scChIL-seq) method relies on the transposition of the DNA component of ChIL probes into regions proximal to antibody-bound histone marks of interest. The ChIL probe comprised a secondary antibody conjugated to a double-stranded DNA sequence containing a T7 promoter, primer sequence for library preparation, and Tn5 binding sequence. Following transposition of the DNA component of the ChIL probe, *in situ* transcription of labeled regions is performed with T7 RNA polymerase, then RNA extracted, and library preparation conducted. This method has a high signal-to-noise ratio, however, is low-throughput.	(Harada et al. 2019)
Chromatin accessibility and nucleosome occupancy		
scDNase-seq	The DNase-seq protocol was adapted for fluorescence-activated cell sorted single-cells in a 96-well plate. This method is low-throughput.	(Jin et al. 2015)
scATAC-seq	Several methods for single-cell ATAC sequencing have been reported including those that use combinatorial indexing, array-based microfluidic platforms, or droplet microfluidics. Key ATAC steps (cell lysis, tagmentation, barcoding, and amplification) are shared across all single-cell ATAC methods. scATAC-seq using droplet microfluidics is high-throughput, has a relatively simple workflow, and is commercially available. This method involves transposition of pooled nuclei followed by the encapsulation of individual nuclei within a single droplet where cell-specific barcoding of accessible chromatin occurs. Barcoded DNA fragments are then pooled, PCR amplified, and sequenced.	(Satpathy et al. 2019)

(Continued)

Table 15.1 (Continued)

Chromatin interactions		
scHi-C	Adapted the conventional "bulk" Hi-C method so that ligation of adaptors (and barcodes) occurs prior to nuclear lysis. Thus, scHi-C performs *in situ* chromatin cross-linking, restriction enzyme digest, biotin labeling, and ligation, followed by the isolation of individual nuclei and subsequent lysis, purification of interaction fragments, and PCR amplification. This method is low-throughput.	(Nagano et al. 2013)
sciHiC-seq	Single-cell combinatorial indexing Hi-C is a high-throughput method that involves sequential rounds of pooled nuclei barcoding and redistribution, which mitigate the need to isolate individual nuclei. Cells are fixed, lysed, digested with restriction enzymes *in situ* restriction, and a collection of nuclei distributed across 96 wells. Well-specific barcodes are introduced via ligation of indexed biotinylated adaptors, all intact nuclei pooled and proximity ligated, then nuclei are redistributed into wells at a lower density to ensure a low probability of two same-indexed nuclei being present in the same well. Ligation introduces a second well-specific barcode prior to affinity purification and library amplification.	(Ramani et al. 2017)
Multi-omics		
CITE-seq	High-throughput method that combines epitope and transcriptome information. Cells are incubated with barcoded antibodies that recognize target epitopes on the cell surface. Barcodes can be used to distinguish between different antibodies (different barcodes on different antibodies) and also between treatment conditions (a single antibody that is uniquely barcoded for each treatment condition). Labeled cells then undergo a modified method of droplet-microfluidics scRNA-seq, whereby the antibody barcode is captured, indexed, and sequenced.	(Stoeckius et al. 2017)
scMT-seq	Single-cell methylome and transcriptome sequencing. Individual nuclei are isolated, RNA extracted for Smart-seq2, and DNA extracted for scRRBS-seq. Provides high coverage over CpG-rich regions.	(Hu et al. 2016)
scM&T-seq	Simultaneously profiles of genome-wide DNA methylation and gene expression. Single cells are sorted into individual wells where RNA and DNA extractions occur. Single-cell bisulfite libraries are generated using the scPBAT method. Improved throughput in comparison to scMT-seq.	(Angermueller et al. 2016)
scNMT-seq	Single-cell nucleosome, genome-wide methylation, and transcription sequencing. Single cells are lysed and accessible DNA is methylated with a GpC methyltransferase. RNA from individual cells is captured and sequenced using Smart-seq2. DNA is isolated and undergoes scBS-seq library preparation and sequencing.	(Clark et al. 2018)
scCOOL-seq	Measures chromatin accessibility, nucleosome positioning, DNA methylation, copy number variation, and ploidy simultaneously from a single cell. This method is adapted from NOME-seq and PBAT-seq and is low-throughput.	(Guo et al. 2017)
iscCOOL-seq	Single-cell multi-omics method that simplified and improved upon the scCOOL-seq protocol. High-throughput and improved mapping efficacy.	(Gu et al. 2019)
scNOME-seq	Measures DNA methylation and chromatin accessibility and nucleosome occupancy. Low-throughput method adapted from "bulk" NOME-seq workflow, whereby after treatment with a GpC methyltransferase, individual nuclei are isolated prior to nuclear lysis, bisulfite conversion, PCR amplification, and library preparation.	(Pott 2017)
Sn-m3C-seq	Provides chromatin conformation and DNA methylation status from individual cells. Pooled fixed nuclei are digested with restriction enzymes and proximity ligated, then intact nuclei are isolated and DNA bisulfite converted, randomly primed and extended, barcoded and amplified.	(Lee et al. 2019)
SNARE-seq	High-throughput droplet-based single-cell method that measures gene expression and chromatin accessibility. Nuclei are permeabilized and tagmented with Tn5 transposase, then individual nuclei are encapsulated within a single droplet that simultaneously barcodes the mRNA and tagmented DNA. Barcoded fragments are pooled, then RNA and DNA extracted and separate library preparation and sequencing performed.	(Chen et al. 2019a)

and recently developed selective inhibitors of BD1 and BD2 have revealed that they play distinct roles in the recruitment of BRD4 to chromatin (Gilan et al. 2020).

Further layers of complexity result from the generally weak correlation between changes in the distribution of a particular epigenetic mark and gene expression (Figure 15.2). HMAs such as azacitidine and decitabine inhibit DNMTs and cause loss of DNA methylation on a genome-wide basis; however, their effects on transcription are much more selective (Klco et al. 2013). Consequently, the reasons why some tumors are significantly more sensitive to HMAs than others have remained elusive. Inhibitors of EZH2 are another example of

Table 15.2 Epigenetic drugs used for the treatment of cancer.

Target	Drug example	Disease	Effect on chromatin	Effect on gene expression	References
DNMT1	Azacitidine, decitabine	T-cell lymphoma, multiple myeloma	Global hypomethylation	Context dependent	(Sato et al. 2017)
Brd4	AZD5153 I-BET762	B-cell lymphoma, multiple myeloma	Global eviction from chromatin. Selective removal from super-enhancers	↓ *c-Myc, Irf4, Bcl2, Cdk6*	(Dawson et al. 2011; Lovén et al. 2013)
EZH2	Tazemetostat GSK126	B-cell lymphoma, multiple myeloma	Global loss of H3K27me3	Lymphoma- ↑*Irf4, Prdm1, Cdkn1a, Cdkn2b* Myeloma- ↓ *c-Myc, Irf4*, Prdm1, *Xbp1*	(Tremblay-LeMay et al. 2018; Julia and Salles 2021)
Menin	VTP50469	Mixed lineage leukemia rearranged acute lymphoblastic leukemia	Global eviction of menin, loci-specific eviction of Dot1l, MLL1, ↓ H3K79me	↓ *Mef2c, Meis1, Jmjd1c*	(Krivtsov et al. 2019)
Dot1l	EPZ-5676	Mixed lineage leukemia rearranged acute lymphoblastic leukemia	Global loss of H3K79me. Eviction from enhancer regions	↓ *Hoxa9, Meis1,*	(Daigle et al. 2013)
IDH2	Enasidenib	T-cell lymphoma	↑ 5-Hydoxymethylcytosine	Unknown	NCT02273739
HDACi	Romidepsin Vorinostat Panobinostat	T-cell lymphoma, multiple myeloma	↑ Chromatin accessibility	↑ Cell cycle arrest, apoptosis genes	(Imai et al. 2016)
P300	A-485	Multiple myeloma	↓ Chromatin accessibility	↓ *c-Myc, Irf4, Prdm1*	(Hogg et al. 2021)

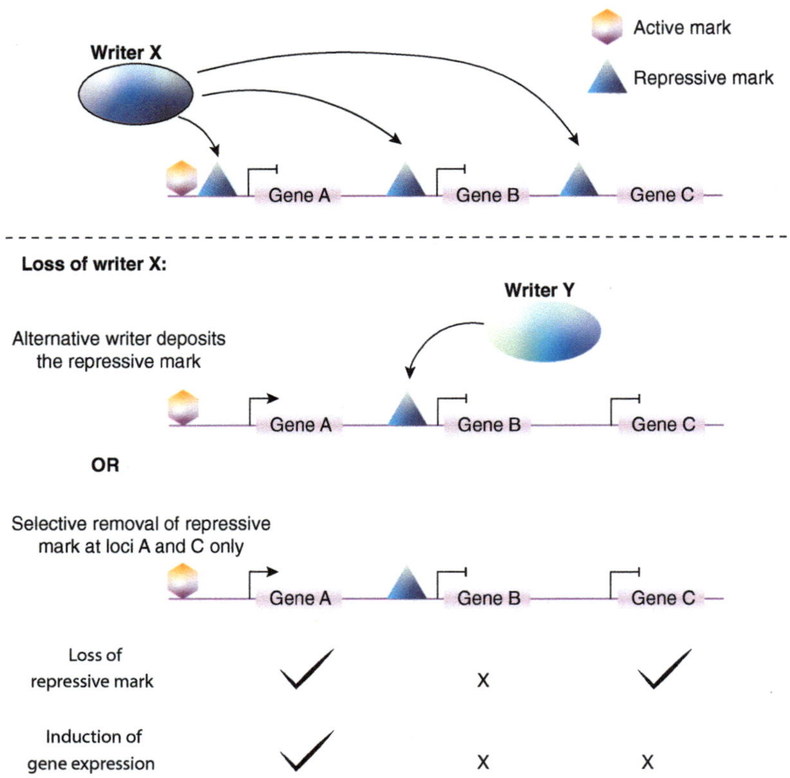

Figure 15.2 The complexity between an epigenetic mark and gene expression. Schematic depicting that loss of a specific epigenetic writer (X) that deposits a repressive mark (triangle) does not always correspond gene expression. Following loss of writer X, depletion of the repressive mark, and maintenance of the active mark upstream of gene A resulted in the induction of gene expression. The repressive mark was not lost from locus B, and thus gene B remained repressed. A possible explanation for this is that another writer (Y) was able to deposit the repressive mark, or that loss of writer X resulted in the loss of the repressive mark from specific loci. At locus C, the loss of the repressive mark does not result in the induction of gene expression.

epigenetic drugs with an apparent disconnect. EZH2 is a component of polycomb repressive complex 2 (PRC2) that deposits the histone PTM H3K27me3 associated with gene silencing. EZH2 inhibitors cause global reduction in H3K27me3, but as with HMAs, the transcriptional programs activated by drug treatment vary, even between relatively closely related B-cell lymphoma cell lines (McCabe et al. 2012). Indeed, in resistant cells, EZH2 inhibition largely fails to reactivate gene expression despite loss of histone methylation that is comparable to that observed in sensitive cells (McCabe et al. 2012).

Incomplete understanding of the molecular events triggered by epigenetic drugs, especially *in vivo*, continues to be a major stumbling block on the path to effective clinical deployment. The time to disease response can vary significantly depending on drug class, with the efficacy of some compounds manifesting only after months of treatment (DiNardo et al. 2018). In the absence of obvious biomarkers and extensive assessment of the effects of a drug on the epigenome and transcriptome of malignant cells, it has been difficult to address even the most fundamental questions about its activity in patients. Notably, however, recent technological advancements have now enabled the incorporation of such measurements to be incorporated into clinical trials, providing important insights into response and resistance (Wang et al. 2021).

It is also notable that, with the exception of EZH2 and mutant IDH1/2 inhibitors, the targets of most other epigenetic drugs do not carry frequent activating mutations in cancer and are also widely expressed in normal tissues. The purported basis for the therapeutic window of these drugs is the apparent "transcriptional addiction" of tumor cells (Bradner et al. 2017). It is certainly true that core transcriptional programs which are essential to sustain disease can be shut off by the removal of chromatin bound factors such as BRD4 (Chapuy et al. 2013; Zuber et al. 2011), Menin (Krivtsov et al. 2019), DOT1L (Bernt et al. 2011), EZH2 (Herviou et al. 2019), and P300/CBP (Hogg et al. 2021), leading to cell death or terminal differentiation. However, most of what we know about these processes has come from studying cancer cell lines or murine models that do not adequately represent the complexity of human cancer. As has become apparent, cancers are extremely epigenetically heterogenous and endowed with a high degree of plasticity, enabling adaptation to therapeutic pressure (Marine et al. 2020).

Beyond the cell-autonomous effects that epigenetic drugs exert on cancer cells is their influence on anti-tumor immunity. Immunostimulatory effects have been reported for histone deacetylase (HDAC) and BRD4 inhibitors in lymphoma models that likely contribute to their overall efficacy (Hogg et al. 2017; West et al. 2014). Conversely, suppression of EZH2 appears to dampen host immunity by stimulating the production of myeloid-derived suppressor cells (MDSCs) from normal hematopoietic progenitors. A greater appreciation of these factors is required to convert the partial responses often observed with epigenetic drugs into deep and long-lasting remissions.

Concluding Remarks

Our rapidly increasing knowledge of chromatin biology coupled with advancements in medicinal chemistry has opened up tremendous possibilities for development of new anti-cancer drugs. The next decade is likely to see a further increase in novel targets and novel first-in-class inhibitors. A major challenge for the field is to identify contexts where these compounds are most likely to make a meaningful impact. As discussed above and elsewhere in this book, epigenetic alterations in cancer are highly complex and may result for a range of reasons including perturbations in upstream metabolic or signaling pathways. As such, patient selection needs to be based on a comprehensive understanding of not only entire proteins but also the individual functional domains within them. As with other targeted drugs, it is unlikely that single-agent treatment can overcome the intratumor heterogeneity of complex cancers. Rationally designed combination strategies that seek to exploit novel vulnerabilities exposed as a result of epigenetic reprogramming offer the most promise.

Acknowledgments

This work was supported by funding from the Cancer Council of Victoria and a generous fellowship from the Brazis family.

Must Read References

Bates S.E. (2020). Epigenetic Therapies for Cancer. *N. Engl. J. Med.* 383 (7): 650–663.

Marine, J.-C., Dawson, S.-J., and Dawson, M.A. (2020). Non-genetic mechanisms of therapeutic resistance in cancer. *Nat. Rev. Cancer* 20 (12): 743–756.

Yoshida, H., Lareau, C.A., Ramirez, R.N. et al. (2019). The cis-regulatory atlas of the mouse immune system. *Cell* 176 (4): 897–912. e20.

References

Aberg, K.A. et al. (2017). A MBD-seq protocol for large-scale methylome-wide studies with (very) low amounts of DNA. *Epigenet.* 12 (9): 743–750.

Aihara, H. et al. (2016). Histone H2A T120 phosphorylation promotes oncogenic transformation via upregulation of Cyclin D1. *Mol. Cell* 64 (1): 176–188.

Akalin, A. et al. (2012). Base-pair resolution DNA methylation sequencing reveals profoundly divergent epigenetic landscapes in acute myeloid leukemia. *PLoS Genet.* 8 (6): e1002781–1002716.

Allis, C.D. and Jenuwein, T. (2016). The molecular hallmarks of epigenetic control. *Nat. Rev. Genet.* 17 (8): 487–500. doi: 10.1038/nrg.2016.59.

Angermueller, C. et al. (2016). Parallel single-cell sequencing links transcriptional and epigenetic heterogeneity. *Nat. Methods* 13 (3): 229–232.

Bannister, A.J. and Kouzarides, T. (2011). Regulation of chromatin by histone modifications. *Cell Research* 21 (3): 381–395.

Bartosovic, M. et al. (2021). Single-cell CUT&Tag profiles histone modifications and transcription factors in complex tissues. *Nat. Biotechnol.* 39 (7): 825–835.

Bates, S.E. (2020). Epigenetic therapies for cancer. *N. Engl. J. Med.* 383 (7): 650–663.

Bell, C.C. et al. (2019). Targeting enhancer switching overcomes non-genetic drug resistance in acute myeloid leukaemia. *Nat. Commun.* 10 (1): 2723–2715.

Bernt, K.M. et al. (2011). MLL-rearranged leukemia is dependent on aberrant H3K79 methylation by DOT1L. *Cancer Cell* 20 (1): 66–78.

Bibikova, M. et al. (2011). High density DNA methylation array with single CpG site resolution. *Genomics* 98 (4): 288–295.

Booth, M.J. et al. (2012). Quantitative sequencing of 5-methylcytosine and 5-hydroxymethylcytosine at single-base resolution. *Science* 336 (6083): 934–937.

Bradner, J.E. et al. (2017). Transcriptional addiction in cancer. *Cell* 168 (4): 629–643.

Buenrostro, J.D. et al. (2013). Transposition of native chromatin for fast and sensitive epigenomic profiling of open chromatin, DNA-binding proteins and nucleosome position. *Nature Methods* 10 (12): 1213–1218.

Cancer Genome Atlas Research, N. et al. (2013). The cancer genome atlas pan-cancer analysis project. *Nat. Genet.* 45 (10): 1113–1120.

Carter, B. et al. (2019). Mapping histone modifications in low cell number and single cells using antibody-guided chromatin tagmentation (ACT-seq). *Nat. Commun.* 10 (1): 3747.

Chang, P. et al. (2018). Computational methods for assessing chromatin hierarchy. *Comput. Struct. Biotechnol. J.* 16: 43–53.

Chapuy, B. et al. (2013). Discovery and characterization of super-enhancer-associated dependencies in diffuse large B cell lymphoma. *Cancer Cell* 24 (6): 777–790.

Chen, S. et al. (2019a). High-throughput sequencing of the transcriptome and chromatin accessibility in the same cell. *Nat. Biotechnol.* 37 (12): 1452–1457.

Cheng, Y. et al. (2019b). Targeting epigenetic regulators for cancer therapy: mechanisms and advances in clinical trials. *Signal Transduct. Target. Ther.* 4 (1): 62–39.

Clark, S.J. et al. (1994). High sensitivity mapping of methylated cytosines. *Nucleic Acids Res.* 22 (15): 2990–2997.

Clark, S.J. et al. (2018). scNMT-seq enables joint profiling of chromatin accessibility DNA methylation and transcription in single cells. *Nat. Commun.* 9 (1): 781.

Corces, M.R. et al. (2016). Lineage-specific and single-cell chromatin accessibility charts human hematopoiesis and leukemia evolution. *Nat. Genet.* 48 (10): 1193–1203.

Daigle, S.R. et al. (2013). Potent inhibition of DOT1L as treatment of MLL-fusion leukemia. *Blood* 122 (6): 1017–1025.

Dawson, M.A. et al. (2011). Inhibition of BET recruitment to chromatin as an effective treatment for MLL-fusion leukaemia. *Nature* 478 (7370): 529–533. doi: 10.1038/nature10509.

Dawson, M.A. (2017). The cancer epigenome: concepts, challenges, and therapeutic opportunities. *Science* 355 (6330): 1147–1152.

Dekker, J. et al. (2002). Capturing chromosome conformation. *Science* 295 (5558): 1306–1311.

DiNardo, C.D. et al. (2018). Durable remissions with ivosidenib in IDH1-mutated relapsed or refractory AML. *N. Engl. J. Med.* 378 (25): 2386–2398.

El Kennani, S. et al. (2018). Proteomic analysis of histone variants and their PTMs: strategies and pitfalls. *Proteomes* 6 (3): 29.

Fan, J. et al. (2020). Single-cell transcriptomics in cancer: computational challenges and opportunities. *Exp. Mol. Med.* 52 (9): 1452–1465.

Frommer, M. et al. (1992). A genomic sequencing protocol that yields a positive display of 5-methylcytosine residues in individual DNA strands. *Proc. Natl Acad. Sci.* 89 (5): 1827–1831.

Gilan, O. et al. (2020). Selective targeting of BD1 and BD2 of the BET proteins in cancer and immunoinflammation. *Science* 368 (6489): 387–394.

Glass, J.L. et al. (2017). Epigenetic identity in AML depends on disruption of nonpromoter regulatory elements and is affected by antagonistic effects of mutations in epigenetic modifiers. *Cancer Dis.* 7 (8): 868–883.

Gu, C. et al. (2019). Integrative single-cell analysis of transcriptome, DNA methylome and chromatin accessibility in mouse oocytes. *Cell Res.* 29 (2): 110–123.

Gu, H. et al. (2010). Genome-scale DNA methylation mapping of clinical samples at single-nucleotide resolution. *Nat. Methods* 7 (2): 133–136.

Guo, F. et al. (2017). Single-cell multi-omics sequencing of mouse early embryos and embryonic stem cells. *Cell Res.* 27 (8): 967–988.

Guo, H. et al. (2015). Profiling DNA methylome landscapes of mammalian cells with single-cell reduced-representation bisulfite sequencing. *Nat. Protoc.* 10 (5): 645–659.

Han, L. et al. (2017). Bisulfite-independent analysis of CpG island methylation enables genome-scale stratification of single cells. *Nucleic Acids Res.* 45 (10): e77.

Harada, A. et al. (2019). A chromatin integration labelling method enables epigenomic profiling with lower input. *Nat. Cell Biol.* 21 (2): 287–296.

Herviou, L. et al. (2019). EZH2 is overexpressed in transitional preplasmablasts and is involved in human plasma cell differentiation. *Leukemia* 33 (8): 2047–2060.

Hogg, S.J. et al. (2017). BET-bromodomain inhibitors engage the host immune system and regulate expression of the immune checkpoint ligand PD-L1. *Cell Rep.* 18 (9): 2162–2174. doi: 10.1016/j.celrep.2017.02.011.

Hogg, S.J. et al. (2020). Targeting the epigenetic regulation of antitumour immunity. *Nat. Rev. Drug Dis.* 1–25. doi: 10.1038/s41573-020-0077-5.

Hogg, S.J. et al. (2021). Targeting histone acetylation dynamics and oncogenic transcription by catalytic P300/CBP inhibition. *Mol. Cell* 81 (10): 2183–2200.e2113.

Hu, Y. et al. (2016). Simultaneous profiling of transcriptome and DNA methylome from a single cell. *Genome Biol.* 17 (1): 88.

Hu, Y. and Ma, W. (2021). EnHiC: learning fine-resolution Hi-C contact maps using a generative adversarial framework. *Bioinform.* 37: i272–i279.

Huang, H. et al. (2015). Quantitative proteomic analysis of histone modifications. *Chem. Rev.* 115 (6): 2376–2418.

Huang, Y. et al. (2012). The anti-CMS technique for genome-wide mapping of 5-hydroxymethylcytosine. *Nat. Protoc.* 7 (10): 1897–1908.

Imai, Y. et al. (2016). Action mechanisms of histone deacetylase inhibitors in the treatment of hematological malignancies. *Cancer Sci.* 107 (11): 1543–1549.

Islam, S. et al. (2014). Quantitative single-cell RNA-seq with unique molecular identifiers. *Nat. Methods* 11 (2): 163–166.

Jiang, Y. et al. (2013). Mechanisms of epigenetic deregulation in lymphoid neoplasms. *Blood* 121 (21): 4271–4279.

Jin, W. et al. (2015). Genome-wide detection of DNase I hypersensitive sites in single cells and FFPE tissue samples. *Nature* 528 (7580): 142–146.

Julia, E. and Salles, G. (2021). EZH2 inhibition by tazemetostat: mechanisms of action, safety and efficacy in relapsed/refractory follicular lymphoma. *Future Oncol.* 17 (17): 2127–2140.

Kandoth, C. et al. (2013). Mutational landscape and significance across 12 major cancer types. *Nature* 502 (7471): 333–339.

Kawashima, S.A. et al. (2010). Phosphorylation of H2A by Bub1 prevents chromosomal instability through localizing shugoshin. *Science* 327 (5962): 172–177.

Kaya-Okur, H.S. et al. (2019). CUT&Tag for efficient epigenomic profiling of small samples and single cells. *Nat. Commun.* 1–10. doi: 10.1038/s41467-019-09982-5.

Keller, L. et al. (2021). Clinical relevance of blood-based ctDNA analysis: mutation detection and beyond. *Br. J. Cancer* 124 (2): 345–358.

Kempfer, R. and Pombo, A. (2020). Methods for mapping 3D chromosome architecture. *Nat. Rev. Genetics* 21 (4): 207–226.

Klco, J.M. et al. (2013). Genomic impact of transient low-dose decitabine treatment on primary AML cells. *Blood* 121 (9): 1633–1643.

Klemm, S.L. et al. (2019). Chromatin accessibility and the regulatory epigenome. *Nat. Rev. Genetics* 20 (4): 207–220.

Krivtsov, A.V. et al. (2019). A Menin-MLL inhibitor induces specific chromatin changes and eradicates disease in models of MLL-rearranged leukemia. *Cancer Cell* 36 (6): 660–673.e611.

Ku, W.L. et al. (2019). Single-cell chromatin immunocleavage sequencing (scChIC-seq) to profile histone modification. *Nat. Methods* 16 (4): 323–325.

Lara-Astiaso, D. et al. (2014). Immunogenetics. Chromatin state dynamics during blood formation. *Science* 345 (6199): 943–949.

Lee, D.-S. et al. (2019). Simultaneous profiling of 3D genome structure and DNA methylation in single human cells. *Nat. Methods* 16 (10): 999–1006.

Lim, B. et al. (2020). Advancing cancer research and medicine with single-cell genomics. *Cancer Cell* 37 (4): 456–470.

Lio, C.-W.J. and Rao, A. (2019). TET enzymes and 5hmC in adaptive and innate immune systems. *Front. Immunol.* 10: 210.

Lister, R. et al. (2009). Human DNA methylomes at base resolution show widespread epigenomic differences. *Nature* 462 (7271): 315–322.

Liu, Y. et al. (2019). A practical guide for DNase-seq data analysis: from data management to common applications. *Brief. Bioinform.* 20 (5): 1865–1877.

Lovén, J. et al. (2013). Selective inhibition of tumor oncogenes by disruption of super-enhancers. *Cell* 153 (2): 320–334.

Lu, C. and Thompson, C.B. (2012). Metabolic regulation of epigenetics. *Cell Metab.* 16 (1): 9–17.

Marine, J.-C. et al. (2020). Non-genetic mechanisms of therapeutic resistance in cancer. *Nat. Rev. Cancer* 20 (12): 743–756.

Marzluff, W.F. et al. (2008). Metabolism and regulation of canonical histone mRNAs: life without a poly(A) tail. *Nat. Rev. Genetics* 9 (11): 843–854.

McCabe, M.T. et al. (2012). EZH2 inhibition as a therapeutic strategy for lymphoma with EZH2-activating mutations. *Nature* 492 (7427): 108–112.

Mehrmohamadi, M. et al. (2018). Distinct chromatin accessibility profiles of lymphoma subtypes revealed by targeted cell free DNA profiling. *Blood* 132: 672–672.

Meissner, A. et al. (2005). Reduced representation bisulfite sequencing for comparative high-resolution DNA methylation analysis. *Nucleic Acids Res.* 33 (18): 5868–5877.

Meyers, R.M. et al. (2017). Computational correction of copy number effect improves specificity of CRISPR–Cas9 essentiality screens in cancer cells. *Nat. Genet.* 49 (12): 1779–1784.

Miura, F. et al. (2012). Amplification-free whole-genome bisulfite sequencing by post-bisulfite adaptor tagging. *Nucleic Acids Res.* 40 (17): e136.

Mulqueen, R.M. et al. (2018). Highly scalable generation of DNA methylation profiles in single cells. *Nat. Biotechnol.* 36 (5): 428–431.

Nagano, T. et al. (2013). Single-cell Hi-C reveals cell-to-cell variability in chromosome structure. *Nature* 502 (7469): 59–64.

Nair, S.S. et al. (2011). Comparison of methyl-DNA immunoprecipitation (MeDIP) and methyl-CpG binding domain (MBD) protein capture for genome-wide DNA methylation analysis reveal CpG sequence coverage bias. *Epigenetics* 6 (1): 34–44.

Nakato, R. and Sakata, T. (2021). Methods for ChIP-seq analysis: a practical workflow and advanced applications. *Methods* 187: 44–53.

Navin, N. et al. (2011). Tumour evolution inferred by single-cell sequencing. *Nature* 472 (7341): 90–94.

Olova, N. et al. (2018). Comparison of whole-genome bisulfite sequencing library preparation strategies identifies sources of biases affecting DNA methylation data. *Genome Biol.* 19 (1): 33–19.

Pott, S. (2017). Simultaneous measurement of chromatin accessibility, DNA methylation, and nucleosome phasing in single cells. *eLife* 6.

Qu, K. et al. (2017). Chromatin accessibility landscape of cutaneous T cell lymphoma and dynamic response to HDAC inhibitors. *Cancer Cell* 32 (1): 27–41.e24. doi: 10.1016/j.ccell.2017.05.008.

Ramani, V. et al. (2017). Massively multiplex single-cell Hi-C. *Nat. Methods* 14 (3): 263–266.

Rendeiro, A.F. et al. (2016). Chromatin accessibility maps of chronic lymphocytic leukaemia identify subtype-specific epigenome signatures and transcription regulatory networks. *Nat. Commun.* 7 (1): 11938.

Ribeiro, M.L. et al. (2019). Recent advances in the targeting of epigenetic regulators in B-cell non-Hodgkin lymphoma. *Front. Genetics* 10: 986.

Robertson, G. et al. (2007). Genome-wide profiles of STAT1 DNA association using chromatin immunoprecipitation and massively parallel sequencing. *Nat. Methods* 4 (8): 651–657.

Rotem, A. et al. (2015). Single-cell ChIP-seq reveals cell subpopulations defined by chromatin state. *Nat. Biotechnol.* 33 (11): 1165–1172.

Sato, T. et al. (2017). DNA hypomethylating drugs in cancer therapy. *Cold Spring Harb. Perspect Med.* 7 (5).

Satpathy, A.T. et al. (2019). Massively parallel single-cell chromatin landscapes of human immune cell development and intratumoral T cell exhaustion. *Nat. Biotechnol.* 37 (8): 925–936.

Schmitt, A.D. et al. (2016). Genome-wide mapping and analysis of chromosome architecture. *Nat. Rev. Mol. Cell Biol.* 17 (12): 743–755.

Schübeler, D. (2015). Function and information content of DNA methylation. *Nature* 517 (7534): 321–326.

Scourzic, L. et al. (2021). Deciphering the complexity of 3D chromatin organization driving lymphopoiesis and lymphoid malignancies. *Front. Immunol.* 12: 669881–669881.

Serre, D. et al. (2010). MBD-isolated genome sequencing provides a high-throughput and comprehensive survey of DNA methylation in the human genome. *Nucleic Acids Res.* 38 (2): 391–399.

Shen, H. and Laird, P.W. (2013). Interplay between the cancer genome and epigenome. *Cell* 153 (1): 38–55. doi: 10.1016/j.cell.2013.03.008.

Skene, P.J. and Henikoff, S. (2017). An efficient targeted nuclease strategy for high-resolution mapping of DNA binding sites. *eLife* 6.

Slany, R.K. (2016). The molecular mechanics of mixed lineage leukemia. *Oncogene* 35 (40): 5215–5223. doi: 10.1038/onc.2016.30.

Smallwood, S.A. et al. (2014). Single-cell genome-wide bisulfite sequencing for assessing epigenetic heterogeneity. *Nat. Methods* 11 (8): 817–820.

Spainhour, J.C. et al. (2019). Correlation patterns between DNA methylation and gene expression in the cancer genome atlas. *Cancer Informat.* 18: 1176935119828776.

Stirzaker, C. et al. (2014). Mining cancer methylomes: prospects and challenges. *Trends in Genetics* 30 (2): 75–84. doi: 10.1016/j.tig.2013.11.004.

Stoeckius, M. et al. (2017). Simultaneous epitope and transcriptome measurement in single cells. *Nat. Methods* 14 (9): 865–868.

Tang, F. et al. (2009). mRNA-Seq whole-transcriptome analysis of a single cell. *Nat. Methods* 6 (5): 377–382.

Tremblay-LeMay, R. et al. (2018). EZH2 as a therapeutic target for multiple myeloma and other haematological malignancies. *Biomarker Res.* 6: 34.

Ushijima, T. et al. (2021). Mapping genomic and epigenomic evolution in cancer ecosystems. *Science* 373 (6562): 1474–1479.

Wang, F. et al. (2021). Leukemia stemness and co-occurring mutations drive resistance to IDH inhibitors in acute myeloid leukemia. *Nat. Commun.* 12 (1): 2607–2613.

Wang, Q. et al. (2019). CoBATCH for high-throughput single-cell epigenomic profiling. *Mol. Cell* 76 (1): 206–216. e207.

Weber, M. et al. (2005). Chromosome-wide and promoter-specific analyses identify sites of differential DNA methylation in normal and transformed human cells. *Nat. Genet.* 37 (8): 853–862.

West, A.C. et al. (2014). The combination of histone deacetylase inhibitors with immune-stimulating antibodies has potent anti-cancer effects. *OncoImmunology* 1 (3): 377–379.

Yang, A.S. et al. (2004). A simple method for estimating global DNA methylation using bisulfite PCR of repetitive DNA elements. *Nucleic Acids Res.* 32 (3): e38.

Yu, M. et al. (2012). Base-resolution analysis of 5-hydroxymethylcytosine in the mammalian genome. *Cell* 149 (6): 1368–1380.

Zhang, Y. et al. (2021). Single-cell RNA sequencing in cancer research. *J. Exp. Clin. Cancer Res.* 40 (1): 81.

Zhao, Y. and Garcia, B.A. (2015). Comprehensive catalog of currently documented histone modifications. *Cold Spring Harb. Perspect. Biol.* 7 (9): a025064.

Zilionis, R. et al. (2017). Single-cell barcoding and sequencing using droplet microfluidics. *Nat. Protoc.* 12 (1): 44–73.

Zuber, J. et al. (2011). RNAi screen identifies Brd4 as a therapeutic target in acute myeloid leukaemia. *Nature* 478 (7370): 524–528.

16

Clinical Experience with Epigenetic Drugs in Lymphoid Malignancies

Enrica Marchi, Ipsita Pal, and John Sanil Manavalan

Division of Hematology-Oncology, Department of Medicine, University of Virginia Comprehensive Cancer Center, VA, USA

Take Home Messages

- Epigenetic drugs have proven to be effective treatments in select types of lymphoid malignancies, especially the T-cell lymphomas.
- Drugs that affect the epigenome have been shown to sensitize and prime the tumor and the microenvironment to be more sensitive to chemotherapy and select immunotherapies.
- The real benefits of these drugs are likely to reside on the development of combination therapies, either with other epigenetic agents or traditional therapies.

Introduction

In the early twentieth century, the German researcher Theodor Boveri described the basic tenets of tumor biology: cells can turn cancerous when they lose the programming that controls their division and death. This loss usually results from a mutation that disrupts a cell's internal "checks and balances" and changes the order of nucleotides within the DNA code itself. Later, other researchers discovered that cells could become malignant through pathways that are not directly the result of changes in DNA sequence. This alternate path, typically called *epigenetics*, provides the cell with information on how the genetic code should be read and accessed by the cell's machinery. The epigenetic code is written on top of the DNA code, and ultimately plays a role in the activation or repression of genes. The study of epigenetics is a complex topic that has evolved since 1939 when British developmental biologist C.H. Waddington introduced the term. Now, the modern definition covers heritable gene expression changes that are not caused by alterations in the DNA sequence (Esteller 2008). Epigenetics is also a key component of an organism's normal development, from embryonic development through adulthood; dysregulation of the epigenetic machinery can significantly contribute to the origin and progression of human diseases including cancer. Epigenetic mechanisms regulate gene transcription and genomic stability and maintain normal cell growth, development, and differentiation (Bird 2007; Maze 2015). As such, epigenetic regulation is a dynamic and reversible process and epigenetic modifications are carried out by different proteins categorized as writers,erasers, readers, or movers (Bates 2020). Writers add modifications and include DNA methyltransferases (DNMTs), histone lysine methyltransferases (KMTs), and histone acetyltransferases (HATs); erasers, including histone lysine demethylases (KDMs) and histone deacetylases (HDACs), remove post-translational modifications. Recognition that bromodomain and chromodomain proteins "read" acetylated or methylated residues, respectively, led to the term readers. Movers are chromatin-remodeling proteins that move nucleosomes and allow gene transcription. Three out of the four families of epigenetic proteins – readers, writers, and erasers are considered to be druggable targets.

Epigenome and Cancer

Epigenetic processes comprise inherited, somatic, and reversible changes in gene expression in cancer cells. DNA methylation, histone modification (acetylation, methylation, phosphorylation, etc.), and non-coding RNAs are the major epigenetic mechanisms that control gene activity leading

Precision Cancer Therapies: Targeting Oncogenic Drivers and Signaling Pathways in Lymphoid Malignancies: From Concept to Practice, Volume 1, First Edition. Edited by Owen A. O'Connor, Stephen M. Ansell, and John F. Seymour.

to a number of cancers (Baylin and Jones 2016). Most cancer subtypes exhibit both hypermethylation of certain DNA sequences and hypomethylation of others relative to appropriate controls that account for the tissue specificity of DNA methylation (Ehrlich 2009; Feinberg and Vogelstein 1983). Specifically, hypermethylation of the promoter and enhancer region of tumor suppressor genes is a frequent event in cancer cells (Greger 1989). Genome-wide DNA hypomethylation is observed in cancer cells leading to chromosomal instability (Eden 2003), aberrant gene expression (Berdasco and Esteller 2010), and loss of imprinting (Wilson et al. 2007). A wide family of enzymes known as the DNMT regulates DNA methylation. The DNMTs are typically defined as DNMT1, DNMT1b, DNMT1o, DNMT1p, DNMT2, DNMT3A, DNMT3b and its isoforms, and DNMT3L (Monk et al. 1991).

Apart from methylation, histone modification is another process that plays an important role in cancer. Histone modifications control the active and inactive state of chromatin which ultimately influences gene expression. All of these epigenetic changes, labeled as "first hits" of tumorigenesis, occur before the development of cancer and are necessary for any genetic changes in a cancer cell (Plass 2013). Epigenetic changes are present in all human cancers and are now known to cooperate with genetic alterations to drive the cancer phenotype. Cancer genetics and epigenetics are inextricably linked in generating the malignant phenotype; epigenetic changes can cause mutations in genes, and, conversely, mutations are frequently observed in genes that modify the epigenome. Owing to the well-established role of epigenetic dysregulation in the origin and progression of cancer, lot of research effort has been invested in the development of epigenetic drugs as cancer therapeutics.

At present, eight agents affecting four discrete epigenetic targets (DNMT, HDAC, EZH2, and IDH1/2 inhibitors) have been approved by the US Food and Drug Administration (FDA) for the treatment of diverse hematologic malignancies (Table 16.1). In addition, a wide range of epigenetic-based drugs are undergoing investigation in clinical trials around the world. While we will describe in detail the clinical data with these different classes of epigenetic drugs, it is clear that the available agents, either alone or in combination, can have a far reaching impact on gene transcription. For example, the hypomethylating agents (HMAs) azacytidine and decitabine, which are indicated for the treatment of myelodysplastic syndromes (MDS) and acute myeloid leukemia (AML) with low blast percentage (Cashen 2010; Fenaux 2010; Garcia-Manero 2013), inhibit methylation of CpG islands leading to fine regulation of transcription. The HDAC inhibitors, which include drugs like vorinostat, romidepsin, belinostat, and panobinostat are approved for the treatment of patients with progressive or recurrent T-cell lymphomas (TCLs) like cutaneous T-cell lymphoma (CTCL) and peripheral T-cell lymphoma (PTCL) (Duvic 2007; O'Connor 2015; Olsen 2007) and multiple myeloma (panobinostat in combination with bortezomib). More recently, three additional epigenetic drugs were approved for hematologic malignancies, including: the IDH2 inhibitor, enasidenib, for patients with relapsed or refractory (R/R) AML whose disease harbors specific mutations in the *IDH2* gene (FDA approved in 2017) (Stein 2017); the IDH1 inhibitor, ivosidenib for the same indication, in patients whose tumors harbor specific mutations in the *IDH1* gene (FDA approved in 2021) (Abou-Alfa 2020), and the EZH2 inhibitor, tazemetostat for patients with R/R follicular lymphoma (FL) whose tumors are positive for EZH2 mutations and who have received at least two lines of prior therapies (FDA approved in 2020) (Morschhauser 2020). In this chapter, we will discuss the approved epigenetic agents in hematologic malignancies and some of the ongoing cutting-edge research, focusing on rational combination of different epigenetic agents.

Different Epigenetic Classes of Drugs in Hematologic Malignancies

DNMT Inhibitors

As discussed above and in other chapters, promoter hypermethylation and genome-wide hypomethylation play an essential role in the regulation of gene expression, likely leading to inactivation of tumor suppression genes (Esteller 2008; Nishiyama and Nakanishi 2021) and genomic instability, respectively (Cunningham 1998; Gama-Sosa 1983; Moore et al. 2013). DNMT1, DNMT3A, and DNMT3B are the three different DNMTs that catalyze DNA methylation through the addition of a methyl group from S-adenosyl-L-methionine on to the C5-position of cytosines to form 5-methylcytosine (5mC). DNMT1 is responsible for the maintenance of DNA methylation during replication by functioning as a substrate for hemi-methylated CpG dinucleotides (Robertson 2005). *De novo* methylation is carried out by DNMT3A and DNMT3B during embryogenesis and germ cell development (Okano 1999). DNA demethylation is carried out by ten-eleven translocation (TET) enzymes, such as TET2, which converts 5-methylcytosine to 5-hydroxymethylcytosine (5-hmC) (Rasmussen and Helin 2016). DNA HMAs can revert the gene silencing of tumor suppressor genes by targeting the DNMT activity and play an important role in novel epigenetic drug development (Lopez-Serra and Esteller 2012). DNMT inhibitors can be categorized into two types based on their chemical structure, namely, nucleoside analogs and non-nucleoside analogs. Nucleosides analogs are primarily derivatives of cytidine and inhibit DNMT through the formation of covalent bonds between DNA-cytosine methyltransferase

Table 16.1 FDA-approved epigenetic agents in hematologic malignancies.

Drug	Class	Conditions approved for	Year of approval
Azacytidine	DNMT inhibitor	Myelodysplastic syndrome Chronic myelomonocytic leukemia Acute myeloid leukemia	2004 2020
Decitabine	DNMT inhibitor	Myelodysplastic syndrome	
Vorinostat	HDAC (class I and class II) inhibitor	Advanced primary cutaneous T-cell lymphoma	2006
Romidepsin	HDAC (class I and class II) inhibitor	Cutaneous T-cell lymphoma	2009
Belinostat	Pan-HDAC inhibitor	Relapsed or refractory peripheral T-cell lymphoma (PTCL)	2014
Panobinostat	Pan-HDAC inhibitor	Relapsed multiple myeloma	2015
Tazemetostat	EZH2 inhibitor	Relapsed or refractory (R/R) follicular lymphoma	2020
Ivosidenib	IDH1 inhibitor	Newly diagnosed acute myeloid leukemia with an IDH1 mutation	2019
Enasidenib	IDH2 inhibitor	Relapsed or refractory AML and an IDH2 gene mutation	2017

and DNA-containing cytosine (Santi et al. 1984). The DNMT inhibitors (or hypomethylators) azacytidine and decitabine represent the first class of epigenetic-modulating drugs to be approved by the FDA. These drugs are pyrimidine nucleoside analogs of cytosine that are incorporated into DNA and form covalent bonds between the 5-azacytosine ring and the DNMT enzyme, thus causing irreversible DNMT inactivation (Esteller 2008; Siedlecki 2006). Major disadvantage of using these drugs include their poor bioavailability and chemical instability (Gros 2012). In comparison with nucleoside analogs, non-nucleoside analogs are less likely to be incorporated into DNA and hence offer a safer way to target DNA methylation. Among the non-nucleoside compounds several natural compounds have been identified such as genistein (Meeran et al. 2010), (−)-epigallocatechin 3-O-gallate (EGCG) (Fang 2003), and laccaic acid A (Fagan 2013). Other than natural compounds, repurposed drugs such as hydralazine (anti-hypertensive) and procaine (anesthetic agent) target the catalytic region of DNMT1 and DNMT3A (Arce 2006; Segura-Pacheco 2003), respectively (Cornacchia 1988). Novel inhibitors such as phthalimido-l-tryptophan (RG108) that block the active site of DNMT1 (Brueckner 2005) and the quinolone-based compound SGI-1027 (Datta 2009) have also been reported as non-nucleoside DNMT inhibitors. Unfortunately, non-nucleoside DNMT inhibitors showed much lower potency compared to the nucleoside DNMT inhibitors and their mechanism of action is not well investigated (Seidel 2012).

5-Azacytidine and Decitabine

HMAs like azacytidine and decitabine have been shown to reverse transcriptional repression secondary to hypermethylation. Azacytidine and decitabine induce their hypomethylating effects by irreversibly binding to DNMTs, which lead to proteolytically mediated degradation of the drug-DNMT complex depleting their protein levels (Stresemann and Lyko 2008). Although both drugs target DNMTs, their chemistry and pharmacology are distinctly different, with decitabine containing a deoxyribose structure, while azacytidinecomprised a ribose backbone. Because of this subtle biochemical difference, decitabine is 100% incorporated into DNA following tri-phosphorylation catalyzed by deoxycytidine kinase, deoxycytidylate kinase, and diphosphokinase while azacytidine is predominately integrated into RNA (80–90%), with only 10–20% being incorporated into DNA, as it requires an additional enzymatic step to convert the ribose to deoxyribose, a reaction catalyzed by ribonucleotide reductase (Stresemann and Lyko 2008). Due to these differences in their biochemical pharmacology, it is clear that the effects of azacytidine and decitabine are quite unique, and that these differences can have profound impacts on their mechanisms of action at the genetic level. The specific and detailed mechanism of action is still being researched.

Experiences in Lymphoid Malignancy

Recurrent mutations in various epigenetic genes have been recently described in specific subtypes of non-Hodgkin's lymphoma (Cairns 2012; Clozel 2013). These mutations can play a role in the pathogenesis of the disease and agents modulating DNA and histone methylation, such as inhibitors of DNMT, EZH2, and HDAC, have demonstrated promising clinical results. Lymphomas derived from the germinal center (GC) diffuse large B-cell lymphoma (DLBCL), FL, and subtypes of PTCL including angioimmunoblastic T-cell lymphoma (AITL), and T follicular helper (TFH-PTCL) are characterized by significant epigenetic dysregulation. In an effort to target these derangements, DNMT inhibitors have been investigated alone and in combination as a means of improving response to chemotherapy in DLBCL patients, or in combination with other epigenetic agents in the treatment of PTCL.

The addition of DNMT inhibitors to standard chemotherapy has been evaluated in several phase 1/2 trials in patients with diffuse large B-cell lymphoma (DLBCL). In 2011, 10 patients with RR lymphoma (four DLBCL, three follicular lymphoma (FL), one Hodgkin's lymphoma (HL), one small lymphocytic lymphoma (SLL), one cutaneous T-cell lymphoma (CTCL) were treated with escalating doses of azacytidine prior to chemotherapy with cyclophosphamide, vincristine, and rituximab (Martin 2017). In this trial, one patient maintained a complete response (CR) for seven months, while another maintained a partial response (PR) for six months. Grade 3/4 toxicities included neutropenia, thrombocytopenia, anemia, nausea, bacteremia, abscess, and hypoalbuminemia. Subsequent trials have evaluated the role of DNMT inhibitors in newly diagnosed DLBCL. Twelve patients with newly diagnosed DLBCL received escalating doses of azacytidine in advance of R-CHOP (Clozel 2013). Azacytidine was administered subcutaneously (SQ) at escalating doses for five days, followed by chemotherapy. Nearly 91% (11/12) of patients had CRs, and more significantly 10 patients remained in remission at a median follow-up of 13 months. In 2017, oral azacytidine in combination with R-CHOP was utilized in a similar cohort of 33 patients with both DLBCL and FL (Martin 2017). Here, 97% (32/33) of patients responded, and the estimated one-year progression-free survival (PFS) was 86%. Interestingly, those with higher IPI scores had a similar estimated PFS to those with low IPI scores (84% vs. 89%). All patients, however, experienced grade 3 or 4 neutropenia, with four developing neutropenic fever, two with dose-limiting toxicities at the highest dose levels (reactivation of hepatitis C and prolonged neutropenia), and six requiring modifications of planned therapy. Decitabine was used in a larger, similarly structured trial (Zhang 2019). A total of 58 patients with treatment-naive DLBCL received escalating doses of decitabine prior to receiving R-CHOP. Of 35 evaluable patients at time of analysis, 30/35 patients (86%) responded, with 26 CRs and 4 PRs. At a median follow-up of 12 months, 25 patients remained in remission. Grade 3 or higher hematological toxicities were common, with neutropenia generally occurring for a short duration during the first cycle of treatment. No major hematological adverse events (AE) or death related to AEs occurred. These studies establish that priming with DNMT inhibitors can prolong survival in high IPI score DLBCLs and FLs. In contrast to other studies involving epigenetic regulators, these trials focus on treatment-naive patients, demonstrating a role for HMAs even in this early stage of newly diagnosed DLBCL. Durability of responses compared with R-CHOP monotherapy will still need to be assessed in a randomized fashion. In addition, attention to the molecular drivers of disease subtype must be evaluated. Just as has been performed in the analysis of Bruton's tyrosine kinase (BTK) inhibitors in DLBCL, understanding the biology that might be most sensitive to DNMT inhibitors will be imperative for this treatment strategy to be successful. Clinical trials assessing DNMT inhibitors in combination with salvage chemotherapy in R/R DLBCLs are ongoing; some examples include azacytidine in combination with R-ICE (NCT03450343) and decitabine combined with R $\pm$ DHAP (NCT03579082). To date, 15 patients were enrolled and 13 patients were evaluable. Of these patients the overall response rate (ORR) was 53.8% with one patient achieving a CR. The median time to disease progression, however, was only 2.5 months. An additional trial aims to evaluate the safety and efficacy of priming with low-dose decitabine followed by GVD (gemcitabine, vinorelbine, and doxorubicin) chemotherapy and the anti-PD-1 antibody (SHR-1210) in R/R primary mediastinal B-cell lymphoma. If a recommended phase 2 dose is identified, the addition of decitabine priming phase will be evaluated (NCT03346642). Finally, the role of DNMT inhibitors for the treatment of DLBCL is being evaluated in a randomized trial (NCT03579082) where patients are treated with R-DHAP with or without decitabine.

Several early clinical experiences have suggested that the use of DNMT inhibitors as monotherapy could also lead to significant responses in specific subtypes of PTCL, namely, AITL and TFH PTCL (Lemonnier 2018). Nineteen patients with R/R TCLs were treated with azacytidine SQ, with six patients also receiving infusions of rituximab for Epstein–Barr virus (EBV) positivity. Twelve of the 19 patients had AITL, and the ORR for these patients was 75% (9/12), with five CRs. Only two of the AITL patients experienced progression, at 86 and 499 days, respectively. Eight of the AITL patients were noted to have TET2 mutations, all of whom responded to therapy. The remaining seven patients in the cohort, who had other subtypes of TCL, were non-responsive to therapy, with only one PR. AEs included hematologic toxicities, polyneuropathy, and diarrhea (Delarue 2016). Combinations of the HMA, azacytidine or decitabine, have also been shown to be synergistic with HDAC inhibitors in pre-clinical models of TCL (Marchi 2015; Scotto 2021). Based on these findings, a phase 1/2 trial with oral azacytidine has been led by our group. In this study, 25 TCL patients (11 newly diagnosed, 14 R/R, 17 with AITL or TFH-subtype PTCL) were treated with oral azacytidine 300 mg daily from days 1 to 14, romidepsin at 14 mg/m^2 dosed on days 8, 15, and 22, administered on a 35-day cycle (Falchi 2021; O'Connor 2019). Of 19 evaluable patients, the ORR was 68% (13/19), with 42% CR (8/19). Response rates were comparable across newly diagnosed and R/R patients. Of the 11 evaluable patients with AITL or PTCL-TFH, there were 10 responses, with six CRs. A total of 90% (9/10) of patients with TET2 mutations responded. AEs included hematologic toxicities, lung infection, and febrile neutropenia, with no patients discontinuing therapy due to an AE. PFS of patients on trial was 7.9 months. While it appeared that the number of mutations in epigenetic genes was higher in patients that responded to treatment, a clear correlation with the presence of TET2 mutation and response to treatment remains to be established. Currently, a randomized phase 2B clinical trial comparing the combination of oral azacytidine and romidepsin versus standard of care in patients with R/R PTCL is accruing patients (*NCT04747236*). This trial aims to establish and compare PFS for the combination of azacytidine and romidepsin versus standard of care. Azacytidine is also being evaluated in a first-line, phase 2, single-arm trial in combination with CHOP chemotherapy for patient with PTCL. This trial is currently enrolling patients (NCT03542266) and preliminary result of the first 20 patients enrolled was presented at the 2021 ASH meeting (Ruan 2020). Finally, based on the preclinical observation that HMAs could sensitize the tumor and the microenvironment to immune-checkpoint inhibitors, several clinical trials are currently investigating this concept and assessing the role of combination of DNMT inhibitors with chemotherapy regimens, or immunotherapy. In addition, the role of decitabine in combination with pembrolizumab, or in combination with pralatrexate and decitabine, has been investigated in a phase 1B trial in patient with R/R PTCL and CTCL. The preliminary result of the trial on the first 13 patients enrolled has been presented (*NCT03240211*) (Marchi 2020).

Experiences in AML and MDS

While clearly not a lymphoid malignancy, early experiences with DNMT3 inhibitors were essentially entirely focused on myeloid diseases, and thus may serve as a frame of reference for how to study these agents in lymphoma. HMAs have been deployed for years for myeloid hematologic malignancies and have become the standard therapy for patients with high-risk MDS (HR-MDS) or AML who are not candidates for allogeneic HSCT and intensive chemotherapies (Gf 2020). Azacytidine and decitabine are lower intensity chemotherapy agents and have been approved to treat MDS by the FDA. On 1 September 2020, the FDA approved oral azacytidine for the maintenance treatment of patients with AML. As describe above, these two agents are slightly different in structure: azacytidine is a ribonucleoside, while decitabine is a deoxyribonucleoside (Lyko and Brown 2005) but they both act by depletion of DNMT. Clinical data suggests that azacytidine is more effective than decitabine (Fenaux 2010). Observational studies of these two agents have shown similar efficacy and toxicity profiles in the treatment of refractory anemia with excessive blasts (MDS-RAEB) (Salim 2016). Compared with conventional care regimens (CCR), both azacytidine and decitabine have shown delayed progression to AML (Fenaux 2009; Kantarjian 2006; Lübbert 2011). However, only azacytidine has shown a significant advantage in OS compared with CCR (median OS, 24.5 vs. 15 months, respectively) in patients with HR-MDS and AML with 20–30% marrow blasts (Fenaux 2009), establishing it as the first-line treatment of choice for those patients who are unfit for transplant.

Up to now, direct comparison of azacytidine and decitabine has been performed in rare, randomized trials, leading to the choice dilemma of these two agents for patients and physicians. Several meta-analyses have been conducted to compare the efficacy and safety of azacytidine and decitabine in MDS or AML patients. None of them made a comparison in HR-MDS and AML. Comparatively, these experiences in the lymphoid malignancies is much earlier, and more research needs to be conducted in order to better appreciate the differences between these two hypomethylating drugs, and how they impact the tumor microenvironment, and synergize with more conventional agents used in the disease.

Guadecitabine

Guadecitabine, a next-generation HMA, is a dinucleotide antimetabolite of a decitabine linked via phosphodiester bond to guanosine. Guadecitabine prolongs the exposure of tumor cells to the active metabolite, decitabine, leading to an enhanced uptake of decitabine into the DNA of rapidly dividing cancer cells. Guadecitabine is also resistant to degradation by cytidine deaminase. A study (Phase 1/2) with an aim to determine the genomic and epigenomic predictors of response to guadecitabine in R/R AML was recently completed. The study results indicated a 17% response rate to guadecitabine (two CR, three CR with CRi or CR with CRp) in the phase 1 component and 23% (14 CR, 9 CRi/CRp) in phase 2. Peripheral blood blasts and hemoglobin were identified as predictors of response and cytogenetics, gene expression, RAS mutations, and hemoglobin as predictors of survival (NCT01261312). Recently, the efficacy and safety of guadecitabine was evaluated in phase 3 study (ASTRAL-1 study) in adults with previously untreated AML. The patients selected were ineligible for intensive induction chemotherapy. The study design involved the administration of guadecitabine, delivered (SC, 60 mg/m^2/day for five days) in combination with either azacytidine (IV or SC 75 mg/m^2/day, seven days), decitabine (IV 20 mg/m^2/day, five days), or low-dose cytarabine (SC 20 mg b.i.d., 10 days), administered in 28-day cycles. The results of this investigation revealed that primary endpoints of CR rate or OS were not met (NCT02348489) Recently, Astex and Otsuka announced the evaluation results of guadecitabine in phase 3 ASTRAL-2 and ASTRAL-3 studies in patients with previously treated AML and MDS or CML. Based on the result of this trial, guadecitabine did not improve the OS and the study was unable to meet the primary endpoint. Once again, while interesting in myeloid diseases, there is essentially no experience with this agent in lymphoid malignancies.

HDAC Inhibitors

HDACs are essential for gene transcriptional activities. The alternation of HDACs expression, mutation, and/or inappropriate recruitments has been discovered in a broad range of tumors contributing to the tumorigenesis through a serial of biological pathways. More recently, it has been shown that aberrant expression of HDACs plays a central role in the pathogenesis of various subtypes of PTCL (Marquard 2009). HDACs, therefore, are a promising cancer therapeutic target. Based on their sequence homology, HDAC family consisting of 11 HDACs can be grouped into four enzyme classes: class I (HDAC1, HDAC2, HDAC3, and HDAC8), class II (HDAC4, HDAC5, HDAC6, HDAC7, HDAC9, and HDAC10), class III (SIRT1, SIRT2, SIRT3, SIRT4, SIRT5, SIRT6, and SIRT7), and class IV (HDAC11). Unlike their name, the deacetylase activity of HDACs is not specific to histones only. HDAC catalyzes the removal of acetyl groups from acetylated lysine residues in histones, resulting in changes in chromatin condensation and ultimately modulation of gene expression, which induces many of the cellular effects seen following exposure to inhibitors of these enzymes. Most HDAC inhibitors are pan-HDAC inhibitors, implying they inhibit both class I (HDACs 1, 2, 3, 8) and class II (HDACs 4, 5, 6, 7, 9, 10) HDACs. In addition, they inhibit the sole class IV HDAC referred to as HDAC 11. The clinically available HDAC inhibitors do not inhibit class III HDACs (sirtuins or SIRTs). Notably, in addition to inhibiting the deacetylation of HDAC, HDAC inhibitors can influence the acetylation status of non-histone proteins such as cytoplasmic proteins acetylation, influencing their post-translational state and subsequent function (Janke and Montagnac 2017).

The approval of belinostat adds to the list of HDAC inhibitors that have been approved for PTCL that also include romidepsin for CTCL and PTCL, vorinostat for CTCL, and chidamide, only approved in China for PTCL. Here, we discuss FDA-approved HDAC inhibitors in terms of their functional mechanism establishing the anti-tumor effects and potential clinical applications including the synergistic effects in combinational treatment.

Vorinostat

Vorinostat was the first HDAC inhibitor approved for the treatment of any malignancy. Also known as suberoylanilide hydroxamic acid (SAHA), vorinostat is an orally available HDAC inhibitor with activity against class I and class II HDACs (Kelly et al. 2003, 2005). In a panel of CTCL cell lines, exposure to vorinostat led to acetylation of histones, BAX, STAT6, and caspase-3, and triggered higher rates of apoptosis in peripheral blood mononuclear cells isolated from CTCL patients as compared to healthy donors (Zhang 2005). Vorinostat was first approved in CTCL after phase 2 and phase 2a studies demonstrated an objective response rate (ORR) of 24.2% and 29.5 %, respectively, with a time to progression (TTP) of 12–20 weeks (Duvic 2007; Olsen 2007).

Romidepsin

Romidepsin is a macrolide small molecule belonging to a family of bicyclic peptides, which selectively inhibits class I and to a lesser extent class II HDACs. Romidepsin was approved by the FDA in 2009 for treatment of CTCL and in 2011 for the treatment relapsed and refractory PTCL [Celgene Corporation (2014). Istodax (romidepsin) package insert. Retrieved from http://www.istodax.com/pdfs istodax_packageinsert.pdf]. The results of two separate phase 2 clinical trials formed the basis of this approval in R/R PTCL. In the first study, Piekarz and colleagues enrolled 47 patients with various subtypes of PTCL, including PTCL not otherwise specified (NOS), angioimmunoblastic, ALK-negative ALCL, and enteropathy-associated TCL (Piekarz et al. 2011). All of these patients had received prior therapy with a median of three prior treatments (range 1–11) and 18 (38%) patients had previously undergone autologous stem cell transplantation (SCT). The ORR was 38%, with CRs in 8 of the 45 patients. Responses were seen across the spectrum of subtypes enrolled, and the median DOR was 8.9 months (range 2–74). Patients with AITL, of which there were six cases enrolled, were noted to have a lower response rate, and only one patient achieved a response, albeit a sustained PR for 23 months. It is unclear why this aggressive subtype of PTCL responded less well to romidepsin; however, the sample size was small, and responses were more robust in future trials. Common toxicities included nausea, fatigue, transient thrombocytopenia, and neutropenia. In registration study, a larger registration-directed trial, 130 patients with PTCL, whose disease had failed to respond to at least one prior systemic therapy, were enrolled (Coiffier 2012, 2014). An independent review confirmed an ORR of 25%, including 15% of patients who achieved a CR or complete response unconfirmed (CRu). Similar response rates were seen across a variety of subset analyses, including number of prior therapies, presence of a prior SCT, and refractoriness to the most recent therapy. The median DOR was 17 months, and of the 19 patients who achieved CR/CRu, 17 (89%) continued to remain progression-free at a median follow-up of 13.4 months. Although the study population was not as diverse or as heavily treated as the one accrued in the PROPEL study, responses were seen in many of the subtypes, including PTCL-NOS (29%), AITL (33%), and ALK-negative ALCL (24%) (Coiffier 2014). A recent update published longer durations of response on the order of 22.3 months and median PFS and OS times of 4 and 11.3 months, respectively. The median DOR for all responders measured at 28 months was not reached for those who achieved a CR or CRu. Remarkably, even patients with a lack of response or a transient response to prior therapy achieved durable responses. None of the baseline characteristics examined in the subgroup analysis, including heavy pretreatment, response to prior therapy, and advanced disease, barred long-term responses to romidepsin.

Based on the result of these two trials, romidepsin received accelerated approval from the US FDA for patients with R/R PTCL. Bristol Myers Squibb subsequently conducted a confirmatory phase 3 study evaluating romidepsin plus CHOP (Ro-CHOP) versus CHOP in front-line for patients with PTCL. Unfortunately, the trial did not meet the primary efficacy endpoint of PFS, so, based on the negative result of the post-marketing confirmatory trial, romidepsin for R/R patients with PTCL was withdrawn from the market. Presently, romidepsin remains on the market only for patients with R/R CTCL.

Belinostat

Belinostat, *N*-hydroxy-3-[3-(phenylsulfamoyl) phenyl] prop-2-enamide, is a low-molecular-weight HDAC inhibitor with a sulfonamide–hydroxamide structure. Similar to vorinostat, the hydroxamate region of belinostat chelates zinc, a necessary element for the HDAC family of enzymes to properly function. Belinostat is a pan-HDAC inhibitor, inhibiting classes I, II, and IV HDAC isoforms with nanomolar potency. In July 2014, the FDA granted accelerated approval to belinostat for the treatment of patients with relapsed and/or refractory PTCL, making it the latest HDAC inhibitor to be approved. In March 2015, Foss and colleagues published the results of an open-label, multicenter phase 2 study of belinostat in 53 patients with relapsed and refractory PTCL or CTCL who failed at least one prior systemic therapy (Foss 2015). Patients were treated with belinostat given as 1000 mg/m^2 intravenously for five days on a 21-day cycle. A total of 24 patients with PTCL, 40% of whom had stage IV disease at the time of enrollment, had already received a median of three prior systemic therapies. A total of 29 patients with CTCL had received a median of one prior skin-directed therapy (range 0–4) and four prior systemic therapies (range 1–9); 55% had stage IV disease. The ORRs were 25% (PTCL) and 14% (CTCL). Treatment-related AEs occurred in 77% of patients and primarily included nausea (43%), vomiting (21%), infusion site pain (13%), and dizziness (11%). Treatment-related serious AEs included one grade 5 ventricular fibrillation; grade 4 thrombocytopenia; grade 3 peripheral edema, apraxia, paralytic ileus, and pneumonitis; and grade 2 jugular vein thrombosis. Subsequently, O'Connor and colleagues published the results of the pivotal phase 2 BELIEF trial (O'Connor 2015). In this study, 129 patients with R/R PTCL who relapsed after or were refractory to at least one prior systemic therapy received treatment with belinostat 1000 mg/m^2 daily on days 1–5 on a 21-day cycle. The ORR in the 120 evaluable patients was 25.8%, including 13 (10.8%) patients with CR and 18 (15%) patients with PR. The median DOR was 13.6 months, with the longest ongoing response currently reaching more than 36 months. Median PFS and OS were 1.6 and 7.9 months, respectively. Twelve of the enrolled patients underwent SCT after belinostat monotherapy. Similar to other HDAC inhibitors, the most common grade 3/4 AEs involved anemia (10.8%), thrombocytopenia (7%), dyspnea (6.2%), and neutropenia (6.2%). Subjects with AITL did surprisingly well with 46% of these patients showing response to treatment. It is important to recognize, however, that the subset analysis of this heterogeneous population was not designed to explore the effectiveness of belinostat in this specific subpopulation of patients. These data further emphasize the need for future disease-focused investigation with HDAC inhibitors in the T-cell malignancies.

EZH2 Inhibitors

EZH2 is a histone methyl transferase enzyme responsible for methylating lysine 27 (mono-, di-, and trimethylation) in histone H3 (H3K27). H3K27me3 is more frequently interlinked with transcriptional repression, and it is a significant epigenetic phenomenon during tissue development and stem cell fate determination. Specifically, functioning of EZH2 in biological processes occurs through three types of mechanism, including PRC2-dependent H3K27 methylation, PRC2-dependent non-histone protein methylation, and PRC2-independent gene transactivation (Herviou 2016). As such, EZH2 works as a master regulator of cell cycle progression, autophagy, and apoptosis, promotes DNA damage repair, and inhibits cellular senescence (Ito 2018; Nutt 2020; Yao 2016). In view of the aforementioned notions, it is clear that EZH2 plays an important role in cell lineage determination and relative signaling pathways. This enzyme has been found to be overexpressed in wide varieties of cancer, such as prostate (Varambally 2002), gastric (Qiu 2020), breast (Bachmann 2006), bladder (Martínez-Fernández 2015), lung (Chang and Hung 2012), and pancreatic cancers (Ougolkov et al. 2008). In this context, EZH2-targeting therapies, at present, have garnered significant attention for the treatment of many types of cancer. Till now, tazemetostat stands as the only approved EZH2 inhibitor for advanced epithelioid sarcoma (Italiano 2018) and R/R FL that are EZH2 mutation positive (Morschhauser 2020).

Tazemetostat was recently investigated in a phase 2 trial in patients with wild and mutant EZH2, relapsed, FL. The result of the study showed ORR of 69% (31 of 45 patients) in the EZH2 mutant cohort and 35% (19 of 54 patients) in the EZH2 WT cohort. CRs were observed in six (13%) patients in the EZH2 mutant cohort and two (4%) patients in the EZH2 WT cohort. The median duration of response was 10.9 months and 13.0 months in the EZH2 mutant cohort and EZH2WT cohort, respectively. The result of this trial supported the FDA approval of tazemetostat in EZH2 mutated, R/R FL (Morschhauser 2020).

Various additional EZH2 inhibitors are being evaluated at preclinical and early clinical stages. The details of selected important EZH2 inhibitors are mentioned in Table 16.2. It is

Table 16.2 Novel epigenetic drugs in clinical trial.

Target	Drug	Cancer types	Trial id
HDAC inhibitor	Abexinostat	Follicular lymphoma, diffuse large B-cell lymphoma, non-Hodgkin's lymphoma, mantle cell lymphoma	NCT03934567 (FL), NCT03936153 (DLBCL), NCT04024696 (NHL), NCT00724984 (FL, MCL), NCT00562224 (NHL, HL, CLL, MM)
	Givinostat	Chronic myeloproliferative diseases, chronic myeloproliferative neoplasms, refractory/relapsed lymphocytic leukemia	NCT00606307 (CMD), NCT01761968, NCT00792831 (CLL)
	Tinostamustine	Relapsed/refractory multiple myeloma, relapsed/refractory Hodgkin's lymphoma, relapsed/refractory peripheral T-cell lymphoma (PTCL), relapsed/refractory cutaneous T-cell lymphoma (CTCL), and relapsed/refractory T-cell prolymphocytic leukemia (T-PLL)	NCT02576496 (PTCL, CTCL, T-PLL, MM), NCT03687125 (MM)
	Entinostat	Leukemia, multiple myeloma and plasma cell neoplasm, myelodysplastic syndromes, relapsed or refractory Hodgkin's lymphoma	NCT00015925 (AML, CML, ALL, MM, MDS), NCT00866333 (R/R-HL), NCT00020579 (lymphoma), NCT00015925 (MM, MDS, AML/ALL/CLL)
	Mocetinostat	Myelodysplastic syndromes, acute myelogenous leukemia, Hodgkin's lymphoma, refractory chronic lymphocytic leukemia, relapsed and refractory diffuse large B-cell lymphoma, and follicular lymphoma	NCT00324129 (R/R AML/ALL, MDS), NCT00374296 (AML, MDS), NCT00358982 (HL), NCT00324194 (AML/ALL, MDS), NCT00431873 (CLL), NCT02282358 (R/R DLBCL, FL)
EZH2 inhibitor	CPI-0209	Peripheral T-cell lymphoma, diffuse large B-cell lymphoma	NCT04104776
	PF-06821497	Follicular lymphoma	NCT03460977
	Valemetostat	Relapsed or refractory adult T-cell leukemia/lymphoma, relapse/refractory B-cell lymphoma, relapsed/refractory peripheral T-cell lymphoma	NCT04102150 (R/R A-TLL), NCT04842877 (R/R BCL), NCT04703192 (R/R PTCL, A-TLL)

noteworthy to mention that a homolog of EZH2, EZH1, is present in a non-canonical PRC2 complex. As such, EZH1 complements EZH2 in mediating H3K27 methylation and is also endowed with HMT activity. In light of this disclosure, it is highly anticipated that simultaneous inhibition of EZH1/EZH2 that can be attained via dual EZH1/EZH2 inhibitors might exert more potent anti-cancer effects (Shen 2008).

Valemetostat is a novel, potent, and selective dual inhibitor of EZH2 and EZH1 that has demonstrated anti-tumor activity against hematologic malignancies, especially TCL, including R/R adult T-cell leukemia/lymphoma (ATL) in a phase 1 study. Preliminary efficacy data from 45 patients with R/R PTCL and 14 with R/R ATL demonstrated ORR of 54.5% and 57.1%, with a CR of 12% and 4%, respectively. Valemetostat resulted in a ≥50% ORR, with potentially durable responses both in R/R PTCL and R/R ATL (EHA 2021. Abstract S218).

Valemetostat activity in PTCL is currently being explored in a global, pivotal phase 2 trial in patient with R/R PTCL in the United States (NCT04703192) and R/R ATL in Japan (Foss 2021).

At present, a number of EZH2 inhibitors are under development and evaluation in early phase clinical trials (Table 16.2).

Summary

Over the past couple of decades, it is clear particular classes of drug targeting different aspects of cancer cell biology have found an important therapeutic place. For example, drugs targeting DNMT3 have now been established as standard of care for patients with myeloid diseases like AML and MDS, and are only of late being studied with some promise in patients with lymphoma. In this context, two strategies have emerged. First, the concept of using the HMA as a priming strategy in DLBCL prior to traditional chemotherapy has shown some promise, though these regimens have been associated with significant hematologic toxicity and will ultimately require randomized studies to better understand. Alternatively, HMAs are clearly synergistic with HDAC inhibitors, and are producing significant and durable remission in PTCL, in particular those subtypes that tend to have more dysregulation of genes like TET2 and IDH, like AITL and PTCL-TFH subtypes. Finally, EZH2 inhibitors so far have been approved for patients with FL, and seem to produce better outcomes for those patients with EZH2 mutations, though tazemetostat is approved for patients with FL who do not carry an EZH2 mutation but who also do not have any other options available to them. Albeit preliminary, there is a suggestion that EZH2 inhibitors have activity in PTCL. Clearly, it so far appears PTCL may be a disease where these various drugs in combination, or in combination with various immunologic agents like PD-1 antibodies, can have a significant impact. Clearly appreciating this activity in the context of the underlying mutational landscape and histology will be required to advance these treatments in the most optimal way possible.

Must Read References

Esteller, M. (2008). Epigenetics in cancer. *N. Engl. J. Med.* 358 (11): 1148–1159.

Scotto, L. et al. (2021). targeting the T-cell lymphoma epigenome induces cell death, cancer testes antigens, immune-modulatory signaling pathways. *Mol. Cancer Ther.* 20 (8): 1422–1430.

Baylin, S.B. and Jones, P.A. (2016). Epigenetic Determinants of Cancer. *Cold Spring Harb. Perspect. Biol.* 8 (9).

References

Abou-Alfa, G.K. et al. (2020). Ivosidenib in IDH1-mutant, chemotherapy-refractory cholangiocarcinoma (ClarIDHy): a multicentre, randomised, double-blind, placebo-controlled, phase 3 study. *Lancet Oncol.* 21 (6): 796–807.

Arce, C. et al. (2006). Hydralazine target: from blood vessels to the epigenome. *J. Transl. Med.* 4: 10.

Bachmann, I.M. et al. (2006). EZH2 expression is associated with high proliferation rate and aggressive tumor subgroups in cutaneous melanoma and cancers of the endometrium, prostate and breast. *J. Clin. Oncol.* 24 (2): 268–273.

Bates, S.E. (2020). Epigenetic therapies for cancer. *N. Engl. J. Med.* 383 (7): 650–663.

Baylin, S.B. and Jones, P.A. (2016). Epigenetic determinants of cancer. *Cold Spring Harb. Perspect. Biol.* 8 (9).

Berdasco, M. and Esteller, M. (2010). Aberrant epigenetic landscape in cancer: how cellular identity goes awry. *Dev. Cell* 19 (5): 698–711.

Bird, A. (2007). Perceptions of epigenetics. *Nat.* 447 (7143): 396–398.

Brueckner, B. et al. (2005). Epigenetic reactivation of tumor suppressor genes by a novel small-molecule inhibitor of human DNA methyltransferases. *Cancer Res.* 65 (14): 6305–6311.

Cairns, R.A. et al. (2012). IDH2 mutations are frequent in angioimmunoblastic T-cell lymphoma. *Blood* 119 (8): 1901–1903.

Cashen, A.F. et al. (2010). Multicenter, phase II study of decitabine for the first-line treatment of older patients with acute myeloid leukemia. *J. Clin. Oncol.* 28 (4): 556–561.

Chang, C.J. and Hung, M.C. (2012). The role of EZH2 in tumour progression. *Br. J. Cancer* 106 (2): 243–247.

Clozel, T. et al. (2013). Mechanism-based epigenetic chemosensitization therapy of diffuse large B-cell lymphoma. *Cancer Discov.* 3 (9): 1002–1019.

Coiffier, B. et al. (2012). Results from a pivotal, open-label, phase II study of romidepsin in relapsed or refractory peripheral T-cell lymphoma after prior systemic therapy. *J. Clin. Oncol.* 30 (6): 631–636.

Coiffier, B. et al. (2014). Romidepsin for the treatment of relapsed/refractory peripheral T-cell lymphoma: pivotal study update demonstrates durable responses. *J. Hematol. Oncol.* 7: 11.

Cornacchia, E. et al. (1988). Hydralazine and procainamide inhibit T cell DNA methylation and induce autoreactivity. *J. Immunol.* 140 (7): 2197–2200.

Cunningham, J.M. et al. (1998). Hypermethylation of the hMLH1 promoter in colon cancer with microsatellite instability. *Cancer Res.* 58 (15): 3455–3460.

Datta, J. et al. (2009). A new class of quinoline-based DNA hypomethylating agents reactivates tumor suppressor genes by blocking DNA methyltransferase 1 activity and inducing its degradation. *Cancer Res.* 69 (10): 4277–4285.

Delarue, R. et al. (2016). Treatment with hypomethylating agent 5-azacytidine induces sustained response in angioimmunoblastic T cell lymphomas. *Blood* 128 (22): 4164.

Duvic, M. et al. (2007). Phase 2 trial of oral vorinostat (suberoylanilide hydroxamic acid, SAHA) for refractory cutaneous T-cell lymphoma (CTCL). *Blood* 109 (1): 31–39.

Eden, A. et al. (2003). Chromosomal instability and tumors promoted by DNA hypomethylation. *Science* 300 (5618): 455.

Ehrlich, M. (2009). DNA hypomethylation in cancer cells. *Epigenomics* 1 (2): 239–259.

Esteller, M. (2008). Epigenetics in cancer. *N. Engl. J. Med.* 358 (11): 1148–1159.

Fagan, R.L. et al. (2013). Laccaic acid A is a direct, DNA-competitive inhibitor of DNA methyltransferase 1. *J. Biol. Chem.* 288 (33): 23858–23867.

Falchi, L. et al. (2021). Combined oral 5-azacytidine and romidepsin are highly effective in patients with PTCL: a multicenter phase 2 study. *Blood* 137 (16): 2161–2170.

Fang, M.Z. et al. (2003). Tea polyphenol (-)-epigallocatechin-3-gallate inhibits DNA methyltransferase and reactivates methylation-silenced genes in cancer cell lines. *Cancer Res.* 63 (22): 7563–7570.

Feinberg, A.P. and Vogelstein, B. (1983). Hypomethylation distinguishes genes of some human cancers from their normal counterparts. *Nat.* 301 (5895): 89–92.

Fenaux, P. et al. (2009). Efficacy of azacitidine compared with that of conventional care regimens in the treatment of higher-risk myelodysplastic syndromes: a randomised, open-label, phase III study. *Lancet Oncol.* 10 (3): 223–232.

Fenaux, P. et al. (2010). Azacitidine prolongs overall survival compared with conventional care regimens in elderly patients with low bone marrow blast count acute myeloid leukemia. *J. Clin. Oncol.* 28 (4): 562–569.

Foss, F. et al. (2015). A phase II trial of Belinostat (PXD101) in patients with relapsed or refractory peripheral or cutaneous T-cell lymphoma. *Br. J. Haematol.* 168 (6): 811–819.

Foss, F.M. et al. (2021). A global phase 2 study of valemetostat tosylate (Valemetostat) in patients with relapsed or refractory (R/R) peripheral T-cell lymphoma (PTCL), Including R/R Adult T-Cell Leukemia/Lymphoma (ATL) - Valentine-PTCL01. *Blood* 138 (Supplement 1): 2533–2533.

Gama-Sosa, M.A. et al. (1983). The 5-methylcytosine content of DNA from human tumors. *Nucleic Acids Res* 11 (19): 6883–6894.

Garcia-Manero, G. et al. (2013). Randomized open-label phase II study of decitabine in patients with low- or intermediate-risk myelodysplastic syndromes. *J. Clin. Oncol.* 31 (20): 2548–2553.

Gf, S. (2020). In MDS, is higher risk higher reward? *Hematology Am. Soc. Hematol. Educ. Program*. 2019 2019: 381–390. *Hematology Am. Soc. Hematol. Educ. Program* 2020 (1): 680.

Greger, V. et al. (1989). Epigenetic changes may contribute to the formation and spontaneous regression of retinoblastoma. *Hum. Genet.* 83 (2): 155–158.

Gros, C. et al. (2012). DNA methylation inhibitors in cancer: recent and future approaches. *Biochimie* 94 (11): 2280–2296.

Herviou, L. et al. (2016). EZH2 in normal hematopoiesis and hematological malignancies. *Oncotarget* 7 (3): 2284–2296.

Italiano, A. et al. (2018). Tazemetostat, an EZH2 inhibitor, in relapsed or refractory B-cell non-Hodgkin lymphoma and advanced solid tumours: a first-in-human, open-label, phase 1 study. *Lancet Oncol.* 19 (5): 649–659.

Ito, T. et al. (2018). Regulation of cellular senescence by polycomb chromatin modifiers through distinct DNA damage- and histone methylation-dependent pathways. *Cell Rep.* 22 (13): 3480–3492.

Janke, C. and Montagnac, G. (2017). Causes and consequences of microtubule acetylation. *Curr. Biol.* 27 (23): R1287–r1292.

Kantarjian, H. et al. (2006). Decitabine improves patient outcomes in myelodysplastic syndromes: results of a phase III randomized study. *Cancer* 106 (8): 1794–1803.

Kelly, W.K. et al. (2003). Phase I clinical trial of histone deacetylase inhibitor: suberoylanilide hydroxamic acid administered intravenously. *Clin. Cancer Res.* 9 (10 Pt 1): 3578–3588.

Kelly, W.K. et al. (2005). Phase I study of an oral histone deacetylase inhibitor, suberoylanilide hydroxamic acid, in patients with advanced cancer. *J. Clin. Oncol.* 23 (17): 3923–3931.

Lemonnier, F. et al. (2018). Treatment with 5-azacytidine induces a sustained response in patients with angioimmunoblastic T-cell lymphoma. *Blood* 132 (21): 2305–2309.

Lopez-Serra, P. and Esteller, M. (2012). DNA methylation-associated silencing of tumor-suppressor microRNAs in cancer. *Oncogene* 31 (13): 1609–1622.

Lübbert, M. et al. (2011). Low-dose decitabine versus best supportive care in elderly patients with intermediate-or high-risk myelodysplastic syndrome (MDS) ineligible for intensive chemotherapy: final results of the randomized phase III study of the European organisation for research and treatment of cancer leukemia group and the German MDS study group. *J. Clin. Oncol.* 29 (15): 1987–1996.

Lyko, F. and Brown, R. (2005). DNA methyltransferase inhibitors and the development of epigenetic cancer therapies. *J. Natl. Cancer Inst.* 97 (20): 1498–1506.

Marchi, E. et al. (2015). The combination of hypomethylating agents and histone deacetylase inhibitors produce marked synergy in preclinical models of T-cell lymphoma. *Br. J. Haematol. 171 (2): 215–226.*

Marchi, E. et al. (2020). The Integration of PD1 blockade with epigenetic therapy is highly active and safe in heavily treated patients with T-cell lymphoma (PTCL) and cutaneous T-cell lymphoma (CTCL). *J. Clin. Oncol.* 38 (15_suppl): 8049–8049.

Marquard, L. et al. (2009). Histone deacetylase 1, 2, 6 and acetylated histone H4 in B- and T-cell lymphomas. *Histopathol.* 54 (6): 688–698.

Martin, P. et al. (2017). A phase I, open label, multicenter trial of oral Azacitidine (CC-486) Plus R-CHOP in patients with high-risk, previously untreated diffuse large B-cell lymphoma, Grade 3B follicular lymphoma, or transformed lymphoma. *Blood* 130: 192.

Martínez-Fernández, M. et al. (2015). EZH2 in bladder cancer, a promising therapeutic target. *Int. J. Mol. Sci.* 16 (11): 27107–27132.

Maze, I. et al. (2015). Critical role of histone turnover in neuronal transcription and plasticity. *Neuron* 87 (1): 77–94.

Meeran, S.M., Ahmed, A., and Tollefsbol, T.O. (2010). Epigenetic targets of bioactive dietary components for cancer prevention and therapy. *Clin. Epigenet.* 1 (3–4): 101–116.

Monk, M., Adams, R.L., and Rinaldi, A. (1991). Decrease in DNA methylase activity during preimplantation development in the mouse. *Development* 112 (1): 189–192.

Moore, L.D., Le, T., and Fan, G. (2013). DNA methylation and its basic function. *Neuropsychopharmacol.* 38 (1): 23–38.

Morschhauser, F. et al. (2020). Tazemetostat for patients with relapsed or refractory follicular lymphoma: an open-label, single-arm, multicentre, phase 2 trial. *Lancet Oncol.* 21 (11): 1433–1442.

Nishiyama, A. and Nakanishi, M. (2021). Navigating the DNA methylation landscape of cancer. *Trends Genet.* 37 (11): 1012–1027.

Nutt, S.L. et al. (2020). EZH2 function in immune cell development. *Biol. Chem.* 401 (8): 933–943.

O'Connor, O.A. et al. (2015). Belinostat in patients with relapsed or refractory peripheral T-cell lymphoma: results of the pivotal phase II BELIEF (CLN-19) study. *J. Clin. Oncol.* 33 (23): 2492–2499.

O'Connor, O.A. et al. (2019). Oral 5-azacytidine and romidepsin exhibit marked activity in patients with PTCL: a multicenter phase 1 study. *Blood* 134 (17): 1395–1405.

Okano, M. et al. (1999). DNA methyltransferases Dnmt3a and Dnmt3b are essential for de novo methylation and mammalian development. *Cell* 99 (3): 247–257.

Olsen, E.A. et al. (2007). Phase IIb multicenter trial of vorinostat in patients with persistent, progressive, or treatment refractory cutaneous T-cell lymphoma. *J. Clin. Oncol.* 25 (21): 3109–3115.

Ougolkov, A.V., Bilim, V.N., and Billadeau, D.D. (2008). Regulation of pancreatic tumor cell proliferation and chemoresistance by the histone methyltransferase enhancer of zeste homologue 2. *Clin. Cancer Res.* 14 (21): 6790–6796.

Piekarz, R.L. et al. (2011). Phase 2 trial of romidepsin in patients with peripheral T-cell lymphoma. *Blood* 117 (22): 5827–5834.

Plass, C. et al. (2013). Mutations in regulators of the epigenome and their connections to global chromatin patterns in cancer. *Nat. Rev. Genet.* 14 (11): 765–780.

Qiu, B.Q. et al. (2020). Long non-coding RNA PSMA3-AS1 promotes malignant phenotypes of esophageal cancer by modulating the miR-101/EZH2 axis as a ceRNA. *Aging (Albany NY)* 12 (2): 1843–1856.

Rasmussen, K.D. and Helin, K. (2016). Role of TET enzymes in DNA methylation, development, and cancer. *Genes Dev.* 30 (7): 733–750.

Robertson, K.D. (2005). DNA methylation and human disease. *Nat. Rev. Genet.* 6 (8): 597–610.

Ruan, J. et al. (2020). Multi-center phase II study of oral azacitidine (CC-486) plus CHOP as initial treatment for peripheral T-cell lymphoma (PTCL). *Blood* 136 (Supplement 1): 33–34.

Salim, O. et al. (2016). Azacitidine versus decitabine in patients with refractory anemia with excess blast-Results of multicenter study. *Leuk. Res.* 45: 82–89.

Santi, D.V., Norment, A., and Garrett, C.E. (1984). Covalent bond formation between a DNA-cytosine methyltransferase and DNA containing 5-azacytosine. *Proc. Natl. Acad. Sci. U.S.A.* 81 (22): 6993–6997.

Scotto, L. et al. (2021). Targeting the T-cell lymphoma epigenome induces cell death, cancer testes antigens, immune-modulatory signaling pathways. *Mol. Cancer Ther.* 20 (8): 1422–1430.

Segura-Pacheco, B. et al. (2003). Reactivation of tumor suppressor genes by the cardiovascular drugs hydralazine and procainamide and their potential use in cancer therapy. *Clin. Cancer Res.* 9 (5): 1596–1603.

Seidel, C. et al. (2012). Chromatin-modifying agents in anti-cancer therapy. *Biochimie* 94 (11): 2264–2279.

Shen, X. et al. (2008). EZH1 mediates methylation on histone H3 lysine 27 and complements EZH2 in maintaining stem cell identity and executing pluripotency. *Mol. Cell* 32 (4): 491–502.

Siedlecki, P. et al. (2006). Discovery of two novel, small-molecule inhibitors of DNA methylation. *J. Med. Chem.* 49 (2): 678–683.

Stein, E.M. et al. (2017). Enasidenib in mutant IDH2 relapsed or refractory acute myeloid leukemia. *Blood* 130 (6): 722–731.

Stresemann, C. and Lyko, F. (2008). Modes of action of the DNA methyltransferase inhibitors azacytidine and decitabine. *Int. J. Cancer* 123 (1): 8–13.

Varambally, S. et al. (2002). The polycomb group protein EZH2 is involved in progression of prostate cancer. *Nat.* 419 (6907): 624–629.

Wilson, A.S., Power, B.E., and Molloy, P.L. (2007). DNA hypomethylation and human diseases. *Biochim. Biophys. Acta* 1775 (1): 138–162.

Yao, Y. et al. (2016). Downregulation of enhancer of zeste homolog 2 (EZH2) is essential for the induction of autophagy and apoptosis in colorectal cancer cells. *Genes (Basel)* 7 (10).

Zhang, C. et al. (2005). Selective induction of apoptosis by histone deacetylase inhibitor SAHA in cutaneous T-cell lymphoma cells: relevance to mechanism of therapeutic action. *J. Invest. Dermatol.* 125 (5): 1045–1052.

Zhang, M. et al. (2019). Decitabine plus r-chop in patients with newly diagnosed diffuse large b-cell lymphoma: interim results of a phase I/II study. *Hematol. Oncol.* 37: 528-528.

17

Future Prospects for Targeting the Epigenome in Lymphomas

Yusuke Isshiki and Ari Melnick

Division of Hematology and Oncology, Joan and Sanford I Weill Department of Medicine, Weill Cornell Medicine, New York, NY, USA

Take Home Messages

- Aberrant epigenetic programming is hallmark of most B-cell and T-cell lymphomas, providing ample opportunity for impactful implementation of epigenetic therapies that counteract this process.
- Precision targeting of the epigenome requires specific and well-defined direct evidence that biological response is caused by an epigenetic effect that lymphomas are dependent on.
- Although there are currently few precision epigenetic therapies in the clinic, many such drugs are in development and could become important cornerstones of lymphoma therapeutic regimens.
- Precision epigenetic therapies are mostly well tolerated and often combine well and synergize with other standard or novel therapeutic agents, such as BH3 mimetics.
- Epigenetic therapies enhance the immunogenicity of lymphoma cells, and in certain cases may also enhance host anti-lymphoma immune response proving a strong rationale for combination with immunotherapies.

Introduction

Epigenetic regulation is colloquially defined as molecular mechanisms controlling gene expression and other genomic functions that are not encoded by the genome. Over the years, epigenetic mechanisms have emerged as an appealing and target-rich therapeutic space for the treatment of B-cell and T-cell lymphomas. This was initially driven in part due to the success of histone deacetylase (HDAC) inhibitors in treating T-cell lymphomas (Bates 2020), although the basis of this efficacy is still unknown. On the other hand, mutational profiling has revealed that somatic mutations in chromatin modifiers and transcription factors are a hallmark of follicular lymphoma (FL) and diffuse large B-cell lymphomas (DLBCL) (Reddy et al. 2017). Importantly mutations in epigenetic modifiers are also prevalent in T-cell lymphomas such as angioimmunoblastic T-cell lymphomas (AITL) (Tari et al. 2021), and occur to some extent in most lymphomas. DLBCLs were recently categorized into subtypes based on somatic mutation profiles, all of which generally have epigenetic/transcriptional mutations (Chapuy et al. 2018; Wright et al. 2020). This has naturally raised the expectation of developing precision therapies for these tumors. Here we will review some of the emerging epigenetic targets and epigenetic therapies with potential to significantly advance the lymphoma therapeutic landscape. Given the many subtypes of lymphomas it is impossible to cover the whole field, so we focus mostly on DLBCL and FL, which are the two most common entities.

Emerging Epigenetic Therapies

EZH2- and PRC2-targeted Therapies Are Emerging as Potential Cornerstone Therapies for Lymphomas

EZH2 is a H3K27 methyltransferase that mediates epigenetic silencing, dependent on its integration into the multi-protein polycomb repressive complex 2 (PRC2) for its enzymatic activity. EZH2 mediates H3K27 methylation in a processive manner, which means that as PRC2 slides along chromatin it causes H3K27 methylation over long stretches of nucleosomes. EZH2 is essential for development of the germinal center B-cells from which most FLs and DLBCLs arise and is highly expressed in lymphomas, pointing to potential for

Precision Cancer Therapies: Targeting Oncogenic Drivers and Signaling Pathways in Lymphoid Malignancies: From Concept to Practice, Volume 1, First Edition. Edited by Owen A. O'Connor, Stephen M. Ansell, and John F. Seymour.

wild-type EZH2 to drive "non-oncogene addiction" in these tumors (Beguelin et al. 2013; Caganova et al. 2013; Velichutina et al. 2010). Lymphoma dependency on wild-type EZH2 is linked to its repressing cell cycle checkpoint and B-cell terminal differentiation genes (Beguelin et al. 2013, 2017; Caganova et al. 2013; Velichutina et al. 2010). EZH2 mediates these effects by adding the H3K27me3 mark to promoters of active genes marked by H3K4me3, thus creating bivalent chromatin (H3K27me3 + H3K4me3) that transiently represses expression of affected genes, but can be rapidly reversed when B-cells exit the germinal center reaction (Beguelin et al. 2013).

EZH2 is normally inefficient at mediating H3K27 trimethylation. However, the canonical $EZH2^{Y641}$ somatic mutations observed in FL and DLBCL confer far greater H3K27me3 activity and yield significant increase in H3K27me3 abundance (Sneeringer et al. 2010). This causes aberrant repression of an additional ~2000 promoters not normally repressed by EZH2, including many genes involved in recognition and response to T-cells (Beguelin et al. 2020). This enables EZH2 mutant B-cells to escape from the requirement for T-cell help, and instead induces them to become dependent on follicular dendritic cells thus forming an aberrant immune niche with typical histological characteristics of FLs (Beguelin et al. 2020). In DLBCLs, there is further progression of the EZH2 mutant epigenetic program resulting in broad silencing of *MHC II* genes and an immune-depleted microenvironment (Ennishi et al. 2019). Notably, EZH2 inhibitor treatment in mice with $EZH2^{Y641F}$ mutant lymphomas recruited a rich infiltrate of $CD4^+$ and granzyme B^+ cytotoxic $CD8^+$ cells, followed by long-term remission (Takata et al. 2022).

Tazemetostat, the first selective EZH2 inhibitor, is FDA (Food and Drug Administration) approved for use in relapsed/refractory FL with or without EZH2 mutation (Morschhauser et al. 2020). However, two inhibitors (valemetostat and CPI-0209) currently in clinical trials target both EZH2 and its close homolog EZH1. Dual targeting has been claimed to overcome partial compensation of EZH2 inhibition by EZH1 and hence yield a more potent therapeutic effect (Yamagishi et al. 2019). Although it remains to be seen if such results can be confirmed, clinical trials of these agents are ongoing for B-cell and T-cell lymphomas and will provide valuable insight into this question. Similarly, PRC2 function can also be abrogated by compounds that block the interaction of PRC2 subunit EED with H3K27me3, which is required for EZH2 and EZH1 activities. An EED inhibitor called MAK683 is currently in clinical trials for patients with B-cell lymphomas (Huang et al. 2022). Tazemetostat was more active in FL than DLBCL patients, even though primary human DLBCL cells are quite sensitive to high doses *in vivo* (Scholze et al. 2020). It will be of interest to see whether total PRC2 suppression yields a greater effect in DLBCL, as well as other lymphomas where pre-clinical activity is reported such as mantle cell lymphoma (MCL), chronic lymphocytic leukemia (CLL), and T-cell lymphoma (Chartomatsidou et al. 2019; Li et al. 2019; Pikman et al. 2020).

SETD2, a Novel Therapeutic Target for DLBCLs

SETD2 is the sole histone methyltransferase that catalyzes H3K36me3, a histone mark located throughout actively transcribed gene bodies (Lam and Chen 2022), where it plays important roles in DNA damage sensing, splicing, and prevention of spurious intragenic transcripts (Lam and Chen 2022). A few studies suggest there are also non-histone SETD2 targets (Lam and Chen 2022). *SETD2* genetic lesions occur in ~5% of DLBCL patients and are almost always heterozygous missense or nonsense mutations (Leung et al. 2022). H3K36me3 plays a particularly vital role in B-cells, where it was recently shown to protect the non-template strand of DNA from being heavily mutated by activation-induced cytosine deaminase (AICDA) during the germinal center reaction (Leung et al. 2022). Accordingly, primary murine and human *SETD2* mutant DLBCLs featured a higher burden of somatic mutations and structural variants as compared to *SETD2* wild-type lymphomas (Leung et al. 2022). Most strikingly, CRISPR editing of *SETD2* failed to yield homozygous clones in most DLBCL cell lines, suggesting that *SETD2* is essential for the survival of DLBCLs and explaining why *SETD2* mutations are almost always heterozygous in the DLBCL context (Leung et al. 2022). Along these lines, a highly potent and specific clinical grade SETD2 inhibitor was recently developed (Lampe et al. 2021), which is highly active against DLBCLs *in vitro* and *in vivo* (Totman et al. 2021), and is currently in its first in man clinical trial (NCT05121103). The mechanism through which SETD2 inhibitors suppress DLBCLs remains unknown and must be investigated to properly position these therapeutic agents and interpret outcomes from clinical trials.

LSD1, a Case of Bait and Switch

LSD1 is a flavin adenine dinucleotide (FAD)-dependent amine oxidase family demethylase that specifically removes H3K4 monomethylation, a mark required for gene enhancer functionality (Zhang et al. 2021). In germinal center B-cells, LSD1 is required to repress enhancers of transiently repressed immune signaling genes that are later activated by the histone methyltransferase KMT2D upon exit from the germinal center reaction (Hatzi et al. 2019). LSD1 knockout impaired development of DLBCLs in mice and LSD1 knockdown has anti-proliferative effects against DLBCL cell lines (Hatzi et al. 2019), suggesting a potential role for LSD1 inhibitors for DLBCL patients. Several specific and potent LSD1 inhibitors are in clinical trials, and in pre-clinical studies were active against acute myeloid leukemias (AMLs) (Zhang et al. 2021). Surprisingly LSD1 inhibitors had no activity against DLBCL cells, and further study revealed that loss of histone demethylase activity was not sufficient for anti-lymphoma activity, which required loss of both enzymatic and the "tower" protein interaction domain (Hatzi et al. 2019). This suggests that LSD1 degraders might still be active against DLBCLs and are worth pursuing.

TET2 is a dioxygenase that oxidizes 5′methylcytosine to 5′hydroxymethylcytosine (5hmC) primarily at gene enhancers. TET2 loss-of-functions occur in myeloid and lymphoid malignancies and are extremely common in AITL (Tari et al. 2021). Loss of TET2 results aberrant gene repression primarily due to loss of 5hmC at gene enhancers and to a lesser extent to hypermethylation of gene promoters (Rampal et al. 2014). Translational studies conducted in primary human AML cells showed that LSD1 inhibitors were especially highly active against TET2 mutant patient specimens (Duy et al. 2019). The reason for this was that TET2 deficiency resulted in loss of enhancer 5hmC, which in turn led to aberrant recruitment of LSD1 to enhancers regulating important tumor suppressors (Duy et al. 2019). TET2 mutations are extremely common in AITL (Tari et al. 2021). If similar effects occur in AITL, then LSD1 inhibitors might have significant therapeutic impact in this setting.

A Surprising Indication for KDM5 Histone Demethylase Inhibitors

The KDM5 family consists of four Jumonji domain histone demethylases that primarily demethylate H3K4me3, a mark associated with active gene promoters (Harmeyer et al. 2017). It has not proven easy to generate compounds with strong selective inhibition of KDM5 Jumonji domains, although several such small molecules have been developed over the years (Heward et al. 2021). A surprising role for KDM5 inhibitors was recently discovered as an approach to rescue aberrant transcriptional repression caused by the common loss-of-function *KMT2D* mutation in lymphomas (Heward et al. 2021). On the surface this might seem unexpected, since *KMT2D* loss-of-function results in loss of H3K4me1 whereas KDM5 inhibitors prevent demethylation of H3K4me3. However, Heward et al. reasoned that inhibiting KDM5 demethylases would alter H3K4 methylation dynamics to restore expression of genes that would normally become repressed due to KMT2D loss-of-function. Indeed, using three different KDM5 inhibitors they showed that KDM5 inhibitors were selectively more active against *KMT2D* mutant than *KMT2D* wild-type DLBCLs *in vitro* and *in vivo*, could reverse aberrant silencing of immune signaling genes caused by *KMT2D* mutation, and synergized with MCL1 inhibitors (Heward et al. 2021). These data point to KDM5 inhibitors as a potential precision therapy for *KMT2D* mutant lymphomas and an emerging opportunity once these compounds reach clinical trials.

New Opportunities Provided by Emerging Histone Deacetylase Inhibitors

Ever since HDACs were shown to mediate oncogenic transcriptional repression by leukemia fusion proteins, there has been great interest in such compounds. There are 11 members of the HDAC family of enzymes, which regulate thousands of proteins through lysine acetylation, all of which could be potentially affected by these drugs. Most HDAC inhibitors block the function of multiple HDACs, making it difficult to conclusively define how these drugs work against cancer cells (Bates 2020). As of yet, there is no conclusive evidence that HDAC inhibitors mediate their clinical effects at the epigenetic level in lymphomas or via a long list of other molecular actions including DNA damage. These pleiotropic effects likely explain why HDAC inhibitors are associated with significant toxicities (Bates 2020). Although at the chromatin level HDACs primarily repress genes through histone deacetylation, HDAC inhibitors do not induce a predominant transcriptional activation signal. Therefore, it may not be strictly accurate to label multi-HDAC inhibitors as "epigenetic therapy." Yet the fact that HDAC inhibitors have proven activity against T-cell lymphomas underlines the need for continued research into exactly why these tumors respond, since perhaps there might be a more specific way to deliver the beneficial effects of these drugs (O'Connor et al. 2019).

One such approach involves targeting specific HDAC isoforms, among which HDAC3 is the most specifically tied to epigenetic effects. HDAC3 has to date only co-purified with co-repressor complexes containing the NCOR1 or NCOR2 scaffold adaptor proteins and is inactive in the absence of these co-repressors, which allosterically induce its enzymatic activity (Stengel et al. 2019; You et al.2013). In germinal center B-cells, HDAC3 is a critical cofactor for BCL6 and FOXO1 in deacetylating enhancers for immune signaling and antigen presentation genes (Jiang et al. 2017; Stengel et al. 2019). These enhancers are later reactivated by the CREBBP histone acetyltransferase upon immune synapse signaling (Jiang et al. 2017). However, CREBBP is frequently inactivated by missense or truncation mutations in FLs and DLBCLs, which leave HDAC3 unopposed in repressing enhancers, a situation that causes *CREBBP* mutant lymphomas to becoming addicted to HDAC3 (Jiang et al. 2017; Mondello et al. 2020).

HDAC3-selective inhibitors have anti-proliferative effect against GCB-DLBCLs, and are most potently effective against those with *CREBBP* mutations (Jiang et al. 2017; Mondello et al. 2020). In contrast multi-HDAC inhibitors are cytotoxic to lymphoma cells without regard to their somatic mutation profiles (Mondello et al. 2020). Unlike multi-HDAC inhibitors, HDAC3 inhibitors almost exclusively induce transcriptional activation, including MHC class II genes (Mondello et al.

2020). HDAC3 inhibitors induced recruitment of CD4 and CD8 cells into primary murine BCL6-dependent lymphomas and caused lymphoma cells to trigger an MHCI/II-dependent T-cell cytotoxic response, suggesting that perhaps a major determinant of their efficacy is to restore host immune clearance of lymphoma cells (Mondello et al. 2020). TET2 loss-of-function also made DLBCL cells selectively sensitive to HDAC3 inhibition, apparently because loss of enhancer 5hmC also impairs CREBBP activity (Dominguez et al. 2018). This is conceptually similar to the effect of LSD1 in repressing enhancers in TET2-deficient AML patients. Given that HDAC3 inhibitors lack the toxicity of multi-HDAC inhibitors, they may be well-suited components of multi-modality therapeutic regimens.

Sirtuins, the "Other HDACs," Potential Therapeutic Targets in B-cell Lymphomas

Sirtuins comprise a class of NAD-dependent lysine deacetylases and deacylases, about which little is known in the lymphoma context. The most studied are the class I sirtuins (SIRT1, SIRT2, and SIRT3). Using niacinamide to suppress general sirtuin function in combination with multi-HDAC inhibitors resulted in synergistic toxicity to lymphoma cells and prompted a clinical trial with this combination with some responses observed (Amengual et al. 2013). Compounds with selective but not highly potent activity against SIRT2 induced toxicity against lymphoma cells (Chowdhury et al. 2020). It is not clear whether the effect targeting SIRT1 or SIRT2 is through epigenetic mechanisms at present. An shRNA screen of the seven sirtuins in DLBCL cell lines showed that the strongest dependency was for SIRT3, an exclusively mitochondrial sirtuin (Li et al. 2019). SIRT3 inhibitors potently killed DLBCLs *in vitro* and *in vivo* (Li et al. 2019). Notably, targeting SIRT3 resulted in profound histone deacetylation, which was most likely secondary to severe reduction in AcetylCoA caused by impaired TCA cycle function and was of uncertain epigenetic impact (Li et al. 2019). Overall, it remains unclear if inhibitors of nuclear sirtuins will have efficacy as a form of epigenetic targeted therapy.

Histone Acetyltransferase Inhibitors, Lacking Selectivity but with Activity in Lymphomas

The closely related CREBBP and P300 histone acetyltransferases are considered as therapeutic targets in multiple tumor types. Both mediate H3K27 and H3K18 acetylation to primarily activate enhancers and play partially non-overlapping roles in the germinal reaction (Meyer et al. 2019). However, CREBBP and EP300 have numerous non-histone targets as well, so it is not always easy to ascertain which downstream effects are directly a consequence of their actions on histones. A number of small molecule inhibitors have been developed targeting either their histone acetyl transferase (HAT) domains or bromodomains (He et al. 2021), although without apparent strong selectivity for either CREBBP or P300. Of note, a recent study showed that *CREBBP* mutant lymphomas may exhibit synthetic lethality to CREBBP/P300 inhibitors, presumably because of their strong dependence on residual HAT activity (Meyer et al. 2019). Given the potentially deleterious effect of combined CREBBP and EP300 loss-of-function there is concern that dual inhibitors may result in significant toxicities. Hence, there is a great need for selective inhibitors.

Is There a Potential Role for BET Inhibitors for Lymphoma?

The bromo- and extraterminal (BET) domain protein BRD4 was proposed as an epigenetic therapeutic target in light of its role in binding to acetylated histones and contributing to transcriptional activation of genes such as MYC (Spriano et al. 2020). The effect of BRD4 was suggested to be more evident at clustered enhancers or super-enhancers, reflecting the higher abundance of H3K27acetylation at such sites (Spriano et al. 2020). BET inhibitors were shown to impair expression of genes controlled by enhancers and super-enhancers in DLBCL, although *in vivo* activity was modest (Chapuy et al. 2013). BET inhibitors were initially claimed to represent a way to target MYC, a key oncogenic transcription factor that supports metabolic fitness of tumor cells. However, subsequent studies showed lack of concordance between effects on MYC and anti-tumor efficacy and that MYC downregulation did not explain the activity of these compounds (Spriano et al. 2020). BET inhibitors are not unique in downregulating MYC, which is induced by many drugs such as chemotherapeutics, HDAC inhibitors, and others (Pei et al. 2016). Downregulation of MYC may actually represent a survival mechanism for tumor cells as they go into a quiescent/diapause-like state to recover from exposure to toxic challenges (Dhimolea et al. 2021; Duy et al. 2021; Rehman et al. 2021), and BET inhibitors apparently made tumor cells more resistant to chemotherapy (Dhimolea et al. 2021). Several groups have identified alternative mechanisms through which BET inhibitors may have anti-lymphoma efficacy, such as reduction of phosphorylated IKKb and hence reduced nuclear factor-κB (NF-κB) activity in ABC-DLBCL cell lines, among many others (Ceribelli et al. 2014; Spriano et al. 2020). Given their broad role in supporting transcription, BET inhibitors are fairly toxic in humans, roughly similar to HDAC inhibitors (Spriano et al. 2020). Consistent with the *in vivo* pre-clinical data, the activity of this class of compounds in lymphomas is modest, but may still have a future if they can be combined with other modalities such as checkpoint inhibitors (Hogg et al. 2017) where there could be relatively little cross-toxicity. Another promising development is the creation of BET degrader small molecules that may have greater specificity for BRD4 and have quite potent anti-lymphoma activity (Fiskus et al. 2021; Spriano et al. 2020).

DNA Methyltransferase Inhibitors Are Increasingly Relevant for Treatment of Lymphomas

DNA methyltransferases DNMT1, DNMT3a, and DNMT3b add methyl groups at CpG dinucleotides (5′mC) throughout the genome. When located at gene promoters 5′methylcytosine (5mC) is linked to repression of genes, whereas at other regulatory elements it can have various other functional impacts such as creating or abolishing binding sites for transcription factors (Duy et al. 2020). Aberrant cytosine methylation patterning is a hallmark of all cancers, and has many context-specific functions (Duy et al. 2020). Aberrant DNA hypermethylation is linked to silencing of general and cell context-specific tumor suppressors, whereas heterogeneity of cytosine methylation within a given tumor is linked to fitness and inferior outcome (Duy et al. 2020). Nucleoside analog DNA methyltransferase inhibitors (DNMTis) such as 5′azacytidine and decitabine were the earliest epigenetic therapies, and proposed to mediate their therapeutic effect through incorporation into DNA, irreversibly binding to DNA methyltransferases (DNMTs) and consequent reduction in cytosine methylation, among other actions (Pechalrieu et al. 2017). One of the complexities of interpreting data generated with these compounds is that they function as DNA-damaging chemotherapy drugs within the dose range that is used for parenteral administration of these compounds (Pechalrieu et al. 2017). However, this can be avoided by use of low nanomolar concentrations of drugs such as 5′azacytidine or decitabine. In the clinic, this can be achieved by using the oral versions of these drugs (CC-486 and cedazuridine–decitabine [C-DEC]), which have lower peak concentrations and more sustained exposure of cells to demethylating doses (Garcia-Manero et al. 2022; Martin et al. 2022; Patel et al. 2021).

Clinical translation of these drugs for lymphoma was initiated based on pre-clinical experiments showing that nanomolar (demethylating) doses of DNMTi caused chemotherapy-resistant DLBCL cell lines to be rendered sensitive to clinically achievable concentrations of drugs like doxorubicin (Clozel et al. 2013). This was due to demethylation of a small set of genes aberrantly hypermethylated and silenced in high-risk DLBCLs, the most critical of which was SMAD1 (Clozel et al. 2013). Preventing SMAD1 de-repression prevented DNMTi chemosensitization, whereas its ectopic expression induced chemosensitization even in the absence of DNMTi (Clozel et al. 2013). These data were independently confirmed by Stelling et al. (2019). Sequential biopsies performed in a phase 1 clinical trial of 5′azacytidine showed that primary DLBCL cells at diagnosis were resistant to doxorubicin, but became sensitive after the first cycle of DNMTi, concordant with SMAD1 demethylation (Clozel et al. 2013). These mechanistic data and promising early phase clinical results justified initiation of phase 3 clinical trial of CC-486 for newly diagnosed older DLBCL patients in combination with R-miniCHOP (NCT04799275).

A novel role for DNMTi was revealed by studies performing either CRISPR or small molecule screening to convert Epstein–Barr virus positive (EBV+) lymphoma cells from the poorly immunogenic latency I state to the latency III state expressing immunoreactive proteins such as LMP1 (Dalton et al. 2020; Guo et al. 2020). The strikingly convergent studies revealed the strongest CRISPR signal for DNMT1 and its partner protein UHRF1, whereas decitabine was by far the most potent small molecule inducer of latency III (Dalton et al. 2020; Guo et al. 2020). Hence, DNMTi could be used in the clinic to convert EBV lymphomas into an immunogenic state where they can be recognized and attacked by host immune or engineered T-cells. DNMTi are also relevant to T-cell lymphomas, where the frequent mutation of TET2 could potentially provide a rational basis response to these inhibitors (Cogan et al. 2020). Looking to the future, a recent report presented a novel DNMT1-specific inhibitor that does not incorporate into DNA, allowing for greater target engagement and efficacy (Pappalardi et al. 2021). If compounds like these are able to be used in humans, there is potential for significant therapeutic benefit, and easier integration into combination clinical trials such as those underway for B-cell and T-cell lymphomas.

Nucleosome Remodeling Complex Inhibitors

BAF (**B**RG1/BRM-**a**ssociated **f**actor) complexes are multi-subunit protein assemblies that play a critical role in organizing the spatial distribution of nucleosomes throughout the genome. All BAF complexes have ATPase subunits that power movement or disassembly of nucleosomes, which is important for transcriptional regulation, DNA repair, and other processes (Wanior et al. 2021). There are three general classes of BAF complexes: BAF, polybromo BAF (pBAF), and non-canonical BAF (ncBAF), defined based on subunit preference and each with distinct general and cell context-specific dependent functions (Wanior et al. 2021). Presumed inactivating BAF subunit gene mutations are highly recurrent across many tumor types. The most commonly mutated subunits in lymphomas are ARID1A (**AT** **r**ich **i**nteracting **d**omain 1A), and SMARCA4 (**SW**I/**SN**F **R**elated, **M**atrix **A**ssociated, **A**ctin Dependent **R**egulator Of **C**hromatin, Subfamily **A**, Member **4**) (Chapuy et al. 2018; Reddy et al. 2017; Wright et al. 2020). ARID1A is a BAF-specific subunit that anchors the BAF complex, binds to DNA, and has allosteric functions. SMARCA4 is an ATPase subunit that can assemble into any of the BAF complexes (Wanior et al. 2021). Very little is known regarding the contribution of BAF mutations to lymphomagenesis, although one report suggested that they could induce resistance to ibrutinib and venetoclax treatment in MCL (Agarwal et al. 2019).

Given that BAF mutations confer loss-of-function the design of therapeutic approaches is not straightforward. However, it has been shown that SMARCA4 mutant lymphomas are heavily dependent on the other BAF ATPase SMARCA2, and that targeting SMARCA2 yields a synthetic lethal effect (Hoffman et al. 2014). Tool compounds are being developed targeting the SMARCA2 ATPase or bromodomain, as well as PROTACs to degrade SMARCA2 (Wanior et al. 2021). In a similar manner, loss of ARID1B is synthetic lethal in ARID1A mutant tumors (Helming et al. 2014; Mullen et al. 2021). BAF mutations lead to synthetic lethalities toward therapeutic agents targeting PARP1, protein kinases, and others (Wanior et al. 2021). Of note, polycomb and BAF complexes have opposing functions during development and it was shown that ARID1A mutation makes ovarian cancer cells more responsive to EZH2 inhibition (Bitler et al. 2015). However, it is not clear to what extent this might occur in lymphomas and other tumors. Hence, BAF-targeted epigenetic therapy holds promise but remains understudied in the lymphoma context.

Precision Epigenetic Therapy

Having reviewed emerging epigenetic therapies for lymphoma, it is worth considering in which cases the label of "epigenetic therapy" is precisely accurate, given that the epigenome will react to a broad palette of signals, environment cues, and toxins. Hence, many drugs can be considered as "epigenetic therapies" in the sense that they can induce therapeutically relevant epigenetic responses. Even compounds targeted to *bona fide* epigenetic regulatory proteins may have on-target non-epigenetic effects given that many of these enzymes can covalently modify non-histone proteins. For example, EZH2 was suggested to regulate actin polymerization and T-cell receptor signaling, whereas SETD2 was shown to methylate lysine residues of microtubules during cytokinesis (Dobenecker et al. 2018; Park et al. 2016; Su et al. 2005). To rigorously predict, define, and interpret the benefit of targeting epigenetic mechanisms it is useful to consider what might constitute "precision epigenetic therapy." We propose the following general principles:

1) *Hits a well-defined and mostly epigenetic-specific target.* Several highly specific and potent small molecules target EZH2, LSD1, and SETD2 (Duy et al. 2020; Lampe et al. 2021; Zhang et al. 2021), and the best documented functions of these chromatin modifiers are linked to their effects on histone methylation. Examples of drugs that may not meet this criterion are the multi-HDAC and PRMT5 inhibitors (Bates 2020; Zhu and Rui 2019). Multi-HDACi results in acetylation of hundreds of nuclear and cytoplasmatic proteins (Bates 2020). PRMT5 is a symmetric arginine methyltransferase that methylates several arginine residues on histones 3 and 4 but likewise is present throughout cytoplasm and nucleus and has many targets (Zhu and Rui 2019). Both classes of drugs have a multitude of effects, and have not been shown to mediate their therapeutic actions through effects on the epigenome. This does not mean that such drugs have no clinical utility, only that their effects cannot currently be interpreted as being mediated through epigenetic mechanisms.
2) *Achieves full target engagement at clinically relevant doses, without off-target effects.* In pre-clinical studies, compounds are often given at doses that exceed what is achievable in humans either because of toxicity, off-target effects, or due to pharmacokinetic and formulation issues. The plasticity of the epigenome confers on cells the ability to tolerate short periods of disruption, and it is thought that sustained and thorough target engagement is usually important. Evaluating this in the clinic is challenging since the biochemical impact of these drugs can vary between cell types so that non-tumor tissues may not be suitable as surrogates. Drugs such as multi-HDACi or BETi that may be quite toxic at full target engagement might not meet this criterion (Bates 2020; Doroshow et al. 2017).
3) *The target drives a well-defined epigenetic dependency in specific lymphomas.* Although novel therapeutics can succeed empirically without a solid biomedical rationale, achieving efficacy is more likely when there is a rigorous scientific basis for translation. Unfortunately, there are few epigenetic examples thus far in lymphomas. The best documented is the use of EZH2-targeted therapy for patients with EZH2 gain-of-function mutations. Moreover, given that EZH2 is a lineage factor for germinal center B-cells these compounds are also active in EZH2 WT germinal center-derived lymphomas. SMAD1 hypermethylation and silencing in DLBCL causes chemotherapy resistance. DNMTis can rescue SMAD1 expression and sensitize lymphomas to chemotherapies (Clozel et al. 2013; Stelling et al. 2019). *CREBBP* mutation leads to dependency on HDAC3, the enzymatic function of which is mostly linked to its effects on histones, and hence greater responsiveness to HDAC3-selective inhibitors (Jiang et al. 2017; Mondello et al. 2020). Loss of CREBBP function also mediates synthetic lethality to HAT inhibitors (Meyer et al. 2019). KMT2D loss-of-function or mutation results in sensitivity of DLBCLs to KDM5 inhibitors (Heward et al. 2021).
4) *Patients can be selected based on biomarker that indicates dependency on a specific epigenetic mechanism.* Reciprocal

to point (3) there are several genetic biomarkers that can enrich for likely responders include EZH2, *CREBBP*, and *KMT2D* mutations as noted above (Heward et al. 2021; Jiang et al. 2017; Meyer et al. 2019; Mondello et al. 2020). Given that TET2 loss-of-function mimics some of the effects of CREBBP mutation, HDAC3 inhibitors were also more active in this setting in pre-clinical studies (Dominguez et al. 2018). KMT2D mutations are potential biomarkers to guide use of KDM5 inhibitors (Heward et al. 2021). SMAD1 hypermethylation may be a biomarker for use of DNMTi in DLBCLs and Hodgkin's lymphoma (Clozel et al. 2013; Gerlach et al. 2021; Stelling et al. 2019). Perhaps the most precise biomarkers for epigenetic therapies are the somatic mutations in IDH1 and IDH2, which were shown to cause aberrant epigenetic programming and are reversed by use of mutant-specific inhibitors (Cerchione et al. 2021; Figueroa et al. 2010). As of yet, there are few such examples and it remains critical for pre-clinical studies to use the right primary lymphoma systems to nominate candidate biomarkers to guide the use of these agents.

Maximizing the Impact of Emerging Epigenetic Therapies

Rational Combination of Epigenetic Agents

The epigenome is composed of many layers of interdependent and interactive biochemical information encoded by dozens of histone post-translational modifications, cytosine modifications, chromatin accessibility patterns, and three-dimensional architectural positioning. Plasticity and adaptability are hallmarks of the epigenome, and are essential to life since this permits cells to rapidly adapt their phenotype to changes in their environment, extracellular signals, toxic exposures, etc. The highly interconnected nature of the epigenome makes it so that disruption or change of any specific biochemical mechanism will have significant repercussions on the rest of the layers of the epigenome. This principle is dramatically illustrated by the example of somatic mutations in linker histone 1 isoforms, which are highly recurrent in germinal center-derived lymphomas (FLs and DLBCLs) (Yusufova et al. 2021). Loss of histone 1 isoforms in germinal center B-cells causes major shifts in chromatin accessibility and profound changes in histone modifications such as H3K27me3, H3K36me2, and H3K9me3, resulting in transcriptional activation of stem cell genes that are normally inaccessible to differentiated B-cells (Yusufova et al. 2021).

Thus, any specific perturbation induced by chromatin modifier mutations should be expected to affect various other epigenetic layers. As noted earlier, TET2 mutation in DLBCL results in loss of enhancer 5hmC, gain of 5mC, loss of H3K27acetyl, and perhaps other layers that were not examined (Dominguez et al. 2018; Rosikiewicz et al. 2020). *This is significant because a single therapeutic agent is unlikely to restore all affected epigenetic layers and hence may not yield the expected benefit.* We propose that maximal impact may require rational combination of epigenetic therapies, based on solid mechanistic science. For example, in the case of TET2, it may be desirable to combine HDAC3 and DNMT inhibitors to restore the enhancer H3K27acetylation and demethylate silenced gene promoters. This scenario is further complicated by the fact that lymphomas often have more than one epigenetic modifier mutation. For example, CREBBP and KMT2D mutations frequently occur together in FL and GCB-DLBCL, suggesting that HDAC3 and KDM5 inhibitors might be appropriate to test in this setting.

Rational Combination with Immunotherapies

When considering combinatorial therapy of epigenetic targeted therapies with immunotherapies, it is important to consider the potential for epigenetic therapies to make lymphoma cells more immunogenic, as well as their potential to either enhance or disrupt anti-lymphoma immune responses. In terms of the latter, there is increasing evidence showing how epigenetic instructions control or modulate T-cell-dependent immune responses, pointing to both opportunities and hazards of epigenetic targeted therapies with respect to the immune system. For example, during differentiation of effector $CD8^+$ T-cells, effector T-cell associated genes repressed by cytosine methylation and H3K27me3 in naive T-cells are activated by acquisition of active histone marks such as H3K4me3 and H3K9ac. Reciprocally, memory T-cell associated transcription factors active in naive T-cells are silenced by gain of repressive histone marks and reduction of active marks (Henning et al. 2018). Persistent T-cell activation in chronic infections or cancer leads to an exhausted phenotype where cytotoxic and proliferative activity of effector T-cells are epigenetically attenuated (Wherry and Kurachi 2015). Thus, epigenetic mechanisms dynamically regulate $CD8^+$ T-cell differentiation upon antigen encounter.

Notably, $CD8^+$ T-cell specific deletion of *Dnmt3a* results in increased memory CD8 T-cell differentiation and reduced terminal effector T-cell differentiation. This is due in part through upregulation of memory T-cell-related genes repressed by cytosine methylation during effector T-cell differentiation (Ladle et al. 2016). Along these lines combination of PD-1 checkpoint inhibitor camrelizumab plus decitabine in relapsed/refractory Hodgkin's lymphoma yielded superior survival compared with camrelizumab alone. Increased circulating memory T-cells after combination therapy was associated with superior survival (Liu et al. 2021). DNMTi may also improve the outcome of immune checkpoint blockade therapy through the de-repression of type I IFN signaling in tumors to activate anti-tumor T-cell response (Gonda et al. 2020; Stone et al. 2017). This is proposed to occur in part through re-activation of endogenous retroviral elements and consequent viral mimicry responses (Chen et al. 2021).

Chimeric antigen receptor (CAR) T-cell therapy is now a standard therapy for patients with relapsed/refractory B-cell lymphomas. Several studies suggested that genetic ablation or pharmacological inhibition of DNMT improve CAR-T cell activity. Exposing T-cells to decitabine before manufacturing CAR-T cells increases memory CAR-T cells (Wang et al. 2021), suggesting that DNMTi may promote memory $CD8^+$ T-cell differentiation. This may be related to the role of cytosine methylation in favoring exhaustion of cytotoxic T-cells, since inhibition of DNMT1 prevents exhaustion and prolongs CAR-T cell cytotoxic activity (Prinzing et al. 2021; Wang et al. 2021). DNMTi also enhances cytotoxic efficacy of CAR-T cells against B-ALL by increasing CAR-T cell/tumor cell conjugation through the upregulation of T-cell co-stimulatory ligands on leukemia cells (Xu et al. 2021). Favorable cytosine methylation profiles in CAR-T cells was associated with the enrichment of naive or memory CAR-T cells, high CR rate, and prolonged overall survival (Garcia-Prieto et al. 2022). Gain of cytosine methylation at T memory genes limits the cytotoxic activity of CAR-T cells by inducing CAR-T cell exhaustion (Zebley et al. 2021).

DNMT1 plays an important role in maintaining T regulatory cells (Tregs) by repressing pro-inflammatory genes through cytosine methylation, and Dnmt1 knockout mice develop lethal autoimmune disease due to Treg dysfunction (DuPage et al. 2015). This suggests additional utility of DNMTi to inhibit Treg functions, which can otherwise limit the efficacy of immunotherapies (Deng et al. 2020; Gattinoni et al. 2005; Togashi et al. 2019). Finally, epigenetic silencing of virus-specific antigens is an important immune escape mechanism in viral-associated lymphomas. For example, DNMT1 represses the expression of EBV-specific antigens in B-cell lymphoma cells and hence impairs recognition by EBV-specific cytotoxic T-cells (Guo et al. 2020). Along these lines decitabine treatment of EBV+ lymphoma cells restores expression of EBV antigens and enhances the presentation of virus-specific peptides on MHC. As a result, decitabine treatment sensitized EBV+ lymphoma cells to lysis by EBV-specific cytotoxic T-cells (Dalton et al. 2020). Collectively, there is a strong rationale for using DNMTi to potentiate immunotherapies and it seems warranted to develop further clinical trials with proper correlative studies to test these concepts in lymphomas.

EZH2 plays complex roles in the immune system. Ablation of EZH2 in $CD8^+$ T-cells was shown to inhibit effector T-cell development and increases memory $CD8^+$ T-cell by activating memory T-cell-related genes (Gray et al. 2017). EZH2 is expressed in exhausted $CD8^+$ T-cells, suggesting a possible role in these cells (Schietinger et al. 2016). On the other hand, EZH2 phosphorylation downstream of AKT, which inhibits EZH2 activity resulted in induction of effector T-cell differentiation and related gene sets (He et al. 2017). EZH2 may play roles in both Th1 and Th2 differentiation. For example, EZH2 represses the Th1 master regulatory transcription factor T-BET (Tumes et al. 2013). IFN-γ signaling induces H3K27 demethylase JMJD3 and de-represses T-BET by antagonizing EZH2, which promotes Th1 differentiation and IFN-γ production (Li et al. 2014). EZH2 also represses Th2 transcription factor Gata3, and deletion of EZH2 in naive CD4 T-cells enhanced Th2 cell differentiation and functions (Tumes et al. 2013). EZH2 cooperates with BCL6 in supporting formation of T follicular helper (TFH) cells by repressing p19ARF and Cdkn2a, and loss of EZH2 impairs TFH transcriptional programming and TFH formation (Li et al. 2018). Finally, Treg-specific deletion of EZH2 reduces the number of $FOXP3^+$ cells, and leads to spontaneous autoimmunity (DuPage et al. 2015; Yang et al. 2015).

These data make it difficult to predict exactly how EZH2 inhibitors might help or hinder immunotherapies. On the one hand, tazemetostat attenuated cytotoxic effects of non-exhausted CAR-T cells through reduction of H3K27me3 at exhaustion genes (Weber et al. 2021), although we have not seen this in our unpublished data. Moreover, in B-cell lymphomas EZH2 inhibition enhanced anti-tumor natural killer (NK) cell response through upregulation of CD58, a co-stimulatory receptor that binds to CD2 (Otsuka et al. 2020), suggesting that EZH2i may enhance NK cell-based immunotherapies such as CAR-NK cells. Although it is still unclear how EZH2 inhibition might enhance efficacy of immune checkpoint blockade in lymphoma, it was shown that EZH2i induces MHCI/II and PRAME expression in DLBCLs (Dersh et al. 2021; Ennishi et al. 2019; Takata et al. 2022). Pre-clinical studies in solid tumors show that EZH2i synergizes the efficacy of PD1, PDL1, or CTLA4 blockade by enhancing the infiltration of $CD4^+$ and $CD8^+$ T-cells and reducing Tregs in the tumor microenvironment (Goswami et al. 2018; Peng et al. 2015; Zhou et al. 2020; Zingg et al. 2017). This will be further addressed by a currently open clinical trial combining EZH2 with checkpoint blockade for solid tumors (NCT04388852).

HDAC3 is reported to inhibit the expression of cytotoxic proteins in effector $CD8^+$ T-cells, and *Hdac3* KO $CD8^+$ T-cells were not able to persist after antigen stimulation (Tay et al. 2020). However, this may be due to a scaffolding effect of HDAC3 rather than its enzymatic function, since HDAC3-selective inhibitors enhance recruitment of T-cells, drive potent MHC-dependent cytotoxic T-cell responses against primary DLBCLs (Mondello et al. 2020; Takata et al. 2022) Indeed, the combination of HDAC3 inhibitor BRD3308 with PDL1 blockade enhanced IFN-γ production, recruitment of $CD4^+$ and $CD8^+$ cells into DLBCLs in a syngeneic mouse model, and yielded significantly enhanced anti-lymphoma compared to either drug along (Mondello et al. 2020).

In conclusion, DNMTi, EZH2i, and HDAC3i have potential to combine favorably with immunotherapies such as checkpoint inhibitors, CAR-T cells and bispecific T-cell engaging antibodies. It thus warranted to continue to rigorously investigate the potential benefit of such epigenetic inhibitors in combination with immunotherapies for B-cell lymphomas. Multi-HDACs are also being tested for these kinds of activities although it is important to note the caveats raised earlier.

Conclusions

Taken together, there is strong mechanistic rationale for deployment of precision epigenetic therapies in B- and T-cell lymphomas and promising pre-clinical and clinical data. Although very few precision epigenetic targeted therapies have made it to the clinic at this point, many are in development and it is anticipated that there will be opportunity to test a wide variety of such therapies relevant to lymphoma in the near future. Critical to this venture is rigorous testing of such agents with the most state-of-the-art lymphoma model systems such as genetically engineered immunocompetent mice with syngeneic primary lymphomas reflecting the human disease, and/or PDX specimens grown in organoids or most ideally in humanized immunocompromised mice. Given the favorable impact of combining epigenetic targeted therapies with immunotherapies and targeted agents such as BH3 mimetics, it is of special interest to build these drugs into multi-modality regimens for first-line therapy of lymphomas, using regimens with low dose or even no cytotoxic agents. Overall, we believe that this new and emerging therapeutic field is likely to become of central importance to lymphoma standard of care in the future.

Acknowledgments

AMM is supported by NCI R35 CA220499, NCI P01 CA220499, NCI R01 CA234561, R01 CA266279, LLS SCOR 7021–20, and LLS TRP 6605–20.

Disclosures

AMM consulting for Treeline, Epizyme, Astra Zeneca, Daichi Sankyo, BMS, ExoTherapeutics, Janssen. Research funding from Epizyme, Astra Zeneca, Janssen.

Major Papers

Duy,C., Beguelin, W. and Melnick. A.(2020). **Epigenetic mechanisms in leukemias and lymphomas**. *Cold. Spring. Harb. Perspect. Med.* 10 (12.): 32014848. PMCID: PMC7706582. doi: 10.1101/cshperspect.a034959.

Bates, S. E. (2020). **Epigenetic therapies for cancer.** *N. Engl. J. Med.* 383 (7): 650–663. 32786190. doi: 10.1056/NEJMra1805035.

Must Read References

Bates, S.E. (2020). Epigenetic therapies for cancer. *N. Engl. J. Med.* 383 (7): 650–663.

Clozel, T., Yang, S., Elstrom, R.L., Tam, W., Martin, P., Kormaksson, M. et al. (2013). Mechanism-based epigenetic chemosensitization therapy of diffuse large B-cell lymphoma. *Cancer Discov.* 3 (9): 1002-1019.

Gonda, T.A., Fang, J., Salas, M., Do, C., Hsu, E., Zhukovskaya, A. et al. (2020). A DNA hypomethylating drug alters the tumor microenvironment and improves the effectiveness of immune checkpoint inhibitors in a mouse model of pancreatic cancer. *Cancer Res.* 80 (21): 4754-4767.

References

Agarwal, R., Chan, Y.C., Tam, C.S., Hunter, T., Vassiliadis, D. et al. (2019). Dynamic molecular monitoring reveals that SWI-SNF mutations mediate resistance to ibrutinib plus venetoclax in mantle cell lymphoma. *Nat. Med.* 25 (1): 119–129.

Amengual, J.E., Clark-Garvey, S., Kalac, M., Scotto, L., Marchi, E. et al (2013). Sirtuin and pan-class I/II deacetylase (DAC) inhibition is synergistic in preclinical models and clinical studies of lymphoma. *Blood* 122 (12): 2104–2113.

Bates, S.E. (2020). Epigenetic therapies for cancer. *N. Engl. J. Med.* 383 (7): 650–663.

Beguelin, W., Popovic, R., Teater, M., Jiang, Y., Bunting, K.L. et al. (2013). EZH2 is required for germinal center formation and somatic EZH2 mutations promote lymphoid transformation. *Cancer Cell* 23 (5): 677–692.

Beguelin, W., Rivas, M.A., Calvo Fernandez, M.T., Teater, M., Purwada, A. et al. (2017). EZH2 enables germinal centre formation through epigenetic silencing of CDKN1A and an Rb-E2F1 feedback loop. *Nat. Commun.* 8 (1): 877.

Beguelin, W., Teater, M., Meydan, C., Hoehn, K.B., Phillip, J.M. et al. (2020). Mutant EZH2 induces a pre-malignant lymphoma niche by reprogramming the immune response. *Cancer Cell* 37 (5): 655–73 e11.

Bitler, B.G., Aird, K.M., Garipov, A., Li, H., Amatangelo, M. et al. (2015). Synthetic lethality by targeting EZH2 methyltransferase activity in ARID1A-mutated cancers. *Nat. Med.* 21 (3): 231–238.

Caganova, M., Carrisi, C., Varano, G., Mainoldi, F., Zanardi, F. et al. (2013). Germinal center dysregulation by histone methyltransferase EZH2 promotes lymphomagenesis. *J. Clin. Invest.* 123 (12): 5009–5022.

Cerchione, C., Romano, A., Daver, N., DiNardo, C., Jabbour, E.J. et al. (2021). IDH1/IDH2 Inhibition in acute myeloid leukemia. *Front. Oncol.* 11: 639387.

Ceribelli, M., Kelly, P.N., Shaffer, A.L., Wright, G.W., Xiao, W. et al. (2014). Blockade of oncogenic IkappaB kinase activity in diffuse large B-cell lymphoma by bromodomain and extraterminal domain protein inhibitors. *Proc. Natl. Acad. Sci. U. S. A.* 111 (31): 11365–11370.

Chapuy, B., McKeown, M.R., Lin, C.Y., Monti, S., Roemer, M.G. et al. (2013). Discovery and characterization of super-enhancer-associated dependencies in diffuse large B cell lymphoma. *Cancer Cell* 24 (6): 777–790.

Chapuy, B., Stewart, C., Dunford, A.J., Kim, J., Kamburov, A. et al. (2018). Molecular subtypes of diffuse large B cell lymphoma are associated with distinct pathogenic mechanisms and outcomes. *Nat. Med.* 24 (5): 679–690.

Chartomatsidou, E., Ntoufa, S., Kotta, K., Rovida, A., Akritidou, M.A. et al. (2019). Inhibition of EZH2 and immune signaling exerts synergistic antitumor effects in chronic lymphocytic leukemia. *Blood Adv.* 3 (12): 1891–1896.

Chen, R., Ishak, C.A., and De Carvalho, D.D. (2021). Endogenous retroelements and the viral mimicry response in cancer therapy and cellular homeostasis. *Cancer Discov.* 11 (11): 2707–2725.

Chowdhury, S., Sripathy, S., Webster, A., Park, A., Lao, U. et al (2020). Discovery of selective SIRT2 inhibitors as therapeutic agents in B-cell lymphoma and other malignancies. *Molecules* 25 (3).

Clozel, T., Yang, S., Elstrom, R.L., Tam, W., Martin, P. et al. (2013). Mechanism-based epigenetic chemosensitization therapy of diffuse large B-cell lymphoma. *Cancer Discov.* 3 (9): 1002–1019.

Cogan, J.C., Liu, Y., and Amengual, J.E. (2020). Hypomethylating agents in lymphoma. *Curr. Treat. Options Oncol.* 21 (8): 61.

Dalton, T., Doubrovina, E., Pankov, D., Reynolds, R., Scholze, H. et al. (2020). Epigenetic reprogramming sensitizes immunologically silent EBV+ lymphomas to virus-directed immunotherapy. *Blood* 135 (21): 1870–1881.

Deng, Q., Han, G., Puebla-Osorio, N., Ma, M.C.J., Strati, P. et al. (2020). Characteristics of anti-CD19 CAR T cell infusion products associated with efficacy and toxicity in patients with large B cell lymphomas. *Nat. Med.* 26 (12): 1878–1887.

Dersh, D., Phelan, J.D., Gumina, M.E., Wang, B., Arbuckle, J.H. et al. (2021). Genome-wide screens identify lineage- and tumor-specific genes modulating MHC-I- and MHC-ii-restricted immunosurveillance of human lymphomas. *Immunity* 54 (1): 116–31 e10.

Dhimolea, E., de Matos Simoes, R., Kansara, D., Al'Khafaji, A., Bouyssou, J. et al (2021). An embryonic diapause-like adaptation with suppressed myc activity enables tumor treatment persistence. *Cancer Cell* 39 (2): 240–56 e11.

Dobenecker, M.W., Park, J.S., Marcello, J., McCabe, M.T., Gregory, R. et al. (2018). Signaling function of PRC2 is essential for TCR-driven T cell responses. *J. Exp. Med.* 215 (4): 1101–1113.

Dominguez, P.M., Ghamlouch, H., Rosikiewicz, W., Kumar, P., Beguelin, W. et al. (2018). TET2 deficiency causes germinal center hyperplasia, impairs plasma cell differentiation, and promotes B-cell lymphomagenesis. *Cancer Discov.* 8 (12): 1632–1653.

Doroshow, D.B., Eder, J.P., and LoRusso, P.M. (2017). BET inhibitors: a novel epigenetic approach. *Ann. Oncol.* 28 (8): 1776–1787.

DuPage, M., Chopra, G., Quiros, J., Rosenthal, W.L., Morar, M.M. et al. (2015). The chromatin-modifying enzyme Ezh2 is critical for the maintenance of regulatory T cell identity after activation. *Immunity* 42 (2): 227–238.

Duy, C., Beguelin, W., and Melnick, A. (2020). Epigenetic mechanisms in leukemias and lymphomas. *Cold Spring Harb. Perspect. Med.* 10 (12).

Duy, C., Li, M., Teater, M., Meydan, C., Garrett-Bakelman, F.E. et al (2021). Chemotherapy induces senescence-like resilient cells capable of initiating AML recurrence. *Cancer Discov.* 11 (6): 1542–1561.

Duy, C., Teater, M., Garrett-Bakelman, F.E., Lee, T.C., Meydan, C. et al (2019). Rational targeting of cooperating layers of the epigenome yields enhanced therapeutic efficacy against AML. *Cancer Discov.* 9 (7): 872–889.

Ennishi, D., Takata, K., Beguelin, W., Duns, G., Mottok, A. et al (2019). Molecular and genetic characterization of MHC deficiency identifies EZH2 as therapeutic target for enhancing immune recognition. *Cancer Discov.* 9 (4): 546–563.

Figueroa, M.E., Abdel-Wahab, O., Lu, C., Ward, P.S., Patel, J. et al (2010). Leukemic IDH1 and IDH2 mutations result in a hypermethylation phenotype, disrupt TET2 function, and impair hematopoietic differentiation. *Cancer Cell* 18 (6): 553–567.

Fiskus, W., Mill, C.P., Perera, D., Birdwell, C., Deng, Q. et al (2021). BET proteolysis targeted chimera-based therapy of novel models of Richter transformation-diffuse large B-cell lymphoma. *Leukemia* 35 (9): 2621–2634.

Garcia-Manero, G., Dohner, H., Wei, A.H., La Torre, I., Skikne, B. et al (2022). Oral Azacitidine (CC-486) for the treatment of myeloid malignancies. *Clin. Lymphoma Myeloma. Leuk.* 22 (4): 236–250.

Garcia-Prieto, C.A., Villanueva, L., Bueno-Costa, A., Davalos, V., Gonzalez-Navarro, E.A. et al (2022). Epigenetic profiling and response to CD19 chimeric antigen receptor T-cell therapy in B-cell malignancies. *J. Natl. Cancer Inst.* 114 (3): 436–445.

Gattinoni, L., Klebanoff, C.A., Palmer, D.C., Wrzesinski, C., Kerstann, K. et al. (2005). Acquisition of full effector function in vitro paradoxically impairs the in vivo antitumor efficacy of adoptively transferred CD8+ T cells. *J. Clin. Invest.* 115 (6): 1616–1626.

Gerlach, M.M., Stelling-Germani, A., Wu, T.C., Newrzela, S., Doring, C. et al. (2021). SMAD1 promoter hypermethylation and lack of SMAD1 expression in Hodgkin lymphoma: a potential target for hypomethylating drug therapy. *Haematologica* 106 (2): 619–621.

Gonda, T.A., Fang, J., Salas, M., Do, C., Hsu, E. et al (2020). A DNA hypomethylating drug alters the tumor microenvironment and improves the effectiveness of immune checkpoint inhibitors in a mouse model of pancreatic cancer. *Cancer Res.* 80 (21): 4754–4767.

Goswami, S., Apostolou, I., Zhang, J., Skepner, J., Anandhan, S. et al. (2018). Modulation of EZH2 expression in T cells improves efficacy of anti-CTLA-4 therapy. *J. Clin. Invest.* 128 (9): 3813–3818.

Gray, S.M., Amezquita, R.A., Guan, T., Kleinstein, S.H., and Kaech, S.M. (2017). Polycomb repressive complex 2-mediated chromatin repression guides effector CD8(+) T cell terminal differentiation and loss of multipotency. *Immunity* 46 (4): 596–608.

Guo, R., Zhang, Y., Teng, M., Jiang, C., Schineller, M. et al (2020). DNA methylation enzymes and PRC1 restrict B-cell Epstein-Barr virus oncoprotein expression. *Nat. Microbiol.* 5 (8): 1051–1063.

Harmeyer, K.M., Facompre, N.D., Herlyn, M., and Basu, D. (2017). JARID1 histone demethylases: emerging targets in cancer. *Trends Cancer* 3 (10): 713–725.

Hatzi, K., Geng, H., Doane, A.S., Meydan, C., LaRiviere, R. et al. (2019). Histone demethylase LSD1 is required for germinal center formation and BCL6-driven lymphomagenesis. *Nat. Immunol.* 20 (1): 86–96.

He, S., Liu, Y., Meng, L., Sun, H., Wang, Y. et al. (2017). Ezh2 phosphorylation state determines its capacity to maintain CD8(+) T memory precursors for antitumor immunity. *Nat. Commun.* 8 (1): 2125.

He, Z.X., Wei, B.F., Zhang, X., Gong, Y.P., Ma, L.Y. et al. (2021). Current development of CBP/p300 inhibitors in the last decade. *Eur. J. Med. Chem.* 209: 112861.

Helming, K.C., Wang, X., Wilson, B.G., Vazquez, F., Haswell, J.R. et al. (2014). ARID1B is a specific vulnerability in ARID1A-mutant cancers. *Nat. Med.* 20 (3): 251–254.

Henning, A.N., Roychoudhuri, R., and Restifo, N.P. (2018). Epigenetic control of CD8(+) T cell differentiation. *Nat. Rev. Immunol.* 18 (5): 340–356.

Heward, J., Konali, L., D'Avola, A., Close, K., Yeomans, A. et al. (2021). KDM5 inhibition offers a novel therapeutic strategy for the treatment of KMT2D mutant lymphomas. *Blood* 138 (5): 370–381.

Hoffman, G.R., Rahal, R., Buxton, F., Xiang, K., McAllister, G. et al. (2014). Functional epigenetics approach identifies BRM/SMARCA2 as a critical synthetic lethal target in BRG1-deficient cancers. *Proc. Natl. Acad. Sci. U. S. A.* 111 (8): 3128–3133.

Hogg, S.J., Vervoort, S.J., Deswal, S., Ott, C.J., Li, J. et al. (2017). BET-bromodomain inhibitors engage the host immune system and regulate expression of the immune checkpoint ligand PD-L1. *Cell Rep.* 18 (9): 2162–2174.

Huang, Y., Sendzik, M., Zhang, J., Gao, Z., Sun, Y. et al (2022). Discovery of the clinical candidate MAK683: an EED-directed, allosteric, and selective PRC2 inhibitor for the treatment of advanced malignancies. *J. Med. Chem.* 65 (7): *5317–5333*.

Jiang, Y., Ortega-Molina, A., Geng, H., Ying, H.Y., Hatzi, K. et al. (2017). CREBBP inactivation promotes the development of HDAC3-dependent lymphomas. *Cancer Discov.* 7 (1): 38–53.

Ladle, B.H., Li, K.P., Phillips, M.J., Pucsek, A.B., Haile, A. et al. (2016). De novo DNA methylation by DNA methyltransferase 3a controls early effector CD8+ T-cell fate decisions following activation. *Proc. Natl. Acad. Sci. U. S. A.* 113 (38): 10631–10636.

Lam, U.T.F. and Chen, E.S. (2022). Molecular mechanisms in governing genomic stability and tumor suppression by the SETD2 H3K36 methyltransferase. *Int. J. Biochem. Cell Biol.* 144: 106155.

Lampe, J.W., Alford, J.S., Boriak-Sjodin, P.A., Brach, D., Cosmopoulos, K. et al. (2021). Discovery of a first-in-class inhibitor of the histone methyltransferase SETD2 suitable for preclinical studies. *ACS Med. Chem. Lett.* 12 (10): 1539–1545.

Leung, W., Teater, M., Durmaz, C., Meydan, C., Chivu, A. et al. (2022). SETD2 haploinsufficiency enhances germinal center-associated AICDA somatic hypermutation to drive B cell lymphomagenesis. Cancer Discovery, In Press.

Li, F., Zeng, Z., Xing, S., Gullicksrud, J.A., Shan, Q. et al. (2018). Ezh2 programs TFH differentiation by integrating phosphorylation-dependent activation of Bcl6 and polycomb-dependent repression of p19Arf. *Nat. Commun.* 9 (1): 5452.

Li, M., Chiang, Y.L., Lyssiotis, C.A., Teater, M.R., Hong, J.Y. et al. (2019). Non-oncogene addiction to SIRT3 plays a critical role in lymphomagenesis. *Cancer Cell* 35 (6): 916–31 e9.

Li, Q., Zou, J., Wang, M., Ding, X., Chepelev, I. et al. (2014). Critical role of histone demethylase Jmjd3 in the regulation of CD4+ T-cell differentiation. *Nat. Commun.* 5: 5780.

Li, W., Bi, C., Han, Y., Tian, T., Wang, X. et al. (2019). Targeting EZH1/2 induces cell cycle arrest and inhibits cell proliferation through reactivation of p57(CDKN1C) and TP53INP1 in mantle cell lymphoma. *Cancer Bio.l Med.* 16 (3): 530–541.

Liu, Y., Wang, C., Li, X., Dong, L., Yang, Q. et al. (2021). Improved clinical outcome in a randomized phase II study of anti-PD-1 camrelizumab plus decitabine in relapsed/refractory Hodgkin lymphoma. *J. Immunother. Cancer* 9 (4).

Martin, P., Bartlett, N.L., Chavez, J.C., Reagan, J.L., Smith, S.M. et al. (2022). Phase 1 study of oral azacitidine (CC-486) plus R-CHOP in previously untreated intermediate- to high-risk DLBCL. *Blood* 139 (8): 1147–1159.

Meyer, S.N., Scuoppo, C., Vlasevska, S., Bal, E., Holmes, A.B. et al. (2019). Unique and shared epigenetic programs of the CREBBP and EP300 acetyltransferases in germinal center B cells reveal targetable dependencies in lymphoma. *Immunity* 51 (3): 535–47 e9.

Mondello, P., Tadros, S., Teater, M., Fontan, L., Chang, A.Y. et al. (2020). Selective inhibition of HDAC3 targets synthetic vulnerabilities and activates immune surveillance in lymphoma. *Cancer Discov.* 10 (3): 440–459.

Morschhauser, F., Tilly, H., Chaidos, A., McKay, P., Phillips, T. et al. (2020). Tazemetostat for patients with relapsed or refractory follicular lymphoma: an open-label, single-arm, multicentre, phase 2 trial. *Lancet Oncol.* 21 (11): 1433–1442.

Mullen, J., Kato, S., Sicklick, J.K., and Kurzrock, R. (2021). Targeting ARID1A mutations in cancer. *Cancer Treat Rev.* 100: 102287.

O'Connor, O.A., Falchi, L., Lue, J., Marchi, E., Kinahan, C. et al. (2019). Targeting the peripheral T-cell lymphoma (PTCL) epigenome with oral 5-azacytidine and romidepsin produces phase 1 study of oral 5-azacytidine and romidepsin produces marked lineage specific activity in patients with chemotherapy resistant disease: a multicenter phase 1 study. *Blood.* 134 (17): 1395–1405.

Otsuka, Y., Nishikori, M., Arima, H., Izumi, K., Kitawaki, T. et al. (2020). EZH2 inhibitors restore epigenetically silenced CD58 expression in B-cell lymphomas. *Mol. Immunol.* 119: 35–45.

Pappalardi, M.B., Keenan, K., Cockerill, M., Kellner, W.A., Stowell, A. et al. (2021). Discovery of a first-in-class reversible DNMT1-selective inhibitor with improved tolerability and efficacy in acute myeloid leukemia. *Nat. Cancer.* 2 (10): 1002–1017.

Park, I.Y., Powell, R.T., Tripathi, D.N., Dere, R., Ho, T.H. et al. (2016). Dual chromatin and cytoskeletal remodeling by SETD2. *Cell* 166 (4): 950–962.

Patel, A.A., Cahill, K., Saygin, C., and Odenike, O. (2021). Cedazuridine/decitabine: from preclinical to clinical development in myeloid malignancies. *Blood Adv.* 5 (8): 2264–2271.

Pechalrieu, D., Etievant, C., and Arimondo, P.B. (2017). DNA methyltransferase inhibitors in cancer: from pharmacology to translational studies. *Biochem. Pharmacol.* 129: 1–13.

Pei, Y., Liu, K.W., Wang, J., Garancher, A., Tao, R. et al. (2016). HDAC and PI3K antagonists cooperate to inhibit growth of MYC-driven medulloblastoma. *Cancer Cell.* 29 (3): 311–323.

Peng, D., Kryczek, I., Nagarsheth, N., Zhao, L., Wei, S. et al. (2015). Epigenetic silencing of TH1-type chemokines shapes tumour immunity and immunotherapy. *Nature* 527 (7577): 249–253.

Pikman, Y., Conway, A.S., Robichaud, A.L., Kitara, S., Church, A.J. et al. (2020). Targeting EZH2 for the treatment of hepatosplenic T-cell lymphoma. *Blood Adv.* 4 (7): 1265–1269.

Prinzing, B., Zebley, C.C., Petersen, C.T., Fan, Y., Anido, A.A. et al. (2021). Deleting DNMT3A in CAR T cells prevents exhaustion and enhances antitumor activity. *Sci. Transl. Med.* 13 (620): eabh0272.

Rampal, R., Alkalin, A., Madzo, J., Vasanthakumar, A., Pronier, E. et al. (2014). DNA hydroxymethylation profiling reveals that WT1 mutations result in loss of TET2 function in acute myeloid leukemia. *Cell Rep.* 9 (5): 1841–1855.

Reddy, A., Zhang, J., Davis, N.S., Moffitt, A.B., Love, C.L. et al. (2017). Genetic and functional drivers of diffuse large B cell lymphoma. *Cell* 171 (2): 481–94 e15.

Rehman, S.K., Haynes, J., Collignon, E., Brown, K.R., Wang, Y. et al. (2021). Colorectal cancer cells enter a diapause-like DTP state to survive chemotherapy. *Cell* 184 (1): 226–42 e21.

Rosikiewicz, W., Chen, X., Dominguez, P.M., Ghamlouch, H., Aoufouchi, S. et al. (2020). TET2 deficiency reprograms the germinal center B cell epigenome and silences genes linked to lymphomagenesis. *Sci. Adv.* 6 (25): eaay5872.

Schietinger, A., Philip, M., Krisnawan, V.E., Chiu, E.Y., Delrow, J.J. et al. (2016). Tumor-specific T cell dysfunction is a dynamic antigen-driven differentiation program initiated early during tumorigenesis. *Immunity* 45 (2): 389–401.

Scholze, H., Stephenson, R.E., Reynolds, R., Shah, S., Puri, R. et al. (2020). Combined EZH2 and Bcl-2 inhibitors as precision therapy for genetically defined DLBCL subtypes. *Blood Adv.* 4 (20): 5226–5231.

Sneeringer, C.J., Scott, M.P., Kuntz, K.W., Knutson, S.K., Pollock, R.M. et al. (2010). Coordinated activities of wild-type plus mutant EZH2 drive tumor-associated hypertrimethylation of lysine 27 on histone H3 (H3K27) in human B-cell lymphomas. *Proc. Natl. Acad. Sci. U. S. A.* 107 (49): 20980–20985.

Spriano, F., Stathis, A., and Bertoni, F. (2020). Targeting BET bromodomain proteins in cancer: the example of lymphomas. *Pharmacol Ther.* 215: 107631.

Stelling, A., Wu, C.T., Bertram, K., Hashwah, H., Theocharides, A.P.A. et al (2019). Pharmacological DNA demethylation restores SMAD1 expression and tumor suppressive signaling in diffuse large B-cell lymphoma. *Blood Adv.* 3 (20): 3020–3032.

Stengel, K.R., Bhaskara, S., Wang, J., Liu, Q., Ellis, J.D. et al. (2019). Histone deacetylase 3 controls a transcriptional network required for B cell maturation. *Nucleic Acids Res.* 47 (20): 10612–10627.

Stone, M.L., Chiappinelli, K.B., Li, H., Murphy, L.M., Travers, M.E. et al. (2017). Epigenetic therapy activates type I interferon signaling in murine ovarian cancer to reduce immunosuppression and tumor burden. *Proc. Natl. Acad. Sci. U. S. A.* 114 (51): E10981–E90.

Su, I.H., Dobenecker, M.W., Dickinson, E., Oser, M., Basavaraj, A. et al. (2005). Polycomb group protein ezh2 controls actin polymerization and cell signaling. *Cell* 121 (3): 425–436.

Takata, K., Chong, L.C., Ennishi, D., Aoki, T., Li, M.Y. et al. (2022). Tumor associated antigen PRAME exhibits dualistic functions that are targetable in diffuse large B-cell lymphoma. *J. Clin. Invest. 132 (10): e145343.*

Tari, G., Lemonnier, F., and Morschhauser, F. (2021). Epigenetic focus on angioimmunoblastic T-cell lymphoma: pathogenesis and treatment. *Curr. Opin. Oncol.* 33 (5): 400–405.

Tay, R.E., Olawoyin, O., Cejas, P., Xie, Y., Meyer, C.A. et al (2020). Hdac3 is an epigenetic inhibitor of the cytotoxicity program in CD8 T cells. *J. Exp. Med.* 217 (7).

Togashi, Y., Shitara, K., and Nishikawa, H. (2019). Regulatory T cells in cancer immunosuppression – implications for anticancer therapy. *Nat. Rev. Clin. Oncol.* 16 (6): 356–371.

Totman, J., Brach, D., Motwani, V., Howe, S., Deutschman, E. et al. (2021). Pharmacologic inhibition of the histone methyltransferase SETD2 with EZM0414 as a novel therapeutic strategy in relapsed or refractory multiple myeloma and diffuse large B-cell lymphoma. *ASH Annual Meeting Abstract* 1142.

Tumes, D.J., Onodera, A., Suzuki, A., Shinoda, K., Endo, Y. et al. (2013). The polycomb protein Ezh2 regulates differentiation and plasticity of CD4(+) T helper type 1 and type 2 cells. *Immunity* 39 (5): 819–832.

Velichutina, I., Shaknovich, R., Geng, H., Johnson, N.A., Gascoyne, R.D. et al. (2010). EZH2-mediated epigenetic silencing in germinal center B cells contributes to proliferation and lymphomagenesis. *Blood* 116 (24): 5247–5255.

Wang, Y., Tong, C., Dai, H., Wu, Z., Han, X. et al. (2021). Low-dose decitabine priming endows CAR T cells with enhanced and persistent antitumour potential via epigenetic reprogramming. *Nat. Commun.* 12 (1): 409.

Wanior, M., Kramer, A., Knapp, S., and Joerger, A.C. (2021). Exploiting vulnerabilities of SWI/SNF chromatin remodelling complexes for cancer therapy. *Oncogene* 40 (21): 3637–3654.

Weber, E.W., Parker, K.R., Sotillo, E., Lynn, R.C., Anbunathan, H. et al. (2021). Transient rest restores functionality in exhausted CAR-T cells through epigenetic remodeling. *Science* 372 (6537).

Wherry, E.J. and Kurachi, M. (2015). Molecular and cellular insights into T cell exhaustion. *Nat Rev Immunol* 15 (8): 486–499.

Wright, G.W., Huang, D.W., Phelan, J.D., Coulibaly, Z.A., Roulland, S. et al (2020). A probabilistic classification tool for genetic subtypes of diffuse large B cell lymphoma with therapeutic implications. *Cancer Cell* 37 (4): 551–68 e14.

Xu, N., Tse, B., Yang, L., Tang, T.C.Y., Haber, M. et al. (2021). Priming leukemia with 5-azacytidine enhances CAR T cell therapy. *Immunotargets Ther.* 10: 123–140.

Yamagishi, M., Hori, M., Fujikawa, D., Ohsugi, T., Honma, D. et al. (2019). Targeting excessive EZH1 and EZH2 activities for abnormal histone methylation and transcription network in malignant lymphomas. *Cell Rep.* 29 (8): 2321–37 e7.

Yang, X.P., Jiang, K., Hirahara, K., Vahedi, G., Afzali, B. et al. (2015). EZH2 is crucial for both differentiation of regulatory T cells and T effector cell expansion. *Sci. Rep.* 5: 10643.

You, S.H., Lim, H.W., Sun, Z., Broache, M., Won, K.J. et al. (2013). Nuclear receptor co-repressors are required for the histone-deacetylase activity of HDAC3 in vivo. *Nat. Struct. Mol. Biol.* 20 (2): 182–187.

Yusufova, N., Kloetgen, A., Teater, M., Osunsade, A., Camarillo, J.M. et al. (2021). Histone H1 loss drives lymphoma by disrupting 3D chromatin architecture. *Nature* 589 (7841): 299–305.

Zebley, C.C., Brown, C., Mi, T., Fan, Y., Alli, S. et al. (2021). CD19-CAR T cells undergo exhaustion DNA methylation programming in patients with acute lymphoblastic leukemia. *Cell Rep.* 37 (9): 110079.

Zhang, S., Liu, M., Yao, Y., Yu, B., and Liu, H. (2021). Targeting LSD1 for acute myeloid leukemia (AML) treatment. *Pharmacol Res.* 164: 105335.

Zhou, L., Mudianto, T., Ma, X., Riley, R., and Uppaluri, (2020). Targeting EZH2 enhances antigen presentation, antitumor immunity, and circumvents anti-PD-1 resistance in head and neck cancer. *Clin. Cancer Res.* 26 (1): 290–300.

Zhu, F. and Rui, L. (2019). PRMT5 in gene regulation and hematologic malignancies. *Genes. Dis.* 6 (3): 247–257.

Zingg, D., Arenas-Ramirez, N., Sahin, D., Rosalia, R.A., Antunes, A.T. et al (2017). The histone methyltransferase Ezh2 controls mechanisms of adaptive resistance to tumor immunotherapy. *Cell Rep.* 20 (4): 854–867.

Section V

Targeting the B-cell Receptor (BCR)

18

The Pathologic Role of BCR Dysregulation in Lymphoid Malignancies

Jan A. Burger

Department of Leukemia, The University of Texas MD Anderson Cancer Center, Houston, TX, USA

Take Home Messages

- B-cell receptor signaling is indispensable for normal B-cell development and adaptive immunity.
- In some B-cell leukemias and lymphomas, the malignant B-cells utilize BCR signaling for growth and survival.
- The mechanism of activation of BCR signaling includes continuous BCR stimulation by microbial antigens and/or autoantigens that are present in the tissue microenvironment, oncogenic mutations within the BCR complex or downstream signaling components, and ligand-independent tonic BCR signaling.

Introduction: The BCR in Normal and Malignant B Lymphocytes

The principal function of the B-cell receptor (BCR), a transmembrane receptor located on the cell surface of B lymphocytes, is to regulate B-cell development and, in mature B-cells, to generate antigen-specific immune responses based on the capacity of B-cells to recognize a great diversity of potential antigens via their unique BCRs (Melchers 2015). For example, the maturation of B lymphocytes from precursor B-cells requires the expression of a functional precursor BCR (pre-BCR). Loss-of-function mutations in components of the BCR (μ heavy chain, CD79A, and CD79B) or downstream signaling molecules such as Bruton's tyrosine kinase (BTK) or the adapter protein B-cell linker protein (BLNK) arrest B-cell development, leading to human immune-deficiencies characterized by agammaglobulinemia and the absence of mature B-cells (reviewed in Pieper et al. (2013) and Smith (2017)). Developing B-cells undergo recombination of distinct immunoglobulin (IG) heavy and light chain variable (V), diversity (D; for heavy chains only), and joining (J) genes, which makes the human BCR repertoire incredibly large, containing approximately 10^{16}–10^{18} unique BCR IG sequences (Dekosky et al. 2015; Kaplinsky and Arnaout 2016). Successful V(D)J recombination leads to the expression of functional BCR molecules of IgM and IgD isotypes on the surface of naive B-cells, allowing for antigen recognition, which in turn allows for the generation of antigen-specific antibody responses. Once activated by antigen, B-cells multiply and mature in germinal centers (GC) within secondary lymphoid organs (SLOs) by two distinct molecular mechanism, somatic hypermutation (SHM) and class-switch recombination (CSR) (De Silva and Klein 2015). SHM is characterized by the introduction of mutations within rearranged BCR IG genes at rates of 10^{-5}–10^{-3} mutations per base pair per generation (10^6-fold higher than spontaneous mutations occurring elsewhere in the genome) (Di Noia and Neuberger 2007; Peled et al. 2008). CSR replaces the constant heavy chain genes (IGHC) from IGHM/IGHD to IGHG or IGHE or IGHA, switching IG production from IgM/IgD to IgG, IgE, or IgA isotypes, without altering the antigen specificity (Stavnezer and Schrader 2014). Ultimately, positively selected GC B-cells give rise to memory B-cells with high-affinity BCRs and long-lived plasma cells. Plasma cells can home to the bone marrow or reside in SLOs, where they secrete antibodies.

BCR Signaling

The BCR generates two types of signal: a continuous low-strength signal termed "tonic," mediated by PI3Kα and PI3Kδ, thought to be independent of antigen binding, and an "activated" BCR signal in response to antigen binding, which activates downstream signaling to induce proliferation,

Precision Cancer Therapies: Targeting Oncogenic Drivers and Signaling Pathways in Lymphoid Malignancies: From Concept to Practice, Volume 1, First Edition. Edited by Owen A. O'Connor, Stephen M. Ansell, and John F. Seymour.

survival, and differentiation of B-cells. More specifically, BCR triggering causes conformational changes within the BCR complex that allows SRC family kinases to phosphorylate CD79A, CD79B, and spleen tyrosine kinase (SYK). After the phosphorylation of the cytoplasmic domains of the BCR co-receptor CD19 by LYN, phosphatidylinositol-3-kinase (PI3K) is recruited and activated, generating phosphatidylinositol-(3,4,5)-triphosphate (PIP3), a lipid second messenger molecule. PIP3 is essential for BTK recruitment and PLCγ2 activation, linking the function of PI3K with Ca^{2+} signaling and downstream activation of AKT and mammalian target of rapamycin (mTOR). Combined BTK and PI3K-dependent signaling regulate B-cell metabolism, proliferation, DNA repair, survival, cytoskeleton remodeling, and migration (Okkenhaug 2013). PI3Kδ is the form predominantly expressed by hematopoietic cells and plays a critical role in B-cell homeostasis and function (Okkenhaug and Vanhaesebroeck 2003). The importance of the BCR-related kinases BTK, SYK, PI3Kδ, and the phospholipase PLCγ2 for antigen-dependent BCR signaling was corroborated in mouse models, which demonstrated defective BCR signaling and function in the absence of each of these signaling components (Table 18.1) (Fruman et al. 2000). Downstream pathway activation results in calcium mobilization, and RAS and MAPK activation. Activation of phospholipase Cγ2 (PLCγ2), protein kinase Cβ (PKCβ), and caspase recruitment domain-containing protein 11 (CARD11) recruits BCL-10 and mucosa-associated lymphoid tissue lymphoma translocation 1 (MALT1) into a multiprotein CARD11–BCL-10-MALT1 (CBM) complex that activates nuclear factor-κB (NF-κB) signaling via IκB kinase (IKK) (Davis et al. 2010; Shaffer et al. 2012).

BCR Signaling in B-cell Malignancies

Many mechanism of normal B-cell humoral immunity has been co-opted by malignant B-cells, including BCR signaling and engagement with T helper cells (T_H cells) in the tissue microenvironment, supporting B-cell proliferation and survival (Rui et al. 2011), see Figures 18.1 and 18.2. The expressed IGHV provides clues to the antigen

Table 18.1 Consequences of genetic or pharmacological alteration of BCR signaling-related kinases.

Kinase	Gene deletion/mutation	Activating receptors in B-cells	Function in CLL	Inhibitor(s)	Effects of pharmacological inhibition
Bruton's tyrosine kinase (BTK)	In humans: X-linked agammaglobulinemia (XLA, Bruton's agammaglobulinemia); in mice: X-linked immunodeficiency (xid) (Smith 2017)	BCR, integrins, chemokine receptors	Survival, proliferation and migration, BCR signaling, chemokine secretion (CCL3, CCL4)	**Ibrutinib (Imbruvica)** **Acalabrutinib (Calquence)** **Zanubrutinib (Brukinsa)**	Ig levels generally remain stable, IgA levels can increase (Byrd et al. 2013; Sun et al. 2015), vaccine responses to novel antigens are altered (Pleyer et al. 2021). No increase in serious infections (Coutre et al. 2017) except mild cases of *Pneumocystis jiroveci* pneumonia (PJP) (Ahn et al. 2016). T-cell compartment diversifies (Yin et al. 2017) and becomes more functional (Long et al. 2017).
PI3Kδ	In humans: rare loss-of-function mutations in the p85α or p110δ subunits of PI3Kδ cause immunodeficiency and immune-mediated pathologies, including colitis (Lucas et al. 2016). Mutations in *PIK3CD* and *PIK3R1* cause a combined immunodeficiency syndrome called activated PI3Kδ syndrome (APDS) (Lucas et al. 2016). In mice: deficient antibody responses, lack of B1 cells and marginal zone B-cells (Okkenhaug et al. 2002)	BCR, integrins, chemokine receptors	CLL cell survival and migration, chemokine secretion (CCL3, CCL4)	**Idelalisib (Zydelig)** **Duvelisib (Copiktra)** also blocks PI3Kγ Umbralisib (Ukoniq)	Inhibition with idelalisib can be complicated by immune-mediated hepatitis, colitis, and pneumonitis; increased numbers of infections were seen when given in combination with other agents.

(Continued)

Table 18.1 (Continued)

Kinase	Gene deletion/mutation	Activating receptors in B-cells	Function in CLL	Inhibitor(s)	Effects of pharmacological inhibition
Spleen tyrosine kinase (SYK)	In mice: severe defect of B lymphopoiesis (Turner et al. 1995)	BCR, integrins, chemokine receptors	Survival and migration via BCR and chemokine receptor – signaling, chemokine secretion (CCL3, CCL4)	Fostamatinib (Tavalisse)	Immunological effects of pharmacological SYK inhibition with fostamatinib or GS-9973 have not been analyzed.

Names of FDA-approved kinase inhibitors are highlighted in bold.

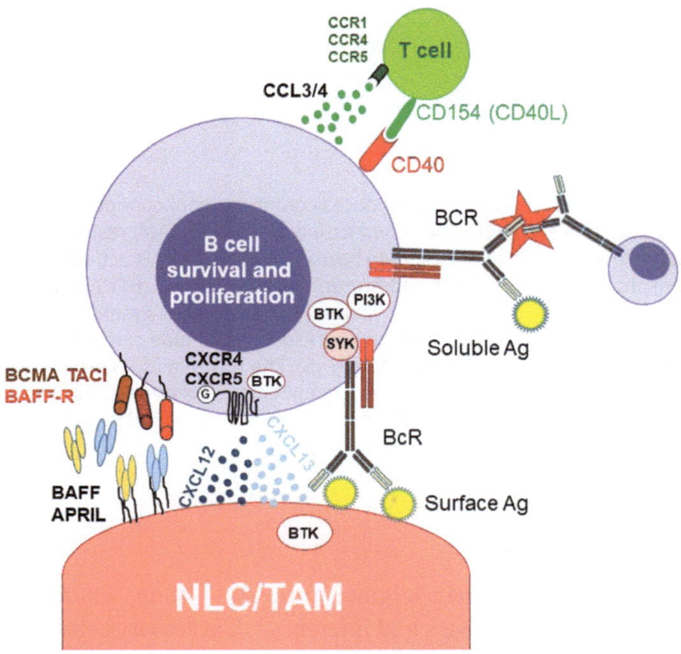

Figure 18.1 **The lymph node microenvironment in CLL.** CLL cells and express surface immunoglobulins (sIG) of the IgM and IgD isotypes, which are the core of the B-cell receptor (BCR) complex. The BCR can bind soluble or cell surface antigens, triggering BCR signaling which in turn activates cytoplasmatic kinases that propagate the signal, including SYK, BTK, and PI3K, favoring CLL cells survival and proliferation. BCR signaling can also be activated by recognition of intrinsic BCR motifs (red star, right side) resulting in autonomous BCR signaling. In CLL, nurse-like cells (NLC) activate BCR signaling via surface antigens; they also express BAFF and APRIL, which can activate corresponding receptors on CLL cells. NLC (and other types of macrophages) also express BTK. Furthermore, activated T-cells support CLL cells growth via cytokines and CD40 ligand (CD154), activating CD40 on CLL cells. BCR-related kinases, such as BTK, are also involved in signaling of chemokine receptors, such as CXCR4 and CXCR5, and adhesion molecules, and, consequently, BTK inhibition downmodulates the function of these tissue-homing receptors. Therefore, CLL cells are released from the lymph node microenvironment into the peripheral blood, once BTK inhibitor therapy is started, causing a transient redistribution lymphocytosis.

specificity of the transformed B-cell. Notably, the IGHV repertoire in several B-cell malignancies is heavily biased, suggesting preferential expansion of B-cells with distinct antigenic specificities (Baliakas et al. 2014; Hadzidimitriou et al. 2011; Stamatopoulos et al. 2017; Young et al. 2015). In chronic lymphocytic leukemia (CLL), the expression of virtually identical BCR clonotypes between different patients, referred to as BCR stereotypy, has been interpreted as evidence for antigen selection (Agathangelidis et al. 2012). Many of the predicted BCR specificities appear directed at autoantigens (Burger and Chiorazzi 2013; Young et al. 2015).

Reactivity of BCRs to autoantigens exposed on apoptotic cells has been reported for CLL and activated B-cell-type-DLBCL (ABC-DLBCL), a subtype of diffuse large B-cell lymphoma (DLBCL). The importance of autoantigen-dependent BCR activation has been shown in CLL (Duhren-von Minden et al. 2012) and ABC-DLBCL (Young et al. 2015) by expressing CLL- or lymphoma cell-derived BCRs in cell lines. This finding led to the demonstration that CLL- or lymphoma-derived BCRs can bind self-antigens, including structural elements within the framework region (FR), a subdivision of the IGHV region (Duhren-von Minden et al. 2012; Young et al. 2015).

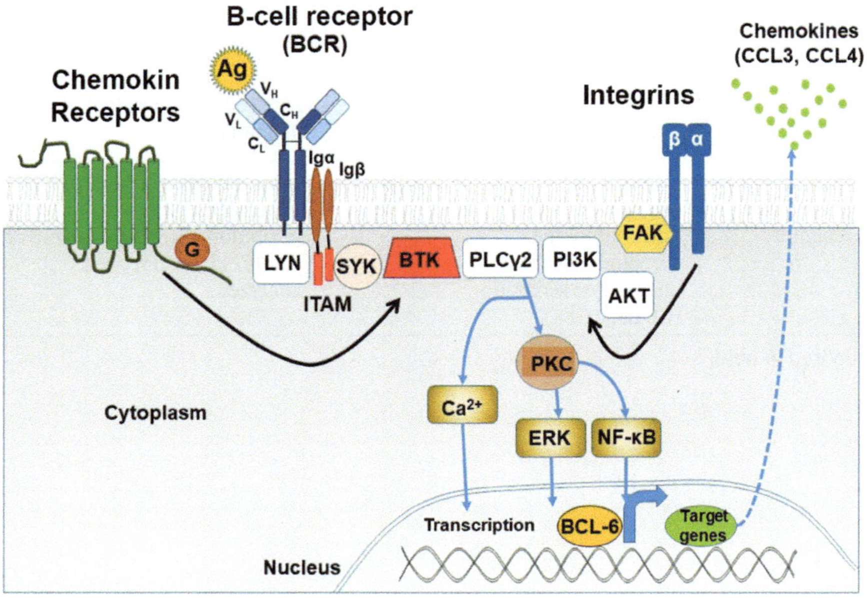

Figure 18.2 **The B-cell receptor signaling pathway.** Antigen binding by the B-cell receptor (BCR) induces conformational changes and the assembly of a signaling complex that induces phosphorylation of immunoreceptor tyrosine-based activation motif (ITAM) residues on the cytoplasmic tails of CD79A (also known as Igα) and CD79B (also known as Igβ). In turn, spleen tyrosine kinase (SYK) is activated, which is followed by the activation of B-cell linker protein (BLNK), phospholipase Cγ2 (PLCγ2), and Bruton's tyrosine kinase (BTK). BLNK allows SYK to phosphorylate BTK, while LYN also directly phosphorylates BTK. Tonic BCR signaling via the PI3K pathway is essential for the survival of mature B-cells and subtypes of B-cell non-Hodgkin's lymphoma (B-NHL). Further downstream responses include calcium (Ca^{2+}) mobilization, and activation of protein kinase C (PKC), the RAS-MAPK pathway and nuclear factor-κB (NF-κB). The positive BCR co-receptor CD19 contributes to the activation of the PI3K-AKT pathway and to the induction of survival. In chronic lymphocytic leukemia (CLL), the downstream signaling response causes downregulation of the transcriptional repressor *BCL6*, and promotes transcription in the nucleus, including that of C-C motif chemokine 3 (*CCL3*) and *CCL4* chemokine genes, which are then translated and secreted.

B-cell Proliferation in Secondary Lymphatic Organs (SLOs)

T-cell-dependent antibody responses require an orchestrated interaction of B-cells, T-cells, and antigen-presenting cells (APCs) which occurs in the SLOs (i.e. lymph nodes and spleen). The process of B-cell selection, expansion, and differentiation starts by B-cell activation via antigen, either in the form of soluble antigen within the lymphatic fluid or as antigen presented to the B-cells by APC (macrophages, dendritic cells, follicular dendritic cells [FDC]), followed by B-cell engagement with antigen-specific T_H cells (De Silva and Klein 2015; Sage and Sharpe 2015; Victora and Nussenzweig 2012). Only B-cells which interact with T-cells move onward to form early GCs (secondary follicles). As the GC matures, dark and light zones are formed, containing densely packed centroblasts and CXC-chemokine ligand $(CXCL12)^+$ fibroblastic reticular cells within the dark zone, versus smaller centrocytes, along with T follicular helper (T_{FH}) and $CXCL13^+$ FDC in the light zones. Centroblasts first undergo SHM in the dark zone resulting in the diversification of the BCR repertoire, a prerequisite for subsequent selection of B-cells carrying high-affinity BCRs. B-cells then migrate to the light zone, where they become centrocytes and interact with accessory cells (FDC and T_{FH} cells) for selection that is part of the antibody affinity maturation process. CSR and differentiation into memory B and plasma cell precursors also occur the light zone of the GC.

Like antigen-selected normal B-cells, CLL cells also proliferate primarily in secondary lymphatic tissues, where they form "proliferation centers," previously referred to as "pseudofollicles." CLL cells in proliferation centers express the proliferation marker Ki-67, a finding confirmed by deuterium labeling in patients which established that CLL cells proliferate primarily in the SLO (Herndon et al. 2017). In the microenvironment of SLO, CLL cells are in intimate contact with T-cells (Patten et al. 2008), monocyte-derived nurse-like cells (NLC) (Bhattacharya et al. 2011; Burkle et al. 2007) which are comparable to lymphoma-associated macrophages in other B-cell lymphomas, mesenchymal stromal cells (MSCs) (Ruan et al. 2006), and extracellular matrix (ECM) factors, such as hyaluronan or fibronectin. Gene expression profiling of CLL cells revealed that BCR and NF-κB signaling are activated in the lymph nodes, but not in other compartments (blood and bone marrow) (Herishanu et al. 2011), strongly supporting that BCR signaling is the central disease driver in CLL.

In proliferative centers, CLL cells are interspersed with large numbers of T_H cells (Patten et al. 2008), and in particular Ki67$^+$ proliferating CLL cells co-localized with T-cells, suggesting that T-cells contribute to the pathogenesis by fostering CLL cell growth (Patten et al. 2008). Growth of primary CLL cells in immune-deficient mice requires the presence of activated autologous T-cells (Bagnara et al. 2011; Patten et al. 2016). Chemokines are thought to regulate the engagement between CLL cells and T-cells (Ghia et al. 2002). For example, upon BCR engagement with antigen, both normal B-cells and CLL cells secrete C-C motif chemokine 3 (CCL3; also known as MIP1α) and CCL4 (also known as MIP1β) (Burger et al. 2009; Krzysiek et al. 1999), which in turn attract T-cells for cognate T cell–B cell interactions. CLL cells in proliferative centers produce higher concentrations of CCL3 than CLL cells outside of the proliferative centers, and lymph node specimens from patients in whom the CLL cells express higher amounts of the CCL3 protein are more densely infiltrated by T-cells (Hartmann et al. 2016), supporting the concept of BCR signaling-driven attraction of T-cells via chemokines.

Another cell type that can support malignant B-cells in SLO is specialized macrophages (i.e. NLC in CLL or tumor-associated macrophages/TAM in other lymphomas). NLC can activate a number of pathways by secreting chemokines (CXCL12 and CXCL13) (Burger et al. 2000; Burkle et al. 2007), expressing tumor necrosis factor (TNF) family members (B-cell activating factor [BAFF] and a proliferation-inducing ligand [APRIL]) (Nishio et al. 2005), and ligands for the BCR (Binder et al. 2010; Hacken et al. 2017). Gene expression studies have revealed that BCR signaling is the most prominent pathway activated in CLL cells upon contact with NLC (Burger et al. 2009). In support of a crucial role for NLC in CLL progression, deletion of LYN kinase disables the "nursing" function of macrophages, resulting in delayed disease progression in a mouse CLL model (Nguyen et al. 2016). Accordingly, targeting of macrophages, either by colony-stimulating factor 1 receptor (CSF1R) signaling blockade using clodrolip (the bisphosphonate known as clodronate encapsulated in liposomes) (Galletti et al. 2016) or by deletion of migration inhibitory factor (MIF) (Reinart et al. 2013), was also shown to delay leukemia development in other CLL mouse models. In follicular lymphoma (FL), gene expression studies revealed that T-cell and macrophage-derived expression signatures, rather than lymphoma cell signatures, determine the outcome of the disease when treatment was based on chemotherapy (Dave et al. 2004). With the introduction of rituximab the impact of TAM on FL prognosis is less prominent (reviewed in Gouni et al. (2021)). FL cells associate with T_H cells, especially T_{FH} cells, MSCs, FDCs, and macrophages (Kridel et al. 2012).

The BCR Complex in Malignant B-cells

CLL

In CLL, BCR signaling in SLOs appears to be the major factor driving proliferation. Mutations in the BCR or downstream signaling components, as identified in DLBCL (Davis et al. 2010), are absent (Philippen et al. 2010) or rarely present (Thompson et al. 1997) in CLL. Surface IgM (sIgM) molecules are downregulated on CLL cells *in vivo* but recover *in vitro*, providing evidence of engagement with putative antigens *in vivo* (Mockridge et al. 2007). Furthermore, the bias in IGHV gene usage and association of certain IGHV genes with specific IGHD and IGHJ segments ("stereotyped BCRs") (Stamatopoulos et al. 2017) argue for antigen-dependent BCR activation as a dominant mechanism in CLL. In CLL, the number of somatic mutations in the clonal IGHV genes is used to distinguish patients with "unmutated" CLL (U-CLL, with 98% or more sequence homology with the germline sequence) from those with "mutated" CLL (M-CLL, with less than 98% sequence homology) (Hamblin et al. 1999; Rassenti et al. 2008). Patients with M-CLL (50–60% of cases) generally experience indolent disease, whereas those with U-CLL (40–50% of cases) typically have more rapid disease progression, adverse genetic features, clonal evolution, and experience less benefit from chemotherapy-based treatments (Damle et al. 1999; Hamblin et al. 1999). Interestingly, BTK inhibitor therapy overcomes the negative prognostic impact of U-CLL, based on longer follow-up of M-CLL and U-CLL patients treated with ibrutinib (Burger et al. 2020). IGHV gene SHM stratus is stable in individual patients, in contrast to other prognostic markers (i.e. cytogenetics) (Rosenquist et al. 2017), and provides clues about the origin of CLL. U-CLL probably derives from a B-cell that has not experienced a "GC-like" reaction, whereas M-CLL derives from a mature B-cell subset with acquired SHM during a "GC-like" reaction (Kipps et al. 2017; Seifert et al. 2012).

The presence or absence of acquired SHM translates into higher or lower antigen selectivity and affinity of the BCR, respectively. Examples of the restricted reactivity of BCR from M-CLL are binding to the Fc-tail of IgG (so-called "rheumatoid factors") or to β-(1,6)-glucan, an antigenic determinant of yeast (Hoogeboom et al. 2013). In contrast, low-affinity BCR from patients with U-CLL are polyreactive, i.e. they can recognize various foreign and autoantigens, such as vimentin, myosin, or rheumatoid factors present in the tissue microenvironment (Burger and Chiorazzi 2013). Furthermore, U-CLLs have a higher BCR signaling capacity which has been linked to a higher expression of ζ-associated protein of 70 kDa (ZAP-70) (Chen et al. 2005, 2002), and lower expression of myristoylated alanine-rich C-kinase substrate (MARCKS) (Beckmann et al. 2021). Collectively, these data support the concept of antigen-driven selection and expansion of CLL clones, which determines the pace of disease progression and disease aggressiveness. Likewise, in a significant fraction of patients with mantle cell lymphoma (MCL), the malignant B-cells express hypermutated IGHV and use a restricted IGHV repertoire, with a similar prognostic impact as in CLL (Hadzidimitriou et al. 2011; Navarro et al. 2012; Xochelli et al. 2015), indicating that the concept of antigen selection also applies to MCL (Hadzidimitriou et al. 2011). Further, ABC-DLBCL cells express BCRs with restricted antigen specificities (Young et al. 2015). Thus, antigenic stimulation and clonal selection play a role in several mature B-cell malignancies.

BCR Signaling in DLBCL

DLBCL is a highly heterogeneous disease, in which the malignant B-cells carry frequent mutations, many of which can function as genetic drivers of the disease (Chapuy et al. 2018; Schmitz et al. 2018; Shaffer et al. 2012). Based on gene expression studies, two subtypes of DLBCL were identified that are linked to BCR signaling, the germinal center B cell-like (GCB) and activated B cell-like (ABC) subtypes of DLBCL. Gene expression of ABC-DLBCL cells resembles that of normal B-cells activated though the BCR (Alizadeh et al. 2000), and is initiated by autoantigens triggering the BCR. Specifically, BCRs from ABC-DLBCL can be triggered by self-antigens present in the tissue microenvironment, by surface N-acetyl-lactosamine glycans, or epitopes present in the Ig heavy chain of the BCR itself. While ABC-DLBCL cases typically express BCRs of the IgM isotype, promoting survival and mitogenic signaling through the NF-κB pathway, GCB-DLBCL commonly expresses BCRs of the IgG isotype, linked to differentiation rather than cell proliferation.

BCR signaling in ABC-DLBCL activates NF-κB through a signaling cascade of SYK, BTK, and protein kinase C (PKC)-β to generate the CARD11–BCL10–MALT1 adaptor complex, which in turn activates IκB kinase. In contrast, "tonic," low-level BCR signaling does not require high-affinity antigen binding, triggers PI3K, and is important for survival of GCB-DLBCL cells. When treated with chemo-immunotherapy (CIT), patients with ABC-DLBCL have inferior prognosis, but can respond to ibrutinib (Wilson et al. 2015), especially in cases of ABC-DLBCL carrying the myeloid differentiation primary response 88 (*MYD88*)^{L265P} mutation or mutations in *CD79B* (80% response rate). Ibrutinib-responsiveness in ABC-DLBCL is linked with a multiprotein supercomplex formed by MYD88, TLR9, and the BCR, termed the My-T-BCR supercomplex (Phelan et al. 2018), and has chronic active BCR signaling resulting in PI3K and NF-κB pathway activation (Davis et al. 2010). Mechanism of BCR pathway activation in ABC-DLBCL includes antigen-dependent BCR triggering and mutations of components of the BCR itself or in downstream signaling molecules that enhance or inhibit BCR signaling and activation of the NF-κB pathway (i.e. MYD88, TNFAIP3, CD79A/B, and CARD11).

CD79B mutations, which occur in about 30% of ABC-DLBCL cases, enhance BCR signaling by preventing BCR internalization, inhibiting negative BCR regulators such as LYN, and increasing surface IgM expression. Another common mutation in ABC-DLBCL affects the adaptor protein MYD88 that is critical for NF-κB activation downstream of Toll-like receptors (TLRs) (Ngo et al. 2011). TLR signaling is part of innate immune responses and cooperative signaling between TLR and BCR pathways can enhance NF-κB activation and suppress tolerance of autoreactive B-cells (Leadbetter et al. 2002; Wilson et al. 2015). *MYD88 L265P* mutations frequently occur in DLBCL patients who also harbor *CD79B* mutations. *MYD88 L265P* mutations have also been recognized as a hallmark genetic lesion in Waldenstrom's macroglobulinemia (WM) (Treon et al. 2012).

A critical role for antigen-dependent BCR activation in ABC-DLBCL, in addition to acquired somatic mutations in signaling components, is supported by the observations that *CD79* mutations cannot autonomously activate BCR signaling and that BCRs on these lymphoma cells form BCR clusters resembling BCR complexes on normal, antigen-triggered B-cells (Davis et al. 2010; Tolar et al. 2009). Moreover, up to a third of ABC-DLBCLs express the Ig variable heavy chain 4–34 (VH4-34), usually associated with reactivity to autoantigens (Young et al. 2015). Furthermore, ABC-DLBCL cell lines express specific VH sequences which can react with motifs of the BCR itself or with antigens released during apoptotic cell death (Young et al. 2015).

GCB-DLBCL cell lines are not dependent on NF-κB activation or BTK signaling, nor do these tumor cell lines display clustering of cell surface BCR molecules (Davis et al. 2010). However, DLBCL cell lines with low NF-κB activity can be sensitive to SYK inhibition (Chen et al. 2008, 2013). GCB-DLBCL dependency on tonic BCR signaling has been proposed, based on the following findings. First, forced activation of AKT rescued BCR-dependent GCB-DLBCL cell lines from knockdown of SYK or CD19 (Chen et al. 2013). Second, in contrast to ABC-DLBCL (Young et al. 2015), the replacement of the antigen-binding site of the BCR in GCB-DLBCL had no effect on tonic signaling (Havranek et al. 2017). In keeping with a critical role for tonic PI3K-AKT signaling in GCB-DLBCL, inactivation of the negative regulator of PI3K signaling *PTEN* is common in primary GCB-DLBCL (Chen et al. 2013) but not in ABC-DLBCL (Lenz et al. 2008). Inactivation of PTEN can maintain tonic survival signals in the absence of effective BCR signaling (Havranek et al. 2017), a mechanism that may explain the relatively low response rate to SYK inhibition in GCB-DLBCL (Friedberg et al. 2010).

Tonic BCR Signaling in Burkitt's Lymphoma

Burkitt's lymphoma (BL) is a rare, aggressive B-cell malignancy which is derived from GC B-cells and is transformed by a translocation of the c-Myc oncogene into the H chain locus of the BCR (Dalla-Favera et al. 1982). In contrast to antigen-dependent activated BCR signaling, antigen-independent tonic BCR signaling supports survival of malignant B-cells primarily through the PI3K-AKT-mTOR pathway. Using RNAi screens, the survival of BL cell lines was shown to require BCR expression, SYK and PI3K signaling, but not the activation of NF-κB (Schmitz et al. 2014, 2012). Furthermore, a BL mouse model suggested that BCR expression is required for BL cell survival (Varano et al. 2017). CRISPR/Cas9-medited deletion of BCR-related molecules in a BL cell line, Ramos, showed that the fitness of the Ramos B-cells requires the expression of the CD19 and the Igβ subunit of the BCR (He et al. 2018). Interestingly, the mode of BCR signaling in BL resembles that observed in GCB-DLBCL, being NF-κB-independent, but requiring on PI3K/mTOR signaling with CD19 use as an adaptor (Phelan et al. 2018) and resembling "tonic" BCR signaling, originally described in normal murine B-cells (Lam et al. 1997). However, the concept of BL driven by oncogenic coupling of MYC and PI3K-AKT activity, based on the potentiating effect of PI3K activation on MYC-dependent B-cell lymphomagenesis in a murine BL model, was challenged by lack of sensitivity of BL cells to AKT knockdown or inhibition, in contrast to GCB DLBCL cells, arguing against a growth-promoting role for the PI3K-AKT axis in BL (Gehringer et al. 2020).

BCR Signaling in Follicular Lymphoma (FL)

FL, an indolent B-cell malignancy derived from GC B-cells, characteristically carries the t(14;18) (q32;q21) translocation, which places *BCL2* gene into the IGHC locus, resulting in BCL2 overexpression. Despite the loss of one Ig allele through the t(14;18), FL cells retain surface expression of a functional BCR. Ongoing IGHV SHM results in a wide variety of FL subclones in each patient, carrying distinct IGHV sequences. Moreover, FL cells express unusual, mannosylated glycans in the antigen-binding site of the BCR (N-glycosylation sites) (Kuppers and Stevenson 2018; Odabashian et al. 2020) which allows for interactions with lectins present in the FL microenvironment. For example, the lectin dendritic cell-specific ICAM-3-grabbing nonintegrin (DC-SIGN), expressed by macrophages in FL tissue, induces a persistent signaling for FL survival/proliferation, providing an explanation for the negative prognostic impact of macrophage tissue infiltration in FL (Dave et al. 2004). In addition, triggering by other autoantigens, such as vimentin, BCR cross-reactivity with microbial antigens, or mutations affecting BCR pathway members have been suggested to activate the BCR signaling in FL (Krysiak et al. 2017).

BCR Signaling in Mantle Cell Lymphoma (MCL) and Marginal Zone Lymphoma (MZL)

MCL cell characteristically has the t(11;14)(q13;q32) translocation which places the *CCDN1* gene into the IGHC gene locus, resulting in cyclin D1 overexpression. Lymphoma cells from mostly MCL patients have unmutated IGHV, a minority (~30%) have mutated IGHV (Navarro et al. 2012). A pathogenic role of the BCR in MCL is suggested by stereotyped BCRs detected in ~10% of MCL patients (Hadzidimitriou et al. 2011), as well as activation of BCR pathway molecules in MCL cells. BCR signaling can regulate survival of leukemia MCL cells via NF-κB signaling, upregulating anti-apoptotic factors and cytokines, and signaling via PI3K, AKT, GSK-3β inhibition, and β-catenin stabilization (Saba et al. 2016).

Marginal zone lymphoma (MZL) is typically subclassified into three distinct subtypes, comprising: nodal (NMZL), extranodal or mucosa-associated (MALT lymphoma), and primary splenic (SMZL). MZL was one of the first B-cell malignancies in which antigen selection during transformation and/or continued antigenic drive by microorganisms was demonstrated to trigger the development and expansion of the malignant B-cells. Specific examples are the development of MALT lymphomas in the context of chronic *Helicobacter pylori* infection (Wotherspoon et al. 1993), hepatitis C virus (HCV) promoting SMZL, *Borrelia* spp. in cutaneous MZL (Cerroni et al. 1997), and *Chlamydia psittaci* in ocular adnexal MZL (Ferreri et al. 2004). Beside infection, chronic autoantigen stimulation contributes to the development MALT lymphomas of the salivary gland and thyroid in patients with Sjögren's syndrome or Hashimoto's thyroiditis, respectively. MZL cells typically express somatically mutated IGHV genes and stereotyped BCR is common in MZL. Despite a common association between MZL and infection, the infectious agent does not appear to commonly trigger the BCR on MZL directly, but rather seems to play a co-stimulatory role.

Targeting BCR Signaling

Normal and malignant B-cells contain kinases that are essential for transmitting signals from surface receptors into the cytoplasm, regulating B-cell survival and proliferation. The most important kinases are SYK, BTK, and PI3 kinase isoforms, especially PI3K delta (PI3Kδ). These kinases are essential for BCR signaling, but also transmit signaling from chemokine receptors (i.e. CXCR4 and CXCR5) and adhesion molecules, which regulate B-cell trafficking and tissue homing. The type of BCR signaling co-opted by a particular lymphoma subtype determines the sensitivity to small molecule inhibitors. B-cell malignancies relying on BCR-driven NF-κB activation can be sensitive to inhibitors of BTK (Davis et al. 2010), IKK (Davis et al. 2010), or MALT1 (Dai et al. 2017; Fontan et al. 2012). In contrast, B-cell malignancies relying on tonic signaling can respond to SYK and/or PI3K-AKT signaling inhibition (Chen et al. 2013; Schmitz et al. 2014; Szydlowski et al. 2016).

Inhibitors of SYK (Friedberg et al. 2010), BTK (Byrd et al. 2013), and PI3Kδ (Furman et al. 2014; Gopal et al. 2014) have been developed over the last 15 years. The BTK inhibitor ibrutinib is currently approved for treatment of patients with CLL, MCL, WM, and MZL, while the PI3Kδ inhibitor idelalisib is approved for patients with relapsed CLL (in combination with rituximab, a monoclonal antibody targeting the B-cell antigen CD20) and FL. The following discussion is focused on these two approved first-in-class agents because they are well characterized in terms of preclinical and clinical activities. Both drugs have remarkable therapeutic efficacy in patients with CLL (Byrd et al. 2013; Furman et al. 2014), MCL (Kahl et al. 2014; Wang et al. 2013), FL (Gopal et al. 2014), MZL (Noy et al. 2017), and WM (Treon et al. 2015), while responses are uncommon or restricted to subsets of patients in other B-cell malignancies, such as DLBCL (Wilson et al. 2015). Importantly, the overall response rates (ORR) and durability of responses to BTK and PI3Kδ inhibitors differ substantially between different B-cell malignancies. Most patients with CLL (Burger et al. 2020; Byrd et al. 2019, 2020a; Sharman et al. 2019a, b) and WM (Castillo et al. 2021; Treon et al. 2021; Wagner-Johnston et al. 2021) have long remissions with both classes of inhibitors. In relapsed and refractory MCL, both BTK and PI3Kδ inhibitors achieve high initial response rates, though the median progression-free survival (PFS) is vastly different for the two drugs, being 13.9 months (Wang et al. 2013) for ibrutinib and only 3.7 months for idelalisib (Kahl et al. 2014), both of which are considerably shorter than for patients with CLL treated with these same agents. In patients with DLBCL, responses are limited to the ABC subtype, and the duration of response is typically only a few months (Wilson et al. 2015).

On the one hand, the substantial differences in response rates and response duration between different B-cell malignancies may reflect the variable dependencies on BCR signaling and/or interactions with the microenvironment. On the other hand, the genetic background and the degree of genetic instability are likely to contribute to the activation of pathways that can overcome BTK or PI3Kδ inhibition. Cyclin-dependent kinase 4 (CDK4)-driven proliferation of ibrutinib-resistant MCL cells represents an example for this type of escape mechanism (Chiron et al. 2014), which can clinically be addressed by ibrutinib combination therapy with the CDK4 inhibitor palbociclib, with encouraging early clinical trial data (Martin et al. 2019).

The indolent lymphomas, comprising CLL, FL, MZL, and most cases of MCL, are incurable with chemotherapy (Sehn 2016). In these types of lymphoma, BCR signaling inhibitors have become an attractive option for patients relapsing after CIT, or have replaced CIT, as in CLL, based on a series of randomized trials in which ibrutinib or acalabrutinib was compared to standard CIT. BCR signaling inhibitors have also been added to standard chemotherapy-based regimens in the hope of extending the duration of response. In contrast, a majority of patients with DLBCL can be cured with chemotherapy (Miller et al. 2016), normally given together with CD20 monoclonal antibodies (i.e. R-CHOP) (Coiffier et al. 2002). However, the ABC subset has a higher relapse risk and inferior survival when compared to the GCB DLBCL subtype with standard chemotherapy-based treatment (Alizadeh et al. 2000). Thus, the addition of BCR pathway inhibitors to standard chemotherapy regimens has been investigated with the goal of increasing the cure rate of patients with DLBCL. Unfortunately, the studies completed to date have not demonstrated any benefit in adding BTKi to conventional chemotherapy in DLBCL. For example, in the randomized PHOENIX study, ibrutinib plus R-CHOP did not improve event-free survival (EFS) or PFS in non-GCB DLBCL in the overall patient population, with significant survival benefit in younger patients, but no survival benefit and increased toxicity in patients over the age of 60 years (Younes et al. 2019), compared to R-CHOP alone. Newer DLBCL subclassifications based on genetic alterations (Chapuy et al. 2018; Schmitz et al. 2018) demonstrate the complexity of DLBCL and may in future DLBCL trials better define which subsets beyond ABC versus GCB DLBCL benefit from the addition of BKT inhibitors or other targeted agents.

Bruton's Tyrosine Kinase (BTK) Inhibitors

BTK is a non-receptor tyrosine kinase of the Tec family that is primarily expressed in hematopoietic cells, particularly in B lymphocytes, but not in T-cells or plasma cells. BTK is critical for B-cell development, based on the findings that humans and mice lacking functional BTK due to function null mutations lack mature blood B-cells and IGs (patients with X-linked agammaglobulinemia/XLA) or have defective B-cell signaling (mice with X-linked immunodeficiency/xid) (Smith 2017). After activation of the BCR, BTK becomes activated by upstream kinases, including LYN and SYK. Besides its role in BCR signaling, BTK also transmits signals from chemokine receptors and adhesion molecules (integrins) (de Gorter et al. 2007; Spaargaren et al. 2003), CD19, CD38, CD40, tumor necrosis family receptors (TNFR), and TLRs. Its role in signaling of the chemokine receptors and adhesion molecules is of particular translational and clinical interest, because it is the basis for redistribution of tissue CLL cells and MCL cells into the peripheral blood during the first weeks of treatment (Burger and Montserrat 2013), a characteristic clinical activity of the BTK inhibitors, which can also be seen with SYK and PI3K inhibitors.

Ibrutinib

Ibrutinib, a selective irreversible (covalent) BTK inhibitor (Honigberg et al. 2010) which entered the clinic in 2009, is administered orally once daily In frontline CLL therapy, ibrutinib induces durable long-term remissions, whereas patients with relapsed/refractory disease over time can progress and develop resistance (Byrd et al. 2020b). High-risk CLL patients with del(17p) and/or complex karyotype who received prior CIT are at a particularly high risk of developing resistance over time. Efficacy and safety of ibrutinib in the frontline CLL setting were established in the RESONATE-2 trial, which compared ibrutinib with chlorambucil in older patients with untreated CLL or small lymphocytic lymphoma (SLL) (Burger et al. 2020, 2015). After a follow-up of 60 months, PFS and overall survival (OS) were significantly greater in the ibrutinib-treated patients (five-year PFS/OS: 70/83% vs. 12/68% with chlorambucil). Importantly, the PFS of patients with high-risk features (11q deletion, and/or unmutated IGHV genes) was not different from low-risk patients, indicating that ibrutinib treatment was able to overcome the negative prognostic impact these high-risk features. Along the same lines, the long-term outcome of treatment-naive CLL patients with *TP53* alterations is also substantially better compared to historic cohorts of patients treated with CIT, with a reported six-year PFS of 60% (Sivina et al. 2021) or 61% (Ahn et al. 2020) and OS of 79% (Ahn et al. 2020; Sivina et al. 2021). A series of randomized trials confirmed significant PFS benefit in CLL patients receiving ibrutinib alone or in combination with CD20 antibodies when compared to low, intermediate or higher intensity CIT regimen (i.e. chlorambucil + anti-CD20 [Moreno et al. 2019], bendamustine & rituximab (BR) [Woyach et al. 2018], and fludarabine, cyclophosphamide & rituximab (FCR) [Shanafelt et al. 2019]). Diarrhea, bruising, musculoskeletal discomfort, atrial fibrillation, and arterial hypertension are side effects that appear to be less frequent with the newer BTK inhibitors.

Acalabrutinib

Acalabrutinib, like ibrutinib, is an irreversible BTK inhibitor which covalently binds Cys-481 in the ATP binding pocket of BTK, blocking BCR signaling through BTK. Acalabrutinib has higher selectivity for BTK than ibrutinib and does not inhibit epidermal growth factor receptor (EGFR), interleukin-2 inducible tyrosine kinase (ITK), or tyrosine kinase expressed in hepatocellular carcinoma (TEC) kinase, which are partially inhibited by ibrutinib (Byrd et al. 2016). There appears to be advantages with acalabrutinib compared to ibrutinib in terms of better tolerability due to reduced off-target kinase inhibition, which could reduce bleeding and atrial fibrillation and other cardiac events, as suggested by cross-trial comparisons and in a recent randomized trial that compared acalabrutinib with ibrutinib in the relapsed disease setting (Byrd et al. 2021). Acalabrutinib, which requires an acidic environment for optimal bioabsorption, can cause headaches, typically at the beginning of therapy. The headaches are usually minor and generally self-limited, without requiring medical treatment, but often responding to caffeine. A phase 1/2 study demonstrated high response rates in patients with relapsed/refractory CLL (Byrd et al. 2016). ELEVATE-TN was a three-arm randomized study that compared acalabrutinib plus obinutuzumab to acalabrutinib monotherapy to obinutuzumab plus chlorambucil in patients with treatment-naive CLL (Sharman et al. 2019a). After a median follow-up of 28.3 months, acalabrutinib monotherapy or in combination with obinutuzumab significantly improved PFS compared to obinutuzumab plus chlorambucil. The ASCEND trial compared acalabrutinib monotherapy with the investigator's choice of rituximab plus either idelalisib or bendamustine in relapsed/refractory CLL. After a median follow-up of 22 months, acalabrutinib significantly prolonged PFS compared with idelalisib or bendamustine with estimated 18-month PFS rates of 82% for acalabrutinib versus 48% for the idelalisib- or bendamustine-treated patients (Ghia et al. 2020). In a first head-to-head comparison of two BTK inhibitors (acalabrutinib vs. ibrutinib) in relapsed CLL patients, acalabrutinib demonstrated comparable activity as ibrutinib, with fewer cardiovascular side effects (all-grade atrial fibrillation 9.4% vs. 16.0%) (Byrd et al. 2021).

BTK Inhibitors with Anti-CD20 Antibodies

The addition of rituximab to chemotherapy regimen substantially improved outcome of patients with CLL and other B-cell malignancies. In contrast, when rituximab was combined with ibrutinib in patients with CLL there was no PFS benefit seen in two randomized trials (Burger et al. 2019; Woyach et al. 2018). Obinutuzumab, on the other hand, when combined with acalabrutinib, improved PFS over acalabrutinib monotherapy (estimated 24-month PFS of 93% vs. 87%), a rather small and perhaps clinically insignificant difference, noting the study was not specifically powered for this comparison (Sharman et al. 2020). A potential explanation could come from preclinical studies that investigated potential antagonism between ibrutinib and rituximab, based on the off-target activity of ibrutinib inhibiting ITK (Dubovsky et al. 2013), which is expressed in natural killer (NK) and T-cells. In preclinical models, it was noted that ibrutinib can antagonize rituximab's anti-lymphoma activity, based on its interference with FcR-stimulated antibody-dependent cell-mediated cytotoxicity (ADCC) (Kohrt et al. 2014). However, the relative contribution and importance of NK cells, monocytes, or other effector cells for CD20 antibody-mediated killing of B-cells remains controversial. What argues against the relevance of these preclinical findings is the fact that the rituximab induced faster disease clearance from the peripheral blood and deeper remissions when combined with ibrutinib (Burger et al. 2019), indicating that ibrutinib does not play an antagonistic role when combined with rituximab in the clinical setting. Obinutuzumab has been shown to be more effective than rituximab in CLL (Goede et al. 2014), and, therefore, the 6% PFS difference noted in the acalabrutinib plus obinutuzumab trial, in my assessment, points toward higher efficacy of obinutuzumab as compared with rituximab, rather than being based on higher BTK selectivity and lack of ITK inhibition by acalabrutinib.

Zanubrutinib

Zanubrutinib, another covalent BTK inhibitor, is more BTK-selective than ibrutinib which has demonstrated high response rates and favorable safety in a phase 1/2 trial in CLL/SLL patients (Tam et al. 2019). Results from a phase 2 trial among 109 treatment-naive CLL patients with del(17p) reported a high ORR of 94.5% with a complete response rate of 3.7% and an estimated 18-month PFS and OS of 88.6% and 95.1%, respectively (Tam et al. 2019). Grade ≥3 adverse events included neutropenia (12.9%) and pneumonia (3.7%), while atrial fibrillation was uncommon. The phase 3 ASPEN study compared the efficacy and safety of ibrutinib with zanubrutinib in 201 patients with WM, and demonstrated similar PFS and OS in both arms, and a trend, albeit not statistically significant, for deeper responses and fewer cardiac side effects with zanubrutinib (all grade atrial fibrillation: 2% vs. 15% with ibrutinib), although neutropenia was slightly more common with zanubrutinib (Tam et al. 2019). Zanubrutinib is approved by the FDA for WM, MZL, and MCL; CLL registration studies are ongoing.

Pirtobrutinib

The reversible BTK binding mechanism, as with ibrutinib, acalabrutinib, and zanubrutinib, can result in the outgrowth of resistant subclones which frequently carry a mutated cysteine (C481) at the ibrutinib binding site, with a C481 to serine substitution being the most common resistance mutation. To overcome this resistance mechanism, non-covalent BTK inhibitors such as pirtobrutinib were found to be effective when C481 was mutated (Estupinan et al. 2021). This concept translated well in the clinical setting, where pirtobrutinib (LOXO-305), a selective and reversible BTK inhibitor, was tested in a phase 1/2 trial in 323 patients with relapsed/refractory B-cell malignancies, including 121 CLL patients who were previously treated with an irreversible BTK inhibitor (Mato et al. 2021). Among these CLL patients, pirtobrutinib induced responses in 62%, with similarly high response rates in BTK inhibitor-resistant or intolerant patients (ORR 67% and 52%, respectively). Patients with *BTK* C481 mutation or *BTK* wild-type also had similar response rates.

Idelalisib

Idelalisib (GS-1101, CAL-101) is an orally available reversible inhibitor of the PI3K δ isoform, which is primarily expressed in hematopoietic cells and plays a central role in normal B-cell development and function, transducing signals from the BCR as well as from receptors for cytokines, chemokines, and integrins. Drugs in this class inhibit the catalytic subunit of PI3K, causing a decrease in phosphorylation of several downstream targets including AKT. The predominant effects of idelalisib include inhibition of BCR signaling, affecting leukemia cell survival and proliferation, along with disrupted migration and homing of CLL cells and other elements of the crosstalk between CLL cells and their microenvironment. For example, redistribution lymphocytosis, similarly to ibrutinib, was commonly seen in patients with CLL and SLL (Brown et al. 2014), which were less frequently observed in patients with FL and MZL (Flinn et al. 2014). A randomized phase 3 clinical trial of idelalisib plus rituximab versus placebo and rituximab in relapsed/refractory patients with CLL demonstrated substantial superiority of the idelalisib arm (Furman et al. 2014). A phase 2 clinical trial of idelalisib monotherapy in patients with relapsed indolent lymphoma reported an ORR of 57%, with a median PFS of 11 months, supporting the approval of idelalisib plus rituximab for relapsed CLL and FL (Brown et al. 2014). A series of idelalisib combination trials raised safety concerns due to increased toxicity, including hepatotoxicity, infections (mostly pulmonary infections and sepsis) (Zelenetz et al. 2017), as well as rashes (Smith et al. 2017). Opportunistic infections (cytomegalovirus [CMV] and *Pneumocystis jiroveci* pneumonia [PJP]) were found to be more frequent in idelalisib in combination with CD20 antibodies (Jones et al. 2017). Second-generation PI3K inhibitors are currently being explored; duvelisib (IPI-145) (Dong et al. 2014), an inhibitor targeting the γ and δ isoforms of PI3K, and umbralisib (TGR-1202) (Burris et al. 2018; Locatelli et al. 2016), a selective PI3Kδ and casein kinase 1ε inhibitor structurally different from idelalisib, have entered advanced stages of clinical development in B-cell malignancies. Details on these drugs, their pharmacology and clinical data, and approved FDA indications are reviewed in detail in other chapters.

Conclusions

Targeted therapies with BTK and PI3K inhibitors have fundamentally changed our treatment paradigm for patients with CLL, MCL, WM, MZL, and FL. These developments have put a spotlight on the role of BCR signaling in B-cell lymphoma and leukemia. Indeed, the targets of these drugs, BTK and PI3K isoforms, are kinases that play important roles in BCR signaling. Consequently, BCR-driven proliferation and survival of malignant B-cells may be the primary target of these agents. However, it is also increasingly evident that these agents have broader effects, not only within the malignant B-cells but also in the tissue microenvironment. First, they also affect the function of other cell surface receptors, such as the signaling of chemokine receptors and adhesion molecules, that regulate cooperatively the tissue homing of B-cells (de Gorter et al. 2007; Spaargaren et al. 2003). Second, they target and modulate the function of other cells within the microenvironment, such as macrophages, that carry BTK (Gunderson et al. 2016) and PI3K (Galletti et al. 2016). The effects on homing receptor function and signaling are particularly noteworthy and clinically relevant in patients with CLL, as it is accompanied by a rapid-onset redistribution lymphocytosis along with often dramatic shrinkage of lymph nodes and enlarged spleen due to egress of malignant B-cells from the lymphoid tissue into the peripheral blood. Hence, an additional mechanism of action of these agents may be anoikis, i.e. cell death by detachment from a supportive microenvironment. BTK and PI3K inhibitors cause redistribution lymphocytosis, thereby removing CLL cells from their supportive tissue milieu that activates a multitude of pro-survival pathways. CLL is the disease with the highest response rates and the most durable remissions with these agents, as compared to other B-cell malignancies (Advani et al. 2013; Byrd et al. 2015; Flinn et al. 2014; Furman et al. 2014). Additionally, CLL cells are mobilized more effectively by BTK and PI3K inhibitors from the SLO into the PB than any other type of malignant B-cells (Byrd et al. 2013; Chang et al. 2013; Flinn et al. 2014), supporting this additional mechanism.

Today, we are successfully using treatments for B-cell malignancies that target BCR signaling, activated by interactions between malignant B-cells and their tissue microenvironment, rather than by oncogenic transformation. The success of the BTK and PI3K inhibitors has and will continue to ignite further enthusiasm into this area of research, where studies of the crosstalk between malignant B-cells and their microenvironment will likely uncover additional successful therapeutic targets in the near future.

Acknowledgments

This chapter was supported by the generous philanthropic contributions to The University of Texas MD Anderson Cancer Center Moon Shots Program™, the CLL Global Research Foundation, and in part by the MD Anderson Cancer Support Grant CA016672.

Conflict of Interest

Jan A. Burger received research funding from Pharmacyclics, Gilead, AstraZeneca, BeiGene, and speaker fees from Janssen.

Must Read References

Burger, J.A. and Montserrat, E. (2013). Coming full circle: 70 years of chronic lymphocytic leukemia cell redistribution, from glucocorticoids to inhibitors of B-cell receptor signaling. *Blood* 121: 1501–1509.

De Silva, N.S. and Klein, U. (2015). Dynamics of B cells in germinal centres. *Nat. Rev. Immunol.* 15: 137–148.

Okkenhaug, K. and Vanhaesebroeck, B. (2003). PI3K in lymphocyte development, differentiation and activation. *Nat. Rev. Immunol.* 3: 317–330.

References

Advani, R.H., Buggy, J.J., Sharman, J.P., Smith, S.M., Boyd, T.E. et al. (2013). Bruton tyrosine kinase inhibitor ibrutinib (PCI-32765) has significant activity in patients with relapsed/refractory B-cell malignancies. *J. Clin. Oncol.* 31: 88–94.

Agathangelidis, A., Darzentas, N., Hadzidimitriou, A., Brochet, X., Murray, F. et al. (2012). Stereotyped B-cell receptors in one-third of chronic lymphocytic leukemia: a molecular classification with implications for targeted therapies. *Blood* 119: 4467–4475.

Ahn, I.E., Jerussi, T., Farooqui, M., Tian, X., Wiestner, A. et al. (2016). Atypical Pneumocystis jirovecii pneumonia in previously untreated patients with CLL on single-agent ibrutinib. *Blood* 128: 1940–1943.

Ahn, I.E., Tian, X., and Wiestner, A. (2020). Ibrutinib for chronic lymphocytic leukemia with TP53 alterations. *N. Engl. J. Med.* 383: 498–500.

Alizadeh, A.A., Eisen, M.B., Davis, R.E., Ma, C., Lossos, I.S. et al. (2000). Distinct types of diffuse large B-cell lymphoma identified by gene expression profiling. *Nature* 403: 503–511.

Bagnara, D., Kaufman, M.S., Calissano, C., Marsilio, S., Patten, P.E. et al. (2011). A novel adoptive transfer model of chronic lymphocytic leukemia suggests a key role for T lymphocytes in the disease. *Blood* 117: 5463–5472.

Baliakas, P., Hadzidimitriou, A., Sutton, L.A., Minga, E., Agathangelidis, A. et al. (2014). Clinical effect of stereotyped B-cell receptor immunoglobulins in chronic lymphocytic leukaemia: a retrospective multicentre study. *Lancet. Haematol.* 1: e74–84.

Beckmann, L., Berg, V., Dickhut, C., SUN, C., Merkel, O. et al. (2021). MARCKS affects cell motility and response to BTK inhibitors in CLL. *Blood* 138: 544–556.

Bhattacharya, N., Diener, S., Idler, I.S., Barth, T.F., Rauen, J. et al. (2011). Non-malignant B cells and chronic lymphocytic leukemia cells induce a pro-survival phenotype in CD14+ cells from peripheral blood. *Leukemia* 25: 722–726.

Binder, M., Lechenne, B., Ummanni, R., Scharf, C., Balabanov, S. et al. (2010). Stereotypical chronic lymphocytic leukemia B-cell receptors recognize survival promoting antigens on stromal cells. *PLoS One* 5: e15992.

Brown, J.R., Byrd, J.C., Coutre, S.E., Benson, D.M., Flinn, I.W. et al. (2014). Idelalisib, an inhibitor of phosphatidylinositol 3-kinase p110delta, for relapsed/refractory chronic lymphocytic leukemia. *Blood* 123: 3390–3397.

Burger, J.A., Barr, P.M., Robak, T., Owen, C., Ghia, P. et al. (2020). Long-term efficacy and safety of first-line ibrutinib treatment for patients with CLL/SLL: 5 years of follow-up from the phase 3 RESONATE-2 study. *Leukemia* 34: 787–798.

Burger, J.A. and Chiorazzi, N. (2013). B cell receptor signaling in chronic lymphocytic leukemia. *Trends. Immunol.* 34: 592–601.

Burger, J.A. and Montserrat, E. (2013). Coming full circle: 70 years of chronic lymphocytic leukemia cell redistribution, from glucocorticoids to inhibitors of B-cell receptor signaling. *Blood* 121: 1501–1509.

Burger, J.A., Quiroga, M.P., Hartmann, E., Burkle, A., Wierda, W.G. et al. (2009). High-level expression of the T-cell chemokines CCL3 and CCL4 by chronic lymphocytic leukemia B cells in nurselike cell cocultures and after BCR stimulation. *Blood* 113: 3050–3058.

Burger, J.A., Sivina, M., Jain, N., Kim, E., Kadia, T. et al. (2019). Randomized trial of ibrutinib vs ibrutinib plus rituximab in patients with chronic lymphocytic leukemia. *Blood* 133: 1011–1019.

Burger, J.A., Tedeschi, A., Barr, P.M., Robak, T., Owen, C. et al. (2015). Ibrutinib as initial therapy for patients with chronic lymphocytic leukemia. *N. Engl. J. Med.* 373: 2425–2437.

Burger, J.A., Tsukada, N., Burger, M., Zvaifler, N.J., Dell'aquila, M. et al. (2000). Blood-derived nurse-like cells protect chronic lymphocytic leukemia B cells from spontaneous apoptosis through stromal cell-derived factor-1. *Blood* 96: 2655–2663.

Burkle, A., Niedermeier, M., Schmitt-graff, A., Wierda, W.G., Keating, M.J. et al. (2007). Overexpression of the CXCR5 chemokine receptor, and its ligand, CXCL13 in B-cell chronic lymphocytic leukemia. *Blood* 110: 3316–3325.

Burris, H.A., 3RD, Flinn, I.W., Patel, M.R., Fenske, T.S., Deng, C. et al. (2018). Umbralisib, a novel PI3Kdelta and casein kinase-1epsilon inhibitor, in relapsed or refractory chronic lymphocytic leukaemia and lymphoma: an open-label, phase 1, dose-escalation, first-in-human study. *Lancet. Oncol.* 19: 486–496.

Byrd, J.C., Furman, R.R., Coutre, S.E., Burger, J.A., Blum, K.A. et al. (2015). Three-year follow-up of treatment-naive and previously treated patients with CLL and SLL receiving single-agent ibrutinib. *Blood* 125: 2497–2506.

Byrd, J.C., Furman, R.R., Coutre, S.E., Flinn, I.W., Burger, J.A. et al. (2020a). Ibrutinib treatment for first-line and relapsed/refractory chronic lymphocytic leukemia: final analysis of the pivotal phase Ib/II PCYC-1102 study. *Clin. Cancer Res.* 26: 3918–3927.

Byrd, J.C., Furman, R.R., Coutre, S.E., Flinn, I.W., Burger, J.A. et al. (2013). Targeting BTK with ibrutinib in relapsed chronic lymphocytic leukemia. *N. Engl. J. Med.* 369: 32–42.

Byrd, J.C., Harrington, B., O'Brien, S., Jones, J.A., Schuh, A. et al. (2016). Acalabrutinib (ACP-196) in relapsed chronic lymphocytic leukemia. *N. Engl. J. Med.* 374: 323–332.

Byrd, J.C., Hillmen, P., Ghia, P., Kater, A.P., Chanan-khan, A. et al. (2021). Acalabrutinib versus ibrutinib in previously treated chronic lymphocytic leukemia: results of the first randomized phase III trial. *J. Clin. Oncol.* 39: 3441–3452.

Byrd, J.C., Hillmen, P., O'Brien, S., Barrientos, J.C., Reddy, N.M. et al. (2019). Long-term follow-up of the RESONATE phase 3 trial of ibrutinib vs ofatumumab. *Blood* 133: 2031–2042.

Byrd, J.C., Wierda, W.G., Schuh, A., Devereux, S., Chaves, J.M. et al. (2020b). Acalabrutinib monotherapy in patients with relapsed/refractory chronic lymphocytic leukemia: updated phase 2 results. *Blood* 135: 1204–1213.

Castillo, J.J., Meid, K., Gustine, J.N., Leventoff, C., White, T. et al. (2021). Long-term follow-up of ibrutinib monotherapy in treatment-naive patients with Waldenstrom macroglobulinemia. *Leukemia*. doi.org/10.1038/s41375-021-01417-9

Cerroni, L., Zochling, N., Putz, B., and Kerl, H. (1997). Infection by borrelia burgdorferi and cutaneous B-cell lymphoma. *J. Cutan. Pathol.* 24: 457–461.

Chang, B.Y., Francesco, M., De Rooij, M.F., Magadala, P., Steggerda, S.M. et al. (2013). Egress of CD19(+)CD5(+) cells into peripheral blood following treatment with the bruton tyrosine kinase inhibitor ibrutinib in mantle cell lymphoma patients. *Blood* 122: 2412–2424.

Chapuy, B., Stewart, C., Dunford, A.J., KIM, J., Kamburov, A. et al. (2018). Author correction: molecular subtypes of diffuse large B cell lymphoma are associated with distinct pathogenic mechanisms and outcomes. *Nat. Med.* 24: 1290–1291.

Chen, L., Apgar, J., Huynh, L., Dicker, F., Giago-mcgahan, T. et al. (2005). ZAP-70 directly enhances IgM signaling in chronic lymphocytic leukemia. *Blood* 105: 2036–2041.

Chen, L., Monti, S., Juszczynski, P., Daley, J., Chen, W. et al. (2008). SYK-dependent tonic B-cell receptor signaling is a rational treatment target in diffuse large B-cell lymphoma. *Blood* 111: 2230–2237.

Chen, L., Monti, S., Juszczynski, P., Ouyang, J., Chapuy, B. et al. (2013). SYK inhibition modulates distinct PI3K/AKT-dependent survival pathways and cholesterol biosynthesis in diffuse large B cell lymphomas. *Cancer Cell* 23: 826–838.

Chen, L., Widhopf, G., Huynh, L., Rassenti, L., Rai, K.R. et al. (2002). Expression of ZAP-70 is associated with increased B-cell receptor signaling in chronic lymphocytic leukemia. *Blood* 100: 4609–4614.

Chiron, D., Di Liberto, M., Martin, P., Huang, X., Sharman, J. et al. (2014). Cell-cycle reprogramming for PI3K inhibition overrides a relapse-specific C481S BTK mutation revealed by longitudinal functional genomics in mantle cell lymphoma. *Cancer Discov.* 4: 1022–1035.

Coiffier, B., Lepage, E., Briere, J., Herbrecht, R., Tilly, H. et al. (2002). chop chemotherapy plus rituximab compared with chop alone in elderly patients with diffuse large-b-cell lymphoma. *N. Engl. J. Med.* 346: 235–242.

Coutre, S.E., Furman, R.R., Flinn, I.W., Burger, J.A., Blum, K. et al. (2017). Extended treatment with single-agent ibrutinib at the 420 mg dose leads to durable responses in chronic lymphocytic leukemia/Small lymphocytic lymphoma. *Clin. Cancer Res.* 23: 1149–1155.

Dai, B., Grau, M., Juilland, M., Klener, P., Horing, E. et al. (2017). B-cell receptor-driven MALT1 activity regulates MYC signaling in mantle cell lymphoma. *Blood* 129: 333–346.

Dalla-Favera, R., Bregni, M., Erikson, J., Patterson, D., Gallo, R.C. et al. (1982). Human c-myc onc gene is located on the region of chromosome 8 that is translocated in Burkitt lymphoma cells. *Proc. Natl. Acad. Sci. U S A.* 79: 7824–7827.

Damle, R.N., Wasil, T., Fais, F., Ghiotto, F., Valetto, A. et al. (1999). Ig V gene mutation status and CD38 expression as novel prognostic indicators in chronic lymphocytic leukemia. *Blood* 94: 1840–1847.

Dave, S.S., Wright, G., Tan, B., Rosenwald, A., Gascoyne, R.D. et al. (2004). Prediction of survival in follicular lymphoma based on molecular features of tumor-infiltrating immune cells. *N. Engl. J. Med.* 351: 2159–2169.

Davis, R.E., Ngo, V.N., Lenz, G., Tolar, P., Young, R.M. et al. (2010). Chronic active B-cell-receptor signalling in diffuse large B-cell lymphoma. *Nature* 463: 88–92.

de Gorter, D.J., Beuling, E.A., Kersseboom, R., Middendorp, S., Van Gils, J.M. et al. (2007). Bruton's tyrosine kinase and phospholipase Cgamma2 mediate chemokine-controlled B cell migration and homing. *Immunity* 26: 93–104.

De Silva, N.S. and Klein, U. (2015). Dynamics of B cells in germinal centres. *Nat. Rev. Immunol.* 15: 137–148.

Dekosky, B.J., Kojima, T., Rodin, A., Charab, W., Ippolito, G.C. et al. (2015). In-depth determination and analysis of the human paired heavy- and light-chain antibody repertoire. *Nat. Med.* 21: 86–91.

Di Noia, J.M. and Neuberger, M.S. (2007). Molecular mechanisms of antibody somatic hypermutation. *Annu. Rev. Biochem.* 76: 1–22.

Dong, S., Guinn, D., Dubovsky, J.A., Zhong, Y., Lehman, A. et al. (2014). IPI-145 antagonizes intrinsic and extrinsic survival signals in chronic lymphocytic leukemia cells. *Blood* 124: 3583–3586.

Dubovsky, J.A., Beckwith, K.A., Natarajan, G., Woyach, J.A., Jaglowski, S. et al. (2013). Ibrutinib is an irreversible molecular inhibitor of ITK driving a Th1-selective pressure in T lymphocytes. *Blood* 122: 2539–2549.

Duhren-von Minden, M., Ubelhart, R., Schneider, D., Wossning, T., Bach, M.P. et al. (2012). Chronic lymphocytic leukaemia is driven by antigen-independent cell-autonomous signalling. *Nature* 489: 309–312.

Estupinan, H.Y., Berglof, A., Zain, R., and Smith, C.I.E. (2021). Comparative analysis of BTK inhibitors and mechanisms underlying adverse effects. *Front Cell Dev. Biol.* 9: 630942.

Ferreri, A.J., Guidoboni, M., Ponzoni, M., De Conciliis, C., Dell'oro, S. et al. (2004). Evidence for an association between chlamydia psittaci and ocular adnexal lymphomas. *J. Natl. Cancer Inst.* 96: 586–594.

Flinn, I.W., Kahl, B.S., Leonard, J.P., Furman, R.R., Brown, J.R. et al. (2014). Idelalisib, a selective inhibitor of phosphatidylinositol 3-kinase-delta, as therapy for previously treated indolent non-Hodgkin lymphoma. *Blood* 123: 3406–3413.

Fontan, L., Yang, C., Kabaleeswaran, V., Volpon, L., Osborne, M.J. et al. (2012). MALT1 small molecule inhibitors specifically suppress ABC-DLBCL in vitro and in vivo. *Cancer Cell* 22: 812–824.

Friedberg, J.W., Sharman, J., Sweetenham, J., Johnston, P.B., Vose, J.M. et al. (2010). Inhibition of syk with fostamatinib disodium has significant clinical activity in non-Hodgkin lymphoma and chronic lymphocytic leukemia. *Blood* 115: 2578–2585.

Fruman, D.A., Satterthwaite, A.B., and Witte, O.N. (2000). Xid-like phenotypes: a B cell signalosome takes shape. *Immunity* 13: 1–3.

Furman, R.R., Sharman, J.P., Coutre, S.E., Cheson, B.D., Pagel, J.M. et al. (2014). Idelalisib and rituximab in relapsed chronic lymphocytic leukemia. *N. Engl. J. Med.* 370: 997–1007.

Galletti, G., Scielzo, C., Barbaglio, F., Rodriguez, T.V., Riba, M. et al. (2016). Targeting macrophages sensitizes chronic lymphocytic leukemia to apoptosis and inhibits disease progression. *Cell Rep.* 14: 1748–1760.

Gehringer, F., Weissinger, S.E., Moller, P., Wirth, T., and Ushmorov, A. (2020). Physiological levels of the PTEN-PI3K-AKT axis activity are required for maintenance of Burkitt lymphoma. *Leukemia* 34: 857–871.

Ghia, P., Pluta, A., Wach, M., Lysak, D., Kozak, T. et al. (2020). ASCEND: phase III, randomized trial of acalabrutinib versus idelalisib plus rituximab or bendamustine plus rituximab in relapsed or refractory chronic lymphocytic leukemia. *J. Clin. Oncol.* 38: 2849–2861.

Ghia, P., Strola, G., Granziero, L., Geuna, M., Guida, G. et al. (2002). Chronic lymphocytic leukemia B cells are endowed with the capacity to attract CD4+, CD40L+ T cells by producing CCL22. *Eur. J. Immunol.* 32: 1403–1413.

Goede, V., Fischer, K., Busch, R., Engelke, A., Eichhorst, B. et al. (2014). Obinutuzumab plus chlorambucil in patients with CLL and coexisting conditions. *N. Engl. J. Med.* 370: 1101–1110.

Gopal, A.K., Kahl, B.S., De Vos, S., Wagner-Johnston, N.D., Schuster, S.J. et al. (2014). PI3Kdelta inhibition by idelalisib in patients with relapsed indolent lymphoma. *N. Engl. J. Med.* 370: 1008–1018.

Gouni, S., Marques-piubelli, M.L., and Strati, P. (2021). Follicular lymphoma and macrophages: impact of approved and novel therapies. *Blood Adv.* 5: 4303–4312.

Gunderson, A.J., Kaneda, M.M., Tsujikawa, T., Nguyen, A.V., Affara, N.I. et al. (2016). Bruton tyrosine kinase-dependent immune cell cross-talk drives pancreas cancer. *Cancer Discov.* 6: 270–285.

Hacken, E.T., Gounari, M., Back, J.W., Shimanovskaya, E., Scarfo, L. et al. (2017). Calreticulin as a novel B-cell receptor antigen in chronic lymphocytic leukemia. *Haematologica.* 102: e394–e396.

Hadzidimitriou, A., Agathangelidis, A., Darzentas, N., Murray, F., Delfau-larue, M.H. et al. (2011). Is there a role for antigen selection in mantle cell lymphoma? Immunogenetic support from a series of 807 cases. *Blood* 118: 3088–3095.

Hamblin, T.J., Davis, Z., Gardiner, A., Oscier, D.G., and Stevenson, F.K. (1999). Unmutated Ig V(H) genes are associated with a more aggressive form of chronic lymphocytic leukemia. *Blood* 94: 1848–1854.

Hartmann, E.M., Rudelius, M., Burger, J.A., and Rosenwald, A. (2016). CCL3 chemokine expression by chronic lymphocytic leukemia cells orchestrates the composition of the microenvironment in lymph node infiltrates. *Leuk. Lymphoma* 57: 563–571.

Havranek, O., Xu, J., Kohrer, S., Wang, Z., Becker, L. et al. (2017). Tonic B-cell receptor signaling in diffuse large B-cell lymphoma. *Blood.* 130 (8): 995–1006.

He, X., Klasener, K., Iype, J.M., Becker, M., Maity, P.C. et al. (2018). Continuous signaling of CD79b and CD19 is required for the fitness of Burkitt lymphoma B cells. *EMBO. J.* 37.

Herishanu, Y., Perez-galan, P., Liu, D., Biancotto, A., Pittaluga, S. et al. (2011). The lymph node microenvironment promotes B-cell receptor signaling, NF-kappaB activation, and tumor proliferation in chronic lymphocytic leukemia. *Blood* 117: 563–574.

Herndon, T.M., Chen, S.S., Saba, N.S., Valdez, J., Emson, C. et al. (2017). Direct in vivo evidence for increased proliferation of CLL cells in lymph nodes compared to bone marrow and peripheral blood. *Leukemia.* 31 (6): 1340–1347.

Honigberg, L.A., Smith, A.M., Sirisawad, M., Verner, E., Loury, D. et al. (2010). The Bruton tyrosine kinase inhibitor PCI-32765 blocks B-cell activation and is efficacious in models of autoimmune disease and B-cell malignancy. *Proc. Natl. Acad. Sci. U S A.* 107: 13075–13080.

Hoogeboom, R., Van Kessel, K.P., Hochstenbach, F., Wormhoudt, T.A., Reinten, R.J. et al. (2013). A mutated B cell chronic lymphocytic leukemia subset that recognizes and responds to fungi. *J. Exp. Med.* 210: 59–70.

Jones, J.A., Robak, T., Brown, J.R., Awan, F.T., Badoux, X. et al. (2017). Efficacy and safety of idelalisib in combination with ofatumumab for previously treated chronic lymphocytic leukaemia: an open-label, randomised phase 3 trial. *Lancet. Haematol.* 4: e114–e126.

Kahl, B.S., Spurgeon, S.E., Furman, R.R., Flinn, I.W., Coutre, S.E. et al. (2014). A phase 1 study of the PI3Kdelta inhibitor idelalisib in patients with relapsed/refractory mantle cell lymphoma (MCL). *Blood* 123: 3398–3405.

Kaplinsky, J. and Arnaout, R. (2016). Robust estimates of overall immune-repertoire diversity from high-throughput measurements on samples. *Nat. Commun.* 7: 11881.

Kipps, T.J., Stevenson, F.K., Wu, C.J., Croce, C.M., Packham, G. et al. (2017). Chronic lymphocytic leukaemia. *Nat. Rev. Dis. Primers.* 3: 17008.

Kohrt, H.E., Sagiv-barfi, I., Rafiq, S., Herman, S.E., Butchar, J.P. et al. (2014). Ibrutinib antagonizes rituximab-dependent NK cell-mediated cytotoxicity. *Blood* 123: 1957–1960.

Kridel, R., Sehn, L.H., and Gascoyne, R.D. (2012). Pathogenesis of follicular lymphoma. *J. Clin. Invest.* 122: 3424–3431.

Krysiak, K., Gomez, F., White, B.S., Matlock, M., Miller, C.A. et al. (2017). Recurrent somatic mutations affecting B-cell receptor signaling pathway genes in follicular lymphoma. *Blood* 129: 473–483.

Krzysiek, R., Lefevre, E.A., Zou, W., Foussat, A., Bernard, J. et al. (1999). Antigen receptor engagement selectively induces macrophage inflammatory protein-1 alpha (MIP-1 alpha) and MIP-1 beta chemokine production in human B cells. *J. Immunol.* 162: 4455–4463.

Kuppers, R. and Stevenson, F.K. (2018). Critical influences on the pathogenesis of follicular lymphoma. *Blood* 131: 2297–2306.

Lam, K.P., Kuhn, R., and Rajewsky, K. (1997). In vivo ablation of surface immunoglobulin on mature B cells by inducible gene targeting results in rapid cell death. *Cell* 90: 1073–1083.

Leadbetter, E.A., Rifkin, I.R., Hohlbaum, A.M., Beaudette, B.C., Shlomchik, M.J. et al. (2002). Chromatin-IgG complexes activate B cells by dual engagement of IgM and Toll-like receptors. *Nature* 416: 603–607.

Lenz, G., Wright, G.W., Emre, N.C., Kohlhammer, H., Dave, S.S. et al. (2008). Molecular subtypes of diffuse large B-cell lymphoma arise by distinct genetic pathways. *Proc. Natl. Acad. Sci. U S A.* 105: 13520–13525.

Locatelli, S.L., Careddu, G., Inghirami, G., Castagna, L., Sportelli, P. et al. (2016). The novel PI3K-delta inhibitor TGR-1202 enhances brentuximab Vedotin-induced Hodgkin lymphoma cell death via mitotic arrest. *Leukemia* 30: 2402–2405.

Long, M., Beckwith, K., Do, P., Mundy, B.L., Gordon, A. et al. (2017). Ibrutinib treatment improves T cell number and function in CLL patients. *J. Clin. Invest.* 127: 3052–3064.

Lucas, C.L., Chandra, A., Nejentsev, S., Condliffe, A.M., and Okkenhaug, K. (2016). PI3Kdelta and primary immunodeficiencies. *Nat. Rev. Immunol.* 16: 702–714.

Martin, P., Bartlett, N.L., Blum, K.A., Park, S., Maddocks, K. et al. (2019). A phase 1 trial of ibrutinib plus palbociclib in previously treated mantle cell lymphoma. *Blood* 133: 1201–1204.

Mato, A.R., Shah, N.N., Jurczak, W., Cheah, C.Y., Pagel, J.M. et al. (2021). Pirtobrutinib in relapsed or refractory B-cell malignancies (BRUIN): a phase 1/2 study. *Lancet.* 397: 892–901.

Melchers, F. (2015). Checkpoints that control B cell development. *J. Clin. Invest.* 125: 2203–2210.

Miller, K.D., Siegel, R.L., Lin, C.C., Mariotto, A.B., Kramer, J.L. et al. (2016). Cancer treatment and survivorship statistics, 2016. *CA Cancer J. Clin.* 66: 271–289.

Mockridge, C.I., Potter, K.N., Wheatley, I., Neville, L.A., Packham, G. et al. (2007). Reversible anergy of sIgM-mediated signaling in the two subsets of CLL defined by VH-gene mutational status. *Blood* 109: 4424–4431.

Moreno, C., Greil, R., Demirkan, F., Tedeschi, A., Anz, B. et al. (2019). Ibrutinib plus obinutuzumab versus chlorambucil plus obinutuzumab in first-line treatment of chronic lymphocytic leukaemia (iLLUMINATE): a multicentre, randomised, open-label, phase 3 trial. *Lancet. Oncol.* 20: 43–56.

Navarro, A., Clot, G., Royo, C., Jares, P., Hadzidimitriou, A. et al. (2012). Molecular subsets of mantle cell lymphoma defined by the IGHV mutational status and SOX11 expression have distinct biologic and clinical features. *Cancer Res.* 72: 5307–5316.

Ngo, V.N., Young, R.M., Schmitz, R., Jhavar, S., Xiao, W. et al. (2011). Oncogenically active MYD88 mutations in human lymphoma. *Nature* 470: 115–119.

Nguyen, P.H., Fedorchenko, O., Rosen, N., Koch, M., Barthel, R. et al. (2016). LYN kinase in the tumor microenvironment is essential for the progression of chronic lymphocytic leukemia. *Cancer Cell* 30: 610–622.

Nishio, M., Endo, T., Tsukada, N., Ohata, J., Kitada, S. et al. (2005). Nurselike cells express BAFF and APRIL, which can promote survival of chronic lymphocytic leukemia cells via a paracrine pathway distinct from that of SDF-1alpha. *Blood* 106: 1012–1020.

Noy, A., De Vos, S., Thieblemont, C., Martin, P., Flowers, C.R. et al. (2017). Targeting bruton tyrosine kinase with ibrutinib in relapsed/refractory marginal zone lymphoma. *Blood* 129: 2224–2232.

Odabashian, M., Carlotti, E., Araf, S., Okosun, J., Spada, F. et al. (2020). IGHV sequencing reveals acquired N-glycosylation sites as a clonal and stable event during follicular lymphoma evolution. *Blood* 135: 834–844.

Okkenhaug, K. (2013). Signaling by the phosphoinositide 3-kinase family in immune cells. *Annu. Rev. Immunol.* 31: 675–704.

Okkenhaug, K., Bilancio, A., Farjot, G., Priddle, H., Sancho, S. et al. (2002). Impaired B and T cell antigen receptor signaling in p110delta PI 3-kinase mutant mice. *Science* 297: 1031–1034.

Okkenhaug, K. and Vanhaesebroeck, B. (2003). PI3K in lymphocyte development, differentiation and activation. *Nat. Rev. Immunol.* 3: 317–330.

Patten, P.E., Buggins, A.G., Richards, J., Wotherspoon, A., Salisbury, J. et al. (2008). CD38 expression in chronic lymphocytic leukemia is regulated by the tumor microenvironment. *Blood* 111: 5173–5181.

Patten, P.E., Ferrer, G., Chen, S.S., Simone, R., Marsilio, S. et al. (2016). Chronic lymphocytic leukemia cells diversify and differentiate in vivo via a nonclassical Th1-dependent, Bcl-6-deficient process. *JCI Insight* 1.

Peled, J.U., Kuang, F.L., Iglesias-ussel, M.D., Roa, S., Kalis, S.L. et al. (2008). The biochemistry of somatic hypermutation. *Annu. Rev. Immunol.* 26: 481–511.

Phelan, J.D., Young, R.M., Webster, D.E., Roulland, S., Wright, G.W. et al. (2018). A multiprotein supercomplex controlling oncogenic signalling in lymphoma. *Nature* 560: 387–391.

Philippen, A., Diener, S., Zenz, T., Dohner, H., Stilgenbauer, S. et al. (2010). SYK carries no activating point mutations in patients with chronic lymphocytic leukaemia (CLL). *Br. J. Haematol.* 150: 633–636.

Pieper, K., Grimbacher, B., and Eibel, H. (2013). B-cell biology and development. *J. Allergy. Clin. Immunol.* 131: 959–971.

Pleyer, C., Ali, M.A., Cohen, J.I., Tian, X., Soto, S. et al. (2021). Effect of bruton tyrosine kinase inhibitor on efficacy of adjuvanted recombinant hepatitis B and zoster vaccines. *Blood* 137: 185–189.

Rassenti, L.Z., Jain, S., Keating, M.J., Wierda, W.G., Grever, M.R. et al. (2008). Relative value of ZAP-70, CD38, and immunoglobulin mutation status in predicting aggressive disease in chronic lymphocytic leukemia. *Blood* 112: 1923–1930.

Reinart, N., Nguyen, P.H., Boucas, J., Rosen, N., Kvasnicka, H.M. et al. (2013). Delayed development of chronic lymphocytic leukemia in the absence of macrophage migration inhibitory factor. *Blood* 121: 812–821.

Rosenquist, R., Ghia, P., Hadzidimitriou, A., Sutton, L.A., Agathangelidis, A. et al. (2017). Immunoglobulin gene sequence analysis in chronic lymphocytic leukemia: updated ERIC recommendations. *Leukemia* 31: 1477–1481.

Ruan, J., Hyjek, E., Kermani, P., Christos, P.J., Hooper, A.T. et al. (2006). Magnitude of stromal hemangiogenesis correlates with histologic subtype of non-Hodgkin's lymphoma. *Clin. Cancer Res.* 12: 5622–5631.

Rui, L., Schmitz, R., Ceribelli, M., and Staudt, L.M. (2011). Malignant pirates of the immune system. *Nat. Immunol.* 12: 933–940.

Saba, N.S., Liu, D., Herman, S.E., Underbayev, C., Tian, X. et al. (2016). Pathogenic role of B-cell receptor signaling and canonical NF-kappaB activation in mantle cell lymphoma. *Blood* 128: 82–92.

Sage, P.T. and Sharpe, A.H. (2015). T follicular regulatory cells in the regulation of B cell responses. *Trends Immunol.* 36: 410–418.

Schmitz, R., Ceribelli, M., Pittaluga, S., Wright, G., and Staudt, L.M. (2014). Oncogenic mechanisms in Burkitt lymphoma. *Cold Spring Harb. Perspect Med.* 4.

Schmitz, R., Wright, G.W., Huang, D.W., Johnson, C.A., Phelan, J.D. et al. (2018). Genetics and pathogenesis of diffuse large B-cell lymphoma. *N. Engl. J. Med.* 378: 1396–1407.

Schmitz, R., Young, R.M., Ceribelli, M., Jhavar, S., Xiao, W. et al. (2012). Burkitt lymphoma pathogenesis and therapeutic targets from structural and functional genomics. *Nature* 490: 116–120.

Sehn, L.H. (2016). Introduction to a review series: the paradox of indolent B-cell lymphoma. *Blood* 127: 2045–2046.

Seifert, M., Sellmann, L., Bloehdorn, J., Wein, F., Stilgenbauer, S. et al. (2012). Cellular origin and pathophysiology of chronic lymphocytic leukemia. *J. Exp. Med.* 209: 2183–2198.

Shaffer, A.L., 3RD, Young, R.M., and Staudt, L.M. (2012). Pathogenesis of human B cell lymphomas. *Annu. Rev. Immunol.* 30: 565–610.

Shanafelt, T.D., Wang, X.V., Kay, N.E., Hanson, C.A., O'Brien, S. et al. (2019). Ibrutinib-rituximab or chemoimmunotherapy for chronic lymphocytic leukemia. *N. Engl. J. Med.* 381: 432–443.

Sharman, J.P., Banerji, V., Fogliatto, L.M., Herishanu, Y., Munir, T. et al. (2019a). ELEVATE TN: phase 3 study of acalabrutinib combined with obinutuzumab (O) or alone vs O plus chlorambucil (Clb) in patients (Pts) with treatment-naive chronic lymphocytic leukemia (CLL). *Blood* 134: 31-31.

Sharman, J.P., Coutre, S.E., Furman, R.R., Cheson, B.D., Pagel, J.M. et al. (2019b). Final results of a randomized, phase iii study of rituximab with or without idelalisib followed by open-label idelalisib in patients with relapsed chronic lymphocytic leukemia. *J. Clin. Oncol.* 37: 1391–1402.

Sharman, J.P., Egyed, M., Jurczak, W., Skarbnik, A., Pagel, J.M. et al. (2020). Acalabrutinib with or without obinutuzumab versus chlorambucil and obinutuzmab for treatment-naive chronic lymphocytic leukaemia (ELEVATE TN): a randomised, controlled, phase 3 trial. *Lancet.* 395: 1278–1291.

Sivina, M., Kim, E., Wierda, W.G., Ferrajoli, A., Jain, N. et al. (2021). Ibrutinib induces durable remissions in treatment-naive patients with CLL and 17p deletion/TP53 mutations. *Blood.* 138 (24): 2589–2592.

Smith, C.I. (2017). From identification of the BTK kinase to effective management of leukemia. *Oncogene* 36: 2045–2053.

Smith, S.M., Pitcher, B.N., Jung, S.H., Bartlett, N.L., Wagner-Johnston, N. et al. (2017). Safety and tolerability of idelalisib, lenalidomide, and rituximab in relapsed and refractory lymphoma: the alliance for clinical trials in oncology A051201 and A051202 phase 1 trials. *Lancet. Haematol.* 4: e176–e182.

Spaargaren, M., Beuling, E.A., Rurup, M.L., Meijer, H.P., Klok, M.D. et al. (2003). The B cell antigen receptor controls integrin activity through Btk and PLCgamma2. *J. Exp. Med.* 198: 1539–1550.

Stamatopoulos, K., Agathangelidis, A., Rosenquist, R., and GHIA, P. (2017). Antigen receptor stereotypy in chronic lymphocytic leukemia. *Leukemia.* 31: 282–291.

Stavnezer, J. and Schrader, C.E. (2014). IgH chain class switch recombination: mechanism and regulation. *J. Immunol.* 193: 5370–5378.

Sun, C., Tian, X., Lee, Y.S., Gunti, S., Lipsky, A. et al. (2015). Partial reconstitution of humoral immunity and fewer infections in patients with chronic lymphocytic leukemia treated with ibrutinib. *Blood* 126: 2213–2219.

Szydlowski, M., Kiliszek, P., Sewastianik, T., Jablonska, E., Bialopiotrowicz, E. et al. (2016). FOXO1 activation is an effector of SYK and AKT inhibition in tonic BCR signal-dependent diffuse large B-cell lymphomas. *Blood* 127: 739–748.

Tam, C.S., Trotman, J., Opat, S., BURGER, J.A., Cull, G. et al. (2019). Phase 1 study of the selective BTK inhibitor zanubrutinib in B-cell malignancies and safety and efficacy evaluation in CLL. *Blood* 134: 851–859.

Thompson, A.A., Talley, J.A., Do, H.N., Kagan, H.L., Kunkel, L. et al. (1997). Aberrations of the B-cell receptor B29 (CD79b) gene in chronic lymphocytic leukemia. *Blood* 90: 1387–1394.

Tolar, P., Hanna, J., Krueger, P.D., and Pierce, S.K. (2009). The constant region of the membrane immunoglobulin mediates B cell-receptor clustering and signaling in response to membrane antigens. *Immunity* 30: 44–55.

Treon, S.P., Meid, K., Gustine, J., Yang, G., XU, L. et al. (2021). Long-term follow-up of ibrutinib monotherapy in symptomatic, previously treated patients with Waldenstrom macroglobulinemia. *J. Clin. Oncol.* 39: 565–575.

Treon, S.P., Tripsas, C.K., Meid, K., Warren, D., Varma, G. et al. (2015). Ibrutinib in previously treated waldenstrom's macroglobulinemia. *N. Engl. J. Med.* 372: 1430–1440.

Treon, S.P., Xu, L., Yang, G., Zhou, Y., Liu, X. et al. (2012). MYD88 L265P somatic mutation in Waldenstrom's macroglobulinemia. *N. Engl. J. Med.* 367: 826–833.

Turner, M., Mee, P.J., Costello, P.S., Williams, O., Price, A.A. et al. (1995). Perinatal lethality and blocked B-cell development in mice lacking the tyrosine kinase Syk. *Nature* 378: 298–302.

Varano, G., Raffel, S., Sormani, M., Zanardi, F., Lonardi, S. et al. (2017). The B-cell receptor controls fitness of MYC-driven lymphoma cells via GSK3beta inhibition. *Nature* 546: 302–306.

Victora, G.D. and Nussenzweig, M.C. (2012). Germinal centers. *Annu. Rev. Immunol.* 30: 429–457.

Wagner-Johnston, N.D., Schuster, S.J., Devos, S., Salles, G., Jurczak, W.J. et al. (2021). Outcomes of patients with up to 6 years of follow-up from a phase 2 study of idelalisib for relapsed indolent lymphomas. *Leuk. Lymphoma.* 62: 1077–1087.

Wang, M.L., Rule, S., Martin, P., Goy, A., Auer, R. et al. (2013). Targeting BTK with ibrutinib in relapsed or refractory mantle-cell lymphoma. *N. Engl. J. Med.* 369: 507–516.

Wilson, W.H., Young, R.M., Schmitz, R., Yang, Y., Pittaluga, S. et al. (2015). Targeting B cell receptor signaling with ibrutinib in diffuse large B cell lymphoma. *Nat. Med.* 21: 922–926.

Wotherspoon, A.C., Doglioni, C., Diss, T.C., Pan, L., Moschini, A. et al. (1993). Regression of primary low-grade B-cell gastric lymphoma of mucosa-associated lymphoid tissue type after eradication of Helicobacter pylori. *Lancet.* 342: 575–577.

Woyach, J.A., Ruppert, A.S., Heerema, N.A., Zhao, W., Booth, A.M. et al. (2018). Ibrutinib regimens versus chemoimmunotherapy in older patients with untreated CLL. *N. Engl. J. Med.* 379: 2517–2528.

Xochelli, A., Sutton, L.A., Agathangelidis, A., Stalika, E., Karypidou, M. et al. (2015). Molecular evidence for antigen drive in the natural history of mantle cell lymphoma. *Am. J. Pathol.* 185: 1740–1748.

Yin, Q., Sivina, M., Robins, H., Yusko, E., Vignali, M. et al. (2017). Ibrutinib therapy increases t cell repertoire diversity in patients with chronic lymphocytic leukemia. *J. Immunol.* 198: 1740–1747.

Younes, A., Sehn, L.H., Johnson, P., Zinzani, P.L., HONG, X. et al. (2019). Randomized phase III trial of ibrutinib and rituximab plus cyclophosphamide, doxorubicin, vincristine, and prednisone in Non-Germinal center B-cell diffuse large B-cell lymphoma. *J. Clin. Oncol.* 37: 1285–1295.

Young, R.M., Wu, T., Schmitz, R., Dawood, M., Xiao, W. et al. (2015). Survival of human lymphoma cells requires B-cell receptor engagement by self-antigens. *Proc. Natl. Acad. Sci. U S A.* 112: 13447–13454.

Zelenetz, A.D., Barrientos, J.C., Brown, J.R., Coiffier, B., Delgado, J. et al. (2017). Idelalisib or placebo in combination with bendamustine and rituximab in patients with relapsed or refractory chronic lymphocytic leukaemia: interim results from a phase 3, randomised, double-blind, placebo-controlled trial. *Lancet. Oncol.* 18: 297–311.

19

Pharmacologic Features of Drugs Targeting Bruton's Tyrosine Kinase (BTK)

Joel McCay and John G. Gribben

Centre for Haemato-Oncology, Barts Cancer Institute, Queen Mary University of London, London, UK

Take Home Messages

- Bruton's tyrosine kinase (BTK) is a crucial signaling protein that links B-cell antigen receptor signaling to the activation, proliferation, and survival of B-cells.
- The development of very specific small-molecule BTK inhibitors has made BTK an important therapeutic target in the treatment of B-cell malignancies and autoimmune diseases.
- Here, we discuss the role of BTK in BCR signaling and the current status of BTK inhibition in B-cell malignancies and autoimmunity.

Introduction

In order to appreciate the merits of targeting BTK, it is crucial to understand the complex network of signaling pathways that interface with BTK leading to its activation. These pathways in their composite play an absolutely essential role in governing the proliferation and survival of B-lymphocytes, be they normal or malignant. Bruton's tyrosine kinase (BTK) is one of the five members of the highly conserved family of cytoplasmic tyrosine kinase expressed in hepatocellular carcinoma (TEC) kinases (Tomlinson et al. 2004). The TEC family of kinases is expressed primarily on hematopoietic cells. The five members of the family are interleukin-2 inducible T-cell Kinase (ITK), BTK, resting lymphocyte kinase (RLK), TEC, and bone marrow-expressed kinase (BMX). None of the TEC family kinases contain the C-terminal regulatory phosphorylation site that is considered critical for controlling the function of SRC family kinases. The gene encoding BTK was discovered as the gene affected in patients with X-linked agammaglobulinemia (XLA) (Tsukada et al. 1993; Vetrie et al. 1993).

BTK is of vital importance in cell signaling and ultimately B-cell proliferation and survival. BTK phosphorylation is directly impacted by B-cell receptor (BCR) signaling. Conformational changes in the various domains of the protein lead to a cascade of protein binding, kinase activation, and signaling. The functional outcome of this signaling process is activation of a transcriptional pathway important in B-cell survival that predominantly influences nuclear factor (NF)-κB. It is due to the lack of functional BTK protein in XLA patients that mature B-cells and antibodies are almost completely absent. BCR signaling abnormalities in kinases downstream of the BCR have been demonstrated to be defective or abnormally activated in numerous autoimmune disorders and malignancies (Corneth et al. 2016; Kil et al. 2012; Morel 2010). Furthermore, in human autoimmune diseases, genetic susceptibility loci include genes encoding BCR signaling molecules.

The role of BTK signaling in the survival and proliferation of clonal B-cells is pivotal, an observation underscored by the effects of BTK inhibitors (BTKis) in chronic lymphocytic leukemia (CLL). Upon BCR activation, BTK is recruited to the cell surface membrane before various kinases are activated.

Lck/Yes novel tyrosine kinase (LYN) and spleen tyrosine kinase (SYK) recruitment to the cell surface allows for concomitant activation of the CD79a/b transmembrane receptor via phosphorylation of the motif residues on the cytoplasmic tails. This activation leads to further intracellular kinase activation, such as phosphoinositide 3-kinases (PI3K), SYK, and phosphatidylinositol 4,5-bisphosphate (PIP2), which phosphorylates BTK. Activation of BTK via this pathway leads to the sequential activation of other kinases and proteins downstream of BTK (Jiang et al. 2019; Lu et al. 2009; Martin et al. 2013; McCay and Gribben 2022; Palma et al. 2021; Thompson 2020). One of these downstream enzymes is phospholipase Cγ2 (PLCγ2). As the primary target of BTK, PLCγ2 phosphorylation leads to inositol triphosphate (IP3) generation, a messenger protein responsible for intracellular calcium influx (Takata and Kurosaki 1996). Calcium influx triggers multiple different transcriptional pathways such as Rat sarcoma virus (RAS) signaling-dependent extracellular signal-regulated kinases (ERK) 1/2 phosphorylation or NF-κB resulting in B-cell survival and proliferation (Figure 19.1)

Precision Cancer Therapies: Targeting Oncogenic Drivers and Signaling Pathways in Lymphoid Malignancies: From Concept to Practice, Volume 1,
First Edition. Edited by Owen A. O'Connor, Stephen M. Ansell, and John F. Seymour.

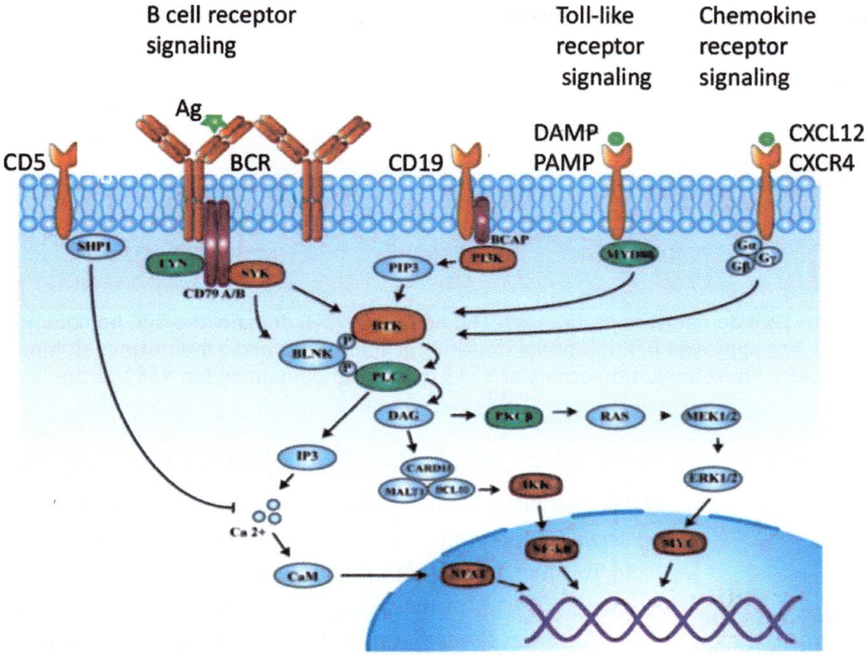

Figure 19.1 The central role of BTK in B-cell signaling. B-cell signaling showing the role of BTK following BCR stimulation via antigen leading to cell surface recruitment of the kinases LYN and SYK binding to the cytoplasmic tail of CD79a/b. BTK is then phosphorylated via PIP3 which is activated via PI3K before BTK phosphorylates PLCγ2 which leads to multiple paths responsible for gene regulation and cell survival and proliferation.

(Hendriks et al. 2014; Jiang et al. 2019; Kil et al. 2012; Lu et al. 2009; Martin et al. 2013; McCay and Gribben 2022; Palma et al. 2021; Takata and Kurosaki 1996; Thompson 2020). Observed effects of B-cell-depleting therapy in patients with significant autoimmune disease as well as in B-cell malignancies have informed the development of successful B-cell-targeted therapies such as the BCL2 inhibitor venetoclax or the BTK inhibitors ibrutinib, acalabrutinib, and zanubrutinib.

While the crystallographic structure of any full-length auto-inhibited TEC family kinase is still lacking, in 2015 a fragment containing three of the domains of BTK was successfully crystallized. This allowed the first glimpse into the three-dimensional representation of how the TEC kinase domains are spatially arranged (Wang et al. 2015). The SRC-module of BTK comprised the SH3-SH2-kinase fragment crystallized as a domain swapped dimer (DSD) with the domain swapping occurring in the SH2 portion of the fragment (Wang et al. 2019). While the functional significance of the DSD is unknown, each half of the DSD adopts an auto-inhibitory conformation. The SH3 and SH2 domains assemble on the back of the kinase domain with the SH2-linker region contacting both the SH3 and kinase domain N-lobe (Joseph et al. 2017; von Raussendorf et al. 2017). This domain arrangement and auto-inhibitory changes described resemble SRC kinases despite the absence of the SRC regulatory tail in the TEC family.

The *BTK* gene at position Xq21. 3-q22 encodes for a 659 amino acid protein, and to date has been shown to have over 400 mutations (Gene Ontology Classifications 2022; Jiang et al. 2019; von Raussendorf et al. 2017). The protein is made of five domains with varying roles between the N terminus and C terminus (Figure 19.2). The five domains from N to C terminus and their roles include:

1) the pleckstrin homology (PH) domain – responsible for protein recruitment to the cell surface following the binding of intracellular phosphatidylinositol lipids, such as PIP3
2) the proline-rich TEC homology (TH) domain – responsible for protein stability via its zinc-finger motif
3) the two SRC homology (SH) domains SH3 and SH2 – responsible for protein–protein interactions as well as binding of proline-rich regions. Autophosphorylation of the SH3 domain at point Y233 leads to conformational change and activation of the binding domain. Binding of B-cell linker proteins such as BLNK following phosphorylation by SYK also occurs at the SH2 domain
4) the catalytic domain – this domain is phosphorylated at position Y551 by either LYN or SYK and this results in autophosphorylation of the SH3 domain at the Y233 position. The currently approved BTKi work by covalently binding at the C481 occupying the ATP binding site.

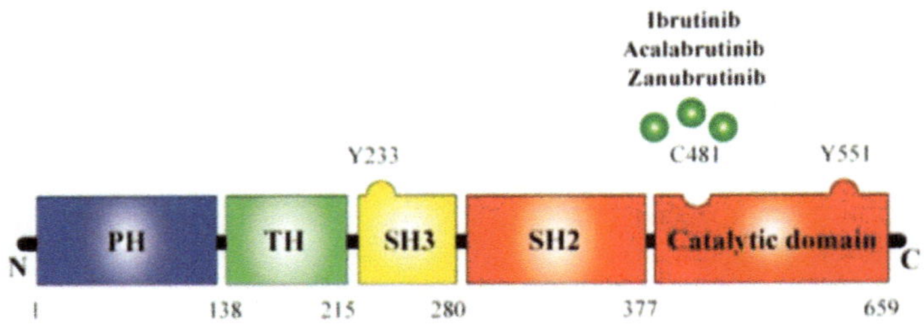

Figure 19.2 Schematic structure of BTK.
BTK is composed of five domains: pleckstrin homology (PH) domain, the proline-rich TEC homology (TH) domain, the SRC homology (SH) domains SH3 and SH2, and the catalytic domain. The approved BTK inhibitors ibrutinib, acalabrutinib, and zanubrutinib all bind to the same site in the catalytic domain at position C481. Phosphorylation occurs at Y233 in the SH3 domain and at Y551 in the catalytic domain.

BTK and B-cell Activating Factor Receptor (BAFFR) Signaling

BCR signaling and B-cell activating factor (BAFF) are the two most important components involved in B-cell survival and proliferation. BAFF is a cytokine of the tumor necrosis factor (TNF) ligand family (Lam et al. 1997) and its role is to activate and bind to three receptors B-cell maturation antigen (BCMA), transmembrane activator and CAML interactor (TACI), and BAFF receptor (BAFFR) which are responsible for canonical and non-canonical activation of NF-κB.

Activation of these pathways induces B-cell survival in a direct and indirect fashion by reducing pro-apoptotic factors or by increasing BAFFR expression, respectively, as well as supporting plasma cell differentiation (Craxton et al. 2005; Stadanlick et al. 2008). These signals in combination can impact on B-cell selection and ultimately lead to a pro-inflammatory phenotype. BTK and BAFF overexpression was shown to lead to Sjögren's syndrome or systemic lupus erythematous (SLE) in mice and a pro-inflammatory cytokine profile and immune cell populations (Rip et al. 2018; Stadanlick et al. 2008). BAFF overexpression in human cells increases autoimmune reactive B-cells allowing for maturation and proliferation within lymph node germinal centers, further promoting an autoimmune phenotype (Moisini and Davidson 2009).

BTK in Cell Signaling Pathways

BTK expression is not limited to B-cells and is present in other hematopoietic cell lines including granulocytes, macrophages, and erythroid cells (Craxton et al. 2005; Gene Ontology Classifications 2022; Lam et al. 1997; Rip et al. 2018; Stadanlick et al. 2008). Although BTK expression has been reported in T-cells in murine models, it is now generally accepted that these cells do not express BTK protein commonly in humans (de Weers et al. 1993; Schmidt et al. 2004). BTK also plays a role in many other key immune signaling pathways, including FcR signaling, chemokine receptors, and Toll-like receptor (TLR) pathways.

A role of BTK in mediating FcR signaling is seen in both autoimmune disease and malignant disease. Macrophages express the FcR in various subtypes and upon activation of the receptor can trigger antibody-mediated events as well as impact on other surrounding cells (Chang et al. 2011; Chiu et al. 2002). FcεR activation promotes histamine release mediated by BTK in mast cells leading to inflammation and enhanced antigen presentation to T-cells, as seen in rheumatoid arthritis patients. Inhibition of BTK in these individuals leads to reduced B- and myeloid cell numbers which are known to worsen disease phenotype (Luo et al. 2010). In malignancy, expression of BTK has been shown to increase polarization of macrophages toward an M2 phenotype which is more associated with cancer cell development and metastatic disease. Overexpression of BTK in tumor-associated macrophages leads to upregulation of FcR and inhibition of CD8+ cytotoxic T-cells within the tumor microenvironment (TME) of certain cancer types (Di Paolo et al. 2011; Wang et al. 2021).

TLRs are expressed on a number of innate immune cells including macrophages, dendritic cells, and fibroblasts (Colado et al. 2018). BTK plays a role in many TLR signaling pathways, including TLR 7 and 9, and in the development of autoimmunity (Kawasaki and Kawai 2014). Though not directly involved in TLR receptor signaling to the extent that is seen in BCR signaling, it plays a vital role as a linker protein, much like the role of BLNK in the SH2 domain of BTK. BTK is responsible for facilitating the binding of myeloid differentiation primary response 88 (MyD88) and MyD88 adaptor-like (MAL) to TLR by recruitment of these proteins to the cell surface (Colado et al. 2018; Kawasaki and Kawai 2014; Rip et al. 2019; Wang et al. 2021). This leads to activation of the NF-κB pathway as well as production of pro-inflammatory cytokines and enhanced B-cell survival. Specific TLR can also impact on B-cell expression of BAFF, leading to increased cell proliferation and survival (Abu-Rish et al. 2013). MAL phosphorylation has been shown to be inhibited by BTKi in TLR2 and 4 signaling (Gray et al. 2006).

Multiple chemokines have been shown to be influenced by BTK in normal physiology as well as in disease. The chemokine CXCL12, which is highly expressed in lymph nodes and bone marrow cells, activates BTK following binding to its target receptor CXCR4 (de Gorter et al. 2007). The role of CXCR4 is important in cell adhesion and migration via pathways involving PLCγ2 and AKT. Other chemokines like CCL3 and CCL4 are upregulated in mantle cell lymphoma (MCL) following BCR activation. Treatment with BTKi such as ibrutinib, acalabrutinib, or zanubrutinib was found to suppress these chemokines as well as other cell populations within the TME, including human marrow stromal cells that are associated with tumor cell migration and metastasis highlighting the important role BTK has on tumor biology and progression (Staversky et al. 2018; Turley et al. 2015).

It is clear that the role of BTK in numerous cell-signaling pathways across various cells of the innate and adaptive immune system is not only a mechanism for disease development but also a target for therapeutic intervention.

BTK Inhibitor Development and Mechanisms of Action

The fundamental mechanism of action of the approved BTK inhibitors is by irreversibly binding to the ATP binding site of the kinase domain on BTK via a covalent bond. This bond occurs at amino acid C481 and classifies these kinase inhibitors as type VI (Davids and Brown 2014). Other classes of kinase inhibitors such as I–IV are reversible inhibitors that bind either directly or indirectly to impact the ATP binding site (Roskoski 2016). In attempts to overcome off-target side effects and the emerging resistance patterns seen with ibrutinib, several selective second-generation BTK inhibitors have been developed. Acalabrutinib and zanubrutinib are novel next-generation BTK inhibitors that also irreversibly bind to the C481 residue of BTK, but they have greater selectivity and fewer off-target effects compared to ibrutinib (Wu et al. 2016). These subtle changes impact drug half-life, dosage, and the clinical side effect profiles. Of note patients with comorbidities such as hypertension or atrial fibrillation may benefit from the BTK inhibitor acalabrutinib over ibrutinib due to its increased selectivity and reduced incidence of these side effects (Wu et al. 2016).

An observed benefit of covalent inhibitors is their ability to reach higher and more sustained levels of BTK occupancy, compared with reversible inhibitors that need to be present in the circulation at persistent high levels to allow for effective sustained inhibition. Newer drugs such as rilzabrutinib bind to C481 in the same covalent manner, although with selectively prolonged occupancy of BTK due to structural optimization, its binding is reversible, potentially reducing side effects in selected patient groups (Langrish et al. 2021). Pirtobrutinib is another new reversible BTKi classified as a type II kinase inhibitor. Its mechanism of action is not via covalent binding to C481 but through preventing phosphorylation of Y551 residue of the catalytic domain more proximal to the C terminus. This is achieved by reversible binding at a region adjacent to the ATP binding site, comprised three residues known as the H3 pocket (Aslan et al. 2022).

Before widespread use of ibrutinib several compounds were developed showing a direct correlation between B-cell apoptosis and BTK occupancy *in vitro* (Mahajan et al. 1999). Though there is limited clinical information for many of these compounds, some have been shown to impair Janus kinase 2 signaling significantly *in vitro*, making many of these compounds less specific for BTK inhibition (van den Akker et al. 2004). Further development of more specific compounds by numerous laboratories and groups leads to the development of PCI-29732, a kinase which demonstrated significant inhibition of BTK, though not exclusively selective for this kinase (Honigberg et al. 2010). More recent data has shown that PCI-29732 has benefits in enhancing efficacy of conventional chemotherapy in cell lines (Ge et al. 2018). Building on this work leads to the development of PCI-32765, which showed 1:1 occupancy of the BTK protein which was irreversible (Brown 2013). In time, PCI-32765 would later be renamed ibrutinib. Since these initial discoveries over 100 clinical trials have been completed with ibrutinib, with over 200 trials now ongoing (clinicaltrials.gov. n.d.; clinicaltrials.gov. n.d.).

BTK Inhibitors in Malignancy

BTKi in CLL/SLL and Waldenstrom's macroglobulinemia. Ibrutinib obtained US Food and Drug Administration (FDA) approval in 2013 for MCL patients, and subsequently for CLL patients upon successful phase 2 trials (Byrd et al. 2013; Niemann et al. 2016; Wang et al. 2013). Multiple BTKis currently have approval for use in other B-cell malignancies such as Waldenstrom's macroglobulinemia (WM) and marginal zone lymphoma (MZL) (Castillo et al. 2022; www.imbruvicahcp.com. n.d.; Oncology Times 2017; www.nice.org.uk. n.d.).

The strongest evidence for the importance of BCR-mediated signaling in B-cell malignancies comes from the observed clinical benefit of pathway inhibitors downstream of the BCR, such as BTKi in CLL. The phosphorylation of kinases such as LYN, SYK, BTK, and PI3K leads to activation of NF-κB and CLL cell survival and proliferation (Rickert 2013; Seda and Mraz 2015; Takata and Kurosaki 1996). Downregulation of these kinases significantly delayed the onset and slowed the growth of CLL in the Eμ-TCL1 CLL mouse model but still initiated lymphomagenesis. BTK deficiency *in vivo* halted tumor formation, whereas overexpression of BTK increased tumor incidence and mortality (Baptista et al. 2021). BTKis have also shown that some of their off-target effects may be beneficial in altering the TME in CLL. Loss of immune inhibitory checkpoint cell surface molecules as well as improved B-to-T-cell synapse formation were observed in ibrutinib-treated patients suggesting that the effect of BTKis is not limited to tumor cell apoptosis only (Byrd et al. 2014).

Numerous trials in CLL including the RESONATE and RESONATE 2 studies showed the improved outcomes of CLL patients compared with anti-CD20 antibody therapy and chemoimmunotherapy (CI), respectively. Both trials showed marked improvement in overall response rates (ORR), progression-free survival (PFS), and overall survival (OS) across more than five years of follow-up (Burger et al. 2020; Castillo et al. 2019). The landmark RESONATE trial led to FDA approval of ibrutinib for CLL/SLL patients in 2014. Subsequent studies have demonstrated superiority of ibrutinib to chemotherapy leading to approval of BTKis as first-line treatment in CLL and they are now being explored in combination therapy with anti-CD20 monoclonal antibodies, chemotherapy, and BCL2 inhibitors. Ibrutinib is a successful treatment in untreated symptomatic WM patients, especially in CXCR4 wild-type patients, offering an effective tolerable treatment in a disease with mean age of onset of 70 years (Castillo et al. 2019). More recently Zanubrutinib has also been approved for use in WM.

BTK inhibitors in diffuse large B-cell Lymphoma (DLBCL). DLBCL is the most common non-Hodgkin's lymphoma (NHL) worldwide. Although this disease is generally chemotherapy sensitive with five-year survival rates of 70–80% for low-risk disease, high-risk and relapsed/refractory disease remain a significant problem (Lacy et al. 2020). New prognostication strategies as well as improved molecular diagnostics have led to better risk stratification of disease and improved selection of treatment pathways. Classification of DLBLCL can be analyzed in various ways including *de novo* versus transformed, cytogenetic, and molecular abnormalities (i.e. "double" or "triple" hit lymphomas) or via the cell-of- origin of the B-cell itself (i.e. germinal center B-cell [GCB], activated B-cell [ABC], and unclassifiable). ABC and GCB differ in their molecular mutations and cell signaling pathways, which ultimately impact on disease characteristics and prognosis. The ABC subtype relies on BCR signaling and is associated with mutations in caspase recruitment domain family member 11 (CARD11), CD79a/b, and MYD88 mutations as well as increased NF-κB activation (Goy et al. 2019). The GCB subtype is primarily associated with PI3K/AKT activation rather than NF-κB which points to the role that BTKi may play in the treatment of the ABC subtype in the future. While pre-clinical data exists establishing a role for ibrutinib in inducing apoptosis of ABC-DLBCL, especially when employed in combination therapy, a randomized phase 3 trial (the PHOENIX Study) failed to confirm the benefit of adding ibrutinib to R-CHOP (Younes et al. 2019). It is conceivable that more precise genotyping and molecular profiling of patients using the newer molecular classification schemes may improve the ability to select for patients most likely to benefit from the addition of a BTK inhibitor.

Mantle cell, follicular and marginal zone lymphoma. Other B-cell malignancies in which various BTKi are FDA approved for treatment include MCL, follicular lymphoma (FL), and MZL.

MCL is a rare subtype of NHL with a hallmark chromosomal translocation t(11:14) leading to overexpression of cyclin D1 (Merolle et al. 2018). As is the case in other B-cell malignancies, MCL cells show increased expression of intracellular kinases such as PI3K which drives BTK activation (Advani et al. 2013). Disease phenotype ranges from indolent disease to those with high-grade aggressive disease requiring aggressive chemotherapy. Given the age of onset of many MCL patients is greater than 50 years, with advanced disease at presentation, the option for high-dose therapy is not always feasible. Initial studies on the use of ibrutinib in patients with high-risk relapsed disease were shown to be beneficial with response rates of 60% and BTK occupancy maintained for 24 hours (Wang et al. 2015). Larger studies lead to the approval of ibrutinib in relapsed MCL and new evidence showing its durability and tolerability in the disease (de Claro et al. 2015, 2018).

FL is a germinal center B-cell malignancy which is largely indolent, and treatment is reserved for those with advanced, symptomatic, or transformed disease (Kumar et al. 2021). It is characterized by chromosome translocation t(14:18) leading to overexpression of BCL2, an anti-apoptotic protein involved in B-cell survival (Bartlett et al. 2018). Multiple signaling pathway mutations are observed in FL such as NF-κB, *CARD11*, and MYD*88*. The use of single-agent ibrutinib in FL was observed to improve outcomes and responses in patients, especially in those with rituximab sensitive disease (Dangi-Garimella 2014). Interestingly, CARD11 mutations were described as a risk factor from development of ibrutinib resistance.

MZL is commonly associated with infections such as *Helicobacter pylori* or other chronic inflammatory states (Merolle et al. 2018). It can present as nodal, extra-nodal, or splenic disease with most cases being indolent and responding well to antibiotic therapy for those with associated infection. In the cases of high-risk disease (i.e. *TP53* deletion, t(11:18) or chromosomal abnormalities such as deletion 7q), CI may be need. Options for those who relapse, have a poor performance status, or have resistant disease remain limited. FDA approval of ibrutinib for MZL previously treated with one prior anti-CD20 therapy was granted in 2017 based on the significant findings relating to improved PFS compared to standard chemotherapy regimens (Mhibik et al. 2019).

BTK Inhibitors in Solid Cancers

Though some evidence for the benefit of ibrutinib has been shown in pancreatic cancer, with tumor regression and immune cell restoration, the clinical data is yet to show any discernable benefit. Further research and development on treatment regimes, especially in cancer cells expressing high levels of immune checkpoint blockade molecules, such as metastatic melanoma, may harbor a role for BTKi in the future.

BTK Inhibitors in Autoimmune Diseases

The off-target effects of ibrutinib on BTK in other cell types as well as its effects in other TEC kinases such as ITK in T-cells may contribute to improved tumor cell detection and apoptosis. These phenomena are well documented in CLL with effects on the TME as well as the impact on humoral immunity (Montalban et al. 2019). The tumor cell mechanisms which allow for immune evasion and progression include T-cell exhaustion, immunosuppressive cytokine profiles, and upregulation of inhibitory cell surface molecules such as programmed cell death receptor 1 (PD-1). BTKis restore these changes though they can cause immune side effects such as polyarthralgia and skin reactions (Davids and Brown 2014; Roskoski 2016; Wu et al. 2016). Given these off-target effects with ibrutinib the use of such kinase inhibitors in autoimmune disease might be expected to lead to worsening of disease phenotype. Despite this, more targeted specific kinase inhibitors have been developed for the use in autoimmune diseases including multiple sclerosis (MS) and rheumatoid arthritis (RA) (Bartlett et al. 2018). Evobrutinib, a selective inhibitor of BTK, binds covalently to the kinase with high occupancy as well as CNS penetration. Given the underlying mechanism of chronic BCR stimulation via antigen and cytokine release, the inhibitor has shown reduced number of enhancing lesions via MRI compared to placebo in this phase 2 trial. These early results in MS as well as other studies studying selective BTKi in SLE and RA offer a new paradigm of treatment for these chronic debilitating disorders.

Mechanisms of Resistance

The most common mechanism of BTKi resistance is the well-documented mutation C481S within the catalytic domain which prevents BTKi binding (Woyach et al. 2014; Mato et al. 2021; Smith and Burger 2021). Reasons for development of resistance are still not fully understood but variation in degree of BTK occupancy may be an important factor. Other mutations downstream of BTK, such as in PLCγ2, play a role in resistance development but are less common, and usually co-exist with BTK C481S. Other important factors involved in increased frequency of development of BTKi resistance include disease genotype (i.e. complex cytogenetics), specific molecular mutations (CARD11 in FL patients), and the transcriptional pathway activated within the B-cell. Notably, it has been observed that BTK resistance mutations have been observed in the NF-κB arm of signaling but not in the PI3K-RAS-MAPK pathway.

Despite the development of these mutations, a number of next-generation inhibitors are in clinical development, such as pirtobrutinib. Phase 2/3 data has shown the safety of pirtobrutinib, a reversible selective inhibitor which non-covalently binds to BTK. Its safety and maintained efficacy was observed in a cohort of CLL/SLL and MCL patients with BTKi intolerance or resistance (Miklos et al. 2017).

Finally, the origin from which the BTK mutation has occurred appears to directly affect malignant cell clonal expansion, and multiple resistance mutations can develop within subclones. Those with direct BTK mutations compared to PLCy2 or CARD11 mutations were found to have a larger clonal population size as well as higher allelic burden present. BTK and downstream mutations can also exist in the same clone or within subclones which may lead to the development of newer resistance patterns or refractory/progressive disease.

Summary

BTK plays a role within the B-cell and is vital in normal BCR signaling to maintain cell survival. It is now considered the gateway to cancer cell proliferation in B-cell malignancies and as a driver of autoreactive B-cells in chronic inflammatory disorders. Given the worldwide use of BTKi as a first-line treatment in multiple B-cell malignancies, it is likely that their use will increase with time. New research in their use in doublet and triplet therapy for CLL as a first-line standard of care could carve out their role as the backbone of treatment in multiple B-cell malignancies. More long-term studies assessing their benefit as maintenance therapy are needed, and may lead to increased use of BTKi in the not-so-distant future. It is important to consider the challenges and hurdles that come with any new treatment such as unwanted side effects and development of drug resistance. Despite these challenges, the introduction of more selective agents such as acalabrutinib, zanubrutinib, and pirtobrutinib offers hope for better treatment plans and care for an often already heavily treated population. There is still a lot of research to be done on the clinical role they can play in DLBCL and in chronic inflammatory and autoimmune disorders before they can be hailed with the same success as seen in CLL and MCL. Finally, promising evidence is emerging in their role in treatment of chronic graft versus host disease (GvHD) in hemopoietic stem cell transplant (Waller et al. 2019). With the vast array of benefits described following BTKi treatment it is important that research continues in order to improve our patient's quality and quantity of life.

Must Read References

Burger, J.A., Barr, P.M., Robak, T. et al. (2020). Long-term efficacy and safety of first-line ibrutinib treatment for patients with CLL/SLL: 5 years of follow-up from the phase 3 RESONATE-2 study. *Leukemia* 34: 787–798.

Mato, A.R., Shah, N.N., Jurczak, W. et al. (2021 March 6). Pirtobrutinib in relapsed or refractory B-cell malignancies (BRUIN): a phase 1/2 study. *Lancet* 397 (10277):892–901.

McCay, J. and Gribben, J.G. (2022 April). The role of BTK inhibitors on the tumor microenvironment in CLL. *Leuk. Lymphoma* 23: 1–10.

Wang, M.L., Blum, K.A., Martin, P. et al. (2015).Long-term follow-up of MCL patients treated with single-agent ibrutinib: updated safety and efficacy results. *Blood* 126 (6): 739–745.

References

Abu-Rish, E.Y., Amrani, Y., and Browning, M.J. (2013). Toll-like receptor 9 activation induces expression of membrane-bound B-cell activating factor (BAFF) on human B cells and leads to increased proliferation in response to both soluble and membrane-bound BAFF. *Rheumatology* 52 (7): 1190–1201.

Advani, R.H., Buggy, J.J., Sharman, J.P. et al. (2013). Bruton tyrosine kinase inhibitor ibrutinib (PCI-32765) has significant activity in patients with relapsed/refractory B-cell malignancies. *J. Clin. Oncol.* 31: 88–94.

Aslan, B., Kismali, G., Iles, L.R. et al. (2022). Pirtobrutinib inhibits wild-type and mutant Bruton's tyrosine kinase-mediated signaling in chronic lymphocytic leukemia. *Blood Cancer J.* 12 (80).

Baptista, M.J., Baskar, S., Gaglione, E.M. et al. (2021). Select antitumor cytotoxic CD8+ T clonotypes expand in patients with chronic lymphocytic leukemia treated with ibrutinib. *Clin. Cancer Res.: An Official J. Am. Ass. Cancer Res.* [online] 27 (16): 4624–4633.

Bartlett, N.L., Costello, B.A., LaPlant, B.R. et al. (2018). Single-agent ibrutinib in relapsed or refractory follicular lymphoma: a phase 2 consortium trial. *Blood* 131 (2): 182–190.

Brown, J.R. (2013 March). Ibrutinib (PCI-32765), the first BTK (Bruton's tyrosine kinase) inhibitor in clinical trials. *Curr. Hematol. Malig. Rep.* 8 (1): 1–6.

Burger, J.A., Barr, P.M., Robak, T. et al. (2020). Long-term efficacy and safety of first-line ibrutinib treatment for patients with CLL/SLL: 5 years of follow-up from the phase 3 RESONATE-2 study. *Leukemia* 34: 787–798.

Byrd, J.C., Brown, J.R., O'Brien, S. et al. (2014). Ibrutinib versus ofatumumab in previously treated chronic lymphoid leukemia. *N. Engl. J. Med.* 371 (3): 213–223.

Byrd, J.C., Furman, R.R., Coutre, S.E. et al. (2013). Targeting BTK with ibrutinib in relapsed chronic lymphocytic leukemia. *N. Engl. J. Med.* 369 (1): 32–42.

Castillo, J.J., Meid, K., Gustine, J.N. et al. (2022). Long-term follow-up of ibrutinib monotherapy in treatment-naive patients with Waldenstrom macroglobulinemia. *Leukemia* 36: 532–539.

Castillo, J.J., Xu, L., Gustine, J.N. et al. (2019 November). CXCR4 mutation subtypes impact response and survival outcomes in patients with Waldenström macroglobulinaemia treated with ibrutinib. *Br. J. Haematol.* 187 (3): 356–363.

Chang, B.Y., Huang, M.M., Francesco, M. et al. (2011). The Bruton tyrosine kinase inhibitor PCI-32765 ameliorates autoimmune arthritis by inhibition of multiple effector cells. *Arthritis Res. Ther.* 13 (4): R115.

Chiu, C.W., Dalton, M., Ishiai, M. et al. (2002). BLNK: molecular scaffolding through 'cis'-mediated organization of signaling proteins. *EMBO J.* 21 (23): 6461–6472.

clinicaltrials.gov. (n.d.). *Search of: ibrutinib | Completed Studies - List Results - ClinicalTrials.gov.* [online] Available at: https://clinicaltrials.gov/ct2/results?term=ibrutinib&Search=Apply&recrs=e&age_v=&gndr=&type=&rslt= (accessed 27 July 2022).

clinicaltrials.gov. (n.d.).*Search of: ibrutinib | Recruiting, Active, not recruiting, Enrolling by invitation Studies - List Results -clinicaltrials.gov.* [online] Available at: https://clinicaltrials.gov/ct2/results?term=ibrutinib&Search=Apply&recrs=a&recrs=f&recrs=d&age_v=&gndr=&type=&rslt= (Accessed 27 July 2022).

Colado, A., Genoula, M., Cougoule, C. et al. (2018). Effect of the BTK inhibitor ibrutinib on macrophage- and γδ T cell-mediated response against Mycobacterium tuberculosis. *Blood Cancer J.* [Online] 8 (11): 1–6. Available at: www.nature.com/articles/s41408-018-0136-x (accessed 23 July 2022).

Corneth, O.B.J., Klein Wolterink, R.G.J., and Hendriks, R.W. (2016). BTK Signaling in B cell differentiation and autoimmunity. *Curr. Top Microbiol. Immunol.* 393: 67–105.

Craxton, A., Draves, K.E., Gruppi, A. et al. (2005). BAFF regulates B cell survival by downregulating the BH3-only family member Bim via the ERK pathway. *J. Exp. Med.* 202 (10): 1363–1374.

Dangi-Garimella, S. (2014 March). FDA grants accelerated approval for ibrutinib for CLL. *Am. J. Manag. Care* 20 (5Spec No.): E10.PMID: 25618623).

Davids, M.S. and Brown, J.R. (2014 May). Ibrutinib: a first in class covalent inhibitor of Bruton's tyrosine kinase. *Future Oncol.* 10 (6): 957–967.

de Claro, R.A., McGinn, K.M., Verdun, N. et al. (2015 Aug 15). FDA approval: ibrutinib for patients with previously treated mantle cell lymphoma and previously treated chronic lymphocytic leukemia. *Clin. Cancer Res.* 21 (16): 3586–3590.

de Gorter, D.J., Beuling, E.A., Kersseboom, R. et al. (2007). Bruton's tyrosine kinase and phospholipase Cgamma2 mediate chemokine-controlled B cell migration and homing. *Immunity* 26 (1): 93–104.

de Weers, M., Verschuren, M.C., Kraakman, M.E. et al. (1993). The Bruton's tyrosine kinase gene is expressed throughout B cell differentiation, from early precursor B cell stages preceding immunoglobulin gene rearrangement up to mature B cell stages. *Eur. J. Immunol.* 23 (12): 3109–3114.

Di Paolo, J.A., Huang, T., Balazs, M. et al. (2011). Specific Btk inhibition suppresses B cell- and myeloid cell-mediated arthritis. *Nat. Chem. Biol.* 7 (1): 41–50.

Ge, C., Wang, F., Cui, C. et al. (2018). PCI29732, a bruton's tyrosine kinase inhibitor, enhanced the efficacy of conventional chemotherapeutic agents in ABCG2-overexpressing cancer cells. *Cell Physiol. Biochem.* 48: 2302–2317.

Gene Ontology Classifications. (2022). http://www.informatics.jax.org/go/marker/MGI:88216#tabular

Goy, A., Ramchandren, R., Ghosh, N. et al. (2019). Ibrutinib plus lenalidomide and rituximab has promising activity in relapsed/refractory non-germinal center B-cell-like DLBCL. *Blood* 134: 1024–1036.

Gray, P., Dunne, A., Brikos, C. et al. (2006). MyD88 adapter-like (Mal) is phosphorylated by Bruton's Tyrosine Kinase during TLR2 and TLR4 signal transduction. *J. Biol. Chem.* 281 (15): 10489–10495.

Hendriks, R.W., Yuvaraj, S., and Kil, L.P. (2014). Targeting Bruton's tyrosine kinase in B cell malignancies. *Nat. Rev. Cancer* 14 (4): 219–232.

Honigberg, L.A., Smith, A.M., Sirisawad, M. et al. (2010 July 20). The Bruton tyrosine kinase inhibitor PCI-32765 blocks B-cell activation and is efficacious in models of autoimmune disease and B-cell malignancy. *Proc. Natl. Acad. Sci. U.S.A.* 107 (29): 13075–13080.

(2017 February 25). Ibrutinib Approved for Marginal Zone Lymphoma Patients. Oncology Times 39 (4): 19. doi: 10.1097/01.COT.0000513328.33415.48.

Jiang, S.H., Athanasopoulos, V., Ellyard, J.I. et al. (2019). Functional rare and low frequency variants in BLK and BANK1 contribute to human lupus. *Nat. Commun.* 10 (1): 2201.

Joseph, R.E., Wales, T.E., Fulton, D.B. et al. (2017). Achieving a graded immune response: BTK adopts a range of active/inactive conformations dictated by multiple interdomain contacts. *Structure* 25 (10): 1481–1494.e4.

Kawasaki, T. and Kawai, T. (2014). Toll-like receptor signaling pathways. *Front. Immunol.* 5 (461): doi: 10.3389/fimmu.2014.00461.

Kil, L.P., de Bruijn, M.J., van Nimwegen, M. et al. (2012). Btk levels set the threshold for B-cell activation and negative selection of autoreactive B cells in mice. *Blood* 119 (16): 3744–3756.

Kumar, E., Pickard, L., and Okosun, J. (2021). Pathogenesis of follicular lymphoma: genetics to the microenvironment to clinical translation. *Br. J. Haematol.* 194: 810–821.

Lacy, S.E., Barrans, S.L., Beer, P.A. et al. (2020). Targeted sequencing in DLBCL, molecular subtypes, and outcomes: a haematological malignancy research network report. *Blood* 135 (20): 1759–1771.

Lam, K.P., Kuhn, R., and Rajewsky, K. (1997). In vivo ablation of surface immunoglobulin on mature B cells by inducible gene targeting results in rapid cell death. *Cell* 90 (6): 1073–1083.

Langrish, C.L., Bradshaw, J.M., Francesco, M.R. et al. (2021 Apr 1). Preclinical efficacy and anti-inflammatory mechanisms of action of the Bruton Tyrosine Kinase inhibitor rilzabrutinib for immune-mediated disease. *J. Immunol.* 206 (7): 1454–1468.

Lu, R., Vidal, G.S., Kelly, J.A. et al. (2009). Genetic associations of LYN with systemic lupus erythematosus. *Genes Immun.* 10 (5): 397–403.

Luo, Y., Pollard, J.W., and Casadevall, A. (2010). Fcγ receptor cross-linking stimulates cell proliferation of macrophages via the ERK pathway. *J. Biol. Chem.* 285 (6): 4232–4242.

Mahajan, S., Ghosh, S., Sudbeck, E.A. et al. (1999). Rational design and synthesis of a novel anti-leukemic agent targeting Bruton's tyrosine kinase (BTK), LFM-A13 [alpha-cyano-beta-hydroxy-beta-methyl-N-(2, 5-dibromophenyl) propenamide]*J. Biol. Chem.* 274: 9587–9599.

Martin, J.E., Assassi, S., Diaz-Gallo, L.M. et al. (2013). A systemic sclerosis and systemic lupus erythematosus pan-meta-GWAS reveals new shared susceptibility loci.*Hum. Mol. Genet.* 22 (19): 4021–4029.

Mato, A.R., Shah, N.N., Jurczak, W. et al. (2021 Mar 6). Pirtobrutinib in relapsed or refractory B-cell malignancies (BRUIN): a phase 1/2 study. *Lancet* 397 (10277): 892–901.

McCay, J. and Gribben, J.G. (2022 April). The role of BTK inhibitors on the tumor microenvironment in CLL. *Leuk. Lymphoma* 23: 1–10.

Merolle, M.I., Ahmed, M., Nomie, K. et al. (2018 March 27). The B cell receptor signaling pathway in mantle cell lymphoma. *Oncotarget* 9 (38): 25332–25341.

Mhibik, M., Wiestner, A., and Sun, C. (2019). Harnessing the effects of BTKi on T cells for effective immunotherapy against CLL. *Int. J. Mol. Sci.* 21 (1): 68.

Miklos, D., Cutler, C.S., Arora, M. et al. (2017). Ibrutinib for chronic graft-versus-host disease after failure of prior therapy. *Blood* 130 (21): 2243–2250.

Moisini, I. and Davidson, A. (2009). BAFF: a local and systemic target in autoimmune diseases. *Clin. Exp. Immunol.* 158 (2): 155–163.

Montalban, X., Arnold, D.L., Weber, M.S. et al. (2019). Placebo-controlled trial of an oral BTK inhibitor in multiple sclerosis. *N. Engl. J. Med.* 380 (25): 2406–2417.

Morel, L. (2010). Genetics of SLE: evidence from mouse models. *Nat. Rev. Rheumatol.* 6 (6): 348–357.

Niemann, C.U., Herman, S.E., Maric, I. et al. (2016). Disruption of in vivo chronic lymphocytic leukemia tumor-microenvironment interactions by ibrutinib–findings from an investigator-initiated phase II study. *Clin. Cancer Res.* 22: 1572–1582.

Palma, M., Mulder, T.A., and Österborg, A. (2021 July). BTK inhibitors in chronic lymphocytic leukemia: biological activity and immune effects. *Front. Immunol.* 1 (12): 686768.

(2020). Pan-London Haemato-Oncology Clinical Guidelines Lymphoid Malignancies Part 2: Diffuse Large B-Cell Lymphoma. [online] Available at: https://www.kingshealthpartners.org/assets/000/003/343/Pan_London_DLBCL_Guidelines_Jan_2020_original.pdf (accessed 26 July 2022).

(2018). Pan-London Haemato-Oncology Clinical Guidelines Lymphoid Malignancies Part 3: Follicular Lymphoma. [online] Available at: https://rmpartners.nhs.uk/wp-content/uploads/2018/11/PanLondon_FL_Guidelines_Sept2018_v2.pdf (accessed 26 July 2022).

(2020). Pan-London Haemato-Oncology Clinical Guidelines Lymphoid Malignancies Part 5: Less Common Lymphoid Malignancies. [online] Available at: https://rmpartners.nhs.uk/wp-content/uploads/2020/01/Pan-London-Less-Common-Guidelines-Jan-2020.pdf (accessed 26 July 2022).

Rickert, R. (2013). New insights into pre-BCR and BCR signalling with relevance to B cell malignancies. *Nat. Rev. Immunol.* 13: 578–591. https://doi.org/10.1038/nri3487.

Rip, J., de Bruijn, M.J.W., Appelman, M.K. et al. (2019). Toll-like receptor signaling drives Btk-mediated autoimmune disease. *Front. Immunol.* 10.

Rip, J., Van Der Ploeg, E.K., Hendriks, R.W. et al. (2018). The role of Bruton's tyrosine kinase in immune cell signaling and systemic autoimmunity. *Crit. Rev. Immunol.* 38 (1): 17–62.

Roskoski, R., Jr. (2016 January). Classification of small molecule protein kinase inhibitors based upon the structures of their drug-enzyme complexes. *Pharmacol. Res.* 103: 26–48.

Schmidt, U., van den Akker, E., Parren-van Amelsvoort, M. et al. (2004). Btk is required for an efficient response to erythropoietin and for SCF-controlled protection against TRAIL in erythroid progenitors. *J. Exp. Med.* 199 (6): 785–795.

Seda, V. and Mraz, M. (2015 March). B-cell receptor signalling and its crosstalk with other pathways in normal and malignant cells. *Eur. J. Haematol.* 94 (3): 193–205.

Smith, C.I.E. and Burger, J.A. (2021 Jun 10). Resistance mutations to BTK inhibitors originate from the NF-κB but Not From the PI3K-RAS-MAPK Arm of the B cell receptor signaling pathway. *Front. Immunol.* 12: 689472.

Stadanlick, J.E., Kaileh, M., Karnell, F.G. et al. (2008). Tonic B cell antigen receptor signals supply an NF-kappaB substrate for prosurvival BLyS signaling. *Nat. Immunol.* 9 (12): 1379–1387.

Staversky, R.J., Byun, D.K., Georger, M.A. et al. (2018). The chemokine CCL3 regulates myeloid differentiation and hematopoietic stem cell numbers. *Sci. Rep.* [Online] 8 (1): 14691. Available at: https://www.nature.com/articles/s41598-018-32978-y.

Takata, M. and Kurosaki, T. (1996). A role for Bruton's tyrosine kinase in B cell antigen receptor-mediated activation of phospholipase C-gamma 2. *J. Exp. Med.* 184 (1): 31–40.

Thompson, P.A. (2020). Occupy BTK: the key to controlling CLL. *Blood* 136 (1): 4–6.

Tomlinson, M.G., Kane, L.P., Su, J. et al. (2004). Expression and function of Tec, Itk, and Btk in lymphocytes: evidence for a unique role for Tec. *Mol. Cell Biol.* 24 (6): 2455–2466.

Tsukada, S., Saffran, D.C., Rawlings, D.J. et al. (1993). Deficient expression of a B cell cytoplasmic tyrosine kinase in human X-linked agammaglobulinemia. *Cell* 72 (2): 279–290.

Turley, S.J., Cremasco, V., and Astarita, J.L. (2015). Immunological hallmarks of stromal cells in the tumour microenvironment. *Nat. Rev. Immunol.* 15 (11): 669–682.

van den Akker, E., van Dijk, T.B., Schmidt, U. et al. (2004 May). The Btk inhibitor LFM-A13 is a potent inhibitor of Jak2 kinase activity. *Biol. Chem.* 385 (5): 409–413.

Vetrie, D., Vorechovsky, I., Sideras, P. et al. (1993). The gene involved in X-linked agammaglobulinaemia is a member of the src family of protein-tyrosine kinases. *Nature* 361 (6409): 226–233.

von Raussendorf, F., de Ruiter, A., and Leonard, T.A. (2017). A switch in nucleotide affinity governs activation of the Src and Tec family kinases. *Sci. Rep.* 7: 17405.

Waller, E.K., Miklos, D., Cutler, C. et al. (2019). Ibrutinib for chronic graft-versus-host disease after failure of prior therapy: 1-year update of a phase 1b/2 study. Biol. *Blood Marrow Transplant.* 25: 2002–2007.

Wang, H., Yung, M.M.H., Ngan, H.Y.S. et al. (2021). The impact of the tumor microenvironment on macrophage polarization in cancer metastatic progression. *Int. J. Mol. Sci.* [Online] 22 (12): 6560. Available at: https://pubmed.ncbi.nlm.nih.gov/34207286 (accessed 23 July 2022).

Wang, M.L., Blum, K.A., Martin, P. et al. (2015). Long-term follow-up of MCL patients treated with single-agent ibrutinib: updated safety and efficacy results. *Blood* 126 (6): 739–745.

Wang, M.L., Rule, S., Martin, P. et al. (2013). Targeting BTK with ibrutinib in relapsed or refractory mantle-cell lymphoma. *N. Engl. J. Med.* 369 (6): 507–516.

Wang, Q., Pechersky, Y., Sagawa, S. et al. (2019). Structural mechanism for Bruton's tyrosine kinase activation at the cell membrane. *Proc. Natl. Acad. Sci. U.S.A.*

Wang, Q.I., Vogan, E.M., Nocka, L.M. et al. (2015). Autoinhibition of Bruton's tyrosine kinase (Btk) and activation by soluble inositol hexakisphosphate. *Elife* 4.

Woyach, J.A., Furman, R.R., Liu, T.M. et al. (2014). Resistance mechanisms for the Bruton's tyrosine kinase inhibitor ibrutinib. *N. Engl. J. Med.* 370 (24): 2286–2294.

Wu, J., Zhang, M., and Liu, D. (2016 March). Acalabrutinib (ACP-196): a selective second-generation BTK inhibitor. *J. Hematol. Oncol.* 9 (9): 21.

(n.d.). *Marginal Zone Lymphoma Treatment | IMBRUVICA® (ibrutinib) | HCP.* [online] Available at: www.imbruvicahcp.com. https://www.imbruvicahcp.com/mzl#:~:text=IMBRUVICA%C2%AE%20(ibrutinib)%20is%20a (accessed 27 July 2022).

(n.d.). *Overview | Ibrutinib for treating Waldenstrom's macroglobulinaemia | Guidance | NICE.* [online] Available at: www.nice.org.uk. https://www.nice.org.uk/guidance/ta795 (accessed 27 July 2022).

Younes, A., Sehn, L.H., Johnson, P. et al. (2019 May 20). PHOENIX investigators. Randomized phase III trial of ibrutinib and rituximab plus cyclophosphamide, doxorubicin, vincristine, and prednisone in non-germinal center B-cell diffuse large B-cell lymphoma. *J. Clin. Oncol.* 37 (15): 1285–1295.

20

Clinical Experience with Drugs Targeting Bruton's Tyrosine Kinase (BTK)

Julia Aronson[1], Anthony R. Mato[1], Catherine C. Coombs[2], Prioty Islam[3], Lindsey E. Roeker[1], and Toby Eyre[4]

[1] Memorial Sloan Kettering Cancer Center, New York, NY, USA
[2] University of North Carolina, Chapel Hill, NC, USA
[3] Levine Cancer Center, Raleigh, NC, USA
[4] University of Oxford, Oxford, UK

Take Home Messages

- Bruton's tyrosine kinase (BTK) inhibitors have revolutionized the care of patients with CLL and other B-cell malignancies.
- The originally approved BTK inhibitors are all considered covalent irreversible inhibitors of BTK (ibrutinib, acalabrutinib, zanubrutinib), while the newest BTK inhibitor is reversible (PIRTOBRUTINIB).
- The first approved BTK inhibitor, ibrutinib, is associated with a variety of toxicities thought to be related to its lack of selectivity, while acalabrutinib and zanubrutinib appear to have less toxicity owing to their improved selectivity.
- While highly effective, BTK inhibitors do not produce high rates of undetectable minimal residual disease.
- Combination of BTK inhibitor with other targeted drugs like venetoclax or anti-CD20 monoclonal antibodies appears to provide an incremental improvement in efficacy with some increases toxicity.

Introduction: Chronic Lymphocytic Leukemia (CLL)

The management of CLL has been revolutionized by the development of agents that target B-cell receptor signaling. While several key targets of this pathway have been identified, Bruton's tyrosine kinase (BTK) is the most clinically relevant target identified in this pathway to date. At this time, two covalent inhibitors of BTK (BTKi, ibrutinib and acalabrutinib) have been FDA approved for the treatment of CLL/SLL in the front-line and relapsed settings, and several others are in development. The first BTKi, ibrutinib, was approved for the treatment of CLL in 2014 in the relapsed/refractory (R/R) setting and soon thereafter in the front-line setting for patients with deletion of chromosome 17p (del17p). Today, it is approved for the treatment of all CLL patients who meet iwCLL (International Workshop on CLL) criteria for CLL-directed therapy either as monotherapy or in combination with anti-CD20 monoclonal antibodies (rituximab, obinutuzumab). Ibrutinib has directly led to a paradigm shift in the management of CLL by improving survival outcomes against several agents including ofatumumab, chlorambucil, bendamustine/rituximab (BR), fludarabine/cyclophosphamide/rituximab (FCR), and chlorambucil/obinutuzumab. Yet, clinical outcomes with this molecule are somewhat limited by discontinuations due to adverse events (AEs) and clinical/molecular resistance. Our approach to this following section will be to describe the clinical experience of ibrutinib in CLL by highlighting its strengths and limitations. Thereafter, we will critically examine other BTKis that are approved or in development to assess how they may contribute to the advancement of the field for patients and address the limitations associated with the first-in-class BTKi, ibrutinib.

Ibrutinib: Clinical Trials

Ibrutinib demonstrated impressive clinical activity in the initial phase 1b-2 study published in 2013 by Byrd et al. In a heavily pre-treated patient population (median four prior therapies), most of whom did not have any standard of care options, the overall response rate (ORR) to ibrutinib was 71%, and these responses were remarkably durable (estimated 26-month progression-free survival [PFS] and overall survival [OS] were 75% and 83%, respectively). In the 28 patients with del(17p) CLL, the estimated 26-month PFS and OS were 57% and 70%, respectively. From a safety perspective, ibrutinib was well tolerated (4% discontinuation rate due to AEs), and, interestingly, safety signals for BTKi-associated AEs, such as atrial fibrillation (AF) and bleeding, were not observed in this early single-arm study. Subsequently, ibrutinib was compared to chlorambucil and ofatumumab in randomized phase 3 studies in the front-line and R/R settings.

In the phase 3 RESONATE study, ibrutinib was compared to ofatumumab in patients with R/R CLL with the primary endpoint being PFS (Byrd et al. 2014). This was also a heavily

Precision Cancer Therapies: Targeting Oncogenic Drivers and Signaling Pathways in Lymphoid Malignancies: From Concept to Practice, Volume 1, First Edition. Edited by Owen A. O'Connor, Stephen M. Ansell, and John F. Seymour.

pre-treated, high-risk population (median three prior therapies, del(17p) 32%). Ibrutinib demonstrated superior PFS (hazard ratio (HR) 0.22, $p < 0.001$) and OS (HR 0.43, $p = 0.005$) compared with ofatumumab. This study led to the approval of ibrutinib in the R/R setting. In the phase 3 RESONATE-2 study, ibrutinib was compared to chlorambucil in the front-line setting with the primary endpoint being PFS (Burger et al. 2015). Ibrutinib again demonstrated a superior PFS (HR 0.16, $p < 0.001$) and OS (HR 0.16, $p = 0.001$) advantage over chlorambucil, leading to its front line approval for all patients with CLL. From a safety perspective, the randomized design of the RESONATE and RESONATE-2 studies provided important insights into the AE profile unique to BTKi. AEs unique to ibrutinib (vs. control) included AF, bleeding-related events, hypertension, arthralgia, and infection.

Prior to the development of ibrutinib, treatment with chemoimmunotherapy, namely, FCR, was considered the most effective combination therapy for management of patients with CLL in the front-line and relapse/refractory settings. In the phase 3 E1912 trial, ibrutinib in combination with rituximab (IR) was compared with FCR in a young previously untreated population of patients with CLL, the primary endpoint again being PFS (Shanafelt et al. 2019). Overall, IR exhibited superior three-year PFS (HR 0.35, $p < 0.001$) and three-year OS (HR 0.17, $p < 0.001$) compared to FCR. However, when analyzed as subgroups, there was a notable distinction between treatment groups. In patients with IGHV (immunoglobulin heavy chain variable region)-unmutated CLL, IR remained superior to FCR (three-year PFS: 90.7% vs. 62.5%, respectively; HR 0.26, 95% CI 0.14–0.51, $p < 0.0001$), whereas for patients with IGHV-mutated disease, there was no significant difference in PFS (three-year PFS: 87.7% vs. 88%, respectively; HR 0.44, 95% CI 0.14–1.36, $p = 0.07$). From a safety perspective, this trial similarly highlighted the unique AE profile of ibrutinib seen in the RESONATE/RESONATE-2 studies. AEs distinctive to the IR group (vs. FCR) included cardiac arrhythmias, in particular AF (7.4% vs. 3.2%) and hypertension (18.8% vs. 8.2%).

Ibrutinib as monotherapy and in combination with rituximab (IR) was compared to the fixed duration chemoimmunotherapy combination of BR in the Alliance A041202 phase 3 trial (Woyach et al. 2018). Study participants were an untreated, older CLL patient population (median age 71 years, range 65–89 years). In terms of the primary endpoint, ibrutinib monotherapy or IR demonstrated superior two-year PFS compared with BR (HR 0.39, $p < 0.001$ and HR 0.38, $p < 0.001$, respectively). Interestingly, there was no significant difference in PFS between the ibrutinib and IR groups (HR 1.00, $p = 0.49$). Unlike the E1912 study, no OS benefit was observed for the ibrutinib-containing arms as compared to BR. Regarding the AE profile for the ibrutinib-based therapy in this older population of patients, infection, AF, and hypertension were noted to have higher occurrences compared to the BR group.

In the phase 3 iLLUMINATE trial, the combination of ibrutinib and obinutuzumab (IO) was compared to the combination of chlorambucil and obinutuzumab with the primary endpoint being PFS (Moreno et al. 2019). This was a previously untreated, high-risk population (del(17p) 12%, unmutated IGHV 62%). IO showed an improved 30-month PFS compared with chlorambucil and obinutuzumab (79% and 31%, respectively; HR 0.26, $p < 0.0001$). However, a major limitation of this trial design is that it lacked an ibrutinib monotherapy arm, therefore making it hard to judge the relative contribution of obinutuzumab to ibrutinib monotherapy. This limitation is particularly relevant given the findings of the Alliance A041202 trial where rituximab did not demonstrate a PFS benefit when added to ibrutinib as compared to ibrutinib alone.

Ibrutinib: Real-world Evidence

Thus far, we have focused on describing the data from large, prospective randomized clinical trials (RCTs) to highlight the clinical activity and AEs as associated with ibrutinib. However, RCTs often include a study population which may not reflect the patients who are most commonly receiving ibrutinib in clinical practice. The use of real-world evidence (RWE) studies is increasingly enhancing our understanding of targeted therapies in clinical practice by lending further insights into ibrutinib's AE profile, clinical outcomes, and sequencing of therapies following ibrutinib. While the literature for this topic is extensive and has been previously reviewed by the authors, we have included some key RWE examples to highlight important observations (Islam and Mato 2020).

Several RWE studies have reported higher rates of AEs and discontinuation for ibrutinib in clinical practice as compared to RCTs. Mato et al. led a US-based RWE study to characterize AEs leading to ibrutinib discontinuation in clinical practice in 616 patients (87% R/R, 13% first-line) (Mato et al. 2018). In contrast to ibrutinib's low discontinuation rates on initial reports of clinical trials, in this study 41% of patients discontinued ibrutinib with a median time to discontinuation of approximately six to seven months. In contrast to the initial reports for all of the clinical trials highlighted thus far in this review, AEs were the most common reason for discontinuation in all settings (63% of discontinuations in first-line and 50% of discontinuations in R/R settings). The most common AEs leading to discontinuation included arthralgia and AF. New AEs leading to discontinuation such as pneumonitis were also observed and subsequently further described in a case series (Mato et al. 2016). The authors concluded that a wider range of AEs and a higher rate of discontinuation (majority due to AE) defined ibrutinib's experience in clinical practice in contrast to the experiences reported in clinical trials.

Recently updated long-term five-year follow-up data from the RESONATE-2 now shows discontinuation rates in line with the RWE experiences (42%) with AE being the most common reason for discontinuation (~50% of discontinuations) (Burger et al. 2020). While AEs are the most common reason for ibrutinib's discontinuation in all settings, progression of disease (POD) is the second most common reason for discontinuation. Recent observations reported by Woyach et al. have provided important insight in the ibrutinib's most common mechanisms of resistance in patients with CLL including most frequently mutations at the BTK C481 amino acid residue which impair ibrutinib's binding to BTK and less commonly downstream activating mutations in PLCgamma2 (Woyach et al. 2014).

A major limitation of the RESONATE-2 study was the exclusion of patients with poor-risk disease as defined by the presence of a deletion of chromosome 17p (del17p). Similarly, the ECOG 1912 study excluded patients with del(17p), while the iLLUMINATE and Alliance A041202 studies included a small minority of patients with del(17p). Therefore, there are limited prospective data for ibrutinib's activity in a patient population with traditionally the poorest prognosis, particularly in the front-line setting. To address this data gap, Mato et al. performed an international real-world retrospective cohort study of 391 CLL patients treated with ibrutinib monotherapy in the front-line setting including 29.8% of patients with del(17p) and 20% with *TP53* mutation (Islam and Mato 2019). Of note, while the ORR was similar for the del(17p) group versus non-del(17p) patients, the PFS and OS were inferior for the del(17p) cohort (PFS 87% vs. 92% at one year, OS 89% vs. 95% at one year). This RWE study highlights an unmet need in CLL which is not evident from ibrutinib's RCTs due to limited enrollment of this patient population and lack of studies dedicated to CLL patients with poor-risk disease in the front-line setting.

In summary, while ibrutinib has changed the standard of care for all CLL patients by improving survival outcomes in every clinical scenario in which it has been tested, our review of the literature has also identified the following limitations: (i) a unique AE profile related to on- and off-target effects; (ii) high rates of AEs leading to drug discontinuation; and (iii) well-defined mechanisms of resistance leading to drug discontinuation. In the next section of the chapter, we will examine whether next-generation covalent inhibitors of BTK or first in class non-covalent inhibitors of BTK can address these limitations and possibly further improve patient outcomes when treated with a BTKi.

Acalabrutinib

In 2016, Byrd et al. reported on acalabrutinib, a highly selective inhibitor of BTK, as a potentially safer and efficacious therapy for R/R CLL (Byrd et al. 2015). In the phase 1–2 study of a small, heavily pre-treated, high-risk population (N = 61, median three prior therapies, del(17p) 31%, unmutated IGHV 75%), acalabrutinib administered at a dose of 100 mg orally twice daily (b.i.d.) demonstrated an impressive ORR of 95% (100% for patients with del(17p)) with only two progression or death events noted for the entire cohort (median follow-up of approximately 14 months). The AE profile of acalabrutinib was distinct in that no events of AF or major hemorrhage were noted, though hypertension occurred in 20% of patients. Headache (43%), diarrhea (39%), and weight gain (26%) were the most frequently noted all-grade AEs. Although this study lacked a control arm to accurately determine unique AEs attributed to acalabrutinib (vs. control) and no head-to-head data versus ibrutinib was available at this time, the early phase data was encouraging as acalabrutinib was noted to be well tolerated without any obvious compromise in efficacy. Similar to progression events on ibrutinib, C481 mutations appeared to be the most frequently observed mechanism of resistance to acalabrutinib (Woyach et al. 2019). Subsequently, acalabrutinib has been compared to clinically relevant controls in RCTs in both the front-line and R/R settings, leading to its FDA approvals for all patients with CLL.

In the phase 3 ELEVATE-TN study, acalabrutinib as monotherapy and in combination with obinutuzumab (AO) was compared to the combination of chlorambucil and obinutuzumab (CO) in an untreated CLL patient population (unmutated IGHV 63%, del(17p) 9%, *TP53mut* 11%). The primary endpoint was PFS between the AO and CO arms, and a secondary endpoint included PFS between acalabrutinib monotherapy and CO. Both AO and acalabrutinib monotherapy demonstrated superior 24-month PFS compared to CO (93%, 87%, and 47%, respectively; $p < 0.0001$) (Sharman et al. 2020). Similar improvements in PFS were seen in a subgroup analyses between AO and CO, including unmutated IGHV (91% and 31%), del(17p) CLL (88% and 22%), and *TP53* mutated disease (95% and 19%). Additionally, an important observation was that the estimated PFS for AO was superior to acalabrutinib monotherapy at 24 months. From a safety perspective, neutropenia and infection were the most prevalent high-grade AEs across all treatment groups, while headache and diarrhea were noted to have higher occurrences in both acalabrutinib groups compared to CO. BTKi AEs of clinical interest including AF, ventricular arrhythmias, major bleeding, and hypertension were infrequent events (all occurring in <10% of patients). Of note, arthralgia (range 15.1–21.9%) and any grade bleeding (39–43%, most frequently contusion) were frequent events. In a four-year follow-up to ELEVATE-TN, the estimated 48-month OS rates for AO, acalabrutinib monotherapy, and CO were 93%, 88%, and 88% (p = 0.06), respectively, with a greater complete response (CR) rate with AO (26.8%) compared to CO (12.4%) (Sharman et al. 2021). The most important finding from the updated data from ELEVATE-TN was the maintained difference in PFS for the AO versus acalabrutinib monotherapy arms at 48 months (87 vs. 78%, $p = 0.03$) confirming for the first time the relative beneficial contribution for an anti-CD20 monoclonal antibody in addition to a BTKi in the front-line setting. At a median follow-up of 46.9 months the discontinuation rates for acalabrutinib and AO were 30.7% and 25.1%, respectively, with AEs being the most common reason for discontinuation (~13%).

In the R/R setting, acalabrutinib monotherapy was compared to investigators choice of either BR or idelalisib–rituximab (Idela-R) in the phase 3 ASCEND trial (Ghia et al. 2020). This trial is particularly important because it represents the first head-to-head comparison of two targeted inhibitors in the R/R setting with the primary endpoint being PFS. At a median follow-up of 16.1 months, PFS was 83% in the acalabrutinib group and 56% in the investigators choice group resulting in a significantly longer PFS in the acalabrutinib arm versus control (HR 0.31, $p < 0.001$). The estimated 12-month PFS for acalabrutinib was 88%. Acalabrutinib was well tolerated with the three most common AEs, grades 3–4 AEs being neutropenia, anemia, and pneumonia. In the acalabrutinib arm, any grade AF, bleeding, and hypertension were noted to occur in 5%, 26%, and 3% of patients, respectively.

Comprehensive data on the AE profile of acalabrutinib came from an integrated safety analysis of 1040 CLL patients treated with acalabrutinib (65% R/R, 35% front line). In this study, acalabrutinib was found to be well tolerated. The most common all-grade AEs were headache 38% and diarrhea 37% (Furman et al. 2021). Notably, the rate of AF was low at 4% and hypertension was observed in 8%. The overall discontinuation rate for acalabrutinib due to AE was 9%, while 17% discontinued due to POD (median follow-up 24.6 months). Rogers et al. (2021) have also studied acalabrutinib in patients with progression of CLL who were previously intolerant to ibrutinib. In this study, acalabrutinib was well tolerated with a discontinuation rate due to AE of 17%.

Ibrutinib Versus Acalabrutinib

ELEVATE-RR was an open-label, randomized, non-inferiority phase 3 trial comparing acalabrutinib with ibrutinib in patients with R/R CLL (Byrd et al. 2021). The primary endpoint was independent-review committee (IRC)-assessed PFS. A total of 533 patients were randomized, and with a median follow-up of 40.9 months, acalabrutinib was deemed non-inferior to ibrutinib, both achieving a median PFS of 38.4 months (HR 1.00; 95% CI 0.79–1.27). All-grade AF, a key secondary endpoint, was lower for acalabrutinib-treated patients, seen in 9.4% compared to 16.0% of ibrutinib-treated patients ($p = 0.02$). Other key secondary endpoints did not differ between acalabrutinib and ibrutinib, including rates of grade ≥3 infections (30.8% vs. 30.0%) and Richter's transformation (3.8% vs. 4.9%). Further, median OS for both arms was not reached and did not differ. Discontinuations of therapy due to AEs occurred in 14.7% of acalabrutinib-treated patients and 21.3% of ibrutinib-treated patients. In this first head-to-head trial of BTKis in CLL, acalabrutinib appears to have an improved safety profile without compromising efficacy.

Zanubrutinib in CLL

Zanubrutinib is a selective, covalent BTKi that is not yet FDA approved for treatment of CLL, although approved for mantle cell lymphoma (MCL), marginal zone lymphoma (MZL), and Waldenstrom's macroglobulinemia (WM) with ongoing studies that have demonstrated activity in the treatment of CLL in the front-line and R/R settings. The ongoing SEQUOIA phase 3 study includes three cohorts of patients with CLL who require front-line therapy. Two of these cohorts selectively enrolled patients with del(17p), which is notable given that these high-risk individuals had not been extensively/exclusively studied in prior front-line trials of covalent BTKis. One cohort of patients with del(17p), in which patients receive zanubrutinib monotherapy, has now fully accrued. While follow-up is limited (7.0 months in the efficacy analysis, 6.3 months in the safety analysis), the ORR is 92.2%. The most common AEs are contusion in 20%, rash in 11%, upper respiratory tract infection in 10%, and nausea in 10% (Tam et al. 2019). Outcomes from the first cohort, which randomized treatment naive patients without del(17p) to zanubrutinib versus BR, and the third cohort, which includes patients with del(17p) receiving zanubrutinib and venetoclax in combination, have not yet been reported.

The phase 3 ALPINE study included 415 patients with R/R CLL, who were randomized to receive continuous zanubrutinib versus ibrutinib. The primary endpoint for this study was ORR. Notably partial response with lymphocytosis was not included as a response in this study. The first interim analysis included 15 months median follow-up and demonstrated that ORR was significantly higher with zanubrutinib than ibrutinib (78.3% vs. 62.5%). Importantly, while the 12-month PFS (95% vs. 84%) and OS (97% vs. 93%) rates were also higher for zanubrutinib than ibrutinib (Hillmen et al. 2021), the AE profile for zanubrutinib demonstrated a decreased risk of AF as compared to ibrutinib.

Pirtobrutinib in CLL

Pirtobrutinib (LOXO-305) is a novel, oral, non-covalent, reversible BTKi under development. Its novel binding mechanism at the ATP binding pocket is not dependent on presence of a wild-type C481 residue which contrasts it with the available covalent BTKis including ibrutinib, acalabrutinib, and zanubrutinib, which share the same resistance mechanisms. Pirtobrutinib thus far has been studied in the phase 1/2 BRUIN trial which included 170 patients with CLL/SLL in the safety population, of whom 139 patients were efficacy evaluable as of the most recent data cut (27 September 2020) (Mato et al. 2021). Safety data across all patients included in this study (N = 323) was favorable with only three adverse effects seen in >10% of patients (fatigue, diarrhea, contusion) and infrequent grade ≥3 adverse effects (most common grade ≥3 event was neutropenia which occurred in 32 patients). Five patients (1%) discontinued treatment due to an AE, a rate that compares favorably with other BTKis. No dose-limited toxicities (DLT) were reported and no maximum tolerated dose (MTD) was reached. Subsequently, 200 mg once daily was selected as the dose for further development. In this heavily pretreated cohort (median of three prior therapies), the ORR for pirtobrutinib was 63%, similar to the subset of patients with prior BTKi exposure (median of four prior therapies) with a 62% ORR. Responses appeared to deepen over time with an 86% ORR for patients on drug for ≥10 months. Pirtobrutinib represents the first BTKi to have clinical activity following progression on a covalent BTKi and therefore could potentially fill a major area of unmet need for patients with CLL. Pirtobrutinib's ongoing development in CLL has now been extended to phase 3 trials examining its role in the R/R and front-line settings (NCT04666038, NCT04965493, NCT05023980).

BTK Inhibition in Indolent B-cell non-Hodgkin's Lymphoma

In addition to CLL where BTK inhibition has represented a cornerstone of modern therapy, BTKis are effective and key licensed standard therapies in a range of indolent non-Hodgkin's lymphoma (NHL) entities.

Mantle Cell Lymphoma (MCL)

MCL is an uncommon, heterogenous form of NHL that is most common in males and typically occurs in the seventh decade. Three BTKis are approved for use in R/R MCL following pivotal phase 2 clinical trials. Ibrutinib (administered at a dose of 560 mg daily) was the initial BTKi to be approved following unprecedented responses. Among 111 heavily treated MCL patients, the ORR and CR rate were 68% and 21%, respectively (Wang et al. 2013). Median PFS and 18-month OS were 13.9 and 58%, respectively. Substantial PFS benefit (median PFS 14.6 months vs. 6.2 months; HR 0.43; $p < 0.0001$) was subsequently documented in the RAY trial, where patients received ibrutinib or temsirolimus in randomized fashion (Dreyling et al. 2016).

Acalabrutinib is a second-generation BTKi with reduced "off-target" kinase inhibition. A total of 124 patients with R/R MCL (median of two prior lines) received acalabrutinib monotherapy in the pivotal phase 2 trial. ORR by positron electron topography (PET/CT) was 81% (CR 40%) (Wang et al. 2018). Longer follow-up demonstrated a median duration of response (DOR) of 26 months, a median PFS of 20 months, and an estimated 24-month OS rate of 72.4% (Wang et al. 2019).

Zanubrutinib (160 mg b.i.d.) is the most recently approved second-generation covalent BTKi based on the results of a phase 2, single-arm trial of 86 R/R MCL patients conducted in China (Song et al. 2020). PET/CT assessed ORR was 84% and CR 68.6%. Median DOR and PFS were 19.5 and 22.1 months, respectively. There were only three major bleeding events, and no cases of AF.

Across these pivotal studies, patients with blastoid morphology, *TP53* mutations, and a high Ki67% proliferation index have an inferior ORR and PFS compared to patients without these features. For example, 13.9% (20/144) of patients tested for *TP53* in a pooled ibrutinib analysis had *TP53* mutated MCL. These 20 patients had a significantly inferior ORR (55.0% vs. 70.2%), median PFS (4.0 vs. 12.0 months), and median OS (10.3 vs. 33.6 months) compared to those with unmutated *TP53*. Additionally, depth of response, DOR, and overall PFS and OS are generally superior in patients receiving BTKi – specifically ibrutinib – at first relapse compared to later relapse (Rule et al. 2019).

To date, no RCTs have compared first- and second-generation BTKis in R/R MCL. Ongoing RCTs are assessing the role of front-line covalent BTK inhibition in MCL. Single-arm front-line studies suggest high levels of efficacy in low-risk populations. Fifty younger MCL patients receiving front-line ibrutinib-R has been recently reported, with an ORR and five-year PFS of 90% (CR of 62%) and 88%, respectively (Jain et al. 2020). Despite this impressive activity, a spectrum of grade 3–4 toxicities was reported as follows: atrial fibrillation at 22%, diarrhea at 14%, fatigue at 18%, and myalgia at 14%. Whether second- or next-generation BTKis will improve tolerability and survival in this setting remains to be determined.

Pirtobrutinib has also been studied in patients with MCL resistant to first- or second-generation covalent BTKis. In one such study, among 56 heavily pre-treated MCL patients (median three prior lines, 93% prior covalent BTKi, 98% prior anti-CD20, 92% prior chemotherapy) treated with pirtobrutinib, the initial ORR was 52% (14 CR, 12 PR) in the phase 1/2 BRUIN trial (Mato et al. 2021; Wang et al. 2020). An ORR of 52% was also in those who had received a prior covalent BTKi. The early safety profile of pirtobrutinib is impressive with only 1.5% of patients discontinuing due to AEs and <1% developing AF. A large, international randomized trial of pirtobrutinib versus investigators choice of covalent BTKi (BRUIN-MCL-321, NCT04662255) has recently commenced.

Historically, MCL patients who failed a BTKi have exhibited a poor survival. Over recent years, more encouraging activity has been documented in the post-BTKi space, with venetoclax, R-BAC (rituximab, bendamustine, cytarabine), and particularly anti-CD19 chimeric antigen receptor T-cell (CAR-T) therapy demonstrating high efficacy (Eyre et al. 2019; McCulloch et al. 2020; Wang et al. 2020).

Waldenstrom's Macroglobulinemia (WM)

Pivotal trials have demonstrated high levels of efficacy in WM, an uncommon indolent B-cell malignancy typically affecting the bone marrow and spleen. It is associated with secretion of an IgM paraprotein, and often carries MYD88(L265P) and CXCR4 mutations. Ibrutinib was approved in R/R WM following a phase 2 trial of 63 patients who received 420 mg daily until progression or unacceptable toxicity (Treon et al. 2015). The ORR was 90.5%, and the major response rate (MRR) was 73.0%, with highest ORR documented in patients with MYD88(L265P) and CXCR4(WT) (100% ORR and 91.2% MRR). The estimated two-year PFS was 69.1%. Ibrutinib is also approved in combination with rituximab in front-line and R/R WM following the randomized INNOVATE trial where 150 symptomatic WM patients received ibrutinib–rituximab or placebo plus rituximab (Dimopoulos et al. 2018). At 30 months the PFS was 82% with ibrutinib–rituximab versus 28% with placebo–rituximab (HR 0.20; $p < 0.001$), a benefit independent of the MYD88 or CXCR4 genotype. Improvement in cytopenias and depth of response was also significantly greater in the ibrutinib arm. AF and hypertension were observed in 12% and 13% of patients, respectively.

Phase 2 trials have also demonstrated high efficacy for acalabrutinib and zanubrutinib in WM (Owen et al. 2020; Trotman et al. 2020). In one study, 122 patients received acalabrutinib with a reported ORR of 93% in front-line (n = 14) and 86% in R/R patients (n = 92). Three-year follow-up of a phase 1/2 trial of zanubrutinib monotherapy (160 mg b.i.d. [n = 50] or 320 mg once daily [n = 23]) demonstrated an ORR of 95.9% and the VGPR/CR rate was 45.2%. Depth of response increased over time: VGPR/CR 20.5% at 6 months and 43.8% at 24 months. The estimated three-year PFS was 80.5%. The ASPEN RCT is the first published trial in B-cell malignancies to directly compare two covalent BTKis (Tam et al. 2020). Patients with MYD88 L265P-mutated WM were randomized 1:1 to ibrutinib (n = 98) or zanubrutinib (n = 101) monotherapy. The primary endpoint was the proportion achieving CR or VGPR (very good partial remission) by independent review. Twenty-nine (28%) zanubrutinib patients and 19 (19%) ibrutinib patients achieved a VGPR, a non-statistically significant difference ($p = 0.09$). Although the study did not meet its primary endpoint and PFS rates were similar, significantly less cardiovascular toxicity (15% vs. 2% rate of AF), fewer dose reductions (ibrutinib 23% vs. zanubrutinib 14%), and AEs leading to treatment discontinuation (ibrutinib 9% vs. zanubrutinib 4%) were noted in the zanubrutinib arm.

Marginal Zone Lymphoma (MZL)

MZL is an uncommon NHL defined by distinct subtypes with nodal, extranodal, and splenic involvement. While data with BTKis is more scarce, a pivotal international phase 2 trial with ibrutinib monotherapy has been reported (Noy et al. 2017). Patients with histologically confirmed MZL of all subtypes who received ≥1 prior line with an anti-CD20 antibody-containing regimen received 560 mg ibrutinib daily until progression or unacceptable toxicity. The primary endpoint was ORR. Sixty-three patients (median 66 years, median two prior lines) achieved an ORR of 48% initially and 58% with longer follow-up. The median PFS was 15.7 months. ORRs were 63%, 47%, and 62% for extranodal, nodal, and splenic subtypes, respectively. Recent exploratory biomarker studies demonstrated that nuclear factor-κB (NF-κB) pathway gene mutations correlated with improved outcomes (Noy et al. 2020). Preliminary results of the MAGNOLIA phase 2 trial of zanubrutinib monotherapy have been reported (Opat et al. 2020). Sixty-eight patients were treated (median age 70 years, median two prior lines). At a short median follow-up of 6.8 months, the investigator-assessed ORR was 60% (CR 15%). Responses were observed in all subtypes; ORR was 58%, 64%, 58%, and 50% in extranodal, nodal, splenic, and undefined subtypes, respectively.

CNS Involvement with B-cell Malignancies

BTKis are able to cross the blood–brain barrier. Although no prospective trials have been performed, ibrutinib has demonstrated clear efficacy in CNS involvement by MCL or WM (Bing–Neel syndrome). Eighty-four patients with CNS involvement of MCL were retrospectively collected in one international series (Rusconi et al. 2020). Acknowledging the limitations of a non-randomized or fully balanced study design, 26 patients who received ibrutinib achieved superior CR rates ((42% vs. 22%, $p = 0.02$)) and OS (one-year OS: 59% vs. 25%; HR = 0.39, $p = 0.011$) when compared to the 28 patients receiving blood–brain barrier-penetrating immunochemotherapy. A separate international, retrospective series of 28 patients receiving ibrutinib for Bing–Neel syndrome demonstrated a best symptomatic response of 85%, improvement or resolution of radiological abnormalities in 83%, and CSF (cerebrospinal fluid) clearance in 47% (Castillo et al. 2019). Two-year event-free survival with ibrutinib was 80% and five-year OS was 86%.

Real-world Data

In contrast to the breath of the practice-informing real-world evidence series published in CLL, data outlining BTKi experience of other indolent B-cell malignancies from routine clinical practice is limited. A large recent series (n = 211) from the United Kingdom where ibrutinib is uniformly prescribed at first relapse demonstrated an ORR of 69% (CR 27%) in patients with a median age of 73 years (McCulloch et al. 2021). The median PFS was 17.8 months and median OS 23.9 months. In contrast to CLL series, drug-related AEs leading to dose reductions occurred in only 10% and discontinuation only in 5%. The MANTLE-FIRST consortium analyzed outcomes of second-line therapies in 261 patients (21% rituximab–bendamustine, 29% R-BAC, 19% ibrutinib, 31% others) (Visco et al. 2021). Overall, ibrutinib and R-BAC were associated with improved median PFS-2 (24 and 25 months, respectively), compared to rituximab–bendamustine (13 months) or others (7 months). Ibrutinib was associated with superior outcomes in those with early POD to front-line therapy, but in those with later POD, there was little difference since between ibrutinib and bendamustine-based therapy.

Conclusions

BTKis have radically changed the treatment landscape for patients with CLL given improvement in survival demonstrated in multiple randomized studies. Data on ibrutinib demonstrate excellent efficacy with durable remissions, though toxicity remains common, particularly in real-world series. Second-generation BTKis, including FDA approved acalabrutinib and investigational zanubrutinib, are more selective for BTK with less off-target effects to address toxicity issues associated with ibrutinib. In direct comparison with ibrutinib, it appears that acalabrutinib/zanubrutinib is associated with lower rate of atrial fibrillation and zanubrutinib is associated with lower discontinuation due to toxicity. Efficacy of acalabrutinib and ibrutinib appears to be equivalent, while zanubrutinib has demonstrated superior PFS with limited follow-up. Pirtobrutinib is a non-covalent BTKi under development, which has demonstrated an impressive safety profile and ability to overcome BTK resistance mutations that can arise with covalent BTKi use. Finally, we have reviewed the more modest, though still important, body of literature supporting the role of BTKis in other B-cell malignancies.

Must Read References

Burger, J.A. et al. (2015). Ibrutinib as initial therapy for patients with chronic lymphocytic leukemia. *N. Engl. J. Med.* 373 (25): 2425–2437.

Mato, A.R. et al. (2021). Pirtobrutinib in relapsed or refractory B-cell malignancies (BRUIN): a phase 1/2 study. *The Lancet* 397 (10277): 892–901.

Woyach, J.A. et al. (2014). Resistance mechanisms for the Bruton's Tyrosine Kinase inhibitor Ibrutinib. *N. Engl. J. Med.* 370 (24): 2286–2294.

References

Burger, J.A. et al. (2015). Ibrutinib as initial therapy for patients with chronic lymphocytic leukemia. *N. Engl. J. Med.* 373 (25): 2425–2437.

Burger, J.A. et al. (2020). Long-term efficacy and safety of first-line ibrutinib treatment for patients with CLL/SLL: 5 years of follow-up from the phase 3 RESONATE-2 study. *Leukemia* 34 (3): 787–798.

Byrd, J.C. et al. (2013). Targeting BTK with ibrutinib in relapsed chronic lymphocytic leukemia. *N. Engl. J. Med.* 369 (1): 32–42.

Byrd, J.C. et al. (2014). Ibrutinib versus ofatumumab in previously treated chronic lymphoid leukemia. *N. Engl. J. Med.* 371 (3): 213–223.

Byrd, J.C. et al. (2015). Acalabrutinib (ACP-196) in relapsed chronic lymphocytic leukemia. *N. Engl. J. Med.* 374 (4): 323–332.

Byrd, J.C. et al. (2021). First results of a head-to-head trial of acalabrutinib versus ibrutinib in previously treated chronic lymphocytic leukemia. *J. Clin. Oncol.* 39 (15_suppl): 7500–7500.

Castillo, J.J. et al. (2019). Ibrutinib for the treatment of Bing-Neel syndrome: a multicenter study. *Blood* 133 (4): 299–305.

Dimopoulos, M.A. et al. (2018). Phase 3 trial of Ibrutinib plus Rituximab in Waldenström's Macroglobulinemia. *N. Engl. J. Med.* 378 (25): 2399–2410.

Dreyling, M. et al. (2016). Ibrutinib versus temsirolimus in patients with relapsed or refractory mantle-cell lymphoma: an international, randomised, open-label, phase 3 study. *Lancet* 387 (10020): 770–778.

Eyre, T.A. et al. (2019). Efficacy of venetoclax monotherapy in patients with relapsed, refractory mantle cell lymphoma after Bruton tyrosine kinase inhibitor therapy. *Haematologica* 104 (2): e68–e71.

Furman, R.R. et al. (2021). Pooled analysis of safety data from clinical trials evaluating acalabrutinib monotherapy in mature B-cell malignancies. *Leukemia* 35 (11): 3201–3211.

Ghia, P. et al. (2020). ASCEND: phase III, randomized trial of acalabrutinib versus idelalisib plus rituximab or bendamustine plus rituximab in relapsed or refractory chronic lymphocytic leukemia. *J. Clin. Oncol.* 38 (25): 2849–2861.

Hillmen, P. et al. (2021). First interim analysis of alpine study: results of a phase 3 randomized study of zanubrutinib vs ibrutinib in patients with relapsed/refractory chronic lymphocytic leukemia/small lymphocytic lymphoma. In *Proceedings of the 2021 European Hematology Association Virtual Congress*.

Islam, P. and Mato, A.R. (2019). Real-world evidence for chronic lymphocytic leukemia in the era of targeted therapies. *Cancer J. (Sudbury, Mass.)* 25 (6): 442.

Islam, P. and Mato, A.R. (2020). Utilizing Real-World Evidence (RWE) to improve care in chronic lymphocytic leukemia: challenges and opportunities. *Current Hematologic Malignancy Rep.* 15 (4): 254–260.

Jain, P. et al. (2020). Combination of ibrutinib with rituximab (IR) in previously untreated older patients with mantle cell lymphoma (MCL)-a phase II clinical trial. *Blood* 136: 41–42.

Mato, A.R. et al. (2016). Ibrutinib-induced pneumonitis in patients with chronic lymphocytic leukemia. *Blood, J. Am. Soc. Hematol.* 127 (8): 1064–1067.

Mato, A.R. et al. (2018). Toxicities and outcomes of 616 ibrutinib-treated patients in the United States: a real-world analysis. *Haematologica* 103 (5): 874.

Mato, A.R. et al. (2021). Pirtobrutinib in relapsed or refractory B-cell malignancies (BRUIN): a phase 1/2 study. *The Lancet* 397 (10277): 892–901.

McCulloch, R. et al. (2020). Efficacy of R-BAC in relapsed, refractory mantle cell lymphoma post BTK inhibitor therapy. *Br. J. Haematol.* 189 (4): 684–688.

McCulloch, R. et al. (2021). Ibrutinib for mantle cell lymphoma at first relapse: a United Kingdom real-world analysis of outcomes in 211 patients. *Br. J. Haematol.* 193 (2): 290–298.

Moreno, C. et al. (2019). Ibrutinib plus obinutuzumab versus chlorambucil plus obinutuzumab in first-line treatment of chronic lymphocytic leukaemia (iLLUMINATE): a multicentre, randomised, open-label, phase 3 trial. *The Lancet Oncol.* 20 (1): 43–56.

Noy, A. et al. (2017). Targeting Bruton tyrosine kinase with ibrutinib in relapsed/refractory marginal zone lymphoma. *Blood* 129 (16): 2224–2232.

Noy, A. et al. (2020). Durable ibrutinib responses in relapsed/refractory marginal zone lymphoma: long-term follow-up and biomarker analysis. *Blood Adv.* 4 (22): 5773–5784.

Opat, S. et al. (2020). Efficacy and safety of zanubrutinib in patients with relapsed/refractory marginal zone lymphoma: initial results of the MAGNOLIA (BGB-3111-214) trial. *Blood* 136: 28–30.

Owen, R.G. et al. (2020). Acalabrutinib monotherapy in patients with Waldenström macroglobulinemia: a single-arm, multicentre, phase 2 study. *Lancet Haematol.* 7 (2): e112–e121.

Rogers, K.A. et al. (2021). Phase II study of acalabrutinib in ibrutinib-intolerant patients with relapsed/refractory chronic lymphocytic leukemia. *Haematologica* 106 (9): 2364–2373.

Rule, S. et al. (2019). Ibrutinib for the treatment of relapsed/refractory mantle cell lymphoma: extended 3.5-year follow up from a pooled analysis. *Haematologica* 104 (5): e211–e214.

Rusconi, C., Cheah, C., and Tucker, D. (2020). Ibrutinib compared to immuno-chemotherapy for central nervous system relapse of mantle cell lymphoma: a report from Fondazione Italiana Linfomi (FIL) and European Mantle Cell Lymphoma Network (EMCLN). *HemaSphere* 4: S1.

Shanafelt, T.D. et al. (2019). Ibrutinib–rituximab or chemoimmunotherapy for chronic lymphocytic leukemia. *N. Engl. J. Med.* 381 (5): 432–443.

Sharman, J.P. et al. (2020). Acalabrutinib with or without obinutuzumab versus chlorambucil and obinutuzumab for treatment-naive chronic lymphocytic leukaemia (ELEVATE-TN): a randomised, controlled, phase 3 trial. *The Lancet* 395 (10232): 1278–1291.

Sharman, J.P. et al. (2021). CLL-139: acalabrutinib±obinutuzumab vs obinutuzumab+ chlorambucil in treatment-naïve chronic lymphocytic leukemia: ELEVATE-TN 4-year follow-up. *Clin. Lymphoma Myeloma and Leuk.* 21: S318–S319.

Song, Y. et al. (2020). Treatment of patients with relapsed or refractory mantle-cell lymphoma with Zanubrutinib, a selective inhibitor of Bruton's Tyrosine Kinase. *Clin. Cancer Res.* 26 (16): 4216–4224.

Tam, C.S. et al. (2019). Efficacy and safety of zanubrutinib in patients with treatment-naive chronic lymphocytic leukemia (CLL) or Small Lymphocytic Lymphoma (SLL) with Del(17p): initial results from arm C of the Sequoia (BGB-3111-304) trial. *Blood* 134 (Supplement_1): 499–499.

Tam, C.S. et al. (2020). A randomized phase 3 trial of zanubrutinib vs ibrutinib in symptomatic Waldenström macroglobulinemia: the ASPEN study. *Blood* 136 (18): 2038–2050.

Treon, S.P. et al. (2015). Ibrutinib in previously treated Waldenström's macroglobulinemia. *N. Engl. J. Med.* 372 (15): 1430–1440.

Trotman, J. et al. (2020). Zanubrutinib for the treatment of patients with Waldenström macroglobulinemia: 3 years of follow-up. *Blood* 136 (18): 2027–2037.

Visco, C. et al. (2021). Outcomes in first relapsed-refractory younger patients with mantle cell lymphoma: results from the MANTLE-FIRST study. *Leukemia* 35 (3): 787–795.

Wang, M. et al. (2018). Acalabrutinib in relapsed or refractory mantle cell lymphoma (ACE-LY-004): a single-arm, multicentre, phase 2 trial. *Lancet* 391 (10121): 659–667.

Wang, M. et al. (2019). Durable response with single-agent acalabrutinib in patients with relapsed or refractory mantle cell lymphoma. *Leukemia* 33 (11): 2762–2766.

Wang, M. et al. (2020). LOXO-305, a next generation, highly selective, non-covalent BTK inhibitor in previously treated mantle cell lymphoma, Waldenström's macroglobulinemia, and other non-Hodgkin lymphomas: results from the phase 1/2 BRUIN study. *Blood* 136: 8–10.

Wang, M. et al. (2020). KTE-X19 CAR T-cell therapy in relapsed or refractory mantle-cell lymphoma. *N. Engl. J. Med.* 382 (14): 1331–1342.

Wang, M.L. et al. (2013). Targeting BTK with ibrutinib in relapsed or refractory mantle-cell lymphoma. *N. Engl. J. Med.* 369 (6): 507–516.

Woyach, J. et al. (2019). Resistance to acalabrutinib in CLL is mediated primarily by BTK mutations. *Blood* 134 (Supplement_1): 504–504.

Woyach, J.A. et al. (2014). Resistance mechanisms for the bruton's tyrosine kinase inhibitor ibrutinib. *N. Engl. J. Med.* 370 (24): 2286–2294.

Woyach, J.A. et al. (2018). Ibrutinib regimens versus chemoimmunotherapy in older patients with untreated CLL. *N. Engl. J. Med.* 379 (26): 2517–2528.

21

Promising Combinations of BTK Inhibitors with Other Targeted Agents

Nicholas J. Schmidt, Michael E. Williams, and Craig A. Portell

Hematology/Oncology Division, University of Virginia Cancer Center, Charlottesville, VA, USA

Take Home Messages

- While BTK inhibitor (BTKi) monotherapy remains integral to the treatment paradigm of various lymphoid malignancies, these agents are limited in their ability to reliably induce complete remission, the development of resistance mutations, and the need for an indefinite treatment course.
- Combinatorial regimens adding targeted agents in conjunction with BTKi aim to address these limitations of BTKi monotherapy.
- Currently, BTKi plus anti-CD20 monoclonal antibodies provide the most mature data from large, randomized studies in support of their use in CLL, MCL, and WM.
- BCL2 inhibition with venetoclax plus BTKi has shown marked clinical synergy and deep remissions, particularly in CLL, though additional follow-up is needed to fully define a role in the treatment paradigm.
- Inhibitors of CDK 4/6, PI3Kδ, the proteasome, ROR1, mTOR, SYK, and HDAC have demonstrated preclinical and/or early phase clinical synergy with BTKi. Clinical studies are currently enrolling in order to elucidate the role of these combinations in the future treatment landscape.

Introduction

Bruton's tyrosine kinase inhibitors (BTKis) are established as critical agents in the treatment paradigm for many B-cell malignancies, improving outcomes and survival even among those with historically poor responses to traditional immunochemotherapy. This therapeutic class provides an oral, targeted, non-chemotherapeutic option for treatment in either the frontline or relapsed/refractory (R/R) settings for many lymphoid malignancies. While these agents are effective and generally well tolerated as monotherapy, there are important limitations when combining BTKi with other targeted agents. In this chapter, we focus primarily on combinatorial therapies employing BTKi with other agents, as well as their current and potential future use in the treatment of chronic lymphocytic leukemia (CLL), mantle cell lymphoma (MCL), and Waldenstrom's macroglobulinemia (WM).

Limitations of BTK Inhibitor Monotherapy

Across the spectrum of lymphoid malignancies, BTKi monotherapy achieves low rates of complete remission (CR). In the PCYC-1104 phase 2 study that led to the first accelerated approval of ibrutinib in 2013 for relapsed MCL, only 21% of patients achieved a CR (Wang et al. 2013). Six-year follow-up from the initial RESONATE trial of ibrutinib in previously treated CLL found that while the overall response rate was 91%, only 11% of patients achieved either CR or CRi (CR with incomplete marrow recovery) with ibrutinib monotherapy (Munir et al. 2019).

Additionally, and in light of the tendency for these agents to induce only partial remission (PR), and in order to maintain treatment response, BTKi therapy is generally continued indefinitely until disease progression or unacceptable toxicity. This is supported by data in CLL that has demonstrated an improvement in CR rates with longer term ibrutinib therapy. Five-year follow-up of the PCYC-1102/1103 study of single-agent ibrutinib for patients with CLL noted an increase in CR rates in previously untreated patients from 11% at a median follow-up of 35.2 months to 29% at five years (O'Brien et al. 2018). Another example can be found in the six-year final analysis of the RESONATE study mentioned above, in which an observed CR/CRi rate at two years of 5.6% rose to

Precision Cancer Therapies: Targeting Oncogenic Drivers and Signaling Pathways in Lymphoid Malignancies: From Concept to Practice, Volume 1, First Edition. Edited by Owen A. O'Connor, Stephen M. Ansell, and John F. Seymour.

11% at five years (Munir et al. 2019). Though still a modest CR rate, the results support the paradigm of continuing ibrutinib indefinitely when utilized as a single agent in previously treated patients.

Central to the investigation of combinatorial therapies are BTKi resistance mechanisms. Woyach et al. (2017) found resistance mutations BTK C481S or upregulation of PLCG2 in 85% (40/46) of patients with disease progression on ibrutinib. Overcoming known mechanisms of resistance is a critical principle underlying the importance of combination regimens with BTKi.

While BTKi monotherapy is highly effective in achieving disease response, it appears that these therapies have a cytostatic mechanism of action. Thus, a high rate of CR is not seen and relapses may progress quickly, supporting the need for continued therapy as a mainstay of BTKi monotherapy. The potential to achieve deep therapeutic responses, and to convert an indefinite treatment course to time-limited therapy, has motivated investigators to develop synergistic combination regimens. Rational selection of these agents focused on overcoming resistance mechanisms then becomes the major consideration.

Identifying Synergistic Combinations

Given the above rationale for combinatorial therapy involving BTKis and additional targeted agents, the next challenge is to rationally identify appropriate candidates for co-administration with BTKi. Critical to this process is selecting partner therapeutic classes which demonstrate synergy with BTKi. Potential synergistic targets are evaluated in the preclinical setting via *in vitro* combinatorial drug screening and *in vivo* murine models. Axelrod et al. (2014) tested 14 different agents, including drugs targeting PI3K, SYK (spleen tyrosine kinase), mTOR (mammalian target of rapamycin), BCL2 (B-cell lymphoma 2), and proteasome inhibitors in conjunction with ibrutinib. Partner agents were each introduced to MCL cell lines at three separate doses in combination with ibrutinib at either 6, 12, or 21 micromolar concentrations in a standard 3 × 3 matrix. Percent cytotoxicity and synergy were then assessed for each combination. The highest degree of synergistic cytotoxicity with ibrutinib was observed with proteasome inhibitors (both bortezomib and carfilzomib) as well as the BCL2 inhibitor venetoclax. The combination of carfilzomib and ibrutinib was further assessed in MCL mouse models. Animals treated with the combination exhibited a significantly longer overall survival (OS) than those administered ibrutinib alone.

The promising results of drug screening led to the development of phase 1/2 clinical trials evaluating co-administration of proteasome inhibitors with ibrutinib in MCL (Cohen et al. 2019; Lee et al. 2020a). Following identification of a combination of interest in the preclinical setting, development of early phase clinical trials requires defining the optimal dosing, pharmacodynamics, and safety profiles of these agents in clinical practice. Treatment regimens that remain of interest following these studies often translate to larger randomized trials that may ultimately establish new standards of care. This pattern of development from the preclinical setting to the clinical stage will be evident in many of the promising therapy combinations discussed throughout this chapter.

Combinations of BTK Inhibitors and Targeted Drugs as the Standard of Care

BTKi + Anti-CD20 Monoclonal Antibodies

While many combinatorial therapies are presently under investigation, current US Food and Drug Administration (FDA) approvals specific to concurrent use of targeted agents are primarily limited to BTKi with anti-CD20 monoclonal antibodies (Table 21.1). The landmark studies leading to these approvals in WM, CLL, and MCL are discussed below. Given the importance of routine assessment of additive toxicity profiles when discussing combination regimens, rates of serious adverse events in these trials will also be highlighted.

Waldenstrom's Macroglobulinemia – iNNOVATE Study

WM achieved the first approval for combination of these drug classes following the results of the iNNOVATE trial (Dimopoulos et al. 2018). Preceding this landmark study, preclinical data had demonstrated synergy between these drug classes (Zhang et al. 2014). A critical component in the development of this trial was the discovery that MYD88 and CXCR4 status are predictive of a response to BTKi monotherapy (Treon et al. 2015). In this study, the highest response rates with single-agent ibrutinib were observed in the MYD88 mutated/CXCR4 wild-type population, while lowest response rates were seen in patients with MYD88 wild-type/CXCR4 wild-type.

The iNNOVATE phase 3 randomized, placebo-controlled trial enrolled 150 patients in a 1:1 fashion to either receive ibrutinib 420 mg daily plus rituximab 375 mg/m^2 weekly in weeks 1–4 and 17–20 or rituximab (with identical dosing scheme) plus placebo (Dimopoulos et al. 2018). Previously untreated patients (45%), as well as those with recurrent disease (55%), were included in this study. The primary endpoint was progression-free survival (PFS). Thirty-month PFS was 82% in the ibrutinib–rituximab group compared to 28% in the rituximab–placebo arm ($p < 0.001$). By way of comparison, the five-year PFS (median follow-up 59 months) with single-agent ibrutinib in an R/R patient population was 54% (Treon et al. 2021). Importantly, the iNNOVATE PFS benefit was preserved in the less favorable MYD88 and CXCR4 subgroups, which were not seen in the monotherapy study. Secondary endpoints of major response rate, defined as CR, VGPR (very

Table 21.1 Current FDA approvals for BTKi + anti-CD20 monoclonal antibodies.

Date of FDA approval	Regimen	Disease	Line of therapy	Landmark study	Landmark PFS
08/2018	IBR + R	WM	FL or R/R	iNNOVATE	30 mo: 82% (IBR + R) vs. 28% (R)
01/2019	IBR + O	CLL	FL	iLLUMINATE	30 mo: 79% (IBR + O) vs. 31% (Clb + O)
11/2019	Acala ± O	CLL	FL	ELEVATE-TN	Estimated 30 mo: 90% (Acala + O) vs. 82% (Acala) vs. 34% (Clb + O)
04/2020	IBR + R	CLL	R/R	E1912	36 mo: 89.4% (IBR + R) vs. 72.9% (FCR)

Abbreviations: Acala = acalabrutinib; Clb = chlorambucil; CLL = chronic lymphocytic leukemia; FCR = fludarabine, cyclophosphamide, rituximab; FL = first-line; IBR = ibrutinib; mo = months; O = obinutuzumab; R = rituximab; R/R = relapsed/refractory; WM = Waldenstrom's macroglobulinemia.

good partial remission), or PR (72% vs. 32%), as well as overall response rate (92% vs. 47%) were also statistically significant favoring ibrutinib–rituximab. Additionally, responses to ibrutinib–rituximab were durable, with 92% ongoing at two years in contrast to 47% in the rituximab–placebo arm. A significant improvement in both the rate and magnitude of IgM response was also seen with ibrutinib–rituximab, and at four weeks following treatment initiation the median IgM level was 56% lower than pretreatment baseline with combination therapy versus 6% higher in the rituximab–placebo group.

Regarding the safety profile, grade ≥3 atrial fibrillation (12% vs. 1%) and hypertension (13% vs. 4%) occurred more frequently with combination therapy. Importantly, the rate of IgM flare at treatment onset was significantly reduced in the ibrutinib–rituximab group compared to rituximab–placebo (8% vs. 47%). No patient in the ibrutinib–rituximab arm underwent plasmapheresis, while this was required in 12 patients in the rituximab–placebo group.

In retrospect, this study would have been more informative by comparing ibrutinib plus placebo to ibrutinib plus rituximab. However, it was based on this study, which did demonstrate an impressive and durable response with a reasonable toxicity profile, that the combination of ibrutinib and rituximab was approved by the FDA in August 2018 for treatment of WM in both the frontline and relapsed settings.

Chronic Lymphocytic Leukemia (CLL)

The approval of ibrutinib in 2014 based on the RESONATE study (Byrd et al. 2014) revolutionized the CLL treatment paradigm. Whereas prior standards of care consisted primarily of cytotoxic chemotherapy with or without immunotherapy, the utility of BTKis ushered in an era of frontline targeted therapies for treatment of this disease. Based on previously noted limitations of BTKis as monotherapy as well as the established preclinical synergy, the addition of anti-CD20 immunotherapy represented an attempt to improve upon this groundbreaking paradigm shift from traditional cytotoxic agents to targeted regimens.

Ibrutinib + Obinutuzumab – iLLUMINATE Study

Multiple pivotal studies have evaluated combinations of anti-CD20 therapy with BTKi in the treatment of CLL. The iLLUMINATE trial (Moreno et al. 2019) led to the first FDA approval of combination therapy with these drug classes in CLL. This phase 3 study enrolled 229 patients who were randomized 1:1 to receive either ibrutinib 420 mg daily plus obinutuzumab or chlorambucil plus obinutuzumab, each for six cycles in total. The trial met its primary endpoint, with an estimated 30-month PFS of 79% in the ibrutinib/obinutuzumab arm versus 31% for chlorambucil/obinutuzumab. This PFS benefit (median PFS NR (not reached) vs. 14.7 months) was also demonstrated in patients with high-risk disease, defined by the presence of deletion 17p or 11q, TP53 mutation, or an unmutated IGHV (immunoglobulin heavy chain variable region). Complete responses, including CRi, were documented in 91% of patients in the ibrutinib plus obinutuzumab arm compared with 81% receiving chlorambucil and obinutuzumab. The high CR rate seen with ibrutinib plus obinutuzumab is of particular interest given previously described low CR rates with single-agent BTKi therapy. Responses appeared durable, with the median duration of response not reached in the ibrutinib/obinutuzumab arm versus 18.1 months for chlorambucil/obinutuzumab. Rates of grade 3 or 4 adverse events did not differ significantly between the two groups (68% vs. 70%). However, serious adverse events of any grade were observed in 58% of patients (65/113) treated with ibrutinib/obinutuzumab versus 35% (40/115) of patients receiving chlorambucil/obinutuzumab, though it is important to note that patients in the ibrutinib arm were on therapy for a median

2.5 years versus only 5.1 months with chlorambucil and obinutuzumab, and therefore had more time on therapy to develop adverse effects.

Acalabrutinib + Obinutuzumab – ELEVATE TN Study

Acalabrutinib in combination with obinutuzumab was assessed in the ELEVATE-TN trial (Sharman et al. 2020). This phase 3 study enrolled 535 patients with previously untreated CLL and randomized 1:1:1 into three arms: acalabrutinib alone, acalabrutinib with obinutuzumab, or chlorambucil plus obinutuzumab. As in iNNOVATE and iLLUMINATE, the primary outcome was PFS. PFS at median follow-up of 28 months was not reached in the acalabrutinib plus obinutuzumab group versus 22.6 months with chlorambucil and obinutuzumab (HR [hazard ratio] 0.10). Of note, the median PFS was also not reached in the acalabrutinib alone group. Overall response rates were highest with acalabrutinib plus obinutuzumab (94%) versus acalabrutinib alone (85%) and chlorambucil plus obinutuzumab (79%). Complete responses were seen in 13% of patients receiving acalabrutinib and obinutuzumab versus 5% with chlorambucil and obinutuzumab, and in only one patient with acalabrutinib alone. Grade ≥3 toxicities were observed in 70% of patients in both acalabrutinib plus obinutuzumab as well as chlorambucil plus obinutuzumab groups. Nearly 80% of patients receiving either acalabrutinib plus obinutuzumab or acalabrutinib alone remained on therapy at two years.

To assess comparative efficacy and toxicities, acalabrutinib was recently evaluated by the ELEVATE-RR study (Byrd et al. 2021), a non-inferiority trial randomizing patients with R/R, high-risk CLL to acalabrutinib 100 mg b.i.d. versus ibrutinib 420 mg daily. Median PFS as well as OS did not differ in the two treatment arms, but the rates of atrial fibrillation (9.4% vs. 16%), hypertension (9.4% vs. 23.2%), and bleeding events (38% vs. 51.3%) were all significantly lower with acalabrutinib than ibrutinib. Additionally, treatment discontinuation due to treatment-related adverse events was demonstrated in 14.7% of patients taking acalabrutinib versus 21.3% taking ibrutinib. Ongoing and planned combination regimens employing newer generation covalent and non-covalent BTKis will explore the efficacy and improved side effect profiles of these more recently developed agents (Table 21.3).

Ibrutinib + Rituximab: A Tale of Two Trials

The Alliance A041202 and the E1912 trials juxtapose conflicting data regarding the utility of ibrutinib plus rituximab in CLL (Table 21.2; Shanafelt et al. 2019; Woyach et al. 2018).

The Alliance A041202 trial was a three-arm, phase 3 study which enrolled 547 patients with previously untreated CLL over the age of 65 years (Woyach et al. 2018). Patients were randomized in a 1:1:1 ratio to treatment with bendamustine plus rituximab (BR), ibrutinib plus rituximab, or ibrutinib alone, with PFS as the primary endpoint. Median PFS was not reached in either of the ibrutinib-containing groups; the estimated two-year PFS was 74% with BR versus 88% with ibrutinib plus rituximab and 87% with ibrutinib alone. Importantly, there was no significant difference between the PFS demonstrated with ibrutinib combined with rituximab versus ibrutinib monotherapy or in OS among all three arms of the study. The CR rate was higher with BR (26%) than ibrutinib alone (7%) or ibrutinib with rituximab (12%), which was also true for the achievement of minimal residual disease (MRD) negativity, which was documented in 8% of patients treated with BR versus 1% and 4%, respectively, for ibrutinib alone or in combination with rituximab. Grade ≥3 hematologic adverse events were seen in 61% of patients treated with BR versus 41% with ibrutinib alone and 39% with ibrutinib plus rituximab. Non-hematologic grade ≥3 adverse events were observed in 63% of patients receiving BR versus 74% with either ibrutinib arm. The rates of secondary malignancies were similar in the three groups, though non-significantly higher with ibrutinib plus rituximab (13%, 13%, 16%). Richter's transformation was noted in one patient treated with BR and two patients treated with ibrutinib plus rituximab. Patient deaths occurring either during treatment or in the subsequent 30 days following treatment discontinuation were seen in two patients (1%) receiving BR, 13 (7%) on ibrutinib, and 13 (7%) treated with ibrutinib plus rituximab. Unexplained or unwitnessed death occurred in two

Table 21.2 Comparison of the alliance A041202 and E1912 trials.

Ibrutinib + Rituximab trials in untreated CLL	Study arms	Key inclusion	Key exclusion	Estimated PFS	Overall survival
Alliance A041202	1. BR	Age ≥65 yr	None	1. 74%	1. 95%
	2. IBR alone	Any cytogenetics		2. 88%	2. 90%
	3. IBR + Ritux			3. 87%	3. 94%
E1912	1. FCR	Age ≤70 yr	17p deletion	1. 72.9%	1. 91.5%
	2. IBR + Ritux			2. 89.4%	2. 98.8%

Abbreviations: CLL = chronic lymphocytic leukemia; BR = bendamustine/rituximab; FCR = fludarabine, cyclophosphamide, rituximab; IBR = ibrutinib; PFS = progression-free survival; yr = year.

(1%) patients treated with BR versus seven (4%) and four (2%) patients treated with ibrutinib and ibrutinib plus rituximab, respectively.

The phase 3 E1912 trial enrolled 529 patients under the age of 70 years randomized 2:1 to treatment with ibrutinib plus six cycles of monthly rituximab versus six cycles of fludarabine, cyclophosphamide, and rituximab (FCR) (Shanafelt et al. 2019). Ibrutinib was continued indefinitely until disease progression. Of note, patients with 17p deletion were excluded from this study as they were not recommended to get FCR at the time of study. The three-year PFS (primary study endpoint) was 89.4% in the ibrutinib–rituximab group versus 72.9% in the FCR group (HR for death or progression 0.35). Interestingly, on planned subgroup analysis this PFS benefit was only seen in the IGHV-unmutated cohort. As a secondary endpoint, OS was also significantly improved in the ibrutinib–rituximab group with a three-year OS of 98.8% versus 91.5% for the FCR arm (HR for death 0.17). Rates of complete response (CR 17.2% vs. 30.3%) and MRD negativity (8.3% vs. 59.2%), however, were significantly lower in the ibrutinib plus rituximab arm compared with FCR. Overall incidence of grade ≥3 adverse effects did not differ between the two groups (80.1% vs. 79.7%). Grade ≥3 neutropenia was documented more frequently in the FCR arm (44.9% vs. 25.6%), while grade ≥3 hypertension (8.2% vs. 18.8%), hemorrhagic events (0% vs. 1.1%), and cardiac toxicity (0.9% vs. 6.5%) occurred more frequently in the ibrutinib–rituximab group. Additionally, there was one sudden death in a patient receiving ibrutinib plus rituximab. Overall, there were 10 deaths during the observation period in the FCR group versus four in the ibrutinib–rituximab arm, noting the different cohort sizes due to the 1:2 randomization.

Alliance A04212 Versus E1912: The Role of Ibrutinib + Rituximab in CLL

In comparing the results of these concurrent trials, it is important to note the different patient populations assessed as well as differences in trial design. While the Alliance study enrolled patients over the age of 65 years, the E1912 trial included only patients under the age of 70 years. Patients with 17p deleted CLL, a subgroup that has been associated with a poorer prognosis, were excluded from the E1912 trial but included in Alliance A041202. Additionally, planned subgroup analysis demonstrated that the PFS benefit observed in favor of combination ibrutinib and rituximab was driven primarily by the cohort of patients with IGHV-unmutated disease. The long-term efficacy of FCR and the potential for deep, sustained remissions in 17p-intact, IGHV-mutated CLL have been previously demonstrated (Chai-Adisaksopha and Brown 2017), and the success of FCR in this cohort may contribute to the lack of a PFS benefit for ibrutinib-containing regimens in this subgroup.

The most obvious difference in design between the two trials is that while the Alliance study was a three-arm trial which included an ibrutinib monotherapy group, the E1912 only administered ibrutinib in combination with rituximab without a monotherapy comparator arm. Therefore, while a major conclusion from the Alliance study was the lack of benefit conferred by the addition of rituximab to ibrutinib, the E1912 trial could only conclude that the combination granted a PFS and OS benefit over FCR chemotherapy for the population studied.

Based on the results of these studies, it is reasonable to consider ibrutinib with rituximab in the frontline setting for patients under the age of 65 years with IGHV unmutated CLL without 17p deletion given the statistically significant improvement in PFS and OS demonstrated by the E1912 trial in this population. Given the lack of PFS or OS benefit achieved with the addition of rituximab to ibrutinib monotherapy in the Alliance A041202 trial, as well as the potential for additional adverse events with concurrent use, this combination should be used with some caution in patients over the age of 70 years.

Mantle Cell Lymphoma

While there has not been a disease-specific FDA approval to date for the combination of ibrutinib plus an anti-CD20 antibody in MCL, there is data supporting efficacy and safety in the second-line setting. In a phase 2 single-arm, single-center study performed at MD Anderson Cancer Center (Wang et al. 2016), 50 patients with R/R MCL were enrolled and received ibrutinib 560 mg daily with rituximab 375 mg/m^2 weekly for four weeks, monthly for six months, and then every other month for a total of two years. Objective response rate (ORR), the primary endpoint, was observed in 88% of patients, 44% of whom achieved a CR. In contrast, single-agent ibrutinib in this patient population previously demonstrated an ORR of 67% with 23% of patients achieving CR (Wang et al. 2016). The safety profile was largely consistent with prior studies of ibrutinib, with the most prominent adverse event of atrial fibrillation in 14% (7/50) of patients on this study leading to therapy discontinuation in 6% (3/50).

Integration of ibrutinib plus rituximab into frontline treatment was evaluated in the Window-1 trial (Wang et al. 2019). This phase 2 single-center trial enrolled 131 previously untreated MCL patients. Patients received ibrutinib and rituximab in combination for either 12 cycles of therapy or until a CR was achieved, and then received four cycles R-hyperCVAD (hyperfractionated cyclophosphamide/vincristine/adriamycin/dexamethasone) alternating with R-high-dose methotrexate plus high-dose cytarabine. Induction therapy in transplant eligible patients using a hyperCVAD-based regimen versus BR was previously evaluated by the S1106 trial (Chen et al. 2017). While both BR and hyperCVAD demonstrated similarly high response rates, there was significantly more toxicity associated with hyperCVAD. Of particular importance given the standard of care for ASCT (autologous stem cell transplant) following induction, approximately one-third of patients who received hyperCVAD failed to collect sufficient cells for transplant. An attempt to mitigate the significant toxicity observed with intensive chemotherapy represented a rationale for investigating a partially chemotherapy-free induction by the Window-1 trial. Overall response rate following the first phase of therapy with ibrutinib–rituximab was 95% (CR 21%), which rose to 100% (and CR 94%) following completion of the second phase of therapy with the hyperCVAD-based regimen. As expected with a chemotherapy-free first phase, rates of grades 3–4 myelosuppression were low (4%). Interestingly, there were no patients who experienced grades 3–4 atrial fibrillation or bleeding events while treated with ibrutinib.

BTKi and BCL2 Inhibitors

CLL

With respect to emerging partners for combinatorial therapy with BTKis, targeting BCL2 ranks among the most promising to date. In fact, BCL2 inhibitors have been previously championed as the ideal synergistic agent to pair with ibrutinib based on preclinical profiling (Cervantes-Gomez et al. 2015). Venetoclax is currently the clinically relevant agent in this class, and was approved by the FDA for treatment of CLL in 2016. As previously referenced, preclinical studies have demonstrated marked synergistic cytotoxicity between ibrutinib and venetoclax (Deng et al. 2017; Jayappa et al. 2017). Two recent studies, CAPTIVATE and GLOW, established the efficacy of ibrutinib and venetoclax in the frontline setting for CLL, while justifying the potential for a fixed-duration treatment option in this disease (Kater et al. 2022; Tam et al. 2019).

CAPTIVATE Study

The CAPTIVATE trial (Tam et al. 2019) was a phase 2 multicenter study which enrolled patients with previously untreated CLL. Each received single-agent ibrutinib 420 mg daily for three cycles followed by concurrent administration with venetoclax using a dose ramp up from 20 up to 400 mg daily over five weeks to mitigate the risk of tumor lysis syndrome (TLS). This study included a cohort using MRD testing to guide risk-adapted therapy as well as a cohort for which fixed-duration therapy was planned irrespective of MRD status.

In the cohort guided by MRD testing, MRD was assessed in the peripheral blood following cycles 6, 9, and 12. Therapy was continued for 12 cycles in total, at which time MRD was also assessed by bone marrow biopsy. Patients with undetectable MRD on bone marrow biopsy following 12 cycles and for at least three months in the peripheral blood (comprising 58% of the initial study population) were then randomized 1:1 to continued treatment with ibrutinib versus placebo (Wierda et al. 2021). The primary endpoint for the MRD negative population was one-year disease-free survival (DFS), which did not significantly differ between patients receiving placebo (95.3%) versus those who continued ibrutinib (100%). Patients with persistent MRD positivity (or for those who had demonstrated undetectable MRD for less than three months) were continued on venetoclax plus ibrutinib, after which undetectable MRD rates on bone marrow analysis improved from 32% at the time of randomization to 54%. The 30-month PFS was approximately 95% across all groups irrespective of MRD status, a testament to the activity of this regimen in CLL. From a safety perspective, the most common grades 3–4 adverse events were neutropenia (36%), thrombocytopenia (5%), and hypertension (10%), largely consistent with expected toxicities observed with the independent use of venetoclax or ibrutinib.

In the fixed-duration cohort, ibrutinib plus venetoclax was also administered for a total of 12 cycles, with the same lead-in detailed above. The primary endpoint for this group was CR rate. Complete response was achieved in 55% of patients, 89% of whom have remained in CR for greater than one year with additional follow-up pending (Ghia et al. 2021). PFS (95%) and OS (98%) were also reported as secondary outcomes. Neutropenia (33%) and hypertension (6%) were again the two most common grades 3–4 adverse events, and were observed with similar frequency to the MRD-driven cohort as reported above.

GLOW Trial

While the CAPTIVATE study enrolled fit patients under the age of 65 years, the GLOW trial included only patients over 65 years or adult patients with additional medical comorbidities defined as a Cumulative illness rating scale (CIRS) score over 6 or evidence of renal dysfunction with a creatinine clearance <70 ml/min (Kater et al. 2022). In contrast to the phase 2 CAPTIVATE trial, GLOW is a phase 3 study which enrolled 106 previously untreated CLL patients who were randomized 1:1 to receive 12 cycles of ibrutinib plus venetoclax (with same dosing and ibrutinib lead-in/venetoclax ramp-up schedule used in the CAPTIVATE trial detailed above) versus six cycles of chlorambucil plus obinutuzumab. The primary endpoint was PFS, which at median follow-up of 27.7 months was significantly improved with ibrutinib–venetoclax compared to chlorambucil–obinutuzumab (NR vs. 21 months, HR 0.216). Rates of MRD at three months after treatment (51.9% vs. 17.1%) as well as CR determined by an independent review committee (38.7% vs. 11.4%) were also significantly higher with ibrutinib plus venetoclax. Grade ≥3 adverse events with ibrutinib plus venetoclax were similar to the results in CAPTIVATE, with neutropenia (34.9%), diarrhea (10.4%), and hypertension (7.5%) observed most frequently.

Relapsed/Refractory CLL – CLARITY Study

While the CAPTIVATE and GLOW trials demonstrated the potential for ibrutinib and venetoclax in the frontline setting, the prospect of using this combination regimen for relapsed disease is also intriguing. The CLARITY study, a phase 2 trial enrolling 53 patients, administered ibrutinib plus venetoclax for one year with the primary endpoint of MRD negativity at 12 months (Hillmen et al. 2018). Bone marrow samples obtained at 12 months on therapy revealed no morphologic evidence of CLL in 81% of patients and MRD testing was negative in 36% of patients. Radiographic CR/CRi by CT was also achieved in 51% of patients. As in the frontline studies cited above, neutropenia and diarrhea were the adverse effects most frequently observed in this trial.

Ibrutinib plus Venetoclax in CLL

The CAPTIVATE, GLOW, and CLARITY trials all present encouraging data regarding the efficacy and safety of ibrutinib plus venetoclax for CLL in the frontline (CAPTIVATE, GLOW) and relapsed (CLARITY) settings. In comparison to relatively low CR rates cited for single-agent ibrutinib, the combination of these agents is not only able to induce CR at a significantly higher rate but also demonstrates the ability to produce deep, and in some cases MRD-negative, remissions which appear durable. Toxicities observed were largely as expected given the independent profiles of these two agents, without significant additive adverse events recorded. Additionally, three cycles of ibrutinib lead-in prior to initiation of venetoclax appeared to decrease patients' risk for TLS based on the presence of high tumor burden at the time of treatment initiation. Reduction of TLS risk from high to moderate/low was cited in 90% of patients in CAPTIVATE (Tam et al. 2019) and 84.6% in GLOW (Kater et al. 2022). Given the risk of clinically significant TLS with venetoclax in patients with high tumor burden, which can result in death if not closely monitored and prospectively managed (Roberts et al. 2016), TLS mitigation represents a benefit in favor of this scheduled sequential introduction of these agents. Overall, these phase 2 studies confirm the combination of ibrutinib with venetoclax as a highly promising regimen in CLL, although further confirmatory study is needed before moving to standard therapy. Ideally, the combination of ibrutinib plus venetoclax should be compared to a BTKi + CD20 antibody or venetoclax + CD20 antibody to define new standards of treatment. In addition, longer follow-up is needed to define durability of responses and response to subsequent treatment upon disease progression.

Mantle Cell Lymphoma

As in CLL, preclinical studies demonstrating synergy between BCL2 and BTK inhibitors was paramount in promoting clinical trial investigations into this combination (Axelrod et al. 2014; Cervantes-Gomez et al. 2015; Jayappa et al. 2017). Optimal dosing of ibrutinib and venetoclax in combination for MCL remains a matter of some debate, particularly given that both agents are metabolized through CYP3A4. A phase 1/1b dose-finding study enrolling 35 patients supported dosing of this regimen for relapsed disease was ibrutinib 420 mg with venetoclax 200 mg daily (Portell et al. 2019). In this study, while response rates remained the same despite higher dosing regimens, rates of toxicity were noted to increase. This is in contrast to two additional studies, which will be reviewed in this section, utilizing ibrutinib 560 mg and venetoclax 400 mg as the target doses.

Frontline for Mantle Cell Lymphoma – OASIS Trial (Step C)

The OASIS trial was a multicenter phase 1/2 study investigating the combination of ibrutinib with both venetoclax and obinutuzumab (le Gouill et al. 2019). This trial was divided into three steps, with steps A and B evaluating the above combination in R/R MCL, and step C enrolling patients with previously untreated MCL. All three agents were started with cycle one and continued for a total of two years (23 cycles). Ibrutinib was initiated at 560 mg daily and venetoclax dosing was gradually increased via a dose ramp-up to mitigate TLS to a target dose of 400 mg daily. Following two cycles of therapy all 15 patients enrolled achieved at least a PR, with 7/15 in CR/CRi at that time. Of note, particularly given uncertainties in optimal dosing of this combination, only 7/15 patients completed all six planned cycles of therapy. Those who did complete six cycles achieved CR as well as undetectable MRD. Long-term follow-up of this patient population is pending, and further evaluation of this combination in the frontline setting is needed.

Relapsed/Refractory Mantle Cell Lymphoma – AIM and SYMPATICO Studies

While the role of ibrutinib plus venetoclax for MCL as frontline therapy continues to be evaluated, the utility of this combination may be more relevant in the relapsed setting. AIM was a phase 2 study administering ibrutinib 560 mg daily in combination with venetoclax 400 mg daily for patients with R/R MCL (Tam et al. 2018). In total, 24 patients with very poor-risk MCL were enrolled with the primary endpoint of CR rate at week 16. Radiographic CR by CT imaging was achieved in 42% of patients on this study compared to a reported rate of 9% with ibrutinib monotherapy (Wang et al. 2013). PET (positron emission tomography)-negative CR with ibrutinib plus venetoclax was 62%. The most common adverse events were diarrhea (83% any grade, 12% grade ≥3), fatigue (75%, 12%), and nausea/vomiting (71%, 0%). Additionally, grade ≥3 neutropenia was seen in 33% of patients, and serious adverse events were reported in 58% of patients.

The SYMPATICO study is a phase 3 trial evaluating ibrutinib plus venetoclax for patients with R/R MCL (Wang et al. 2021). Data from the safety run-in arm of the study included 21 patients all receiving ibrutinib 560 mg daily plus venetoclax with standard ramp-up in cycle 1 to a target dose of 400 mg daily. This combination boasted high ORR (81%) and CR rate (62%), with 11 patients who had measurable MRD at baseline achieving MRD negativity. Given the acceptable safety-run in, the study proceeded to a double-blind randomization comparing ibrutinib plus venetoclax with ibrutinib plus placebo, also in the R/R setting, data from which is now pending.

The role of combined ibrutinib and venetoclax in both the frontline and R/R settings continues to evolve. Presently, this combination in MCL is best used in a clinical trial setting pending read-out of and longer term follow-up from the OASIS and SYMPATICO trials.

The Future: Ongoing Clinical Trials and Additional BTKi Combinations of Interest

With the exception of the ELEVATE-TN trial (acalabrutinib plus obinutuzumab), all of the combinatorial therapies discussed to this point have utilized ibrutinib, owing to its status as the first-in-class BTKi. While there is continued interest in investigation of synergistic partners with ibrutinib, several ongoing and planned clinical trials have used other BTKi. As previously referenced, acalabrutinib and zanubrutinib are second-generation agents with a more favorable side-effect profile as monotherapy in comparison to ibrutinib (Byrd et al. 2021). Additionally, the recently presented ASPEN trial demonstrated a significantly lower rate of any-grade atrial fibrillation (2% vs. 15%, $p = 0.0005$), as well as non-statistically significant lower incidences of hemorrhage and hypertension, with zanubrutinib in comparison to ibrutinib in patients with WM (Wang et al. 2021). In light of studies demonstrating favorable adverse effect profiles of second-generation BTKi, these agents are appealing for combination with other targeted agents and may favorably modulate potential additive or overlapping toxicities. Tables 21.3a and 21.3b are a list of active clinical trials investigating combinatorial therapy with BTKis in CLL and MCL. This list is not intended to be all-inclusive in such a rapidly moving field, but rather to provide a snapshot of the landscape of current investigation in this domain.

As can be concluded from this sampling of trials, the landscape of treatment remains dynamic. While the highest quality data currently exists in support of the combination of BTKi with either anti-CD20 monoclonal antibodies or venetoclax, other therapeutic classes have demonstrated synergy with BTKi in the preclinical and/or early phase clinical arena. We will now review several of these potential synergistic partner drug classes in greater detail.

BTKi + CDK4/6 Inhibitors

The cyclin-dependent kinases (CDKs) are critical regulators of the cell cycle, and CDKs 4 and 6 can be targeted with the inhibitors abemaciclib, ribociclib, and palbociclib. Preclinical analysis has shown that CDK 4/6 inhibition can sensitize MCL cells to BTK inhibition with ibrutinib (Chiron et al. 2014). Of these agents, palbociclib has been previously evaluated in MCL, both as a single agent (Leonard et al. 2012) as well as in combination with ibrutinib (Martin et al. 2019). While the phase 1b study by Leonard et al. enrolled 12 patients and demonstrated a response rate to single-agent palbociclib of only 18%, the more recent phase 1b study by Martin et al. evaluating ibrutinib plus palbociclib observed an ORR of 67% and a CR rate of 37% (Martin et al. 2019). Rash was the primary dose-limiting toxicity (DLT), and other grade ≥3 toxicities included neutropenia (41%), thrombocytopenia (30%), hypertension (15%), and pulmonary infections (11%). Given the improvement in response rates with combination therapy, the AFT-32 phase 2 trial is further evaluating this combination in MCL.

BTKi + PI3Kδ Inhibitors

The phosphatidylinositol-3 kinase delta isoform (PI3Kδ) is an essential component of the B-cell receptor (BCR) signaling pathway (Miller et al. 2015). Given the importance of PI3Kδ to BCR signaling, concurrent inhibition of this family of kinases and BTK were hypothesized to work synergistically. Combinatorial drug screening confirmed this hypothesis, demonstrating *in vitro* synergistic cytotoxicity with ibrutinib in diffuse large B-cell lymphoma (DLBCL) (Griner et al. 2014). Synergy between these two drug classes has been further evaluated in the preclinical setting in CLL murine models (Niemann et al. 2017). This study administered acalabrutinib and a novel PI3K inhibitor (ACP-319), each as single agents as well as in combination, to TCL1-192 cell-injected mice. Survival of the mice receiving the combination was approximately two weeks longer than those treated with single-agent therapy. Kapoor et al. (2019) demonstrated that concurrent PI3K inhibition aided in bypassing ibrutinib resistance through the upregulation of nuclear transcription factor FOXO3a.

Demonstration of the synergistic relationship between these drug classes in the preclinical setting has resulted in the development of several clinical trials assessing the safety and efficacy of these combinations. The first to assess this combination was a phase 1b study of the PI3Kδ inhibitor umbralisib plus ibrutinib in patients with R/R CLL or MCL (Davids et al. 2019). A total of 42 patients received ibrutinib at standard doses (420 mg for CLL, 560 mg for MCL) together with umbralisib at either 400, or 600, or 800 mg. With respect to the primary outcomes of maximum-tolerated dose (MTD) and DLTs, there were no DLT documented, and the MTD of umbralisib was not reached. Serious adverse events were observed in 29% of patients, with the most frequent adverse effects of any grade being diarrhea (52%), infection (50%), and transaminitis (24%). Overall response rate was 90% in CLL (29% CR) and 67% in MCL (19% CR). All patients in CR continued to have persistent MRD positivity on bone marrow biopsy. Based on this study, the recommended phase 2 dose

Table 21.3(a) Combination targeted agents in CLL: selected clinical trials in 2021–2022.

Clinical trial ID	Study name (if applicable)	Phases	Line of therapy	Combinations tested
NCT03701282	EA9161	Phase 3	FL	IBR + O vs. IBR + VEN + O
NCT03737981	Alliance A041702	Phase 3	FL	IBR + O vs. IBR + VEN + O
NCT04608318	CLL17	Phase 3	FL	IBR vs. VEN + O vs. VEN + IBR
NCT03836261	ACE-CL-311	Phase 3	FL	FCR vs. Acala + VEN vs. Acala + VEN + O
NCT03824483	—	Phase 2	FL CLL or MCL	Zanu + VEN + O
NCT04639362	NEXT STEP	Phase 2	FL	IBR + VEN + O
NCT03868722	PreVent-ACaLL	Phase 2	FL	Acala + VEN
NCT04230304	DIRECT	Phase 2	R/R	IBR + Dara
NCT04458610	—	Phase 2	FL	Zanu + R
NCT04502394	KRT-232–111	Phase 1b/2	R/R CLL or DLBCL	Acala + KRT-232
NCT03479268	—	Phase 1	R/R CLL or NHL	IBR + Pevonedistat
NCT03088878	—	Phase 2	FL CLL	IBR + Cirmtuzumab vs. IBR
NCT04277637	—	Phase 1	B-cell malignancies	Zanu + BGB-11417

Abbreviations: Acala = acalabrutinib; BGB-11417 = novel BCL2 inhibitor; CLL = chronic lymphocytic leukemia; Dara = daratumumab; DLBCL = diffuse large B-cell lymphoma; FL = front-line; IBR = ibrutinib; KRT-232 = novel MDM2 inhibitor; MCL = mantle cell lymphoma; NHL = non-Hodgkin's lymphoma; O = obinutuzumab; R = rituximab; R/R = relapsed/refractory; VEN = venetoclax; Zanu = zanubrutinib.

Table 21.3(b) Combination targeted agents in MCL: selected clinical trials in 2021–2022.

Clinical trial ID	Study name (if applicable)	Phases	Line of therapy	Combinations tested
NCT04002297	BGB 3111–306	Phase 3	FL	Zanu + R vs. BR
NCT03323151	PrE0404	Phase 2	R/R	IBR + Ixazomib
NCT04115631	EA4181	Phase 2	FL	BR + Acala vs. BR + Ara-C vs. BR + Ara-C + Acala
NCT04783415	-	Phase 2	FL	Acala + Umbra + Ublituximab
NCT04484012	-	Phase 2	R/R	Acala + CD19 CAR-T
NCT04234061	TARMAC	Phase 2	R/R, TP53 mutated	IBR + Tisagenlecleucel
NCT03478514	AFT-32	Phase 2	R/R	IBR + Palbociclib
NCT03863184	-	Phase 2	FL	Acala + Lenalidomide + Rituximab
NCT03946878	-	Phase 2	R/R MCL	Acala + VEN
NCT03684694	ADCT 402–103	Phase 1/2	R/R MCL or DLBCL	IBR + Loncastuximab tesirine
NCT03939182	-	Phase 1	R/R MCL or DLBCL	IBR + Abexinostat
NCT04783415	-	Phase 1	R/R	IBR + Copanlisib

Abbreviations: Acala = acalabrutinib; BR = bendamustine + rituximab, DLBCL = diffuse large B-cell lymphoma; FL = front-line; IBR = ibrutinib; MCL = mantle cell lymphoma; R = rituximab; R/R = relapsed/refractory; VEN = venetoclax.

of umbralisib was 800 mg, which is being employed in an ongoing phase 2 trial with acalabrutinib, umbralisib, and the anti-CD20 ublituximab (see Table 21.3b, NCT04783415). Interestingly, two patients with CLL who had received prior ibrutinib were included on this study, and each achieved a partial response with the combination therapy. Though a small sample size, in the context of the previously discussed laboratory evidence that concurrent PI3K inhibition can aid in the overcoming of ibrutinib resistance, this remains a point for follow-up in larger studies of the combination.

BTKi + Proteasome Inhibitors

Proteasome inhibitors, including bortezomib, carfilzomib, and ixazomib, are utilized in various multidrug regimens for the treatment of multiple myeloma, MCL, and WM. Previously referenced combinatorial drug testing identified that carfilzomib and ixazomib exhibited preclinical synergy with ibrutinib (Axelrod et al. 2014). Interestingly, carfilzomib displayed the strongest synergy with ibrutinib in this analysis and gave rise to a phase 1 trial combining these two agents (Lee et al. 2020a). This small study included only eight patients, the accrual for which may have been adversely impacted by both the presence of concurrent trials as well as a rather arduous infusion schedule (carfilzomib was administered by IV infusion on days 1, 2, 8, 9, 15, and 16). As this study was closed due to low patient accrual, determination of MTD was not achieved. Importantly, however, one of the eight patients on this study died with invasive fungal pneumonia, which was an unexpected consequence of this combination. Though no additional safety signals were demonstrated in this small population, careful monitoring will be required in future investigation. The accessibility barrier posed by infusional carfilzomib therapy is mitigated by use of ixazomib, an oral proteasome inhibitor; however, attention to safety with this combination in light of prior experience will also be paramount. Ixazomib in combination with ibrutinib for MCL is being evaluated by the phase 2 PrE0404 study (Cohen et al. 2019). Given the aforementioned synergy between BTKi and proteasome inhibitors, it will be important to follow the results of this trial to aid in determination of the activity and safety of this regimen in MCL.

Ibrutinib + Cirmtuzumab, an Anti-ROR1 Monoclonal Antibody

Preclinical studies have demonstrated synergy between ibrutinib and cirmtuzumab in mouse models (Liu et al. 2020). Cirmtuzumab is a first-in-class monoclonal antibody targeting ROR1, a receptor tyrosine kinase present on malignant cells but not found on normal cells, and has been studied in combination with ibrutinib in a phase 1b/2 trial enrolling 46 patients with CLL or R/R MCL (Lee et al. 2020b). Thus far, initial safety and efficacy data have been presented, with a continued expansion arm in the MCL population as well as a randomized phase 2 study of ibrutinib monotherapy versus cirmtuzumab plus ibrutinib in CLL (NCT03088878) forthcoming. There were no unexpected adverse events from the initial phase 1b analysis, and high rates of overall and complete response were recorded for both MCL (ORR 83%, CR 50%) and CLL (ORR 92%, CR 85%). The high rates of CR are encouraging, particularly in comparison to aforementioned historical data with ibrutinib monotherapy (Tam et al. 2018; Wang et al. 2013). The pending results of the head-to-head ibrutinib versus ibrutinib plus cirmtuzumab will be helpful in further elucidating the role of this regimen in the CLL treatment paradigm.

BTKi + mTOR Inhibitors

The mTOR is a molecular complex which plays an integral role in the regulation of many pathways known to be important in cancer biology, including the PI3K/AKT pathway (Zou et al. 2020). There has also been evidence of pathologic activation of mTOR in B-cell acute lymphoblastic leukemia (B-ALL) and non-Hodgkin's lymphoma (NHL) (Lee et al. 2016). Involvement of mTOR in BCR-adjacent regulation identifies agents targeting this complex as potential candidates to partner with BTKi. A study of the novel BTK inhibitor PLS-123 in conjunction with everolimus exhibited synergistic cytotoxicity *in vitro* as well as in murine models *in vivo* (Li et al. 2018). The synergistic relationship between these drug classes has also been demonstrated in DLBCL mice treated with vistusertib and acalabrutinib in combination (Ezell et al. 2014). Based on the results of this study, a phase 1/2 trial combining these agents in DLBCL was initiated; however, this trial was terminated early by the sponsor after initial data demonstrated that addition of vistusertib did not provide clinical benefit (Collins et al. 2021). This lack of benefit was attributed to pharmacodynamic analysis demonstrating variable target modulation of TORC2/pAKT by vistusertib. While this does not rule out the possibility of clinical relevance of this synergistic relationship, it does illustrate the continued need for more effective therapies in this drug class.

BTKi + SYK Inhibitors

Like PI3K, the SYK is another critical component of BCR signaling (Mócsai et al. 2010). Additionally, pro-survival signaling between SYK and mutated MYD88 has been demonstrated on laboratory examination of bone marrow samples from patients with WM (Munshi et al. 2020). This study also investigated the combination of ibrutinib with the SYK inhibitors trametinib and entospletinib and found synergistic induction of apoptosis in MYD88-mutated WM and DLBCL cell lines. Both currently active and recently published clinical trials are investigating the combination of these drug classes. A phase 1b study combined the second-generation BTKi tirabrutinib with either entospletinib (SYK inhibitor) or idelalisib (PI3Kδ inhibitor) in patients with R/R CLL (Danilov et al. 2020). Twenty-nine patients received tirabrutinib alone, 14 received tirabrutinib/idelalisib, and 10 received tirabrutinib/entospletinib. Safety was the primary endpoint of this study, and no DLT was observed in any of the above cohorts. Grade ≥3 adverse events across all groups were neutropenia (23%), diarrhea (2%), and upper respiratory tract infection (2%). Overall response rates were high in all cohorts (83% for tirabrutinib, 93% for tirabrutinib/idelalisib, and 100% for tirabrutinib/entospletinib), while CR rates remained low (two patients total for tirabrutinib monotherapy and one for each combination). Given the primary aim of this study and the small sample size, this trial was not powered to demonstrate superiority of combinatorial therapy compared to tirabrutinib alone. Importantly, this trial does provide a foundation that combinations of BTKi and PI3K or SYK inhibitors have a reasonable safety profile and activity in CLL warranting further study.

BTKi + HDAC Inhibitors

Histone deacetylases (HDAC) are a class of enzymes that modulate nuclear transcription (Gallinari et al. 2007) which has been primarily used in T-cell lymphomas. Newer agents such as abexinostat have also shown activity in CLL (Evens et al. 2016). Additionally, preclinical studies have demonstrated that BTK is partially regulated by micro-RNAs that may serve as potential targets for HDAC inhibitors (Bottoni et al. 2016). This same study also demonstrated synergistic activity of abexinostat and ibrutinib in CLL even with a known BTKC481S resistance mutation, opening the potential for this combination to overcome a known mechanism of ibrutinib resistance. A phase 1 trial enrolling patients with MCL or DLBCL (NCT03939182) is investigating concurrent administration of abexinostat with ibrutinib.

Ibrutinib + Selinexor

Selinexor is a nuclear exportin-1 (XPO1) inhibitor used in the treatment of R/R multiple myeloma and DLBCL (Kasamon et al. 2021). With regard to the BTK pathway, preclinical studies have demonstrated synergistic cytotoxicity between selinexor and ibrutinib in murine CLL models even in the presence of a BTKC481S resistance mutation (Hing et al. 2015). A phase 1 study of selinexor plus ibrutinib including patients with CLL, DLBCL, and MCL observed a disease control rate of 81%, with 33% of patients reaching a CR or PR (Stephens et al. 2019). Two patients on study experienced DLTs (profound fatigue in both cases) and discontinued therapy, and five patients died on study, with three deaths attributed to disease progression and two to infectious etiologies. Importantly, contrasted with other studies in this chapter, this trial also included patients with R/R DLBCL as well as Richter's transformation. Additionally, 69% of patients on this study were heavily pretreated and had received at least three prior lines of therapy. Despite these limitations, there was clinical activity displayed by this combination that warrant further exploration.

Conclusions

As referenced throughout this chapter, investigation into novel combinatorial therapies involving BTKi for the treatment of lymphoid malignancies is a dynamic field with an ever-changing landscape. The emergence of ibrutinib provided a crucial targeted agent, and BTKi monotherapy has continued to be a mainstay of treatment for CLL, MCL, and WM. Despite the importance of BTKi to the current standards of care, their limitations include the need for indefinite therapy, the development of resistance, and the low frequency of CR. While BTKis remain an integral part of the treatment paradigm for these diseases, clinical trials continue to define the role of synergistic therapies alongside BTKi in improving response rates and patient outcomes. BTKi in combination with anti-CD20 monoclonal antibodies currently provide the greatest breadth of high-quality data, although recent trials combining venetoclax with BTKi (GLOW, CAPTIVATE) are likely to emerge into the standard of care for CLL. Additionally, particularly in light of improved toxicity profiles with newer generation BTKi, there is continued investigation into combining acalabrutinib and zanubrutinib with agents previously used concurrently with ibrutinib. Based on demonstrated preclinical synergy with ibrutinib, targeted agents from other therapeutic classes are in various phases of clinical development. While many were discussed in this chapter, this field is constantly evolving, and new agents under development may prove valuable for integration into various treatment regimens. Taken together, combinations of BTKi with other targeted agents promise continued improvement in outcomes and survival for patients with B-cell malignancies.

Must Read References

Dimopoulos, M.A., Tedeschi, A., Trotman, J. et al. (2018). Phase 3 trial of ibrutinib plus rituximab in Waldenström's macroglobulinemia. *N. Engl. J. Med.* 378: doi: 10.1056/NEJMoa1802917.

Sharman, J.P., Banerji, V., Fogliatto, L.M. et al. (2019). ELEVATE TN: phase 3 study of acalabrutinib combined with obinutuzumab (O) or alone vs O plus chlorambucil (Clb) in patients (Pts) with treatment-naive chronic lymphocytic leukemia (CLL). *Blood* 134: doi: 10.1182/blood-2019–128404.

References

Axelrod, M., Ou, Z., Brett, L.K. et al. (2014). Combinatorial drug screening identifies synergistic co-targeting of Bruton's tyrosine kinase and the proteasome in mantle cell lymphoma. *Leukemia* 28: doi: 10.1038/leu.2013.249.

Bottoni, A., Rizzotto, L., Lai, T.-H. et al. (2016). Targeting BTK through microRNA in chronic lymphocytic leukemia. *Blood* 128: 3101–3112. doi: 10.1182/BLOOD-2016-07-727750.

Byrd, J.C., Brown, J.R., O'Brien, S. et al. (2014). Ibrutinib versus ofatumumab in previously treated chronic lymphoid leukemia. *N. Engl. J. Med.* 371: 213–223. doi: 10.1056/NEJMOA1400376.

Byrd, J.C., Hillmen, P., Ghia, P. et al. (2021). *First results of a head-to-head trial of acalabrutinib versus ibrutinib in previously treated chronic lymphocytic leukemia.* 39: 7500–7500. doi: 10.1200/JCO.2021.39.15_SUPPL.7500.

Cervantes-Gomez, F., Lamothe, B., Woyach, J.A. et al. (2015). Pharmacological and protein profiling suggests venetoclax (ABT-199) as optimal partner with ibrutinib in chronic lymphocytic leukemia. *Clin. Cancer Res.* 21: doi: 10.1158/1078-0432.CCR-14-2809.

Chai-Adisaksopha, C. and Brown, J.R. (2017). FCR achieves long-term durable remissions in patients with IGHV-mutated CLL. *Blood* 130: 2278–2282. doi: 10.1182/BLOOD-2017-07-731588.

Chen, R.W., Li, H., Bernstein, S.H. et al. (2017). RB but not R-HCVAD is a feasible induction regimen prior to auto-HCT in frontline MCL: results of SWOG Study S1106. *Br. J. Haematol.* 176: 759–769. doi: 10.1111/BJH.14480.

Chiron, D., Liberto, M.D., Martin, P. et al. (2014). Cell-cycle reprogramming for PI3K inhibition overrides a relapse-specific C481S BTK mutation revealed by longitudinal functional genomics in mantle cell lymphoma. *Cancer Discov.* 4: 1022–1035. doi: 10.1158/2159-8290.CD-14-0098.

Cohen, J.B., Portell, C.A., Hamadani, M. et al. (2019). A phase I/II study of ibrutinib and ixazomib in relapsed/refractory mantle cell lymphoma: prE0404. *Blood* 134: doi: 10.1182/blood-2019-127494.

Collins, G.P., Clevenger, T.N., Burke, K.A. et al. (2021). A phase 1/2 study of the combination of acalabrutinib and vistusertib in patients with relapsed/refractory B-cell malignancies. doi: 10.1080/10428194.2021.1938027.

Danilov, A.V., Herbaux, C., Walter, H.S. et al. (2020). Phase Ib study of tirabrutinib in combination with idelalisib or entospletinib in previously treated chronic lymphocytic leukemia. *Clin. Cancer Res.* 26: 2810–2818. doi: 10.1158/1078-0432.CCR-19-3504.

Davids, M.S., Kim, H.T., Nicotra, A. et al. Society, B.C.R.P. of the L. and L. (2019). Umbralisib in combination with ibrutinib in patients with relapsed or refractory chronic lymphocytic leukaemia or mantle cell lymphoma: a multicentre phase 1–1B study. *The Lancet. Haematology* 6: e38. doi: 10.1016/S2352-3026(18)30196-0.

Deng, J., Isik, E., Fernandes, S.M. et al. (2017). Bruton's tyrosine kinase inhibition increases BCL-2 dependence and enhances sensitivity to venetoclax in chronic lymphocytic leukemia. *Leukemia* 31 (10): 2075–2084.

Dimopoulos, M.A., Tedeschi, A., Trotman, J. et al. (2018). Phase 3 trial of ibrutinib plus rituximab in Waldenström's macroglobulinemia. *N. Engl. J. Med.* 378: doi: 10.1056/NEJMoa1802917.

Evens, A.M., Balasubramanian, S., Vose, J.M. et al. (2016). A phase I/II multicenter, open-label study of the oral histone deacetylase inhibitor abexinostat in relapsed/refractory lymphoma. *Clin. Cancer Res.* 22: 1059–1066. doi: 10.1158/1078-0432.CCR-15-0624.

Ezell, S.A., Mayo, M., Bihani, T. et al. (2014 Jul 15). Synergistic induction of apoptosis by combination of BTK and dual mTORC1/2 inhibitors in diffuse large B cell lymphoma. *Oncotarget* 5 (13): 4990–5001. doi: 10.18632/oncotarget.2071.

Gallinari, P., Marco, S.D., Jones, P. et al. (2007). HDACs, histone deacetylation and gene transcription: from molecular biology to cancer therapeutics. *Cell Res.* 17 (3): 195–211. doi: 10.1038/sj.cr.7310149.

Ghia, P., Allan, J.N., Siddiqi, T. et al. (2021). Fixed-duration (FD) first-line treatment (tx) with ibrutinib (I) plus venetoclax (V) for chronic lymphocytic leukemia (CLL)/small lymphocytic lymphoma (SLL): primary analysis of the FD cohort of the phase 2 captivate study. 39: 7501–7501. doi: 10.1200/JCO.2021.39.15_SUPPL.7501.

Griner, L.A.M., Guha, R., Shinn, P. et al. (2014). High-throughput combinatorial screening identifies drugs that cooperate with ibrutinib to kill activated B-cell–like diffuse large B-cell lymphoma cells. *Proc. Natl. Acad. Sci.* 111: 2349–2354. doi: 10.1073/PNAS.1311846111.

Hillmen, P., Rawstron, A., Brock, K. et al. (2018). Ibrutinib plus venetoclax in relapsed/refractory CLL: results of the bloodwise TAP clarity study. *Blood* 132: 182–182. doi: 10.1182/BLOOD-2018-182.

Hing, Z.A., Mantel, R., Beckwith, K.A. et al. (2015). Selinexor is effective in acquired resistance to ibrutinib and synergizes with ibrutinib in chronic lymphocytic leukemia. *Blood* 125: 3128–3132. doi: 10.1182/BLOOD-2015-01-621391.

Jayappa, K.D., Portell, C.A., Gordon, V.L. et al. (2017). Microenvironmental agonists generate de novo phenotypic resistance to combined ibrutinib plus venetoclax in CLL and MCL. *Blood Advances* 1: 933–946. doi: 10.1182/BLOODADVANCES.2016004176.

Kapoor, I., Li, Y., Sharma, A. et al. (2019). Resistance to BTK inhibition by ibrutinib can be overcome by preventing FOXO3a nuclear export and PI3K/AKT activation in B-cell lymphoid malignancies. *Cell Death Dis.* 10: doi: 10.1038/s41419-019-2158-0.

Kasamon, Y.L., Price, L.S.L., Okusanya, O.O. et al. (2021). FDA approval summary: selinexor for relapsed or refractory diffuse large B-cell lymphoma. *The Oncologist* 26: 879–886. doi: 10.1002/ONCO.13859.

Kater, A.P., Owen, C., Moreno, C. et al. (2022). Fixed-duration ibrutinib-venetoclax in patients with chronic lymphocytic leukemia and comorbidities. *NEJM Evid.* 1 (7).

le Gouill, S., Morschhauser, F., Bouabdallah, K. et al. (2019). Ibrutinib, venetoclax plus obinutuzumab in newly diagnosed mantle cell lymphoma patients. *Blood* 134: 1530–1530. doi: 10.1182/BLOOD-2019-125681.

Lee, H.J., Schmelz, J.L., Cramer, F. et al. (2020a). A phase I study of carfilzomib in combination with ibrutinib for relapsed refractory mantle cell lymphoma. *Br. J. Haematol.* 188: e94–e98. doi: 10.1111/BJH.16378.

Lee, H.J., Choi, M.Y., Siddiqi, T. et al. (2020b). *Clinical activity of cirmtuzumab, an anti-ROR1 antibody, in combination with ibrutinib: interim results of a phase Ib/II study in mantle cell lymphoma (MCL) or chronic lymphocytic leukemia (CLL).* 38: 8036–8036. doi: 10.1200/JCO.2020.38.15_SUPPL.8036.

Lee, J.S., Vo, T., and Fruman, D.A. (2016). Targeting mTOR for the treatment of B cell malignancies. *Br. J. Clin. Pharmacol.* 82: 1213. doi: 10.1111/BCP.12888.

Leonard, J.P., LaCasce, A.S., Smith, M.R. et al. (2012). Selective CDK4/6 inhibition with tumor responses by PD0332991 in patients with mantle cell lymphoma. *Blood* 119: 4597–4607. doi: 10.1182/BLOOD-2011-10-388298.

Li, J., Wang, X., Xie, Y. et al. (2018). The mTOR kinase inhibitor everolimus synergistically enhances the anti-tumor effect of the Bruton's tyrosine kinase (BTK) inhibitor PLS-123 on Mantle cell lymphoma. *Int. J. Cancer* 142: doi: 10.1002/ijc.31044.

Liu, Z., Liu, J., Zhang, T. et al. (2020). Destabilization of ROR1 enhances activity of Ibrutinib against chronic lymphocytic leukemia in vivo. *Pharmacol.Res.* 151: 104512. doi: 10.1016/J.PHRS.2019.104512.

Martin, P., Bartlett, N.L., Blum, K.A. et al. (2019). A phase 1 trial of ibrutinib plus palbociclib in previously treated mantle cell lymphoma. *Blood* 133: 1201–1204. doi: 10.1182/BLOOD-2018-11-886457.

Miller, B.W., Przepiorka, D., Claro, R.A. et al. (2015). FDA approval: idelalisib monotherapy for the treatment of patients with follicular lymphoma and small lymphocytic lymphoma. *Clin. Cancer Res.* 21: 1525–1529. doi: 10.1158/1078-0432.CCR-14-2522.

Mócsai, A., Ruland, J., and Tybulewicz, V.L.J. (2010). The SYK tyrosine kinase: a crucial player in diverse biological functions. *Nat. Rev. Immunol.* 10 (6): 387–402. doi: 10.1038/nri2765.

Moreno, C., Greil, R., Demirkan, F. et al. (2019). Ibrutinib plus obinutuzumab versus chlorambucil plus obinutuzumab in first-line treatment of chronic lymphocytic leukaemia (iLLUMINATE): a multicentre, randomised, open-label, phase 3 trial. *The Lancet Oncology* 20: doi: 10.1016/S1470-2045(18)30788-5.

Munir, T., Brown, J.R., O'Brien, S. et al. (2019). Final analysis from RESONATE: up to six years of follow-up on ibrutinib in patients with previously treated chronic lymphocytic leukemia or small lymphocytic lymphoma. *Am. J. Hematol.* 94: 1353. doi: 10.1002/AJH.25638.

Munshi, M., Liu, X., Chen, J.G. et al. (2020). SYK is activated by mutated MYD88 and drives pro-survival signaling in MYD88 driven B-cell lymphomas. *Blood Cancer J.* 10 (1): 1–11. doi: 10.1038/s41408-020-0277-6.

Niemann, C.U., Mora-Jensen, H.I., Dadashian, E.L. et al. (2017). Combined BTK and PI3Kδ inhibition with acalabrutinib and ACP-319 improves survival and tumor control in CLL mouse model. *Clin. Cancer Res.* 23: 5814–5823. doi: 10.1158/1078-0432.CCR-17-0650.

O'Brien, S., Furman, R.R., Coutre, S. et al. (2018). Single-agent ibrutinib in treatment-naïve and relapsed/refractory chronic lymphocytic leukemia: a 5-year experience. *Blood* 131: 1910–1919. doi: 10.1182/BLOOD-2017-10-810044.

Portell, C.A., Wages, N.A., Kahl, B.S. et al. (2019). Multi-institution phase I/Ib continual re-assessment study to identify the optimal dose of of ibrutinib (IBR) and venetoclax (VEN) in relapsed or refractory mantle cell lymphoma (MCL). *Blood* 134: 1535–1535. doi: 10.1182/BLOOD-2019-128788.

Roberts, A.W., Davids, M.S., Pagel, J.M. et al. (2016). *Targeting BCL2 with venetoclax in relapsed chronic lymphocytic leukemia.* 374: 311–322.doi: 10.1056/NEJMoa1513257.

Shanafelt, T.D., Wang, X.V., Kay, N.E. et al. (2019). Ibrutinib–rituximab or chemoimmunotherapy for chronic lymphocytic leukemia. *N. Engl. J. Med.* 381: doi: 10.1056/NEJMoa1817073.

Sharman, J.P., Egyed, M., Jurczak, W. et al. (2020). Acalabrutinib with or without binutuzumab versus chlorambucil and obinutuzmab for treatment-naïve chronic lymphocytic leukaemia (ELEVATE TN): a randomised, controlled, phase 3 trial. *Lancet* 395: 1278–1291.

Stephens, D.M., Huang, Y., Agyeman, A. et al. (2019). Selinexor combined with ibrutinib demonstrates tolerability and efficacy in advanced B-cell malignancies: a phase I study. *Blood* 134: 4310–4310. doi: 10.1182/BLOOD-2019-124544.

Tam, C.S., Anderson, M.A., Pott, C. et al. (2018). Ibrutinib plus venetoclax for the treatment of mantle-cell lymphoma. *N. Engl. J. Med.* 378: 1211–1223. doi: 10.1056/NEJMOA1715519.

Tam, C.S., Siddiqi, T., Allan, J.N. et al. (2019). Ibrutinib (Ibr) plus venetoclax (Ven) for first-line treatment of chronic lymphocytic leukemia (CLL)/small lymphocytic lymphoma (SLL): results from the MRD cohort of the phase 2 Captivate study. *Blood* 134: 35–35. doi: 10.1182/BLOOD-2019-121424.

Treon, S.P., Meid, K., Gustine, J. et al. (2021). Long-term follow-up of ibrutinib monotherapy in symptomatic, previously treated patients with Waldenström macroglobulinemia. *J. Clini. Oncol.* 39 (6): 565–575. doi: 10.1200/JCO.20.00555.

Treon, S.P., Xu, L., and Hunter, Z. (2015). MYD88 mutations and response to ibrutinib in Waldenström's macroglobulinemia. *N. Engl. J. Med.* 373: 584–586. doi: 10.1056/NEJMC1506192.

Wang, M.L., Jain, P., Lee, H.J. et al. (2019). Frontline treatment with ibrutinib plus rituximab (IR) followed by short course R-hypercvad/MTX is extremely potent and safe in patients (age ≤ 65 years) with mantle cell lymphoma (MCL) – results of phase-II window-1 clinical trial. *Blood* 134: doi: 10.1182/blood-2019-126044.

Wang, M.L., Lee, H., Chuang, H. et al. (2016). Ibrutinib in combination with rituximab in relapsed or refractory mantle cell lymphoma: a single-centre, open-label, phase 2 trial. *The Lancet Oncology* 17: 48–56. doi: 10.1016/S1470-2045(15)00438-6.

Wang, M., Ramchendren, R., Chen, R. et al. (2021). Concurrent ibrutinib plus venetoclax in relapsed/refractory mantle cell lymphoma: the safety run-in of the phase 3 SYMPATICO study. *J. Hematol. Oncol.* 14: 179.

Wang, M.L., Rule, S., Martin, P. et al. (2013). Targeting BTK with ibrutinib in relapsed or refractory mantle-cell lymphoma. *N. Engl. J. Med.* 369: 507–516. doi: 10.1056/NEJMOA1306220.

Wierda, W.G., Allan, J.N., Siddiqi, T. et al. (2021). Ibrutinib plus venetoclax for first-line treatment of chronic lymphocytic leukemia: primary analysis results from the minimal residual disease cohort of the randomized phase II captivate study. *J. Clin. Oncol.* 39: 3853–3865.

Woyach, J.A., Ruppert, A.S., Guinn, D. et al. (2017). *BTK* ^{C481S} -mediated resistance to ibrutinib in chronic lymphocytic leukemia. *J. Cli. Oncol.* 35: doi: 10.1200/JCO.2016.70.2282.

Woyach, J.A., Ruppert, A.S., Heerema, N.A. et al. (2018). Ibrutinib regimens versus chemoimmunotherapy in older patients with untreated CLL. *N. Engl. J. Med.* 379: doi: 10.1056/NEJMoa1812836.

Zhang, L., Zhang, H., Zhao, D. et al. (2014). Anti-CD20 and B-cell receptor-mediated growth inhibition and apoptosis: a preclinical study of ibrutinib and rituximab combination therapy in mantle cell lymphoma in vitro and in vivo. *Blood* 124: doi: 10.1182/blood.V124.21.1774.1774.

Zou, Z., Tao, T., Li, H. et al. (2020). mTOR signaling pathway and mTOR inhibitors in cancer: progress and challenges. *Cell Biosci.* 10 (1): 1–11. doi: 10.1186/S13578-020-00396-1.

Section VI

Protein Degraders and Membrane Transport Inhibitors

22

The Biological Basis for Targeting Protein Turnover in Malignant Cells

Robert Z. Orlowski

Departments of Lymphoma & Myeloma, and Experimental Therapeutics, The University of Texas MD Anderson Cancer Center, 1515 Holcombe Blvd., Unit 429, Houston, TX 77030, USA

Take Home Messages

- Targeting protein turnover has proven to be an important therapeutic opportunity across a variety of hematologic malignancies.
- Novel drugs in these classes, and novel agents with other activities that modulate protein turnover, will continue to be an important and even expanding part of our strategy against a number of lymphoid malignancies moving forward.
- Three proteasome inhibitors are currently approved for multiple myeloma, including bortezomib, carfilzomib, and ixazomib, while bortezomib is also approved for mantle cell lymphoma.
- Key pharmacologic differences include their chemistry, mechanisms of target inhibition and reversibility, drug administration and half-life, and metabolism, with the latter potentially impacting dosing in patients with hepatic and renal failure.
- Key pharmacologic differences include their potency in inducing degradation of cereblon E3 ligase client proteins such as Ikaros and Aiolos, and the renal elimination of lenalidomide, which therefore requires dose adjustment in the setting of renal insufficiency.

Introduction

Abnormalities of protein metabolism have been known to be a key feature of lymphoid malignancies for nearly two centuries. Indeed, one of the first such descriptions of cancer in general came from Henry Bence Jones, an English physician and chemist who reported on the presence of "a new animal substance occurring in the urine of a patient labouring under mollities ossium" in 1850 (Jones 1850). These abnormal immunoglobulin-derived light chains still bear his name to this day, and are commonly seen in patients with multiple myeloma (MM) and related plasma cell dyscrasias, where the neoplastic cells are terminally differentiated from lymphoid precursors. More than a century later, protein turnover was identified as a key component of cancer-associated cachexia (Lundholm et al. 1978), which was first described by the English ophthalmologist John Zachariah Laurence in 1858, though the association of chronic disease with cachexia was first noted by Hippocrates and colleagues at his school on the Greek island of Kos. Given this brief historical background, it is perhaps noteworthy that the first chemotherapeutic agent specifically designed to directly target protein turnover to achieve a regulatory approval was the proteasome inhibitor (PI) bortezomib for relapsed and/or refractory myeloma (Orlowski et al. 2002; Richardson et al. 2003, 2005). Even more ironically, PIs were first conceived of as agents to combat cancer cachexia given the role of increased activity of the ubiquitin–proteasome pathway in this setting (Temparis et al. 1994) before their direct anti-myeloma activity was appreciated. Currently, there are two drug classes used against lymphoid malignancies that specifically target protein turnover, which include PIs and immunomodulatory agents (IMiDs®). This chapter will review the pharmacology of the three PIs and the three IMiDs® that are currently in routine clinical use for lymphoid malignancies. Also, this chapter will briefly touch on new drugs in these two classes that are currently under development, and also on some new drug classes that impact protein turnover and may in the future find their way to the clinic.

Biological Basis for Targeting Protein Turnover

Regulated intracellular proteolysis in eukaryotes occurs predominantly through the ubiquitin–proteasome pathway. Through ubiquitination, which is typically catalyzed by the coordinated activity of an E1 ubiquitin activating enzyme, and E2 ubiquitin conjugating enzyme, and an E3 ubiquitin ligase, target proteins are marked for proteolysis through

Precision Cancer Therapies: Targeting Oncogenic Drivers and Signaling Pathways in Lymphoid Malignancies: From Concept to Practice, Volume 1, First Edition. Edited by Owen A. O'Connor, Stephen M. Ansell, and John F. Seymour.

poly-ubiquitination of specific lysine residues (Ciechanover 2017). Aaron Ciechanover, Avram Hershko, and Irwin Rose were awarded the Nobel Prize in Chemistry in 2004 for the discovery and characterization of this process. Target proteins are then degraded through the constitutive proteasome, which consists of a 20S core particle with three different catalytic activities encoded in the β1, β2, and β5 subunits, along with two 19S (also known as PA700) cap structures to form the 26S proteasome (Tanaka 2009). These three sets of unique subunits allow cleavage of proteins after acidic amino acids (the post-glutamyl peptide hydrolyzing [PGPH] activity, also known as the caspase-like activity), after basic amino acids (the trypsin-like activity), and after hydrophobic amino acids (the chymotrypsin-like activity [ChT-L]) (Orlowski and Wilk 2000). As a result, proteins with various primary sequences can be degraded into oligopeptides, which are then further cleaved to their constituent amino acids by amino- and carboxy-peptidases. Degradation can also occur in some cell types through an immunoproteasome in which the core particle has the β1, β2, and β5 subunits replaced by low molecular mass protein 2 (LMP2), multicatalytic endopeptidase complex subunit 1 (MECL1), and LMP5, respectively (Ferrington and Gregerson 2012). Another difference between the two is that the immunoproteasome 20S core can be combined with either the 19S/PA700 cap or with an 11S/PA28 cap. While the first PIs were generated as laboratory tool compounds to examine the activity of the proteasome (Orlowski et al. 1991, 1993; Orlowski and Michaud 1989; Vinitsky et al. 1992), later studies demonstrated both *in vitro* and *in vivo* anti-tumor efficacy, prompting interest developing clinically deliverable drugs targeting the proteasome as potential anti-cancer agents (Manasanch and Orlowski 2017; Voorhees et al. 2003).

Approved Drugs Targeting Ubiquitin–Proteasome Pathway

Based on strong pre-clinical validation, and clinical trials ranging from phase 1 safety through phases 2I and 3 efficacy trials, there are now three approved PIs in the United States, including bortezomib, carfilzomib, and ixazomib (Figure 22.1). These Food and Drug Administration (FDA) approvals are exclusively in patients with lymphoid malignancies, including patients with MM ranging from the newly diagnosed (NDMM) (for bortezomib) to the relapsed/refractory setting (RRMM) (for bortezomib, carfilzomib, and ixazomib), and mantle cell lymphoma (MCL; bortezomib) who have had at least one prior therapy (Table 22.1). Two of these PIs, including bortezomib and ixazomib, are dipeptide boronic acids that form a single covalent bond with the N-terminal threonine which serves as the active site of the proteasome subunits responsible for subsequent nucleophilic attack on the target peptide bond. In contrast, carfilzomib is an epoxyketone that forms two covalent bonds with the active site threonine, which results in irreversible inhibition. While bortezomib can be used as a single agent for MCL, and both bortezomib and carfilzomib can be used alone for RRMM, the use of the latter two is mostly in combinations with other drugs to form more active doublet, triplet, and, very recently, even quadruplet regimens. Please be referred to Chapter 24, or one of several recent review articles, for more detailed discussion regarding the current uses of these agents in myeloma (Cowan et al. 2022; Kunacheewa and Orlowski 2019) and elsewhere.

Pharmacologic Mechanisms of Proteasome Inhibitors

Key pharmacologic features of bortezomib, carfilzomib, and ixazomib are summarized in Table 22.1 (Baljevic and Orlowski 2019), and are notable for roughly similar plasma protein binding and large volumes of distribution, but quite different elimination half-lives. These factors, however, do not typically influence decisions about drug selection and dosing. Similarly, though the reversibility of proteasome inhibition is different between the boronic acids and the epoxyketone, recovery of proteasome function after carfilzomib occurs with only a modest delay, possibly due to synthesis and assembly of new proteasomes. Finally, all three are at least to some extent substrates for P-glycoprotein (P-gp), some pre-clinical studies suggest a role for P-gp in resistance to bortezomib and carfilzomib (Verbrugge et al. 2012), and P-gp inhibition may in some models enhance PI efficacy. However, the clinical relevance of this to patient care is unclear, and these considerations also do not guide drug use.

Among factors that may influence drug selection, metabolism of the boronic acids occurs through the hepatic cytochrome

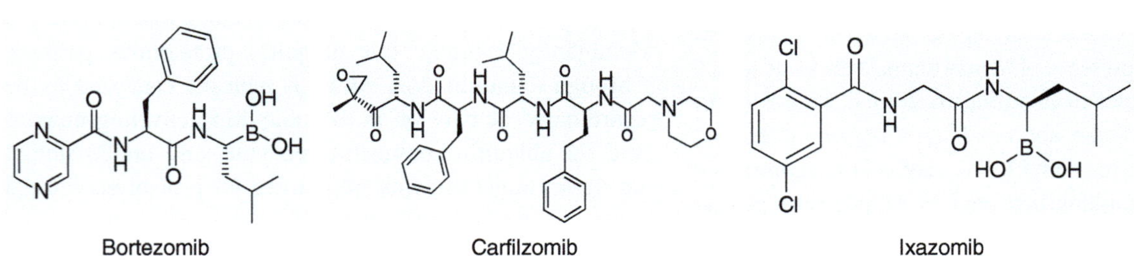

Figure 22.1 Chemical structure of the three proteasome inhibitors currently in routine clinical use, including bortezomib, carfilzomib, and ixazomib.

Table 22.1 Key pharmacologic features of bortezomib, carfilzomib, and ixazomib*.

	Bortezomib	Carfilzomib	Ixazomib
Regulatory approvals	NDMM, RRMM, RR MCL	RRMM	RRMM
Chemistry	Dipeptide boronic acid	Tetrapeptide epoxyketone	Dipeptide boronic acid
Amino acid sequence mimicked by drug	Phe-Leu	Phe-Leu-Phe-Leu	Phe-Leu
Proteasome target activity	ChT-L, PGPH	ChT-L	ChT-L
Mechanism of action	Direct inhibitor	Direct inhibitor	Prodrug that requires hydrolysis to active agent
Administration	i.v. or s.c.	i.v.	p.o.
Reversibility of target inhibition	Slowly reversible	Irreversible	Reversible
Volume of distribution (liters)	721–1 270	28	543
Plasma protein binding (%)	83	97–98	99
Half-life elimination (hours)	76–108	<0.5	228
P-glycoprotein substrate	Yes	Yes	Low affinity
Drug metabolism	Hepatic (via CYPs)	Peptidase cleavage, epoxide hydrolysis	Hepatic (via CYPs)

*Abbreviations: ChT-L = chymotrypsin-like activity; CYPs = cytochrome P450 system; i.v. = intravenous; Leu = leucine; NDMM = newly diagnosed myeloma; PGPH = peptidyl-glutamyl peptide hydrolyzing activity (also known as the caspase-like activity); Phe = phenylalanine; p.o. = oral; RR MCL = relapsed and/or refractory mantle cell lymphoma; RRMM = relapsed and/or refractory myeloma; s.c. = subcutaneous.

P450 system, and bortezomib dosing may need to be reduced in some patients with severe liver disease (LoRusso et al. 2012). In the case of carfilzomib, pharmacokinetic studies showed patients with mild and moderate hepatic impairment had only an ~20–50% higher carfilzomib area under the curve compared to patients with normal hepatic function (Brown et al. 2017), suggesting dosing of carfilzomib probably can be maintained in this setting. Renal impairment is frequently seen in the context of myeloma patients, and studies have supported the safety of both bortezomib (Zhu and Chen 2016) and carfilzomib (Badros et al. 2013) in this setting without the need for dose adjustments, while ixazomib should be dose reduced to 3 mg compared to a standard dose of 4 mg (Gupta et al. 2016). Also, the route of administration is quite relevant, since ixazomib is orally bioavailable and is most often given once weekly on weeks of treatment, providing greater patient convenience. Bortezomib can be administered once or twice weekly either intravenously or subcutaneously during treatment weeks, and doses are given at least three days apart if twice weekly dosing is selected. For bortezomib, the subcutaneous route is more often used due to increased convenience and a decrease in some associated toxicities, especially peripheral sensory neuropathy (Moreau et al. 2011). Carfilzomib, in contrast, is only available for intravenous administration to be given once or twice weekly, with the latter often on consecutive days.

Direct comparisons of the efficacy of these drugs that might guide dosing are limited, but some studies have compared them in a head-to-head fashion. In the relapsed and/or refractory setting, the ENDEAVOR trial compared carfilzomib (20 mg/m^2 on days 1 and 2 of cycle 1; 56 mg/m^2 thereafter on days 8, 9, 15, and 16 of cycle 2, and at this higher dose for all days starting at cycle 2 of each 28-day cycle) with dexamethasone to bortezomib (1.3 mg/m^2; intravenous bolus or subcutaneous injection) with dexamethasone (Dimopoulos et al. 2016). The median progression-free survival (PFS) was 18.7 months in the carfilzomib group versus 9.4 months in the bortezomib group at a pre-planned interim analysis (hazard ratio [HR] 0.53 [95% confidence interval [CI] 0.44–0.65]; $p < 0.0001$). It is unlikely that pharmacologic differences between the two agents contributed to these findings, though the ability to dose carfilzomib on consecutive days, along with its irreversible binding to catalytically active proteasome subunits, was felt to possibly provide an advantage due to a longer duration of proteasome inhibition. However, several other studies that compared the two PIs did not show an efficacy difference, including the phase 3 CLARION study that compared carfilzomib with melphalan and prednisone (KMP) to bortezomib with melphalan and prednisone (VMP) in transplant-ineligible NDMM (Facon et al. 2019). While KMP showed a slightly higher response rate, the median PFS was 22.3 months with KMP versus 22.1 months with VMP (HR 0.906; 95% CI, 0.746–1.101; $p = 0.159$). Similarly, the phase 3 ENDURANCE study compared carfilzomib with lenalidomide and dexamethasone (KRD) to bortezomib with lenalidomide and dexamethasone (VRD) in NDMM patients who did not have an intention to immediately undergo autologous stem cell transplantation (Kumar et al. 2020). Here, the median PFS was 34.6 months (95% CI 28.8–37.8) in the KRD group and 34.4 months in the VRD group (HR 1.04, 95% CI 0.83–1.31; $p = 0.74$).

Other Proteasome Inhibitors

The efficacy of carfilzomib validated epoxyketones as an active class of PIs, but this drug's poor oral bioavailability and metabolic stability limited its use to the parenteral route. An effort to develop an oral version led to the discovery of oprozomib, a tripeptide epoxyketone (Figure 22.2) that has entered clinical trials but is not yet approved. One phase 1/2 study focused on patients with myeloma and the related lymphoid disorder Waldenstrom's macroglobulinemia. This reported response rates ranging from 25% to 41% in different dosing cohorts among myeloma patients, and 47% to 71% in Waldenstrom's (Ghobrial et al. 2019). However, exploration of these different dosing regimens was prompted in part by frequent grade 3 or higher gastrointestinal adverse events, including diarrhea, nausea, and vomiting. A second phase 1b/2 study looking at oprozomib with dexamethasone in relapsed and/or refractory myeloma (Hari et al. 2019) similarly reported promising response rates, including 46.4% among patients with bortezomib-refractory disease, but significant gastrointestinal side effects, which ultimately limited its potential.

A second PI that entered clinical trials for lymphoid malignancies is marizomib, a naturally occurring agent (Figure 22.2) isolated from the marine actinomycete *Salinospora tropica*. This drug can target all three proteasome activities, making it distinct from the other PIs discussed so far that typically inhibit predominantly the ChT-L activity only. As a single agent, marizomib was examined in RRMM and showed only marginal activity, with 6% and 11% of patients achieving at least a minimal response with two different schedules (Richardson et al. 2016). Adverse events that were unique to this drug included dizziness and hallucinations, which were likely a result, at least in part, of this agent's ability to cross the blood–brain barrier (Di et al. 2016). Another study of marizomib (Harrison et al. 2016) similarly described an 11% response rate among 27 efficacy-evaluable RRMM patients on one schedule, and a single complete response in one patient with transformed marginal zone lymphoma (MZL). More recently, a study combining marizomib with pomalidomide and dexamethasone has been reported (Spencer et al. 2018), and showed an overall response rate and clinical benefit rate of 53% (19/36) and 64% (23/36), respectively. However, further development of both oprozomib and marizomib in lymphoid cancers has been halted, and there are no active clinical trials currently enrolling patients.

Immunomodulatory Drugs Affecting Protein Turnover

Background

Thalidomide is the first member of this drug class (Figure 22.3), whose original use as a treatment for morning sickness in pregnant women led to an international tragedy as it induced birth defects in approximately 10 000 babies from the late 1950s to the early 1960s (Zhou et al. 2013). The first report of its benefits in what is now one of its approved uses came from a small case series of six patients with lepromatous leprosy where thalidomide was used as a sedative and led to improvement in erythema nodosum-like skin lesions (Sheskin 1965). Studies demonstrating its anti-angiogenic properties (D'Amato et al. 1994) provided the hypothesis that

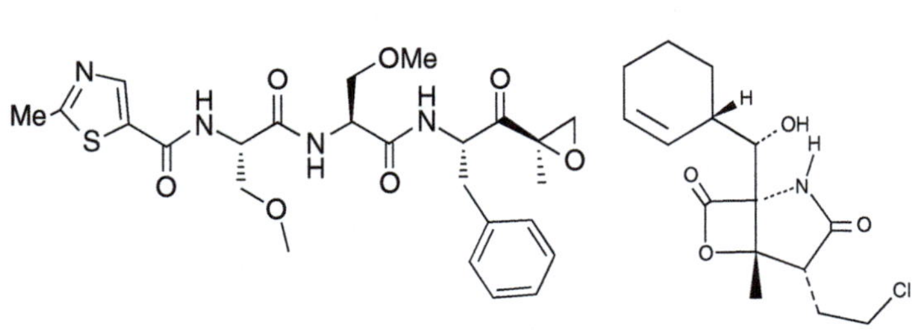

Figure 22.2 Chemical structure of two novel proteasome inhibitors previously in clinical development, including oprozomib and marizomib.

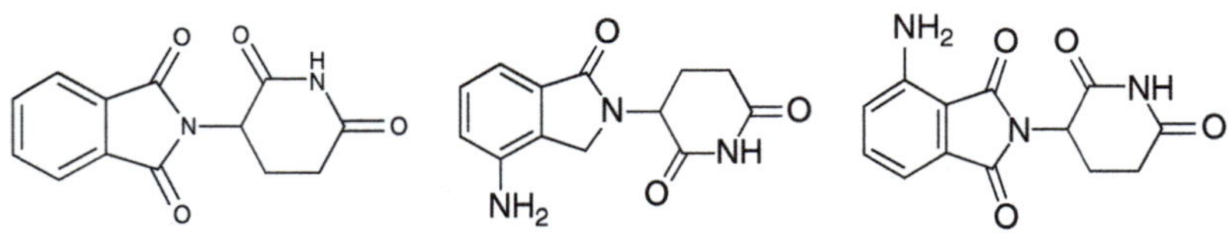

Figure 22.3 Chemical structure of the three immunomodulatory agents currently in routine clinical use, including thalidomide, lenalidomide, and pomalidomide.

led to its first evaluation in myeloma, where thalidomide was shown to have substantial activity in that it reduced monoclonal protein levels in 78% of patients (Singhal et al. 1999), and helped to usher in the novel drug era. The impact of this drug on protein turnover was later identified during studies of its teratogenicity, which showed that it bound to cereblon (CRBN), a component of an E3 ligase complex with damaged DNA binding protein 1 and Cullin 4A (Ito et al. 2011, 2010). This ligase proved to be important for limb outgrowth and expression of the fibroblast growth factor FGF8, while thalidomide bound to CRBN and inhibiting its ubiquitin ligase activity. Additional analogs of thalidomide have since been developed, motivated in part by the desire to reduce some of its associated toxicities, including sedation and constipation. Studies of their mechanisms of action, including of lenalidomide and pomalidomide (Figure 22.3), confirmed that CRBN binding is a key to their anti-cancer activity (Lopez-Girona et al. 2012; Zhu et al. 2011). Importantly, binding of these and other CRBN-targeted molecules to the originally identified thalidomide binding domain can lead to varied downstream effects, with degradation of different client proteins that can modify the resulting phenotypic effects. For example, lenalidomide binding leads to degradation predominantly of Ikaros family zinc finger 1 (IKZF1; Ikaros) and Ikaros family zinc finger 3 (IKZF3; Aiolos) (Jan et al. 2021). In contrast, CC-885 (Matyskiela et al. 2016) and BTX306 (Zou et al. 2020) induce recruitment of G1 to S phase transition 1 (GSPT1) to CRBN through a surface turn containing a glycine residue at a key position, leading to its degradation.

Presently Approved Immunomodulatory Drugs

As with PIs, there are three approved IMiDs® in the United States: thalidomide, lenalidomide, and pomalidomide (Figure 22.3). These FDA approvals are largely in lymphoid malignancies, including for several patient populations with MM ranging from NDMM (for thalidomide [THAL] and lenalidomide [LEN]) to the maintenance (LEN) and RRMM settings (LEN and pomalidomide [POM]) (Table 22.2). Notably, these drugs are most commonly used in rationally designed combinations to take advantage of both their direct anti-tumor effects and ability to modulate immune effector cells in the tumor microenvironment. Commonly used regimens include the IMiDs® with all three PIs, and also with monoclonal antibodies targeting either CD38 (daratumumab and isatuximab) or signaling lymphocytic activation molecule family member 7 (elotuzumab) (Kumar et al. 2017; Rajkumar and Kumar 2020). Thalidomide retains its approval for erythema nodosum leprosum, but its use against myeloma in the United States has waned due to the availability of the more potent and generally better tolerated agents LEN and POM. LEN is also approved for management of patients with myelodysplastic syndrome who have the 5q chromosomal deletion, where this drug induces Casein kinase 1α (CK1α) degradation and differentially impacts 5q-deleted cells because these bear haploinsufficiency for CK1α (List et al. 2018). Finally, LEN is also approved for relapsed and/or refractory MCL, and in combination with the anti-CD20 antibody rituximab for follicular lymphoma (FL) and MZL. Please consult one of several recent review articles for more detailed coverage of the current uses of these agents in myeloma (Cowan et al. 2022; Kunacheewa and Orlowski 2019) and elsewhere.

Pharmacologic Mechanisms of Currently Approved Immunomodulatory Drugs

Some of the key pharmacologic properties of THAL, LEN, and POM (Chen et al. 2017; Gay et al. 2013; Teo et al. 2004) are summarized in Table 22.2. Since many of these compounds incorporate an either unchanged or derivatized phthalimide group from THAL, there are several common characteristics such as a short time to maximum plasma concentration after an oral dose, a large volume of distribution, and low to moderate plasma protein binding. LEN tends to be eliminated more rapidly than either THAL or POM, and one early trial examined both once daily and twice daily dosing (Richardson et al. 2006). However, the latter was associated with increased myelosuppression, prompting the current use of once daily dosing for all three drugs. There are also differences in the ability of the three drugs to act as substrates for P-gp, but there is no known clinical relevance of these characteristics.

The chief factor that does influence drug dosing is the presence of renal failure, in the setting of which there is similar pharmacokinetics of THAL and, even though clearance is doubled during dialysis, no dosing changes or supplemental drug dosing is recommended (Eriksson et al. 2003). Similarly, POM has been found to be safe and effective without dose adjustment in patients with RRMM and either moderate or severe renal insufficiency (Dimopoulos et al. 2018). However, total and renal LEN clearance dramatically declines with worsening renal impairment and, since the majority of the drug is secreted in an unmetabolized form, dose adjustment is mandatory for patients with a creatinine clearance below 60 ml/min (Chen et al. 2007). For patients who present with myeloma-associated renal dysfunction and then see an improvement in their function, a subsequent dose increase of LEN may be warranted. Finally, the three approved IMiDs® do show some differences in their susceptibility to metabolism by hepatic enzymes, but no safety and efficacy studies focusing on patients with hepatic impairment have been performed, so caution is suggested in their use in the setting of hepatic impairment.

Randomized comparisons of the efficacy of these drugs that might guide dosing have not been performed, in part because they tend to have unique regulatory approvals in different

Table 22.2 Key pharmacologic features of thalidomide, lenalidomide, and pomalidomide*.

	Thalidomide	Lenalidomide	Pomalidomide
Regulatory approvals	ENL; NDMM	FL and MZL; MCL; MDS; NDMM, MT MM, RRMM	RRMM
Administration	p.o.	p.o.	p.o.
Time to maximum plasma concentration (Tmax; hours)	3–4	1	2.5–3
Volume of distribution (liters)	70–120	74–91	74–138
Plasma protein binding (%)	55–65 Some binding to α1 acid glycoprotein	40	12–44
Half-life elimination (hours)	5.5–7.3	2.8–3.3	6–8
Metabolism	Minimally metabolized by CYP; non-enzymatic spontaneous hydrolytic cleavage at physiologic pH opening glutarimide and phthalimide rings	Not a CYP substrate; non-enzymatic hydrolysis in aqueous solutions and hepatocytes due to hydrolytic cleavage of glutarimide ring	Enzymatic hydrolysis (hepatic CYP3A4 and 1A2 via hydroxylation and glucuronidation) and non-enzymatic hydrolysis
P-glycoprotein substrate	No	Weak	Yes
Excretion	Products of spontaneous hydrolysis mostly excreted in the urine	Renal (~70–90% as unchanged lenalidomide)	Urine (73% of the dose) as metabolites (41%) or hydrolysis products (25%)

*Abbreviations: CYP = cytochrome P450 system; ENL = erythema nodosum leprosum; FL = follicular lymphoma; MCL = mantle cell lymphoma; MDS = myelodysplastic syndrome; MT MM = maintenance therapy in multiple myeloma; MZL = marginal zone lymphoma; NDMM = newly diagnosed multiple myeloma; p.o. = oral; RRMM = relapsed and/or refractory myeloma; s.c. = subcutaneous.
Data was obtained, where possible, from studies in patients with lymphoid malignancies.

combinations that do not easily allow for direct comparisons. Since LEN was first FDA approved for MM in 2006 at a time when THAL was already available, and several studies showed the efficacy of LEN in at least some patients with disease that had progressed on THAL, these two drugs were initially used in this sequence to maximize patient treatment options. Later, as the generally better tolerability and improved efficacy of LEN became apparent, it has widely supplanted THAL in the United States, and POM is now typically used after prior LEN as it does show efficacy in this setting. This is also supported by a variety of studies which have compared the *in vitro* and/or *in vivo* potency of the three and found POM to be greater than LEN, and THAL to be the weakest (for example Jones et al. (2016)). However, it should be pointed out that formal randomized trials studying the various possible sequences have not been performed, leaving open the possibility that individual patients may benefit from reusing a prior agent, especially if it is given in a new combination, or of even using a less potent drug in the above sequence.

Other Cereblon Modulating Agents

The cereblon E3 ligase modulating (CELMoD®) agent CC-220 (Figure 22.4), now known as iberdomide, was originally discovered in an effort to find novel agents which would induce more rapid degradation of Ikaros and Aiolos (Matyskiela et al. 2018). More recent pre-clinical studies have suggested that it can retain activity in models of LEN- and POM-resistance in myeloma with dysregulated CRBN levels (Bjorklund et al. 2020), supporting that it could be a good addition to our therapeutic armamentarium against this disease. A first-in-human study healthy subjects described a terminal half-life of 9–13 hours and dose-dependent immunomodulatory effects on B-cell and T-cells, as well as grade 3 neutropenia that led to the introduction of a "dosing holiday" (Ye et al. 2021). Safety and efficacy studies of iberdomide have been reported in patients with systemic lupus erythematosus, since Ikaros and Aiolos are associated with immune cell development and lupus pathobiology. Iberdomide appeared to be safe, and to improve the Physician's Global Assessment and Cutaneous Lupus Erythematosus Disease Area and Severity Index (CLASI) activity scores (Furie et al. 2022). This activity was confirmed in a recently reported phase 2 trial which used the systemic lupus erythematosus responder index, prompting the authors to call for larger trials with longer follow-up (Merrill et al. 2022). Multiple studies are underway in myeloma patients ranging from smoldering and NDMM on one end of the spectrum to RRMM on the other, and in various combinations.

A second CELMoD® of note is CC-92480 (Figure 22.4), now known as mezigdomide, which, like iberdomide, was

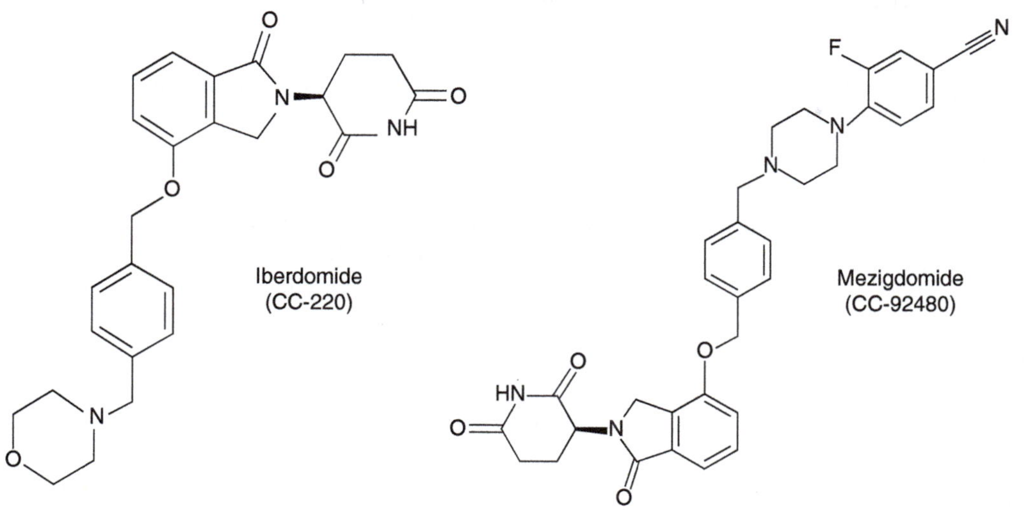

Figure 22.4 Chemical structure of two novel Cereblon modulating agents currently in clinical development, including iberdomide and mezigdomide.

determined to show more rapid Aiolos degradation than LEN or POM and to be active in LEN-refractory models (Hansen et al. 2020). Pharmacokinetic studies in rats supported the possibility of very good oral bioavailability, and identified oxidative dealkylation and amide hydrolysis as the key metabolic pathways (You and Pang 2021). As is the case for iberdomide, several phases 1 and 2 studies with different combinations are underway using mezigdomide in both NDMM and RRMM, but data from these trials of iberdomide or mezigdomide has not yet appeared in peer-reviewed publications, and are eagerly anticipated.

Conclusions

PIs and immunomodulatory drugs ushered in a novel era for myeloma therapy that started the ongoing process of transitioning away from an older generation of cytotoxic drugs. Similarly, in FL, lenalidomide with rituximab has been shown to provide similar outcomes for patients compared to rituximab with a cytotoxic chemotherapy agent (Morschhauser et al. 2018). Moreover, through careful use of physiologically relevant *in vitro* and *in vivo* model systems to better understand their mechanisms of action, these agents have been developed in a rational fashion to maximize their efficacy while improving patient reported outcomes and minimizing toxicities. As a result, outcomes in myeloma have improved dramatically, and they have contributed to a doubling to tripling of the overall survival of newly diagnosed patients. Though none of the six currently approved drugs would any longer be considered novel, they continue to provide important clinical benefits to patients worldwide, and will likely remain parts of our standard of care for many years. Even more importantly, their success validated the therapeutic benefit of targeting intracellular proteolysis as a strategy against diverse cancers. As a result, they have inspired development of an ever enlarging array of novel(er) drug classes, such as CELMoDs® and proteolysis-targeting chimeric molecules, the latter of which are reviewed in a subsequent chapter. Thus, despite the fact that it has now been more than 20 years since the first clinical trials of drugs specifically designed to modulate intracellular proteolysis in lymphoid malignancies were started, it seems safe to state that we have not yet fully leveraged their ability to make a difference for our patients, and that they will be part of our armamentarium when we can cure all of them.

Acknowledgments

R.Z.O., the Florence Maude Thomas Cancer Research Professor, would like to acknowledge support from the Leukemia & Lymphoma Society (SCOR-12206-17), the Dr. Miriam and Sheldon G. Adelson Medical Research Foundation, and the Paula and Rodger Riney Foundation.

Must Read References

Ciechanover, A. (2017). Intracellular protein degradation: from a vague idea thru the lysosome and the ubiquitin-proteasome system and onto human diseases and drug targeting. *Best Pract. Res. Clin. Haematol.* 30: 341–355.

Manasanch, E.E., Orlowski, R.Z. (2017). Proteasome inhibitors in cancer therapy. *Nat. Rev. Clin. Oncol.* 14: 417–433.

Jan, M., Sperling, A.S., Ebert, B.L. (2021). Cancer therapies based on targeted protein degradation – lessons learned with lenalidomide. *Nat. Rev. Clin. Oncol.* 18: 401–417.

References

Badros, A.Z., Vij, R., Martin, T. et al. (2013). Carfilzomib in multiple myeloma patients with renal impairment: pharmacokinetics and safety. *Leukemia* 27 (8): 1707–1714.

Baljevic, M. and Orlowski, R.Z. (2019). Pharmacodynamics and pharmacokinetics of proteasome inhibitors for the treatment of multiple myeloma. *Expert. Opin. Drug Metab. Toxicol.* 15: 459–473.

Bjorklund, C.C., Kang, J., Amatangelo, M. et al. (2020). Iberdomide (CC-220) is a potent cereblon E3 ligase modulator with antitumor and immunostimulatory activities in lenalidomide- and pomalidomide-resistant multiple myeloma cells with dysregulated CRBN. *Leukemia* 34: 1197–1201.

Brown, J., Plummer, R., Bauer, T.M. et al. (2017). Pharmacokinetics of carfilzomib in patients with advanced malignancies and varying degrees of hepatic impairment: an open-label, single-arm, phase 1 study. *Exp. Hematol. Oncol.* 6: 27.

Chen, N., Lau, H., Kong, L. et al. (2007). Pharmacokinetics of lenalidomide in subjects with various degrees of renal impairment and in subjects on hemodialysis. *J. Clin. Pharmacol.* 47: 1466–1475.

Chen, N., Zhou, S., and Palmisano, M. (2017). Clinical pharmacokinetics and pharmacodynamics of lenalidomide. *Clin. Pharmacokinet.* 56: 139–152.

Ciechanover, A. (2017). Intracellular protein degradation: from a vague idea thru the lysosome and the ubiquitin-proteasome system and onto human diseases and drug targeting. *Best Pract. Res. Clin. Haematol.* 30: 341–355.

Cowan, A.J., Green, D.J., Kwok, M. et al. (2022). Diagnosis and management of multiple myeloma: a review. *JAMA* 327: 464–477.

D'Amato, R.J., Loughnan, M.S., Flynn, E. et al. (1994). Thalidomide is an inhibitor of angiogenesis. *Proc. Natl. Acad. Sci. U. S. A.* 91: 4082–4085.

Di, K., Lloyd, G.K., Abraham, V. et al. (2016). Marizomib activity as a single agent in malignant gliomas: ability to cross the blood-brain barrier. *Neuro. Oncol.* 18: 840–848.

Dimopoulos, M., Weisel, K., van de Donk, N. et al. (2018). Pomalidomide plus low-dose dexamethasone in patients with relapsed/refractory multiple myeloma and renal impairment: results from a phase II trial. *J. Clin. Oncol.: Off. J. Am. Soc. Clin. Oncol.* 36: 2035–2043.

Dimopoulos, M.A., Moreau, P., Palumbo, A. et al. (2016). Carfilzomib and dexamethasone versus bortezomib and dexamethasone for patients with relapsed or refractory multiple myeloma (ENDEAVOR): a randomised, phase 3, open-label, multicentre study. *Lancet Oncol.* 17: 27–38.

Eriksson, T., Hoglund, P., Turesson, I. et al. (2003). Pharmacokinetics of thalidomide in patients with impaired renal function and while on and off dialysis. *J. Pharm. Pharmacol.* 55: 1701–1706.

Facon, T., Lee, J.H., Moreau, P. et al. (2019). Carfilzomib or bortezomib with melphalan-prednisone for transplant-ineligible patients with newly diagnosed multiple myeloma. *Blood* 133: 1953–1963.

Ferrington, D.A. and Gregerson, D.S. (2012). Immunoproteasomes: structure, function, and antigen presentation. *Prog. Mol. Biol. Transl. Sci.* 109: 75–112.

Furie, R.A., Hough, D.R., Gaudy, A. et al. (2022). Iberdomide in patients with systemic lupus erythematosus: a randomised, double-blind, placebo-controlled, ascending-dose, phase 2a study. *Lupus. Sci. Med.* 9.

Gay, F., Mina, R., Troia, R. et al. (2013). Pharmacokinetic evaluation of pomalidomide for the treatment of myeloma. *Expert. Opin. Drug Metab. Toxicol.* 9: 1517–1527.

Ghobrial, I.M., Vij, R., Siegel, D. et al. (2019). A phase Ib/II study of oprozomib in patients with advanced multiple myeloma and Waldenstrom macroglobulinemia. *Clin. Cancer Res.: An Off. J. Am. Ass. Cancer Res.* 25: 4907–4916.

Gupta, N., Hanley, M.J., Harvey, R.D. et al. (2016). A pharmacokinetics and safety phase 1/1b study of oral ixazomib in patients with multiple myeloma and severe renal impairment or end-stage renal disease requiring haemodialysis. *Br. J. Haematol.* 174: 748–759.

Hansen, J.D., Correa, M., Nagy, M.A. et al. (2020). Discovery of CRBN E3 ligase modulator CC-92480 for the treatment of relapsed and refractory multiple myeloma. *J. Med. Chem.* 63: 6648–6676.

Hari, P., Paba-Prada, C.E., Voorhees, P.M. et al. (2019). Efficacy and safety results from a phase 1b/2, multicenter, open-label study of oprozomib and dexamethasone in patients with relapsed and/or refractory multiple myeloma. *Leuk. Res.* 83: 106172.

Harrison, S.J., Mainwaring, P., Price, T. et al. (2016). Phase I clinical trial of marizomib (NPI-0052) in patients with advanced malignancies including multiple myeloma: study NPI-0052-102 final results. *Clin. Can. Res.: An Off. J. Am. Ass. Can. Res.* 22: 4559–4566.

Ito, T., Ando, H., and Handa, H. (2011). Teratogenic effects of thalidomide: molecular mechanisms. *Cell. Mol. Life Sci.* 68: 1569–1579.

Ito, T., Ando, H., Suzuki, T. et al.(2010). Identification of a primary target of thalidomide teratogenicity. *Science* 327: 1345–1350.

Jan, M., Sperling, A.S., and Ebert, B.L. (2021). Cancer therapies based on targeted protein degradation – lessons learned with lenalidomide. *Nat. Rev. Clin. Oncol.* 18: 401–417.

Jones, H.B. (1850). Some account of a new animal substance occurring in the urine of a patient labouring under mollities ossium. *Edinb. Med. Surg. J.* 74: 357–368.

Jones, R.J., Iempridee, T., Wang, X. et al. (2016). Lenalidomide, thalidomide, and pomalidomide reactivate the epstein-barr virus lytic cycle through phosphoinositide 3-kinase signaling and ikaros expression. *Clin. Cancer Res.: An Off. J. Am. Ass. Cancer Res.* 22: 4901–4912.

Kumar, S.K., Jacobus, S.J., Cohen, A.D. et al. (2020). Carfilzomib or bortezomib in combination with lenalidomide and dexamethasone for patients with newly diagnosed multiple myeloma without intention for immediate autologous stem-cell transplantation (ENDURANCE): a multicentre, open-label, phase 3, randomised, controlled trial. *Lancet Oncol.* 21: 1317–1330.

Kumar, S.K., Rajkumar, V., Kyle, R.A. et al. (2017). Multiple myeloma. *Nat. Rev. Dis. Primers.* 3: 17046.

Kunacheewa, C. and Orlowski, R.Z. (2019). New drugs in multiple myeloma. *Annu. Rev. Med.* 70: 521–547.

List, A., Ebert, B.L., and Fenaux, P. (2018). A decade of progress in myelodysplastic syndrome with chromosome 5q deletion. *Leukemia* 32: 1493–1499.

Lopez-Girona, A., Mendy, D., Ito, T. et al. (2012). Cereblon is a direct protein target for immunomodulatory and antiproliferative activities of lenalidomide and pomalidomide. *Leukemia* 26: 2326–2335.

LoRusso, P.M., Venkatakrishnan, K., Ramanathan, R.K. et al. (2012). Pharmacokinetics and safety of bortezomib in patients with advanced malignancies and varying degrees of liver dysfunction: phase I NCI organ dysfunction working group study NCI-6432. *Clini. Cancer Res.: An Off. J. Am. Ass. Cancer Res.* 18: 2954–2963.

Lundholm, K., Edstrom, S., Ekman, L. et al. (1978). A comparative study of the influence of malignant tumor on host metabolism in mice and man: evaluation of an experimental model. *Cancer* 42: 453–461.

Manasanch, E.E. and Orlowski, R.Z. (2017). Proteasome inhibitors in cancer therapy. *Nat. Rev. Clin. Oncol.* 14: 417–433.

Matyskiela, M.E., Lu, G., Ito, T. et al. (2016). A novel cereblon modulator recruits GSPT1 to the CRL4(CRBN) ubiquitin ligase. *Nature* 535: 252–257.

Matyskiela, M.E., Zhang, W., Man, H.W. et al. (2018). A cereblon modulator (CC-220) with improved degradation of ikaros and aiolos. *J. Med. Chem.* 61: 535–542.

Merrill, J.T., Werth, V.P., Furie, R. et al. (2022). Phase 2 trial of iberdomide in systemic lupus erythematosus. *N. Engl. J. Med.* 386: 1034–1045.

Moreau, P., Pylypenko, H., Grosicki, S. et al. (2011). Subcutaneous versus intravenous administration of bortezomib in patients with relapsed multiple myeloma: a randomised, phase 3, non-inferiority study. *Lancet Oncol.* 12: 431–440.

Morschhauser, F., Fowler, N.H., Feugier, P. et al. (2018). Rituximab plus lenalidomide in advanced untreated follicular lymphoma. *N. Engl. J. Med.* 379: 934–947.

Orlowski, M., Cardozo, C., Hidalgo, M.C. et al. (1991). Regulation of the peptidylglutamyl-peptide hydrolyzing activity of the pituitary multicatalytic proteinase complex. *Biochemistry* 30: 5999–6005.

Orlowski, M., Cardozo, C., and Michaud, C. (1993). Evidence for the presence of five distinct proteolytic components in the pituitary multicatalytic proteinase complex. Properties of two components cleaving bonds on the carboxyl side of branched chain and small neutral amino acids. *Biochemistry* 32: 1563–1572.

Orlowski, M. and Michaud, C. (1989). Pituitary multicatalytic proteinase complex. Specificity of components and aspects of proteolytic activity. *Biochemistry* 28: 9270–9278.

Orlowski, M. and Wilk, S. (2000). Catalytic activities of the 20 S proteasome, a multicatalytic proteinase complex. *Arch. Biochem. Biophys.* 383: 1–16.

Orlowski, R.Z., Stinchcombe, T.E., Mitchell, B.S. et al. (2002). Phase I trial of the proteasome inhibitor PS-341 in patients with refractory hematologic malignancies. *J. Clin. Oncology: Of. J. Am. Soc. Clin. Oncol.* 20: 4420–4427.

Rajkumar, S.V. and Kumar, S. (2020). Multiple myeloma current treatment algorithms. *Blood Cancer J.* 10: 94.

Richardson, P.G., Barlogie, B., Berenson, J. et al. (2003). A phase 2 study of bortezomib in relapsed, refractory myeloma. *N. Engl. J. Med.* 348: 2609–2617.

Richardson, P.G., Blood, E., Mitsiades, C.S. et al. (2006). A randomized phase 2 study of lenalidomide therapy for patients with relapsed or relapsed and refractory multiple myeloma. *Blood* 108: 3458–3464.

Richardson, P.G., Sonneveld, P., Schuster, M.W. et al. (2005). Bortezomib or high-dose dexamethasone for relapsed multiple myeloma. *N. Engl. J. Med.* 352: 2487–2498.

Richardson, P.G., Zimmerman, T.M., Hofmeister, C.C. et al. (2016). Phase 1 study of marizomib in relapsed or relapsed and refractory multiple myeloma: NPI-0052-101 Part 1. *Blood* 127: 2693–2700.

Sheskin, J. (1965). Thalidomide in the treatment of lepra reactions. *Clin. Pharmacol. Ther.* 6: 303–306.

Singhal, S., Mehta, J., Desikan, R. et al. (1999). Antitumor activity of thalidomide in refractory multiple myeloma. [see comments] [published erratum appears in N Engl J Med 2000 Feb 3;342(5):364]. *N. Engl. J. Med.* 341: 1565–1571.

Spencer, A., Harrison, S., Zonder, J. et al. (2018). A phase 1 clinical trial evaluating marizomib, pomalidomide and low-dose dexamethasone in relapsed and refractory multiple myeloma (NPI-0052-107): final study results. *Br. J. Haematol.* 180: 41–51.

Tanaka, K. (2009). The proteasome: overview of structure and functions. *Proc. Jpn. Acad., Ser. B, Phys. Biol. Sci.* 85: 12–36.

Temparis, S., Asensi, M., Taillandier, D. et al. (1994). Increased ATP-ubiquitin-dependent proteolysis in skeletal muscles of tumor-bearing rats. *Cancer Res.* 54: 5568–5573.

Teo, S.K., Colburn, W.A., Tracewell, W.G. et al. (2004). Clinical pharmacokinetics of thalidomide. *Clin Pharmacokinet.* 43: 311–327.

Verbrugge, S.E., Assaraf, Y.G., Dijkmans, B.A. et al. (2012). Inactivating PSMB5 mutations and P-glycoprotein (multidrug resistance-associated protein/ATP-binding cassette B1) mediate resistance to proteasome inhibitors: ex vivo efficacy of (immuno)proteasome inhibitors in mononuclear blood cells from patients with rheumatoid arthritis. *J. Pharmacol. Exp. Ther.* 341: 174–182.

Vinitsky, A., Michaud, C., Powers, J.C. et al. (1992). Inhibition of the chymotrypsin-like activity of the pituitary multicatalytic proteinase complex. *Biochemistry* 31: 9421–9428.

Voorhees, P.M., Dees, E.C., O'Neil, B. et al. (2003). The proteasome as a target for cancer therapy. *Clin. Cancer Res.: An Off. J. Am. Ass. Cancer Res.* 9: 6316–6325.

Ye, Y., Gaudy, A., Schafer, P. et al. (2021). First-in-human, single- and multiple-ascending-dose studies in healthy subjects to assess pharmacokinetics, pharmacodynamics, and safety/tolerability of iberdomide, a novel cereblon E3 ligase modulator. *Clin. Pharmacol. Drug Dev.* 10: 471–485.

You, W. and Pang, J. (2021). Pharmacokinetics, bioavailability and metabolism of CC-92480 in rat by liquid chromatography combined with electrospray ionization tandem mass spectrometry. *Biomed. Chromatogr.* 35: e5139.

Zhou, S., Wang, F., Hsieh, T.C. (2013). Thalidomide-a notorious sedative to a wonder anticancer drug. *Curr. Med. Chem.* 20: 4102–4108.

Zhu, W. and Chen, W. (2016). Bortezomib-based treatment for multiple myeloma patients with renal impairment: a systematic review and meta-analysis of observational studies. *Medicine (Baltimore)* 95: e5202.

Zhu, Y.X., Braggio, E., Shi, C.X. et al. (2011). Cereblon expression is required for the antimyeloma activity of lenalidomide and pomalidomide. *Blood* 118: 4771–4779.

Zou, J., Jones, R.J., Wang, H. et al. (2020). The novel protein homeostatic modulator BTX306 is active in myeloma and overcomes bortezomib and lenalidomide resistance. *J. Mol. Med.* 98: 1161–1173.

23

Preclinical Overview of Drugs Affecting Protein Turnover in Multiple Myeloma

Giada Bianchi[1], *Matthew Ho*[2], *and Kenneth C. Anderson*[3]

[1] *Amyloidosis Program, Division of Hematology, Department of Medicine, Brigham and Women's Hospital, Harvard Medical School, Boston, MA, USA*
[2] *Department of Internal Medicine, Mayo Clinic, Rochester, MN, USA*
[3] *LeBow Institute for Myeloma Therapeutics and Jerome Lipper Multiple Myeloma Center, Department of Medical Oncology, Dana Farber Cancer Institute, Harvard Medical School, Boston, MA, USA*

Take Home Messages

- Multiple myeloma (MM) cells have high baseline proteotoxic stress owing to genomic instability and near universal aneuploidy, as well as a significant burden of misfolded proteins resulting from an augmented rate of immunoglobulin synthesis. This characteristic makes it the prototypic cancer model for studying proteotoxicity.
- MM cells rely on a highly efficient and interconnected network of protein quality control pathways whose functions include folding, sequestration, and/or degradation of misfolded proteins (protein homeostasis or proteostasis network). Based on this biology, targeting of proteostasis is a promising therapeutic approach alone or in combination with other proteostasis-targeting agents such as proteasome inhibitors.
- Proteasome inhibition is able to induce a potent anti-MM immune response through immunogenic cell death (ICD) while at the same time preserving HLA class I peptide generation.
- Based on the ability of immunomodulatory drugs to hijack the cereblon E3 ligase, a new class of PROTACs (called degronimids) is currently in preclinical development in MM, which allows us to target hitherto undruggable targets such as transcription factors and epigenetic regulators.

Introduction

Given the importance of the proteostasis network on the survival of multiple myeloma (MM) cells, this disease has become the prototypical model to study the many interactions that govern protein homeostasis, as well as the targeted drugs that might affect that biology. High-dose chemotherapy followed by autologous stem cell transplant (ASCT); improvement in supportive care aimed at reducing bone events and infectious complications; and the clinical use of multidrug regimens incorporating proteasome inhibitors (PIs), immunomodulatory drugs (IMiDs), and immunotherapy agents have resulted in steady improvements in the outcome of MM patients (Usmani and Chiosis 2011). Over the last decade alone, the approval of 11 novel agents and a thriving drug pipeline have led to a significant evolution of the treatment landscape in MM (Fok et al. 2018; Fricker 2020). Despite the use of highly effective combination treatment, MM remains incurable and the treatment of relapsed or refractory MM (RRMM) remains challenging, especially in patients with high-risk, triple-class (i.e. PI, IMiD, and monoclonal antibody) refractory disease.

Drug resistance remains an obstacle to cure, and there is significant ongoing basic and translational research aimed at developing novel and effective molecularly targeted and immunotherapy agents, and designing combination therapies capable of overcoming drug resistance. One such area of active

Precision Cancer Therapies: Targeting Oncogenic Drivers and Signaling Pathways in Lymphoid Malignancies: From Concept to Practice, Volume 1, First Edition. Edited by Owen A. O'Connor, Stephen M. Ansell, and John F. Seymour.

research focuses on targeting protein turnover. Cellular protein synthesis is intrinsically error-prone, and misfolded proteins need to be removed to prevent accumulation of toxic, misfolded proteins (Wirth et al. 2020). Furthermore, it has been clearly shown that genomic instability, a hallmark of many types of cancer, also contributes to proteotoxic stress, rendering MM cells especially prone to proteotoxicity (Besse et al. 2021; Jan et al. 2021; Li and Song 2020; Wirth et al. 2020; Xiong et al. 2021). The baseline proteotoxic stress experienced by MM cells has been shown by our group and others to account for the exquisite sensitivity of MM cells to PI treatment. PIs are presently a mainstay of MM treatment in all stages of therapy, including induction, consolidation, and maintenance, in both newly diagnosed and relapsed or refractory (R/R) settings. However, most patients invariably become refractory to PIs over the course of their treatment, which is associated with a negative impact on their overall outcome. In this chapter, we provide an overview of the protein handling machinery, discuss our current understanding of the mechanisms driving PI resistance, and review treatments (both approved and experimental) used to sensitize MM cells to PIs, with a focus on therapies targeting protein homeostasis. We also discuss the role of PI in the era of immunotherapy, and look at promising therapies that are on-the-horizon in MM.

Overview of Protein Handling in MM

Cellular protein synthesis is error-prone, and it is estimated that more than 30% of newly synthesized proteins in eukaryotic cells are misfolded and undergo proteasomal degradation within minutes of protein translation (Gu et al. 2020). These misfolded proteins comprised mainly defective ribosomal proteins (DRiPs), which are the byproducts of mistakes during protein synthesis that arise as a consequence of DNA mutations, damaged mRNAs, misincorporation of amino acids, early termination of translation, and pervasive translation (Fassmannová et al. 2020; Gu et al. 2020). Accumulation of misfolded proteins within the secretory pathway triggers endoplasmic reticulum (ER) stress that, if not adequately and rapidly mitigated, induces apoptosis (Baranowska et al. 2016). Other contributors to elevated proteotoxic stress in cancer include aneuploidy (a consequence of genomic instability), hypoxia, oxidative (and reductive) stress, and nutrient deprivation; all of which have been implicated as key activators of the integrated stress response (ISR), a cytoprotective response to proteotoxic stress (Jagannathan et al. 2015; Kawaguchi et al. 2011; Wang et al. 2018). As such, cancer cells must cope with heightened degrees of proteotoxic stress in order to survive.

MM is the prototypical proteotoxic-stressed cancer: due to pervasive genomic instability and near universal aneuploidy, as well as a significant burden of misfolded proteins resulting from augmented rates of immunoglobulin synthesis, MM cells are characterized by baseline proteotoxicity (Imai et al. 2019; Li et al. 2014). The overabundance of misfolded proteins overwhelms the capacity of the ER protein folding machinery, and hence MM cells rely on the intricated proteostasis network to ensure that these dangerous polypeptides are either folded, degraded, or sequestered to maintain homeostasis and guarantee survival (Figure 23.1) (Gulla et al. 2021; Ramakrishnan and Kumar 2018).

Molecular Chaperones in Protein Folding

Chaperone proteins, such as heat shock protein 70 and 90 (HSP70, HSP90), are key components of the proteostasis network and play an active role in MM survival, progression, drug resistance, and immune evasion (Figure 23.1a) (Hoang et al. 2009; Oyake et al. 1996). Specifically, it has been shown that chaperone proteins interact with multiple client proteins involved in oncogenic signaling pathways and help mitigate proteotoxic stress through facilitation of protein folding, rendering them attractive targets in MM (Di et al. 2016; Feng et al. 2013; Nishimura et al. 2019). HSP90 also facilitates chaperone-mediated autophagy (CMA), and inhibition of HSP90 has been found to reduce CMA activity (Brancolini and Iuliano 2020). NVP-HSP990 and TAS-116 are HSP90 inhibitors in preclinical development that have shown promising synergism with the PI bortezomib (Table 23.1) (Li et al. 2011; Nandi et al. 2006). The HSP90 inhibitors tanespimycin, retaspimycin, and KW-2478 have been evaluated in phase 1/2 clinical trials, but have not advance to later stages of development largely due to their limited therapeutic index (García-Santisteban et al. 2013; Schubert et al. 2000). More recently, heat shock factor 1 (HSF1), the "master regulator" of the heat shock response (HSR), has emerged as a promising therapeutic target in MM, with the premise that targeting an upstream regulator of HSP expression would abrogate compensatory upregulation of individual chaperones (Richardson et al. 2005). HSF1 knockdown in MM cell lines led to decreased expression of HSP70, HSP90, and HSP20 family proteins, and the HSF1 inhibitors CCT251236 and KRIBB11 demonstrated anti-MM activity in a human myeloma xenograft model, with little toxicity to healthy peripheral blood mononuclear cells (PBMCs) (Richardson et al. 2005).

Ubiquitin–Proteasome System (UPS)

At the core of the protein clearance network in eukaryotic cells is the ubiquitin–proteasome system (UPS) (Figure 23.1b) (Wirth et al. 2020). Misfolded proteins are first marked for degradation via sequential conjugation of ubiquitin (Ub) moieties by a three-enzyme cascade involving E1 (activating),

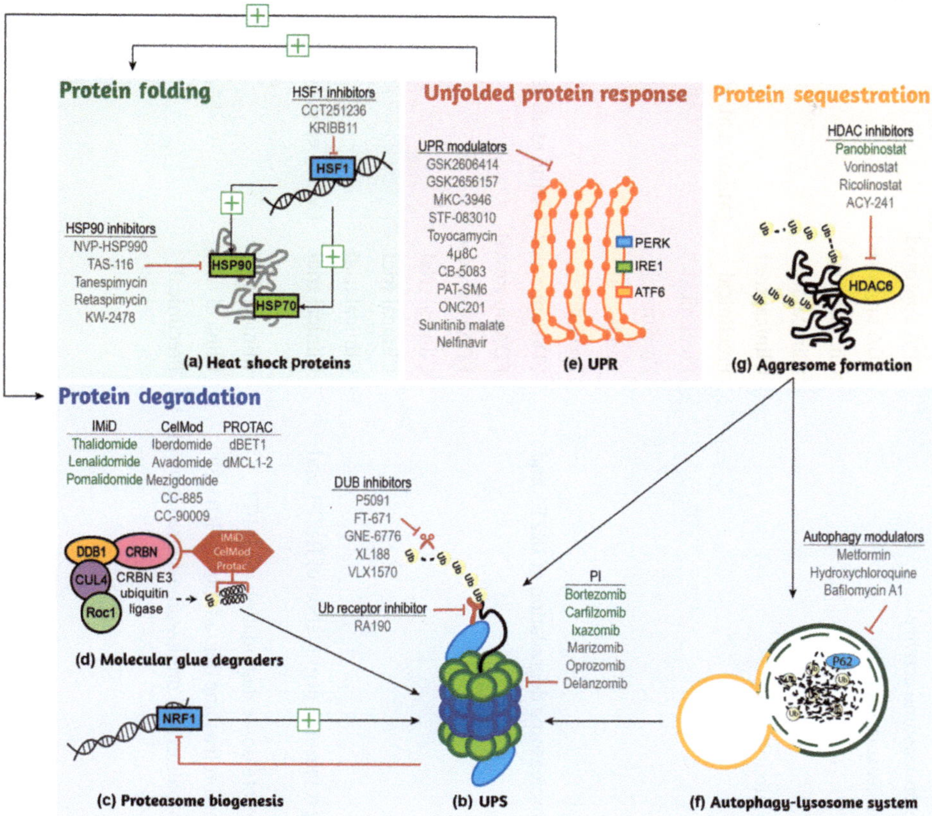

Figure 23.1 Overview of protein handling pathways in MM and the drugs targeting them. MM cells display high levels of baseline proteotoxic stress and are therefore dependent on a highly efficient and interconnected network of protein quality control pathways to maintain proteostasis. Misfolded proteins are either refolded, degraded, or sequestered through the various pathways highlighted. The various FDA-approved and experimental therapies targeting each respective pathway are highlighted in green and gray, respectively.

E2 (conjugating), and E3 (ligating) enzymes to polyubiquitin chains (Baird et al. 2017). Polyubiquitinated (polyUb) target proteins are then translocated to the 26S proteasome, a 2.4 MDa, ATP-dependent, multi-domain proteolytic complex responsible for the bulk degradation of most misfolded or aged cellular proteins. The proteasome is composed of a central, barrel-shaped 20S catalytic particle (CP) containing three distinct, ATP-dependent proteolytic activities, flanked at one or both ends by 19S regulatory particle(s) (RPs), containing proteins participating in substrate recognition, unfolding, and proteasome gate opening. Among these are Ub binding proteins (UBPs), RPN10, RPN13, and/or RNP11, whose function is to recognize and bind polyUb proteins (Auner et al. 2013; Catley et al. 2006; Chauhan et al. 2012). Target proteins are then unfolded and threaded into the 20S channel for degradation (Chauhan et al. 2012). Although Ub is required to target proteins to the proteasome, it can also sterically hinder the subsequent translocation of target proteins through the narrow pore formed by the 19S cap into the CP and needs to be recycled to ensure a constant-free Ub pool (Neri and Bahlis 2013; Walter and Ron 2011). Deubiquitinating enzymes (DUBs) are a large family of enzymes responsible for cleavage of Ub moiety. Proteasome-associated DUBs (i.e. ubiquitin-specific peptidase 14 [USP14], UCH37/UCHL5, RPN11/POH1) are embedded in the 19S RP (Neri and Bahlis 2013; Saavedra-García et al. 2020). In contrast to RPN11, which mainly acts on committed substrates and functions to promote degradation, UCH37 and USP14 can also rescue proteins from degradation prior to their unfolding (Chauhan et al. 2012). USP14 has also been shown to suppress proteasome activity independent of its deubiquitinating ability (Chauhan et al. 2012).

The 20S cylindrical-shaped CP is formed by two outer heptameric α rings and two inner heptameric β rings comprises three main catalytic subunits: the β1 (caspase-like activity), β2 (trypsin-like activity), and β5 (chymotrypsin-like activity) subunits (Townsend et al. 2009). In eukaryotic cells, secretory or transmembrane proteins that do not achieve a timely or adequate folding are retro-translocated via the Sec61 translocon from the ER to the cytosol, where they undergo

Table 23.1 Therapies targeting protein handling pathways in MM.

Drug class	Drug name	Mechanism of action	Status	References
HSP inhibitors	Tanespimycin	HSP90 inhibitor	Clinical trial	(D'Arcy et al. 2011)
	Retaspimycin		Clinical trial	
	KW-2478		Clinical trial	
	TAS-116		Preclinical	
	NVP-HSP990		Preclinical	
	CCT251236	HSF1 inhibitor	Preclinical	(Richardson et al. 2005)
	KRIBB11		Preclinical	
PI	Bortezomib	Reversible boronate acid inhibitor of chymotrypsin-like proteasome activity	FDA approved	(Meister et al. 2007)
	Carfilzomib	Irreversible epoxyketone-based inhibitor of chymotrypsin-like proteasome activity	FDA approved	
	Ixazomib	Reversible oral boronate acid inhibitor of chymotrypsin-like proteasome activity	FDA approved	
	Delanzomib		Clinical trial	
	Oprozomib		Clinical trial	
	Marizomib	Irreversible salinosporamide inhibitor of all three proteasome subunits	Clinical trial	
DUB inhibitors	P5902	USP7 inhibitor	Preclinical	(Milan et al. 2016)
	FT-671		Preclinical	
	GNE-6776		Preclinical	
	XL188		Preclinical	
	VLX1570	USP14 and UCH37 inhibitor	Preclinical	
Molecular glue degraders	Thalidomide	Binds the E3 ligase cereblon to cause polyubiquitination and proteasome degradation of IKZF1 and IKZF3	FDA approved	(Altun et al. 2005)
	Lenalidomide		FDA approved	
	Pomalidomide		FDA approved	
	Iberdomide		Clinical trial	
	Avadomide		Clinical trial	
	Mezigdomide		Clinical trial	
	CC-885	Binds the E3 ligase cereblon to cause polyubiquitination and proteasome degradation of IKZF1 and GSPT1	Clinical trial	(Milan et al. 2016)
	CC-90009	Binds the E3 ligase cereblon to cause polyubiquitination and proteasome degradation of GSPT1	Clinical trial	
	Indisulam	Binds to the E3 ligase DCAF15 to cause polyubiquitination and proteasome degradation of RBM39	Clinical trial	
	CR8	Binds to the CUL4 adaptor protein DDB1 to cause polyubiquitination and proteasome degradation of cyclin K	Preclinical	

PROTACs	dBET1	Binds to the E3 ligase cereblon to cause polyubiquitination and proteasome degradation of BRD4	Preclinical	(Neuse et al. 2020)
	dMCL1-2	Binds to the E3 ligase cereblon to cause polyubiquitination and proteasome degradation of MCL1	Preclinical	
	Compound C3		Preclinical	
UPR modulators	GSK2606414	Induces ER stress through inhibition of PERK activity	Preclinical	(Suraweera et al. 2012)
	GSK2656157	Induces ER stress through inhibition of IRE1a activity	Preclinical	
	MKC-3946		Preclinical	
	STF-083010		Preclinical	
	Toyocamycin		Preclinical	
	4μ8C		Preclinical	
	CB-5083	Induces ER stress by inhibiting ERAD	Clinical trial	
	PAT-SM6	Induces ER stress by inhibiting GRP78	Clinical trial	
	ONC201	Induces ER stress by activating ATF4 and CHOP signaling	Clinical trial	
	Sunitinib malate	Induces ER stress by inhibiting XBP1 splicing	Clinical trial	
	Nelfinavir	Induces UPR through IRE1/XBP1, PERK/eIF2a, and ATF6 signaling	Clinical trial	(Bondeson and Crews, 2017)
HIV-protease		Disrupts DDI2-mediated proteolytic activation of NRF1		(Kisselev et al. 1999; Parzych et al. 2019)
Autophagy modulators	Hydroxychloroquine	Inhibition of autophagy by increased lysosomal pH	Preclinical	(Glick et al. 2010)
	Bafilomycin A	Inhibition of autophagy by prevention of autophagosome/lysosome fusion	Preclinical	(Driessen et al. 2018)
	Metformin	Depending on circumstances, may induce or suppress autophagy to cause apoptosis	Clinical trial	(Michallet et al. 2011; Driscoll and Chowdhury 2012)
HDACi	Panobinostat	Broad spectrum HDAC inhibitor that synergizes with PI and dexamethasone	FDA approved	(Lehrbach and Ruvkun 2016)
	Ricolinostat	Selective HDAC6 inhibitor that inhibits aggresome formation, induces ROS generation, ER stress, and apoptosis	Clinical trial	

Abbreviations: ATF = activating transcription factor; BRD4 = bromodomain containing protein 4; CHOP = C/EBP homologous protein; CUL4 = cullin 4; DDB1 = damage-specific DNA binding protein 1; DDI2 = DNA damage inducible 1 homolog 2; DUB1 = deubiquitinating enzyme; eIF2a = eukaryotic translation initiation factor 2 a; ER = endoplasmic reticulum; ERAD = endoplasmic reticulum-associated degradation; GRP78 = glucose regulatory protein 78; GSPT1 = G to S phase transition 1; HDAC = histone deacetylase; HDACi = histone deacetylase inhibitor; HSF1 = heat shock transcription factor 1; HSP90 = heat shock protein (90 kDa); IRE1a = inositol-requiring enzyme 1 a; IKZF = Ikaros zinc finger; MCL1 = myeloid cell leukemia 1; PERK = protein kinase RNA-like ER kinase; NRF1 = nuclear factor erythroid-derived 2-related factor 1; PI = proteasome inhibitor; PROTAC = proteolysis targeting chimera; RBM39 = RNA binding motif protein 39; ROS = reactive oxidative species; UPR = unfolded protein response; XBP1 = X-box binding protein 1.

proteasome-dependent degradation. This process is collectively known as ER-associated degradation (ERAD) (Guang et al. 2019).

Constitutive proteasome subunits can be replaced by their IFN-γ-inducible counterparts (β1i or LMP2, β2i or MECL-1, and β5i or LMP7) during infection or inflammation, to assemble into the immunoproteasome (Lee et al. 2021). Both constitutive and immunoproteasome participate in antigen presentation by providing peptides to be mounted on MHC class I (Wang and Chan 2006). Similar to other immune cells, MM cells express abundant immunoproteasomes (Lonial and Boise 2011; Mimura et al. 2012). Studies have shown that cancer cells with misfolded protein overload due to mammalian target of rapamycin complex 1 (mTORC1) overactivation (which triggers protein synthesis by inhibiting 4E-BPs and activating S6K1) become reliant on the immunoproteasome for survival (Chauhan et al. 2006; Vangala et al. 2014). The phosphoinositide 3-kinase (PI3K)/protein kinase B (AKT)/mTOR pathway is activated in a large proportion of MM patients, and plays an important role in the MM cell survival, proliferation, and chemoresistance within the context of the bone marrow (BM) microenvironment (Coux et al. 1996; Motosugi and Murata 2019). Other mutations commonly (e.g. RAS) and less commonly (e.g. PTEN and TSC1) implicated in MM have also been shown to promote immunoproteasome formation to protect cells from excessive proteotoxic stress (Vangala et al. 2014).

Drugs Targeting the UPS

Proteasome Inhibitors

There are currently three Food and Drug Administration (FDA) approved PIs (i.e. bortezomib, carfilzomib, and ixazomib) and three PIs undergoing clinical trials (i.e. marizomib, oprozomib, and delanzomib) (Table 23.1) (Meister et al. 2007). Developed in the mid-1990s as a tool to study protein degradation, the first-in-class PI for clinical use, bortezomib, proved to be an extremely powerful anti-cancer drug (Chen et al. 2021; Lamberto et al. 2017). Furthermore, the clinical use of bortezomib for the treatment of MM established this disease as a paradigm of PI-sensitive cancer. PIs can be classified into three groups based on their chemical structure and active moiety: (i) boronates, (ii) epoxyketones, and (iii) γ-lactam-β-lactones (salinosporamide) (Wirth et al. 2020). Bortezomib is a reversible PI with a peptide-like backbone and boronate warhead that targets the chymotryptic-like (β5), and to a lesser extent the caspase-like (β1), activity of the proteasome (Chen et al. 2021; Meister et al. 2007; Zhang et al. 2016). Carfilzomib and oprozomib (orally active) are next-generation PIs with peptide-like backbones and epoxyketone warheads that covalently bond to the threonine residue at the chymotrypsin-like active site to irreversibly inhibit the proteasome (Meister et al. 2007). Ixazomib and delanzomib are orally bioavailable PIs, peptide-like, boronic acids structurally related to bortezomib (Xu et al. 2012). Marizomib, unlike the other PIs discussed, is a naturally occurring salinosporamide isolated from *Salinispora* bacteria, and contains a bicyclic β-lactone γ-lactam (Meister et al. 2007). It is an irreversible inhibitor of all three catalytic subunits of the proteasome. Due to its lipophilicity, marizomib is able to cross the blood–brain barrier, raising concerns for potential central nervous system (CNS) toxicity, and also providing the opportunity to redirect the use of this compound to treat CNS myeloma and glioblastoma, with clinical trials currently ongoing (Chen et al. 2017; Kuhn et al. 2009).

PI activity in MM is mediated via pleiotropic molecular mechanisms that directly target the cancer cell as well as the BM microenvironment. PIs alter the pathogenetic BM niche via anti-osteoclast, anti-angiogenic, and pro-osteoblastic activities. At the level of MM cells, PIs have been demonstrated to inhibit proliferation and induce intrinsic and extrinsic apoptosis pathways; inhibit nuclear factor-kappaB (NF-κB) pathway and DNA repair mechanisms; as well as induce c-Jun NH2-terminal kinase (JNK), terminal unfolded protein response (UPR), HSR, and proteotoxic stress (Aronson and Davies 2012; Kyle and Rajkumar 2008; Ramakrishnan and Kumar 2018). By virtue of their nature as professional immunoglobulin synthesizing cells, MM cells are especially prone to improper protein folding and baseline proteotoxic stress (Seifert et al. 2010). Pharmacological blockade of the proteasome would then result in select cytotoxicity against MM cells, proportional to their higher degree of proteotoxic stress. Consistent with this hypothesis, reduced immunoglobulin synthesis and/or increased proteasomal activity mediate PI resistance in MM cells; while pharmacological disruption of protein folding via ER stressor, inhibition of ERAD, and/or decreased proteasomal activity sensitize MM cells to PI (Brüning et al. 2009; Hanna et al. 2003; Kobayashi et al. 1999; Mimura et al. 2012), MM cells characterized by lower proteotoxicity due to increased proteasome capacity and/or decreased proteasome load are characterized by intrinsic resistance to PIs, a phenomenon observed in 30–40% of MM patients when treated with either bortezomib or carfilzomib as single agents (Fan et al. 2021; Kumar et al. 2011; Nakatogawa et al. 2009; Park et al. 2004; Rodriguez-Gonzalez et al. 2008). Hypothesizing that irreversible proteasomal inhibition and/or broader blockade of all three catalytic activities of the proteasome would overcome bortezomib resistance in the clinic, next-generation PIs were developed. Although these agents could overcome bortezomib resistance in a proportion of patients, severe adverse events not previously noted with bortezomib were noted. Specifically, rare but significant cardiovascular and renal events were reported in carfilzomib-treated patients, while neurologic and renal events were observed in patients receiving marizomib in early phase clinical studies (Andrews et al. 1993; Bejarano and Cuervo 2010; Fok et al. 2018; Negrini et al. 2010; Yong et al. 2016).

Inhibitors of Deubiquitinating Enzymes (DUB)

Ubiquitination is a critical post-translational modification in a multitude of cellular processes including DNA repair and proteolysis (Lu et al. 2014). Ub has eight amino groups (M1, K6, K11, K27, K29, K33, K48, and K63) which allow the formation of up to eight different polyUb chain linkages through its seven lysine (K) residues or N-terminus methionine (M1) (Lu et al. 2014). Adding to the complexity is the ability to form polyubiquitin chains with homotypic (uniform) or heterotypic (mixed) linkages (Lu et al. 2014). Homotypic K48 polyUb typically signals proteasome degradation, while homotypic K63 polyUb plays a role in intracellular signaling, DNA repair, and the endosomal–lysosomal system (Lu et al. 2014). On the other hand, heterotypic K11/K48, K29/K48, and K48/K63 chains have also been implicated in proteasome degradation, while M1/K63 chains function in non-proteasomal pathways to regulate the immune response (Akyol et al. 2006; Gupta et al. 2007; Johnston and Samant 2021; Obeng et al. 2006; Pakos-Zebrucka et al. 2016; Siegel et al. 2012; Wang et al. 2009).

DUBs are a large family of enzymes responsible for Ub removal and recycling from polyUb proteins. They have been extensively studied for their key role in maintaining proteostasis, with a particular interest in targeting them as anti-cancer therapy. Within the 19S proteasome, RPN10 and RPN13 act as Ub receptors to bind K48 polyUb chains with high affinity on the one hand, and recruit proteasome-associated DUBs (e.g. UCH37) to facilitate polyUb removal and thus target degradation on the other hand (Ohtake et al. 2018). *In vitro* studies have shown that inhibition or silencing of RPN11, RPN13, UCH37, USP1, and USP7 individually has potent anti-MM activity, even in the bortezomib-resistant setting (De Gassart et al. 2016; Meyer and Rape 2014; Richardson et al. 2020; Samant et al. 2018; Yun et al. 2017). Targeting of RPN13, UCH37, and USP7 leads to UPS impairment without direct inhibition of proteasome catalytic subunits, which induces both caspase-dependent and UPR-associated apoptosis in primary MM cells and MM cell lines, including those that are bortezomib-resistant (De Gassart et al. 2016; Richardson et al. 2020; Samant et al. 2018; Yun et al. 2017). Interestingly, inhibition or knockdown of RPN13 in plasmacytoid dendritic cells (pDCs) increased expression of CD80, CD83, and CD86, leading to pDC activation and boosting MM-specific cytotoxic T lymphocyte (CTL) and natural killer (NK) cell activity (Vij et al. 2012). Furthermore, inhibition of RPN13 increases pDC calnexin expression, which upregulates costimulatory molecules, cytokines/chemokines, adhesion molecules, and immune signaling pathways (Dimopoulos et al. 2013; Vij et al. 2012). There are a few USP7 inhibitors (e.g. P5091, FT-671, GNE-6776, and XL188) undergoing pre-clinical evaluation (Chang et al. 2018; Jacob et al. 2017; Taniguchi et al. 2002; Yun et al. 2017). The USP14 and UCH37 inhibitor VLX1570 in combination with dexamethasone was evaluated in a phase 1 study in R/RMM (NCT02372240) (Ho et al. 2019). Although anti-MM activity was noted at doses ≥0.6 mg/kg, fatal pulmonary toxicity occurred in two patients receiving 1.2 mg/kg, and the study was terminated (Ho et al. 2019).

USP1 regulates both the Fanconi anemia (FA) interstrand cross-link (ICL) repair pathway and the homologous recombination (HR) DNA double-stranded break (DSB) repair pathway (Hebert et al. 2010; Liang et al. 2019). Preclinical studies have shown that USP1 is overexpressed in MM cells compared to healthy donor plasma cells, and that an inverse correlation exists between USP1 expression and overall and event-free survival in MM patients (Meyer and Rape 2014). Knockdown or pharmacologic inhibition of USP1 triggers caspase-dependent apoptosis in MM cells, and demonstrates synergistic cytotoxicity with histone deacetylase 6 (HDAC6) inhibition, bortezomib, and IMiDs *in vitro* (Meyer and Rape 2014). Mechanistically, USP1 inhibition prevents deubiquitination of FA pathway proteins including Ub-FANCD2, Ub-FANCI, and Ub-PCNA (Meyer and Rape 2014). Monoubiquitination of the FANCI-FANCD2 heterodimer (ID2 complex) by UBE2T (E2 conjugating enzyme) and the FA-core complex (large multi-component E3 ligase), as well as timely deubiquitination of FANCD2 and FANCI by the USP1-UAF1 complex, are critical for ICL repair (Lopez-Girona et al. 2012). During ICL repair, monoubiquitinated ID2 is also able to activate HR to repair DNA DSBs arising from the nucleolytic processing of the DNA cross-link by recruiting HR factors (e.g. BRCA2 and RAD51) (Wang et al. 2004, 2009; Lemonidis et al.; Liang et al. 2016). USP1 also binds DNA with a specificity toward replication fork-like DNA structures, and is thought to play a role in targeting the RAD51AP1-UAF1-USP1 complex to stressed and damaged replication forks (Iurlaro and Munoz-Pinedo 2016). Despite this, *in vitro* studies show that USP1 DNA binding activity may be dispensable for the DNA strand invasion step of RAD51-dependent HR (Cavenagh et al. 2017). Unexpectedly, USP1 inhibition in MM cells decreased RAD51 foci formation, suggesting that HR mechanisms in MM cells can be abrogated by targeting USP1 (Lopez-Girona et al. 2011; Meyer and Rape 2014). It will be of particular interest to determine whether USP1 facilitates RAD51 DNA strand invasion in MM cells or regulates a separate step of RAD-51-dependent HR.

Targeting Proteasome Biogenesis

One potential mechanism of both intrinsic and acquired PI resistance is enhanced *de novo* proteasome biogenesis leading to increased proteasome activity (Figure 23.1c) (Cenci and Sitia 2007). We and others have shown that preconditioning with low, non-toxic doses of PI leads to increased proteasome pool and acquisition of PI resistance (Nishimura et al. 2019; San-Miguel et al. 2014; Wertz et al. 2015) Furthermore, proteomics data in MM cells adapted for long-term survival in PI-containing culture media showed less dependency on the proteasome itself (Ito et al. 2010). Studies in yeast identified RPN4 as a 26S proteasome-associated protein that also binds to the proteasome-associated control element (PACE), a conserved sequence motif in the promoter region of all proteasome subunit genes and some proteasome assembly chaperone genes (Cenci and Sitia 2007). However, there are no mammalian orthologs of RPN4 or the PACE sequence, and the expression of proteasome subunits in mammalian cells is regulated by several distinct transcription factors including nuclear transcription factor Y (NF-Y), which bind to the CCAAT motif in the promoter of six CP subunit genes (α2, α5, α7, β3, β4, and β6), five RP subunit genes (*Rpt1*, *Rpt5*, *Rpt6*, *Rpn10*, and *Rpn11*), and the p28 assembly chaperone (Cenci and Sitia 2007; Chen et al. 2011). Forkhead box protein O4 (FOXO4) and signal transducer and activator of transcription 3 (STAT3) have also been shown to separately regulate RPN6 and β5, respectively (Borjan et al. 2020; Cenci and Sitia 2007). However, seminal work has shown that nuclear factor erythroid-derived 2-related factor 1 (NRF1) is the master regulator of proteasome biogenesis in mammalian systems. In fact, NRF1 is the gatekeeper of the proteasome stress response (PSR), a homeostatic, compensatory response triggered by proteasome insufficiency aimed at increasing proteasome capacity (Braunlin et al. 2021). NRF1 belongs to a family of six cap "n" collar basic leucine zipper (CNC-bZIP) transcription factors including NRF2, NRF3, nuclear factor erythroid 2 (NF-E2) p45 subunit, BTB and CNC homolog 1 (BACH 1), and BACH 2 (Cenci and Sitia 2007; David et al. 2005; Hideshima et al. 2009; Qiao and Zhang 2009; Rowinsky et al. 2020; Zhang et al. 2007). Although both NRF1 and NRF2 recognize the 5′-RTGACTCAGC-3′ consensus sequence present in all 33 proteasome subunit genes, proteasome gene expression has been shown to be predominantly regulated by the former (Hideshima et al. 2003). Studies in cancer have demonstrated that NRF2 has the ability to induce proteasome expression in a p53-dependent manner (McConkey 2017). Under physiologic conditions of adequate proteasome function, newly synthesized NRF1 is imported into the ER, glycosylated and retro-translocated to the cytosol where it undergoes rapid proteasomal degradation via ERAD (Cenci et al. 2006; El Arfani et al. 2018). However, when the proteasome activity is insufficient to process the load of polyUb proteins, NRF1 is stabilized, deglycosylated by N-glycanase 1 (NGLY1), and proteolytically cleaved by the aspartic protease DNA damaged inducible 1 homolog 2 (DDI2). Cleaved NRF1 (and possibly also full-length, unprocessed isoform) translocates to the nucleus where it becomes transcriptionally active by dimerization with small MAF proteins, activating complex transcriptional programs that include proteasome subunit transcription (Cenci and Sitia 2007; Donnelly and Storchova 2015). In our recent work, we showed that MM cells are dependent on NRF1/DDI2-mediated PSR for survival and that knockout of either genes results in decreased proteasome biogenesis, increased sensitivity to PI, and loss of viability (Braunlin et al. 2021). Targeting the PSR pathway therefore represents a potential therapeutic approach to overcome PI resistance. Inhibition or knockout of NGLY1, DDI2, or NRF1 both potentiated PI activity in MM cell lines and reduced plasmacytoma formation in an *in vivo* mouse model (Braunlin et al. 2021; Han et al. 2008). However, no known inhibitor of NRF1 or DDI2 has been identified and a model drug targeting NGLY1 is in early preclinical development. While it does not appear that the protease inhibitor nelfinavir directly binds DDI2, recent studies have shown that nelfinavir disrupts DDI2-mediated proteolytic activation of NRF1 and synergizes with PI in the setting of blockade of export of newly synthesized proteins from the ER and activating the UPR (Besse et al. 2017; Kisselev et al. 1999; Kisselev and Goldberg 2001; Meiners et al. 2003; Parzych et al. 2019; Walerych et al. 2016). Consistent with this, nelfinavir demonstrated promising clinical activity when used in combination with bortezomib and dexamethasone in heavily pretreated patients with bortezomib and/or IMiD refractory MM (Singh et al. 2011).

Molecular Glue Degraders and Proteolysis-targeting Chimera (PROTACs)

The IMiD thalidomide and its derivatives, lenalidomide and pomalidomide, are FDA approved oral agents for the treatment of MM. Cereblon (CRBN) has been identified as the molecular target mediating IMiD-associated MM cytotoxicity (Figure 23.1d). Together with DNA damage-binding protein 1 (DDB1), CRBN is the substrate receptor of the cullin 4 ring E3 ubiquitin ligase complex ($CRL4^{CRBN}$), which polyubiquitinates proteins to mark them for degradation. IMiDs such as lenalidomide act as a molecular glue to bind $CRL4^{CRBN}$ on the one hand and IKZF1 (Ikaros) and IKZF3 (Aiolos) on the other hand to enhance $CRL4^{CRBN}$-mediated IKZF1 and IKZF3 proteasome degradation (Adams 2004; Kroemer et al. 2013). Loss of IKZF3, in particular, results in downregulation of interferon regulatory factor 4 (IRF4), an essential gene that regulates other pro-survival genes including *MYC*, *CDK6*, and *CASP*, as well as several proteins involved in nuclear transport and protein folding such as KPNA2, NUP153, and *DNAJA2* (Krönke et al. 2014; Turnbull et al. 2017; Yu et al. 2004). IKZF1 and IKZF3 are also transcriptional repressors of interleukin 2 (IL-2), which may account for the T-cell immunostimulatory properties of IMiDs (Liang et al. 2020; Yamamoto et al. 2021).

Based on the understanding of IMiD-related targeted proteolysis, a new class of high-affinity cereblon E3 ligase modulators (CelMoDs) has been developed for maximal and rapid degradation of IKZF1 and IKZF3, with greater potency and specificity than IMiDs. A number of CelMods are currently in clinical trial (Table 23.1), and early results show promising activity, even in heavily pretreated lenalidomide and pomalidomide refractory MM (Chowdhury and Enenkel 2015). Another class of targeted protein degraders is proteolysis targeting chimeras (PROTACs), which are heterobifunctional small molecules with two binding motifs separated by a linker. These heterobifunctional molecules bind to an E3 ubiquitin ligase on one site and a specific protein of interest (POI) on the other site (Khong and Spencer 2011). There are currently a few IMiD-based PROTACs (also degronimids) in preclinical development in MM, which allow us to target protein previously considered to be undruggable targets, such as the transcriptional and epigenetic regulator bromodomain-containing protein 4 (BRD4) and the anti-apoptotic protein myeloid cell leukemia 1 (MCL1) (Table 23.1) (Neuse et al. 2020).

Endoplasmic Reticulum (ER) Stress and the Unfolded Protein Response (UPR)

Integral to the survival of MM cells is their ability to mitigate ER stress, which occurs when the protein-folding capacity of the ER becomes overwhelmed (Zhang et al. 2014). To prevent proteotoxicity, the ERAD pathway targets misfolded ER proteins out to the cytosol for proteasomal degradation (Emmerich et al. 2013). If or when the misfolded protein load exceeds the cellular thresholds (regardless of whether they accumulate within or outside the ER), the resultant ER stress induces activation of the tripartite UPR (activating transcription factor 6 [ATF6], inositol-requiring enzyme 1 [IRE1], and protein kinase RNA-like ER kinase [PERK] pathways) (Figure 23.1e) (Emmerich et al. 2013). Under physiologic conditions, the three arms of the UPR function as parallel feedback loops to mitigate ER stress. PERK (and downstream phosphorylation of eukaryotic initiation factor-2α [eIF2α]) and IRE1α (and downstream splicing of X-box binding protein 1 [XBP1]) mRNA activation regulates ER expansion and inhibits global protein synthesis; together with XBP1, ATF6 upregulates ER-resident chaperone proteins (e.g. BIP, protein disulphide isomerase [PDI], and GRP94) to enhance ER protein folding capacity (Emmerich et al. 2013). However, in the setting of prolonged or irremediable stress that overwhelms cellular compensatory ability to maintain proteostasis, the UPR functions as a molecular switch to trigger the terminal UPR and apoptosis through the PERK-ATF4-CHOP-GADD34 pathway (Bianchi et al. 2015; Emmerich et al. 2013).

Drugs Targeting the UPR

The impact of UPR activation on PI sensitivity is complex. For example, spliced XBP1 (XBP1s) is a key transcription factor that drives terminal differentiation of B lymphocytes to plasma cells (Brüning et al. 2009). Mature MM cells with higher expression of XBP1s secrete more antibodies and are more sensitive to PI compared to XBP1s-negative MM cells arrested at pre-plasmablast stage (Brüning et al. 2009; Das et al. 2017). However, in terminally differentiated MM cells, XBP1s can serve a cytoprotective role by increasing chaperone transcription and promoting ERAD, thus decreasing unfolded protein load and resulting in PI resistance (Bianchi et al. 2015). Consistent with this effect, knockdown of XBP1 has been shown to result in stress-induced MM apoptosis and increased sensitivity to PI (Leung-Hagesteijn et al. 2013; Soriano et al. 2016). Additionally, IRE1α endoribonuclease domain-specific inhibitors (e.g. MKC-3946) have also been studied as a way to disrupt XBP1 splicing and activate the terminal UPR through the PERK-ATF4-CHOP-GADD34 pathway (Kuhn et al. 2007). ER stressors such as tunicamycin, thapsigargin, and brefeldin A have demonstrated good, single-agent *in vitro* anti-MM activity and strong synergism in combination with PIs. However, their clinical use is limited by unanticipated untoward toxicities reducing their therapeutic index (Chang et al. 2015; Grice and Nathan 2016; Ramakrishnan and Kumar 2018; Song et al. 2016). ERAD inhibitors (e.g. eeyarestatin 1, DBeQ, and OSSL_325096) targeting p97-dependent retro-translocation have been shown in preclinical studies to synergize with PI in both PI-sensitive and resistant MM cell lines and patient-derived MM cells, with only minor toxicity observed in untransformed, non-secretory control cells (Kobayashi et al. 1999; Manton et al. 2016). However, early phase clinical trials with the first-generation p97 inhibitor CB-5083 were halted due to safety concerns. Clinical protocols with a second-generation p97 inhibitor are currently underway in hematologic malignancies.

Autophagy and Aggresome Pathways

There is *in vitro* evidence of close interplay between the proteasome and alternative proteolytic pathways, such as aggresomes or autophagy, as proteasomal inhibition induces formation of aggresomes and stimulates autophagy-mediated protein degradation (Koizumi et al. 2016; Lin et al. 2008; Milner et al. 2013). Aggresomes and authophagy thus represent a potential escape pathway and resistance mechanism to PI (Lee et al. 2003; Moi et al. 1994; Santo et al. 2012; Shaffer et al. 2008).

Autophagy is a highly conserved self-degradative, energy-recycling pathway that mediates lysosomal digestion of organelles, intracellular pathogens, and misfolded proteins in response to stressors such as nutrient and energy deprivation, ER stress, and hypoxia (Chan et al. 1993). In mammalian cells, there are three main types of autophagy, namely, macroautophagy (Figure 23.1f), microautophagy, and CMA, among which macroautophagy (hereon referred to as autophagy) is the most extensively studied (Liu et al. 2019; Saxton and Sabatini 2017). There are two types of autophagy, bulk (non-selective) and selective (Neefjes et al. 2011). Bulk autophagy begins with the non-selective engulfment of bulk cytoplasm by a developing phagophore and ends with the formation of the autolysosome and degradation by lysosomal hydrolases (Itakura and Mizushima 2010; Saxton and Sabatini 2017; Wang et al. 2016). Selective autophagy refers to the specific elimination of cargo bound to autophagy receptors and is classified according to the cargo involved (e.g. mitochondria [mitophagy], peroxisomes [pexophagy], ribosomes [ribophagy], and aggresomes [aggrephagy]) (Couillault et al. 2012). Some degree of basal autophagy is necessary in MM to alleviate proteotoxic stress by limiting immunoglobulin secretion and providing an alternative proteolytic pathway through crosstalk between the UPS, autophagy, and the UPR (Driessen et al. 2018; Shaffer et al. 2008; Suzuki et al. 2015; Yun et al. 2016). Despite this, combined inhibition of the proteasome and autophagy has reported inconsistent results, ranging from synergism to antagonism (Suzuki et al. 2015). One explanation is that although basal autophagy is protective, prolonged and overwhelming autophagy triggers autophagic cell death (Mimura et al. 2012; Tomlin et al. 2017).

As alluded to earlier, misfolded proteins that fail chaperone-mediated protein folding are transferred to the UPS and autophagy pathways for protein degradation. However, biophysical limitations (e.g. complex proteins structures may not always be sufficiently unfolded to enter the narrow proteasome CP) and/or overload of these protein clearance systems may lead to an excess of misfolded proteins that can be sequestered in spatially constricted sites (e.g. aggresomes or juxtanuclear quality control compartment [JUNQ]) for further triage (Won et al. 2019). Aggresomes are juxtanuclear structures containing accumulated polyUb proteins, which typically occur in response to proteotoxic stress (Figure 23.1g) (Chauhan et al. 2005). HDAC6 is responsible for aggresome formation by binding polyUb proteins with high affinity and dynein motor complexes, mediating shuttling of polyUb proteins toward the microtubule organizing center (MTOC) where they are sequestered within aggresomes (Chauhan et al. 2005). Following this, aggresomal protein clearance may be mediated by selective autophagy in a process involving p62/SQSTM1 and HDAC6 and/or the proteasome (Won et al. 2019). Preclinical studies show that HDAC6 inhibition is able to overcome PI resistance and synergizes with both PIs and IMiDs (Lamy et al. 2013; Mediani et al. 2019). Predicated on this knowledge, HDAC inhibitors have been successfully combined with PI in clinical trials, and HDAC6-specific inhibitors are in clinical development (Guang and Bianchi 2017; Sah et al. 2017).

Targeting Nutrient Metabolism to Enhance Proteotoxic Stress

Perturbation of amino acid, glucose, and lipid metabolism has also been implicated in PI resistance (Catley et al. 2006). Apart from preventing accumulation of misfolded proteins, the UPS also facilitates nutrient conservation through the conversion of misfolded proteins into usable amino acids (Catley et al. 2006). PIs may therefore cause intracellular amino acid shortage as a mechanism of cytotoxicity and trigger the ISR and autophagy to address nutrient scarcity (Catley et al. 2006). Consistent with this, amino acid supplementation is able to rescue cells from PI toxicity without reducing proteasome workload (Tian et al. 2014). The ISR is the main adaptive pathway activated in response to nutrient deprivation and a variety of other stress signals (e.g. viral infection, heme deprivation, and ER stress). Four distinct serine/threonine protein kinases (i.e. GCN2 [nutrient deprivation], PKR [viral infection], HRI [heme deprivation], PERK [ER stress]) act as sensors and these pathways converge on the phosphorylation of eIF2α, which eventually leads to global attenuation of Cap-dependent mRNA translation and preferential translation of genes that alleviate proteotoxic stress (Jagannathan et al. 2015; Leto et al. 2019). While the role of GCN2 has not yet been studied in MM, a pro-survival role has been described in response to UPS disruption in solid cancer cell lines (Ray et al. 2019). MM cells are dependent on glucose uptake and metabolism for survival. Knockdown of glucose transporter 4 (GLUT4) or hexokinase II (HKII) is lethal, and glucose deficiency is associated with increased VCP/p97 dependency and activation of the terminal UPR (Catley et al. 2006). Additionally, elevated glucose metabolism activity as a result of the hypoxic BM microenvironment has been observed in PI resistance (Murai et al. 2011). Various pathways implicated in glucose metabolism, such as hypoxia inducible factor-1α (HIF-1α), HIF-2α, HKII, and lactate dehydrogenase A (LDHA), are upregulated in relapsed and/or PI-refractory MM patients; however, it is unclear if these simply serve as biomarkers of advance-stage disease or rather have a causative effect in MM relapse (Murai et al. 2011). Consistent with this, disruption of LDHA or pyruvate dehydrogenase kinase-1 (PDK-1) signaling has been shown to restore PI sensitivity and have additive cytotoxic effects with bortezomib, respectively (Catley et al. 2006). Interestingly, use of the oral anti-hyperglycemic medication metformin for ≥4 years has been associated with reduced risk of progression from monoclonal gammopathy of undetermined significance (MGUS) to MM (Hussain et al. 2004). The precise mechanism of anti-MM activity of metformin has not been fully elucidated. While metformin has been implicated in autophagy modulation, the studies have been inconsistent about whether metformin induces or suppresses autophagy or what downstream effectors are involved. For example, one study showed that metformin induces autophagy and G0/G1 cell cycle arrest without apoptosis in MM cell lines through AMPK activation and mTORC1 and mTORC2 inhibition (Michallet et al. 2011). On the other hand, a distinct study demonstrated that metformin is also able to suppress bortezomib-induced GRP78-dependent autophagy to enhance bortezomib cytotoxicity (Driscoll and Chowdhury 2012). A phase 1 clinical trial is currently assessing the safety and efficacy of metformin, nelfinavir, and bortezomib in patients with RRMM (NCT03829020).

Tight control of fatty acid and lipid metabolism is also integral to survival and proliferation of MM cells, and this presents a therapeutic opportunity. Disruption of fatty acid synthesis with orlistat or statins was shown to inhibit MM proliferation in preclinical studies (Catley et al. 2006). Additionally, orlistat was also able to sensitize MM cells to bortezomib. Inhibition of β-oxidation or sphingosine kinase 2 (SK2), a lipid kinase involved in sphingolipid metabolism, was also able to inhibit MM proliferation (Catley et al. 2006). These examples highlight the potential utility of laboratory-based repurposing of drugs targeting metabolic pathways for cancer treatment. Advanced clinical studies are highly awaited to assess whether this approach is of therapeutic value.

The Role of Proteasome Inhibition in the Era of Immunotherapy

Immunotherapy has clearly revolutionized treatment of solid and hematologic malignancies, and the prognosis of MM patients has been impacted by the clinical advent of monoclonal antibodies and more recently cellular therapies. The observation that allogeneic stem cell transplantation offers a chance of cure based on graft-versus-myeloma effect has fueled research efforts focused on harnessing the power of the immune system against myeloma to achieve long-term control of the disease (Kategaya et al. 2017). The CD38-targeting antibody daratumumab and the SLAMF7-targeting antibody elotuzumab, the antibody drug conjugate belantamab mafodotin, a distinct CD38-targeting antibody isatuximab in combination with either pomalidomide or carfilzomib, and the first chimeric antigen receptor T-cell idecabtagene vicleucel (BCMA CAR-T) are all immune therapies recently FDA approved to treat RRMM. Moreover, several distinct BCMA CAR-T and bispecific target engagers (BiTEs) are currently in clinical trials in MM and are likely to result in a paradigm shift in the treatment of our patients.

While these agents are effective, they are not curative, and long-term control of the disease continues to be elusive. This is likely the result of both cancer-intrinsic mechanisms, including high genomic instability and clonal heterogeneity, as well as microenvironment-related mechanisms in the context of a cancer permissive BM milieu. Thus, there has been growing research interest in unleashing the immune system by using checkpoint inhibitors such as PD1/PD-L1 inhibitors. Results of early phase clinical trials with these agents have been disappointing (Kategaya et al. 2017). However, ongoing studies are evaluating inhibitors of distinct immune checkpoints or immune agonist proteins (e.g. LAG3 or TIGIT and OX40, respectively) alone or in combination with other drugs in relapsed MM, as well as in precursor diseases (i.e. smoldering MM) (Kategaya et al. 2017).

Recently, it has been shown that PIs are able to induce potent anti-MM immune responses through immunogenic cell death (ICD) (Orlowski et al. 2007). ICD leads to the release of endogenous tumor cell proteins (i.e. damage-associated molecular patterns [DAMPs]) which are translocated to the cell surface of the dying tumor cell, thereby increasing their uptake by dendritic cells for the cross-priming of CD8+ T-cells to stimulate cancer-specific immune responses (Bianchi et al. 2009; Yau et al. 2017). Specifically, *in vitro* experiments showed that MM cells treated with bortezomib released calreticulin (CALR) which is translocated to the cell surface, enhancing apoptotic tumor cell phagocytosis by dendritic cells, leading to CD4+ and CD8+ T-cell expansion selective against MM (Orlowski et al. 2007). *In vivo* experiments further demonstrated that bortezomib inhibited the proliferation of $5TGM1^{WT}$ murine MM cells engrafted in immunocompetent mice to a greater extent compared to those engrafted in immunodeficient mice or immunocompetent mice with 5TGM1 $Calr^{KO}$ tumors (Orlowski et al. 2007). Importantly, re-inoculation of untreated $5TGM1^{WT}$ cells two weeks after bortezomib-induced tumor regression in immunocompetent mice failed to result in tumor engraftment. Separately, vaccination of immunocompetent mice with *in vitro* bortezomib-treated $5TGM1^{WT}$ cells protected the mice from developing tumors on re-challenge with 5TGM1 cells (Orlowski et al. 2007). Importantly, ICD triggered by bortezomib in mice was associated with a type I interferon gene signature; and among MM patients treated with bortezomib, those with a type I interferon gene signature have improved clinical outcome.

Complementary to this, and perhaps somewhat counterintuitive as bortezomib inhibits the immunoproteasome, is a study showing that PIs do not reduce human leukocyte antigen (HLA) class I cell surface presentation even at doses that inhibit up to 80–90% of the chymotrypsin-like proteasome activity (Vij et al. 2012). PI had variable effects on the synthesis rates of individual HLA peptides: although a reduction in the levels of most HLA peptides was seen, the levels of many others were increased, suggesting that the composition of the peptide-MHC class I repertoire may be significantly altered (Vij et al. 2012). It would therefore be interesting to study if prolonged PI exposure (e.g. during bortezomib + lenalidomide maintenance in high-risk patients) can significantly impact the development of long-lasting anti-MM cellular immunity.

Conclusions and Future Perspectives

We live in an exciting time where a better understanding of MM and protein homeostasis biology has catalyzed the development of novel treatment strategies, resulting in a steady and significant improvement in the care and outcome of MM patients. The clinical use of PI and IMiDs as induction, consolidation, and maintenance therapy, with or without high-dose chemotherapy and ASCT, has resulted in a remarkable improvement in median overall survival (OS) for MM patients. Since the landmark approval of bortezomib in 2003, many more novel agents, including immunotherapies such as CAR-T cell therapy, monoclonal antibodies, antibody-drug conjugates (ADCs), have been approved for MM, and have led to unprecedented reduction in risk of progression or death in the RRMM setting. Further improvement in MM patient care will, at least in part, be derived from development of novel drugs targeting: impaired protein synthesis and degradation mechanisms (HDAC6, DUB, and DDI2 inhibitors as well as modulators of the UPR and autophagy); the cancer tolerant, immunosuppressive BM microenvironment (next-generation CAR-T cells, ADCs, and tumor vaccination strategies); as well as genomic instability and impaired DNA repair mechanisms.

Must Read References

Adams, J. (2004 May). The proteasome: a suitable antineoplastic target. *Nat. Rev. Cancer* 4 (5): 349–360.

Bondeson, D.P. and Crews, C.M. (2017 January 6). Targeted protein degradation by small molecules. *Annu. Rev. Pharmacol. Toxicol.* 57: 107–123.

Kisselev, A.F. and Goldberg, A.L. (2001 August). Proteasome inhibitors: from research tools to drug candidates. *Chem. Biol.* 8 (8): 739–758.

Schubert, U., Anton, L.C., Gibbs, J. et al. (2000 April 13). Rapid degradation of a large fraction of newly synthesized proteins by proteasomes. *Nature* 404 (6779): 770–774.

References

Adams, J. (2004 May). The proteasome: a suitable antineoplastic target. *Nat. Rev. Cancer* 4 (5): 349–360.

Akyol, S., Gercel-Taylor, C., Reynolds, L.C. et al. (2006 June). HSP-10 in ovarian cancer: expression and suppression of T-cell signaling. *Gynecol. Oncol.* 101 (3): 481–486.

Altun, M., Galardy, P.J., Shringarpure, R. et al. (2005 September 1). Effects of PS-341 on the activity and composition of proteasomes in multiple myeloma cells. *Cancer Res.* 65 (17): 7896–7901.

Andrews, N.C., Erdjument-Bromage, H., Davidson, M.B. et al. (1993 April 22). Erythroid transcription factor NF-E2 is a haematopoietic-specific basic-leucine zipper protein. *Nature* 362 (6422): 722–728.

Aronson, L.I. and Davies, F.E. (2012). DangER: protein ovERload. Targeting protein degradation to treat myeloma. *Haematologica* 97 (8): 1119–1130.

Auner, H.W., Moody, A.M., Ward, T.H. et al. (2013). Combined inhibition of p97 and the proteasome causes lethal disruption of the secretory apparatus in multiple myeloma cells. *PLoS One* 8 (9): e74415.

Baird, L., Tsujita, T., Kobayashi, E.H. et al. (2017 February 15). A homeostatic shift facilitates endoplasmic reticulum proteostasis through transcriptional integration of proteostatic stress response pathways. *Mol. Cell Biol.* 37 (4).

Baranowska, K., Misund, K., Starheim, K.K. et al. (2016). Hydroxychloroquine potentiates carfilzomib toxicity towards myeloma cells. *Oncotarget* 7 (43): 70845–70856.

Bejarano, E. and Cuervo, A.M. (2010 February). Chaperone-mediated autophagy. *Proc. Am. Thorac. Soc.* 7 (1): 29–39.

Besse, A., Besse, L., Stolze, S.C. et al. (2017). Nelfinavir blocks export of newly synthesized protein from the ER and interacts with ER-resident and mitochondrial proteins in an activity-dependent fashion. *Blood* 130 (Supplement 1): 3074–3074.

Besse, L., Besse, A., Stolze, S.C. et al. (2021). Treatment with HIV-protease inhibitor nelfinavir identifies membrane lipid composition and fluidity as a therapeutic target in advanced multiple myeloma. *Cancer Res.* 81 (17): 4581–4593.

Bianchi, G., Oliva, L., Cascio, P. et al. (2009 March 26). The proteasome load versus capacity balance determines apoptotic sensitivity of multiple myeloma cells to proteasome inhibition. *Blood* 113 (13): 3040–3049.

Bianchi, G., Richardson, P.G., and Anderson, K.C. (2015 June 1). Promising therapies in multiple myeloma. *Blood* 26 (3): 300–310.

Bondeson, D.P. and Crews, C.M. (2017 January 6). Targeted protein degradation by small molecules. *Annu. Rev. Pharmacol. Toxicol.* 57: 107–123.

Borjan, B., Kern, J., Steiner, N. et al. (2020 2020-January-22). Spliced XBP1 levels determine sensitivity of multiple myeloma cells to proteasome inhibitor bortezomib independent of the unfolded protein response mediator GRP78. *Front. Oncol.* 9 (1530).

Brancolini, C. and Iuliano, L. (2020 August 23). Proteotoxic stress and cell death in cancer cells. *Cancers (Basel)* 12 (9).

Braunlin, M., Belani, R., Buchanan, J. et al. (2021 February). Trends in the multiple myeloma treatment landscape and survival: a U.S. analysis using 2011-2019 oncology clinic electronic health record data. *Leuk. Lymphoma* 62 (2): 377–386.

Brüning, A., Burger, P., Vogel, M. et al. (2009 February). Nelfinavir induces the unfolded protein response in ovarian cancer cells, resulting in ER vacuolization, cell cycle retardation and apoptosis. *Cancer Biol. Ther.* 8 (3): 226–232.

Catley, L., Weisberg, E., Kiziltepe, T. et al. (2006 November 15). Aggresome induction by proteasome inhibitor bortezomib and alpha-tubulin hyperacetylation by tubulin deacetylase (TDAC) inhibitor LBH589 are synergistic in myeloma cells. *Blood* 108 (10): 3441–3449.

Cavenagh, J., Oakervee, H., Baetiong-Caguioa, P. et al. (2017 October). A phase I/II study of KW-2478, an Hsp90 inhibitor, in combination with bortezomib in patients with relapsed/refractory multiple myeloma. *Br. J. Cancer* 117 (9): 1295–1302.

Cenci, S., Mezghrani, A., Cascio, P. et al. (2006 Mar 8). Progressively impaired proteasomal capacity during terminal plasma cell differentiation. *EMBO J.* 25 (5): 1104–1113.

Cenci, S. and Sitia, R. (2007 July 31). Managing and exploiting stress in the antibody factory. *FEBS Lett.* 581 (19): 3652–3657.

Chan, J.Y., Han, X.L., and Kan, Y.W. (1993 December 1). Cloning of Nrf1, an NF-E2-related transcription factor, by genetic selection in yeast. *Proc. Natl. Acad. Sci. U.S.A.* 90 (23): 11371–11375.

Chang, S.H., Luo, S., O'Brian, K.K. et al. (2015 January). Association between metformin use and progression of monoclonal gammopathy of undetermined significance to multiple myeloma in US veterans with diabetes mellitus: a population-based retrospective cohort study. *Lancet Haematol.* 2 (1): e30–36.

Chang, T.-K., Lawrence, D.A., Lu, M. et al. (2018 2018/08/16). Coordination between two branches of the unfolded protein response determines apoptotic cell fate. *Mol. Cell* 71 (4): 629–636.e625.

Chauhan, D., Catley, L., Li, G. et al. (2005 November). A novel orally active proteasome inhibitor induces apoptosis in multiple myeloma cells with mechanisms distinct from Bortezomib. *Cancer Cell* 8 (5): 407–419.

Chauhan, D., Hideshima, T., and Anderson, K.C. (2006 October 23). A novel proteasome inhibitor NPI-0052 as an anticancer therapy. *Br. J. Cancer* 95 (8): 961–965.

Chauhan, D., Tian, Z., Nicholson, B. et al. (2012 September 11). A small molecule inhibitor of ubiquitin-specific protease-7 induces apoptosis in multiple myeloma cells and overcomes bortezomib resistance. *Cancer Cell* 22 (3): 345–358.

Chen, B., Retzlaff, M., Roos, T. et al. (2011). Cellular strategies of protein quality control. *Cold Spring Harb. Perspect Biol.* 3 (8): a004374–a004374.

Chen, Q., Cai, D., Li, M. et al. (2017 Aug). The homologous recombination protein RAD51 is a promising therapeutic target for cervical carcinoma. *Oncol. Rep.* 38 (2): 767–774.

Chen, T., Ho, M., Briere, J. et al. (2021 October 14). Multiple myeloma cells depend on the DDI2/NRF1-mediated proteasome stress response for survival. *Blood Adv.* 6 (2): 429–440.

Chowdhury, M. and Enenkel, C. (2015). Intracellular dynamics of the ubiquitin-proteasome-system. *F1000Res* 4: 367.

Couillault, C., Fourquet, P., Pophillat, M. et al. (2012 May 1). A UPR-independent infection-specific role for a BiP/GRP78 protein in the control of antimicrobial peptide expression in C. elegans epidermis. *Virulence* 3 (3): 299–308.

Coux, O., Tanaka, K., and Goldberg, A.L. (1996). Structure and functions of the 20S and 26S proteasomes. *Ann. Rev. Biochem.* 65: 801–847.

D'Arcy, P., Brnjic, S., Olofsson, M.H. et al. (2011 December). Inhibition of proteasome deubiquitinating activity as a new cancer therapy. *Nat. Med.* 17 (12): 1636–1640.

Das, D.S., Das, A., Ray, A. et al. (2017). Blockade of deubiquitylating enzyme USP1 Inhibits DNA repair and triggers apoptosis in multiple myeloma cells. *Clin. Cancer Res.: An Off. J. Am. Ass. Cancer Res.* 23 (15): 4280–4289.

David, E., Sun, S.Y., Waller, E.K. et al. (2005 December 15). The combination of the farnesyl transferase inhibitor lonafarnib and the proteasome inhibitor bortezomib induces synergistic apoptosis in human myeloma cells that is associated with down-regulation of p-AKT. *Blood* 106 (13): 4322–4329.

De Gassart, A., Bujisic, B., Zaffalon, L. et al. (2016). An inhibitor of HIV-1 protease modulates constitutive eIF2α dephosphorylation to trigger a specific integrated stress response. *Proc. Natl. Acad. Sci.* 113 (2): E117–E126.

Di, K., Lloyd, G.K., Abraham, V. et al. (2016 June). Marizomib activity as a single agent in malignant gliomas: ability to cross the blood-brain barrier. *Neuro. Oncol.* 18 (6): 840–848.

Dimopoulos, M., Siegel, D.S., Lonial, S. et al. (2013 October). Vorinostat or placebo in combination with bortezomib in patients with multiple myeloma (VANTAGE 088): a multicentre, randomised, double-blind study. *The Lancet Oncol.* 14 (11): 1129–1140.

Donnelly, N. and Storchova, Z. (2015 April-June). Aneuploidy and proteotoxic stress in cancer. *Mol. Cell Oncol.* 2 (2): e976491.

Driessen, C., Müller, R., Novak, U. et al. (2018). Promising activity of nelfinavir-bortezomib-dexamethasone in proteasome inhibitor-refractory multiple myeloma. *Blood* 132 (19): 2097–2100.

Driscoll, J.J. and Chowdhury, R.D. (2012 December 28). Molecular crosstalk between the proteasome, aggresomes and autophagy: translational potential and clinical implications. *Cancer Lett.* 325 (2): 147–154.

El Arfani, C., De Veirman, K., Maes, K. et al. (2018). Metabolic features of multiple myeloma. *Int. J. Mol. Sci.* 19 (4): 1200.

Emmerich, C.H., Ordureau, A., Strickson, S. et al. (2013). Activation of the canonical IKK complex by K63/M1-linked hybrid ubiquitin chains. *Proc. Natl. Acad. Sci.* 110 (38): 15247.

Fan, Y., Liang, Z., Zhang, J. et al. (2021 February 28). Oral proteasomal inhibitors ixazomib, oprozomib, and delanzomib upregulate the function of organic anion transporter 3 (OAT3): implications in OAT3-mediated drug-drug interactions. *Pharmaceutics* 13 (3).

Fassmannová, D., Sedlák, F., Sedláček, J. et al. (2020). Nelfinavir inhibits the TCF11/Nrf1-mediated proteasome recovery pathway in multiple myeloma. *Cancers* 12 (5): 1065.

Feng, Y., He, D., Yao, Z. et al. (2013 12/24/online). The machinery of macroautophagy. *Cell Res.* 24: 24.

Fok, J.H.L., Hedayat, S., Zhang, L. et al. (2018). HSF1 is essential for myeloma cell survival and a promising therapeutic target. *Clin. Cancer Res.* 24 (10): 2395–2407.

Fricker, L.D. (2020 Jan 6). Proteasome inhibitor drugs. *Annu. Rev. Pharmacol. Toxicol.* 60: 457–476.

García-Santisteban, I., Peters, G.J., Giovannetti, E. et al. (2013 August 10). USP1 deubiquitinase: cellular functions, regulatory mechanisms and emerging potential as target in cancer therapy. *Mol. Cancer* 12: 91.

Glick, D., Barth, S., and Macleod, K.F. (2010 May). Autophagy: cellular and molecular mechanisms. *J. Pathol.* 221 (1): 3–12.

Grice, G.L. and Nathan, J.A. (2016). The recognition of ubiquitinated proteins by the proteasome. *Cell Mol. Life Sci.* 73 (18): 3497–3506.

Gu, Y., Wang, X., Wang, Y. et al. (2020 November). Nelfinavir inhibits human DDI2 and potentiates cytotoxicity of proteasome inhibitors. *Cell Signal* 75: 109775.

Guang, M.H.Z. and Bianchi, G. (2017). Targeting protein synthesis and degradation in multiple myeloma: a look at What's on the horizon. *Am. J. Hematol. Oncol.* 13 (3): 11.

Guang, M.H.Z., Kavanagh, E.L., Dunne, L.P. et al. (2019). Targeting proteotoxic stress in cancer: a review of the role that protein quality control pathways play in oncogenesis. *Cancers* 11 (1): 66.

Gulla, A., Morelli, E., Samur, M.K. et al. (2021). Bortezomib induces Anti–multiple myeloma immune response mediated by cGAS/STING pathway activation. *Blood Cancer Dis.* 2 (5): 468–483.

Gupta, A.K., Li, B., Cerniglia, G.J. et al. (2007 April). HIV protease inhibitor nelfinavir downregulates Akt phosphorylation by inhibiting proteasomal activity and inducing the unfolded protein response. *Neoplasia* 9 (4): 271–278.

Han, S., Wang, B., Cotter, M.J. et al. (2008 February). Overcoming immune tolerance against multiple myeloma with lentiviral calnexin-engineered dendritic cells. *Mol. Ther.* 16 (2): 269–279.

Hanna, J., Leggett, D.S., and Finley, D. (2003). Ubiquitin depletion as a key mediator of toxicity by translational inhibitors. *Mol. Cell. Biol.* 23 (24): 9251–9261.

Hebert, D.N., Bernasconi, R., and Molinari, M. (2010 July). ERAD substrates: which way out? *Semin. Cell Dev. Biol.* 21 (5): 526–532.

Hideshima, T., Ikeda, H., Chauhan, D. et al. (2009 July 30). Bortezomib induces canonical nuclear factor-kappaB activation in multiple myeloma cells. *Blood* 114 (5): 1046–1052.

Hideshima, T., Mitsiades, C., Akiyama, M. et al. (2003 February 15). Molecular mechanisms mediating antimyeloma activity of proteasome inhibitor PS-341. *Blood* 101 (4): 1530–1534.

Ho, M., Patel, A., Hanley, C. et al. (2019). Exploiting autophagy in multiple myeloma. *J. Cancer Metastasis Treat.* 5: 70.

Hoang, B., Benavides, A., Shi, Y. et al. (2009 July). Effect of autophagy on multiple myeloma cell viability. *Mol. Cancer Ther.* 8 (7): 1974–1984.

Hussain, S., Wilson, J.B., Medhurst, A.L. et al. (2004). Direct interaction of FANCD2 with BRCA2 in DNA damage response pathways. *Human Mol. Gene.* 13 (12): 1241–1248.

Imai, Y., Hirano, M., Kobayashi, M. et al.(2019). HDAC inhibitors exert anti-myeloma effects through multiple modes of action. *Cancers* 11 (4): 475.

Itakura, E. and Mizushima, N. (2010 August). Characterization of autophagosome formation site by a hierarchical analysis of mammalian Atg proteins. *Autophagy* 6 (6): 764–776.

Ito, T.A.H., Suzuki, T., Ogura, T. et al. (2010). Identification of a primary target of thalidomide teratogenicity. *Science* 327 (5971): 1345–1350.

Iurlaro, R. and Munoz-Pinedo, C. (2016 July). Cell death induced by endoplasmic reticulum stress. *FEBS J.* 283 (14): 2640–2652.

Jacob, J.A., Salmani, J.M.M., Jiang, Z. et al. (2017 May). Autophagy: an overview and its roles in cancer and obesity. *Clin. Chim. Acta* 468: 85–89.

Jagannathan, S., Abdel-Malek, M.A., Malek, E. et al. (2015 November). Pharmacologic screens reveal metformin that suppresses GRP78-dependent autophagy to enhance the anti-myeloma effect of bortezomib. *Leukemia* 29 (11): 2184–2191.

Jan, M., Sperling, A.S., and Ebert, B.L. (2021 2021/07/01). Cancer therapies based on targeted protein degradation – lessons learned with lenalidomide. *Nat. Rev. Clin. Oncol.* 18 (7): 401–417.

Johnston, H.E. and Samant, R.S. (2021). Alternative systems for misfolded protein clearance: life beyond the proteasome. *The FEBS J.* 288 (15): 4464–4487.

Kategaya, L., Di Lello, P., Rougé, L. et al. (2017 2017/10/01). USP7 small-molecule inhibitors interfere with ubiquitin binding. *Nature* 550 (7677): 534–538.

Kawaguchi, T., Miyazawa, K., Moriya, S. et al. (2011 Mar). Combined treatment with bortezomib plus bafilomycin A1 enhances the cytocidal effect and induces endoplasmic reticulum stress in U266 myeloma cells: crosstalk among proteasome, autophagy-lysosome and ER stress. *Int. J. Oncol.* 38 (3): 643–654.

Khong, T. and Spencer, A. (2011 October). Targeting HSP 90 induces apoptosis and inhibits critical survival and proliferation pathways in multiple myeloma. *Mol. Cancer Ther.* 10 (10): 1909–1917.

Kisselev, A.F., Akopian, T.N., Castillo, V. et al. (1999 September). Proteasome active sites allosterically regulate each other, suggesting a cyclical bite-chew mechanism for protein breakdown. *Mol. Cell* 4 (3): 395–402.

Kisselev, A.F. and Goldberg, A.L. (2001 August). Proteasome inhibitors: from research tools to drug candidates. *Chem. Biol.* 8 (8): 739–758.

Kobayashi, A., Ito, E., Toki, T. et al. (1999 March 5). Molecular cloning and functional characterization of a new Cap'n' collar family transcription factor Nrf3. *J. Biol. Chem.* 274 (10): 6443–6452.

Koizumi, S., Irie, T., Hirayama, S. et al. (2016 August 16). The aspartyl protease DDI2 activates Nrf1 to compensate for proteasome dysfunction. *Elife* 5.

Kroemer, G., Galluzzi, L., Kepp, O. et al. (2013 2013/03/21). Immunogenic cell death in cancer therapy. *Ann. Rev. Immunol.* 31 (1): 51–72.

Krönke, J., Udeshi, N.D., Narla, A. et al. (2014 January 17). Lenalidomide causes selective degradation of IKZF1 and IKZF3 in multiple myeloma cells. *Science* 343 (6168): 301–305.

Kuhn, D.J., Chen, Q., Voorhees, P.M. et al. (2007 November 1). Potent activity of carfilzomib, a novel, irreversible inhibitor of the ubiquitin-proteasome pathway, against preclinical models of multiple myeloma. *Blood* 110 (9): 3281–3290.

Kuhn, D.J., Hunsucker, S.A., Chen, Q. et al. (2009 May 7). Targeted inhibition of the immunoproteasome is a potent strategy against models of multiple myeloma that overcomes resistance to conventional drugs and nonspecific proteasome inhibitors. *Blood* 113 (19): 4667–4676.

Kumar, S.K., Lacy, M.Q., Hayman, S.R. et al. (2011 August). Lenalidomide, cyclophosphamide and dexamethasone (CRd) for newly diagnosed multiple myeloma: results from a phase 2 trial. *Am. J. Hematol.* 86 (8): 640–645.

Kyle, R.A. and Rajkumar, S.V. (2008 Mar 15). Multiple myeloma. *Blood* 111 (6): 2962–2972.

Lamberto, I., Liu, X., Seo, H.S. et al. (2017 Dec 21). Structure-guided development of a potent and selective non-covalent active-site inhibitor of USP7. *Cell Chem. Biol.* 24 (12): 1490–1500.e1411.

Lamy, L., Ngo, V.N., Emre, N.C. et al. (2013 April 15). Control of autophagic cell death by caspase-10 in multiple myeloma. *Cancer Cell* 23 (4): 435–449.

Lee, A.H., Iwakoshi, N.N., Anderson, K.C. et al. (2003 August 19). Proteasome inhibitors disrupt the unfolded protein response in myeloma cells. *Proc. Natl. Acad. Sci. U. S. A.* 100 (17): 9946–9951.

Lee, S.W., Yeon, S.K., Kim, G.W. et al. (2021 January 29). HDAC6-selective inhibitor overcomes bortezomib resistance in multiple myeloma. *Int. J. Mol. Sci.* 22 (3).

Lehrbach, N.J. and Ruvkun, G. (2016 August 16). Proteasome dysfunction triggers activation of SKN-1A/Nrf1 by the aspartic protease DDI-1. *Elife* 5.

Lemonidis, K., Arkinson, C., Rennie, M.L. et al. Mechanism, specificity, and function of FANCD2-FANCI ubiquitination and deubiquitination. *The FEBS J.* 289 (16): 4811–4829.

Leto, D.E., Morgens, D.W., Zhang, L. et al. (2019 2019/01/17/). Genome-wide CRISPR analysis identifies substrate-specific conjugation modules in ER-associated degradation. *Mol. Cell.* 73 (2): 377–389.e311.

Leung-Hagesteijn, C., Erdmann, N., Cheung, G. et al. (2013 September 9). Xbp1s-negative tumor B cells and pre-plasmablasts mediate therapeutic proteasome inhibitor resistance in multiple myeloma. *Cancer Cell* 24 (3): 289–304.

Li, J., Zhu, J., Cao, B. et al. (2014). The mTOR signaling pathway is an emerging therapeutic target in multiple myeloma. *Curr. Pharm. Des.* 20 (1): 125–135.

Li, X., Matilainen, O., Jin, C. et al. (2011 June). Specific SKN-1/Nrf stress responses to perturbations in translation elongation and proteasome activity. *PLoS Genet.* 7 (6): e1002119.

Li, X. and Song, Y. (2020 2020/05/13). Proteolysis-targeting chimera (PROTAC) for targeted protein degradation and cancer therapy. *J. Hematol. Oncol.* 13 (1): 50.

Liang, F., Longerich, S., Miller, A.S. et al. (2016 June 7). Promotion of RAD51-mediated homologous DNA pairing by the RAD51AP1-UAF1 complex. *Cell. Rep.* 15 (10): 2118–2126.

Liang, F., Miller, A.S., Longerich, S. et al. (2019 2019/06/28). DNA requirement in FANCD2 deubiquitination by USP1-UAF1-RAD51AP1 in the Fanconi anemia DNA damage response. *Nat. Commun.* 10 (1): 2849.

Liang, F., Miller, A.S., Tang, C. et al. (2020 June 12). The DNA-binding activity of USP1-associated factor 1 is required for efficient RAD51-mediated homologous DNA pairing and homology-directed DNA repair. *J. Biol. Chem.* 295 (24): 8186–8194.

Lin, J.H., Walter, P., and Yen, T.S.B. (2008). Endoplasmic reticulum stress in disease pathogenesis. *Ann. Rev. Pathol.* 3: 399–425.

Liu, P., Zhao, L., Pol, J. et al. (2019 2019/04/02). Crizotinib-induced immunogenic cell death in non-small cell lung cancer. *Nat. Commun.* 10 (1): 1486.

Lonial, S. and Boise, L.H. (2011 Apr). Farnesyl transferase inhibitors, autophagy, and proteasome inhibition: synergy for all the right reasons. *Autophagy* 7 (4): 448–449.

Lopez-Girona, A., Heintel, D., Zhang, L.H. et al. (2011 Aug). Lenalidomide downregulates the cell survival factor, interferon regulatory factor-4, providing a potential mechanistic link for predicting response. *Br. J. Haematol.* 154 (3): 325–336.

Lopez-Girona, A.M.D., Ito, T., Miller, K. et al. (2012). Cereblon is a direct protein target for immunomodulatory and antiproliferative activities of lenalidomide and pomalidomide. *Leukemia* 26 (11): 2326–2335.

Lu, G., Middleton, R.E., Sun, H. et al. (2014 January 17). The myeloma drug lenalidomide promotes the cereblon-dependent destruction of Ikaros proteins. *Science* 343 (6168): 305–309.

Manton, C.A., Johnson, B., Singh, M. et al. (2016 2016/01/25). Induction of cell death by the novel proteasome inhibitor marizomib in glioblastoma in vitro and in vivo. *Sci. Rep.* 6 (1): 18953.

McConkey, D.J. (2017 January 15). The integrated stress response and proteotoxicity in cancer therapy. *Biochem. Biophys. Res. Commun.* 482 (3): 450–453.

Mediani, L., Guillén-Boixet, J., Vinet, J. et al. (2019). Defective ribosomal products challenge nuclear function by impairing nuclear condensate dynamics and immobilizing ubiquitin. *The EMBO J.* 38 (15): e101341.

Meiners, S., Heyken, D., Weller, A. et al. (2003 Jun 13). Inhibition of proteasome activity induces concerted expression of proteasome genes and de novo formation of Mammalian proteasomes. *J. Biol. Chem.* 278 (24): 21517–21525.

Meister, S., Schubert, U., Neubert, K. et al. (2007 February 15). Extensive immunoglobulin production sensitizes myeloma cells for proteasome inhibition. *Cancer Res.* 67 (4): 1783–1792.

Meyer, H.-J. and Rape, M. (2014 2014/05/08/). Enhanced protein degradation by branched ubiquitin chains. *Cell* 157 (4): 910–921.

Michallet, A.S., Mondiere, P., Taillardet, M. et al. (2011). Compromising the unfolded protein response induces autophagy-mediated cell death in multiple myeloma cells. *PloS one* 6 (10): e25820.

Milan, E., Fabbri, M., and Cenci, S. (2016 May). Autophagy in plasma cell ontogeny and malignancy. *J. Clin. Immunol.* 36 (Suppl 1): 18–24.

Milner, E., Gutter-Kapon, L., Bassani-Strenberg, M. et al. (2013). The effect of proteasome inhibition on the generation of the human leukocyte antigen (HLA) peptidome. *Mol. Cell. Proteom.* 12 (7): 1853–1864.

Mimura, N., Fulciniti, M., Gorgun, G. et al. (2012 June 14). Blockade of XBP1 splicing by inhibition of IRE1alpha is a promising therapeutic option in multiple myeloma. *Blood* 119 (24): 5772–5781.

Mimura, N., Fulciniti, M., Gorgun, G. et al. (2012). Blockade of XBP1 splicing by inhibition of IRE1α is a promising therapeutic option in multiple myeloma. *Blood* 119 (24): 5772–5781.

Moi, P., Chan, K., Asunis, I. et al.(1994 October 11). Isolation of NF-E2-related factor 2 (Nrf2), a NF-E2-like basic leucine zipper transcriptional activator that binds to the tandem NF-E2/AP1 repeat of the beta-globin locus control region. *Proc. Natl. Acad. Sci. U. S. A.* 91 (21): 9926–9930.

Motosugi, R. and Murata, S. (2019 2019-May-01). Dynamic regulation of proteasome expression. *Front. Mol. Biosci.* 6 (30).

Murai, J., Yang, K., Dejsuphong, D. et al. (2011 June). The USP1/UAF1 complex promotes double-strand break repair through homologous recombination. *Mol. Cell Biol.* 31 (12): 2462–2469.

Nakatogawa, H., Suzuki, K., Kamada, Y. et al. (2009 06/03/ online). Dynamics and diversity in autophagy mechanisms: lessons from yeast. *Nat. Rev. Mol. Cell Biol.* 10: 458.

Nandi, D., Tahiliani, P., Kumar, A. et al. (2006 March). The ubiquitin-proteasome system. *J. Biosci.* 31 (1): 137–155.

Neefjes, J., Jongsma, M.L.M., Paul, P. et al. (2011 December). Towards a systems understanding of MHC class I and MHC class II antigen presentation. *Nat. Rev. Immunol.* 11 (12): 823–836.

Negrini, S., Gorgoulis, V.G., and Halazonetis, T.D. (2010 March). Genomic instability–an evolving hallmark of cancer. *Nat. Rev. Mol. Cel.l Biol.* 11 (3): 220–228.

Neri, P. and Bahlis, N.J. (2013 June). Genomic instability in multiple myeloma: mechanisms and therapeutic implications. *Expert Opin. Biol. Ther.* 13 (Suppl 1): S69–82.

Neuse, C.J., Lomas, O.C., Schliemann, C. et al. (2020 2020/11/01). Genome instability in multiple myeloma. *Leukemia* 34 (11): 2887–2897.

Nishimura, N., Radwan, M.O., Amano, M. et al. (2019). Novel p97/VCP inhibitor induces endoplasmic reticulum stress and apoptosis in both bortezomib-sensitive and -resistant multiple myeloma cells. *Cancer Sci.* 110 (10): 3275–3287.

Obeng, E.A., Carlson, L.M., Gutman, D.M. et al. (2006 June 15). Proteasome inhibitors induce a terminal unfolded protein response in multiple myeloma cells. *Blood* 107 (12): 4907–4916.

Ohtake, F., Tsuchiya, H., Saeki, Y. et al. (2018). K63 ubiquitylation triggers proteasomal degradation by seeding branched ubiquitin chains. *Proc. Natl. Acad. Sci.* 115 (7): E1401.

Orlowski, R.Z., Nagler, A., Sonneveld, P. et al. (2007 September 1). Randomized phase III study of pegylated liposomal doxorubicin plus bortezomib compared with bortezomib alone in relapsed or refractory multiple myeloma: combination therapy improves time to progression. *J. Clin. Oncol.* 25 (25): 3892–3901.

Oyake, T., Itoh, K., Motohashi, H. et al. (1996). Bach proteins belong to a novel family of BTB-basic leucine zipper transcription factors that interact with MafK and regulate transcription through the NF-E2 site. *Mol. Cell. Biol.* 16 (11): 6083–6095.

Pakos-Zebrucka, K., Koryga, I., Mnich, K. et al. (2016 October). The integrated stress response. *EMBO Rep.* 17 (10): 1374–1395.

Park, H.R., Tomida, A., Sato, S. et al. (2004 September 1). Effect on tumor cells of blocking survival response to glucose deprivation. *J. Natl. Cancer Inst.* 96 (17): 1300–1310.

Parzych, K., Saavedra-García, P., Valbuena, G.N. et al. (2019). The coordinated action of VCP/p97 and GCN2 regulates cancer cell metabolism and proteostasis during nutrient limitation. *Oncogene* 38 (17): 3216–3231.

Qiao, L. and Zhang, J. (2009 May 29). Inhibition of lysosomal functions reduces proteasomal activity. *Neurosci. Lett.* 456 (1): 15–19.

Ramakrishnan, V. and Kumar, S. (2018 November). PI3K/AKT/ mTOR pathway in multiple myeloma: from basic biology to clinical promise. *Leuk. Lymphoma.* 59 (11): 2524–2534.

Ray, A., Song, Y., Chauhan, D. et al. (2019 2019/08/12). Blockade of ubiquitin receptor Rpn13 in plasmacytoid dendritic cells triggers anti-myeloma immunity. *Blood Cancer J.* 9 (8): 64.

Richardson, P.G., Sonneveld, P., Schuster, M.W. et al. (2005 June 16). Bortezomib or high-dose dexamethasone for relapsed multiple myeloma. *The N. Engl. J. Med.* 352 (24): 2487–2498.

Richardson, P.G., Vangsted, A.J., Ramasamy, K. et al. (2020). First-in-human phase I study of the novel CELMoD agent CC-92480 combined with dexamethasone (DEX) in patients (pts) with relapsed/refractory multiple myeloma (RRMM). *J. Clin. Oncol.* 38 (15_suppl): 8500-8500.

Rodriguez-Gonzalez, A., Lin, T., Ikeda, A.K. et al. (2008 April 15). Role of the aggresome pathway in cancer: targeting histone deacetylase 6-dependent protein degradation. *Cancer Res.* 68 (8): 2557–2560.

Rowinsky, E.K., Paner, A., Berdeja, J.G. et al. (2020 2020/10/01). Phase 1 study of the protein deubiquitinase inhibitor VLX1570 in patients with relapsed and/or refractory multiple myeloma. *Invest. New Drugs* 38 (5): 1448–1453.

Saavedra-García, P., Martini, F., and Auner, H.W. (2020). Proteasome inhibition in multiple myeloma: lessons for other cancers. *Am. J. of Physiol. Cell Physiol.* 318 (3): C451–C462.

Sah, D.P., Tian, G., and Finley, D. (2017). Meddling with fate: the proteasomal deubiquitinating enzymes. *J. Mol. Biol.* 429 (22): 3525–3545.

Samant, R.S., Livingston, C.M., Sontag, E.M. et al. (2018 2018/11/01). Distinct proteostasis circuits cooperate in nuclear and cytoplasmic protein quality control. *Nature* 563 (7731): 407–411.

San-Miguel, J.F., Hungria, V.T., Yoon, S.S. et al. (2014 October). Panobinostat plus bortezomib and dexamethasone versus placebo plus bortezomib and dexamethasone in patients with relapsed or relapsed and refractory multiple myeloma: a multicentre, randomised, double-blind phase 3 trial. *Lancet Oncol.* 15 (11): 1195–1206.

Santo, L., Hideshima, T., Kung, A.L. et al. (2012 March 15). Preclinical activity, pharmacodynamic, and pharmacokinetic properties of a selective HDAC6 inhibitor, ACY-1215, in combination with bortezomib in multiple myeloma. *Blood* 119 (11): 2579–2589.

Saxton, R.A. and Sabatini, D.M. (2017 March 9). mTOR signaling in growth, metabolism, and disease. *Cell* 168 (6): 960–976.

Schubert, U., Anton, L.C., Gibbs, J. et al. (2000 April 13). Rapid degradation of a large fraction of newly synthesized proteins by proteasomes. *Nature* 404 (6779): 770–774.

Seifert, U., Bialy, L.P., Ebstein, F. et al. (2010 August 20). Immunoproteasomes preserve protein homeostasis upon interferon-induced oxidative stress. *Cell* 142 (4): 613–624.

Shaffer, A.L., Emre, N.C., Lamy, L. et al. (2008 July 10). IRF4 addiction in multiple myeloma. *Nature* 454 (7201): 226–231.

Siegel, D.S., Martin, T., Wang, M. et al. (2012 October 4). A phase 2 study of single-agent carfilzomib (PX-171-003-A1) in patients with relapsed and refractory multiple myeloma. *Blood* 120 (14): 2817–2825.

Singh, A.V., Bandi, M., Aujay, M.A. et al. (2011 January). PR-924, a selective inhibitor of the immunoproteasome subunit LMP-7, blocks multiple myeloma cell growth both in vitro and in vivo. *Br. J. Haematol.* 152 (2): 155–163.

Song, Y., Ray, A., Li, S. et al. (2016 September). Targeting proteasome ubiquitin receptor Rpn13 in multiple myeloma. *Leukemia* 30 (9): 1877–1886.

Soriano, G.P., Besse, L., Li, N. et al. (2016 November). Proteasome inhibitor-adapted myeloma cells are largely independent from proteasome activity and show complex proteomic changes, in particular in redox and energy metabolism. *Leukemia* 30 (11): 2198–2207.

Suraweera, A., Münch, C., Hanssum, A. et al. (2012 October 26). Failure of amino acid homeostasis causes cell death following proteasome inhibition. *Mol. Cell* 48 (2): 242–253.

Suzuki, R., Hideshima, T., Mimura, N. et al. (2015 February). Anti-tumor activities of selective HSP90alpha/beta inhibitor, TAS-116, in combination with bortezomib in multiple myeloma. *Leukemia* 29 (2): 510–514.

Taniguchi, T., Garcia-Higuera, I., Andreassen, P.R. et al. (2002). S-phase–specific interaction of the Fanconi anemia protein, FANCD2, with BRCA1 and RAD51. *Blood* 100 (7): 2414–2420.

Tian, Z., D'Arcy, P., Wang, X. et al. (2014 January 30). A novel small molecule inhibitor of deubiquitylating enzyme USP14 and UCHL5 induces apoptosis in multiple myeloma and overcomes bortezomib resistance. *Blood* 123 (5): 706–716.

Tomlin, F.M., Uim, G.-D., Liu, Y.-C. et al. (2017 2017/11/22). Inhibition of NGLY1 inactivates the transcription factor Nrf1 and potentiates proteasome inhibitor cytotoxicity. *ACS Cen. Sci.* 3 (11): 1143–1155.

Townsend, D.M., Manevich, Y., He, L. et al. (2009 October 1). Nitrosative stress-induced s-glutathionylation of protein disulfide isomerase leads to activation of the unfolded protein response. *Cancer Res.* 69 (19): 7626–7634.

Turnbull, A.P., Ioannidis, S., Krajewski, W.W. et al. (2017 2017/10/01). Molecular basis of USP7 inhibition by selective small-molecule inhibitors. *Nature* 550 (7677): 481–486.

Usmani, S.Z. and Chiosis, G. (2011 June). HSP90 inhibitors as therapy for multiple myeloma. *Clin. Lymphoma. Myeloma. Leuk.* 11 (Suppl 1): S77–81.

Vangala, J.R., Dudem, S., Jain, N. et al. (2014 May 2). Regulation of PSMB5 protein and β subunits of mammalian proteasome by constitutively activated signal transducer and activator of transcription 3 (STAT3): potential role in bortezomib-mediated anticancer therapy. *J. Biol. Chem.* 289 (18): 12612–12622.

Vij, R., Siegel, D.S., Jagannath, S. et al. (2012 September). An open-label, single-arm, phase 2 study of single-agent carfilzomib in patients with relapsed and/or refractory multiple myeloma who have been previously treated with bortezomib. *Br. J. Haematol.* 158 (6): 739–748.

Vij, R., Wang, M., Kaufman, J.L. et al. (2012 June 14). An open-label, single-arm, phase 2 (PX-171-004) study of single-agent carfilzomib in bortezomib-naive patients with relapsed and/or refractory multiple myeloma. *Blood* 119 (24): 5661–5670.

Walerych, D., Lisek, K., Sommaggio, R. et al. (2016 August). Proteasome machinery is instrumental in a common gain-of-function program of the p53 missense mutants in cancer. *Nat. Cell. Bio.l* 18 (8): 897–909.

Walter, P. and Ron, D. (2011 November 25). The unfolded protein response: from stress pathway to homeostatic regulation. *Science* 334 (6059): 1081–1086.

Wang, M., Wey, S., Zhang, Y. et al. (2009 September). Role of the unfolded protein response regulator GRP78/BiP in development, cancer, and neurological disorders. *Antioxid. Redox. Signal.* 11 (9): 2307–2316.

Wang, Q., Mora-Jensen, H., Weniger, M.A. et al. (2009 February 17). ERAD inhibitors integrate ER stress with an epigenetic mechanism to activate BH3-only protein NOXA in cancer cells. *Proc. Natl. Acad. Sci. U. S. A.* 106 (7): 2200–2205.

Wang, W. and Chan, J.Y. (2006 July 14). Nrf1 is targeted to the endoplasmic reticulum membrane by an N-terminal transmembrane domain. inhibition of nuclear translocation and transacting function. *J. Biol. Chem.* 281 (28): 19676–19687.

Wang, X., Andreassen, P.R., and D'Andrea, A.D. (2004). Functional interaction of monoubiquitinated FANCD2 and BRCA2/FANCD1 in chromatin. *Mol. Cell. Biol.* 24 (13): 5850–5862.

Wang, X., Mazurkiewicz, M., Hillert, E.K. et al. (2016). The proteasome deubiquitinase inhibitor VLX1570 shows selectivity for ubiquitin-specific protease-14 and induces apoptosis of multiple myeloma cells. *Sci. Rep.* 6: 26979.

Wang, Y., Xu, W., Yan, Z. et al. (2018 March). Metformin induces autophagy and G0/G1 phase cell cycle arrest in myeloma by targeting the AMPK/mTORC1 and mTORC2 pathways. *J. Exp. Clin. Cancer Res.* 37 (1): 63.

Wertz, I.E., Newton, K., Seshasayee, D. et al. (2015 2015/12/01). Phosphorylation and linear ubiquitin direct A20 inhibition of inflammation. *Nature* 528 (7582): 370–375.

Wirth, M., Schick, M., Keller, U. et al. (2020). Ubiquitination and ubiquitin-like modifications in multiple myeloma: biology and therapy. *Cancers* 12 (12): 3764.

Won, H.R., Lee, D.H., Yeon, S.K. et al. (2019 2019/08/01). HDAC6-selective inhibitor synergistically enhances the anticancer activity of immunomodulatory drugs in multiple myeloma. *Int. J. Oncol.* 55 (2): 499–512.

Xiong, S., Chng, W.-J., and Zhou, J. (2021 2021/04/01). Crosstalk between endoplasmic reticulum stress and oxidative stress: a dynamic duo in multiple myeloma. *Cell. Mol. Life Sci.* 78 (8): 3883–3906.

Xu, H., Fu, J., Ha, S.W. et al. (2012 April). The CCAAT box-binding transcription factor NF-Y regulates basal expression of human proteasome genes. *Biochim. Biophys. Acta* 1823 (4): 818–825.

Yamamoto, L., Amodio, N., Gulla, A. et al. (2021 2021-January-27). Harnessing the Immune system against multiple myeloma: challenges and opportunities. *Front. Oncol.* 10 (3160).

Yau, R.G., Doerner, K., Castellanos, E.R. et al. (2017 2017/11/02/). Assembly and function of heterotypic ubiquitin chains in Cell-cycle and protein quality control. *Cell* 171 (4): 918–933.e920.

Yong, K., Cavet, J., Johnson, P. et al. (2016 January). Phase I study of KW-2478, a novel Hsp90 inhibitor, in patients with B-cell malignancies. *Br. J. Cancer* 114 (1): 7–13.

Yu, L., Alva, A., Su, H. et al. (2004 June 4). Regulation of an ATG7-beclin 1 program of autophagic cell death by caspase-8. *Science* 304 (5676): 1500–1502.

Yun, Y.S., Kim, K.H., Tschida, B. et al. (2016 February 18). mTORC1 coordinates protein synthesis and immunoproteasome formation via PRAS40 to prevent accumulation of protein stress. *Mol. Cell* 61 (4): 625–639.

Yun, Z., Zhichao, J., Hao, Y. et al. (2017 August). Targeting autophagy in multiple myeloma. *Leuk. Res.* 59: 97–104.

Zhang, L., Fok, J.H.L., and Davies, F.E. (2014). Heat shock proteins in multiple myeloma. *Oncotarget* 5 (5): 1132–1148.

Zhang, X.D., Baladandayuthapani, V., Lin, H. et al. (2016 May 9). Tight junction protein 1 modulates proteasome capacity and proteasome inhibitor sensitivity in multiple myeloma via EGFR/JAK1/STAT3 signaling. *Cancer Cell* 29 (5): 639–652.

Zhang, Y., Lucocq, J.M., Yamamoto, M. et al. (2007 December 1). The NHB1 (N-terminal homology box 1) sequence in transcription factor Nrf1 is required to anchor it to the endoplasmic reticulum and also to enable its asparagine-glycosylation. *Biochem. J.* 408 (2): 161–172.

24

Clinical Experience on Proteasome Inhibitors in Cancer

Noa Biran, Pooja Phull, and Andre Goy

John Theurer Cancer Center at HMH and Hackensack Meridian School of Medicine, Hackensack, NJ, USA

Take Home Messages

- Protein homeostasis is a tightly regulated process, which, thanks to a better understanding over the last two to three decades, emerged as potential therapeutic target in many conditions, especially in cancer cells, given their increased dependency on protein synthesis. The ubiquitin–proteasome system (UPS) plays a central role in cellular protein homeostasis and appears responsible for the degradation of ~80% of cellular proteins under normal conditions. At the core of the UPS, the proteasome can exist in multiple forms that can change through a dynamically regulated process.
- The development of multiple proteasome inhibitors (PIs), over the last two decades, with bortezomib as lead compound, has been the first success in targeting protein degradation in cancer, in particular in multiple myeloma where it became a foundation in all current standards. A benefit was also confirmed in amyloidosis, while multiple Pis have now been approved in MM to improve on efficacy, decrease resistance, reduce toxicity, or finally improve on convenience with oral agents.
- PI also showed benefit in lymphoma in particular mantle cell lymphoma, where bortezomib was approved both in relapse and in the frontline setting. Among other histological lymphoma subtypes a clinical benefit for bortezomib has also been recognized in rare conditions such as Waldenstrom's macroglobulinemia, CTCL, lymphoblastic lymphoma, plasmablastic lymphoma, and EBV-driven lymphoproliferative disorders as well as GVH.
- The level of success seen with Pis in hematological malignancies has not translated into solid tumors, where despite promising pre-clinical data, Pis have not translated into any meaningful activity.
- A better understanding of mechanisms of resistance (access to cells, level of cells' reliance on proteasome among others) might help expand the opportunities for targeting protein degradation. Several directions are being explored from increasing specificity (through targeting E3 ligases) to targeting other steps/structures in the UPS pathway and eventually new PROteolysis Targeting Chimeras (PROTACs), which rather than acting as a conventional enzyme inhibitor would work by inducing selective intracellular proteolysis on demand.

Introduction to Proteasome Inhibitors (Pis)

One of the hallmarks of tumor cells is greatly increased protein synthesis when compared to normal, non-transformed cells, which appears necessary to support a proliferative state within a tumor. In addition, protein synthesis is inherently an error prone process, with increased rates of mutated proteins in cancer cells. Maintaining proteome homeostasis, or proteostasis, involves complex mechanisms to supervise protein synthesis, protein folding and editing, assure conformational stability, and regulate protein degradation. It is estimated that up to 30% of newly synthesized proteins are degraded by the proteasome within minutes of their translation, which is thought to play a role in recycling of amino acids which is necessary to maintain translation (Schubert et al. 2000). The regulation of protein degradation encompasses vastly complex mechanisms with established redundancies to guarantee protein integrity. If disrupted, unfolded proteins accumulate within the cell, which can lead to proteotoxic stresses that can eventually impair cellular viability. Cellular integrity is maintained by built-in adaptive response mechanisms to proteotoxic stress, which can also be caused by other factors

Precision Cancer Therapies: Targeting Oncogenic Drivers and Signaling Pathways in Lymphoid Malignancies: From Concept to Practice, Volume 1, First Edition. Edited by Owen A. O'Connor, Stephen M. Ansell, and John F. Seymour.

such as hypoxia, oxidative stress, or nutrients deprivation. These cell rescue mechanisms were covered in more detail in previous chapters with a prominent role for molecular chaperones, such as heat shock protein (HSP), which are found upregulated across cancers compared to normal cells, where they have been shown to correlate with poor outcome. There are two major pathways for protein degradation: the ubiquitin–proteasome system (UPS), which appears responsible for degradation of ~80% of cellular proteins under normal conditions (Zhao et al. 2015), and the lysosomal degradation pathway as part of autophagy, an intracellular pathway for bulk protein degradation and removal of damaged organelles by lysosomes (Kenific and Debnath 2015).

Based on its functional characteristics the proteasome has often been referred to as the cell "garbage can," which could also be suggested by its structure. The core 20S proteasome is composed of four stacked units arranged into a cylindrical structure, including two symmetrical outer rings made of seven homologous α subunits and two inner rings comprising seven homologous β subunits. The three subunits β1, β2, and β5 (encoded by the genes *PSMB1*, *PSMB2*, and *PSMB5*, respectively), which are responsible for the proteolytic activity of the proteasome, able to cleave proteins with caspase-like activity (β1), trypsin-like activity (β2), and chymotrypsin-like activity (β5). Substrate proteins are typically degraded to short polypeptides in the range of 3–25 amino acids, which can then be further recycled into individual amino acids by distinct endopeptidases. The UPS is a multistep process, as shown in Figure 24.1, aiming at tagging and then targeting proteins through the 19S proteasome units, which cap the 20S core proteasome, which collectively form the 26S constitutive proteasome (CP). The initial step leads to tagging of a protein with a ubiquitin protein residue from an initial E1 "activating" enzyme, of which there are only two encoded in the genome. The second step involves an E2 ubiquitin conjugating enzyme (~40 individual coded), which adds polyubiquitin chains (at least four residues as a "classic signal for degradation"). The large diversity of E3 enzymes, supported by over 600 individual genes in mammalian cells, confers substrate specificity for final E2 ligase conjugation. The 19S RP unit is divided into two biochemically separable subcomplexes: the "base and the lid." The distal lid contains at least nine proteins that are responsible for ubiquitin binding and removal. One core component of the lid is a Jab1/MPN domain-associated metalloisopeptidase (JAMM) domain-containing protein Rpn11 (*POH1*/*PSMD14*), which couples deubiquitination with degradation. This offers an opportunity for the development of Rpn11 inhibitors such as capzimin inhibitor within the 19S RP (Li et al. 2017), broadening the scope of UPS inhibitors in the future. The base of the 19S RP includes a ring-shaped heterohexamer of ATPases that engage and unfold substrate polypeptides to allow for their translocation into the proteolytic pore of the 20S core unit. Ubiquitin moieties are removed while proteins substrates get eventually recycled into amino acids. Proteasomes are highly preserved structures from yeast to humans and can be found in both cytosol and nucleus. The amount of proteasome engagement in any given cell can vary greatly by cell subtypes, ranging from 20% to over 80% in plasma cells (rapid immunoglobulin turnover). In addition, the process can be inducible depending on the cell's phases and metabolic status or environmental conditions.

Another important alternate form of the proteasome is the "immunoproteasome" (IP). This form of the proteasome incorporates different proteolytic β-subunits (β1i, β2i, and β5i subunits instead of β1, β2, and β5 subunits) within the core 20S structure. The IP is preferentially expressed in cells of the immune system, induced by interferon-γ, and appears to result in different cleavage patterns allowing for peptide presentation via major histocompatibility complex (MHC) class I for example. Therefore, it is hypothesized that specific inhibitors of the IP might be more advantageous in targeting cells of the immune system, which may have indications in the treatment of blood cancers as well as autoimmune diseases. KZR-616 is a first-in-class specific IP inhibitor that has advanced to the stage of clinical trials in autoimmune diseases (Johnson et al. 2018), while M3258 just entered phase 1 in myeloma (Sanderson et al. 2021). Multiple proteasome forms are typically present in a single cell type, including hybrid proteasomes well beyond this review, which can change through a dynamically regulated process, suggesting that the proteasome is optimized for each cell function and over time. Finally, proteasomes are not only a site for proteins degradation, but they are also responsible for protein editing and protein activation, including the conversion of proteins into peptides with biological activity, a phenomenon highly preserved as well from yeasts to humans.

One of the remarkable aspects related to the development of proteasome inhibitors (Pis) is the wonder they were ever developed at all, given their apparent lack of "specificity," and the ubiquitous need for proteasome activity across both normal and malignant cells. The first Pis were developed to treat muscle wasting disorders with a lead compound called MG-132, which also inhibited other proteases in addition to the β5 subunit of the proteasome. The boronic acid derivative bortezomib (initially known as MG-341, and later on as PS-341) showed more favorable specificity toward the chymotrypsin-like activity of the proteasome. Although not successful for the initial indication of muscle wasting, screening of bortezomib through the NCI-60 cancer cell lines panel revealed that the large majority of tumor cell lines were sensitive to PS-341, with an average LC_{50} in the 5–7 nM (Adams 2002). Following initial pre-clinical studies demonstrating increased sensitivity of cancer cells to bortezomib relative to non-malignant cells, several groups started to explore the potential benefit of bortezomib in cancer, with early evidence of activity in myeloma, creating a momentum that has transformed several blood cancers well beyond merely this disease.

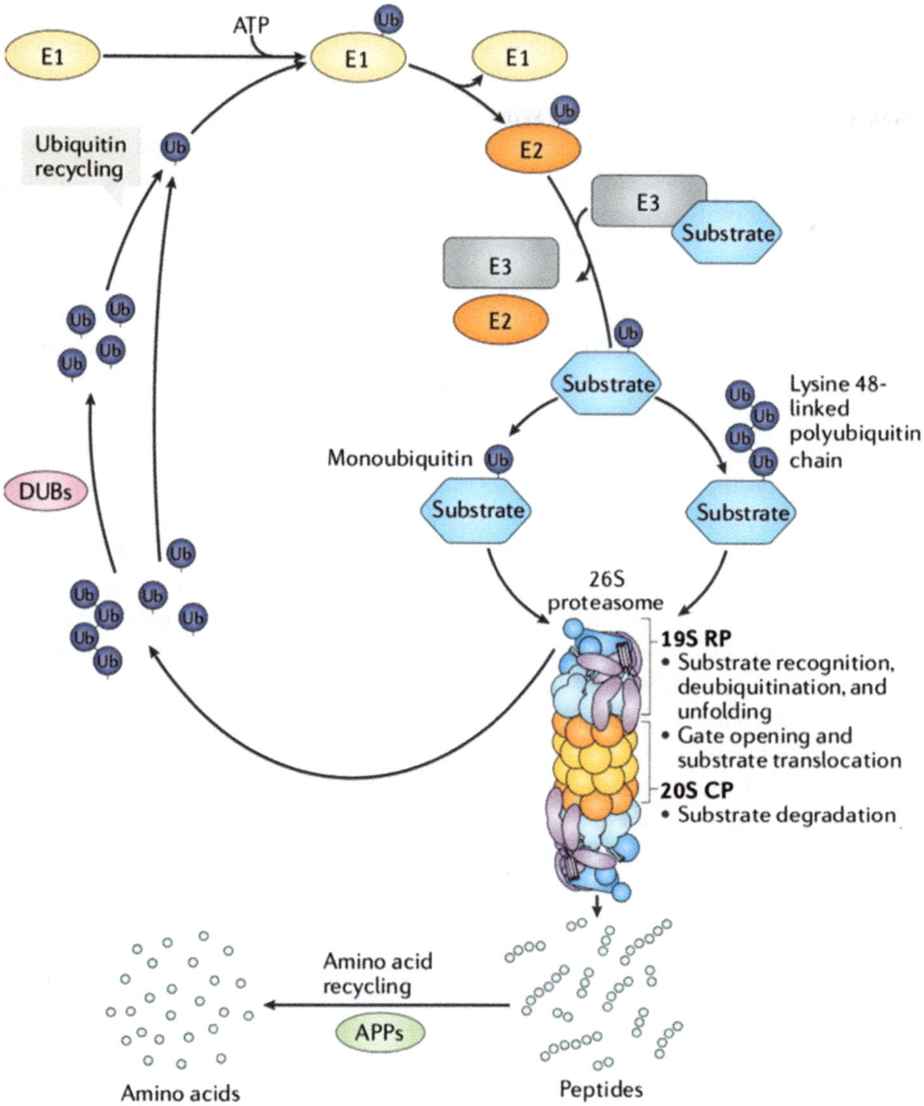

Figure 24.1 The ubiquitin–proteasome system. Ubiquitylation consists of the covalent binding of ubiquitin (Ub) to lysine residues exposed at the surface of targeted substrates. Ub is first activated by the ubiquitin-activating enzyme (E1) in the presence of ATP, before being bound to E1. The ubiquitin is then transferred from E1 to the ubiquitin-conjugating enzyme (E2). A ubiquitin ligase (E3) (which carries specificity) recruits the ubiquitin bound E2 enzyme and a substrate to transfer the ubiquitin from E2 to the substrate. The formation of lysine 48-linked polyubiquitin chains, the main signal for proteasomal degradation, is mediated by successive cycles of ubiquitin conjugation. Monoubiquitylation may be sufficient for proteasome targeting though four to six Ub residues are required to targeting to the 19S unit. When targeted to the proteasome, substrates are degraded into short peptides, which are further broken down into amino acids by aminopeptidases. The ubiquitin molecules are usually removed from the substrate by the proteasome by deubiquitylating enzymes (DUBs) before substrate degradation. Released free ubiquitin molecules are recycled for another round of ubiquitylation.

Clinical Activity in Plasma Cell Disorders

Role of Proteasome Inhibition in Plasma Cells: Mechanisms of Action and Mechanisms of Resistance

Pis are preferentially toxic to multiple myeloma (MM) cells due to a number of mechanisms. The exquisite sensitivity of MM cells lies in the fact that inhibition of the proteasome disrupts the degradation of toxic misfolded proteins presumed to derive from high-level immunoglobulin production. The "load versus capacity" model expects that cells with a high proteasome workload and degradative capacity, as is the case for immunoglobulin-producing MM cells, have a higher apoptotic sensitivity to proteasome inhibition (Bianchi et al. 2009). Polyubiquitinated proteins present in patient-derived MM cells seen by intracellular immunostaining correlate with immunoglobulin content and with apoptotic sensitivity to PI. Other notable mechanisms of action that have been proposed for the toxic effects of PI on MM cells include PI-induced endoplasmic reticulum (ER)-stress, disruption of genotoxic stress response mechanisms, and a reduction in pro-survival signaling by nuclear factor-kappaB (NF-κB)

(Mitsiades et al. 2003). Mechanisms of resistance to proteasome inhibition have been identified and will be discussed in more detail later. Mutations within the 20S proteasome, although not frequently observed in MM patients, have been demonstrated through protein structural modeling and functional assays, in which mutations in the Proteasome subunit beta5 (PSMB5) subunit of the 20S proteasome conferred resistance to bortezomib (Zhou and Chng 2019).

Proteasome Inhibitors with Clinical Activity in Multiple Myeloma

Bortezomib

Bortezomib was the first-in-class PI to be introduced into clinical use. It is a dipeptidyl boronic acid-based specific, reversible PI which targets the chymotrypsin- and caspase-like active sites. Bortezomib has minimal effect on trypsin-like activity and induces ER stress response associated with disruption of the unfolded protein response, an important mechanism of action of proteasome inhibition in MM because of the high intrinsic immunoglobulin production of the neoplastic cells (Reddy and Czuczman 2010). Importantly, bortezomib has also been associated with increased osteoblastic activity, decreased osteoclastic activity, and decreased bone resorption (Zangari et al. 2012). Ultimately this has translated into an association with increased bone formation, a phenomenon extremely crucial in a disease characterized by bone loss and diffuse osteolytic bone disease. The safety of bortezomib was initially established in phase 1 studies evaluating patients with relapsed/refractory MM (Orlowski et al. 2002). When administered intravenously (IV) on a twice weekly schedule, the maximum tolerated dose (MTD) was determined to be 1.3 mg/m^2. The dose-limiting adverse events (AEs) were peripheral neuropathy and diarrhea, while myelosuppression was not clinically significant.

Once safety was established, the efficacy of bortezomib was confirmed in large phase 2 studies, which led to high overall response rates (ORR) in patients who had previously progressed on standard cytotoxic therapies. The phase 2 SUMMIT study investigated single-agent bortezomib, showing an ORR of 27% with bortezomib and a median time to progression (TTP) of seven months compared with three months with patients' prior line of therapy (Richardson et al. 2003). This study led to the approval of bortezomib in 2005 for the treatment of relapsed and refractory MM (RRMM). Further phases 2 and 3 studies established the efficacy of bortezomib, first in the relapsed/refractory setting, and subsequently as a subcutaneous (SQ) injection, as re-treatment, in frontline MM, before autologous stem cell transplant and in combination regimens incorporated into conditioning, consolidation, and maintenance therapy. Table 24.1 summarizes the key clinical studies that established the efficacy of bortezomib in patients with MM across all settings of disease.

Table 24.1 Key phase 3 clinical trials utilizing bortezomib-based regimens in patients with multiple myeloma.

Study	Treatment regimen	N	ORR/CR (%)	Outcome duration
VISTA (San Miguel et al. 2008)	VMP vs. MP	344 vs. 338	71/31 35/4	TTP 24 mo; OS 56.4 mo TTP 16.6 mo; OS 43.1 mo
GIMEMA-MM-03–05 (Bringhen et al. 2010; Palumbo et al. 2014)	VMPT-VT VMP Weekly bortez Twice weekly bortezomib	254 257 372 179	89/38 81/24 85/30 86/35	3-yr PFS 54 mo; 3-yr OS 89 mo 3-yr PFS 41 mo; 3-yr OS 87 mo 3-yr PFS 50 mo; 3-yr OS 88 mo 3-yr PFS 47 mo, 3-yr OS 89 mo
IFM 2005–10 (Harousseau et al. 2010)	VD vs. VAD	240 242	78.5/14.8 62.8/6.4	PFS 36 mo; 3-yr OS 81.4 mo PFS 20.7 mo; 3-yr OS 77.4 mo
HOVON-65/GMMG-HD4 (Sonneveld et al. 2010)	PAD induction → Bortezomib maintenance VAD induction → Thalidomide maintenance	371/205 373/239	78/11 77/5	PFS 36 mo; 3-yr OS 78 mo PFS 27 mo; 3-yr OS 70 mo
APEX (Richardson et al. 2007)	Bortez vs. Dex	333 336	43/9 18/<1	Median TTP 6.2 mo; median OS 29.8 mo Median TTP 3.5 mo; median OS 23.7 mo

Abbreviations: CR = complete remission; mo = months; MP = melphalan, prednisone; ORR = overall response rates; OS = overall survival; PAD = bortezomib, doxorubicin, dexamethasone; PFS = progression-free survival; TTP = time to progression; VAD = vincristine, doxorubicin, dexamethasone; VD = bortezomib, dex; VMP = bortezomib, melphalan, prednisone; VMPT-VT = bortezomib, melphalan, prednisone, thalidomide followed by bortezomib, thalidomide; yr = year.

Carfilzomib

Carfilzomib, known as a second-generation PI, is an epoxyketone, and irreversibly binds to the 20S subunit of the proteolytic catalytic core. Like bortezomib, carfilzomib inhibits both the constitutive and IP, but it is structurally and mechanistically distinct from bortezomib, demonstrating sustained inhibition of chymotrypsin-like activity and appears to have a more potent and greater selectivity for the chymotrypsin-like protease compared with bortezomib (Jain et al. 2011). Off-target enzyme activity, specifically toward serine proteases, is minimal. Carfilzomib can trigger cell cycle arrest, induce apoptosis, and activate stress response pathways in MM cell lines, even those resistant to bortezomib. The Food and Drug Administration (FDA) approved carfilzomib in January 2016 for patients with RRMM. Based on promising results observed in early phase 1 clinical studies including PX-171–001 (O'Connor et al. 2009c) and PX-171–002 (Alsina et al. 2012) trials, several phase 2 studies evaluating the efficacy of single-agent carfilzomib were initiated. Key clinical trials which led to the FDA approval of carfilzomib in combination with dexamethasone, immunomodulatory drugs (ImiDS), and anti-CD38 monoclonal antibodies in the relapsed/refractory and upfront settings are shown in Table 24.2.

In 2013, Siegel et al. published safety data for single-agent carfilzomib for 526 patients with advanced MM who participated in four phase 2 studies PX-171–003-AO, PX-171–003-1, PX-171–004, and PX-171–005 (Siegel et al. 2013). The most common Aes of any grade included fatigue (55.5%), anemia (46.8%), and nausea (44.9%). Cardiac Aes of any grade were reported in 22.1% in the grouped analyses – of which 7.2% had cardiac failure, 42.2% dyspnea, and 33.1% renal impairment-related Aes. Notably the incidence of peripheral neuropathy was low overall, at 13.9%, including in patients with baseline peripheral neuropathy (12.7%), and the incidence of

Table 24.2 Key phases 2 and 3 clinical trials utilizing carfilzomib-based regimens in patients with relapsed/refractory and upfront MM.

Trial	Treatment regimen	Phases	N	ORR	Median PFS/ OS (mo)	Carfilzomib dose
Relapsed/Refractory						
PX-171–003 (Siegel et al. 2012)	Carfilzomib single agent	2	266	23.7%	3.7/15.6	20 mg/m^2 first cycle; 27 mg/m^2 cycle 2+
ASPIRE (Siegel et al. 2018)	KRD vs. RD	3	396 396	87.1% 66.7%	26.3/48.3 21.2/40.4	20 mg/m^2 first two doses, then 27 mg/m^2 all subsequent doses
ENDEAVOR (Dimopoulos et al. 2017)	Kd vs. Vd	3	464 465	77% 63%	18.7/47.6 11.2/not reported	20 mg/m^2 IV first two doses, then 56 mg/m^2 dose 3+
ARROW (Moreau et al. 2018)	Once weekly carfilzomib vs. Twice weekly carfilzomib	3	240 238	62.9% 40.8%	11.2/not reported 7.6/not reported	20 mg/m^2 dose 1 then 70 mg/m^2 for all subsequent doses 20 mg/m^2 first two doses, then 27 mg/m^2 for all subsequent doses
CANDOR (Dimopoulos et al. 2020)	DKd vs. Kd	312 154	3	84% 75%	NR/NR 16.6/NR	20 mg/m^2 days 1 and 2 then 56 mg/m^2 for all subsequent doses
IKEMA (Moreau et al. 2021)	IKd vs. Kd	179 123	3	87% 75%	NR/not reported 19.15/not reported	20 mg/m^2 days 1 and 2 then 56 mg/m^2 IV for all subsequent doses
Newly Diagnosed						
FORTE (Gay et al. 2021)	KRD + ASCT vs. KRD × 12 cycles vs. KCD + ASCT	2	158 157 159	97% (sCR 46%) 94% (sCR 44%) 91% (sCR 32%)	4-yr PFS 69% 4-yr PFS 56% 4-yr PFS 51%	20 mg/m^2 on days 1 and 2 then 36 mg/m^2 for all subsequent doses

Abbreviations: ASCT = autologous stem cell transplantation; DKD = daratumumab, carfilzomib, dexamethasone; IKd = isatuximab, carfilzomib, dexamethasone; KCD = carfilzomib, cyclophosphamide, dexamethasone; Kd = carfilzomib/dexamethasone; KRD = carfilzomib, lenalidomide, dexamethasone; mo = months; NR = no reached; ORR = overall response rates; OS = overall survival; PFS = progression-free survival; RD = lenalidomide, dexamethasone; sCR = stringent complete remission; Vd = bortezomib, dexamethasone; yr = year.

discontinuations or dose reductions attributable to Aes was low. In real-world practice, selecting patients <75 years of age and without any serious cardiac comorbidities and optimizing pre- and post-carfilzomib-hydration has significantly mitigated the risk of cardiac-related Aes.

Ixazomib

The long-term use of Pis can be limited by parenteral administration and treatment-related toxicities. Ixazomib, which also inhibits the chymotrypsin-like activity of the β5 subunit of the 20S proteasome, was the first oral PI to enter the clinic. It was FDA approved in November 2015 in combination with lenalidomide and dexamethasone for the treatment of patients with MM who have received at least one prior therapy. Approval was based on the results of the international, multicenter, randomized phase 3 TOURMALINE-MM1 study (Moreau et al. 2016), which demonstrated a statistically significant improvement in progression-free survival (PFS) with ixazomib, lenalidomide, and dexamethasone (IRd) versus placebo-Rd in patients with RRMM (median PFS 20.6 vs. 14.7 months; hazard ratio [HR] 0.74; 95% confidence interval [CI] 0.59–0.94; $p = 0.01$), with limited additional toxicity. The final analysis of the TOURMALINE-MM-1 study, after a median follow-up of over seven years, reported no statistically significant difference in median overall survival (OS). Ixazomib maintenance was evaluated in the phase 3 TOURMALLINE-MM-3 study which enrolled 656 patients and randomly assigned them to receive ixazomib maintenance (N = 395) or placebo (N = 261) following autologous stem cell transplantation (ASCT) (Dimopoulos et al. 2019). The ixazomib arm showed a modest improvement in median PFS, 26.5 months compared to 21.3 months ($p = 0.0023$, 95% CI 0.58–0.89) with placebo, and is therefore not routinely used in the maintenance setting.

Other Oral Proteasome Inhibitors Evaluated for Use in Patients with Multiple Myeloma

Oprozomib

Oprozomib is a tripeptide analog of carfilzomib, is orally bioavailable, and has shown anti-tumor activity comparable with carfilzomib in pre-clinical models (Zhou et al. 2009). The phase 1b/2 study NCG01416428 evaluated single-agent oprozomib in patients with relapsed hematologic malignancy including those with MM and Waldenstrom's macroglobulinemia (WM) (Ghobrial et al. 2016). In the phase 1b portion, the MTD was 300 mg/day when administered on days 1, 2, 8, and 9 of a 14-day cycle or 240 mg/day when administered on days 1–5 of a 14-day cycle. Among response-eligible patients with MM in the phase 2 portion, the ORR was 34% in the 300 mg/day cohort with responses seen even in carfilzomib-refractory patients.

Marizomib (NPI-0052)

Marizomib is a natural lactone compound derived from the marine gram-positive actinomycete bacterium *Salinospora tropica*. Marizomib is unlike both bortezomib and carfilzomib and does not exhibit cross-resistance with other PIs. Preclinical studies have demonstrated that marizomib-induced apoptosis is mediated primarily through activation of caspase-8 mediated signaling pathways (Chauhan et al. 2005) and did not affect viability of bone marrow stromal cells (BMOSCs). A phase 1 study (NPI-0052–102) evaluated the MTD, pharmacokinetics (PK), and pharmacodynamics (PD) of marizomib intravenously on two dosing schedules. The recommended phase 2 dose (RP2D) was 0.7 mg/m^2 over 10 minutes, and most common AEs were fatigue, nausea, diarrhea, and infusion site pain, while the ORR was 11% in 27 efficacy evaluable RRMM patients (Harrison et al. 2016).

Inhibitors of the Immunoproteasome complex

The immunoproteasome is a term that was discovered during studies of antigen presentation on the cell surface for T-cell recognition to stimulate immune response in collaboration with MHC class I molecules. The IP or 20Si differs from the 20S CP in that the proteolytic β5, β2, and β1 subunits are replaced with different subunits (low-molecular mass polypeptide (LMP)-6, LMP-10, MECL1, and LMP2). The IP was named based on its inducibility by interferon-gamma as well as the location of the *β1i* and *β5i* genes in close proximity to other genes of the MHC-II, including the *TAP1* and *TAP2* genes which encode the transporters associated with antigen presentation (Tanaka 1998). The currently approved PIs bortezomib and carfilzomib appear to target both the constitutive and IP s indiscriminately. This may explain, in part, some of the AEs observed, including peripheral neuropathy and gastrointestinal toxicity. It is possible that IP-selective inhibitors may have the ability to maintain the anti-myeloma efficacy, while reducing these toxicities, thereby increasing the therapeutic index. Several promising IP-specific inhibitors have been explored, including IP inhibitors PR-924, an LMP-7-selective tripeptide epoxyketone PI.

Role of Proteasome Inhibitors in Amyloidosis

Systemic (AL) amyloidosis is characterized by organ dysfunction arising from the aberrant deposition of insoluble, misfolded protein into organic tissues. In this subtype of amyloidosis, the implicated protein is composed of light chains secreted by malignant plasma cell clones (Vaxman and Gertz 2019). Given the similarity between the underlying pathophysiology of AL amyloidosis and MM, the management of the former entity has historically been extrapolated from myeloma-based regimens (Dispenzieri et al. 2022).

PIs have been considered a promising therapeutic intervention for AL amyloidosis given that the malignant plasma cells implicated in AL amyloidosis require proteasome activity to counteract light chain-mediated toxicity (Milani and Palladini 2020). Bortezomib is widely used in the upfront management of newly diagnosed AL amyloidosis, as it carries potent single-agent activity that is further enhanced in combination regimens such as with dexamethasone, or cyclophosphamide and dexamethasone, or with melphalan and dexamethasone (Vaxman and Gertz 2019). The more recent ANDROMEDA trial comparing the activity of bortezomib, cyclophosphamide, and dexamethasone with or without daratumumab found improved rates of hematologic complete response as well as improved organ responses favoring the daratumumab arm (Kastritis et al. 2021). Based upon this study, the quadruplet regimen has largely been accepted as the current standard of care in the management of newly diagnosed AL amyloidosis.

The use of carfilzomib has been limited in AL amyloidosis, as it has been associated with an increased risk of hospitalization in these patients, despite demonstrating clear activity in this disease setting (Vaxman and Gertz 2019). This phenomenon is likely due to the risk of cardiotoxicity associated with carfilzomib, as well as the poor tolerance of the concomitant hydration required with this drug, in patients with frequent underlying amyloid-related cardiomyopathy (Hasib Sidiqi and Gertz 2021). The recently published TOURMALINE-AL1 trial demonstrated a 53% hematologic response rate with the combination of ixazomib with dexamethasone in patients with relapsed/refractory disease. This study did not meet its primary endpoint of improved best overall hematologic response rate and OS with ixazomib as compared to physician's choice. However, the authors did note that time-to-event data favored the ixazomib arm, thus indicating that ixazomib has a role in the relapsed/refractory setting where few treatment options are available (Dispenzieri et al. 2022).

Rationale for Combinations w/ Proteasome Inhibitors

One of the earliest PI-based combination regimens used in MM was the addition of the alkylating agent cyclophosphamide to bortezomib and dexamethasone. This regimen has been historically considered a viable regimen in both the newly diagnosed as well as relapsed/refractory settings based on early trials demonstrating an 88% ORR in the upfront setting, and 75% in the relapsed/refractory population (Davies et al. 2007; Reeder et al. 2009).

PI and Cytotoxic Agents

One of the earliest PI-based combination regimens used in MM was the addition of the alkylating agent cyclophosphamide to bortezomib and dexamethasone. This regimen has been historically considered a viable regimen in both the newly diagnosed as well as relapsed/refractory settings based on early trials demonstrating an 88% ORR in the upfront setting, and 75% in the relapsed/refractory population (Davies et al. 2007; Reeder et al. 2009).

Combination of bortezomib with intensive cytotoxic therapy, most often VDT-PACE regimen as mentioned above (bortezomib, dexamethasone, thalidomide, cisplatin, doxorubicin, cyclophosphamide, and etoposide [Lakshman et al. 2017]), remains a highly effective salvage for patients with relapsed disease especially when followed by a consolidative stem cell transplant (Lakshman et al. 2017). While such combinations carry higher toxicities such as myelotoxicity, neutropenic fever, and nephrotoxicity, they do remain effective salvage regimens for patients with relapsed disease, especially when followed by a consolidative stem cell transplant (Lakshman et al. 2017). A similar combination, KD-PACE (a combination of carfilzomib with dexamethasone, cisplatin, doxorubicin, cyclophosphamide, and etoposide), has also been determined to be an effective regimen for patients with MM presenting with aggressive relapse or plasma cell leukemia to achieve disease control prior to consolidative therapy (Alsouqi et al. 2021).

PI + Immunomodulatory Agents (IMIDS)

As discussed above, the landmark phases 1/2 trial exploring the combination of bortezomib with lenalidomide and dexamethasone (VRd) proved this regimen to be both tolerable and effective in patients with newly diagnosed MM, with an 18-month PFS of 75% and OS of 97% (Richardson et al. 2010). A retrospective analysis of 1000 patients with newly diagnosed MM treated with VRd showed that this regimen was associated with a 97.1% ORR after induction therapy and a median PFS of 65 months (Joseph et al. 2020). Though not used as commonly in the current MM management in the United States, both bortezomib and carfilzomib have demonstrated effectiveness in treating both newly diagnosed as well as relapsed/refractory MM when combined with the immunomodulatory agent thalidomide (Rosiñol et al. 2012; Sonneveld et al. 2015).

In patients with newly diagnosed MM, the combination of carfilzomib, lenalidomide, and dexamethasone prior to autologous stem cell transplant demonstrated high efficacy with a 76% stringent complete response rate in the intent-to-treat population and a five-year PFS and OS of 72% and 84%, respectively (Jasielec et al. 2020). The ASPIRE trial compared the effectiveness of lenalidomide and dexamethasone with or without carfilzomib in patients with previously treated MM. This study demonstrated an improved PFS and ORR favoring the addition of carfilzomib to the lenalidomide/dexamethasone backbone. Importantly, in patients who have progressed on bortezomib-based and lenalidomide-based regimens, the combination of carfilzomib with pomalidomide has clear activity with a median time to response of two months, and a median PFS of 18 months (Sonneveld et al. 2018).

For transplant-ineligible patients, ixazomib combined with lenalidomide and dexamethasone (IRd) has been associated with improved complete/very good partial response rates as well as superior PFS compared with lenalidomide/dexamethasone alone (Facon et al. 2021).

PI and Monoclonal Antibodies

Over the past decade, monoclonal antibodies targeting CD38 (daratumumab, isatuximab) and SLAMF7 (elotuzumab) have emerged as effective agents in the treatment of both newly diagnosed as well as relapsed/refractory MM (Lonial et al. 2016). The addition of bortezomib or carfilzomib to the anti-CD38 antibody daratumumab provides effective disease control and improved PFS for patients with relapsed/refractory MM (Chari et al. 2019; Dimopoulos et al. 2020). Bortezomib plus dexamethasone can also be combined with elotuzumab in patients with relapsed/refractory disease, and is associated with improved PFS as compared to that of bortezomib/dexamethasone without the addition of the monoclonal antibody targeting SLAMF7 (Palumbo et al. 2015).

In patients with newly diagnosed MM, the combination of ixazomib with daratumumab is an effective treatment option for frail patients as this regimen has been associated with an ORR of 78% and a median PFS of 13.8 months in this patient population (Stege et al. 2021). More recently, there has been a growing interest in the use of upfront quadruplet regimens for managing patients with newly diagnosed MM. These regimens consist of a PI combined with an immunomodulatory agent, an anti-CD38 monoclonal antibody, and steroid (Goldschmidt et al. 2021; Landgren et al. 2021). Thus far, these trials have demonstrated favorable outcomes with PFS and/or minimal residual disease (MRD), though it should be noted that the utility of MRD has not yet been fully established in myeloma. Furthermore, given the activity of many of these agents at time of relapse, it remains to be seen if these quadruplet regimens are meaningfully associated with improved patients' outcome over time.

PI and HDAC Inhibitors

While histone deacetylase (HDAC) inhibitors have limited single-agent activity, they have improved efficacy when combined with PIs (Bae et al. 2018). There are several proposed mechanisms underlying the synergy between these two drug classes, including the concomitant proteasome and aggresome pathway inhibition, which promote apoptosis of the myeloma cell (Chauhan et al. 2005). The PANORAMA 3 trial reported a 62.2% ORR in patients with relapsed/refractory MM, who were treated with a combination of bortezomib, panobinostat, and dexamethasone, thus indicating this regimen as a promising option for patients with progressive MM (Laubach et al. 2021). Unfortunately, panobinostat was withdrawn from the United States market by the manufacturer in November 2021 (based on deemed "not feasible post-approval studies required by the FDA").

PI and Nuclear Transport Inhibitor Selinexor

Selinexor is an oral drug that reversibly inhibits exportin 1 (XPO1), a protein which has been shown to be upregulated in MM as well as in many other cancers. The phase 1b/2 BOSTON trial comparing the combination of bortezomib and dexamethasone with or without selinexor in patients with relapsed/refractory MM showed significantly improved PFS favoring the addition of selinexor to the PI-based regimen, indicating that this combination is an effective choice in the management of MM patients who have had disease progression after one to three prior lines of therapy (Grosicki et al. 2020).

Future Directions of PI-based Combination Regimens

Given that PIs have clearly been established as a cornerstone of the management of MM, it will be imperative to study the effectiveness of newly emerging anti-myeloma drugs when combined with PIs. For example, the newer B-cell maturation antigen (BCMA)-antibody-drug conjugate, belantamab, will need to be evaluated for potential synergistic activity when combined with PIs. The DREAMM-6 trial evaluating the clinical activity of belantamab in combination with bortezomib and dexamethasone is already underway. Other novel therapies including bispecific T-cell engagers directed at targets such as BCMA (elranatamab, teclistamab), FcRH5 (cevostamab), and GPRC5D (talquetamab) have recently emerged as promising therapeutic options for patients with relapsed/refractory MM (Bahlis et al. 2021; Chari et al. 2020). It remains to be investigated whether combinations of these agents with PIs and other anti-myeloma agents will prove to be safe and effective options for a heavily pretreated MM patient population, and such investigations are currently ongoing (NCT 05050097).

Clinical Activity of Proteasome Inhibitors in Lymphoid Malignancies

Besides MM, bortezomib was evaluated across the board in lymphoid malignancies as summarized in Table 24.3, with diverse results observed and the most impact seen in mantle cell lymphoma (MCL).

Clinical Activity of Bortezomib (BTZ) in Mantle Cell Lymphoma (MCL)

Bortezomib Phase 2 in R/R MCL Led to Early Approval

The early phase 1 testing of PS-341, or bortezomib, as first-in-class PI entering the clinic, explored several schedules and dosing (Hamilton et al. 2005) and helped establish the original biweekly schedule, while suggesting early on activity in myeloma and in some cases of lymphomas as well. The single-agent activity of bortezomib in MCL was recognized in two subsequent phase 2 trials in heavily pretreated patients in 2005 (Goy et al. 2005b; O'Connor et al. 2005). In one study, bortezomib was given at 1.5 mg/m^2 twice weekly for 2 weeks (days 1, 4, 8, and 11), followed by a one-week rest period (one cycle), patients were treated until progression

Table 24.3 Relevant studies for bortezomib in lymphoma.

Lymphoma subtype	Clinical activity	Approval	Comments
Mantle cell			
R/R setting	-Two concomitant phase 2 at 1.5 mg/m^2 days 1, 4, 8, 11 q 21 days showed ORR 40–50% (Goy et al. 2005b; O'Connor et al. 2005)		
	- Pivotal trial: BTZ was given at 1.3 mg/m^2 days 1, 4, 8, 11 (q 21 days) leading to 33% ORR and 8% CR rate with median DOR >9 mo (Fisher et al. 2006) and >28 mo in CR-CRu pts (Goy et al. 2009)	- BTZ was approved in 2006 based on the pivotal PINNACLE study	-BTZ became the first FDA approved drug in MCL -Responses were durable in CR/CRu pts although pts stopped therapy after four BTZ cycles post achieving CR-CRu
Frontline	Several combinations w/ R-CHOP type therapy (with slight differences in design and BTZ schedules) showed promising CR rate (Ruan et al. 2011) and PFS (Till et al. 2016)		
	- The benefit of R-CHOP-BTZ was confirmed by LYM-3002 trial, a large, randomized phase 3, comparing R-CHOP with R-CHP therapy (VR-CAP) (Robak et al. 2015) in non-transplant eligible MCL pts	- Led to first frontline regimen FDA approved in MCL in 2014	- VR-CAP led to doubling of median PFS 14.4vs–24.7 mo ($p < 0.001$) and increased CR rate 42vs–53% . ($p = 0.007$) -w/ longer follow-up VR-CAP also translated into > median TTNT (44.5 vs. 24.8 mo; $p < 0.001$) and into three years longer OS (90.7 vs. 55.7 mo; $p = 0.001$) (Robak et al. 2018)
	Combination w/ R-HyperCVAD led to high CR rate >80% but no difference in median TTF (55 mo not different than historical controls) (Romaguera et al. 2010)	NA	Other studies w/ VcR-CVAD, (Kahl et al. 2012) and/or HDT-ASCT in MCL (Chang et al. 2018) suggested also better outcome than historical controls
	RiBVD (rituximab, bendamustine, bortezomib at 1.3 mg/m^2 on days 1, 4, 8, and 11 and dexamethasone 40 mg on day 2) as first-line treatment in MCL pts ≥65 yr (Gressin et al. 2019)	NA	-With a median follow-up of 52 mo, primary objective was reached with a 24-mo PFS rate of 70%. -87% pts (47/54 pts) were found MRD -ve post induction which highly impacted outcome: 4-yr OS 86.6% vs. 28.6%, in MRD-ve vs. MRD + ve after induction ($p < 0.0001$)
	Based on BR-BTZ feasibility and early results, E1411 study assigned 373 pts into four arms (stratified by MIPI and age) to receive BR ± BTZ 1.3 mg/m^2 days 1, 4, 8, 11 – later amended to 1.6 mg/m^2 days 1, 8, (IV or SQ) for six cycles, followed a second randomization maintenance rituximab vs. rituximab + lenalidomide for 2 yr	NA	-No benefit found for BR-BTZ vs. BR based on ORR 89% vs. 89% and CR 59% vs. 66% and a 2-yr PFS of 74% vs. 79% - Planned correlative, MRD study (by flow and NGS) showed high MRD -ve rate: 87–89% at mid induction and 91–95% post completion of six cycles - MRD status significantly post third cycle impacted outcome, doubling median PFS from 26–29 mo in MRD + ve pts vs. 58.9 mo in MRD -ve pts (Smith et al. 2021)
Maintenance or consolidation post induction in MCL	In CALGB/Alliance 50403 trial, BTZ was used in a randomized phase 2 as consolidation (BC) or maintenance (BM) beginning on day 90 in 151 pts post standard CALGB induction (rituximab + augmented-dose R-CHOP/methotrexate, high-dose cytarabine followed by cyclophosphamide/carmustine/etoposide (CBV) and ASCT)	NA	-Both arms showed a median PFS significantly greater than 4 yr and higher than historical CALGB similar induction study - 8-yr PFS estimates in the BC and BM arms were 54.1% and 64.4%, respectively, and again significantly longer than prior similar trial without BTZ (Kaplan et al. 2020)

(Continued)

Table 24.3 (Continued)

Lymphoma subtype	Clinical activity	Approval	Comments
Mantle cell			
	Another study looked at six cycles of R-CHOP plus BTZ (1.3 mg/m^2 days 1 and 4 of 21-day cycles) followed by BTZ maintenance (1.3 mg/m^2 days 1, 4, 8, and 11 every 3 mo for 2 yr) in 65 newly diagnosed MCL (Till et al. 2016)	NA	2-yr PFS was 62%, and 2-yr OS 85% which appeared favorable comparing to R-CHOP alone (med PFS 12–14 mo)
Follicular lymphoma	-High ORR 70% w/ BTZ single agent in R/R FL in an early phase 2 by O'Connor et al. (2005)	NA	-Also promising activity in R/R FL with BTZ in combination with rituximab (Baiocchi et al. 2011)
	-Provided rationale for international phase 3 trial (LYM-3001) in R/R FL. - 670 pts received R alone (weekly × 4 then monthly × 5) with or without BTZ at 1.6 mg/m^2 on days 1, 8, 15, and 22 of each of 35 cycles maximum -Primary endpoint was PFS by ITT analysis -Randomization was stratified by risk factors	NA	-Patients received a median of five cycles altogether (mostly because of POD) -Though results showed statistically higher ORR (49% vs. 63%; $p < 0.0004$) and CR rate (18% vs. 25%; $p < 0.035$), after a median follow-up of 34.9 mo, there was no difference in median PFS 11.0 vs. 12.8 mo (Coiffier et al. 2011)
	-Other smaller studies looked at combinations w/ R alone or R-CHOP type chemotherapy (Craig et al. 2014)	NA	-Results appeared promising (de Vos et al. 2009) though with some differences based on schedules and dosing used while biweekly schedules seemed greater (Gerecitano et al. 2009; Ribrag et al. 2013)
Diffuse large cell lymphoma			
	-Minimal activity initially observed as single-agent BTZ in R/R DLBCL (only one PR in the original phase 2 from MD Anderson) (Goy et al. 2005a) -Early studies suggested BTZ had preferential activity in R/R ABC subtype, when combined with DA-R-EPOCH (Dunleavy et al. 2009), showing a significantly higher ORR 83% vs. 13% ($p < 0.001$) in the ABC vs. GCB subtypes and longer median OS of 10.8 mo vs. 3.4 mo ($p = 0.003$) - Other phase 2 also suggested that BTZ-R-CHOP alleviated the poor-risk features associated with the ABC (Ruan et al. 2011)	NA	-Earlier combinations studies provided a rationale for the PYRAMID trial, randomized phase 2 R-CHOP w or w/o BTZ in non-GC DLBCL (by Hans-based algorithm/IHC), which showed no benefit: 2-yr PFS 77.6% vs. 82.0% ($p = 0.61$) and no difference in ORR (98% vs. 96%) or 2-yr OS (88.4% vs. 93.0%) (Leonard et al. 2017) -Another study looked at VR-CAP vs. R-CHOP using this time a centrally confirmed IHC in 164 patients but showed no benefit either (Offner et al. 2015) -Next study of BTZ-R-CHOP vs. R-CHOP was REMoDL-B (>1 000 pts) – which evaluated the COO based on GEP (whole genome) (Davies et al. 2019). Study showed no difference either: 30-mo PFS 70.1% vs. 74.3% ($p = 0.28$) for the GC and ABC population, respectively -Of note the control arm as in many other studies with R-CHOP + X showed a 2- to 3-yr PFS of 70–80% in ABC/non-GC subtype, almost twice as expected based on historical controls (due to selection bias during enrollment process, [Maurer et al. 2018])
WM	BTZ single agent induces a PR in approximately 41–60% of patients with R/R WM (Dimopoulos et al. 2010; Treon et al. 2007), while the median PFS was 6–11 mo (Treon et al. 2009)	Used as off-label treatment	
	-In combination with rituximab, major response was seen in 50–83% of patients (Ghobrial et al. 2010)	Used as off-label treatment	

(Continued)

Table 24.3 (Continued)

Lymphoma subtype	Clinical activity	Approval	Comments
Mantle cell			
	-In untreated bortezomib with dexamethasone and rituximab (BDR) led to an ORR of 96% with 22% achieving a CR and/or near CR (Treon et al. 2009)	Used as off-label treatment	-Similar regimen was reported by the European Myeloma Network in previously untreated WM showing also very high ORR at 85% including 3% CR, 7% VGPR, and a median PFS of 43 mo and an OS at 7 yr of 66% (Dimopoulos et al. 2010)
	CyBORD is a regimen well documented in MM and amyloidosis. It was also tested in WM leading to high ORR (defined as at least MR) at 93% (14/15 pts) and the major response rate (defined as at least PR) was observed in eight patients (53%) (Leblebjian et al. 2015)	Used as off-label treatment	Showed high ORR and DOR in untreated WM
	-Carfilzomib, a neuropathy-sparing PI, in comb w/ rituximab and dexamethasone in pts w/ symptomatic WM showed high ORR 87.1% and was not impacted by MYD88 or CXCR4 mutation status (Treon et al. 2014)		
Marginal zone	Small nb of pts w/ MZL enrolled in other studies w/ iNHL (Craig et al. 2014; De Vos et al. 2009)	NA	Showed ORR 50–60%
SLL/CLL	Minimal activity w/ BTZ even looking at different schedules and cohorts (O'Connor et al. 2005; Faderl et al. 2006), or using carfilzomib (Awan et al. 2015)		*Ex vivo* data suggests fresh human plasma containing dietary flavonoid quercetin, blocked CLL cell killing by bortezomib (Wickremasinghe 2008)

Abbreviations: CR = complete response; CRu = complete response unconfirmed; DOR = duration of response; mo = months; nb = number; ORR = overall response rate; pts = patients; yr = years.

of disease (POD) or toxicity unless they achieved a complete remission (CR), in which case then received two additional cycles before being monitored. A total of 26 patients were enrolled, including 15 indolent non-Hodgkin's lymphoma (iNHL) (10 follicular lymphoma [FL], three small lymphocytic lymphoma [SLL], and two marginal zone lymphoma [MZL]) and 11 MCL patients, with a median of three prior therapies (range: 0–5), and by design a maximum of three prior cytotoxics allowed. Out of the 10 evaluable MCL patients, the ORR was 50% (one CRu and four PR), while the ORR reached 77% in FL (7/9 patients, including one CR and one CRu), and 2/2 PR in MZL, but no response observed in SLL (0/3). Of notice, similar activity was seen in relapsed versus refractory MCL (O'Connor et al. 2009a) with an ORR of 50% versus 43%. In the other phase 2 study, bortezomib was administered using a similar schedule of 1.5 mg/m^2 IV on days 1, 4, 8, and 11, every 21 days for a maximum of six cycles. Patients were stratified, based on pre-clinical data into arm A (33 MCL) or arm B (other B-cell non-Hodgkin's lymphoma [NHL]: 12 diffuse large B-cell lymphoma [DLBCL], 5 FL, 3 tFL, 4 SLL, 2 WM, and 1 MZL). In that study, there was no limitation in the number of prior therapies, leading to a median/range number of prior therapies of 3.5 (range: 1–12) in arm A and of 4 (range: 1–12) in arm B. Of notice in the MCL group, over 80% of the patients had prior intensive therapy with R-HyperCVAD and/or HDT followed by ASCT. Out of 29 evaluable MCL patients, 12 responded (six CR and six PR), producing an ORR of 41%, while the ORR was only 19% in arm B. These concomitant studies served as rationale for the PINNACLE study, a global phase 2 trial across 35 centers, which served as pivotal trial for bortezomib approval (Fisher et al. 2006). In that trial, bortezomib was given at a dose of 1.3 mg/m^2 on days 1, 4, 8, and 11 of a 3-week cycle, for up to 17 cycles or four cycles beyond initial reporting of CR/CRu. A total of 155 patients with R/R MCL, with a median age of 65 years, were included after one to two prior lines of therapy (including an anthracycline or mitoxantrone, and rituximab, each ≥1 line). Across the entire population, which received a median of one prior therapy (range: 1–3), bortezomib showed an ORR of 33%, with a CR rate of 8%. Responses typically occurred rapidly with a median time to first response of 1.3 months (i.e. within two cycles). The median PFS was 9.2 months, and the median duration of response (DOR) was 10 months overall, though it extended to over 27 months in patients who achieved a CR (Goy et al. 2009), despite being off therapy (four cycles beyond CR/CRu by study design). The toxicity profile confirmed prior observations from previous phase 2 studies with grade ≥3 AEs consisting of peripheral neuropathy (13%), fatigue (12%), and thrombocytopenia (11%). Longer follow-up confirmed the benefit of single-agent bortezomib in R/R MCL with a median OS of 36 months in responding patients (Goy et al. 2009). A pre-planned exploratory analyses of PINNACLE protocol-specified candidate biomarkers of bortezomib activity was performed by immunohistochemistry (IHC) and included materials available from 73 R/R MCL patients. Consistent with other studies, elevated Ki-67 (≥50% cut-off) was a marker of poor prognosis, demonstrating significant association with shorter TTP and OS. Elevated NF-κB p65 and low PSMA5 expressions demonstrated a trend for better response and were significantly associated with longer TTP, while elevated NF-κB p65 demonstrated a trend toward longer OS. These data were consistent with data from myeloma clinical genomics research, suggesting biomarkers relevance across tumor types (Goy et al. 2010). Based on the PINNACLE data, bortezomib was approved in 2006 in R/R MCL after at least one line of therapy. This was the first novel therapy in R/R MCL, in a population often resistant to standard therapies including high-dose therapy in that setting, while providing also an option to explore new combinations in MCL.

Importing Bortezomib in the Management of MCL

Frontline setting

A small phase 2 study of single-agent BTZ in MCL which included both treated and untreated MCL had shown similar activity with an ORR of 46% in both groups (Belch et al. 2007). However, based on PI mechanisms of action and preclinical data, the logical next step was to combine with existing regimens used in MCL. In an initial prospective phase 1/2 study, bortezomib was combined with R-CHOP in 36 previously untreated MCL patients, using a dose escalation of R-CHOP plus bortezomib (0.7 mg/m^2, 1.0 mg/m^2, 1.3 mg/m^2) on days 1 and 4 for six cycles. This study showed very promising results with an ORR of 91% including 72% CR/CRu and a median PFS of 23 months (Ruan et al. 2011). Similar results were observed in a phase 2 from SWOG, in which R-CHOP was combined with bortezomib (1.3 mg/m^2 on days 1 and 4 of 21 days cycles) followed by bortezomib maintenance (1.3 mg/m^2 days 1, 4, 8, and 11 every three months for two years) (Till et al. 2016). Among the 65 previously untreated MCL patients, the two-year PFS was 62% and OS 85%.

The benefit of BTZ-R-CHOP approach was confirmed in an important study, the LYM-3002 trial, a large randomized phase 3, comparing R-CHOP with R-CHP therapy (VR-CAP), where vincristine was replaced with bortezomib (given IV on days 1, 4, 8, and 11) for 6 to 8 to 21-day cycles and no maintenance, in previously untreated MCL patients and deemed ineligible for HDT and ASCT (Robak et al. 2015). The results, reviewed by an independent committee, were impressive with almost a doubling of the median PFS from 14.4 to 24.7 months after VR-CAP ($p < 0.001$) and a CR rate increased from 42% to 53% versus ($p = 0.007$). The superiority of VR-CAP also translated into a superior median time to next therapy (44.5 vs. 24.8 months [$p < 0.001$]) and with longer follow-up (82 months) into three years longer OS (90.7 months vs. 55.7 months; $p = 0.001$) (Robak et al. 2018). VR-CAP was associated with deeper reduction in tumor volumes across patients, though the benefit overall was most significant in low and intermediate MIPI (Verhoef et al. 2017). The benefit of adding bortezomib was confirmed by the impact of BTZ dose intensity received (≥4.6 mg/m^2/cycle), which revealed a strong predictor for OS post-VR-CAP confirmed in multivariate analysis (Robak et al. 2019). Serious AEs in the LYM-3002 study were observed in 38% and 30% of patients with VR-CAP and R-CHOP, respectively, including increased myelotoxicity in the VR-CAP arm comparing to the R-CHOP arm (grade ≥3 neutropenia 85% vs. 67% and grade ≥3 thrombocytopenia 57% vs. 6%). The LYM-3002 trial proved an instructive example in how to establish a new standard as VR-CAP became the first FDA approved regimen in the management of frontline MCL.

Of interest another *post hoc* analysis focused on a subgroup of 80 patients aged <60 years who did not receive stem cell transplantation despite medical eligibility. Again a benefit of VR-CAP over R-CHOP emerged, revealing a CR-CRu rate of 67% versus 39% and after a 40 months median follow-up, a median PFS (by independent radiology committee) of 32.6 versus 12.0 months, while the median OS was NR versus 47.3 months (Drach et al. 2018). Although these improvements did not reach statistical significance, likely due to small sample size, they illustrated again the benefit of VR-CAP even in a younger ASCT-eligible population. Finally, cost-analysis models in the United Kingdom suggested that VR-CAP brought higher quality-adjusted life year (QALY) gain and was a cost-effective option for previously untreated patients with MCL (Van Keep et al. 2016). VR-CAP was also studied as an induction regimen pre-ASCT combined with alternating high-dose (HD) AraC. The preliminary results demonstrate a CR rate of 86% (Smith et al. 2019) and continue to be studied in larger ongoing trials.

Bortezomib similarly was tested as part of multiple other front-line regimens in both high-dose and dose-intensive settings in younger patients and with standard regimens used in older people. In a phase 1 trial, bortezomib was added to the R-HyperCVAD combination at a fixed dose of 1.3 mg/m^2 IV on days 2 and 5 and using a dose escalation approach (0.7, 1, 1.3 mg/m^2) to the R-M/A regimen. After the initial 20 patients showed no unexpected toxicity (Romaguera et al. 2010), the Bz-R-HyperCVAD/BzR-MA combination was expanded to include 95 newly diagnosed MCL patients. The ORR at end of six cycles was 100% with a CR rate of 82%, while the toxicity profile was not significantly different than what had been previously reported with standard R-HyperCVAD. However, though median OS had not been reached, the median time to treatment failure (TTF) was 55 months, which was not different from the original R-HyperCVAD (Romaguera et al. 2018). An alternative modified version of HyperCVAD (modified hyper-cyclophosphamide, doxorubicin, vincristine, dexamethasone) was also studied in combination with bortezomib (VcR-CVAD) in untreated MCL, using six cycles followed by maintenance rituximab (MR) for two years (Chang et al. 2018). Transplant-eligible patients had the option of ASCT consolidation instead of MR. The primary endpoint was CR rate after VcR-CVAD, while secondary endpoints included ORR, PFS, and OS. For the 75 patients enrolled with a median age of 62 years (range: 40–76), the ORR was 95%, with 68% of patients achieving a CR, again with no unexpected toxicities (Kahl et al. 2012). After a median follow-up of 4.5 years, the three-year PFS and OS were 72% and 88%, respectively, suggesting an advantage comparing to historical controls, with no difference in PFS or OS between patients treated with MR (n = 44) versus ASCT (n = 22) (Chang et al. 2018).

Bendamustine and rituximab (BR) in combination became a commonly used first-line therapy in MCL based on the phase 3 trial StiL NHL1 study, comparing R-CHOP with BR in iNHL and MCL (Rummel et al. 2013). In long-term follow-up, there was an increase of over 12 months in the median PFS from 22 to 35 months in favor of BR versus R-CHOP, with no difference in OS, though combined with its more favorable toxicity profile, BR provided a new backbone for combination with novel agents. A phase 2 study evaluated RiBVD (rituximab, bendamustine, bortezomib at 1.3 mg/m^2 on days 1, 4, 8, and 11 and dexamethasone 40 mg on day 2) as first-line treatment in MCL patients ≥65 years. The study required no maintenance therapy and was designed with the primary endpoint to increase the 18-month PFS rate to 65% or higher. A total of 74 patients (median age of 73 years) received a maximum of six 28-day cycles. With a median follow-up of 52 months, the primary objective was reached with a 24-month PFS rate of 70%. Of notice, neither the MCL prognostic index MIPI nor PET-based response or Ki-67 value (cut off ≥30%) showed a significant prognostic impact on OS. However, after six cycles of treatment, 54 of 59 responding patients were analyzed for peripheral blood MRD. A total of 87% (47/54) of these responding patients were negative, which translated into a highly significant difference in outcome at four years with an OS of 86.6% in patients MRD-ve versus 28.6%, in patients with persistent MRD after induction ($p < 0.0001$). Grades 3–4 toxicities included neutropenia (51%), thrombocytopenia (35%), and lymphopenia (65%) as well as fatigue (18.5%) and neuropathy (15%). These results compared favorably with other regimens producing high MRD negative responders, which are now widely being recognized as an increasingly impactful factor in managing MCL patients (Gressin et al. 2019).

Based on the BR-BTZ feasibility and early results, the US-Canadian Intergroup trial E1411 (conducted between May 2012 and September 2016) randomly assigned 373 patients into four arms (stratified by MIPI and age [</≥60 years]) to receive BR ± bortezomib (bortezomib 1.3 mg/m^2 days 1, 4, 8, 11 – later amended to 1.6 mg/m^2 days 1, 8, IV or SQ) for six cycles, followed (second randomization) by maintenance rituximab versus rituximab + lenalidomide for two years. This study showed no impact with an ORR of 89% versus 89% and CR 59% versus 66% for BR versus BR-BTZ, respectively, and a two-year PFS of 74% versus 79%. However, as a planned correlative, MRD was assessed after cycle 3 of induction (I3), end of induction (EOI), and after four cycles of maintenance (C4) using two methods: clonoSEQ® NGS-based MRD assay (Adaptive Biotechnologies, Seattle, WA) and flow cytometry (FC) (I3 and EOI only) performed at a central laboratory (Mayo Clinic). While NGS may have higher sensitivity, the sensitivity of 10^{-4} obtainable by flow was used as cutoff for both NGS and FC. Results showed high concordance between NGS and FC and showed that at mid induction 87–89% of patients had achieved FC or NGS MRD negative status. This number rose to 91–95% post completion of six cycles. The MRD status post the first three cycles by either NGS or FC had a significant impact on outcome, doubling the median PFS from 26 to 29 months in patients with MRD positive by NGS or FC to 58.9 months in MRD negative patients. Analysis by treatment arm with longer follow-up, as well as comparison with centrally reviewed PET/CTs included in this study, is still ongoing, but at this point, results did not suggest any benefit from the addition of bortezomib to a BR backbone (Smith et al. 2021).

Differences of regimens and schedules used in combining BTZ with chemoimmunotherapy might explain some of the differences seen among studies, in particular studies looking at weekly BTZ schedules as single agent versus biweekly showed clearly less activity (Gerecitano et al. 2009) while most combination studies used a weekly approach based on concern of potential added toxicities. VR-CAP, which used a biweekly standard BTZ dosing, showed clear superiority and offers a new platform for combinations with other new agents, such as the ongoing study of VR-CAP with Bruton's tyrosine kinase inhibitor (BTKi) acalabrutinib.

Bortezomib Role as Maintenance or Consolidation Post Induction

Besides combinations of BTZ with chemoimmunotherapy, others explored the use of BTZ as consolidation or maintenance to prevent the typical recurrence pattern seen after induction in MCL. In one randomized phase 2 trial, from the CALGB/Alliance 50403 trial, bortezomib was used as consolidation (BC) or maintenance (BM). Following augmented-dose R-CHOP/methotrexate, high-dose cytarabine followed by cyclophosphamide/carmustine/etoposide (CBV) autotransplant, and rituximab, patients were randomized to BC (1.3 mg/m^2 IV days 1, 4, 8, 11 of a three-week cycle for four cycles) or BM (1.6 mg/m^2 IV once weekly × 4, every eight weeks for 18 months) beginning on day 90. The primary endpoint was PFS from randomization for each arm. Both BM and BC added toxicities mostly myelosuppression and neuropathy but were manageable. Of the 151 patients enrolled; 118 (80%) underwent ASCT, and 102 (68%) were randomized. Both arms met the primary endpoint, with a median PFS significantly greater than four years ($p < 0.001$). The eight-year PFS estimates in the BC and BM arms were 54.1% and 64.4%, respectively, and were significantly longer for transplanted patients on CALGB/ALLIANCE-50403 compared with those on CALGB-ALLIANCE 59909, prior similar trial without BTZ. PFS and OS were significantly better for those who were MRD-negative post induction (Kaplan et al. 2020). In another study, authors looked at six cycles of R-CHOP plus bortezomib (1.3 mg/m^2 days 1 and 4 of 21-day cycles) followed by bortezomib maintenance (1.3 mg/m^2 days 1, 4, 8, and 11 every three months for two years) in 65 newly diagnosed MCL. The treatment was well tolerated, and toxicities were mainly hematologic and manageable, and grade ≥3 peripheral neuropathy was about 5% (Till et al. 2016). With a median follow-up of 6.8 years, the two-year PFS was 62%, and the two-year OS 85%. Though these results appear favorable comparing to R-CHOP alone (median PFS 12–14 months), there was still a persistent pattern of relapse and the five-year PFS and OS were 28% and 66%, respectively. Of notice, the MIPI scores significantly impacted the two-year PFS but did not predict long-term (≥5 years) PFS. An additional study also looked at bortezomib combination with DA-R-EPOCH this time, followed by maintenance bortezomib versus observation. Treatment was divided into three parts: part A – bortezomib (1.3 or 1.5 mg/m^2) on days 1, 4, 8, and 11 for one cycle; part B – bortezomib (1.3 mg/m^2) on days 1 and 4 of DA-EPOCH-R (as previously described) for six cycles; and part C in which responding patients (CR or PR) after part B were randomized to maintenance bortezomib (1.3 mg/m^2 on days 1, 4, 8, and 11 q 8 weeks for 18 months) or observation. A total of 43 patients were treated with a median PFS of 48 months and a four-year OS of 80%. Maintenance bortezomib (13 patients) or observation (11 patients) had similar PFS ($p = 0.41$) and 1/3 patients required dose reduction because of neuropathy. Another small study (28 patients) looked at combining BTZ and rituximab as maintenance in patients who achieved a CR post induction and HDT-ASCT leading to a promising two-year disease-free survival (DFS) of 90% and two-year OS of 94% (Chen et al. 2018). Adding bortezomib as consolidation and/or maintenance strategy seemed encouraging, particularly in the CALGB study. However, the field has evolved, and the concept of maintenance is now fully established, and part of standard of care in MCL with rituximab in both older and younger patients (Kluin-Nelemans et al. 2020; Le Gouill et al. 2017).

Bortezomib Role in the Management of R/R MCL

The addition of BTZ was concomitantly explored through several combinations in R/R MCL in order to build upon the single-agent observation. First, combining with chemoimmunotherapy regimens aimed at overcoming the poor response of MCL to standard therapies in the R/R setting, due to frequently acquired chemoresistance. BR was combined with BTZ in iNHL including MCL showing an ORR of 71% (Friedberg et al. 2011) or cyclophosphamide and rituximab (21 patients showing an ORR of 74% and 42% CR [Lee et al. 2017]). Another study looked at the feasibility of combining BTZ with fludarabine (both using dose escalation cohorts) followed subsequently by rituximab. Authors reported significant dose-limiting myelosuppression and clinical responses were seen in 11 patients, five of whom were refractory to their most recent treatment regimen (Barr et al. 2009). The LYM-4003 was a phase 1b/2 study combining fludarabine and cyclophosphamide + BTZ in R/R MCL patients for a maximum of six cycles after a lead dose escalation phase to establish safety. A total of 40 patients were enrolled; the ORR was 72% with 31% CRs and the median DOR was 26.3 months comparing favorably with FC alone in that setting (Wang et al. 2021). Finally, BTZ was also combined with cladribine and rituximab in a series which included both treatment naive and R/R iNHL and MCL (Puvvada et al. 2018). The results were impressive overall with 100% ORR and 50% CR in MCL though most of them were treatment naive and the CR rate was not different than previously reported with the R-CdA combination alone in MCL (Spurgeon et al. 2011). Finally, several other studies have been initiated looking at BTZ + FCR, BTZ + Dex, and rituximab plus cytarabine which have not been reported in full just yet. Bortezomib was also combined with cyclophosphamide plus dexamethasone (CY-BorD) showing 13/21 responders (ORR 62%), with four CR (19%) (Sonbol et al. 2018), while a larger phase 2 (57 patients) explored BTZ with cyclophosphamide plus prednisone and rituximab (Cy-BorP) using two different BTZ schedules, weekly (n = 13) and twice weekly (n = 33), showing an ORR of 46% (23% CR/CRu) and 64% (36% CR/CRu), respectively (Gerecitano et al. 2011).

Most of the efforts aiming at expanding BTZ role in R/R MCL have focused on combinations with biological agents. Early on BTZ was combined with rituximab and or dexamethasone in a small series of R/R MCL demonstrating very high

ORR of 82% (13 patients), including 44% of CR (Lamm et al. 2011). Multiple other agents appeared in the MCL field since the approval of BTZ in 2006, providing new opportunities for unique combinations. Combinations of BTZ and lenalidomide were initiated by CALGB with two phases: induction using lenalidomide (days 1–14) plus bortezomib (days 1/4/8/11) every 21 days for eight cycles followed in responding patients by maintenance using the same schedule except BTZ was given on days 1 and 8 only. A total of 53 patients were enrolled after having failed one to five prior therapies, leading to an ORR of 40% with 15% CR. Although seven patients (six of them being CR) had durable remission (median, 3.2 years), all other patients progressed. Given the single-agent activity of BTZ, this was deemed not beneficial combination (Morrison et al. 2015). We reported a small study looking at BCL2 inhibitor obatoclax and bortezomib in R/R MCL, which was deemed feasible but showed no meaningful activity in spite of strong pre-clinical rationale (Goy et al. 2014), although one patient achieved a CR and is still NED to this date. As next step, BTZ was added to ibrutinib, the first BTKi approved in R/R MCL. This study is still ongoing and BTZ is given SQ to reduce neurotoxicity without compromising efficacy as suggested by real-world data (Skarbnik et al. 2017). Carfilzomib, a second-generation PI with proven effectiveness in pre-clinical models and less neurotoxicity in a phase 1 clinical trial (O'Connor et al. 2009b), was tested as single agent in a very limited series of six very heavily pretreated patients (median number of six prior therapies), albeit with no convincing activity (Lee et al. 2019). A small pilot study looked at carfilzomib and ibrutinib in R/R MCL using a dose escalation design which enrolled eight patients, five having failed prior BTKi, a population carrying usually a very poor outcome. The toxicity was manageable and predominantly included AEs manifest as hematological, electrolytes, GI, and fatigue, though there was a grade 5 toxicity with acute pneumonia leading to respiratory failure with blood cultures growing *Candida glabrata* postmortem. Interestingly, there were four responders (all PR), all having failed prior ibrutinib and one patient failed both prior ibrutinib and bortezomib given separately (Lee et al. 2020). Finally, given the promising pre-clinical data of BTZ with HDAC (Paoluzzi et al. 2009), a multicohort study looked at BTZ naive MCL and BTZ exposed either MCL or DLBCL (Yazbeck et al. 2018). Though toxicity was manageable, the efficacy was not convincing with an ORR of 30% of the combination in BTZ naive patients, not different than single-agent BTZ and no real activity observed in the other cohorts.

Clinical Activity of Bortezomib in Indolent Lymphoma (iNHL): Follicular Lymphoma, Marginal Zone, and SLL/CLL Subtypes

Bortezomib showed a high ORR at 70% in R/R FL in an early phase 2 by O'Connor et al. (2005) using a schedule of 1.5 mg/m^2 on days 1, 4, 8, and 11, with of notice a time to response in FL that appeared longer comparing to other histological lymphoma subtypes (O'Connor et al. 2010). The potential for BTZ efficacy in FL was validated in other studies confirming promising activity in R/R FL with BTZ in combination with rituximab in patients receiving a median of three cycles (Baiocchi et al. 2011). Based on these data, a large multicenter international phase 3 trial (LYM-3001) was initiated in R/R FL rituximab-naive or rituximab-sensitive. A total of 670 patients were randomized between R alone (weekly × 4 then monthly × 5) with or without bortezomib at 1.6 mg/m^2 on days 1, 8, 15, and 22 of each of 35 cycles maximum. Randomization was stratified by FLIPI score, previous use of rituximab, time since last therapy, and geographic region while the primary endpoint was PFS by ITT analysis. Patients received a median of five cycles altogether (mostly because of POD). Though results showed statistically higher ORR (49% vs. 63%, $p < 0.0004$) and CR rate (18% vs. 25%, $p < 0.035$), after a median follow-up of 34.9 months, the median PFS was 11.0 months in the rituximab group and 12.8 months in the bortezomib plus rituximab group. Though this difference was statistically significant ($p = 0.039$) and patients with higher risk disease seemed to benefit more from the BTZ-R combination, there was also added toxicity (neutropenia and neuropathy) and the study did not reach magnitude of clinical benefit as the anticipated pre-specified improvement of 33% in PFS and therefore was deemed appropriately not clinically relevant in this setting (Coiffier et al. 2011).

Clearly, a logical extension of these efforts was to explore activity in combination with more traditional chemotherapy agents active in the disease. One of these included a phase 2 trial of bortezomib (1.6 mg/m^2 on days 1 and 8) in combination with R-CHOP (capped vincristine at 1.5 mg per cycle) for up to eight cycles in previously untreated iNHL, included 29 patients: FL (n = 20), MZL (n = 5), and SLL (n = 4). The ORR was 100% with 66% CR and at a median follow-up of 48.7 months, a four-year PFS and OS of 83% and 93%, respectively, while 22/29 patients reported neuropathy (2 patients with Gr 3). By removing vincristine, other studies explored VR-CP or VR-CAP in R/R iNHL including FL using a 1.6 mg/m^2 on days 1 and 8 to improve the toxicity profile. With VR-CP, the ORR was 77%, with 27% CR rate and the median DOR was 21 months, while only one CR and three PR were reported in a small subset of FL with VR-CAP (Craig et al. 2014). As mentioned previously, some of the differences and variable clinical benefit seen with BTZ combinations could be related to differences in BTZ schedule. As a single agent, the best responses were seen in the biweekly versus weekly schedule (Gerecitano et al. 2009; Ribrag et al. 2013). In the combination setting, this was not entirely established and a randomized phase 2 study in R/R FL and MZL explored either bortezomib 1.3 mg/m^2 twice weekly (days 1, 4, 8, and 11; in 21-day cycle for five cycles (arm A)) or bortezomib 1.6 mg/m^2 weekly (days 1, 8, 15, and 22; 35-day cycle, for three cycles (arm B)) plus rituximab 375 mg/m^2 weekly for four weeks (in both arms). A total of 81 patients were enrolled (41 in arm A and 40 in arm B), which revealed an ORR of 49% (14% CR/CRu), a median TTP of 7.0 months, while median DOR was not reached in arm A. In arm B, the ORR was 43% (10% CR/CRu), and the median TTP and DOR were 10.0 and 9.3 months, respectively (de Vos et al. 2009). Though the weekly combination regimen seemed better tolerated, the biweekly regimen might show superior efficacy and durability with regard to clinical benefit. Finally, in a 3 + 3 dose escalation design, carfilzomib was combined with B-R in R/R NHL. The BR-CFZ combination was well tolerated and led to an ORR of 40% with 30% CR in a small series of 10 NHL patients (Kambhampati et al. 2021).

Bortezomib-based combinations have also shown activity in patients with MZL. Several studies mentioned above included small subsets of R/R MZL patients showing efficacy as single agent, supporting the inclusion of MZL in the randomized phase 2 of two different schedules of BTZ with rituximab discussed above (de Vos et al. 2009). The results showed an ORR of 50–60% though numbers were small. While very few studies have focused on the MZL subtype by itself, a phase 2 was dedicated to patients with MALT lymphoma who had not received systemic anti-lymphoma therapy except for *Helicobacter pylori* directed antibiotics (Troch et al. 2009). A total of 16 patients with gastric MALT lymphoma without evidence of large cell transformation were enrolled using days 1, 4, 8, 11 schedules at 1.5 mg/m^2 for a maximum of eight cycles. Results were impressive with an ORR of 80% and 43% CR with only 4/13 progressions at 21 months. While the majority of these patients required dose reduction (GI, neuropathy), the results were promising.

On the other hand, very little activity has been documented in SLL/chronic lymphocytic leukemia (CLL) patients (O'Connor et al. 2005), and a study dedicated to fludarabine failures in 20 CLL patients did not show any responses (Faderl et al. 2006). Another study studied the second-generation PI carfilzomib in R/R CLL or SLL using different cohorts and dose escalation schedules with no significant objective response either among 20 patients enrolled (Awan et al. 2015). *Ex vivo* data revealed that while CLL cells cultured in media containing 10% fetal calf serum successfully underwent apoptosis following exposure to bortezomib, this effect was dramatically decreased in the presence of 50% fresh human plasma. Further studies showed that the dietary flavonoid quercetin, which is present in plasma, blocked CLL cell killing by bortezomib. This action was confirmed by carrying out multiple cellular and molecular assays which showed that bortezomib-induced CLL cell killing occurs via the classic mitochondria-dependent intrinsic apoptotic pathway and that these mechanisms are compromised by quercetin. The blocking effect of flavonoids is attributable to a direct chemical reaction between the boronate moiety of bortezomib and adjacent hydroxyl groups present on some, but not all, flavonoids and such blockade did not apply to myeloma and lymphoma subtypes where BTZ showed maintained activity (Wickremasinghe 2008).

Clinical Activity of Bortezomib in Diffuse Large B-cell Lymphoma (DLBCL)

DLBCL represents over approximately one-third of all lymphomas, which is typically subdivided into one of two main molecular subtypes: the germinal center B-cell like (GCB) and non-germinal center B-cell-like DLBCL (non-GCB DLBCL), the latter of which is associated with an inferior prognosis and survival after first-line chemoimmunotherapy. Minimal activity had been observed as a single-agent bortezomib in R/R DLBCL with only one PR in the original phase 2 from MD Anderson (Goy et al. 2005a). However, early studies suggested that bortezomib had preferential activity in R/R ABC subtype, when combined with DA-R-EPOCH (Dunleavy et al. 2009), showing a significantly higher ORR 83% versus 13% ($p < 0.001$) in the ABC versus GCB subtypes, respectively, as well as a longer median OS of 10.8 months versus 3.4 months ($p = 0.003$). In a study previously mentioned, bortezomib was added to R-CHOP in a phase 2 which included both MCL (36 patients) and DLBCL (40 patients) (Ruan et al. 2011), suggesting that BTZ-R-CHOP alleviated the poor-risk features associated with the ABC subtype, as non-GCB and GCB subtypes showed similar promising results, including an ORR of 100% with 86% CR/CRu and a two-year PFS of 64%. Based on this observation, several new concepts emerged such as the PYRAMID trial, a randomized phase 2 study of R-CHOP with or without bortezomib in non-GC DLBCL as defined by the Hans-based algorithm by IHC (Leonard et al. 2017). After a median follow-up of 34 months, the two-year PFS was 77.6% with R-CHOP and 82.0% with VR-CHOP ($p = 0.61$); there was no difference either in ORR (98% vs. 96%) or two-year OS (88.4% vs. 93.0%). In other words, the outcome in this study for newly diagnosed non-GCB DLBCL was more favorable than expected with R-CHOP and was not significantly improved by adding bortezomib.

Other studies have looked at VR-CAP versus R-CHOP in newly diagnosed non-GC DLBCL, defined this time according to the Hans method but using a centrally confirmed IHC and including 164 patients. There were no significant differences between VR-CAP and R-CHOP for ORR (93.4% vs. 98.6%; $p = 0.11$), CR rate (64.5% vs. 66.2%; $p = 0.80$), two-year PFS (76.2% and 77.1%; $p = 0.76$), or two-year OS rates (80.1% and 79.0%; $p = 0.75$) (Offner et al. 2015). Based on concerns related to the Hans classification (regarding its reproducibility and/or a debatable correlation with gene-expression profiling [GEP] based signatures), a large trial (over 1100 patients) called REMoDL-B used a

GEP (whole genome) approach performed during the first cycle of R-CHOP in order to determine the cell-of-origin (COO) (that is as GC, ABC, or unclassified). Patients were then randomized to either continue with R-CHOP alone or with bortezomib–R-CHOP combination, where BTZ was given at 1.3 mg/m^2 IV or 1.6 mg/m^2 SQ on days 1 and 8 for cycles 2–6 (Davies et al. 2019). Although this was a well-conducted study with real-time molecular characterization for prospective stratification of DLBCL, this study showed no benefit for BTZ combination with no difference in the study primary endpoint or 30-month PFS 70.1% versus 74.3% ($p = 0.28$) for the GC and ABC population, respectively. In essence, several studies have failed to confirm the original hypothesis that bortezomib would improve the outcome of patients with non-GCB DLBCL, which was suggested across several phase 1/2 studies and was supported by an extensive rationale showing that non-GC DLBCL biology relies more on the NF-κB pathway, a well-known target of the PI bortezomib. Such patterns have been seen repeatedly in DLBCL, where in spite of a sound rationale and often robust phase 2 data, larger randomized trials fail to confirm benefit of R-CHOP + X. There can be multiple reasons for this, including schedules differences (BTZ was mostly done weekly on days 1 and 8 or days 1 and 4), which might have been insufficient based on single-agent data (Gerecitano et al. 2009). Another likely explanation is the selection bias introduced in such trials just by the simple fact of being deemed eligible for a trial, or by the time to initiation of therapy, which clearly impacts outcome (Maurer et al. 2018). This delay, through selection bias, explains why the control arm of several of these phase 3 trials showed a three-year PFS almost double what is expected in non-GC patients, and overall, we still have not broken the ceiling of R-CHOP in DLBCL in large randomized trials (Goy 2017).

Bortezomib in Waldenstrom's Macroglobulinemia (WM)

Lymphoplasmacytic cells are also vulnerable to proteasome inhibition and proteasome-targeting therapies have proven clinical efficacy in WM. Bortezomib as a single agent induces a partial response or better in approximately 41–60% of patients with R/RWM (Dimopoulos et al. 2010; Treon et al. 2007), which includes a prompt reduction in IgM of 25% within the first two months of therapy, while the median PFS for patients with R/RWM was 6–11 months (Treon et al. 2009). In combination with rituximab, major response was observed in approximately 50–83% of patients (Ghobrial et al. 2010), though the development of peripheral neuropathy was the main reason for dose reductions or discontinuations, especially in a disease in which baseline WM-related neuropathy is rather common. In patients with untreated WM, Treon et al. (2009) combined bortezomib with dexamethasone and rituximab (BDR) in 23 patients. Responses were rapid and the ORR was 96% with 22% achieving a CR and/or near CR. After a median follow-up of approximately two years, 18/23 patients remained progression free. An "IgM flare" occurred in two patients, both of whom required plasmapheresis. A similar regimen was reported by the European Myeloma Network in previously untreated WM patients showing also very high ORR at 85% including 3% CR, 7% VGPR, and a median PFS of 43 months and an OS at 7 years of 66% (Dimopoulos et al. 2010). However, neurotoxicity led to treatment discontinuations in almost two-thirds of patients.

Carfilzomib, a neuropathy-sparing PI, was evaluated in combination with rituximab and dexamethasone in patients with symptomatic WM without prior exposure to bortezomib and rituximab (Treon et al. 2014). Carfilzomib was administered at 20 mg/m^2 on days 1, 2 then 36 mg/m^2 IV on days 8, 9, 15, 16 and for all subsequent doses. The ORR was 87.1% and was not impacted by MYD88 or CXCR4 mutation status. Peripheral neuropathy occurred in one patient and was grade 2. Carfilzomib offers an effective, neuropathy-sparing PI approach in patients with WM.

Clinical Activity of Bortezomib in Other Lymphomas

T-cell Lymphoma

T-cell lymphoma encompass a very heterogenous group of diseases and single-agent activity was first reported in a series of 15 patients with R/R CTCL with an ORR of 67% including two CR and six PR with relatively durable responses from 7 to 14 months (Zinzani et al. 2007). In systemic T-cell lymphoma, single-agent bortezomib was also evaluated in adult T-cell leukemia/lymphoma (ATL) showing a modest ORR of 6%. Pre-clinical data nevertheless supported combination studies in peripheral T-cell lymphomas (PTCL) and a frontline study combining BTZ (days 1 and 8 at 1.6 mg/m^2) with CHOP (Kim et al. 2012) enrolled 46 patients including PTCL-NOS (n = 16), extranodal NK/T-cell lymphoma, nasal type (ENKTL, n = 10), angioimmunoblastic T-cell lymphoma (AITL, n = 8), ALK-negative anaplastic large-cell lymphoma (ALCL, n = 6), cutaneous T-cell lymphoma (CTCL, n = 5), and hepatosplenic T-cell lymphoma (n = 1). Results were impressive with an ORR of 76% and 65% CR. Of notice PTCL-NOS, AITL, and ALCL showed higher responses with an ORR 87% and CR rate of 73%; however, the three-year OS and PFS were only 47% and 35%, with an unmodified continued pattern of relapse. Another study combined gemcitabine with BTZ in R/R PTCL showing an ORR of 36% and 27% CR, though despite a weekly schedule (days 1 and 8 q 21 days) the regimens was poorly tolerated producing significant myelotoxicity (Evens et al. 2013). Several other combinations supported by pre-clinical models were reported such as BTZ + pralatrexate in older PTCL (1/5 patients achieving a CR) (Lee et al. 2017) as well as a combination of BTZ with the HDAC inhibitor panobinostat. The latter was explored in a phase 2 study of 25 patients who received 20 mg oral panobinostat three times a week together with BTZ 1.3 mg/m^2 twice a week, both for two out of three weeks for up to eight cycles. The ORR was 43% (with 10 responders including five CR), with common treatment-related grades 3–4 AEs including myelotoxicity and GI (diarrhea) (Tan et al. 2015). Carfilzomib was tested in a small phase 1 with 15 heavily pretreated patients (median of five prior therapies), showing only modest activity with an ORR of 13% (one CR and one PR) (Krishnan et al. 2022).

Hodgkin's Lymphoma

Based on the significant activity of gemcitabine in patients with R/R Hodgkin's lymphoma (HL), and the ability of bortezomib to inhibit NF-κB, which plays a critical role in HL biology, a combination of BTZ and gemcitabine was studied in a total of 18 R/R HL patients using BTZ at 1 mg/m^2 on days 1, 4, 8, and 11 plus gemcitabine 800 mg/m^2 on days 1 and 8. The ORR was low at 22% and substantial hepatic toxicity was reported raising additional caution for this combination (Mendler et al. 2008). Another study looked at bortezomib and dexamethasone in relapsed HL, though after 12 patients were enrolled, the study was prematurely closed because no response was observed and a meta-analysis of all four available studies evaluating bortezomib in this population showed no significant benefit of bortezomib (Trelle et al. 2007).

Plasmablastic Lymphoma (PBL)

Plasmablastic lymphoma (PBL) is distinguished from other B-cell lymphomas by the presence of plasmacytic differentiation markers such as CD38, CD138, and MUM1, more commonly seen in immunosuppressed patients, in particular in HIV/AIDS patients, presenting with both oral and extra-oral sites and rapidly progressive tumors with frequent treatment failure with standard DLBCL regimens. Several case reports had revealed impressive activity of bortezomib as single agent in a patient with refractory PBL (Hirosawa et al. 2015) or in combination with rituximab and BTZ in a CD20 positive PBL (Yan et al. 2014). Additional case reports included successful combination with lenalidomide (Marrero et al. 2018) or bortezomib, rituximab, and dexamethasone (Saba et al. 2013). This provided a rationale for combining BTZ with traditional chemotherapy including R-CHOP or R-EPOCH in PBL (Castillo et al. 2015; Dittus et al. 2018). These studies revealed promising and durable responses in a difficult disease, providing a new standard of care in this challenging and orphan disease. A similar hypothesis was generated having established that BTZ could have direct anti-tumor activity and induce lytic activation of Kaposi sarcoma herpesvirus (KSHV). Kaposi sarcoma is also almost solely seen in HIV patients (therefore rarely observed nowadays), and is associated with a very poor outcome. As a single agent, BTZ produced an ORR of 60% as a single agent (all PRs) (Reid et al. 2020).

Lymphoblastic Lymphoma (LL)/Acute Lymphocytic Leukemia (ALL)

Anecdotal reports of efficacy of bortezomib in lymphoblastic lymphoma/acute lymphocytic leukemia (LL/ALL) patients had been reported leading to an array of combinations with intensive ALL inductions both in the pediatric and adult settings. As an example, bortezomib was combined with vincristine, dexamethasone, pegylated asparaginase, and doxorubicin showing acceptable toxicity and a 75% CR rate in B-cell ALL in the R/R setting (Messinger et al. 2012). The Children Oncology Group evaluated the impact of adding bortezomib to reinduction chemotherapy in a total of 135 patients (103 B-ALL, 22 T-ALL, 10 T-LL), showing higher ORR/CR rate as well as achievement of MRD negative status than expected in particular in certain ALL subgroups, such as T-cell ALL, and as per the authors were worthy of further investigation (Horton et al. 2019), and will likely move in the frontline setting pending evaluation in ongoing trials.

EBV Lymphoproliferative Disorders and Other Immunological Conditions

Gamma herpesviruses (GHVs) are responsible for a significant proportion of virus-associated human cancers in particularly lymphoma, which often occur (but not always) in immunocompromised individuals. Methods that employ lytic activation of viruses latently infecting tumors represent a novel strategy of anti-neoplastic therapy. Bortezomib has been shown to be a potent activator of the viral lytic cycle and has demonstrated activity in case reports of Epstein–Barr virus (EBV)-related malignancies including lymphoma and PTLD. Although initial reports implicated the inhibition of the NF-κB pathway, more recent data suggests alternative pathways responsible for bortezomib-mediated lytic induction of GHV viruses. Such hypotheses seem corroborated by small series in combination with chemotherapy (Reid et al. 2012) or other agents including rituximab or HDAC in ongoing trials (Shahid and Prockop 2021). Finally, T-cell chronic active Epstein–Barr virus (CAEBV) is a rare disease in which EBV is present predominantly in T-cells that infiltrate the tissues, with high levels of EBV DNA in the blood, and a rapid course if left untreated toward liver failure and florid symptoms reminiscent of hemophagocytic lymphohistiocytosis. While the only potential for cure is through an allogenic stem cell transplantation, the use of bortezomib and ganciclovir has shown some dramatic responses and could serve as a bridge before cell therapy (Bollard et al. 2007).

Pre-clinical models coupled with the underlying mechanism of action of BTZ in plasma cells which produce elevated levels of immunoglobulin suggest bortezomib might also have a role in autoimmune disorders. Detailed rationale and early clinical results of BTZ efficacy in autoimmune disease are well beyond this chapter, and were reviewed recently elsewhere (Pasquale et al. 2021), including a series of 19 patients with autoimmune hemolytic anemia (AIHA) who had received a single course of bortezomib (at 1.3 mg/m^2 IV on days 1, 4, 8, and 11), leading to six responses (three CR and three PR) for an ORR of 32% and transfusion independence achieved in four additional patients. Among responders, four maintained their response after a median follow-up of 16 months (range: 10–31) while one patient relapsed a year later but obtained a second remission with a second course of bortezomib (Rossi et al. 2018).

Finally, based on a strong rationale, bortezomib has been evaluated in the context of allogenic stem cell transplantation. Early data even suggested decreased incidence of acute graft versus host disease (aGVH) and better immune reconstitution as well as potential for reducing chronic GVH (cGVH) symptoms in steroid refractory patients (Koreth et al. 2012; Pai et al. 2014). However larger trials failed to confirm this observation as single agent, and BTZ has since been combined with other small molecules such as ruxolitinib in cGVH, while third-generation PI such as ixazomib might have more promising efficacy (Pidala et al. 2020), and is being further evaluated in ongoing trials.

Clinical Activity of Proteasome Inhibitors in AML/MDS

Early studies have indicated that bortezomib might be potentially useful in the treatment of acute myeloid leukemia (AML). However, as single agent in R/R AML or in patients unfit for any chemotherapy, only modest activity has been reported (Sarlo et al. 2013). Combination of BTZ in regimens used in managing AML was a logical next step based on preclinical and mechanistic rationale. A combination with the standard 3 + 7 daunorubicin and cytarabine induction chemotherapy resulted in an encouraging remission rate with 65% CR in *de novo* AML (Attar et al. 2013). Other studies explored the addition of BTZ following a dose escalation design together with azacytidine 75 mg/m^2 daily on days 1–7 in R/R AML and showed encouraging results with five responders out of 23 patients (Walker et al. 2014). Bortezomib was also explored in myelodysplastic syndrome (MDS), using subcutaneous bortezomib, in 15 patients who had failed a median of two prior therapies and who were all transfusion dependent. Three patients (20%) showed hematological improvement, while a decrease in ring sideroblasts was observed in 7 out of 10 evaluable patients during treatment. A combination of bortezomib with low-dose AraC (LDAC) in 43 patients with higher risk MDS showed an ORR of 28% (Natarajan-Ame et al. 2012). Finally, combination with lenalidomide or azacytidine in MDS with either bortezomib or even more recently ixazomib might help expand the benefit of PI, although the field of MDS and in particular AML has significantly evolved over the last decade with the approval of numerous novel targeted agents often applying to defined molecular subsets of patients.

Clinical Activity of Proteasome Inhibitors in Solid Tumors

The success of PIs seen in hematological malignancies, particularly in MM and MCL early on, generated a lot of enthusiasm to explore PIs in solid tumors. Not only are these cancers less chemosensitive, but they often acquire resistance over time. Proteasome inhibition impacts multiple pathways that are critical to many of the hallmarks of cancer cells including cell growth and survival, apoptosis as well as metastasis. In addition, during the initial NCI panel testing bortezomib, the drug demonstrates activity across many different subtypes of solid tumors cell lines in the same nM LC50 range as MM cell lines (Adams 2002). However, results overall have been disappointing, with no PI approved so far in any solid tumors (Huang et al. 2014) and very few ongoing trials. Here are some of the directions explored during this process across some key solid tumor cell types.

Extensive pre-clinical studies suggested that bortezomib exhibits anti-tumor activity against multiple solid tumor malignancies (Chen et al. 2011), from NSCLC (Liu et al. 2007) to head and neck squamous cell carcinoma (HNSCC) (Fribley et al. 2004), hepatocellular carcinoma (Chen et al. 2011), melanoma (Qin et al. 2005), prostate cancer (Nikrad et al. 2005), colon cancer (Zhu et al. 2005), renal cell carcinoma (Vaziri et al. 2009), and pancreatic cancer (Nawrocki et al. 2004). However, clinical testing of BTZ as single agent has remained disappointing overall, from NSCLC (Besse et al. 2012; Fanucchi et al. 2006) to recurrent ovarian cancer, unresectable hepatocellular carcinoma (Kim et al. 2012), metastatic colorectal cancer (Mackay et al. 2005), gastric cancers (Shah et al. 2011), melanoma (Markovic et al. 2005), and hormone resistant prostate cancer (Morris et al. 2007), while BTZ in renal cancer showed modest activity in one trial four PR/37 patients (Kondagunta et al. 2004) but only one PR/23 patients in another study (Davis et al. 2004). One limitation is potentially the transient proteasome inhibition obtained with BTZ. Second-generation PIs, in particular irreversible Pis like carfilzomib (at a dosing of 20/36 mg/m^2 IV twice weekly) which are well tolerated, and showed evidence of carfilzomib inhibiting the proteasome in blood cells, though again have demonstrated disappointing anti-tumor activity in 65 patients with advanced solid tumors.

Based on NSCLC xenograft models and pharmacokinetic studies, strategies to enhance BTZ efficacy focused on combination therapies, improving tumor penetration and second-generation PIs. Combination therapies of BTZ with paclitaxel/carboplatin/irinotecan, or even HDAC inhibitor vorinostat, were supported by *in vitro* promising models in NSCLC (Zhao et al. 2015). However, BTZ combined with cisplatin with or without gemcitabine did not improve efficacy in patients with NSCLC (Kontopodis et al. 2016). Since after BTZ treatment, cells accumulate in the radiosensitive G2/M phase of the cell cycle, BTZ was combined with radiation (Cron et al. 2013), albeit with no significant benefit. Second-generation PIs were also tested based on pre-clinical evidence with carfilzomib results in mouse xenograft model of NSCLC cells, revealing a significant survival advantage (Baker et al. 2014) but this did not translate into meaningful clinical activity. Second-generation PI CFZ was found to sensitize breast cancer cells to cytotoxic drugs including doxorubicin in triple negative breast cancer models (Shi et al. 2016) but showed no meaningful activity in the clinic. Furthermore, a study with marizomib and HDAC showed no response in 22 patients in solid tumors (Millward et al. 2012). Finally, alternative delivery models were tested aiming at encapsulating BTZ for improved drug delivery and to overcome the poor penetration of BTZ into lung tumors, but again with no impact on clinical activity (Shen et al. 2014). Together, these results indicate that although PIs display robust activity across solid tumors in the pre-clinical setting, as a single agent in clinical trials or even in combinations, their efficacy has remained very limited. This raises the question of why solid tumor cells carry innate or develop resistance to PIs and how we might be able to address it.

Overcoming Resistance to Proteasome Inhibitors in Cancer and Next Steps in Proteasome Inhibition

The field of PIs has remarkably expanded over the last two decades as summarized in Table 24.4 with second- and third-generation products offering better therapeutic index, higher convenience (oral vs. IV), and expanding the targets beyond the 20S core in the future. However, over time patients typically fail PIs and although the mechanisms underlying BTZ-resistance remain poorly understood, progress has been made in particular for PI in heme malignancies (Gonzalez-Santamarta et al. 2020). Resistance to PIs (especially bortezomib) seen in the lab or in the clinic can occur through multilayered mechanisms. The upregulation of the CP subunit expression, in particular the β5 subunit, leads to increased concentrations of PIs required to achieve sufficient inhibition of chymotrypsin-like proteasome catalytic activity. Point mutations in PSMB5 gene introducing amino acid substitutions in critical positions of the PI-binding pocket of the β5 subunit have been reported, though it is not entirely clear how relevant it is in patients. Besides point mutations, downregulation of IP subunit β5i can help cells escape inhibitory activity of PIs. The cellular extrusion of PIs can be facilitated through the P-glycoprotein (Pgp) drug efflux transporter, though this is mostly relevant for epoxyketone-based PIs. The bulk of resistance seems to be related to activation of pro-survival pathways (such as NF-κB, PI3K/AKT, IGF1) and activation via growth factors and cytokines derived from stromal cells and microenvironment, including the bone marrow. Finally, compensatory mechanisms of proteins degradation through alternate pathways in particular through lysosomes and aggresomes and autophagy can participate in cellular resistance to bortezomib.

As discussed above, the level of success of PIs for hematological malignancies has not translated into solid tumors. Despite encouraging activity and anti-tumor effects of PIs in pre-clinical models of solid tumors, their clinical activity is still very limited. Though several of the mechanisms of resistance might be shared with BTZ, multiple differences with hematological cancers, especially plasma cells, might help explain the overall innate resistance to PI in solid tumors. Constitutive proteasomes are more abundant in solid tumors while in hematological malignancies IPs are much more abundant and constitute an important additional target. The degree of "baseline" engagement of proteasome varies across tissues and is suggested to be higher in MM versus solid tumors, though we do not have yet reliable quantitative and qualitative assessment of constitutive and IP subunits composition in clinical samples. Although the amount on IP in solid tumors is expected to be low, emerging functions of IPs in handling oxidative and toxic stress could hold relevance for PIs combination therapies in solid tumors (Yun et al. 2016). Drug penetration and duration of proteasome inhibition could be addressed by second-generation PIs such as irreversible PIs (carfilzomib, oprozomib) over reversible PIs (BTZ, ixazomib) to ensure prolonged PI, though some of these second-generation PIs might be more sensitive to drug efflux Pgp. Pre-clinical models of enhanced delivery methods through nanoparticles have not translated into any clinical impact yet.

Combinations with other targeted approaches have included cell surface receptors for the death ligand such as TRAIL (Manni et al. 2013), or apoptosis regulators such as MCL1 (with strong evidence in MCL) (Perez-Galan et al. 2011), or Bak with obatoclax based on elegant pre-clinical rational (Perez-Galan et al. 2007), though it did not again translate into a clinical benefit (Goy et al. 2014). However, when combining BTZ together with second-generation BCL2 inhibitor venetoclax, results have been very impressive in MM (Moreau et al. 2017) and such approach is currently evaluated in other tumor types. Studies co-targeting PIs with HDAC inhibitors have also shown great activity in MM and though supported

Table 24.4 Different proteasome inhibitors in the clinic.

Proteasome inhibitor	Active moiety binding	Subunit	Chemical structure	Route	Activity/comments
Bortezomib	Boronate Reversible	$\beta5 > \beta1$ ($\beta5i$)	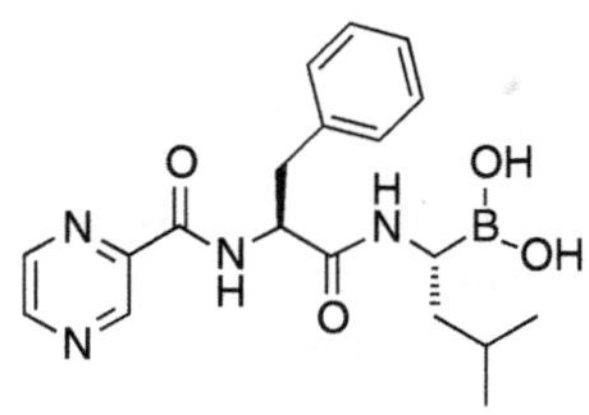	IV SQ	Approved in MM relapse (2003) and frontline Approved in WM Approved in MCL
Carfilzomib	Epoxyketone Irreversible	$\beta5$ ($\beta5i$)	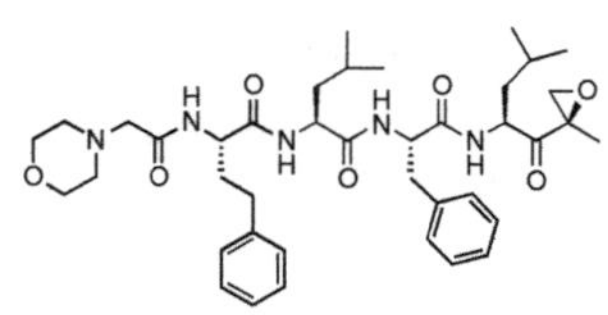	IV	Approved in MM (2016)
Marizomib (NPI-0052)	β-lactone Irreversible	$\beta5 > \beta2 > \beta1$	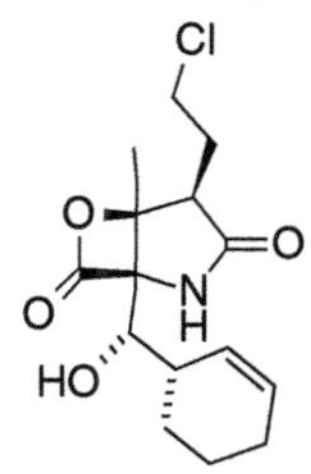	IV	
Delanzomib (CEP18770)	Boronate Reversible	$\beta5 > \beta1$	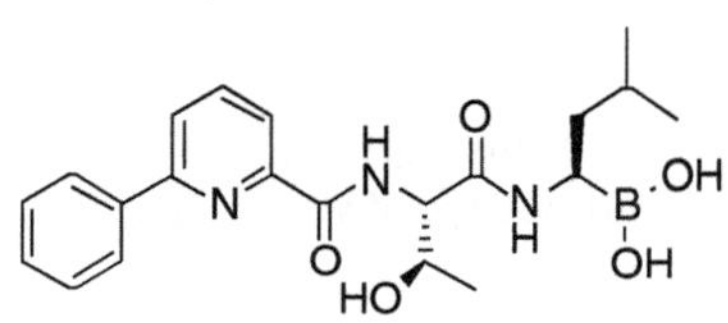	Oral IV	
Ixazomib (MLN9708)	Boronate Reversible	$\beta5 > \beta1$	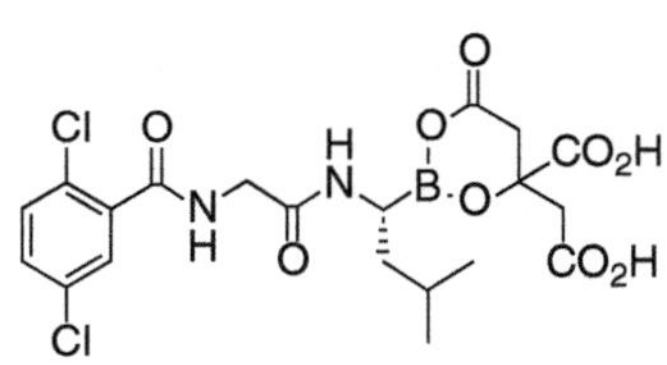	Oral IV	Approved in MM frontline and relapse
Oprozomib (ONX0912)	Epoxyketone Irreversible	$\beta5$ ($\beta5i$)	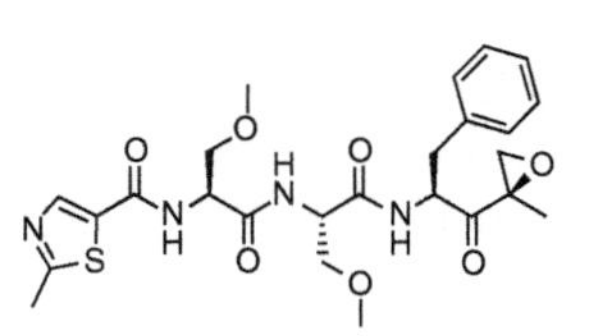	Oral	Approved in relapsed refractory MM
Immunoproteasome inhibitor					
KZR-616 (Zetomipzomib)	Epoxyketone	$\beta5i$	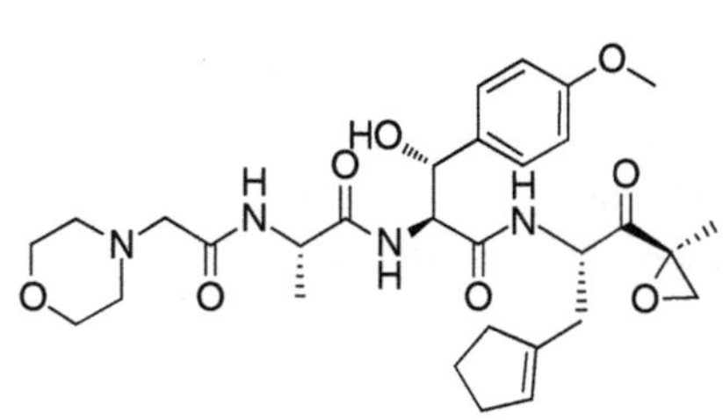	IV	First-in-class IP inhibitor tested in autoimmune diseases
M3258	Reversible	Selective LMP7/$\beta5i$ inhibitor	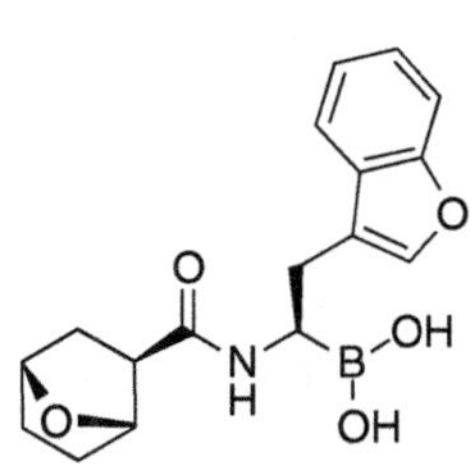	Oral	Phase 1 MM w/ dexamethasone

Abbreviations: MCL = mantle cell lymphoma; MM = multiple myeloma; WM = Waldenstrom's macroglobulinemia.

by pre-clinical data, the same concept exported across other cancers including with second-generation PIs did not translate yet into superior results.

Beyond evaluating next-generation PI inhibitors, strategies to overcome BTZ resistance mechanisms will need to explore PIs that target non-catalytic subunits of the proteasome or other targets in the UPS, such as blocking the deubiquitinases or inhibiting the protein unfolding activity of 19S, most of which is still pre-clinical at this point. On the other hand, bringing some specificity through E3 ligases inhibition could allow to inhibit key pathways in cancer. Targeting the interaction between tumor suppressor p53 and the E3 ligase MDM2 represents, for example, an attractive treatment approach for cancers with wild-type or functional *TP53*. Indeed, several small molecules have been developed and evaluated in various malignancies with early promising results (Konopleva et al. 2020). Finally, neddylation is a post-translational modification that adds a ubiquitin-like protein, NEDD8, to selected substrate proteins, affecting their stability, conformation, subcellular localization, and function. The pharmacologic inhibition of neddylation using a small-molecule inhibitor, MLN4924, does inhibit cullin-RING ubiquitin E3 ligase complexes. It has been since name pevonedistat and has shown promising preliminary results in MM (Shah et al. 2016) and MDS/CMML and is currently evaluated further in ongoing trials.

Disrupting proteins homeostasis, which is clearly an important anti-cancer mechanism, has been challenging and the only success to date has been through inhibitors of the 20S core proteasome, which have transformed the field of MM. Additional activity and benefit have been established over the years in several other blood cancers in particular MCL, WM, ALL, and PBL, though they had less impact than in MM. Nevertheless, this led to a much better understanding of proteins editing and proteins degradation as a multistep and highly complex process. Targeting more specific proteins substrates or pathways in particular p53 might help continue expand this new treatment paradigm across multiple cancer subtypes. Finally, the discovery of PROteolysis TArgeting Chimeras (PROTACs) over 20 years ago has opened an entirely new area of targeted protein degradation (TPD). From the early beginning as chimeric peptides, PROTACs have evolved into potent small molecules that can degrade a variety of intracellular and transmembrane proteins in cells, mice, and more recently in humans, expanding *de facto* TPD well beyond the proteasome. Improved technologies are enabling the development of ligands for "undruggable" proteins and increasing the potential even further for proteins disruption/degradation from the recruitment of new E3 ligases to harnessing the lysosomal degradation and the autophagy pathway, thus potentially enabling the targeted destruction of entire organelles and protein aggregates, and overall pushing the boundaries of drug discovery for the foreseeable future (Bond and Crews 2021; Nalawansha et al. 2020).

Must Read References

Adams, J. (2002). Preclinical and clinical evaluation of proteasome inhibitor PS-341 for the treatment of cancer. *Curr. Opin. Chem. Biol.* 6: 493–500.

O'Connor, O.A., Wright, J., Moskowitz, C. et al. (2005). Phase II clinical experience with the novel proteasome inhibitor bortezomib in patients with indolent non-Hodgkin's lymphoma and mantle cell lymphoma. *J. Clin. Oncol.: Off. J. Am.Soc. Clin. Oncol.* 23: 676–684.

Tan, D., Phipps, C., Hwang, W.Y. et al. (2015). Panobinostat in combination with bortezomib in patients with relapsed or refractory peripheral T-cell lymphoma: an open-label, multicentre phase 2 trial. *Lancet Haematol.* 2: e326–33.

Tanaka, K. (1998). Molecular biology of the proteasome. *Biochem. Biophys. Res. Commun.* 247: 537–541.

References

Adams, J. (2002). Preclinical and clinical evaluation of proteasome inhibitor PS-341 for the treatment of cancer. *Curr. Opin. Chem. Biol.* 6: 493–500.

Alsina, M., Trudel, S., Furman, R.R. et al. (2012). A phase I single-agent study of twice-weekly consecutive-day dosing of the proteasome inhibitor carfilzomib in patients with relapsed or refractory multiple myeloma or lymphoma. *Clin. Cancer. Res.* 18: 4830–4840.

Alsouqi, A., Khan, M., Dhakal, B. et al. (2021). KD-PACE salvage therapy for aggressive relapsed refractory multiple myeloma, plasma cell leukemia and extramedullary myeloma. *Clin. Lymphoma Myeloma. Leuk.* 21: 526–535.

Attar, E.C., Johnson, J.L., Amrein, P.C. et al. (2013). Bortezomib added to daunorubicin and cytarabine during induction therapy and to intermediate-dose cytarabine for consolidation in patients with previously untreated acute myeloid leukemia age 60 to 75 years: CALGB (Alliance) study 10502. *J. Clin. Onco.l* 31: 923–929.

Awan, F.T., Flynn, J.M., Jones, J.A. et al. (2015). Phase I dose escalation trial of the novel proteasome inhibitor carfilzomib in patients with relapsed chronic lymphocytic leukemia and small lymphocytic lymphoma. *Leuk. Lymphoma.* 56: 2834–2840.

Bae, J., Hideshima, T., Tai, Y.T. et al. (2018). Histone deacetylase (HDAC) inhibitor ACY241 enhances anti-tumor activities of antigen-specific central memory cytotoxic T lymphocytes against multiple myeloma and solid tumors. *Leukemia* 32: 1932–1947.

Bahlis, N.J., Raje, N.S., Costello, C. et al. (2021). Efficacy and safety of elranatamab (PF-06863135), a B-cell maturation antigen (BCMA)-CD3 bispecific antibody, in patients with relapsed or refractory multiple myeloma (MM). *J. Clin. Oncol.* 39: 8006–8006.

Baiocchi, R.A., Alinari, L., Lustberg, M.E. et al. (2011). Phase 2 trial of rituximab and bortezomib in patients with relapsed or refractory mantle cell and follicular lymphoma. *Cancer* 117: 2442–2451.

Baker, A.F., Hanke, N.T., Sands, B.J. et al. (2014). Carfilzomib demonstrates broad anti-tumor activity in pre-clinical non-small cell and small cell lung cancer models. *J. Exp. Clin. Cancer Res.* 33: 111.

Barr, P.M., Fu, P., Lazarus, H.M. et al. (2009). Phase I trial of fludarabine, bortezomib and rituximab for relapsed and refractory indolent and mantle cell non-Hodgkin lymphoma. *Br. J. Haematol.* 147: 89–96.

Belch, A., Kouroukis, C.T., Crump, M. et al. (2007). A phase II study of bortezomib in mantle cell lymphoma: the National cancer institute of canada clinical trials group trial IND.150. *An. Oncol.: Off. J. European Soc. Med. Oncol./ESMO* 18: 116–121.

Besse, B., Planchard, D., Veillard, A.S. et al. (2012). Phase 2 study of frontline bortezomib in patients with advanced non-small cell lung cancer. *Lung Cancer* 76: 78–83.

Bianchi, G., Oliva, L., Cascio, P. et al. (2009). The proteasome load versus capacity balance determines apoptotic sensitivity of multiple myeloma cells to proteasome inhibition. *Blood* 113: 3040–3049.

Bollard, C.M., Gottschalk, S., Leen, A.M. et al. (2007). Complete responses of relapsed lymphoma following genetic modification of tumor-antigen presenting cells and T-lymphocyte transfer. *Blood* 110: 2838–2845.

Bond, M.J. and Crews, C.M. (2021). Proteolysis targeting chimeras (PROTACs) come of age: entering the third decade of targeted protein degradation. *RSC Chem. Biol.* 2: 725–742.

Bringhen, S., Larocca, A., Rossi, D. et al. (2010). Efficacy and safety of once-weekly bortezomib in multiple myeloma patients. *Blood* 116: 4745–4753.

Castillo, J.J., Reagan, J.L., Sikov, W.M., and Winer, E.S. (2015). Bortezomib in combination with infusional dose-adjusted EPOCH for the treatment of plasmablastic lymphoma. *Br. J. Haematol.* 169: 352–355.

Chang, J.E., Carmichael, L.L., Kim, K. et al. (2018). VcR-CVAD induction chemotherapy followed by maintenance rituximab produces durable remissions in mantle cell lymphoma: a wisconsin oncology network study. *Clin. Lymphoma. Myeloma. Leuk.* 18: e61–e67.

Chari, A., Martinez-lopez, J., Mateos, M.V. et al. (2019). Daratumumab plus carfilzomib and dexamethasone in patients with relapsed or refractory multiple myeloma. *Blood* 134: 421–431.

Chari, A,B.J., Oriol, A., Van De Donk, N. et al. (2020). A phase 1, first in human study of talquetamab, a G protein-coupled receptor family C group 5 member D(GPRC5D) x CD3 bispecfic antibody, in patients with relapsed and/or refractory multiple myeloma (RRMM). American Society of Hematology, *Blood* 36 (1): 40–41.

Chauhan, D., Catley, L., Li, G. et al. (2005). A novel orally active proteasome inhibitor induces apoptosis in multiple myeloma cells with mechanisms distinct from Bortezomib. *Cancer Cell* 8: 407–419.

Chen, D., Frezza, M., Schmitt, S., and Kanwar, J. Q, P. D. (2011). Bortezomib as the first proteasome inhibitor anticancer drug: current status and future perspectives. *Curr. Cancer Drug Targets.* 11: 239–253.

Chen, R.W., Palmer, J.M., Tomassetti, S. et al. (2018). Multi-center phase II trial of bortezomib and rituximab maintenance combination therapy in patients with mantle cell lymphoma after consolidative autologous stem cell transplantation. *J. Hematol. Oncol.* 11: 87.

Coiffier, B., Osmanov, E.A., Hong, X. et al. (2011). Bortezomib plus rituximab versus rituximab alone in patients with relapsed, rituximab-naive or rituximab-sensitive, follicular lymphoma: a randomised phase 3 trial. *Lancet. Oncol.* 12: 773–784.

Craig, M., Hanna, W.T., Cabanillas, F. et al. (2014). Phase II study of bortezomib in combination with rituximab, cyclophosphamide and prednisone with or without doxorubicin followed by rituximab maintenance in patients with relapsed or refractory follicular lymphoma. *Br. J. Haematol.* 166: 920–928.

Cron, K.R., Zhu, K., Kushwaha, D.S. et al. (2013). Proteasome inhibitors block DNA repair and radiosensitize non-small cell lung cancer. *PLoS One* 8: e73710.

Davies, A., Cummin, T., Barrans, S. et al. (2019). Gene-expression profiling of bortezomib added to standard chemoimmunotherapy for diffuse large B-cell lymphoma (REMoDL-B): an open-label, randomised, phase 3 trial. *Lancet* 20: 649–662.

Davies, F.E., Wu, P., Jenner, M. et al. (2007). The combination of cyclophosphamide, velcade and dexamethasone induces high response rates with comparable toxicity to velcade alone and velcade plus dexamethasone. *Haematologica* 92: 1149–1150.

Davis, N.B., Taber, D.A., Ansari, R.H. et al. (2004). Phase II trial of PS-341 in patients with renal cell cancer: a University of Chicago phase II consortium study. *J. Clin. Oncol.* 22: 115–119.

de Vos, S., Goy, A., Dakhil, S.R. et al. (2009). Multicenter randomized phase II study of weekly or twice-weekly bortezomib plus rituximab in patients with relapsed or refractory follicular or marginal-zone B-cell lymphoma. *J. Clin. Oncol.: Off. J. Am. Soc. Clin. Oncol.* 27: 5023–5030.

Dimopoulos, M., Quach, H., Mateos, M.V. et al. (2020). Carfilzomib, dexamethasone, and daratumumab versus carfilzomib and dexamethasone for patients with relapsed or refractory multiple myeloma (CANDOR): results from a randomised, multicentre, open-label, phase 3 study. *Lancet* 396: 186–197.

Dimopoulos, M.A., Chen, C., Kastritis, E. et al. (2010). Bortezomib as a treatment option in patients with

Waldenstrom macroglobulinemia. *Clin. Lymphoma. Myeloma. Leuk.* 10: 110–117.

Dimopoulos, M.A., Gay, F., Schjesvold, F. et al. (2019). Oral ixazomib maintenance following autologous stem cell transplantation (TOURMALINE-MM3): a double-blind, randomised, placebo-controlled phase 3 trial. *Lancet* 393: 253–264.

Dimopoulos, M.A., Goldschmidt, H., Niesvizky, R. et al. (2017). Carfilzomib or bortezomib in relapsed or refractory multiple myeloma (ENDEAVOR): an interim overall survival analysis of an open-label, randomised, phase 3 trial. *Lancet. Oncol.* 18: 1327–1337.

Dispenzieri, A., Kastritis, E., Wechalekar, A.D. et al. (2022). A randomized phase 3 study of ixazomib-dexamethasone versus physician's choice in relapsed or refractory AL amyloidosis. *Leukemia* 36(1): 225–235.

Dittus, C., Grover, N., Ellsworth, S. et al. (2018). Bortezomib in combination with dose-adjusted EPOCH (etoposide, prednisone, vincristine, cyclophosphamide, and doxorubicin) induces long-term survival in patients with plasmablastic lymphoma: a retrospective analysis. *Leuk. Lymphoma.* 59: 2121–2127.

Drach, J., Huang, H., Samoilova, O. et al. (2018). Efficacy and safety of frontline rituximab, cyclophosphamide, doxorubicin and prednisone plus bortezomib (VR-CAP) or vincristine (R-CHOP) in a subset of newly diagnosed mantle cell lymphoma patients medically eligible for transplantation in the randomized, phase 3 LYM-3002 study. *Leuk. Lymphoma.* 59: 896–903.

Dunleavy, K., Pittaluga, S., Czuczman, M.S. et al. (2009). Differential efficacy of bortezomib plus chemotherapy within molecular subtypes of diffuse large B-cell lymphoma. *Blood* 113: 6069–6076.

Evens, A.M., Rosen, S.T., Helenowski, I. et al. (2013). A phase I/II trial of bortezomib combined concurrently with gemcitabine for relapsed or refractory DLBCL and peripheral T-cell lymphomas. *Br. J. Haematol.* 163: 55–61.

Facon, T., Venner, C.P., Bahlis, N.J. et al. (2021). Oral ixazomib, lenalidomide, and dexamethasone for transplant-ineligible patients with newly diagnosed multiple myeloma. *Blood* 137: 3616–3628.

Faderl, S., Rai, K., Gribben, J. et al. (2006). Phase II study of single-agent bortezomib for the treatment of patients with fludarabine-refractory B-cell chronic lymphocytic leukemia. *Cancer* 107: 916–924.

Fanucchi, M.P., Fossella, F.V., Belt, R. et al. (2006). Randomized phase II study of bortezomib alone and bortezomib in combination with docetaxel in previously treated advanced non-small-cell lung cancer. *J. Clin. Oncol.* 24: 5025–5033.

Fisher, R.I., Bernstein, S.H., Kahl, B.S. et al. (2006). Multicenter phase II study of bortezomib in patients with relapsed or refractory mantle cell lymphoma. *J. Clin. Oncol.: Off. J. Am. Soc. Clin. Oncol.* 24: 4867–4874.

Fribley, A., Zeng, Q., and Wang, C.Y. (2004). Proteasome inhibitor PS-341 induces apoptosis through induction of endoplasmic reticulum stress-reactive oxygen species in head and neck squamous cell carcinoma cells. *Mol. Cell Biol.* 24: 9695–9704.

Friedberg, J.W., Vose, J.M., Kelly, J.L. et al. (2011). The combination of bendamustine, bortezomib, and rituximab for patients with relapsed/refractory indolent and mantle cell non-Hodgkin lymphoma. *Blood* 117: 2807–2812.

Gay, F., Musto, P., Rota-scalabrini, D. et al. (2021). Carfilzomib with cyclophosphamide and dexamethasone or lenalidomide and dexamethasone plus autologous transplantation or carfilzomib plus lenalidomide and dexamethasone, followed by maintenance with carfilzomib plus lenalidomide or lenalidomide alone for patients with newly diagnosed multiple myeloma (FORTE): a randomised, open-label, phase 2 trial. *Lancet. Oncol.* 22: 1705–1720.

Gerecitano, J., Portlock, C., Hamlin, P. et al. (2011). Phase I trial of weekly and twice-weekly bortezomib with rituximab, cyclophosphamide, and prednisone in relapsed or refractory non-Hodgkin lymphoma. *Clin. Cancer Res.: An Off. J. Am. Ass. Cancer Res.* 17: 2493–2501.

Gerecitano, J., Portlock, C., Moskowitz, C. et al. (2009). Phase 2 study of weekly bortezomib in mantle cell and follicular lymphoma. *B. J. Haematol.* 146: 652–655.

Ghobrial, I.M., Hong, F., Padmanabhan, S. et al. (2010). Phase II trial of weekly bortezomib in combination with rituximab in relapsed or relapsed and refractory Waldenstrom macroglobulinemia. *J. Clin. Oncol.* 28: 1422–1428.

Ghobrial, I.M., Savona, M.R., VIJ, R. et al. (2016). Final results from a multicenter, open-label, dose-escalation phase 1b/2 study of single-agent oprozomib in patients with hematologic malignancies. *Blood* 128: 2110.

Goldschmidt, H., Mai, E.K., Nievergall, E. et al. (2021). Addition of isatuximab to lenalidomide, bortezomib and dexamethasone as induction therapy for newly-diagnosed, transplant-eligible multiple myeloma patients: the phase III GMMG-HD7 trial. *Blood* 138: 463-463.

Gonzalez-Santamarta, M., Quinet, G., Reyes-garau, D. et al. (2020). Resistance to the proteasome inhibitors: lessons from multiple myeloma and mantle cell lymphoma. *Adv. Exp. Med. Biol.* 1233: 153–174.

Goy, A. (2017). Succeeding in breaking the R-CHOP ceiling in DLBCL: learning from negative trials. *J. Clin. Oncol.* 35: 3519–3522.

Goy, A., Bernstein, S.H., Kahl, B.S. et al. (2009). Bortezomib in patients with relapsed or refractory mantle cell lymphoma: updated time-to-event analyses of the multicenter phase 2 PINNACLE study. *Ann Oncol.* 20 (3): 520–525.

Goy, A., Bernstein, S.H., Mcdonald, A. et al. (2010). Potential biomarkers of bortezomib activity in mantle cell lymphoma from the phase 2 PINNACLE trial. *Leukemia. Lymphoma.* 51: 1269–1277.

Goy, A., Hernandez-ilzaliturri, F.J., Kahl, B. et al. (2014). A phase I/II study of the pan Bcl-2 inhibitor obatoclax mesylate plus bortezomib for relapsed or refractory mantle cell lymphoma. *Leu.k Lymphoma.* 55: 2761–2768.

Goy, A., Younes, A., Mclaughlin, P. et al. (2005a). Phase II study of proteasome inhibitor bortezomib in relapsed or refractory B-cell non-Hodgkin's lymphoma. *J. Clin. Oncol.* 23: 667–675.

Goy, A., Younes, A., Mclaughlin, P. et al. (2005b). Phase II study of proteasome inhibitor bortezomib in relapsed or refractory B-cell non-Hodgkin's lymphoma. *J. Cli. Oncol.: Off. J. Am. Soc/. Clin. Oncol.* 23: 667–675.

Gressin, R., Daguindau, N., Tempescul, A. et al. (2019). A phase 2 study of rituximab, bendamustine, bortezomib and dexamethasone for first-line treatment of older patients with mantle cell lymphoma. *Haematologica* 104: 138–146.

Grosicki, S., Simonova, M., Spicka, I. et al. (2020). Once-per-week selinexor, bortezomib, and dexamethasone versus twice-per-week bortezomib and dexamethasone in patients with multiple myeloma (BOSTON): a randomised, open-label, phase 3 trial. *Lancet* 396: 1563–1573.

Hamilton, A.L., Eder, J.P., Pavlick, A.C. et al. (2005). Proteasome inhibition with bortezomib (PS-341): a phase I study with pharmacodynamic end points using a day 1 and day 4 schedule in a 14-day cycle. *J. Clin. Oncol.* 23: 6107–6116.

Harousseau, J.L., Attal, M., Avet-loiseau, H. et al. (2010). Bortezomib plus dexamethasone is superior to vincristine plus doxorubicin plus dexamethasone as induction treatment prior to autologous stem-cell transplantation in newly diagnosed multiple myeloma: results of the IFM 2005-01 phase III trial. *J. Clin. Oncol.* 28: 4621–4629.

Harrison, S.J., Mainwaring, P., Price, T. et al. (2016). Phase I clinical trial of marizomib (NPI-0052) in patients with advanced malignancies including multiple myeloma: study NPI-0052-102 final results. *Clin. Cancer Res.* 22: 4559–4566.

Hasib Sidiqi, M. and Gertz, M.A. (2021). Immunoglobulin light chain amyloidosis diagnosis and treatment algorithm 2021. *Blood Cancer J.* 11: 90.

Hirosawa, M., Morimoto, H., Shibuya, R. et al. (2015). A striking response of plasmablastic lymphoma of the oral cavity to bortezomib: a case report. *Biomark. Res.* 3: 28.

Horton, T.M., Whitlock, J.A., LU, X. et al. (2019). Bortezomib reinduction chemotherapy in high-risk ALL in first relapse: a report from the children's oncology group. *Br. J. Haematol.* 186: 274–285.

Huang, Z., Wu, Y., Zhou, X. et al. (2014). Efficacy of therapy with bortezomib in solid tumors: a review based on 32 clinical trials. *Future Oncol.* 10: 1795–1807.

Jain, S., Diefenbach, C., Zain, J., and O'Connor, O.A. (2011). Emerging role of carfilzomib in treatment of relapsed and refractory lymphoid neoplasms and multiple myeloma. *Core Evid.* 6: 43–57.

Jasielec, J.K., Kubicki, T., Raje, N. et al. (2020). Carfilzomib, lenalidomide, and dexamethasone plus transplant in newly diagnosed multiple myeloma. *Blood* 136: 2513–2523.

Johnson, H.W.B., Lowe, E., Anderl, J.L. et al. (2018). Required immunoproteasome subunit inhibition profile for anti-inflammatory efficacy and clinical candidate KZR-616 ((2 S,3 R)- N-((S)-3-(Cyclopent-1-en-1-yl)-1-((R)-2-methyloxiran-2-yl)-1-oxopropan-2-yl)-3-hydroxy-3-(4-methoxyphenyl)-2-((S)-2-(2-morpholinoacetamido)propanamido)propenamide). *J. Med. Chem.* 61: 11127–11143.

Joseph, N.S., Kaufman, J.L., Dhodapkar, M.V. et al. (2020). Long-term follow-up results of lenalidomide, bortezomib, and dexamethasone induction therapy and risk-adapted maintenance approach in newly diagnosed multiple myeloma. *J. Clin. Oncol.* 38: 1928–1937.

Kahl, B., Li, H., Smith, M. et al. (2012). Mature results from ECOG study E1405 – a phase II study of VcR-CVAD with maintenance rituximab for previously untreated mantle cell lymphoma. *Blood* 120: abst # 153.

Kambhampati, S., Fakhri, B., AI, W.Z. et al. (2021). Carfilzomib in combination with bendamustine and rituximab in patients with relapsed or refractory non-hodgkin lymphoma: a phase I trial. *Clin. Lymphoma. Myeloma. Leuk.* 21: 139–146.

Kaplan, L.D., Maurer, M.J., Stock, W. et al. (2020). Bortezomib consolidation or maintenance following immunochemotherapy and autologous stem cell transplantation for mantle cell lymphoma: CALGB/Alliance 50403. *Am. J. Hematol.* 95: 583–593.

Kastritis, E., Palladini, G., Minnema, M.C. et al. (2021). Daratumumab-based treatment for immunoglobulin light-chain amyloidosis. *N. Engl. J. Med.* 385: 46–58.

Kenific, C.M. and Debnath, J. (2015). Cellular and metabolic functions for autophagy in cancer cells. *Trends. Cell Biol.* 25: 37–45.

Kim, S.J., Yoon, D.H., Kang, H.J. et al. Consortium For Improving Survival Of Lymphoma, I. (2012). Bortezomib in combination with CHOP as first-line treatment for patients with stage III/IV peripheral T-cell lymphomas: a multicentre, single-arm, phase 2 trial. *Eur. J. Cancer* 48: 3223–3231.

Kluin-Nelemans, H.C., Hoster, E., Hermine, O. et al. (2020). Treatment of older patients with mantle cell lymphoma (MCL): long-term follow-up of the randomized European MCL elderly trial. *J. Clin. Oncol.* 38: 248–256.

Kondagunta, G.V., Drucker, B., Schwartz, L. et al. (2004). Phase II trial of bortezomib for patients with advanced renal cell carcinoma. *J Clin Oncol* 22: 3720–3725.

Konopleva, M., Martinelli, G., Daver, N. et al. (2020). MDM2 inhibition: an important step forward in cancer therapy. *Leukemia* 34: 2858–2874.

Kontopodis, E., Kotsakis, A., Kentepozidis, N. et al. (2016). A phase II, open-label trial of bortezomib (VELCADE((R))) in combination with gemcitabine and cisplatin in patients with locally advanced or metastatic non-small cell lung cancer. *Cancer Chemother. Pharmacol.* 77: 949–956.

Koreth, J., Stevenson, K.E., Kim, H.T. et al. (2012). Bortezomib-based graft-versus-host disease prophylaxis in HLA-mismatched unrelated donor transplantation. *J. Clin. Oncol.* 30: 3202–3208.

Krishnan, M., Bociek, R.G., Fanale, M. et al. (2022). Phase 1 trial of carfilzomib in relapsed/refractory peripheral T-cell lymphoma. *Ann. Hematol.* 101: 335–340.

Lakshman, A., Singh, P.P., Rajkumar, S.V. et al. (2017). Efficacy of VDT PACE-like regimens in treatment of relapsed/refractory multiple myeloma – a single center experience. *Blood* 130: 3096-3096.

Lamm, W., Kaufmann, H., Raderer, M. et al. (2011). Bortezomib combined with rituximab and dexamethasone is an active regimen for patients with relapsed and chemotherapy-refractory mantle cell lymphoma. *Haematologica* 96: 1008–1014.

Landgren, O., Hultcrantz, M., Diamond, B. et al. (2021). Safety and effectiveness of weekly carfilzomib, lenalidomide, dexamethasone, and daratumumab combination therapy for patients with newly diagnosed multiple myeloma: the MANHATTAN nonrandomized clinical trial. *JAMA Oncol.* 7: 862–868.

Laubach, J.P., Schjesvold, F., Mariz, M. et al. (2021). Efficacy and safety of oral panobinostat plus subcutaneous bortezomib and oral dexamethasone in patients with relapsed or relapsed and refractory multiple myeloma (PANORAMA 3): an open-label, randomised, phase 2 study. *Lancet. Oncol.* 22: 142–154.

Le Gouill, S., Thieblemont, C., Oberic, L. et al. (2017). Rituximab after autologous stem-cell transplantation in mantle-cell lymphoma. *N. Engl. J. Med.* 377: 1250–1260.

Leblebjian, H., Noonan, K., Paba-prada, C. et al. (2015). Cyclophosphamide, bortezomib, and dexamethasone combination in waldenstrom macroglobulinemia. *Am. J. Hematol.* 90: E122–3.

Lee, H.J., Badillo, M., Romaguera, J., and Wang, M. (2019). A phase II study of carfilzomib in the treatment of relapsed/refractory mantle cell lymphoma. *Br. J. Haematol.* 184: 460–462.

Lee, H.J., Romaguera, J.E., Feng, L. et al. (2017). Phase II study of bortezomib in combination with cyclophosphamide and rituximab for relapsed or refractory mantle cell lymphoma. *Oncologist* 22: 549–553.

Lee, H.J., Schmelz, J.L., Cramer, F. et al. (2020). A phase I study of carfilzomib in combination with ibrutinib for relapsed refractory mantle cell lymphoma. *Br. J. Haemato.l* 188: e94–e98.

Leonard, J.P., Kolibaba, K.S., Reeves, J.A. et al. (2017). Randomized phase II study of R-CHOP with or without bortezomib in previously untreated patients with non-germinal center B-cell-like diffuse large B-cell lymphoma. *J. Clin. Oncol.* 35: 3538–3546.

Li, J., Yakushi, T., Parlati, F. et al. (2017). Capzimin is a potent and specific inhibitor of proteasome isopeptidase Rpn11. *Nat. Chem. Biol.* 13: 486–493.

Liu, X., Yue, P., Chen, S. et al. (2007). The proteasome inhibitor PS-341 (bortezomib) up-regulates DR5 expression leading to induction of apoptosis and enhancement of TRAIL-induced apoptosis despite up-regulation of c-FLIP and survivin expression in human NSCLC cells. *Cancer Res.* 67: 4981–4988.

Lonial, S., Durie, B., Palumbo, A., and San-miguel, J. (2016). Monoclonal antibodies in the treatment of multiple myeloma: current status and future perspectives. *Leukemia* 30: 526–535.

Mackay, H., Hedley, D., Major, P. et al. (2005). A phase II trial with pharmacodynamic endpoints of the proteasome inhibitor bortezomib in patients with metastatic colorectal cancer. *Clin. Cancer Res.* 11: 5526–5533.

Manni, S., Brancalion, A., Mandato, E. et al. (2013). Protein kinase CK2 inhibition down modulates the NF-kappaB and STAT3 survival pathways, enhances the cellular proteotoxic stress and synergistically boosts the cytotoxic effect of bortezomib on multiple myeloma and mantle cell lymphoma cells. *PLoS One* 8: e75280.

Markovic, S.N., Geyer, S.M., Dawkins, F. et al. (2005). A phase II study of bortezomib in the treatment of metastatic malignant melanoma. *Cancer* 103: 2584–2589.

Marrero, W.D., Cruz-chacon, A., Castillo, C., and Cabanillas, F. (2018). Successful use of bortezomib-lenalidomide combination as treatment for a patient with plasmablastic lymphoma. *Clin. Lymphoma. Myeloma. Leuk.* 18: e275–e277.

Maurer, M.J., Ghesquieres, H., Link, B.K. et al. (2018). Diagnosis-to-treatment interval is an important clinical factor in newly diagnosed diffuse large B-cell lymphoma and has implication for bias in clinical trials. *J. Clin. Oncol.* 36: 1603–1610.

Mendler, J.H., Kelly, J., Voci, S. et al. (2008). Bortezomib and gemcitabine in relapsed or refractory Hodgkin's lymphoma. *Ann. Oncol.* 19: 1759–1764.

Messinger, Y.H., Gaynon, P.S., Sposto, R. et al. Therapeutic Advances in Childhood, L. and Lymphoma, C. (2012). Bortezomib with chemotherapy is highly active in advanced B-precursor acute lymphoblastic leukemia: therapeutic advances in childhood leukemia & lymphoma (TACL) study. *Blood* 120: 285–290.

Milani, P. and Palladini, G. (2020). Conventional therapy for amyloid light-chain amyloidosis. *Acta. Haematol.* 143: 365–372.

Millward, M., Price, T., Townsend, A. et al. (2012). Phase 1 clinical trial of the novel proteasome inhibitor marizomib with the histone deacetylase inhibitor vorinostat in patients with melanoma, pancreatic and lung cancer based on in vitro assessments of the combination. *Invest. New Drugs* 30: 2303–2317.

Mitsiades, N., Mitsiades, C.S., Richardson, P.G. et al. (2003). The proteasome inhibitor PS-341 potentiates sensitivity of multiple myeloma cells to conventional chemotherapeutic agents: therapeutic applications. *Blood* 101: 2377–2380.

Moreau, P., Chanan-khan, A., Roberts, A.W. et al. (2017). Promising efficacy and acceptable safety of venetoclax plus bortezomib and dexamethasone in relapsed/refractory MM. *Blood* 130: 2392–2400.

Moreau, P., Dimopoulos, M.A., Mikhael, J. et al. (2021). Isatuximab, carfilzomib, and dexamethasone in relapsed multiple myeloma (IKEMA): a multicentre, open-label, randomised phase 3 trial. *Lancet* 397: 2361–2371.

Moreau, P., Masszi, T., Grzasko, N. et al. (2016). Oral ixazomib, lenalidomide, and dexamethasone for multiple myeloma. *N. Engl. J. Med.* 374: 1621–1634.

Moreau, P., Mateos, M.V., Berenson, J.R. et al. (2018). Once weekly versus twice weekly carfilzomib dosing in patients with relapsed and refractory multiple myeloma (A.R.R.O.W.): interim analysis results of a randomised, phase 3 study. *Lancet. Oncol.* 19: 953–964.

Morris, M.J., Kelly, W.K., Slovin, S. et al. (2007). A phase II trial of bortezomib and prednisone for castration resistant metastatic prostate cancer. *J. Urol.* 178: 2378–2383. discussion 2383-4.

Morrison, V.A., Jung, S.H., Johnson, J. et al. (2015). Therapy with bortezomib plus lenalidomide for relapsed/refractory mantle cell lymphoma: final results of a phase II trial (CALGB 50501). *Leuk. Lymphoma.* 56: 958–964.

Nalawansha, D.A., Paiva, S.L., Rafizadeh, D.N. et al. (2020). Retraction of "targeted protein internalization and degradation by ENDosome TARgeting chimeras (ENDTACs)". *ACS Cent. Sci.* 6: 312.

Natarajan-Ame, S., Park, S., Ades, L. et al. (2012). Bortezomib combined with low-dose cytarabine in Intermediate-2 and high risk myelodysplastic syndromes. A phase I/II study by the GFM. *Br. J. Haematol.* 158: 232–237.

Nawrocki, S.T., Sweeney-gotsch, B., Takamori, R., and Mcconkey, D.J. (2004). The proteasome inhibitor bortezomib enhances the activity of docetaxel in orthotopic human pancreatic tumor xenografts. *Mol. Cancer Ther.* 3: 59–70.

Nikrad, M., Johnson, T., Puthalalath, H. et al. (2005). The proteasome inhibitor bortezomib sensitizes cells to killing by death receptor ligand TRAIL via BH3-only proteins Bik and Bim. *Mo.l Cancer Ther.* 4: 443–449.

O'Connor, O.A., Moskowitz, C., Portlock, C. et al. (2009a). Patients with chemotherapy-refractory mantle cell lymphoma experience high response rates and identical progression-free survivals compared with patients with relapsed disease following treatment with single agent bortezomib: results of a multicentre phase 2 clinical trial. *Br. J. Haematol.* 145: 34–39.

O'Connor, O.A., Portlock, C., Moskowitz, C. et al. (2010). Time to treatment response in patients with follicular lymphoma treated with bortezomib is longer compared with other histologic subtypes. *Clin. Cancer Res.* 16: 719–726.

O'Connor, O.A., Stewart, A.K., Vallone, M. et al. (2009b). A phase 1 dose escalation study of the safety and pharmacokinetics of the novel proteasome inhibitor carfilzomib (PR-171) in patients with hematologic malignancies. *Clin. Cancer Res.: An Off. J. Am. Ass. Cancer Res.* 15: 7085–7091.

O'Connor, O.A., Stewart, A.K., Vallone, M. et al. (2009c). A phase 1 dose escalation study of the safety and pharmacokinetics of the novel proteasome inhibitor carfilzomib (PR-171) in patients with hematologic malignancies. *Clin. Cancer Res.* 15: 7085–7091.

O'Connor, O.A., Wright, J., Moskowitz, C. et al. (2005). Phase II clinical experience with the novel proteasome inhibitor bortezomib in patients with indolent non-Hodgkin's lymphoma and mantle cell lymphoma. *J. Clin. Oncol.: Off. J. Am.Soc. Clin. Oncol.* 23: 676–684.

Offner, F., Samoilova, O., Osmanov, E. et al. (2015). Frontline rituximab, cyclophosphamide, doxorubicin, and prednisone with bortezomib (VR-CAP) or vincristine (R-CHOP) for non-GCB DLBCL. *Blood* 126: 1893–1901.

Orlowski, R.Z., Stinchcombe, T.E., Mitchell, B.S. et al. (2002). Phase I trial of the proteasome inhibitor PS-341 in patients with refractory hematologic malignancies. *J. Clin. Oncol.* 20: 4420–4427.

Pai, C.C., Hsiao, H.H., Sun, K. et al. (2014). Therapeutic benefit of bortezomib on acute graft-versus-host disease is tissue specific and is associated with interleukin-6 levels. *Biol. Blood Marrow. Transplant.* 20: 1899–1904.

Palumbo, A., Bringhen, S., Larocca, A. et al. (2014). Bortezomib-melphalan-prednisone-thalidomide followed by maintenance with bortezomib-thalidomide compared with bortezomib-melphalan-prednisone for initial treatment of multiple myeloma: updated follow-up and improved survival. *J. Clin. Oncol.* 32: 634–640.

Palumbo, A., Offidani, M., Pégourie, B. et al. (2015). Elotuzumab plus bortezomib and dexamethasone versus bortezomib and dexamethasone in patients with relapsed/refractory multiple myeloma: 2-year Follow-up. *Blood* 126: 510-510.

Paoluzzi, L., Scotto, L., Seshan, V., and O'Connor, O.A. (2009). Evaluation of the potential of histone deacetylase inhibitors to synergize the antineoplastic effects of the proteasome inhibitor bortezomib in mantle cell lymphoma (MCL). *JCO* 27: abst # 8584.

Pasquale, R., Giannotta, J.A., Barcellini, W., and Fattizzo, B. (2021). Bortezomib in autoimmune hemolytic anemia and beyond. *Ther. Adv. Hematol.* 12: 20406207211046428.

Perez-Galan, P., Mora-jensen, H., Weniger, M.A. et al. (2011). Bortezomib resistance in mantle cell lymphoma is associated with plasmacytic differentiation. *Blood* 117: 542–552.

Perez-Galan, P., Roue, G., Villamor, N. et al. (2007). The BH3-mimetic GX15-070 synergizes with bortezomib in mantle cell lymphoma by enhancing Noxa-mediated activation of Bak. *Blood* 109: 4441–4449.

Pidala, J., Bhatt, V.R., Hamilton, B. et al. (2020). Ixazomib for treatment of refractory chronic graft-versus-host disease: a chronic GVHD consortium phase II trial. *Biol. Blood Marrow Transplant.* 26: 1612–1619.

Puvvada, S.D., Guillen-rodriguez, J., Kumar, A. et al. (2018). Phase 2 open-label study of bortezomib, cladribine, and rituximab in advanced, newly diagnosed, and relapsed/refractory mantle-cell and indolent lymphomas. *Clin. Lymphoma. Myeloma. Leuk.* 18: 58–64.

Qin, J.Z., Ziffra, J., Stennett, L. et al. (2005). Proteasome inhibitors trigger NOXA-mediated apoptosis in melanoma and myeloma cells. *Cancer Res.* 65: 6282–6293.

Reddy, N. and Czuczman, M.S. (2010). Enhancing activity and overcoming chemoresistance in hematologic malignancies with bortezomib: preclinical mechanistic studies. *Ann. Oncol.* 21: 1756–1764.

Reeder, C.B., Reece, D.E., Kukreti, V. et al. (2009). Cyclophosphamide, bortezomib and dexamethasone induction for newly diagnosed multiple myeloma: high response rates in a phase II clinical trial. *Leukemia* 23: 1337–1341.

Reid, E., Nooka, A., Blackmon, J., and Lechowicz, M.J. (2012). Clinical use of rituximab in patients with HIV related lymphoma and multicentric castleman's disease. *Curr Drug Deliv.* 9 (1): 41–51.

Reid, E.G., Suazo, A., Lensing, S.Y. et al. (2020). Pilot trial AMC-063: safety and efficacy of bortezomib in AIDS-associated kaposi sarcoma. *Clin. Cancer Res.* 26: 558–565.

Ribrag, V., Tilly, H., Casasnovas, O. et al. (2013). Efficacy and toxicity of two schedules of bortezomib in patients with recurrent or refractory follicular lymphoma: a randomised phase II trial from the groupe d'Etude des lymphomes de l'Adulte (GELA). *Eur. J. Cancer* 49: 904–910.

Richardson, P.G., Barlogie, B., Berenson, J. et al. (2003). A phase 2 study of bortezomib in relapsed, refractory myeloma. *N. Engl. J. Med.* 348: 2609–2617.

Richardson, P.G., Sonneveld, P., Schuster, M. et al. (2007). Extended follow-up of a phase 3 trial in relapsed multiple myeloma: final time-to-event results of the APEX trial. *Blood* 110: 3557–3560.

Richardson, P.G., Weller, E., Lonial, S. et al. (2010). Lenalidomide, bortezomib, and dexamethasone combination therapy in patients with newly diagnosed multiple myeloma. *Blood* 116: 679–686.

Robak, T., Huang, H., Jin, J. et al. (2015). Bortezomib-based therapy for newly diagnosed mantle-cell lymphoma. *N. Engl. J. Med.* 372: 944–953.

Robak, T., Huang, H., Jin, J. et al. (2019). Association between bortezomib dose intensity and overall survival in mantle cell lymphoma patients on frontline VR-CAP in the phase 3 LYM-3002 study(.). *Leuk. Lymphoma.* 60: 172–179.

Robak, T., Jin, J., Pylypenko, H. et al. (2018). Frontline bortezomib, rituximab, cyclophosphamide, doxorubicin, and prednisone (VR-CAP) versus rituximab, cyclophosphamide, doxorubicin, vincristine, and prednisone (R-CHOP) in transplantation-ineligible patients with newly diagnosed mantle cell lymphoma: final overall survival results of a randomised, open-label, phase 3 study. *Lancet Oncol.* 19: 1449–1458.

Romaguera, J.E., Fayad, L.E., Mclaughlin, P. et al. (2010). Phase I trial of bortezomib in combination with rituximab-hyperCVAD alternating with rituximab, methotrexate and cytarabine for untreated aggressive mantle cell lymphoma. *Br. J. Haematol.* 151: 47–53.

Romaguera, J.E., Wang, M., Feng, L. et al. (2018). Phase 2 trial of bortezomib in combination with rituximab plus hyperfractionated cyclophosphamide, vincristine, doxorubicin, and dexamethasone alternating with bortezomib, rituximab, methotrexate, and cytarabine for untreated mantle cell lymphoma. *Cancer* 124: 2561–2569.

Rosiñol, L., Oriol, A., Teruel, A.I. et al. (2012). Superiority of bortezomib, thalidomide, and dexamethasone (VTD) as induction pretransplantation therapy in multiple myeloma: a randomized phase 3 PETHEMA/GEM study. *Blood* 120: 1589–1596.

Rossi, G., Gramegna, D., Paoloni, F. et al. (2018). Short course of bortezomib in anemic patients with relapsed cold agglutinin disease: a phase 2 prospective GIMEMA study. *Blood* 132: 547–550.

Ruan, J., Martin, P., Furman, R.R. et al. (2011). Bortezomib plus CHOP-rituximab for previously untreated diffuse large B-cell lymphoma and mantle cell lymphoma. *J. Clin. Oncol.: Off. J. Am. Soc. Clin. Oncol.* 29: 690–697.

Rummel, M.J., Niederle, N., Maschmeyer, G. et al. (2013). Bendamustine plus rituximab versus CHOP plus rituximab as first-line treatment for patients with indolent and mantle-cell lymphomas: an open-label, multicentre, randomised, phase 3 non-inferiority trial. *Lancet* 381: 1203–1210.

Saba, N.S., Dang, D., Saba, J. et al. (2013). Bortezomib in plasmablastic lymphoma: a case report and review of the literature. *Onkologie* 36: 287–291.

San Miguel, J.F., Schlag, R., Khuageva, N.K. et al. (2008). Bortezomib plus melphalan and prednisone for initial treatment of multiple myeloma. *N. Engl. J. Med.* 359: 906–917.

Sanderson, M.P., Friese-hamim, M., Walter-bausch, G. et al. (2021). M3258 is a selective inhibitor of the immunoproteasome subunit LMP7 (beta5i) delivering efficacy in multiple myeloma models. *Mol. Cancer Ther.* 20: 1378–1387.

Sarlo, C., Buccisano, F., Maurillo, L. et al. (2013). Phase II study of Bortezomib as a single agent in patients with previously untreated or relapsed/refractory acute myeloid leukemia ineligible for intensive therapy. *Leuk. Res. Treatment* 2013: 705714.

Schubert, U., Anton, L.C., Gibbs, J. et al. (2000). Rapid degradation of a large fraction of newly synthesized proteins by proteasomes. *Nature* 404: 770–774.

Shah, J.J., Jakubowiak, A.J., O'Connor, O.A. et al. (2016). Phase I study of the novel investigational NEDD8-activating enzyme inhibitor pevonedistat (MLN4924) in patients with relapsed/refractory multiple myeloma or lymphoma. *Clin. Cancer Res.* 22: 34–43.

Shah, M.A., Power, D.G., Kindler, H.L. et al. (2011). A multicenter, phase II study of bortezomib (PS-341) in patients with unresectable or metastatic gastric and gastroesophageal junction adenocarcinoma. *Invest. New Drugs* 29: 1475–1481.

Shahid, S. and Prockop, S.E. (2021). Epstein-Barr virus-associated post-transplant lymphoproliferative disorders: beyond chemotherapy treatment. *Cancer Drug Resist.* 4: 646–664.

Shen, J., Song, G., An, M. et al. (2014). The use of hollow mesoporous silica nanospheres to encapsulate bortezomib and improve efficacy for non-small cell lung cancer therapy. *Biomaterials* 35: 316–326.

Shi, Y., Yu, Y., Wang, Z. et al. (2016). Second-generation proteasome inhibitor carfilzomib enhances doxorubicin-induced cytotoxicity and apoptosis in breast cancer cells. *Oncotarget* 7: 73697–73710.

Siegel, D., Martin, T., Nooka, A. et al (2013). Integrated safety profile of single-agent carfilzomib: experience from 526 patients enrolled in 4 phase II clinical studies. *Haematologica* 98: 1753–1761.

Siegel, D.S., Dimopoulos, M.A., Ludwig, H. et al. (2018). Improvement in overall survival with carfilzomib, lenalidomide, and dexamethasone in patients with relapsed or refractory multiple myeloma. *J. Clin. Oncol.* 36: 728–734.

Siegel, D.S., Martin, T., Wang, M. et al. (2012). A phase 2 study of single-agent carfilzomib (PX-171-003-A1) in patients with relapsed and refractory multiple myeloma. *Blood* 120: 2817–2825.

Skarbnik, A.P., Ma, E., Lafeuille, M.H. et al. (2017). Treatment patterns and outcomes with subcutaneous bortezomib in patients with relapsed mantle cell lymphoma: a retrospective, observational study of patient medical records from US community oncology practices. *Leuk. Lymphoma.* 58: 1968–1972.

Smith, M., Jegede, O., Martin, P. et al. (2021). ECOG-ACRIN E1411 randomized phase 2 trial of bendamustine-rituximab (BR)-based induction followed by rituximab (R) ± lenalidomide (L) consolidation for mantle cell lymphoma: effect of adding bortezomib to front-line BR induction on PFS. *JCO* 39: 703.

Smith, S.D., Gandhy, S., Gopal, A.K. et al. (2019). Modified VR-CAP, alternating with rituximab and high-dose cytarabine: an effective pre-transplant induction regimen for mantle cell lymphoma. *Clin. Lymphoma. Myeloma. Leuk.* 19: 48–52.

Sonbol, M.B., Hilal, T., Dueck, A.C. et al. (2018). A phase 2 study of rituximab, cyclophosphamide, bortezomib and dexamethasone (R-CyBorD) in relapsed low grade and mantle cell lymphoma. *Leuk. Lymphoma.* 59: 2128–2134.

Sonneveld, P., Asselbergs, E., Zweegman, S. et al. (2015). Phase 2 study of carfilzomib, thalidomide, and dexamethasone as induction/consolidation therapy for newly diagnosed multiple myeloma. *Blood* 125: 449–456.

Sonneveld, P., Zweegman, S., Cavo, M. et al. (2018). Carfilzomib, pomalidomide and dexamethasone (KPd) in patients with multiple myeloma refractory to bortezomib and lenalidomide. the EMN011 trial. *Blood* 132: 801.

Sonneveld, P.S.-W.I., Van Der Holt, B. et al. (2010). HOVON-65/GMMG-HD4 randomized phase III trial comparing bortezomib, doxorubicin, dexamethasone (PAD) vs VAD followed by high-dose melphalan (HDM) and maintenance with bortezomib or thalidomide in patients with newly diagnosed multiple myeloma. *Blood (ASH Annual Meeting Absracts)* 116: 23–24.

Spurgeon, S.E., Pindyck, T., Okada, C. et al. (2011). Cladribine plus rituximab is an effective therapy for newly diagnosed mantle cell lymphoma. *Leuk. Lymphoma.* 52: 1488–1494.

Stege, C.A.M., Nasserinejad, K., Spek, E.V.D. et al. (2021). Ixazomib, daratumumab, and low-dose dexamethasone in frail patients with newly diagnosed multiple myeloma: the hovon 143 study. *J. Clin. Oncol.* 39: 2758–2767.

Tan, D., Phipps, C., Hwang, W.Y. et al. (2015). Panobinostat in combination with bortezomib in patients with relapsed or refractory peripheral T-cell lymphoma: an open-label, multicentre phase 2 trial. *Lancet Haematol.* 2: e326–33.

Tanaka, K. (1998). Molecular biology of the proteasome. *Biochem. Biophys. Res. Commun.* 247: 537–541.

Till, B.G., Li, H., Bernstein, S.H. et al. (2016). Phase II trial of R-CHOP plus bortezomib induction therapy followed by bortezomib maintenance for newly diagnosed mantle cell lymphoma: SWOG S0601. *Br. J. Haematol.* 172: 208–218.

Trelle, S., Sezer, O., Naumann, R. et al. (2007). Bortezomib in combination with dexamethasone for patients with relapsed Hodgkin's lymphoma: results of a prematurely closed phase II study (NCT00148018). *Haematologica* 92: 568–569.

Treon, S.P., Hunter, Z.R., Matous, J. et al. (2007). Multicenter clinical trial of bortezomib in relapsed/refractory Waldenstrom's macroglobulinemia: results of WMCTG Trial 03-248. *Clin. Cancer Res.* 13: 3320–3325.

Treon, S.P., Ioakimidis, L., Soumerai, J.D. et al. (2009). Primary therapy of Waldenstrom macroglobulinemia with bortezomib, dexamethasone, and rituximab: WMCTG clinical trial 05-180. *J. Clin. Oncol.* 27: 3830–3835.

Treon, S.P., Tripsas, C.K., Meid, K. et al. (2014). Carfilzomib, rituximab, and dexamethasone (CaRD) treatment offers a neuropathy-sparing approach for treating Waldenstrom's macroglobulinemia. *Blood* 124: 503–510.

Troch, M., Jonak, C., Mullauer, L. et al. (2009). A phase II study of bortezomib in patients with MALT lymphoma. *Haematologica* 94: 738–742.

Van Keep, M., Gairy, K., Seshagiri, D. et al. (2016). Cost-effectiveness analysis of bortezomib in combination with rituximab, cyclophosphamide, doxorubicin, vincristine and prednisone (VR-CAP) in patients with previously untreated mantle cell lymphoma. *BMC Cancer* 16: 598.

Vaxman, I. and Gertz, M. (2019). Recent advances in the diagnosis, risk stratification, and management of systemic light-chain amyloidosis. *Acta Haematol.* 141: 93–106.

Vaziri, S.A., Grabowski, D.R., Hill, J. et al. (2009). Inhibition of proteasome activity by bortezomib in renal cancer cells is p53 dependent and VHL independent. *Anticancer Res.* 29: 2961–2969.

Verhoef, G., Robak, T., Huang, H. et al. (2017). Association between quality of response and outcomes in patients with newly diagnosed mantle cell lymphoma receiving VR-CAP versus R-CHOP in the phase 3 LYM-3002 study. *Haematologica* 102: 895–902.

Walker, A.R., Klisovic, R.B., Garzon, R. et al. (2014). Phase I study of azacitidine and bortezomib in adults with relapsed or refractory acute myeloid leukemia. *Leuk. Lymphoma.* 55: 1304–1308.

Wang, X.X., Gao, Y., Jin, J. et al. (2021). Bortezomib in combination with fludarabine plus cyclophosphamide for patients with relapsed or refractory mantle-cell lymphoma: results of the LYM-4003 study. *Ann. Hematol.* 100: 2961–2968.

Wickremasinghe, R.G. (2008). Why is CLL refractory to bortezomib? *Blood* 112: 3540–3541.

Yan, M., Dong, Z., Zhao, F. et al. (2014). CD20-positive plasmablastic lymphoma with excellent response to bortezomib combined with rituximab. *Eur. J. Haematol.* 93: 77–80.

Yazbeck, V., Shafer, D., Perkins, E.B. et al. (2018). A phase II trial of bortezomib and vorinostat in mantle cell lymphoma and diffuse large B-cell lymphoma. *Clin. Lymphoma. Myeloma. Leuk.* 18 (569–575): e1.

Yun, Y.S., Kim, K.H., Tschida, B. et al. (2016). mTORC1 coordinates protein synthesis and immunoproteasome formation via PRAS40 to prevent accumulation of protein stress. *Mol. Cell* 61: 625–639.

Zangari, M., Terpos, E., Zhan, F., and Tricot, G. (2012). Impact of bortezomib on bone health in myeloma: a review of current evidence. *Cancer Treat Rev.* 38: 968–980.

Zhao, J., Zhai, B., Gygi, S.P., and Goldberg, A.L. (2015). mTOR inhibition activates overall protein degradation by the ubiquitin proteasome system as well as by autophagy. *Proc. Natl. Acad. Sci. U. S. A.* 112: 15790–15797.

Zhou, H.-J., Aujay, M.A., Bennett, M.K. et al. (2009). Design and synthesis of an orally bioavailable and selective peptide epoxyketone proteasome inhibitor (PR-047). *J. Med. Chem.* 52: 3028–3038.

Zhou, J. and Chng, W.-J. (2019). Novel mechanism of drug resistance to proteasome inhibitors in multiple myeloma. *World J. Clin. Oncol.* 10: 303–306.

Zhu, H., Zhang, L., DONG, F. et al. (2005). Bik/NBK accumulation correlates with apoptosis-induction by bortezomib (PS-341, Velcade) and other proteasome inhibitors. *Oncogene* 24: 4993–4999.

Zinzani, P.L., Musuraca, G., Tani, M. et al. (2007). Phase II trial of proteasome inhibitor bortezomib in patients with relapsed or refractory cutaneous T-cell lymphoma. *J. Clin. Oncol.* 25: 4293–4297.

25

Targeting Nuclear Protein Transport with XPO Inhibitors in Lymphoma

Farheen Manji, Kyla Trkulja, Rob C. Laister, and John Kuruvilla

Princess Margaret Cancer Centre, University of Toronto, Canada

Take Home Messages

- Nuclear export is a critical cellular process required to maintain cellular homeostasis, which is dysregulated in many cancers, including lymphoma.
- Selective inhibitors of nuclear export such as selinexor target XPO1 by preventing XPO1-cargo protein interactions.
- XPO1 expression is noted to be an adverse prognostic factor in various malignancies. However, no biomarkers for response have been identified for selinexor or other XPO1 inhibitors.
- While early development of XPO1 inhibitors was limited by toxicities, selective inhibitors of nuclear export have shown promise of clinical efficacy and manageable toxicity leading to the approval of selinexor (KPT-330) by the FDA for relapsed/refractory diffuse large B-cell lymphoma with at least two prior lines of therapy.
- The toxicity of selinexor is well described in the multiple myeloma and lymphoma literature with hematologic and GI toxicity the most common. Aggressive supportive care is recommended to prolong duration of treatment and manage side effects.
- In diffuse large B-cell lymphoma, selinexor monotherapy has modest efficacy. Multiple studies are investigating selinexor in combination with chemotherapy or novel agents to try and augment efficacy but toxicity data will be important to understand tolerability of combination therapy.

Introduction

Nuclear-cytoplasmic transport of proteins is essential for normal cellular function but can be disrupted by cancer cells to evade apoptosis and facilitate tumor cell survival and proliferation. As a result, there is growing interest in studying the disruption of nuclear protein transport mechanisms in carcinogenesis as an anti-cancer treatment strategy. One strategy of interest is blockade of the exportin 1 (XPO1), a nuclear export protein, which when dysregulated can suppress key tumor suppressor proteins. This chapter will explore mechanisms of oncogenesis that involve alterations of XPO1 biology and review the key data regarding XPO1 inhibitors in lymphoma. The first-in-class drug targeting this unique process is selinexor (KPT-330), a selective inhibitor of nuclear export (SINE).

XPO1 Biology

The intracellular space of mammalian cells is functionally compartmentalized into distinct locales, in part using membrane bound organelles. The nuclear envelope that separates the cytoplasm and the nucleus is a prototypical example of this phenomenon. The cytoplasm is host to a variety of cellular machineries including the cytoskeleton, secretory machinery, and metabolic enzymes, and is the site of protein translation and folding. The nucleus, on the other hand, houses the genome, the relevant proteins required for duplicating the genome during cell division and maintaining its fidelity in addition to the RNA metabolizing enzymes that generate the templates for protein synthesis. The inability to properly segregate elements of the nuclear and cytoplasmic fractions could be problematic if mislocated proteins interfere with processes in the compartment to which they are mislocalized. In a similar vein, the translocation of proteins away from sites where they are needed to perform critical cellular functions may leave these duties unfulfilled which could lead to loss of function phenotypes. In the case of tumor suppressor proteins, spatiotemporal mislocalization

Precision Cancer Therapies: Targeting Oncogenic Drivers and Signaling Pathways in Lymphoid Malignancies: From Concept to Practice, Volume 1, First Edition. Edited by Owen A. O'Connor, Stephen M. Ansell, and John F. Seymour.

that results in a loss of function represents a potential route to oncogenesis without the need for acquiring mutations. Thus, regulating the transport of the appropriate molecules between the nucleus and the cytoplasm is a key component of cellular homeostasis and, notably, is a process that has been shown to be dysregulated in several cancers including lymphoma.

The nuclear membrane is a semi-selective barrier governed by the nuclear pore complex (NPC) which is permeable to smaller proteins in the range of 40–60 kDa that can freely diffuse through the NPC (Timney et al. 2016). Proteins whose molecular weights exceed this size limit, however, require active, receptor-mediated transport into and out of the nucleus, a process that is tightly regulated by the family of proteins known as the karyopherins (Chook and Süel 2011). Of the 19 known karyopherin-β family members, XPO1 (also known as CRM1) is the best studied and is the target of the novel family of cancer therapeutics known as the SINE compounds. The XPO1 cycle that mediates nuclear export is a tightly regulated, energy-dependent process that is driven by a concentration gradient of RanGTP which is estimated to be a 100-fold higher in the nucleus compared to the cytoplasm and is maintained by nuclear RanGAP which generates RanGTP from RanGDP. This RanGTP concentration gradient is critical to establish the directionality of XPO1's transport activity (Pemberton and Paschal 2005). The interaction of RanGTP with XPO1 in the nucleus stabilizes complex formation between XPO1 and its substrate cargo molecule. This complex is then capable of traversing through the NPC into the cytoplasm. Once in the cytoplasm, the GTP-hydrolyzing enzyme, RanGEF, converts RanGTP onto RanGDP which destabilizes the XPO1 complex and results in the release of the cargo molecule into the cytoplasm (Figure 25.1). While initial estimations pointed to XPO1 being able to facilitate the transport of ~200 proteins, more recent mass spectrometry-based proteomic studies have shown that the XPO1 "exportome" constitutes a panel of over 1000 proteins, though most of these candidate cargo molecules require further validation (Kırlı et al. 2015). The primary mechanism of action associated with XPO1-mediated oncogenesis is believed to be via the nuclear export and subsequent functional inactivation of tumor suppressor proteins that reside in the nucleus (Gravina et al. 2014). Cargo molecules fitting this description that are validated XPO1 targets include, but are not limited to, the well-known tumor suppressors p53, Rb, p21, and p27. As such, the ability of small molecule inhibitors to prevent XPO1-mediated inactivation of nuclear tumor suppressor proteins is likely to be the mechanism by which these inhibitors exert their anti-neoplastic activities.

Our understanding of how XPO1 interacts with various cofactors, cargo proteins, and inhibitors has been greatly aided by a number of structural biology initiatives that have resulted in the generation of high-resolution crystal structures. The full length human XPO1 protein spans 1071 amino acids that fold into 21 repeated Huntington, elongation factor 3, protein phosphatase 2A, TOR1 (HEAT) repeats arranged in circular fashion and taking the form of a ring-like structure (Walker et al. 2021). The top of the ring forms the docking site for RanGTP and RanBP1 which are required to drive the GTP-dependent translocation of the XPO1-cargo complex out of the nucleus. Both the natural product, polyketide leptomycin B (LMB; Figure 25.2b, left), which is a *Streptomyces* sp. secondary metabolite, and the synthetic XPO1 inhibitor selinexor (Figure 25.2b, right) are small molecules that act as potent inhibitors of XPO1 activity. Both molecules alkylate XPO1 by forming a covalent bond with C528 which is located on the outer surface of XPO1, and the covalent modification of XPO1 by selinexor is described as slowly reversible (Sun et al. 2013; Walker et al. 2021). The LMB (Figure 25.2c, left) and selinexor (Figure 25.2c, center) binding sites on XPO1 encompass the same site where the NES sequences for XPO1 cargo molecules bind. This is evident when one compares the crystal structures of the inhibitor and cargo bound forms of XPO1. As an exemplar we show the complex between a 16 residue peptide derived from the XPO1 cargo molecule HDAC5 bound to XPO1 (Figure 25.2c, right). The HDAC5 peptide, like LMB and selinexor, binds to the hydrophobic groove formed between HEAT repeats 11 and 12 on XPO1 (Figure 25.2c, dark blue). This data indicates that the mechanism of action for these two inhibitors is by direct competition for the binding site utilized by XPO1 cargo molecules.

Pre-clinical and Clinical Data

The first XPO1 inhibitor, leptomycin B, was naturally derived from *Streptomyces* and initially used as an antifungal (Nishi et al. 1994). It was noted to target XPO1/CRM1 at Cys528 irreversibly. While anti-tumor activity in pre-clinical models was promising, early phase 1 studies of leptomycin in advanced cancers were halted due to significant toxicity including nausea, vomiting, malaise, and anorexia (Newlands et al. 1996). The second generation of XPO1 inhibitors was developed to covalently interact with Cys528 but with slowly irreversible binding to residues thereby making them more tolerable. The second generation of SINEs includes KPT-185, KPT-251, KPT-276, selinexor, eltanexor, and verdinexor. These agents are all orally bioavailable and selective inhibitors of XPO1; however, selinexor (KPT-330) has shown most promise in clinical data (see Table 25.1).

Phase 1 Evaluation in Non-Hodgkin's Lymphoma

The phase 1 study of selinexor in advanced hematologic malignancies enrolled 79 patients with non-Hodgkin's lymphoma (NHL) (Kuruvilla et al. 2014). The majority

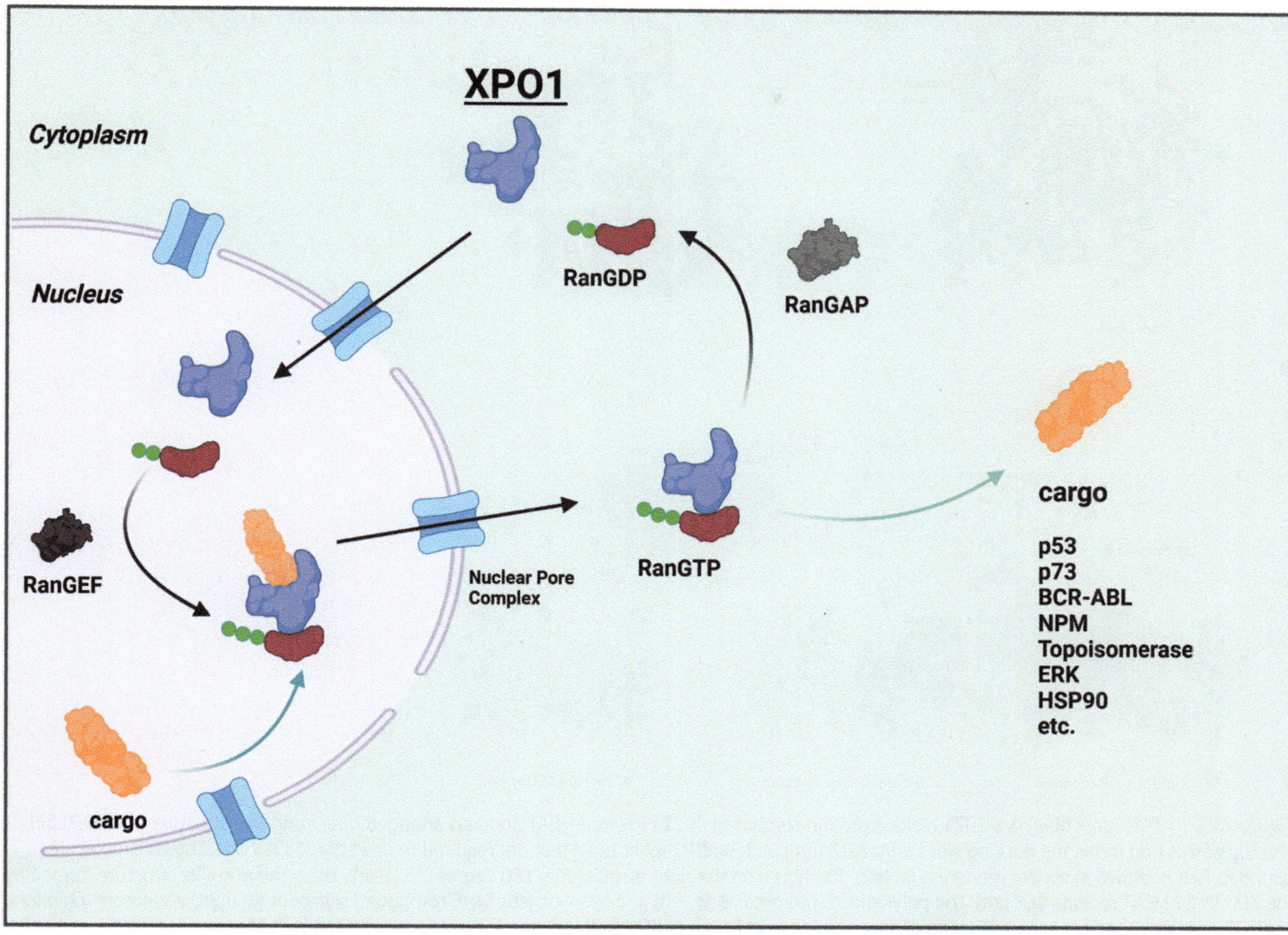

Figure 25.1 The XPO1 cycle mediates the energy-dependent export of cargo molecules from the nucleus to the cytoplasm. RanGTP bound XPO1 interacts with cargo molecules in the nucleus via an interaction between XPO1 and a hydrophobic nuclear export sequence on the target cargo protein. This complex is then capable of traversing through the nuclear pore complex and into the cytoplasm. In the cytoplasm, the cargo molecule is released as RanGAP hydrolyzes RanGTP into RanGDP. Following cargo release XPO1 then translocates back into the nucleus where the cycle can begin anew following the regeneration of RanGTP by RanGEF. (This figure was created using biorender.com).

of patients had diffuse large B-cell lymphoma (DLBCL; n = 43, 54%) followed by follicular lymphoma (FL; n = 9, 12%), Richter transformation (RT) of chronic lymphocytic leukemia (CLL) (n = 8, 10%), CLL (n = 7, 9%), and mantle cell lymphoma (MCL; n = 4, 5%). Additional histologic subtypes enrolled included T-cell lymphoma (cutaneous T-cell lymphoma [CTCL; n = 3] and peripheral T-cell lymphoma [PTCL; n = 3]), Burkitt's lymphoma (BL; n = 1), and marginal zone lymphoma (MZL; n = 1). The study assessed doses ranging from 3 to 80 mg/m^2 in a variety of schedules. The population had several known risk factors of adverse prognosis, including 62% with stage IV disease, 74% with an international prognostic index (IPI) score of 3 or more, 72% with an elevated lactate dehydrogenase (LDH), and 65% over the age of 60 years. Patients had received a median of four prior lines of therapy and 14% of patients with seven or more lines of previous treatment.

The toxicity profile of selinexor in the phase 1 study highlighted several important adverse reactions (Kuruvilla et al. 2014). The eligibility criteria were particularly permissive and allowed patients with broad hematologic parameters (including a platelet count of $\geq 30 \times 10^9/l$, hemoglobin ≥ 8 g/dl, and absolute neutrophil count $\geq 0.8 \times 10^9/l$) enrolled over 13 dose levels. There was one patient in the initial dose escalation that experienced a dose-limiting toxicity (DLT) of grade 4 thrombocytopenia without bleeding. The patient was continued on therapy with platelet transfusions as needed. The most frequent adverse events (AEs) were myelosuppression, gastrointestinal toxicity, and fatigue. Rates of grade 3/4 hematologic toxicity were similar across both studies with the phase 1 study reporting thrombocytopenia (47%), anemia (27%), and neutropenia (32%). There were two patients with treatment-related hematologic serious adverse events

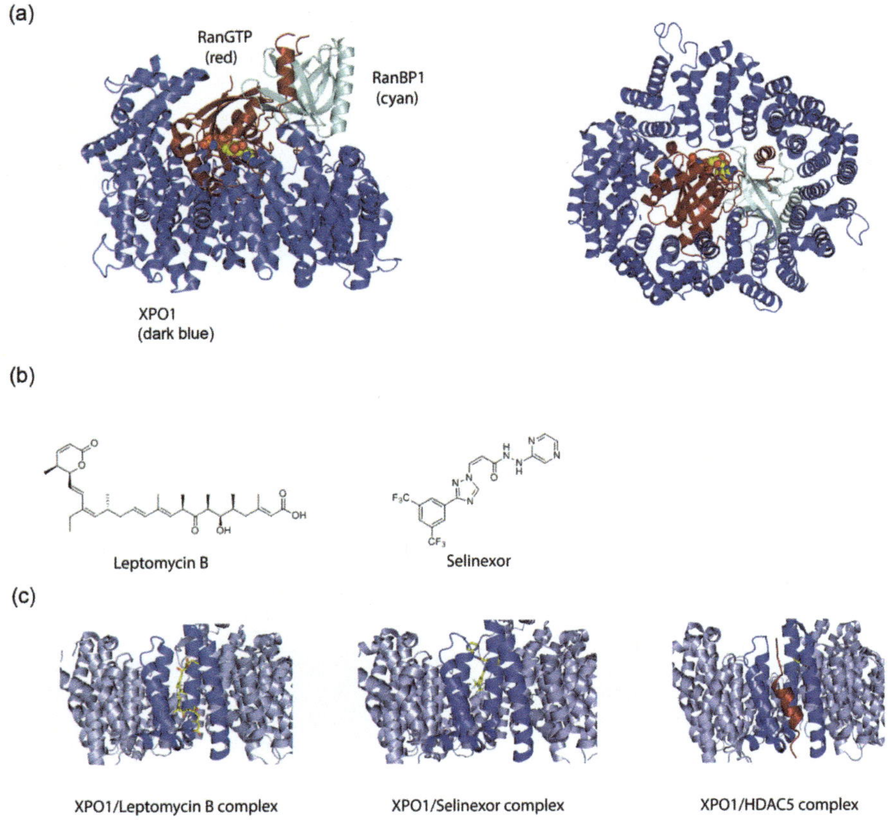

Figure 25.2 XPO1 (dark blue) is a 1071 residue protein composed of 21 repeated HEAT domains arranged into a ring-like structure (PDBID 7L5E). The top of this ring forms the docking site for RanGTP (red) and RanBP1 (light blue) that are required to drive the XPO1 cycle. The GTP molecule bound to Ran is shown in sphere rendering (a; **left**). The figure on the right is rotated by 180 degrees to clearly show the ring-like structure formed by the XPO1's 21 HEAT repeats (**a**; right). The polyketide leptomycin B (**b**; left) and the synthetic SINE compound selinexor (**b**; right) are potent inhibitors of XPO1-mediated nuclear export. Binding of either leptomycin B (**c**; left, PDBID 4HAY) or selinexor (**c**; center, PDBID 7L5E) prevents XPO1's ability to interact with potential cargo proteins by competing for the site on XPO1 that binds the nuclear export sequence. This site is formed by a hydrophobic groove between HEAT repeats 11 and 12 (**c**; dark blue). Both compounds compete for the cargo binding site on XPO1 in part by forming a covalent bond with cysteine 528 (**c**; yellow in stick rendering) that sits atop the groove formed by HEAT domains 11 and 12. For comparison we show the interaction between XPO1 and a 16 amino acid peptide(red) that forms the nuclear export sequence in HDAC5 (**c**; right, PDBID 5UWI).

Table 25.1 Published clinical data on selinexor, alone or in combination.

Regimen	Dose	Phases	Lymphoma	ORR (%)	CR (%)	PR (%)	SD (%)	PD (%)	PFS	OS
Selinexor (Kuruvilla et al. 2014)	3–80 mg/m^2 (Variable schedules)	1b	RR NHL	31	6	26	30	40	NR	NR
Selinexor + RCHOP (Seymour et al. 2021)	60–80 mg weekly with maintenance	1b	Newly diagnosed NHL	100	90	NR	NR	NR	NR	NR
Selinexor (Kalakonda et al. 2020)	60 mg on days 1 and 3	2	RR DLBCL	28	12	17	9	63	mPFS 2.6 mo	mOS 9.1 mo
Selinexor + ibrutinib (Stephens et al. 2019)	30–40 mg	1	RR NHL/CLL	81	12	21	48	15	mPFS 8.9 mo (CLL) and 2.7 mo (NHL)	mOS NR (CLL) and 5.4 mo (NHL)
Selinexor + DICE (Tang et al. 2020)	40–80 mg	1	RR TCL/NKTCL	91	82	NR	NR	NR	NR	NR

Abbreviations: CHOP = cyclophosphamide, doxorubicin, vincristine, prednisone; CLL = chronic lymphocytic leukemia; CR = complete remission; DICE = dexamethasone, ifosfamide, cisplatin, etoposide; DLBCL = diffuse large B-cell lymphoma; mo = months; mOS = median overall survival; mPFS = median progression-free survival; NHL = non-Hodgkin's lymphoma; NKTCL = NK/T-cell lymphoma; NR = not reported; ORR = overall response rate; OS = overall survival; PFS = progression-free survival; PR = partial remission; SD = stable disease; TCL = T-cell lymphoma; PD = progressive disease; RR = relapsed refractory.

(SAEs), one patient with grade 4 anemia who received a blood transfusion and one patient with grade 3 febrile neutropenia. The authors noted a high rate of baseline cytopenias prior to treatment with preexisting thrombocytopenia (15% with platelets $<75 \times 10^9/l$) and neutropenia (13% with ANC $<1.5 \times 10^9/l$) predisposing patients to an increased risk of hematologic toxicity. Gastrointestinal toxicity was particularly common including nausea (66%), anorexia (57%), vomiting (37%), and diarrhea (34%). These were treated with supportive care including anti-emetics (5-HT3 antagonists, D2 antagonists, and dexamethasone). There was a 10% rate of grade 3/4 hyponatremia with two patients being classified as having an SAE. All patients with serious AEs recovered with drug interruption and standard-of-care supportive treatments. With these toxicities, the authors encourage liberal use of supportive care including granulocyte colony-stimulating factor, anti-emetics, and appetite stimulants as needed.

The overall response rate (ORR) in 70 evaluable patients of all NHL subtypes across dose levels was 31%. The complete remission (CR) rate was 6% with 26% partial remission (PR), 30% stable disease (SD), and 40% (PD). Similar ORRs were observed across different dose ranges. The dose ranges were 3–23 mg/m^2 (n = 13, median dose 20 mg/m^2), 30–35 mg/m^2 (n = 28, median dose 35 mg/m^2), and 40–80 mg/m^2 (n = 29, median dose 60 mg/m^2) with respective ORRs of 31%, 39%, and 24%. In the DLBCL cohort, the ORR was 32% with 10% CR and 22% PR. Six patients had MYC and BCL2 and/or BCL6 rearrangements detected by FISH indicating double- or triple-hit lymphoma. The ORR in this genetically high-risk population was 50% (n = 3; one CR and two PR). Based on tolerability and efficacy, 35 mg/m^2 (approximately 60 mg flat dose) was the recommended phase 2 dose.

DLBCL

In the subsequent multicenter randomized phase 2 SADAL study, selinexor was evaluated at a dose either 60 or 100 mg on days 1 and 3 weekly in patients with RR DLBCL who had at least two prior lines of therapy (Kalakonda et al. 2020). Patients were eligible for the study if they had *de novo* or transformed DLBCL, had received two to five lines of prior therapy, and had progressed after or were not eligible for an autologous stem cell transplant (ASCT) with measurable disease based on the Lugano 2014 criteria. For patients who had achieved a CR or PR to their prior therapy, there was an eight-week washout required which was reduced from the originally criterion of 14 weeks. There were 267 patients enrolled in the study for a planned two cohorts of selinexor dosing (60 and 100 mg); however, a preplanned interim analysis of the first 63 patients showed similar efficacy and more favorable toxicity with the 60 mg dose leading to the discontinuation of the 100 mg cohort. Of the 175 patients allocated to the 60 mg arm, 48 were excluded mainly due to protocol changes resulting in 127 patients who received selinexor 60 mg and were included in the modified intention-to-treat and safety populations. The median age of the cohort was 67 years with 45% of patients over the age of 70 years. Most patients had *de novo* DLBCL (n = 94, 74%) with 4% of patients having double- or triple-hit lymphoma. There were a similar number of patients with germinal center B cell-like (GCB) (47%) and non-GCB subtype (50%). The majority of patients had received two prior lines of therapy (n = 75, 59%) and had not undergone ASCT (n = 89, 70%).

The median duration of therapy was nine weeks in evaluable patients with 93% discontinuing due to progressive disease. The ORR was 28% (n = 36, 95% confidence interval [CI] 21–37). This included a CR rate of 12% and PR of 17%. At the median follow-up of 14.7 months, the median progression-free survival (PFS) was 2.6 months and median overall survival (OS) was 9.1 months. In responding patients, the median OS was not reached. The median duration of response (DOR) was 9.3 months (95% CI 4.8–23.0) in the population, which was 4.4 months (95% CI 2.0–not evaluable) for patients in PR, improving to 23 months for patients in CR (95% CI 10.4–23.0). No significant difference in response rate was observed between subgroups including cell of origin, previous ASCT, age, or lines of previous therapy. Based on the results from the SADAL study, selinexor was approved by the US Food and Drug Administration (FDA) for adult patients with relapsed/refractory DLBCL after at least two lines of prior therapy.

In a *post hoc* analysis, patients with lower levels of expression of c-Myc (<40% of cells by immunohistochemistry [IHC]) had better ORR than those with high levels of expression (46.2% vs. 14.8%, $p = 0.012$) (Casasnovas et al. 2022). Patients without the double-expressor phenotype also had a significantly longer median OS compared to those who did (13.7 vs. 5.1 months, hazard ratio [HR] 0.43 [CI 0.23–0.77], $p = 0.004$). Three patients in the study who had progressed after ASCT received selinexor and went on to receive chimeric antigen T-cell receptor (CAR-T) therapy.

Given the single-agent activity and acceptable toxicity profile in DLBCL, there is growing interest in combining selinexor with traditional chemotherapy and/or novel agents. Patients with relapsed/refractory DLBCL have a generally very poor prognosis with response rates of 30–34% to salvage chemotherapy (Crump et al. 2017). As such there is keen interest in improving regimens in this setting by incorporating novel agents. Multiple studies are assessing the combination of selinexor with traditional salvage chemotherapy including ICE (ifosfamide, cisplatin, etoposide),

GDP (gemcitabine, dexamethasone, cisplatin), and DHAOx (dexamethasone, cytarabine, oxaliplatin) (Table 25.2). Selinexor has also been combined with the ibrutinib 420 mg daily in a phase 1 study in patients with CLL/NHL. This included six patients with DLBCL and eight patients with RT. Two of the six patients had responses while the remainder had SD (n = 2) and PD (n = 2). The median PFS was 2.7 months and median OS was 5.4 months. Given the small sample size of the DLBCL cohort and short follow-up, it is not possible to draw conclusions about the efficacy of this combination.

Rituximab, cyclophosphamide, vincristine, doxorubicin, and prednisone (R-CHOP) is the gold standard treatment for newly diagnosed DLBCL. A phase 1b study added selinexor to standard R-CHOP to determine safety, tolerability, maximum tolerated dose (MTD), and the recommended phase 2 dose (Seymour et al. 2021). The study included patients with stage III or IV newly diagnosed DLBCL as well as patients with indolent B-cell lymphomas who had received no prior anthracycline therapy. Dosing of R-CHOP was standard with the addition of selinexor on days 1, 8, and 15 of each cycle at three dose levels: 60 mg, 80 mg, and 100 mg, each followed by maintenance selinexor for one year after. The study enrolled 12 patients, of whom 10 had DLBCL and two had FL. Ten patients were evaluated for efficacy and the ORR was 100% with nine CRs persisting after a median follow-up of 476 days. More discontinuations and dose reductions were noted in the 80 mg cohort and in total 9 of the 12 patients discontinued therapy prior to completing maintenance due to tolerance, non-compliance, and patient preference. Based on tolerance and efficacy, the RP2D is 60 mg of selinexor and will be studied in the multicenter phase 2 study assessing the efficacy of adding selinexor to frontline CHOP in *de novo* and transformed DLBCL (NCT03147885).

High XPO1 expression has been demonstrated to be an adverse prognostic factor in various malignancies, including lymphoma (Gravina et al. 2014). Luo et al. (2018) demonstrated that XPO1 expression was upregulated in DLBCL compared to reactive lymphoid hyperplasia and associated with an advanced clinical stage, high IPI score, and lower OS. Independently, XPO1 expression was associated with worse survival in DLBCL (RR 3.8, $p = 0.006$). Similarly, Deng et al. (2020) demonstrated that high XPO1 expression (>30%) was a negative prognostic factor, being associated with an inferior PFS and OS compared to patients with low XPO1 expression. This difference was also observed in patients with high BCL2 expression and patients with both MYC and BCL2 expression (double-expressor phenotype). XPO1 expression was not significant in impacting OS in patients with double-hit lymphoma. Interestingly, in patients with TP53-mutated DLBCL, high XPO1 showed a trend toward improved PFS, particularly in patients with low BCL2 expression where the difference was statistically significant.

CLL

Selinexor continues to be evaluated in other subtypes of lymphoma where pre-clinical and phase 1 data shows promising early activity. In CLL, where XPO1 mutations are associated predominantly with unmutated IGHV, preclinical models

Table 25.2 Active clinical trials involving selinexor combined with other therapies.

NCT identifier	Regimen	Dose of selinexor	Phases	Lymphoma
NCT02741388	Selinexor + R-DHAOx/ R-GDP	20–80mg	2	RR B-cell lymphoma
NCT02227251	Selinexor	40–60 mg	2b	RR DLBCL
NCT02471911	Selinexor + R-ICE	20–100 mg	1	RR aggressive B-cell lymphoma
NCT03212937	Selinexor + ICE	40 mg	1	PTCL
NCT04442022	R-GDP ± selinexor	40–60 mg	2/3	Transplant/CAR-T ineligible RR DLBCL
NCT02303392	Selinexor + ibrutinib	Not specified	1	RR CLL or aggressive NHL
NCT02436707	Selinexor + R-GDP	40 mg	2	RR aggressive B-cell lymphoma (transplant eligible)
NCT03992339	Selinexor	60 mg	2	RR DLBCL
NCT03147885	Selinexor + R-CHOP	Not specified	1b/2	Newly diagnosed and RR B-cell lymphoma
NCT04640779	Selinexor + choline salicylate	Not specified	1b	RR NHL
NCT03955783	Selinexor + venetoclax	Not specified	1b	High-risk hematologic malignancies including DLBCL

Abbreviations: CHOP = cyclophosphamide, doxorubicin, vincristine and prednisone; DHAOx dexamethasone = cytarabine, oxaliplatin; GDP = gemcitabine, dexamethasone, cisplatin; ICE = ifosfamide, cisplatin, etoposide; R = rituximab.

have shown that selinexor can downregulate BCR signaling and proliferation of malignant cells (Jain et al. 2016; Lapalombella et al. 2012; Zhong et al. 2014). Synergistic effect was also demonstrated *ex vivo* between selinexor and ibrutinib in mouse models where combination therapy was more cytotoxic compared to each agent alone, suggesting inhibition of BCR signaling independent of Bruton's tyrosine kinase (BTK) kinase activity (Hing et al. 2015). In the same study, Hing et al. also demonstrated activity of selinexor in CLL cells with ibrutinib resistance (via BTK C418S mutations), suggesting a potential role for XPO1 inhibition in patients who have failed BTK therapy.

Clinically, the efficacy of selinexor in CLL has been demonstrated in phase 1 studies that included patients with other NHL or hematologic malignancies. In the phase 1 study of selinexor monotherapy in patients with NHL, there were seven patients (9%) who had CLL and eight patients (10%) with RT. Disease characteristics including IGHV status and 17p deletion were not provided in the study. The ORRs for CLL and RT were 33% and 40%, respectively, with no patients achieving CR. In the combination phase 1 study of selinexor and ibrutinib in patients with advanced hematologic malignancies, there were 16 patients (48%) with CLL and 8 patients (24%) with RT (Stephens et al. 2019). Of the CLL patients, all had IGHV unmutated status, 25% had del(17p) and 10 patients had a known BTK mutation. The median number of prior lines of therapy was 3.5 with 11 patients (69%) who had received prior ibrutinib therapy. The ORR was 43% (CR/CRi 12%; PR 31%) with an ORR in patients without prior BTK inhibitor (BTKi) therapy of 100%. With a median follow-up of 5.3 months, the median PFS was 8.9 months and median OS was not reached for patients with CLL. This preliminary phase 1 data suggests activity of the combination as well as safety but larger sample sizes with longer follow-up are needed to assess durability of response.

T-cell Lymphoma

There is limited data on the efficacy of selinexor in T-cell lymphomas (TCL). The phase 1 study of selinexor in advanced malignancies included six patients of whom three had CTCL and three had PTCL. In CTCL, the response rate was only 33% with one PR, while in PTCL one of two responses attained a response (i.e. a PR). A phase 2 study of selinexor in RR PTCL and CTCL was terminated early due to slow enrollment (NCT02314247). A phase 1 study from Tang et al. (2020) combined selinexor at doses of 40–80 mg with dexamethasone, ifosfamide, carboplatin, and etoposide (DICE) in patients with RR PTCL or natural killer (NK)/TCL. Selinexor was given in escalating doses on days 3, 5, and 7 with three dose levels (40, 60, and 80 mg). Eleven patients were enrolled and of the evaluable 10 patients, the OR and CR rates were 91% and 82%, respectively. However, five patients discontinued treatment due to reasons other than PD or lack of response indicating poor tolerability. Conclusions on the efficacy of selinexor in TCL cannot be drawn, necessitating larger studies with longer follow-up which is challenging in uncommon disease groups such as this one.

Mantle Cell Lymphoma

Preclinical experiences have demonstrated broad activity of selinexor in MCL by inducing apoptosis and inhibiting proliferation via downregulation of the nuclear factor-kappaB (NF-κB) pathway (Ming et al. 2018). As seen in CLL, ibrutinib resistance in MCL is related to cytoplasmic retention of proteins implicated in the NF-κB signaling pathway. Ming et al. showed that selinexor induced nuclear retention of such proteins resulting in a greater degree of apoptosis. Additionally, Wang et al. demonstrated the effectiveness of selinexor in ibrutinib-resistant MCL cells lines suggesting a possible role of overcoming or preventing ibrutinib resistance. In clinical studies, the efficacy of selinexor in MCL remains unclear as small numbers of patients have been included in phase 1 studies incorporating multiple lymphoma histologies (Kuruvilla et al. 2014; Stephens et al. 2019).

Toxicity

Selinexor has a fairly established toxicity profile from studies in multiple myeloma (MM) where it is approved by the FDA in combination with dexamethasone for patients who have received at least four prior therapies and in combination with bortezomib and dexamethasone for patients who have received at least one prior therapy (Chari et al. 2019; Grosicki et al. 2020). The pivotal phases 1 and 2 studies of selinexor in lymphoma have shown a similarly consistent toxicity profile that highlights selinexor as a drug with notable side effects but manageable with aggressive supportive care (Kalakonda et al. 2020; Kuruvilla et al. 2014). Though dosing of selinexor varies in MM (100 mg once weekly in combination with bortezomib and dexamethasone, and 80 mg twice weekly in combination with dexamethasone), the common toxicities across both malignancies include cytopenias, GI toxicity, fatigue, anorexia, and hyponatremia.

In the SADAL study, 98% of patients had at least one treatment-emergent adverse event (TEAE) (Kalakonda et al. 2020). Thrombocytopenia, nausea, fatigue, anemia, decreased appetite, diarrhea, constipation, neutropenia, weight loss, vomiting, pyrexia, and asthenia were the most reported TEAE in more than 20% of patients. Grade 3 or higher toxicities were observed with thrombocytopenia (46%), neutropenia (24%), anemia (22%), and fatigue (11%). The rate of febrile neutropenia was 3%. Dose modifications were required for TEAE in 70% of patients, most during the first two cycles. The rate of discontinuation of therapy due to TEAE was 17%. This was consistent with the STORM study in MM where the rate of discontinuation due to TEAE was 18% (Chari et al. 2019). In a *post hoc* analysis, it was reported that the rate of AEs was similar across all subgroups (Casasnovas et al. 2021).

As selinexor is evaluated with chemotherapy and other novel agents, there is emerging information regarding the toxicities associated with combination therapy. Selinexor added to ICE and dexamethasone was evaluated at three dose levels (40, 60, and 80 mg) on days 1, 3, and 5. The most common grade 1/2 toxicities were the same as the monotherapy studies but seen in a larger proportion of patients. Similarly, hematologic toxicities were the most common grade 3/4 AEs but at significantly higher proportions including anemia (82%), thrombocytopenia (82%), and neutropenia (73%). The DLT was thrombocytopenia which was observed in three patients (one at DL1 and two at DL2). There was a high rate of hyponatremia which occurred in 100% of patients with 73% of patients experience a grade 3 event. This is notably higher than the SADAL study which had an 11% incidence of hyponatremia with 8% being grade 3 suggesting this combinatorial toxicity. In the front line, selinexor with RCHOP showed promise with efficacy but with a similar AE profile. There were two DLT in the 60 mg group with patients experiencing grade 3 SVT and grade 3 syncope events. In the 80 mg group, there was one DLT of grade 3 nausea. The majority of AEs were grade 1/2 and included nausea (100%), fatigue (67%), constipation (42%), dizziness (42%), and vomiting (42%). Of the 12 patients enrolled, five discontinued selinexor due to AEs and three required dose reductions.

Recommended management of these toxicities has evolved as selinexor is used more in the real world. The International Myeloma Working Group (IMWG) has published guidelines for clinicians that provide recommendations for monitoring and managing toxicity of selinexor (Mikhael et al. 2020). Particular emphasis is placed on aggressive prophylaxis of nausea with 5-HT3 antagonists and a low threshold to add olanzapine or an NK1R antagonist. The consensus also recommends a strong non-pharmacologic approach to care with frequent assessments early after initiation of selinexor, tracked oral hydration, frequent weigh-ins, and modification of lifestyle factors to improve fatigue. Analysis of a small subcohort of the STORM study showed that patients who received more aggressive supportive care, higher use of anti-emetics as prophylaxis, and frequent assessment of other contributing factors of GI toxicity and fatigue had a lower rate of TEAE-related discontinuation (Chari et al. 2021). This highlights that the toxicity profile of selinexor, while well established, is an important consideration for clinicians when administering it and frequent monitoring and liberal use of supportive care can help mitigate some of the AEs.

Mechanisms of Intrinsic and Acquired Resistance to Selinexor and SINE Compounds

Resistance to selinexor has not yet been rigorously explored in the clinical setting but preclinical data exists to provide insight into potential mechanisms that might explain therapeutic resistance in lymphoma. The XPO1 nuclear export sequences for selinexor, especially the C528 residue, are highly conserved in eukaryotes and the selinexor binding site on XPO1, which also forms the binding site for cargo protein NESs (Neggers et al. 2016). This includes C528 which is the site at which both LMB and selinexor form a covalent bond with XPO1. To date, no mutations have been identified in the XPO1 cargo binding pocket using cell lines that have been made resistant to selinexor by prolonged incubation at gradually increasing doses of drug (Kashyap et al. 2016). This is in contrast to other common classes of drugs such as kinase inhibitors that target the ATP binding cleft where mutations to active site residues involved in drug binding have been identified in several instances both in the laboratory and in clinical specimens (Kashyap et al. 2016). To the best of our knowledge, correlative clinical samples from patients with lack of response or progression following selinexor therapy have not been characterized in depth. However, the selinexor resistant cell lines that have been generated provide some initial clues to inform on potential mechanisms of resistance. These clues may be useful to inform on strategies to overcome resistance to selinexor and other SINE compounds in clinical studies (Crochiere et al. 2015).

Resistance to selinexor has predominantly been studied using other SINE compounds, namely, KPT-185 and KPT-251, which are currently only used as laboratory reagents (Crochiere et al. 2015). These experiments have been performed using the HT-1080 fibrosarcoma cell lines cultured with KPT-185 (Crochiere et al. 2015). The resistant cells have a 130-fold reduction in sensitivity to KPT-185, in addition to a 33-fold reduction in sensitivity to selinexor and a 14-fold reduction in sensitivity to KPT-251. These cells were further characterized to identify pathways or processes that confer resistance to selinexor. Acquired mutations to the drug binding site on XPO1 do not appear to play a role in resistance, as the DNA sequence encompassing these sites was found to be identical when the resistant and parental cell lines were compared. The resistant cells also had similar XPO1 occupancy values for a biotinylated LMB analog, indicating that resistance is not due to reduced drug binding affinity. Thus, it appears that resistance to selinexor is a complex process invoking mechanisms above and beyond simple point mutations to the drug binding site on XPO1 to block drug binding. Additional analyses comparing sensitive and resistant cells showed differences in pathways related to cell adhesion, apoptosis, and inflammation. This suggests that the combined effects of multiply altered pathways appear to be involved in resistance to SINE compounds.

Given that selinexor alkylates C528 on XPO1, it is likely that changes to this residue would result in resistance (Neggers et al. 2016). This is reminiscent of the C481S mutations in BTK that are found in CLL patients that acquire resistance to ibrutinib, the mechanism of action of which proceeds through alkylation of C481 on BTK by the drug. To this end, when C528 in XPO1 was substituted with a serine residue using CRISPR/Cas9 technology, the resultant cells carrying the C528S mutation were two orders of magnitude less sensitive to selinexor (Neggers et al. 2016). This demonstrates that point mutations in XPO1 that confer resistance are possible although they have yet to be observed in clinical samples. Additionally, C528S mutant cells displayed reduced rates of proliferation, suggesting that the C528S mutation, while conferring drug resistance, impacts the overall fitness of the cells (Neggers et al. 2016). Given these observations, it seems unlikely that resistance to selinexor (in combination regimens) by way of the C528S mutation will be of clinical significance as this genetic alteration compromises the fitness of the mutant cells. Nonetheless, how the C528S mutation modulates XPO1 cargo binding and function require further study and lymphoma cell lines harboring this mutation should prove to be a useful tool to better understand the nuances of XPO1 biology in lymphoid malignancies.

Identification and characterization of cases harboring acquired resistance to selinexor in the clinical setting will occur over time as clinicians gain broader experience with the agent. The subsequent analysis of these samples in conjunction with the generation of selinexor resistant lymphoma cell lines will allow us to progressively understand mechanisms of resistance and ultimately address them through novel approaches.

Future Directions

The inhibition of nuclear export is an attractive and emerging therapeutic target in lymphoma but further investigation into the biology of XPO1 and the consequences of XPO1 inhibition are required. In particular, the role of XPO1 in lymphomagenesis, the mechanisms of resistance leading to clinical failure, the potential for synergy with other drug combinations, and the utility of biomarkers to predict response are all facets of XPO1 that remain poorly understood. There is a need to further pursue the underlying biology of XPO1 in the context of potential mechanisms of resistance. This should be an area of active study given how little is known regarding mechanisms of resistance to the drug. While several analyses have been conducted to identify the spectrum of cargo proteins that interact with XPO1, none of these studies have been conducted in lymphoma cells. As it is likely that XPO1 mediates the transfer of different subsets of protein in different malignancies, an understanding of disease-specific XPO1 cargo proteins will shed light on this aspect of XPO1 biology and may be useful to inform on combination strategies that can be translated into the clinic. Finally, while much of the research into the function of XPO1 has focused on the nuclear export of proteins, XPO1 is also known to ferry a variety of RNA molecules out of the nucleus. The identification and biological roles of XPO1's RNA cargo will be another critical piece in further understanding the role of XPO1 in lymphoma. These knowledge gaps aside, selinexor represents a first-in-class, clinically active, synthetic molecule capable of disrupting oncogenic nuclear transport in lymphoma.

In relapsed/refractory DLBCL, selinexor has demonstrated modest efficacy with tolerable toxicity but more clinical data is needed to help clearly define its role in the management of aggressive lymphoma. There is need to evaluate the clinical activity of selinexor in combination with chemotherapy to see if efficacy can be augmented. Such studies are ongoing, including the addition of selinexor to known common salvage regimens such as GDP, ICE, and DHAP/DHAOx. Additionally, there is the synergy with selinexor and other novel agents that has been shown in the preclinical setting and is now being studied in the clinical setting. Specifically, ibrutinib has demonstrated preclinical synergy with selinexor in both MCL and CLL with early clinical results in NHL showing promising efficacy (Hing et al. 2015; Ming et al. 2018; Stephens et al. 2019; Wang et al. 2017). An additional role being explored is the use of selinexor as maintenance therapy. This is being looked at in the frontline setting with RCHOP chemotherapy (NCT03147885) where preliminary data has suggested feasibility of maintenance but concerns due to higher rates of discontinuation due to toxicity. As XPO1 inhibition is studied in various combinations and in various lymphomas, the key factors to its success in the clinical world will be augmenting efficacy while minimizing toxicity. It is clear from the literature thus far that selinexor has a moderate amount of toxicity associated with it, particularly hematologic and GI toxicity (Table 25.1). More experience is emerging that the use of aggressive and liberal supportive care is the key to help minimize interruptions and discontinuations. Additionally, the development of newer generation XPO1 inhibitors is currently ongoing to help mitigate toxicity. Eltanexor (KPT-8602) is a second-generation XPO1 inhibitor with minimal penetration through the blood–brain barrier which in preclinical and animal studies has shown to GI toxicity, including less anorexia and less weight loss. It is currently being studied in certain hematologic malignancies (MM, myelodysplastic syndromes [MDS]) and solid tumors in a phase 1 study (NCT02649790).

The development of XPO1 inhibitors and SINEs has offered scientists and clinicians a novel therapeutic target in malignancies. Over time, improvement in drug development has allowed selective nuclear transport inhibition to be used in hematologic malignancies, particularly MM and lymphoma.

With further understanding of the biology and investigation into novel therapeutic combinations and methods to reduce overall toxicity, XPO1 inhibitors may play a key role in the management of lymphoma.

Must Read References

Kalakonda, N., Maerevoet, M., Cavallo, F. et al. (2020). Selinexor in patients with relapsed or refractory diffuse large B-cell lymphoma (SADAL): a single-arm, multinational, multicentre, open-label, phase 2 trial. *Lancet Haematol.* 7 (7): e511–e22.

Kırlı, K., Karaca, S., Dehne, H.J. et al. (2015). A deep proteomics perspective on CRM1-mediated nuclear export and nucleocytoplasmic partitioning. *Elife* 4.

Kuruvilla, J., Byrd, J.C., Flynn, J.M. et al. (2014). The oral selective inhibitor of nuclear export (SINE) selinexor (KPT-330) demonstrates broad and durable clinical activity in relapsed/refractory non Hodgkin's lymphoma (NHL). *Blood* 124 (21): 396.

Walker, J.S., Hing, Z.A., Harrington, B. et al. (2021). Recurrent XPO1 mutations alter pathogenesis of chronic lymphocytic leukemia. *J. Hematol. Oncol.* 14 (1): 17.

References

Casasnovas, R.O., Follows, G., Zijlstra, J.M. et al. (2022). Comparison of the effectiveness and safety of the oral selective inhibitor of nuclear export, selinexor, in diffuse large B cell Lymphoma Subtypes. *Clin. Lymphoma Myeloma Leuk.* 22 (1): 24–33.

Chari, A., Florendo, E., Mancia, I.S. et al. (2021). Optimal supportive care with selinexor improves outcomes in patients with relapsed/refractory multiple myeloma. *Clin. Lymphoma Myeloma Leuk.* 21 (12): e975–e984.

Chari, A., Vogl, D.T., Gavriatopoulou, M. et al. (2019). Oral selinexor-dexamethasone for triple-class refractory multiple myeloma. *N. Engl. J. Med.* 381 (8): 727–738.

Chook, Y.M. and Süel, K.E. (2011). Nuclear import by karyopherin-βs: recognition and inhibition. *Biochim. Biophys. Acta* 1813 (9): 1593–1606.

Crochiere, M., Kashyap, T., Kalid, O. et al. (2015). Deciphering mechanisms of drug sensitivity and resistance to Selective Inhibitor of Nuclear Export (SINE) compounds. *BMC Cancer* 15: 910.

Crump, M., Neelapu, S.S., Farooq, U. et al. (2017). Outcomes in refractory diffuse large B-cell lymphoma: results from the international SCHOLAR-1 study. *Blood* 130 (16): 1800–1808.

Deng, M., Zhang, M., Xu-Monette, Z.Y. et al. (2020). XPO1 expression worsens the prognosis of unfavorable DLBCL that can be effectively targeted by selinexor in the absence of mutant p53. *J. Hematol. Oncol.* 13 (1): 148.

Gravina, G.L., Senapedis, W., McCauley, D. et al. (2014). Nucleo-cytoplasmic transport as a therapeutic target of cancer. *J. Hematol. Oncol.* 7: 85.

Grosicki, S., Simonova, M., Spicka, I. et al. (2020). Once-per-week selinexor, bortezomib, and dexamethasone versus twice-per-week bortezomib and dexamethasone in patients with multiple myeloma (BOSTON): a randomised, open-label, phase 3 trial. *Lancet* 396 (10262): 1563–1573.

Hing, Z.A., Mantel, R., Beckwith, K.A. et al. (2015). Selinexor is effective in acquired resistance to ibrutinib and synergizes with ibrutinib in chronic lymphocytic leukemia. *Blood* 125 (20): 3128–3132.

Jain, P., Kanagal-Shamanna, R., Wierda, W. et al. (2016). Clinical and molecular characteristics of XPO1 mutations in patients with chronic lymphocytic leukemia. *Am. J. Hematol.* 91 (11): E478–E9.

Kalakonda, N., Maerevoet, M., Cavallo, F. et al. (2020). Selinexor in patients with relapsed or refractory diffuse large B-cell lymphoma (SADAL): a single-arm, multinational, multicentre, open-label, phase 2 trial. *Lancet Haematol.* 7 (7): e511–e22.

Kashyap, T., Argueta, C., Aboukameel, A. et al. (2016). Selinexor, a Selective Inhibitor of Nuclear Export (SINE) compound, acts through NF-kappaB deactivation and combines with proteasome inhibitors to synergistically induce tumor cell death. *Oncotarget* 7 (48): 78883–78895.

Kırlı, K., Karaca, S., Dehne, H.J. et al. (2015). A deep proteomics perspective on CRM1-mediated nuclear export and nucleocytoplasmic partitioning. *Elife* 4.

Kuruvilla, J., Byrd, J.C., Flynn, J.M. et al. (2014). The oral selective inhibitor of nuclear export (SINE) selinexor (KPT-330) demonstrates broad and durable clinical activity in relapsed/refractory non Hodgkin's lymphoma (NHL). *Blood* 124 (21): 396.

Lapalombella, R., Sun, Q., Williams, K. et al. (2012). Selective inhibitors of nuclear export show that CRM1/XPO1 is a target in chronic lymphocytic leukemia. *Blood* 120 (23): 4621–4634.

Luo, B., Huang, L., Gu, Y. et al. (2018). Expression of exportin-1 in diffuse large B-cell lymphoma: immunohistochemistry and TCGA analyses. *Int. J. Clin. Exp. Pathol.* 11 (12): 5547–5560.

Mikhael, J., Noonan, K.R., Faiman, B. et al. (2020). Consensus recommendations for the clinical management of patients with multiple myeloma treated with selinexor. *Clin. Lymphoma Myeloma Leuk.* 20 (6): 351–357.

Ming, M., Wu, W., Xie, B. et al. (2018). XPO1 inhibitor selinexor overcomes intrinsic ibrutinib resistance in mantle cell lymphoma via nuclear retention of IκB. *Mol. Cancer Ther.* 17 (12): 2564–2574.

Neggers, J.E., Vanstreels, E., Baloglu, E. et al. (2016). Heterozygous mutation of cysteine528 in XPO1 is sufficient for resistance to selective inhibitors of nuclear export. *Oncotarget* 7 (42): 68842–68850.

Newlands, E.S., Rustin, G.J., and Brampton, M.H. (1996). Phase I trial of elactocin. *Br. J. Cancer* 74 (4): 648–649.

Nishi, K., Yoshida, M., Fujiwara, D. et al. (1994). Leptomycin B targets a regulatory cascade of crm1, a fission yeast nuclear protein, involved in control of higher order chromosome structure and gene expression. *J. Biol. Chem.* 269 (9): 6320–6324.

Pemberton, L.F. and Paschal, B.M. (2005). Mechanisms of receptor-mediated nuclear import and nuclear export. *Traffic* 6 (3): 187–198.

Seymour, E.K., Khan, H.Y., Li, Y. et al. (2021). Selinexor in combination with R-CHOP for frontline treatment of non-Hodgkin lymphoma: results of a phase I study. *Clin. Cancer Res.* 27 (12): 3307–3316.

Stephens, D.M., Huang, Y., Agyeman, A. et al. (2019). *Selinexor Combined with Ibrutinib Demonstrates Tolerability and Efficacy in Advanced B-cell Malignancies: A Phase I Study*. American Society of Hematology Washington, DC.

Sun, Q., Carrasco, Y.P., Hu, Y. et al. (2013). Nuclear export inhibition through covalent conjugation and hydrolysis of Leptomycin B by CRM1. *Proc. Natl. Acad. Sci. U.S.A.* 110 (4): 1303–1308.

Tang, T., Martin, P., Somasundaram, N. et al. (2020). Phase I study of selinexor in combination with dexamethasone, ifosfamide, carboplatin, etoposide chemotherapy in patients with relapsed or refractory peripheral T-cell or naturalkiller/T-cell lymphoma. Haematol. Online ahead of printl.

Timney, B.L., Raveh, B., Mironska, R. et al. (2016). Simple rules for passive diffusion through the nuclear pore complex. *J. Cell Biol.* 215 (1): 57–76.

Walker, J.S., Hing, Z.A., Harrington, B. et al. (2021). Recurrent XPO1 mutations alter pathogenesis of chronic lymphocytic leukemia. *J. Hematol. Oncol.* 14 (1): 17.

Wang, Y.L., Ming, M., Xie, B. et al. (2017). *XPO1 Inhibitor Selinexor Overcomes Ibrutinib Resistance in Mantle Cell Lymphoma via Nuclear Retention of IκB*. American Society of Hematology Washington, DC.

Zhong, Y., El-Gamal, D., Dubovsky, J.A. et al. (2014). Selinexor suppresses downstream effectors of B-cell activation, proliferation and migration in chronic lymphocytic leukemia cells. *Leukemia* 28 (5): 1158–1163.

26

Heterobifunctional Degraders for the Treatment of Lymphoid Malignancies

Ashwin Gollerkeri, Jared Gollob, and Nello Mainolfi

Kymera Therapeutics, Watertown, MA, USA

Take Home Messages

- Heterobifunctional small molecules are a new class of compounds that enables the development of degraders specific for a target protein of interest.
- Heterobifunctional degraders have several different advantages over traditional small molecule drugs including the ability to access undruggable targets such as transcription factors, to impact enzymatic and scaffolding function or proteins, and to prevent or overcome acquired resistance mutations.
- A number of heterobifunctional degraders targeting key proteins in the development and progression of lymphoma are in early clinical development

Biology of Protein Degraders

Ubiquitin–Proteasome System and Protein Degradation

The ubiquitin–proteasome system (UPS) is the endogenous intracellular mechanism for maintaining protein homeostasis through protein degradation (Figure 26.1a) (modified from Nandi et al. (2006)).

Protein ubiquitination is controlled by E3 ligases, which mediate the polyubiquitination of lysine residues upon recognition and non-covalent binding to the target protein. There are over 600 different E3 ligases, each of which is characterized by its own tissue distribution and protein substrate specificity (Schapira et al. 2019). Examples of E3 ligases include cereblon (CRBN), von Hippel-Lindau (VHL), X-linked inhibitor of apoptosis protein (XIAP), and mouse double minute 2 homolog (MDM2). Proteins that have become ubiquitinated by E3 ligases are marked for subsequent degradation by the proteasome, a protein complex that uses proteases to mediate proteolysis.

Targeted Degraders in Clinical Practice

Protein degraders that are approved and used in the clinic include immunomodulatory "-imide" drugs (IMiDs) such as thalidomide, lenalidomide (LEN), and pomalidomide (POM), as well as the selective estrogen receptor degrader (SERD) fulvestrant. IMiDs are archetypal molecular "glues" that act by binding to CRBN and redirecting it to ubiquitinate neosubstrates including the zinc finger transcription factors Ikaros and Aiolos, leading to the proteasomal degradation of those targets and the subsequent stimulation of a type I interferon response (Krönke et al. 2014; Zhu et al. 2013). IMiDs are commonly used in the treatment of multiple myeloma (MM) and lymphoma, and side effects such as cytopenias, fatigue, and gastrointestinal symptoms are related to on-target effects associated with Ikaros and Aiolos downregulation (Gao et al. 2020; Li et al. 2018; Liu et al. 2019). SERDs like fulvestrant, which is used for the treatment of breast cancer, bind to the estrogen receptor (ER) and induce its ubiquitination and proteasomal degradation (Patel and Bihani 2018). Side effects of fulvestrant are similar to those of other antiestrogen drugs that target the ER (Nathan and Schmid 2017).

Heterobifunctional Small Molecule Degraders

Heterobifunctional small molecules are a new class of compounds that enable the development of degraders specific for a target protein of interest. Whereas IMiDs redirect CRBN toward neosubstrates and SERDs bind to the ER and target it for degradation, heterobifunctional molecules are composed of two ligands mediating non-covalent binding to both an E3 ligase and

Precision Cancer Therapies: Targeting Oncogenic Drivers and Signaling Pathways in Lymphoid Malignancies: From Concept to Practice, Volume 1, First Edition. Edited by Owen A. O'Connor, Stephen M. Ansell, and John F. Seymour.

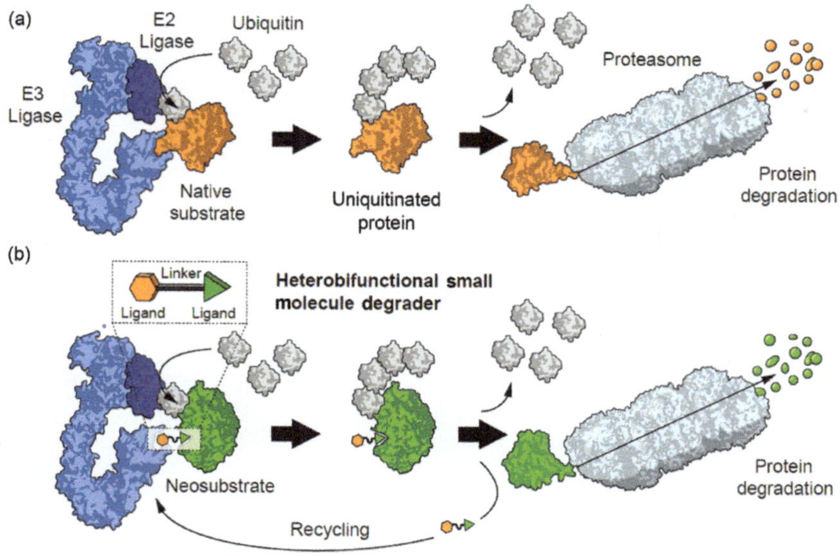

Figure 26.1 UPS-mediated protein degradation (a) and mechanism of action of heterobifunctional small molecule degraders (b).

target protein of interest, respectively, joined together by a chemical linker (Neklesa et al. 2017; Schapira et al. 2019). The heterobifunctional molecule and two proteins form a ternary complex, bringing the E3 ligase in close proximity with a protein that now serves as its neosubstrate, leading to its ubiquitination and degradation and release of the small molecule which then mediates additional rounds of ternary complex formation and protein degradation (Figure 26.1b).

The requirements for stable and productive ternary complex formation contribute to the high level of selectivity that can be achieved with this approach, while the catalytic nature of the mechanism is responsible for its potency (Bondeson et al. 2018). As heterobifunctional molecules have ligands for both an E3 ligase and target protein, they are larger than traditional small molecules, with molecular weight typically in the 600–800 g/mol range.

Scores of heterobifunctional small molecules have been developed as tool compounds against various targets of interest for research purposes, with the majority co-opting either CRBN or VHL (Schapira et al. 2019; Watt et al. 2019). More recently, biotechnology companies like Arvinas, Kymera, C4 Therapeutics, and Nurix have emerged that are focused on using this novel technology to develop drugs for both oncology and non-oncology indications.

Mechanisms of Resistance

Resistance to heterobifunctional degraders could emerge due to alterations in components of the UPS or mutations in the ligand-binding site of the target protein. The latter is less likely, since the catalytic, event-driven mechanism of targeted protein degradation would be less susceptible to changes in ligand binding affinity caused by target protein mutations than the occupancy-driven mechanism of small molecule inhibitors. On the other hand, the experience with IMiDs in MM has shown that acquired resistance to LEN and POM can occur due to alterations in CRBN. In MM, alterations in CRBN, including point mutations, copy losses/structural variations, and splice variants, have been detected in up to 21% of patients who became refractory to LEN and up to 30% who also became refractory to POM. Mutations in Ikaros, Aiolos, and CUL4B have also been found in IMiD-treated MM patients, but at a much lower frequency compared to CRBN alterations (Gooding et al. 2021). In oncology trials using heterobifunctional degraders, it will be important to monitor in tumor tissue for these sorts of genetic changes as well as changes in protein expression levels for whichever E3 ligase is being utilized.

Rationale for Use of Heterobifunctional Degraders in Oncology

Heterobifunctional degraders have the potential to overcome a variety of obstacles to drug development in oncology through a number of different advantages over traditional small molecule drugs (Figure 26.2).

First, they provide a means for drugging undruggable targets such as transcription factors and other oncogenic proteins for which there are no typical small molecule substrate binding regions leading to inhibition of enzymatic activity. Since heterobifunctional small molecules rely on affinity-based interactions rather than functional inhibition of the target protein, they can capitalize on these binding interactions to bring protein target to the UPS system for degradation. The dependency of degrader activity on affinity-based interactions and ternary complex formation also enables enhanced selectivity using existing ligands for targets where avoidance of off-target effects on close homologs is essential for tolerability. This selectivity is further

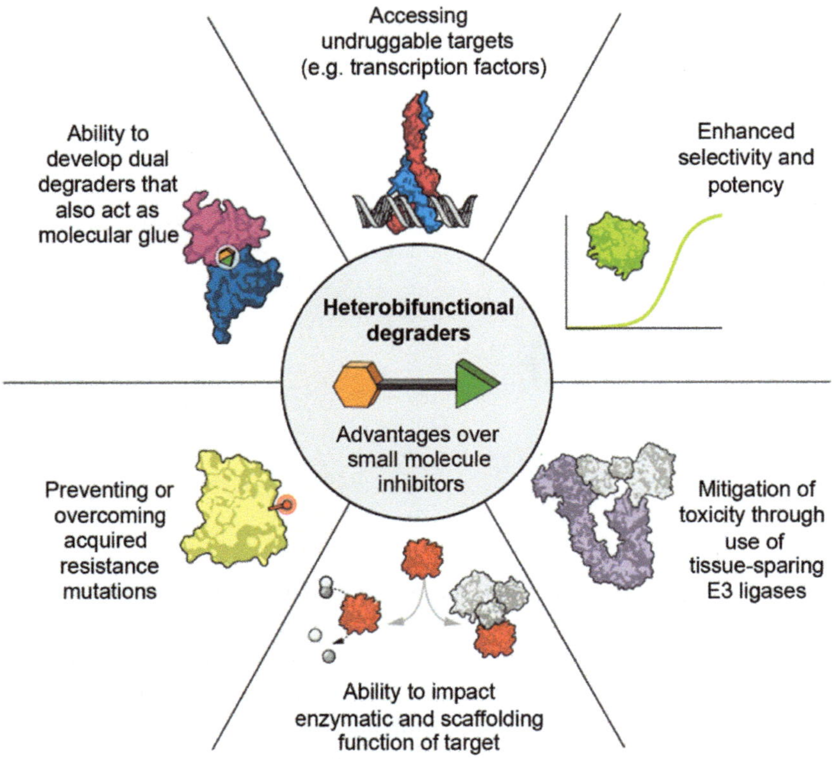

Figure 26.2 Advantages of heterobifunctional small molecule degraders over small molecule inhibitors.

enhanced by the fact that ternary complex-mediated degradation is an event-driven, catalytic mechanism rather than occupancy-driven mechanism, facilitating maximal proteasomal target degradation at sub-stoichiometric drug levels and thereby further minimizing off-target effects and improving safety.

In addition to target selectivity and potency, the safety of heterobifunctional degraders can also be optimized through tissue selectivity by co-opting E3 ligases that are not expressed in target organs of toxicity, such as bone marrow, gastrointestinal tract, and/or kidney (so-called tissue-sparing E3 ligases), but are expressed in the tumors of interest. One example of this is the use of VHL to degrade BCL-xL in order to mitigate the dose-limiting thrombocytopenia associated with small molecule BCL-xL inhibitors. While VHL is ubiquitously expressed by hematologic malignancies and solid tumors, it is not expressed in mature platelets, which are the main target cell of toxicity with BCL-xL inhibitors. Likewise, safety can be improved by co-opting an E3 ligase that is only expressed in a single cell type (so-called tissue-restricted E3 ligases); for example, a B-cell restricted E3 ligase for degraders targeting B-cell lymphomas.

Degraders have a potential advantage over small molecule inhibitors when the function of the target relies on more than one enzymatic activity or is also dependent on protein–protein interactions (i.e. scaffolding function). For example, the DNA repair enzyme Pol Theta is dependent on both its helicase and polymerase activities, whereas signaling downstream of IRAK4 (interleukin-1 receptor-associated kinase 4) is controlled by both its enzymatic activity as well as the scaffolding properties required for myddosome assembly following MYD88 (myeloid differentiation primary response 88) activation. There is also an advantage for a degrader over a small molecule inhibitor when resistance to the inhibitor is driven by mutations within the active binding site. This mode of resistance is common for various tyrosine kinase inhibitors, including EGFR, BCR-ABL, and c-KIT inhibitors, and could either be circumvented or overcome by degraders that bind outside of these mutation hotspots.

Degraders that utilize CRBN also provide the opportunity to incorporate IMiD-like molecular glue activity into a heterobifunctional degrader, thereby creating a triple degrader of Ikaros and Aiolos plus a third target of interest with a mechanistic rationale for combining with the IMiD substrates. Examples of these already in the clinic include Kymera's IRAK4-targeting IRAKIMiD (KT-413) in development for MYD88-mutant diffuse large B-cell lymphoma (DLBCL) and Nurix's Bruton's tyrosine kinase (BTK)-targeting BTK-IMiD (NX-2127) for B-cell malignancies (see section "Development of Heterobifunctional Degraders in Lymphoma" below).

Clinical Experience with Heterobifunctional Degraders

The first heterobifunctional degraders entered the clinic in 2019 in oncology phase 1 studies and provided the first human proof of mechanism for target degradation in tumors and initial anti-tumor proof of concept. These were followed by the first non-oncology, placebo-controlled phase 1 study in healthy volunteers showing dose- and time-dependent target degradation in circulating blood cells. These studies demonstrated oral bioavailability of heterobifunctional degraders and showed that efficacious plasma exposures were safe and well tolerated. These programs continue to progress in the clinic while multiple other programs in oncology have either started enrolling patients or are poised to enter the clinic.

Arvinas Phase 1/2 Trials of PR and ER Degraders

ARV-110

ARV-110 is a potent, selective CRBN-based progesterone receptor (PR) degrader in development for patients with metastatic castration-resistant prostate cancer (mCRPC). In a phase 1 trial of heavily pretreated patients (N = 37), including 82% progressing after prior therapy with the androgen receptor (AR) inhibitors abiraterone and enzalutamide, once daily oral dosing of ARV-110 achieved plasma exposures above thresholds associated with preclinical activity in standard and enzalutamide-resistant prostate cancer models and was associated with prostate-specific antigen (PSA) responses in a subset of patients with AR mutant (40% PSA50) and AR wild-type tumors (13% PSA50). Based on the preliminary activity and favorable safety profile, a phase 2 expansion (N ~ 100) is ongoing to explore development opportunities in earlier-line mCRPC patients and in late-line patients with T878/H875 AR mutations.

ARV-471

ARV-471 is a potent CRBN-based ER degrader in development for patients with metastatic ER positive/human epidermal growth factor receptor 2 (HER2) negative breast cancer. In a phase 1 trial of heavily pretreated patients (N = 21), including 100% whose disease had progressed on prior cyclin-dependent kinase 4/6 (CDK4/6) inhibitor, ARV-471 dosed orally once daily, achieved plasma exposures above thresholds associated with tumor regressions in preclinical models, and was associated with antitumor activity in 4 of 14 eligible patients and a favorable safety profile. An average ER reduction of 62% (maximum of 90%) was observed in paired tumor biopsies from five patients. A phase 2 expansion (N ~ 120) is ongoing for ARV-471 monotherapy as well as combination therapy with the CDK4/6 inhibitor palbociclib.

Kymera Phase 1 Trial of IRAK4 Degrader KT-474

KT-474 is a potent, highly selective, orally administered degrader of IRAK4 in development for toll-like receptor (TLR)/IL-1 receptor (IL-1R)-driven autoimmune and autoinflammatory diseases. IRAK4 is a key component of the myddosome, a multiprotein complex involved in innate immunity that mediates signaling through TLRs and IL-1Rs. The function of IRAK4 is dependent both on its kinase activity and on its scaffolding properties, which are required for the assembly of the myddosome complex following TLR or IL-1R engagement and MYD88 activation. Nuclear factor-kappaB (NF-κB) activation is particularly dependent on the scaffolding function of IRAK4 and is a key driver of cellular proliferation and proinflammatory cytokine and chemokine production mediated by myddosome activation. Full inhibition of IRAK4 signaling therefore requires elimination of the protein, providing a potential advantage to IRAK4 degraders over IRAK4 kinase inhibitors.

Interim results from the single ascending dose (SAD) portion of a randomized, double-blind, placebo-controlled, phase 1 single and multiple ascending dose escalation study in healthy subjects and patients with atopic dermatitis (AD) and hidradenitis suppurativa (HS) showed that single doses of KT-474 were safe and well tolerated, associated with dose-dependent and efficacious plasma exposures, and resulted in dose-dependent IRAK4 degradation in peripheral blood mononuclear cells (PBMC). IRAK4 reduction in PBMC was seen as early as eight hours post-dose and was sustained for at least six days post-dose prior to returning to baseline levels by day 14. Median IRAK4 reduction of 90% was observed at the highest dose tested, with maximum reduction of 94%, demonstrating proof of mechanism for KT-474. The study is continuing enrollment onto the remaining SAD and multiple ascending dose (MAD) portions, where subjects receive 14 daily doses of study drug or placebo. IRAK4 knockdown in skin and in blood along with inflammatory biomarkers will be assessed in both healthy subjects and in AD and HS patients in the MAD portion of the study.

Development of Heterobifunctional Degraders in Lymphoma

A number of heterobifunctional degraders are in early stages of clinical development for the treatment of lymphomas (Table 26.1).

IRAKIMiD Degraders

IRAKIMiDs are triple degraders of IRAK4 and the IMiD substrates Ikaros and Aiolos in development for the treatment of MYD88-mutant DLBCL. Oncogenic mutations in MYD88, most commonly MYD88L265P, have a poor prognosis and occur in approximately 30% of ABC-DLBCL (activated B cell-like DLBCL) and in up to 80% of "ABC-like" primary extranodal lymphomas, including primary central nervous system (CNS) lymphoma. These mutations result in myddosome assembly and constitutive IRAK4-dependent NF-κB pathway activation independent of any engagement of TLRs or IL-1Rs. NF-κB signaling drives tumor cell proliferation

Table 26.1 Heterobifunctional degraders in development for lymphomas.

Compound	Sponsor	Target	Indication	Phase of development
KT-413	Kymera	IRAK4/Ikaros/Aiolos	MYD88-mutant DLBCL	Phase 1 (4Q21)
KT-333	Kymera	STAT3	PTCL, CTCL	Phase 1 (4Q21)
NX-2127	Nurix	BTK/Ikaros/Aiolos	CLL/SLL, FL, DLBCL, MCL, MZL, WM	Phase 1
NX-5948	Nurix	BTK	B-cell malignancies	Preclinical
BGB-16673	BeiGene	BTK	CLL/SLL, MCL, MZL, WM	Phase 1

Abbreviations: BTK = Bruton's tyrosine kinase; CLL = chronic lymphocytic lymphoma; CTCL = cutaneous T-cell lymphoma; DLBCL = diffuse large B-cell lymphoma; FL = follicular lymphoma; IRAK4 = interleukin-1 receptor-associated kinase 4; MCL = mantle cell lymphoma; MYD88 = myeloid differentiation primary response 88; MZL = marginal zone lymphoma; PTCL = peripheral T-cell lymphoma; SLL = small lymphocytic lymphoma; STAT3 = signal transducer and activator of transcription 3; WM = Waldenstrom's macroglobulinemia.

and upregulates the expression of IRF4 (interferon regulatory factor 4) through the transcription factors Ikaros and Aiolos, which in turn further augments NF-κB activation through caspase recruitment domain family member 11 (CARD11) transactivation. IRF4 also inhibits IRF7, which leads to downregulation of type I interferon (IFN) signaling and inhibition of apoptosis, thereby preventing oncogene-induced cell death. The majority of MYD88-mutant DLBCL tumors have one or more additional genotypic alterations that also augment NF-κB signaling and upregulate IRF4 downstream from MYD88/IRAK4, including activating mutations in CD79B and, less frequently, CARD11 mutations or loss of TNFAIP3 (tumor necrosis factor, alpha-induced protein 3). These co-mutations can render MYD88-mutant tumors less dependent on IRAK4 alone for proliferation and survival and provide potential escape mechanisms for IRAK4 inhibition. While inhibiting NF-κB activation by targeting single nodes just downstream of MYD88 or CD79B mutations (IRAK4 and BTK, respectively) would be expected to have some anti-tumor activity, a more robust effect on NF-κB signaling coupled with the restoration of type I IFN signaling could help circumvent tumor escape mechanisms and achieve deeper and more sustained anti-tumor responses across a broader spectrum of genotypes. This therapeutic hypothesis provided the rationale for degrading both IRAK4 and the IMiD substrates Ikaros and Aiolos to maximize NF-κB and IRF4 inhibition for the treatment of MYD88-mutant DLBCL.

KT-413

KT-413 (Kymera Therapeutics) is a heterobifunctional small molecule that co-opts CRBN to mediate IRAK4 ubiquitination and degradation via formation of a ternary complex while also acting as a molecular glue and redirecting CRBN to ubiquitinate and degrade the IMiD substrates Ikaros and Aiolos. In preclinical studies, KT-413 has been shown to be a potent and selective degrader of both IRAK4 and the IMiD substrates Ikaros and Aiolos, with DC50s of 6 nM and 2 nM, respectively. In MYD88-mutant DLBCL cell lines OCI-Ly10 and SUDHL2, KT-413 was more active than the IMiD CC-220 or an IRAK4-selective degrader both in potency and in the maximal level of cell growth inhibition and mechanistically was distinct in its ability to simultaneously block NF-κB signaling and upregulate the type 1 IFN response (Mayo et al. 2021). In multiple cell line-derived and patient-derived MYD88-mutant mouse xenograft models, KT-413 induced complete tumor regressions with intermittent dosing as infrequent as every three weeks and also showed synergistic anti-tumor activity in combination with rituximab or venetoclax (Mayo et al. 2021).

KT-413 will initially be evaluated in patients with relapsed/refractory (R/R) B-cell non-Hodgkin's lymphoma (NHL). The first-in-human study, KT-413–101, is a phase 1, multicenter, dose escalation and expansion study evaluating the safety, tolerability, pharmacokinetics (PK), pharmacodynamics (PD), and clinical activity of KT-413 administered intravenously in patients with R/R B-cell NHL that is planned to be initiated in 2021. The study includes a dose-escalation portion followed by a planned expansion in patients with MYD88-mutant R/R DLBCL. KT-413 may also be assessed subsequently in other MYD88-mutant B-cell lymphomas such as Waldenstrom's macroglobulinemia (WM) and primary central nervous system lymphoma (PCNSL). Once the human safety and PK of KT-413 monotherapy have been assessed, combination trials with standard-of-care agents in DLBCL and other agents with complimentary mechanisms of action are planned.

BTK Degraders

BTK is a non-receptor tyrosine kinase which plays a central role in the signal transduction of the B-cell antigen receptor (BCR) and other cell surface receptors in normal and malignant B lymphocytes (Burger 2019). It belongs to the tyrosine kinase expressed in hepatocellular carcinoma (TeC) protein family which is expressed in most hematopoietic cells and in particular B lymphocytes. BTK is a cytoplasmic protein which, when activated, transmits and amplifies signals from a variety of surface molecules, in particular BCR, that result in activation of the NF-κB signaling pathway (Singh et al. 2017).

BTK activity is critical for survival and proliferation of leukemic B-cells and has been shown to be critical in the pathogenesis of several B-cell malignancies, leading to the development of small molecule BTK inhibitors that have been used successfully to treat patients with chronic lymphocytic lymphoma/small lymphocytic lymphoma (CLL/SLL), WM, mantle cell lymphoma (MCL), and marginal zone lymphoma (MZL).

Although BTK inhibitors are active, they are not considered curative, and therapy-associated resistance mechanisms have been described patients with B-cell malignancies treated with the BTK inhibitor ibrutinib. The resistance mechanisms include the development of BTK mutations that impede binding of ibrutinib as well as additional activating mutations in BTK or other downstream proteins (Singh et al. 2017). In addition, missense mutations within CARD11, a protein downstream of BTK, have been shown to promote BTK-independent activation of NF-κB and thus ibrutinib resistance in DLBCL (Wilson et al. 2015), MCL (Wu et al. 2016), and in primary CNS lymphomas (Grommes et al. 2017). Strategies to overcome or avoid these resistance mechanisms include the development of BTK degraders that can eliminate BTK protein regardless of mutation status, as well as combining this approach with IMiD activity.

NX-2127

NX-2127 (Nurix Therapeutics) is an orally administered, heterobifunctional degrader of BTK and the IMiD substrates Ikaros and Aiolos. Preclinical data supports the activity of NX-2127 in xenograft models harboring BTK mutations conferring clinical resistance to Food and Drug Administration (FDA)-approved agents as well as in models with wild-type BTK. It is currently being evaluated in a phase 1 dose escalation, safety, and tolerability study in patients with R/R B-cell malignancies that was initiated in 2021. Phase 1b expansion cohorts are planned in patients with MCL, MZL, WM, follicular lymphoma (FL), and DLBCL.

NX-5948

NX-5948 is an orally administered heterobifunctional BTK degrader in development for patients with R/R B-cell malignancies. Preclinical data supports NX-5948 activity in tumor models harboring both mutant and wild-type BTK. In addition, there is preclinical evidence that NX-5948 has the ability to cross the blood–brain barrier in animal models. NX-5498 is planned to be in the clinic in 2021.

BGB-16673

BGB-16673 is an orally administered heterobifunctional BTK degrader in development for patients with R/R B-cell malignancies. The first-in-human trial is planned to evaluate BGB-16673 monotherapy in patients with MZL, FL, MCL, CLL/SLL, or WM.

STAT3 Degraders

STAT3 (signal transducer and activator of transcription 3) is a downstream of Janus kinases (JAKs) and belongs to a family of transcription factors responsible for transmitting diverse cytokine and growth factor signals from the cellular membrane to the nucleus to activate genes that are involved in many critical processes such as cell proliferation, differentiation, migration, and apoptosis.

STAT3 is a potentially important target in oncology because it regulates the expression of a variety of genes important in cancer including those controlling cell cycle (e.g. cyclin D1, D2, c-Myc), cell survival (e.g. Bcl-xL, Bcl-2, Mcl-1), and angiogenesis (HIF1α, VEGF) (Furqan et al. 2013). In addition, the STAT family of proteins and STAT3 specifically may be activated by JAK or by upstream receptor tyrosine kinases that are frequently overexpressed or overactivated in a variety of solid tumor cells such as epidermal growth factor receptor (EGFR), fibroblast growth factor receptor (FGFR), hepatocyte growth factor receptor (HGFR), and vascular growth factor receptor (VEGFR), as well as non-receptor tyrosine kinases such as SRC (Yu et al. 2009). In addition to the intrinsic effects on cancer cells, STAT3 also has important immunomodulatory effects on the tumor microenvironment that mediate tumor-induced immunosuppression which contributes to tumor growth and progression (Yu et al. 2009). Aberrantly elevated STAT3 activity is estimated to occur in approximately 70% of human cancers including both hematological malignancies and solid tumors (Johnson et al. 2018). Activating mutations in STAT3 are frequent in large granular lymphocytic leukemia (LGL-L) and subsets of peripheral T-cell lymphoma (PTCL) (Crescenzo et al. 2015; Heavican et al. 2019), and STAT3 pathway hyperactivation is a key driver in anaplastic lymphoma kinase (ALK)+ anaplastic large cell lymphoma (ALCL) and also observed in cutaneous T-cell lymphoma (CTCL) (Litvinov et al. 2016) and subtypes of DLBCL and Hodgkin's lymphoma.

Similar to other transcription factors, selective targeting of STAT3 has been challenging with available modalities. Based on the mechanism of action, it is believed that targeted protein degradation may provide a better opportunity than conventional methods to target difficult-to-drug oncogenic proteins such as STAT3.

KT-333

KT-333 (Kymera Therapeutics) is a potent, highly selective, intravenously administered, heterobifunctional small molecule degrader of STAT3. Pre-clinically, STAT3 degraders have shown anti-tumor activity in mouse xenograft models of ALK+ ALCL and STAT3-mutant ALK–ALCL and anti-proliferative/pro-apoptotic effects in STAT3-mutant natural killer/T-cell (NKT) lymphoma cell lines (Liu et al. 2021). Anti-tumor activity in syngeneic solid tumor and B-cell lymphoma models has also been demonstrated in association with immunomodulatory effects on the tumor microenvironment. KT-333 is currently in development for patients with R/R T-cell lymphomas and LGL-L. The first-in-human study, KT-333–101, is a phase 1, multicenter, dose escalation and expansion study evaluating the safety, tolerability, PK, PD, and clinical activity of KT-333 that is planned to be initiated in 2021. The study includes a dose-escalation portion to be conducted in patients with advanced NHL or solid tumors followed by planned expansions in patients with PTCL, CTCL, LGL-L, and solid tumors. Other potential hematological malignancies under consideration include R/R DLBCL and Hodgkin's lymphoma. Once the human safety and PK of KT-333 monotherapy have been assessed, combination trials with agents with complimentary mechanisms of action are planned.

Conclusions and Future Directions

Heterobifunctional degraders are emerging as a novel therapeutic modality for patients with NHL and other hematological and solid tumor malignancies. Heterobifunctional degraders have multiple advantages compared with small molecule inhibitors, including the ability to target undruggable targets such as transcription factors, greater selectivity and potency, and the ability to inhibit the scaffolding function of proteins. Several degrader compounds are currently being evaluated in solid tumor oncology patients and preliminary results have demonstrated clinical evidence of biological activity and tolerability. Additional clinical evidence supporting the utility of heterobifunctional degraders in oncology is being gathered for multiple different targets in lymphomas through recently initiated clinical trials. Efforts are also ongoing to optimize the therapeutic index of degraders by identifying tumor selective and/or tissue-restricted E3 ligases to minimize toxicity in key organs. Overall, heterobifunctional degraders have the potential to be developed into a novel class of drugs that can be recognized as important therapeutic options in the treatment of NHL and other malignancies.

Must Read References

Nandi, D., Tahiliani, P., Kumar, A., Chandu, D. (2006). The ubiquitin-proteasome system. *J. Biosci.* 31: 137–155.

Neklesa, T.K., Winkler, J.D., Crews, C.M. (2017). Targeted protein degradation by PROTACs. *Phamacol. Ther.* 174: 138–144.

Schapira, M., Calabrese, M.F., Bullock, A.N., Crews, C.M. (2019). Targeted protein degradation: expanding the toolblx. *Nat. Rev. Drug Discov.* 18: 949–963.

References

Bondeson, D.P., Smith, B.E., Burslem, G.M. et al. (2018). Lessons in PROTAC design from selective degradation with a promiscuous warhead. *Cell Chem. Biol.* 25: 78–87.

Burger, J.A. (2019). Bruton tyrosine kinase inhibitors: present and future. *Cancer J.* 25: 386–393.

Crescenzo, R., Abate, F., Lasorsa, E. et al. (2015). Convergent mutations and kinase fusions lead to oncogenic STAT3 activation in anaplastic large cell lymphoma. *Cancer Cell* 27: 516–532.

Furqan, M., Akinleye, A., Mukhi, N. et al. (2013). STAT inhibitors for cancer therapy. *J. Hematol. Oncol.* 6: 90.

Gao, S., Wang, S., and Song, Y. (2020). Novel immunomodulatory drugs and neo-substrates. *Biomark Res.* 8: 2.

Gooding, S., Ansari-Pour, N., Towfic, F. et al. (2021). Multiple cereblon genetic changes are associated with acquired resistance to lenalidomide or pomalidomide in multiple mylemoa. *Blood* 137: 232–237.

Grommes, C., Pastore, A., Palaskas, N. et al. (2017). Ibrutinib unmasks critical role of bruton tyrosine kinase in primary CNS lymphoma. *Cancer Discov.* 7: 1018–1029.

Heavican, T.B., Bouska, A., Yu, J. et al. (2019). Genetic drivers of oncogenic pathways in molecular subgroups of peripheral T-cell lymphoma. *Blood* 133: 1664–1676.

Johnson, D.E., O'Keefe, R.A., and Grandis, J.R. (2018). Targeting the IL-6/JAK/STAT3 signalling axis in cancer. *Nat. Rev. Clin. Oncol.* 15: 234–248.

Krönke, J., Udeshi, N.D., Narla, A. et al. (2014). Lenalidomide causes selective degradation of IKZF1 and IKZF3 in multiple myeloma cells. *Science* 343: 301–305.

Li, S., Fu, J., Wang, H. et al. (2018). IMiD compounds affect $CD34^+$ cell fate and maturation via CRBN-induced IKZF1 degradation. *Blood Adv.* 2: 492–504.

Litvinov, I.V., Shtreis, A., Kobayashi, K. et al. (2016). Investigating potential exogenous tumor initiating and promoting factors for cutaneous T-cell lymphomas (CTCL), a rare skin malignancy. *Oncoimmunology* 5: e1175799.

Liu, J., Song, T., Zhou, W. et al. (2019). A genome-scale CRISPR-Cas9 screening in myeloma cells identifies regulators of immunomodulatory drug sensitivity. *Leukemia* 33: 171–180.

Liu, P., Yang, B., Mayo, M. et al. (2021). Targeting STAT3 with selective protein degraders for the treatment of PTCL. Presented at 13th Annual T-Cell Lymphoma Forum.

Mayo, M., Karnik, R., Klaus, C. et al. (2021). KT-413, a novel IRAKIMiD degrader of IRAK4 and IMiD substrates, has a differentiated MOA that leads to single-agent and combination regressions in MYD88^{MT} lymphoma models. *International Conference on Malignant Lymphoma (ICML)*. abstract #13.

Nandi, D., Tahiliani, P., Kumar, A., and Chandu, D. (2006). The ubiquitin-proteasome system. *J. Biosci.* 31: 137–155.

Nathan, M.R. and Schmid, P. (2017). A review of fulvestrant in breast cancer. *Oncol. Ther.* 5: 17–29.

Neklesa, T.K., Winkler, J.D., and Crews, C.M. (2017). Targeted protein degradation by PROTACs. *Phamacol. Ther.* 174: 138–144.

Patel, H.K. and Bihani, T. (2018). Selective estrogen receptor modulators (SERMs) and selective estrogen receptor degraders (SERDs) in cancer treatment. *Pharmacol. Ther.* 186: 1–24.

Schapira, M., Calabrese, M.F., Bullock, A.N., and Crews, C.M. (2019). Targeted protein degradation: expanding the toolblx. *Nat. Rev. Drug Discov.* 18: 949–963.

Singh, S.P., Pillai, S., de Brujin, M.J.W. et al. (2017). Cell lines generated from a chronic lymphocytic leukemia mouse model exhibit constitutive Btk and Akt signaling. *Oncotarget* 26: 71981–71995.

Watt, G.F., Scott-Stevens, P., and Gaohua, L. (2019). Targeted protein degradation in vivo with proteolysis targeting chimeras: current status and future considerations. *Drug Discov. Today Technol.* 31: 69–80.

Wilson, W.H., Young, R.M., Schmitz, R. et al. (2015). Targeting B cell receptor signaling with ibrutinib in diffuse large B cell lymphoma. *Nat. Med.* 21: 922–926.

Wu, C., de Miranda, N.F., Chen, L. et al. (2016). Genetic heterogeneity in primary and relapsed mantle cell lymphomas: impact of recurrent CARD11 mutations. *Oncotarget* 7: 38180–38190.

Yu, H., Pardoll, D., and Jove, R. (2009). STATs in cancer inflammation and immunity: a leading role for STAT3. *Nat. Rev. Cancer* 9: 798–809.

Zhu, Y.X., Kortuem, K.M., and Stewart, A.K. (2013). Molecular mechanism of action of immune-modulatory drugs thalidomide, lenalidomide and pomalidomide in multiple myeloma. *Leuk. Lymphoma* 54: 683–687.

Section VII

Novel Targets and Therapeutic Prospects in Development

27

Strategies for Targeting the JAK-STAT Pathway in Lymphoid Malignancies

David J. Feith[1,2], Johnson Ung[1,2,], Omar Elghawy[1,2,*], Peibin Yue[3], James Turkson[3], and Thomas P. Loughran Jr[1,2]*

[1] *University of Virginia Cancer Center, University of Virginia School of Medicine, Charlottesville, VA, USA*
[2] *Department of Medicine, Division of Hematology/Oncology, University of Virginia School of Medicine, Charlottesville, VA, USA*
[3] *Department of Medicine, Cedars-Sinai Medical Center, Los Angeles, CA, USA*
[*] *These authors contributed equally*

Take Home Messages

- Cytokine-driven JAK-STAT signaling is a key regulator of lymphocyte proliferation, differentiation, survival, and function.
- JAK-STAT pathway dysregulation has been detected across all lymphoid malignancies via multiple mechanisms including increased cytokine and receptor expression, somatic activating mutations in JAK and STAT proteins, and epigenetic silencing of negative regulators.
- Therapeutics targeting STAT3 and STAT5 exhibit preclinical efficacy in model systems while JAK inhibitors have advanced to early-stage clinical trials in lymphoid malignancies.
- Widespread clinical utility of JAK-STAT targeting agents will require increased development of potent STAT inhibitors with drug-like features, enhanced understanding of disease-specific pathway dependencies, and improved characterization of parallel signaling events and resistance mechanisms to identify efficacious combinatorial therapeutic strategies.

JAK-STAT Signaling and Endogenous Regulators

Cytokine families exhibit well-defined pairing with their associated receptors. These receptor complexes canonically engage with preferred Janus kinase (JAK) and signal transducer and activator of transcription (STAT) family members to propagate intracellular signaling events. However, the system contains substantial redundancy and signaling may proceed via diverse family members across varying biological contexts (Figure 27.1; adapted from and reviewed in Salas et al. (2020), Schwartz et al. (2016), Schwartz et al. (2017), Waldmann and Chen (2017), and You et al. (2020)). Cytokine receptor engagement and complex formation triggers a cascade of intracellular signaling events that culminate in transcriptional activation within the nucleus (Figure 27.2; adapted from and reviewed in Benekli et al. (2009), Harrison (2012), Hu et al. (2021), You et al. (2020)). JAK proteins are recruited to receptor intracellular domains and initiate trans- and auto-phosphorylation events on both components. STAT proteins bind via their Src homology 2 (SH2) domains to phosphotyrosine residues within intracellular receptor domains, thereafter becoming phosphorylated by JAKs on their own tyrosine residues. This represents a canonical readout of STAT protein activation, which precipitates STAT homodimerization and translocation to the nucleus. Activated STATs bind cognate recognition elements within gene promoters to induce transcription. A huge number of STAT-responsive genes have been reported. These may exhibit uniform regulation across cell types or cell-specific responses that are dictated by chromatin architecture (Carpenter and Lo 2014). Target genes include prominent mediators of cellular proliferation (c-Myc, cyclin D1) and survival (Bcl-2, Mcl-1) as well as secreted growth factors and cytokines that condition the microenvironment and mediate immunological processes.

Individual cytokine signaling cascades are typically depicted as a simplistic linear molecular progression from cytokine ligand binding to the receptor to induce a JAK-STAT phosphorylation

Precision Cancer Therapies: Targeting Oncogenic Drivers and Signaling Pathways in Lymphoid Malignancies: From Concept to Practice, Volume 1, First Edition. Edited by Owen A. O'Connor, Stephen M. Ansell, and John F. Seymour.

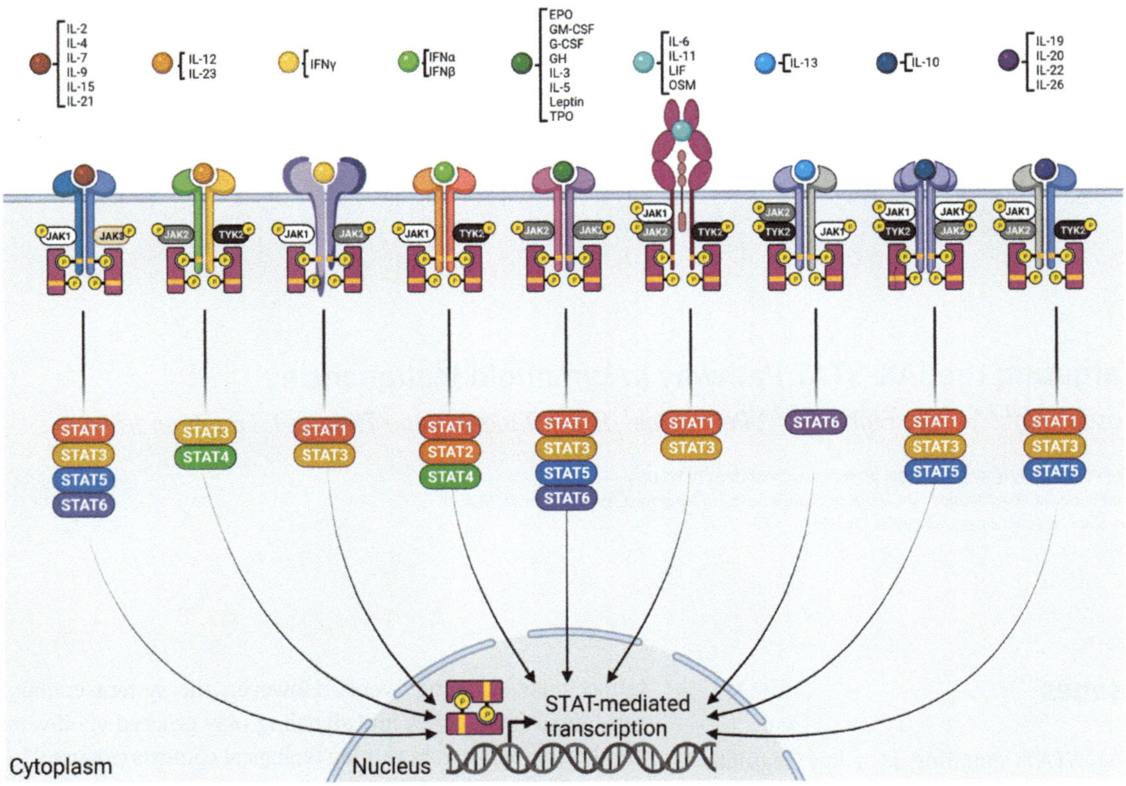

Figure 27.1 **Summary of key mediators of JAK-STAT signaling.** Numerous cytokines and chemokines bind to cell surface receptors to initiate key signaling pathways that regulate lymphocyte proliferation, differentiation, survival, and function. Several JAK-family isoforms (JAK1-3, TYK2) and STAT isoforms (STAT1-6) mediate signal transduction elicited by a multitude of growth factors, cytokines, and hormones. Following receptor activation, specific JAK-family kinases are recruited and undergo multiple phosphorylation events that culminate in the subsequent recruitment and phosphorylation of STAT proteins. Activated STAT dimers translocate to the nuclease to initiate target gene transcription. JAK, Janus kinase; TYK, tyrosine kinase; STAT, signal transducer and activator of transcription; P, phosphate group; IL, interleukin; IFN, interferon; EPO, erythropoietin; TPO, thrombopoietin; GM-CSF, granulocyte-macrophage colony-stimulating factor; G-CSF, granulocyte colony-stimulating factor; GH, growth hormone; LIF, leukemia inhibitory factor; OSM, oncostatin M. Figure created with BioRender.com.

cascade that culminates in target gene transcription. Like most of biology, the reality is dauntingly complex due to: (i) an abundance of bioactive cytokines and chemokines encountered by malignant cells in various microenvironments; (ii) multiple cytokine receptor subtypes and subunits that exhibit shared and specific usage that modulates ligand affinity; (iii) four JAK family proteins (JAK1, JAK2, JAK2, TYK2); (iv) seven STAT family proteins (STAT1, STAT2, STAT3, STAT4, STAT5A, STAT5B, STAT6); (v) multiple proteins that feedback and modulate JAK-STAT signaling; (vi) cell type-specific expression of these signaling components that dictates signaling potential in a given cell, and (vii) cell type-specific chromatin architecture and STAT-specific DNA binding sites that collectively dictate target gene accessibility and expression. Key drivers in lymphoid malignancies include interleukins (IL) that signal through the common gamma-chain (especially IL-2, IL-4, IL-7, and IL-15), IL-6, IL-10 as well as their intracellular signaling components JAK1, JAK2, JAK3, STAT3, and STAT5B.

As in most physiological systems, regulatory proteins provide feedback to prevent overdrive of this signaling pathway. Prominent components of these negative regulatory systems include suppressors of cytokine signaling (SOCS), protein inhibitors of activated STATs (PIAS), and receptor and non-receptor protein tyrosine phosphatases (PTP) (reviewed in Bohmer and Friedrich (2014), Hu et al. (2021), Keewan and Matlawska-Wasowska (2021), and Zhao et al. (2015)). Many of these regulators are also direct STAT transcriptional targets (e.g. CIS, SOCS3). Loss of these components is an alternative mechanism of pathway activation in lymphoid malignancy. For example, studies in large granular lymphocyte (LGL) leukemia report epigenetic silencing of SOCS3 expression (Teramo et al. 2013) as well as DNA hypermethylation in the gene promoter region of protein tyrosine phosphatase receptor type D (PTPRD) of *TET2*-mutated natural killer (NK)-LGL leukemia (Olson et al. 2021).

STAT signaling is also induced via JAK-independent pathways in addition to the canonical cytokine-mediated activation. These include non-receptor tyrosine kinases, receptor tyrosine kinases, and G-protein coupled receptors, such as sphingosine-1-phosphate receptor 1 (S1PR1) (Lee et al. 2010). The alternative activation mechanisms are rife with known drivers of cellular proliferation and survival across the hematologic

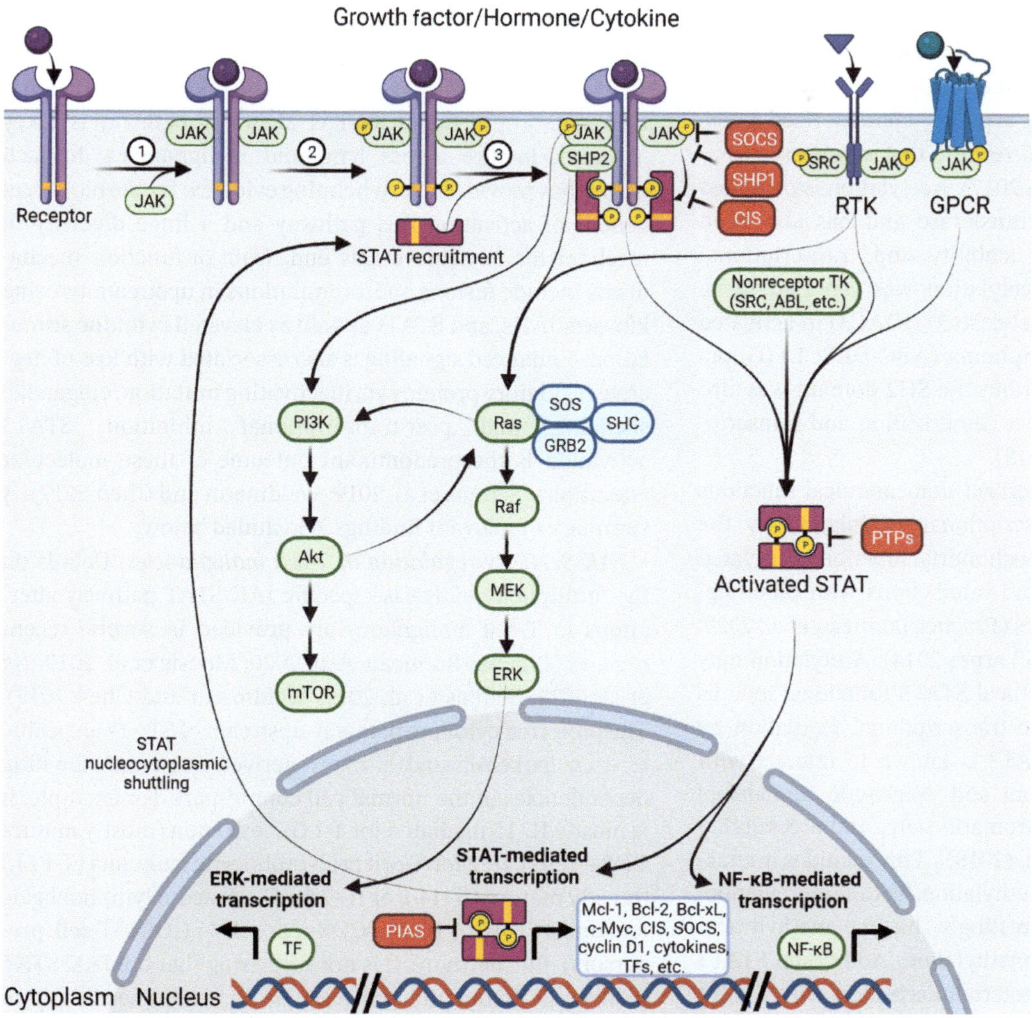

Figure 27.2 **Simplified JAK-STAT signaling and crosstalk with other pathways.** Following receptor activation, JAK-family kinases are recruited to the cytosolic domain of the receptor complex (**1**) and facilitate auto- and/or trans-phosphorylation of tyrosine residues within receptor subunits and JAK proteins (**2**). Specific STAT subunits, dependent on the receptor-JAK combination, are recruited and dock onto the receptor phosphotyrosine residues and activated by JAK phosphorylation (**3**). Activated STATs translocate to the nucleus and participate in STAT-mediated gene transcription while promoting NF-κB transcription. Receptor tyrosine kinases (RTKs), non-receptor TKs, and GPCRs can also activate STATs. JAK activation frequently initiates crosstalk with the PI3K-AKT-mTOR and Ras-Raf-MEK-ERK pathways. Nucleocytoplasmic shuttling of STAT replenishes the cytosol with STAT subunits. Many endogenous proteins negatively regulate JAK-STAT signaling (shown as red symbols). For example, SOCS family proteins (CIS and SOCS1-7) directly bind to JAK and/or the activated receptor to prevent further JAK signaling and STAT recruitment. Endogenous JAK-STAT inhibitors include the PTPs like SHP1, which inhibit JAK-STAT proteins via dephosphorylation. Another notable group of endogenous inhibitors are PIAS proteins, which block DNA binding, recruit transcriptional co-repressors, or promote post-translational modifications of STAT proteins. JAK, Janus kinase; STAT, signal transducer and activator of transcription; RTK, receptor tyrosine kinase; GPCR, G-protein coupled receptor; TF, transcription factor; SOCS, suppressor of cytokine signaling; PTP, protein tyrosine phosphatase; PIAS, protein inhibitor of activated STAT; SHP1, Src homology 2 domain-containing protein tyrosine phosphatase 1. Created with BioRender.com.

malignancies (e.g. ABL proto-oncogene, fms-like receptor tyrosine kinase 3 [FLT3]). Moreover, growth factor/cytokine signaling is known to branch into parallel proliferative and survival pathways such as PI3K/AKT/mTOR, Ras/Raf/MEK/ERK, and nuclear factor-kappaB (NF-κB), a veritable who's who of cancer drivers. Multiple lines of evidence support crosstalk between JAK-STAT and NF-κB signaling including physical interaction, co-localization at promoter elements, and cooperative promotion of various malignancies (Grivennikov and Karin 2010; Lee et al. 2009).

Alternative Regulation and Function of STATs

Post-translational modifications have been detected at specific amino acid residues in STAT3 and STAT5B and are associated with varying functional consequences (Brachet-Botineau et al. 2020). STAT3 can be phosphorylated (Y705, S727), acetylated (K685), or methylated (K140, K180). Similarly, STAT5B can be phosphorylated (Y699, S730), acetylated (K694), sumoylated (K701, K750), or O-GlcNacylated (T92). Phosphorylation at Y705 or Y699 is the canonical signaling readout associated with transcriptional activation. STAT3 phosphorylation at Y705 is also elevated upon acquisition of somatic activating mutations, in particular Y640F. Interestingly, TYK2 mediates a poorly characterized phosphorylation event at the Y640 residue that suppresses transcriptional activity (Mori et al. 2017). Acetylation is mediated by CBP/p300 histone acetyltransferase and has also been reported to enhance dimer stability and transcriptional activity. Moreover, STAT3 acetylation was reported to be regulated by the histone deacetylase 3 (HDAC3) in activated B-cell diffuse large B-cell lymphoma (ABC-DLBCL) (Gupta et al. 2012). Palmitoylation within the SH2 domain was also reported and shown to enhance dimerization and transcriptional activation (Niu et al. 2019).

Additional studies have described non-canonical functions of STAT3 that include transcriptional modulation by the unphosphorylated protein, mitochondrial functions associated with S727 phosphorylation, and interactions with other signaling pathways and organelles (Brachet-Botineau et al. 2020; Majoros et al. 2017; Meier and Larner 2014). Acetylation may also influence these non-canonical STAT3 functions, such as mitochondrial uptake and the transcriptional regulation by unphosphorylated STAT3. STAT3 is known to interact with numerous transcription factors and epigenetic remodelers with widespread impact on chromatin states and accessibility (reviewed in Wingelhofer et al. (2018)). This includes interactions with regulators of DNA methylation, histone methylation, and histone acetylation. Interestingly, histone methyltransferases also mediated STAT3 methylation. Additional STAT3 interacting partners include heterodimerization with STAT1 and STAT5, which may represent an alternative mechanism to integrate physiological signals and/or escape therapeutic targeting (Delgoffe and Vignali 2013). Heterodimerization is influenced by post-translational modifications, receptor subunit composition and/or proximity. Functionally, these heterodimers may represent reservoirs of transcriptionally dead complexes or novel transcriptional complexes with alternative binding to consensus sequences, co-activator proteins, or co-repressor proteins.

These alternate mechanisms to induce STAT phosphorylation and alternative pathways activated downstream of cytokine receptors create daunting challenges for the efficacious and selective targeting of JAK-STAT signaling. In addition, cellular responses to JAK-STAT pathway activation vary depending on cell type, epigenetic state, activity of intersecting pathways, and the magnitude and duration of the signal. Increased understanding of these signaling events in a disease-specific manner is likely to reveal key resistance mechanisms that subvert JAK-STAT inhibitors and to identify dependencies to be targeted for efficacious combinatorial therapeutic regimens.

Dysregulated Cytokine Signaling in Lymphoid Malignancies

Dysregulation of the JAK-STAT signaling pathway is a key hallmark feature across lymphoid malignancies. In fact, nature has provided overwhelming evidence for the biological benefit of activating this pathway and a huge diversity of mechanisms to achieve this end. Gain-of-function mechanisms include fusions and/or mutations in upstream tyrosine kinases, JAKs, and STATs as well as elevated cytokine stimulation. Enhanced signaling is also associated with loss of negative regulatory proteins via inactivating mutation, epigenetic silencing, and post-transcriptional inhibition. STAT3 activation is the predominant outcome of these molecular alterations (Seffens et al. 2019; Waldmann and Chen 2017). A summary of relevant findings is included below.

JAK-STAT dysregulation in T-cell malignancies. Details on the multiplicity of disease-specific JAK-STAT pathway alterations in T-cell malignancy are provided in several recent reviews (Brachet-Botineau et al. 2020; Moosic et al. 2019; Ng et al. 2018; Seffens et al. 2019; Waldmann and Chen 2017). The preferred cytokine pathway upstream of STATs is specific to each leukemia and is likely derived from the signaling dependencies of the normal cell counterpart. For example, it is mostly IL-15 mediated for T-LGL leukemia (mostly mature CD8+ cells), IL-2 for T-cell prolymphocytic leukemia (T-PLL) (mostly mature CD4+), or IL-7 for T-cell acute lymphoblastic leukemia (T-ALL) (CD4−CD8− or CD4+CD8+ T-cell precursors). Furthermore, it is not surprising that the JAK-STAT pathway is frequently activated via increased sensitivity to upstream cytokine stimulation due to upregulated receptor expression (e.g. IL-7R in T-ALL, high affinity IL-2Rα and IL-15Rα in adult T-cell leukemia [ATL]).

The most common somatic variants across T-cell malignancies are activating mutations of STAT3 and STAT5B, in particular the former. Direct STAT3 activation via somatic mutation was an early and straightforward exemplar of the importance of JAK-STAT signaling in T-cell malignancies. The hotspots for STAT3 somatic activating mutations are located within the SH2 domain (Moosic et al. 2019; Seffens et al. 2019; Waldmann and Chen 2017), especially point mutants at residues Y640 and D661. These were first identified in T- and NK-LGL leukemia (Jerez et al. 2012; Koskela et al. 2012) with subsequent detection in additional lymphoid malignancies (Moosic et al. 2019). Mechanistically, these missense mutations are thought to enhance the affinity at the STAT3 homodimer interface to promote persistence of the transcriptionally active state. This is highly reminiscent of the constitutively dimerized and activated STAT3C construct that was utilized in the first demonstration of the transforming potential of STAT3 (Bromberg et al. 1999). Importantly, STAT3 activating mutations have been linked to distinct clinical features and poor prognosis in multiple lymphoid malignancies.

The large number of identified activating mutations, along with identification of inactivating mutations within the SH2 domain, provides an opportunity to identify convergent events to postulate structural implications of varying mutations at particular residues (de Araujo et al. 2019). Various biochemical assays, most commonly STAT3 transcription reporter assays and phospho-STAT3 western blotting, have been utilized to identify increased activation of mutants relative to wild-type. Importantly, functional characterization studies have also identified activating mutations outside of the SH2 domain, included the coiled-coil and DNA binding domain (Andersson et al. 2016; Cheon et al. 2022), and germline gain-of-function variants have been identified within all domains of the protein (Fabre et al. 2019). Additional mechanistic studies showed that upstream cytokine receptor signaling was necessary for survival of ALK− ALCL, the presence of JAK1 and STAT3 somatic activating mutations alone were not sufficient (Chen et al. 2017). Retroviral transduction of bone marrow progenitor cells to drive activated STAT3 protein expression was not sufficient to drive lymphoid malignancy in mice (Dutta et al. 2018). However, a definitive assessment of the ability of STAT3 to drive lymphoid malignancy may require refined genetically engineered mouse models with conditional expression of STAT3 mutants in mature T-cells. Somatic mutation is not a prerequisite for JAK-STAT-driven proliferation and survival signaling. For example, widespread constitutive STAT3 activation was demonstrated in LGL leukemia (Epling-Burnette et al. 2001) over a decade prior to the discovery of somatic activating mutations in approximately a third of LGL leukemia samples (Koskela et al. 2012).

Many alternative mechanisms of JAK-STAT pathway activation have also been described. A number of gene fusions directly impact JAK proteins and/or activate JAK-STAT signaling (e.g. STAT3/JAK2 fusion in indolent T-cell lymphoproliferative disorder of the GI tract [Sharma et al. 2018], JAK2 fusion in T-ALL, ROS1 and TYK2 fusions in ALK− ALCL, and ALK fusions in ALK+ ALCL). Recurrent copy number gains have been detected in multiple JAK and STAT genes, in particular in Sezary's syndrome. Cutaneous T-cell lymphoma (CTCL) is also noteworthy for STAT4 and STAT6 upregulation. Negative regulators of JAK-STAT signaling are frequently inactivated or silenced (e.g. SOCS3 and PTPRD in LGL leukemia, multiple PTPs in aggressive natural killer cell leukemia [ANKL], SOCS1 in extranodal NK/T-cell lymphoma (ENKTCL) [Song et al. 2018], and protein tyrosine phosphatase non-receptor type 1 (PTPN1) in ATL). Collectively, the mutational events, upstream signaling, and loss of feedback regulation combine to activate STAT3 and STAT5B in virtually all T-cell malignancies. JAK1, JAK2, and JAK3 have all been implicated in multiple disease subtypes as well, with somewhat increased evidence for JAK3.

JAK-STAT dysregulation in B-cell malignancies. JAK-STAT signaling pathway mutation and dysregulation have also been reported in B-cell malignancies (reviewed in Rosenquist et al. (2017)). Most notably, aggressive B-cell and DLBCL are characterized by STAT3 and STAT6 mutations. STAT3 activation is detected within the ABC-DLBCL rather than germinal center B-cell (GCB)-DLBCL subtype, and STAT3 targets are highly represented in genes that are differentially expressed between the subtypes (Hardee et al. 2013). Hodgkin's lymphoma (HL) exhibits STAT6, SOCS1, and JAK2 mutations as well as copy number variants that affect JAK1, STAT3, STAT5B, and PTPN1 (Tiacci et al. 2018). STAT6 is also involved in follicular lymphoma whereas B-cell ALL is associated with constitutively activated STAT5B. Mantle cell lymphoma (MCL), marginal zone lymphoma, and chronic lymphocytic leukemia (CLL) exhibit infrequent JAK-STAT mutational events yet pathway activation is detected. In particular, constitutively active STAT3 is strongly linked to CLL pathogenesis, including functional effects on the mitochondria in association with S727 phosphorylation. Multiple myeloma is characterized by IL-6-driven STAT3 activation as well as hypermethylation-mediated silencing of the negative regulators SHP1 (Src homology 2 domain-containing protein tyrosine phosphatase 1) and SOCS1. Therapeutic development and clinical trials in these B-cell diseases have focused on monoclonal antibody (rituximab, anti-CD20), Bruton's tyrosine kinase (BTK; ibrutinib), and Bcl-2 (venetoclax) targeting together with traditional chemotherapy and radiotherapy. However, a number of JAK-STAT-directed approaches are described below.

Strategies to Target the JAK-STAT Pathway

Given the established importance of JAK-STAT signaling in multiple malignant and autoimmune conditions, it is not surprising that this pathway has been the focus of intense drug discovery and development efforts (Figure 27.3; adapted from and reviewed in Benekli et al. (2009), Hu et al. (2021), Johnson et al. (2018), Miklossy et al. (2013), and Waldmann and Chen (2017)). Therapeutic approaches have targeted every level of the pathway from extracellular binding of the receptor to intracellular phosphorylation cascades to nuclear transcription events. They have utilized varying molecular mechanisms including monoclonal antibodies, small molecule kinase inhibitors,

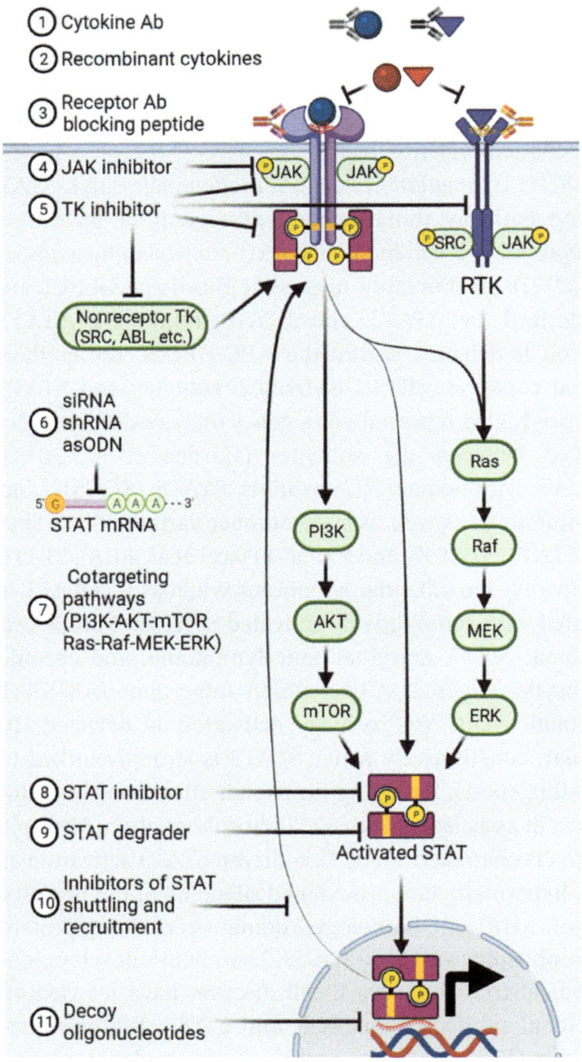

Figure 27.3 Therapeutic avenues for targeting aberrant JAK-STAT signaling in lymphoid malignancies. Drug development efforts have targeted JAK-STAT signaling at every level of the cascade from cytokines to gene expression. These therapeutic strategies include: (**1**) cytokine-directed antibodies; (**2**) receptor-blocking recombinant cytokines; (**3**) receptor-directed antibodies or receptor/cytokine-blocking peptides; (**4**) small molecule JAK inhibitors; (**5**) TK inhibitors; (**6**) STAT mRNA targeting with small interfering RNA, short hairpin RNA, and anti-sense oligodeoxynucleotides; (**7**) co-targeting PI3K-AKT-mTOR or Ras-Raf-MEK-ERK pathways; (**8**) small molecule STAT inhibitors; (**9**) STAT degraders (PROTACs); (**10**) STAT nucleocytoplasmic shuttling inhibitors; (**11**) decoy oligonucleotides. JAK, Janus kinase; STAT, signal transducer and activator of transcription; RTK, receptor tyrosine kinase. Created with BioRender.com.

peptide and small molecule blockers of protein interaction, decoy oligonucleotides, mRNA targeting, and protein degraders. The diversity of these approaches is a consequence of the complexity of JAK-STAT signaling, as described above, as well as the challenges associated with STAT targeting. STATs are notoriously difficult to inhibit because they lack catalytic pockets to serve as high affinity and selective docking sites for potent small molecule inhibitors. In contrast, many groups have identified and optimized small molecule inhibitors of JAK kinase activity with excellent potency and varying isoform selectivity. Thus, the clinical development and testing of JAK inhibitors vastly exceeds that of STAT-targeting approaches. Below, we focus on inhibitors that target JAK and STAT family proteins implicated in the pathogenesis of lymphoid malignancies and describe ongoing and completed clinical trials of these compounds in lymphoid malignancies. STAT3-targeting approaches, which are primarily in preclinical stages, will be discussed first followed by clinical trials of JAK inhibitors.

Direct Targeting Approaches against STAT3

STAT3 is a challenging target for drug discovery and development programs to develop potent and suitable small molecule inhibitors that have clinical utility. This is in part because STAT3 is a transcription factor, and it lacks deep binding pockets amenable to targeting. Thus, the development of small molecule STAT3 inhibitors has faced substantial challenges, including weak potency and lack of suitable drug-like properties. Despite the difficulties, several small molecules have been developed that have shown activity in pre-clinical *in vitro* and *in vivo* models (Debnath et al. 2012; Johnson et al. 2018; Miklossy et al. 2013; Moser et al. 2021). These studies are reviewed below to provide proof-of-concept for the anti-tumor activities of the inhibition of constitutively active STAT3 in diverse cancers, including hematological malignancies (Miklossy et al. 2013; Moser et al. 2021). Moreover, conditional T-cell specific deletion of STAT3 in adult mice led to severely impaired IL-6-induced proliferation (Takeda et al. 1998). Humans with germline STAT3 loss-of-function variants develop normally outside of the predictable immune dysfunction. These genetic findings validate the utility and therapeutic window of STAT3 inhibitor development for lymphoid malignancies.

Oligonucleotide-based Strategies

One of the earliest strategies to target STAT3 was by means of oligonucleotides. Reports of inhibitory effects of oligonucleotide modalities include G-quartet delivered via nanoparticle vehicle to target STAT3, which inhibited tumor growth in the high mobility group A1 (HMGA1) transgenic model of T-cell leukemia (Hillion et al. 2008). Alternative approaches utilized treatment with the STAT3 anti-sense oligonucleotide, AZD9150, which suppressed STAT3 expression and induced anti-tumor activity in lymphoma models (Hong et al. 2015) and has progressed to clinical trials (see below). Moreover, short hairpin (sh)RNA approaches have been proven to inhibit STAT3 function, leading to the reversal of the glycolytic shift, upregulation of latexin tumor suppressor, induction of cancer cell apoptosis, and tumor growth inhibition in the SCC-3 lymphoma model (Akiyama et al. 2015). STAT3-targeting shRNA further induced apoptosis, suppressed STAT3 target gene expression, and blocked tumor-promoting microenvironment, leading to tumor growth inhibition of human ABC-like DLBCL tumors in mice (Scuto et al. 2011). A molecule designed to have a dual-function, CpG-STAT3dODN, which consists of Toll-like receptor 9 (TLR9) agonist (CpG7909) and a high affinity decoy oligonucleotide targeting STAT3 (dODN), was shown to block STAT3 DNA-binding activity, suppress c-Myc and Bcl2L1 expression in human and mouse lymphoma cells, and block growth of human OCI-Ly3 lymphoma in immunodeficient mice and syngeneic A20 lymphoma, and prolong survival (Zhao et al. 2018). CpG-STAT3dODN also induced lymphoma cell-specific CD8/CD4-dependent T-cell immunity (Zhao et al. 2018). Notably, treatment of lymphoma cell lines with the direct STAT3 inhibitor WP1066 suppressed the expression of programmed death-1 (PD-1) ligand 1/2 (PD-L1/2), inhibited lymphoma cell growth, and induced apoptosis (Ma et al. 2017). Thus, multiple lines of evidence demonstrate the direct anti-tumor effects of targeting STAT3 mRNA and its potential to re-engage anti-tumor immune cell function in the tumor microenvironment.

Direct STAT3 Inhibitors as Standalone Agents

Several studies have shown the efficacy of direct STAT3 small molecule inhibitors in select hematological malignancies. Earlier reports showed that STX-0119, which was discovered through virtual screening as a STAT3 dimerization inhibitor, suppressed STAT3 phosphorylation, downregulated STAT3 targets (c-Myc, survivin, cyclin D1, and Bcl-xL), and induced apoptosis. Oral delivery of this compound inhibited *in vivo* human lymphoma growth in subcutaneous xenografts in mice (Ashizawa et al. 2011; Matsuno et al. 2010). Moreover, in preclinical models of ALL and Burkitt's lymphoma, aggressive lymphoid malignancies overexpressing the HMGA1 chromatin remodeling protein, the small molecule direct STAT3 inhibitor, BP-1–102 (Zhang et al. 2012), suppressed STAT3 phosphorylation, reduced expression of STAT3 downstream genes, decreased cell growth, and inhibited tumor growth *in vivo* (Belton et al. 2016). The STAT3 and cancer stem cell inhibitor, napabucasin (BBI-608) (Li et al. 2015), was cytotoxic against non-Hodgkin's lymphoma (NHL) lines, including DLBCL cells, suppressed STAT3 target gene expression including Mcl-1, regulated reactive oxygen species (ROS)-mediated mitogen-activated protein kinase (MAPK) signaling, and inhibited tumor growth *in vivo* both as a single agent and in combination with doxorubicin (Li et al. 2020). In models of nasal-type natural killer/T-cell lymphoma (nasal NKTCL) cells, SNK6, treatment with the small molecule STAT3 inhibitor WP1066 inhibited cell proliferation and induced apoptosis (Geng et al. 2016). Treatment with this compound further suppressed the expression of the downstream targets, c-Myc, cyclin D1, and Bcl-2.

A more recent report showed a new class of molecules that were developed based on the proteolysis targeting chimera (PROTAC) concept. Upon interacting with STAT3, these molecules recruit ubiquitin ligases and enhance STAT3 proteasomal degradation. The PROTAC degrader SD-36 and its hydrolytic product, SD-91, were shown to selectively target STAT3 but not other family members, potently inhibit growth of acute myeloid leukemia (AML) and anaplastic large-cell lymphoma (ALCL) cell lines, induce cell cycle arrest and/or apoptosis, and their delivery *in vivo* led to complete tumor regression in leukemia xenograft models without overt toxicity (Bai et al. 2019; Zhou et al. 2019, 2021).

Natural Product Inhibitors of STAT3

Inhibition of STAT3 activation by natural products has been reported against many cancers, including hematological malignancies (Miklossy et al. 2013). Two flavonoids from a plant source, 4'-methoxy licoflavanone (MLF) and alpinumisoflavone (AIF), demonstrated anti-tumor activity against HL-60 human AML cells, including inhibition of cell proliferation and induction of apoptosis by mechanisms that involved inhibition of STAT3 activation (Kumar et al. 2013). The natural product designated as (R)-5-hydroxy-2-methylchroman-4-one (HMC), a secondary metabolite isolated from an endophytic fungus, inhibited cell proliferation and induce apoptosis of lymphoid and myeloid leukemia lines MOLT-4, HL-60, and K-562 (Pathania et al. 2015). The anti-tumor effects against the leukemia cells occur in part by decreasing the levels of phosphorylated STAT3 through the induction of ubiquitin-dependent degradation (Pathania et al. 2015). The bioflavonoid, quercetin, is reported to inhibit the STAT3, PI3K/AKT, and Wnt/β-catenin pathways as part of the mechanisms leading to suppression of c-FLIP, cyclin D1, and c-Myc expression, and cell death in primary effusion lymphoma (PEL) cells (Granato et al. 2017). The Food and Drug Administration (FDA)-approved anti-microbial agent, atovaquone, has shown inhibitory activity against STAT3 functions. Treatment with atovaquone inhibited STAT3 phosphorylation, presumably by downregulation of cell surface expression of gp130, and STAT3 downstream gene expression in hematological cancer cells, including primary blasts isolated from patients with AML or ALL (Granato et al. 2017). Oral administration of atovaquone inhibited tumor growth and prolonged survival in mouse models of multiple myeloma (Granato et al. 2017). The extended use of atovaquone for *Pneumocystis* prophylaxis in AML patients receiving hematopoietic stem cell transplantation was associated with improved relapse-free survival (Granato et al. 2017).

Chemotherapeutic, Cytotoxic Drugs, and Other Modalities that Directly or Indirectly Inhibit STAT3 Pathway

STAT3 activity has also been implicated as part of the underlying mechanism for anti-tumor effects of chemotherapeutic or cytotoxic agents. In particular, methotrexate, an inhibitor of dihydrofolate reductase (DHFR), has been reported to also inhibit STAT3 activation (Thomas et al. 2015). This STAT3 inhibition was part of the underlying mechanism for methotrexate apoptosis induction in NPM-ALK-positive ALCL (Uchihara et al. 2019). It is unclear how this chemotherapeutic agent suppresses STAT3 activation, beside the observation that cells treated with this agent showed reduced STAT3 phosphorylation (Uchihara et al. 2019). Moreover, the cytotoxic agents DCZ0858 (Lu et al. 2020) and DCZ3301 (Sun et al. 2017), noted as M phase blockers (Hu et al. 2020), have been reported to inhibit the JAK2/STAT3 pathway in DLBCL. This inhibition contributed to the observed anti-proliferative effects *in vitro* and the suppression of tumor growth *in vivo* (Lu et al. 2020; Sun et al. 2017). DCZ3301 inhibited STAT3 phosphorylation by mechanisms involving the suppression of Lck/Yes-related novel protein tyrosine kinases (Lyn) activation (Sun et al. 2017). Treatment with GANT61, an inhibitor of the hedgehog (Hh)/glioma-associated oncogene-1 (GLI1) pathway, was associated with the reduced expression of phosphorylated STAT3 in T-cell lymphomas (Geng et al. 2017), though the mechanism of downregulation of STAT3 signaling is not fully understood. Moreover, the cytotoxic fusion toxin, rGel/BLyS (receptor-mediated delivery of the rGel toxin), was tested against DLBCL and demonstrated STAT3 inhibitory effects. Treatment of DLBCL cells with rGel/BLyS led to IL-6R downregulation, inhibition of STAT3 phosphorylation, reduced STAT3 DNA-binding activity, suppression of STAT3 target gene expression including c-Myc, p21, Mcl-1, and Bcl-xL, accumulation of cells in the sub-G(1) phase of the cell cycle, induction of apoptosis, and inhibition of growth (Lyu et al. 2010). Further, it is reported that persistently active STAT3 co-localizes with elevated expression of sphingosine-1-phosphate receptor 1 (S1PR1), a G-protein-coupled receptor for S1P in the ABC-DLBCL patient specimens (Liu et al. 2012). In this model, shRNA-mediated inhibition of S1PR1 expression altered the expression of STAT3 target genes. Further, treatment with FTY720, a functional antagonist of S1P signaling that is currently in the clinic for other indications, suppressed STAT3 activity and inhibited growth of lymphoma cells *in vitro* and *in vivo* (Lyu et al. 2010). Finally, it was reported that the SIRT1 activators, SRT501 and SRT2183, induced growth arrest and apoptosis associated with deacetylation of STAT3 and NF-κB, and reduced expression of c-Myc, and that SRT2183 treatment reduced the DNA-binding activity of both STAT3 and NF-κB to the promoter of GADD45G in lymphoid cell lines (Scuto et al. 2013).

Inhibition of STAT3 Function in Combination Strategies to Sensitize Tumors and/or Reverse Resistance

Studies have further explored the inhibition of STAT3 function in combination therapeutic strategies with the focus to enhance the anti-tumor activity of other agents and to impair development of resistance. Combination treatment with the JAK1/STAT3 inhibitor, piceatannol, sensitized 2F7 NHL cells to chemotherapies, in part by downregulation of anti-apoptotic Bcl-2 expression (Alas and Bonavida 2003). Treatment of DLBCL cells with the STAT3 inhibitor, STA-21 (Song et al. 2005), synergized with a survivin inhibitor, YM155, to induce apoptosis *in vitro* (Kaneko et al. 2013). Moreover, treatment with WP1066 reversed the IL-6-mediated resistance to the pan-HDAC inhibitors, panobinostat (LBH589) and vorinostat (SAHA), in CLL cells (Lu et al. 2015). In other studies, the STAT3 inhibitor synergized with vorinostat to inhibit growth and induce apoptosis of MCL cells (Lu et al. 2015). In addition, combination treatment with citarinostat (Acy-241), a second-generation, orally administered HDAC6-selective inhibitor, and momelotinib (CYT387), an orally bioavailable JAK-STAT3 signaling inhibitor, led to strong cytotoxicity in lymphoid cell lines that was associated with decreased mitochondrial membrane potential and Bcl-2 and Bcl-xL expression, and induction of activated caspases 9 and 3 (Cosenza et al. 2020). The natural product, cucurbitacin B, enhanced the apoptotic and anti-tumor effects of arsenic trioxide through inhibition of STAT3 phosphorylation in Burkitt's lymphoma Ramos cells (Ding et al. 2017). Studies further showed that while the heat shock protein 90 (Hsp90) inhibitor, luminespib, alone actively suppressed the Y705 phosphorylation of mutant STAT3 and the viability of mutant STAT3 in NK cell lines and LGL leukemia patient samples, the combination of inhibitors of Hsp90, JAK, and mammalian target of rapamycin (mTOR) was more effective at suppressing cell viability than any single agent alone (Kuusanmaki et al. 2017).

A wide variety of modalities are available that interfere with the STAT3 signaling pathway, including those that interact with STAT3 directly and many others that might do so indirectly and by unknown mechanisms. Thus far, the field lacks potent and pharmacologically suitable small molecules that directly inhibit STAT3. However, there is substantial knowledge that has been gained over the years in the strategies to discover suitable STAT3 inhibitors, and the emerging modalities are incorporating new technological concepts, such as the STAT3-targeted PROTACs(Bai et al. 2019). Opportunities remain to develop suitable direct STAT3 inhibitors by way of oligonucleotide-based molecules and small molecule or natural product entities that possess optimum pharmacological properties for clinical application against hematologic malignancies.

Clinical Trials of STAT3 Inhibitors in Lymphoid Malignancy

There are currently no FDA-approved STAT3 inhibitors for lymphoid malignancies. Although hyperactivation of STATs has been implicated in many lymphoid malignancies, limited progress has been made in clinical trials to advance an effective STAT-targeted treatment modality for these cancers. A search of active, completed, or terminated clinical trials registered in ClinicalTrials.gov identified only five STAT inhibitors that have been or are currently being investigated across seven clinical trials in patients with lymphoid malignancies (Table 27.1).

Nearly half of these trials utilized the anti-sense oligonucleotide inhibitor AZD9150. It was well tolerated and achieved preclinical therapeutic levels in several phase 1 trials, but anti-tumor activity was limited. All responses in its first phase 1B trial (NCT01563302) were seen among DLBCL patients, including two complete responses with median duration of response 10.7 months and two partial responses (Reilley et al. 2018). Combination therapy of AZD9150 with anti-PD-L1 checkpoint inhibitor durvalumab in a phase 1 trial (NCT02549651) was not significantly more efficacious with an overall objective response rate of 6.3% with two partial responses (Ribrag et al. 2021). Finally, the efficacy of BTK inhibitor acalabrutinib in a phase 1 trial (NCT03527147) did not improve with addition of AZD9150 compared to acalabrutinib alone and side effects were worse using combination therapy (Abbas and Wierda 2021).

Several other STAT-targeting approaches have progressed to clinical trials in lymphoid malignancy. OPB-51602, a small molecule inhibitor of STAT3 that works through inhibition of complex I and ROS induction, demonstrated efficacy in preclinical models but showed no clear therapeutic response in a phase 1 trial (NCT01344876) (Brambilla et al. 2020; Ogura et al. 2015). OPB-31121, a small molecular inhibitor of STAT3 and STAT5 phosphorylation, was well tolerated among healthy individuals, and results from its phase 1 trial (NCT00511082) in NHL and multiple myeloma have yet to be reported (Brambilla et al. 2015; Hayakawa et al. 2013). Napabucasin is a small molecule STAT3 inhibitor previously shown to eliminate AML cells *in vitro* and *in vivo* via STAT3 pathway inhibition and DNA damage induction (Bi et al. 2019; Zhou et al. 2018). A phase 1 combination trial (NCT02352558) with standard therapy for lymphoid malignancies including 26S proteasome inhibitor bortezomib, receptor tyrosine kinase inhibitor imatinib, and BTK inhibitor ibrutinib was terminated due to insufficient enrollment. Pyrimethamine, an anti-parasitic, has been shown to inhibit STAT3 *in vitro* as well as *in vivo* (Khan et al. 2018). Unfortunately, no objective responses were observed in its phase 1b trial in CLL and SLL (NCT01066663). Half of the patients achieved stable disease while the remainder had progressive disease (Brown et al. 2021).

Targeting STAT5 in Lymphoid Malignancy

The STAT5A and STAT5B transcription factors are also important mediators of malignant transformation, maintenance, and relapse in lymphocytic leukemias (Bandapalli et al. 2014; Kontro et al. 2014; Kucuk et al. 2015; Maurer et al. 2020; Nicolae et al. 2014; Ribeiro et al. 2018). The N642H mutation in the *STAT5B* gene frequently occurs in lymphoid malignancies and mouse studies confirmed its function as a potent leukemic driver (de Araujo et al. 2019; Bandapalli et al. 2014; Klein et al. 2019). Thus, STAT5 inhibitor development is also necessary to improve treatment options for lymphoid malignancies. Despite great efforts to develop STAT5-specific inhibitors, few instances of their evaluation in lymphoid malignancies exist compared to studies characterizing STAT3 inhibitors. Below, we summarize examples of direct STAT5 inhibition in lymphoid malignancies. As previously mentioned, canonical STAT-targeting modalities aim to degrade STAT mRNA, prevent STAT dimerization, DNA binding, transcriptional activity, and/or nucleocytoplasmic shuttling. While STAT3 mRNA-targeting approaches have entered phase 1 clinical trials, STAT5 mRNA-targeting approaches demonstrated only modest effects in proof-of-concept studies (Baśkiewicz-Masiuk et al. 2003). More recently, the emergence of direct STAT degradation using PROTACs provides another STAT-targeting modality. However, the development of PROTACs has been limited to STAT3 with no peer-reviewed reports of STAT5 PROTACs at the time of writing this review (Brachet-Botineau et al. 2020).

Table 27.1 STAT inhibitors tested clinically in lymphoid malignancies.

Drug	Mechanism of action	Disease	Combination Treatment	Phase	NCT number
AZD9150	Anti-sense oligonucleotide inhibitor of STAT3	DLBCL, NHL	None	1/2	NCT01563302
AZD9150	Anti-sense oligonucleotide inhibitor of STAT3	DLBCL	Durvalumab	1	NCT02549651
AZD9150	Anti-sense oligonucleotide inhibitor of STAT3	DLBCL	Acalabrutinib	1	NCT03527147
OPB-51602	Small molecule direct inhibitor of STAT3	NHL, ALL, MM	None	1	NCT01344876
OPB-31121	Small molecule direct inhibitor of STAT3 and STAT5	NHL, MM	None	1	NCT00511082
Napabucasin (BBI608)	Small molecule STAT3 inhibitor	MM, NHL, CLL	Dexamethasone, Bortezomib, Imatinib, or Ibrutinib	1	NCT02352558
Pyrimethamine	Anti-parasitic, inhibits enzyme dihydrofolate reductase	SLL, CLL	None	1/2	NCT01066663

Abbreviations: ALL = acute lymphoblastic leukemia; CLL = chronic lymphocytic leukemia; DLBCL = diffuse large B-cell lymphoma; MM = multiple myeloma; NHL = non-Hodgkin's lymphoma; SLL = small lymphocytic lymphoma.

The STAT5 inhibitor IST5-002, identified using an SH2 domain-specific *in silico* screen, was evaluated in Philadelphia chromosome-positive ALL (Ph+) cell lines and patient samples. Importantly, IST5-002 treatment prevented STAT5 phosphorylation, reduced colony-formation of Ph+ ALL patient samples, and improved overall survival in a cell line xenograft model of Ph+ ALL (Minieri et al. 2018). Despite the promising anti-leukemic effects of IST5-002 in Ph+ ALL, the authors do not address the potential contributory effects of STAT3 inhibition. Dual inhibition of STAT3 and STAT5 with OPB-31121 potently inhibited cell proliferation *in vitro* of ALL, Burkitt's lymphoma, DLBCL, and multiple myeloma cell lines. OPB-31121 treatment reduced leukemic burden *in vivo* while sparing normal human cord blood cells (Hayakawa et al. 2013). Of note, FDA-approved anti-psychotic drugs demonstrate anti-cancer effects via mechanisms involving STAT3 and STAT5 inhibition (Shaw et al. 2021). Repurposing these drugs as a novel therapeutic modality for STAT-addicted lymphoid malignancies shows promise. For example, pimozide, commonly used to treat Tourette's syndrome and schizophrenia, also functions as a STAT5 antagonist. Pimozide reduced STAT5 phosphorylation and decreased proliferation of peripheral T-cell lymphoma (PTCL) cell lines and patient samples *in vitro* (Kiel et al. 2014; Simpson et al. 2018). While very few studies have evaluated direct STAT5-specific inhibitors in lymphoid malignancies, many groups have evaluated STAT5 inhibitors in myeloid leukemias (Brachet-Botineau et al. 2020). One notable example was demonstrated in AML wherein pharmacological inhibition of STAT5 using the novel SH2-targeting compound, AC-4-130, antagonized STAT5 transcriptional activity, induced cell death in cell lines and patient samples while sparing normal CD34+ cells, and reduced leukemic burden *in vivo* (Wingelhofer et al. 2018).

Taken together, there is abundant evidence that STAT proteins, especially STAT3, are hyperactivated via signaling pathway engagement as well as somatic activating mutations in lymphoid malignancy. Preclinical studies have validated the essential role of these therapeutic targets using genetic targeting, tool compounds, and experimental therapeutics. However, clear therapeutic benefit has not been achieved in clinical trials. New agents with improved specificity, potency, and drug-like features may be required to realize the clinical benefit of blocking these key transcription factors.

Clinical Trials of JAK Inhibitors in Lymphoid Malignancies

The clinical development of JAK inhibitors greatly exceeds that of STAT3 inhibitors. The vast majority of FDA approvals and ongoing clinical trials for JAK inhibitors are for myeloproliferative neoplasms (MPN) or autoimmune diseases (rheumatoid arthritis [RA], ulcerative colitis, Crohn's disease). Abundant safety and pharmacokinetic data are available for JAK inhibitors as a result of these studies (Salas et al. 2020; Schwartz et al. 2017; You et al. 2020). Thus far, JAK inhibitors have shown promise in clinical trials for lymphoid malignancies but none have been approved by the FDA.

There are six JAK inhibitors that have been or are currently being investigated across 26 clinical trials in patients with lymphoid malignancies (Table 27.2).

Nearly all small molecule JAK inhibitors exhibit some cross-reactivity due to substantial structural similarity across the JAK family (Hu et al. 2021). Therefore, inhibitors are characterized with respect to the isoform that is most potently inhibited (i.e. IC_{50} value for JAK1, JAK2, JAK3) as well as the specificity relative to other isoforms (i.e. IC_{50} ratio for JAK2/JAK3, JAK1/JAK3). Many of the latest generation inhibitors exhibit low nanomolar IC_{50} values for the primary target. However, these are not strictly exclusive inhibitors of a particular isoform since other family members may still be inhibited with submicromolar potency even when these compounds exhibit several hundred-fold isoform selectivity. In addition, several of these compounds also inhibit other relevant tyrosine kinases (e.g. FLT3 and spleen tyrosine kinase [SYK]). Table 27.2 lists the primary target of each compound.

Ruxolitinib, a JAK1/JAK2 and partial TYK2 inhibitor that was FDA approved in 2011 for use in MPN, by far has the most clinical studies of all the JAK inhibitors. In a phase 2 trial (NCT02015208), ruxolitinib treatment response was not achieved in patients with CLL and the trial was stopped due to the uniformity of biological responses, unexpectedly high incidence of anemia, and no examples of decreased lymphocytosis (Spaner et al. 2016). An additional phase 2 trial (NCT03041636) also did not demonstrate treatment response and was stopped due to poor enrollment. Ruxolitinib showed

Table 27.2 JAK inhibitors tested clinically in lymphoid malignancies.

Drug	Primary target	Disease	Combination treatment	Phases	NCT number
Ruxolitinib	JAK1/JAK2 > TYK2	CLL	None	1/2	NCT02015208
Ruxolitinib	JAK1/JAK2 > TYK2	CLL, SLL	None	2	NCT03041636
Ruxolitinib	JAK1/JAK2 > TYK2	CLL	None	2	NCT02131584
Ruxolitinib	JAK1/JAK2 > TYK2	HL	None	2	NCT02164500
Ruxolitinib	JAK1/JAK2 > TYK2	HL, MLBCL	None	2	NCT01965119
Ruxolitinib	JAK1/JAK2 > TYK2	DLBCL, PTCL	None	2	NCT01431209
Ruxolitinib	JAK1/JAK2 > TYK2	ENKTCL	None	2	NCT02974647
Ruxolitinib	JAK1/JAK2 > TYK2	ATL	None	1/2	NCT01712659
Ruxolitinib	JAK1/JAK2 > TYK2	CLL	Ibrutinib	1/2	NCT02912754
Ruxolitinib	JAK1/JAK2 > TYK2	HL	Nivolumab	1/2	NCT03681561
Ruxolitinib	JAK1/JAK2 > TYK2	ETP-ALL	LVP	1/2	NCT03613428
Ruxolitinib	JAK1/JAK2 > TYK2	ALL	Multiagent chemotherapy	2	NCT02420717
Ruxolitinib	JAK1/JAK2 > TYK2	B-ALL	Multiagent chemotherapy	2	NCT02723994
Ruxolitinib	JAK1/JAK2 > TYK2	T-ALL	Chidamide	1/2	NCT05075681
Itacitinib	JAK1	HL	Everolimus	1/2	NCT03697408
Itacitinib	JAK1	T-PLL	Alemtuzumab	1	NCT03989466
Itacitinib	JAK1	HL	INCB040093	2	NCT02456675
Itacitinib	JAK1	NHL	INCB040093	1	NCT01905813
Itacitinib	JAK1	DLBCL	Ibrutinib	1/2	NCT02760485
Pacritinib	JAK2/FLT3	HL, NHL	None	1	NCT00741871
Pacritinib	JAK2/FTL3	PTCL	None	2	NCT04858256
Pacritinib	JAK2/FTL3	CLL, SLL	Ibrutinib	1/2	NCT02677948
Cerdulatinib	JAK1/JAK2/TYK2/SYK	CLL, SLL, NHL	None	1/2A	NCT01994382
Cerdulatinib	JAK1/JAK2/TYK2/SYK	PTCL, CTCL	None	2B	NCT04021082
Tofacitinib	JAK3/JAK1 > JAK2, TYK2	ENKTCL	Chidamide	2	NCT03598959
Gusacitinib (ASN002)	JAK2/JAK3/TYK2/ SYK > JAK1	DLBCL, FL, MCL, PTCL	None	1/2	NCT02440685

Abbreviations: ALL = acute lymphoblastic leukemia; ATL = adult T-cell leukemia; B-ALL = B-cell acute lymphoblastic leukemia; CLL = chronic lymphocytic leukemia; CTCL = cutaneous T-cell lymphoma; DLBCL = diffuse large B-cell lymphoma; ENKTCL = extranodal NK/T-cell lymphoma; ETP-ALL = early T precursor acute lymphocytic leukemia; FL = follicular lymphoma HL = Hodgkin's lymphoma, LVP = L-asparaginase, vincristine, and prednisone; MCL = mantle cell lymphoma; MLBCL = mediastinal large B-cell lymphoma; NHL = non-Hodgkin's lymphoma; PTCL = peripheral T-cell lymphoma; SLL = small lymphocytic lymphoma; T-ALL = T-cell acute lymphoblastic leukemia; T-PLL = T-cell prolymphocytic leukemia.

promise in a phase 2 trial (NCT02131584) in relieving disease-related CLL symptoms. In particular, 78% of the patients experienced 20% or greater reduction in their mean brief fatigue inventory scores (Jain et al. 2017). Ruxolitinib has also been studied in the treatment of HL. A phase 2 trial (NCT02164500) showed that while ruxolitinib was well tolerated, the overall response rate after six cycles was a mere 9.4% (3/32 patients) (Van Den Neste et al. 2018). All three responders had partial response and 11 patients had transient stable disease. Another phase 2 trial (NCT01965119) confirmed these results showing that ruxolitinib has modest single-agent activity against HL but not mediastinal large B-cell lymphoma (MLBCL) (Kim et al. 2019). One HL patient had complete remission (CR) while 5/13 HL patients had partial remission (PR). All cases of MLBCL progressed after first or second cycle. Ruxolitinib treatment responses were observed in PTCL subtypes in a recent phase 2 biomarker-driven study (NCT01431209) that helped to support a precision therapy approach to JAK-STAT inhibition (Kallam et al. 2019; Moskowitz et al. 2021). Clinical trials to test the efficacy of ruxolitinib in ENKTCL (NCT02974647) and ATL (NCT01712659) are ongoing. Promising responses to ruxolitinib were also observed in two cases of refractory T-LGL leukemia treated off-label (Moignet et al. 2021).

Following these promising single-agent clinical trials, multiple combination therapies with ruxolitinib have been investigated. A phase 2 trial (NCT02912754) showed that ruxolitinib combined with BTK inhibitor ibrutinib suppressed CLL cells effectively (Spaner et al. 2021). Again, however, complete responses with ruxolitinib with or without ibrutinib were not detected. Synergistic effects of ruxolitinib with the anti-PD-1 immunotherapy agent nivolumab are being investigated in a phase 1/2 trial (NCT03681561), which is still recruiting. Ruxolitinib has also been incorporated into the combination treatment schema for various forms of ALL. One preclinical *in vivo* study demonstrated that ruxolitinib enhanced the efficacy of an induction-type regimen consisting of vincristine, dexamethasone, and L-asparaginase in cytokine receptor-like factor 2 (CRLF2)-rearranged Ph-like ALL xenografts (Böhm et al. 2021). Results are pending from a phase 2 trial (NCT03613428) of ruxolitinib with L-asparaginase, vincristine, and prednisone in relapsed/refractory early T-cell precursor (ETP)-ALL, a biologically distinct subtype for which novel therapies are needed. Importantly, ruxolitinib demonstrated activity in murine models in ETP-ALL (Maude et al. 2015). Safety and tolerability were demonstrated for ruxolitinib combined with intensive multiagent chemotherapy in a phase 1 ALL trial (NCT02420717) that demonstrated dose-dependent inhibition of target phosphoproteins and sustained inhibition of phosphorylated STAT5 with continuous ruxolitinib dosing at DL1b (Tasian et al. 2018). Results from the phase 2 portion are still pending. Further phase 2 studies of ruxolitinib with chemotherapy in children with ALL (NCT02723994) and ruxolitinib with HDAC inhibitor chidamide for acute T-cell lymphoblast leukemia/lymphoblastic lymphoma (NCT05075681) are still recruiting. Ruxolitinib has also shown promise in the treatment of ENKTCL in preclinical models in combination with LEE001, believed to be secondary to synergistic combined inhibition of JAK2 and CDK4/6 (Hee et al. 2018). A recent high-throughput matrix screen also identified ruxolitinib in combination with Bcl-2/Bcl-xL inhibitor navitoclax as a candidate for multicomponent therapy for ATL (Zhang et al. 2015).

The next most common JAK inhibitor in clinical trials of lymphoid malignancies is the selective JAK1 inhibitor itacitinib. The combination of itacitinib and everolimus, which binds intracellular protein FKBP-12 to inhibit mTOR, produced an overall response rate (ORR) and CR rate of 79% and 14%, respectively, in a phase 1/2 study (NCT03697408) of heavily pretreated HL patients (Svoboda 2020). Itacitinib is also being tested with alemtuzumab, a selective CD52 antibody and gold standard treatment for T-PLL (Colon Ramos et al. 2021), in an ongoing phase 1 trial (NCT03989466) in T-PLL patients. Itacitinib has also been combined with phosphatidylinositol 3-kinase δ (PI3Kδ) inhibitor INCB040093 in trials of HL (NCT02456675) and NHL (NCT01905813). These studies demonstrated promising activity in select subtypes, with responses of 67% (14/21) in classic HL (vs. 29% with monotherapy) and 31% (4/13) in non-germinal center B-cell-like DLBCL (Phillips et al. 2018). Finally, a phase 1/2 trial (NCT02760485) of itacitinib in combination with BTK inhibitor ibrutinib in subjects with relapsed or refractory DLBCL is still active.

The selective JAK2/FLT3 inhibitor pacritinib has shown promise in treating myelofibrosis and other myeloid malignancies. However, the same efficacy has not been demonstrated in lymphoid malignancies thus far. A phase 1 trial (NCT00741871) of pacritinib in HL or NHL showed that treatment was well tolerated with 9% achieving partial response and 44% stable disease (Younes et al. 2012). A phase 2 trial (NCT04858256) of pacritinib in PTCL patients is active but not yet recruiting. Clinical trials combining pacritinib with other agents used to treat lymphoid malignancies are lacking. The only attempt thus far was a phase 1 combination trial with BTK inhibitor ibrutinib (NCT02677948), which was withdrawn due to the temporary FDA hold of all clinical trials involving pacritinib due to increased incidence of intracranial hemorrhage noted in the PERSIST-1 and PERSIST-2 trials (Mascarenhas et al. 2018; Mesa et al. 2017).

Cerdulatinib is a multikinase inhibitor with greatest potency for JAK1/JAK2/TYK2/SYK. Cerdulatinib inhibited BCR- and IL-4-induced downstream signaling in CLL cells and prevented anti-IgM- and nurse-like cell (NLC)-mediated CCL3/CCL4 production (Blunt et al. 2017). A phase 1/2A study of cerdulatinib (NCT01994382) demonstrated complete JAK and SYK pathway inhibition in whole blood of patients at tolerated exposures in CLL, SLL, and NHL patients (Coffey et al. 2019). Cerdulatinib also showed good tolerability and demonstrated activity in a phase 2A trial (NCT04021082) against both PTCL and CTCL (Horwitz et al. 2018).

Tofacitinib, a pan-JAK/TYK2 inhibitor, has been primarily used in autoimmune conditions. A phase 2 trial (NCT03598959) is currently underway in combination with chidamide, a benzamide-type inhibitor of HDAC isoenzymes 1, 2, 3, and 10. Previous studies showed that mutations of JAK-STAT pathway and histone modification-related genes were detected in 55.9% and 38.2% of ENKTCL cancer samples, respectively (Lee et al. 2015). Tofacitinib clinical activity in LGL leukemia was also identified through an off-label study. Nine LGL leukemia patients with concomitant RA, which is diagnosed in approximately 30% of T-LGL leukemia patients, were treated with the JAK inhibitor tofacitinib that is FDA-approved in RA. All nine were refractory to standard-of-care immunosuppressive agents typically used for LGL leukemia. RA symptoms were improved in 8/9 patients. Leukemia-directed efficacy was shown in 6/9 that also exhibited hematologic responses in LGL leukemia features. Improvement in neutropenia was also observed in 5/7 patients and improvement of anemia in 1/7 patients (Bilori et al. 2015).

Finally, gusacitinib is a pan-JAK/TYK2/SYK inhibitor that has been shown to be safe and tolerable at manageable doses for the treatment of atopic dermatitis. A phase 1 trial (NCT02440685) in lymphoid malignancies was terminated due to a business decision prior to the release of efficacy results (Pavel et al. 2019).

Challenges and Opportunities for Clinical Application of JAK-STAT Targeting Agents

While abundant evidence supports the importance of JAK-STAT signaling in lymphoid malignancies, there is great complexity and redundancy in the cytokines, receptors, and signaling molecules that may drive transformation (Figure 27.1). Lymphoid malignancies are known to exhibit broad heterogeneity in the mechanisms utilized to drive JAK-STAT pathway activation. Therefore, preclinical studies with patient samples and cell lines are essential to identify the key JAK or STAT isoform driver as well as to validate the dependency of each lymphoid malignancy on a particular isoform(s). Thus far, clinical trials of JAK inhibitors in lymphoid malignancies have focused on JAK inhibitors due to their advanced clinical development relative to STAT3-targeting approaches. One potential limitation is that such trials have primarily targeted JAK2 (ruxolitinib) and JAK 1 (itacitinib) with limited focus on JAK3.

It is also important to identify if JAK or STAT family members provide biological redundancy upon treatment with isoform-selective inhibitors. Several JAK inhibitors were shown to be potent and selective in preclinical models and safe in early-stage clinical trials, yet they lack single-agent efficacy. For example, lack of durable response to JAK2 inhibitor was shown to correlate with JAK1 or TYK2 heterodimerization and transactivation of JAK2 (Koppikar et al. 2012). Following this example, it is tempting to speculate that the current push to develop increasingly isoform-specific drugs may reduce the likelihood that these compounds will achieve single-agent efficacy. Nonetheless, this toolbox of selective inhibitors will enable mix-and-match combinatorial therapeutic regimens that are tailored to disease-, subtype-, or even patient-specific signaling networks with refined specificity. These compounds are poised for use in new combinatorial clinical trial regimens upon development of strong biochemical and molecular rationale as well as demonstrated preclinical efficacy.

The branching nature of signaling pathways downstream of membrane receptors also creates a challenge. This observation dictates that potent molecules that hit distal targets may be ineffective if multiple parallel survival signals originate from the same receptor. For example, receptor tyrosine kinases frequently spawn PI3K/AKT and MAPK/ERK signaling in conjunction with STAT3 activation and may also stimulate phosphorylation of STAT1 and STAT5. The single-agent efficacy of even the best STAT3-targeting approaches will be limited by these parallel activation events. More effective blockade of all downstream signaling may be achieved with approaches based on proximal targeting of the cytokine-receptor interaction. For example, a pegylated peptide blocker of the common γc receptor (CD132) effectively blunted IL-2 and IL-15 stimulation of phospho-AKT, ERK, and multiple STATs in LGL leukemia cell lines and patient samples (Wang et al. 2019). Furthermore, the non-canonical functions of STAT3 that are independent of phosphorylation-driven transcriptional activation represent a substantial challenge to most STAT3-targeting approaches. Thus, there is considerable promise around PROTAC degraders with potent drug-like characteristics and demonstrated ability to deplete STAT3 protein. Substantial effort is needed to detail the mechanisms of non-canonical STAT3 functions in order to identify targets for combinatorial therapeutic regimens.

Refined characterization of alternative signaling pathways is likely to identify druggable targets that synergize with JAK-STAT targeting agents. A number of biological targets have emerged to exploit other key therapeutic vulnerabilities in lymphoid malignancies. Common pathways and approaches include the PI3K/AKT/mTOR pathway, survival proteins (Bcl-2 family, survivin), Hsp90 inhibitors, lymphoid signaling pathways (T-cell receptor [TCR] and B-cell receptor [BCR] pathways), and the p53/MDM2/MDMX axis (Dufva et al. 2018; Kuusanmaki et al. 2017; Meyer and Levine, 2014; Ng et al. 2018). Several lines of evidence suggest promising synergy between STAT targeting and immune checkpoint blockade.

STAT3 somatic mutation and activation were shown to induce expression of PD-L1, which may promote immune evasion (Song et al. 2018). The direct STAT3 inhibitor WP1066 suppressed the expression of PD-L1/2 in lymphoma cell lines (Ma et al. 2017). These and additional studies indicate that STAT3 inhibition may enhance immune surveillance by reducing the immunosuppressive microenvironment and inflammation while increasing the function of antigen presenting cells and immune effectors (Yu et al. 2009). Conversely, STAT-targeting approaches may be detrimental in the context of chimeric antigen receptor T-cell (CAR-T)-based therapies that are dependent upon STAT3 and STAT5 signaling. Similarly, off-target STAT targeting could impair IFNγ/STAT1-mediated cancer immune responses.

A close relationship has been identified between STAT3 and STAT5 activation and epigenetic regulatory mechanisms (Wingelhofer et al. 2018). Whole exome sequencing of over 100 T-LGL leukemia samples demonstrated that over half harbored somatic mutations of STAT3. These mutated samples were more likely to exhibit co-mutation of epigenetic regulators that modulate DNA and histone methylation marks (Cheon et al. 2022). Similar widespread mutation of JAK-STAT pathway and epigenetic modifier genes was also reported in breast implant-associated ALCL (Laurent et al. 2020). Cytokine signaling and STAT3 activating mutations were both associated with elevated DNA methyltransferase 1 (DNMT1) and global hypermethylation in LGL leukemia cell and model systems, and STAT3 was found to directly complex with HDAC1 and the histone methyltransferase enhancer of zeste 2 polycomb repressive complex 2 subunit (EZH2) (Kim et al. 2019). Thus, further studies are warranted to characterize STAT3-associated epigenetic modulation as well as the efficacy of combining JAK-STAT inhibitors together with agents that target DNA methylation and/or histone methylation and acetylation marks.

Overall, there remains great optimism around the clinical benefits that could be achieved with potent JAK-STAT targeting approaches that will move cancer treatment away from non-selective cytotoxic chemotherapy. Clinical trials to test these agents remain in the early stages and have disproportionately focused on B-cell diseases despite, arguably, stronger rationale in T-cell malignancies based on existing molecular profiling studies. Substantial medical chemistry approaches are needed to optimize small molecular inhibitors, especially for targeting of STAT3 and other STAT proteins. Preclinical mechanistic studies are needed in cell lines and patient samples to clearly delineate the key targets and JAK-STAT combinations in each lymphoid malignancy. More patient-derived xenograft models are needed as avatars that faithfully recapitulate disease features and heterogeneity. Proper exploitation of these models will narrow the field of combinatorial regimens to identify those that exhibit the greatest efficacy in lymphoid malignancies.

Acknowledgments

This work was supported by the National Institutes of Health under the National Cancer Institute Award Numbers R01CA178393 (TL) and R01CA208851 (JT), and under the National Cancer Institute Research Training Award Number T32CA009109 (JU). The content is solely the responsibility of the authors and does not necessarily represent the official views of the National Institutes of Health. Additional support was provided by LEIDOS Biomedical Research/NCI Contract 19X122Q (JT), Cedars-Sinai Start-up funds (JT), the Bess Family Charitable Fund, the LGL Leukemia Foundation, Dr. Charles and Katharine Hutton Tweedy, William J. Branch, Dr. Szabolcs Szentpetery, and two generous anonymous donors (TL).

Conflict of Interest Disclosures

DF has research funding from AstraZeneca, Dren Bio, Recludix Pharma, and Kymera Therapeutics. TL is on the Scientific Advisory Board and has stock options for Keystone Nano, Bioniz Therapeutics, Dren Bio, Recludix Pharma, and Prime Genomics. TL and DF received honoraria from Kymera Therapeutics. JT is a co-founder of Novella, LLC, which has licensed STAT3 intellectual property. There are no conflicts of interest with the work presented in this manuscript.

Must Read References

Hu, X., Li, J., Fu, M., Zhao, X., Wang, W. (2021). The JAK/STAT signaling pathway: from bench to clinic. *Signal Transduct. Target Ther.* 6 (1): 402.

Schwartz D.M., Kanno, Y., Villarino A., Ward, M., Gadina, M., O'Shea, J.J. (2017). JAK inhibition as a therapeutic strategy for immune and inflammatory diseases. *Nat. Rev. Drug Discov.* 17 (1): 78.

Miklossy, G., Hilliard, T.S., Turkson, J. (2013). Therapeutic modulators of STAT signalling for human diseases. *Nat. Rev. Drug Discov.* 12 (8): 611–629.

References

Abbas, H.A. and Wierda, W.G. (2021). Acalabrutinib: a selective Bruton tyrosine kinase inhibitor for the treatment of B-cell malignancies. *Front Oncol.* 11: 668162.

Akiyama, Y., Iizuka, A., Kume, A. et al. (2015). Effect of STAT3 inhibition on the metabolic switch in a highly STAT3-activated lymphoma cell line. *Cancer Genom. Proteom.* 12 (3): 133–142.

Alas, S. and Bonavida, B. (2003). Inhibition of constitutive STAT3 activity sensitizes resistant non-Hodgkin's lymphoma and multiple myeloma to chemotherapeutic drug-mediated apoptosis. *Clin. Cancer Res.* 9 (1): 316–326.

Andersson, E., Kuusanmaki, H., Bortoluzzi, S. et al. (2016). Activating somatic mutations outside the SH2-domain of STAT3 in LGL leukemia. *Leukemia* 30 (5): 1204–1208.

Ashizawa, T., Miyata, H., Ishii, H. et al. (2011). Antitumor activity of a novel small molecule STAT3 inhibitor against a human lymphoma cell line with high STAT3 activation. *Int. J. Oncol.* 38 (5): 1245–1252.

Bai, L., Zhou, H., Xu, R. et al. (2019). A potent and selective small-molecule degrader of STAT3 achieves complete tumor regression in vivo. *Cancer Cell* 36 (5): 498–511 e417.

Bandapalli, O.R., Schuessele, S., Kunz, J.B. et al. (2014). The activating STAT5B N642H mutation is a common abnormality in pediatric T-cell acute lymphoblastic leukemia and confers a higher risk of relapse. *Haematologica* 99 (10): e188–192.

Baśkiewicz-Masiuk, M., Masiuk, M., and Machaliński, B. (2003). The influence of STAT5 antisense oligodeoxynucleotides on the proliferation and apoptosis of selected human cutaneous T-cell lymphoma cell lines. *Cell Prolif.* 36 (5): 265–278.

Belton, A., Xian, L., Huso, T. et al. (2016). STAT3 inhibitor has potent antitumor activity in B-lineage acute lymphoblastic leukemia cells overexpressing the high mobility group A1 (HMGA1)-STAT3 pathway. *Leuk. Lymphoma.* 57 (11): 2681–2684.

Benekli, M., Baumann, H., and Wetzler, M. (2009). Targeting signal transducer and activator of transcription signaling pathway in leukemias. *J. Clin. Oncol.* 27 (26): 4422–4432.

Bi, S., Chen, K., Feng, L. (2019). et al. Napabucasin (BBI608) eliminate AML cells in vitro and in vivo via inhibition of Stat3 pathway and induction of DNA damage. *Eur. J. Pharmacol.* 855: 252–261.

Bilori, B., Thota, S., Clemente, M.J. et al. (2015). Tofacitinib as a novel salvage therapy for refractory T-cell large granular lymphocytic leukemia. *Leukemia* 29 (12): 2427–2429.

Blunt, M.D., Koehrer, S., Dobson, R.C. et al. (2017). The dual Syk/JAK inhibitor cerdulatinib antagonizes B-cell receptor and microenvironmental signaling in chronic lymphocytic leukemia. *Clin. Cancer Res.* 23 (9): 2313–2324.

Böhm, J.W., Sia, K.C.S., Jones, C. et al. (2021). Combination efficacy of ruxolitinib with standard-of-care drugs in CRLF2-rearranged Ph-like acute lymphoblastic leukemia. *Leukemia* 35 (11): 3101–3112.

Bohmer, F.D. and Friedrich, K. (2014). Protein tyrosine phosphatases as wardens of STAT signaling. *JAKSTAT* 3 (1): e28087.

Brachet-Botineau, M., Polomski, M., Neubauer, H.A. et al. (2020). Pharmacological inhibition of oncogenic STAT3 and STAT5 signaling in hematopoietic cancers. *Cancers (Basel)* 12 (1): 1–48.

Brambilla, L., Genini, D., Laurini, E. et al. (2015). Hitting the right spot: mechanism of action of OPB-31121, a novel and potent inhibitor of the signal transducer and activator of transcription 3 (STAT3). *Mol. Oncol.* 9 (6): 1194–1206.

Brambilla, L., Lahiri, T., Cammer, M. et al. (2020). STAT3 Inhibitor OPB-51602 is cytotoxic to tumor cells through inhibition of complex I and ROS induction. *iScience* 23 (12): 101822.

Bromberg, J.F., Wrzeszczynska, M.H., Devgan, G. et al. (1999). Stat3 as an oncogene. *Cell* 98 (3): 295–303.

Brown, J.R., Walker, S.R., Heppler, L.N. et al. (2021). Targeting constitutively active STAT3 in chronic lymphocytic leukemia: a clinical trial of the STAT3 inhibitor pyrimethamine with pharmacodynamic analyses. *Am. J. Hematol.* 96 (4): E95–E98.

Carpenter, R.L. and Lo, H.W. (2014). STAT3 target genes relevant to human cancers. *Cancers (Basel)* 6 (2): 897–925.

Chen, J., Zhang, Y., Petrus, M.N. et al. (2017). Cytokine receptor signaling is required for the survival of ALK- anaplastic large cell lymphoma, even in the presence of JAK1/STAT3 mutations. *Proc. Natl. Acad. Sci. U.S. A.* 114 (15): 3975–3980.

Cheon, H., Xing, J.C., Moosic, K.B. et al. (2022). Genomic landscape of TCR alpha-beta and TCR gamma-delta T-large granular lymphocyte leukemia. *Blood.* 139 (20): 3058–3072.

Coffey, G.P., Feng, J., Betz, A. et al. (2019). Cerdulatinib pharmacodynamics and relationships to tumor response following oral dosing in patients with relapsed/refractory B-cell malignancies. *Clin. Cancer Res.* 25 (4): 1174–1184.

Colon Ramos, A., Tarekegn, K., Aujla, A. et al. (2021). T-cell prolymphocytic leukemia: an overview of current and future approaches. *Cureus* 13 (2): e13237.

Cosenza, M., Civallero, M., Marcheselli, L. et al. (2020). Citarinostat and Momelotinib co-target HDAC6 and JAK2/STAT3 in lymphoid malignant cell lines: a potential new therapeutic combination. *Apoptosis* 25 (5–6): 370–387.

de Araujo, E.D., Erdogan, F., Neubauer, H.A. et al. (2019). Structural and functional consequences of the STAT5B(N642H) driver mutation. *Nat. Commun.* 10 (1): 2517.

de Araujo, E.D., Orlova, A., Neubauer, H.A. et al. (2019). Structural implications of STAT3 and STAT5 SH2 domain mutations. *Cancers (Basel)* 11 (11).

Debnath, B., Xu, S., and Neamati, N. (2012). Small molecule inhibitors of signal transducer and activator of transcription 3 (Stat3) protein. *J. Med. Chem.* 55 (15): 6645–6668.

Delgoffe, G.M. and Vignali, D.A. (2013). STAT heterodimers in immunity: a mixed message or a unique signal? *JAKSTAT* 2 (1): e23060.

Ding, X., Chi, J., Yang, X. et al. (2017). Cucurbitacin B synergistically enhances the apoptosis-inducing effect of arsenic trioxide by inhibiting STAT3 phosphorylation in lymphoma Ramos cells. *Leuk. Lymphoma.* 58 (10): 2439–2451.

Dufva, O., Kankainen, M., Kelkka, T. et al. (2018). Aggressive natural killer-cell leukemia mutational landscape and drug profiling highlight JAK-STAT signaling as therapeutic target. *Nat. Commun.* 9 (1): 1567.

Dutta, A., Yan, D., Hutchison, R.E. et al. (2018). STAT3 mutations are not sufficient to induce large granular lymphocytic leukaemia in mice. *Br. J. Haematol.* 180 (6): 911–915.

Epling-Burnette, P.K., Liu, J.H., Catlett-Falcone, R. et al. (2001). Inhibition of STAT3 signaling leads to apoptosis of leukemic large granular lymphocytes and decreased Mcl-1 expression. *J. Clin. Invest.* 107 (3): 351–362.

Fabre, A., Marchal, S., Barlogis, V. et al. (2019). Clinical aspects of STAT3 gain-of-function germline mutations: a systematic review. *J. Allergy. Clin. Immunol. Pract.* 7 (6): 1958–1969 e1959.

Geng, L., Li, X., Zhou, X. et al. (2016). WP1066 exhibits antitumor efficacy in nasaltype natural killer/T-cell lymphoma cells through downregulation of the STAT3 signaling pathway. *Oncol. Rep.* 36 (5): 2868–2874.

Geng, L., Lu, K., Li, P. et al. (2017). GLI1 inhibitor GANT61 exhibits antitumor efficacy in T-cell lymphoma cells through down-regulation of p-STAT3 and SOCS3. *Oncotarget* 8 (30): 48701–48710.

Granato, M., Rizzello, C., Gilardini Montani, M.S. et al. (2017). Quercetin induces apoptosis and autophagy in primary effusion lymphoma cells by inhibiting PI3K/AKT/mTOR and STAT3 signaling pathways. *J. Nutr. Biochem.* 41: 124–136.

Grivennikov, S.I. and Karin, M. (2010). Dangerous liaisons: STAT3 and NF-kappaB collaboration and crosstalk in cancer. *Cytokine. Growth Factor Rev.* 21 (1): 11–19.

Gupta, M., Han, J.J., Stenson, M. et al. (2012). Regulation of STAT3 by histone deacetylase-3 in diffuse large B-cell lymphoma: implications for therapy. *Leukemia* 26 (6): 1356–1364.

Hardee, J., Ouyang, Z., Zhang, Y. et al. (2013). STAT3 targets suggest mechanisms of aggressive tumorigenesis in diffuse large B-cell lymphoma. *G3 (Bethesda)* 3 (12): 2173–2185.

Harrison, D.A. (2012). The Jak/STAT pathway. *Cold. Spring. Harb. Perspect. Biol.* 4 (3).

Hayakawa, F., Sugimoto, K., Harada, Y. et al. (2013). A novel STAT inhibitor, OPB-31121, has a significant antitumor effect on leukemia with STAT-addictive oncokinases. *Blood Cancer J.* 3 (11): e166.

Hee, Y.T., Yan, J., Nizetic, D. et al. (2018). LEE011 and ruxolitinib: a synergistic drug combination for natural killer/T-cell lymphoma (NKTCL). *Oncotarget* 9 (61): 31832–31841.

Hillion, J., Dhara, S., Sumter, T.F. et al. (2008). The high-mobility group A1a/signal transducer and activator of transcription-3 axis: an achilles heel for hematopoietic malignancies? *Cancer Res.* 68 (24): 10121–10127.

Hong, D., Kurzrock, R., Kim, Y. et al. (2015). AZD9150, a next-generation antisense oligonucleotide inhibitor of STAT3 with early evidence of clinical activity in lymphoma and lung cancer. *Sci .Transl. Med.* 7 (314): 314ra185.

Horwitz, S.M., Feldman, T.A., Hess, B.T. et al. (2018). The novel SYK/JAK inhibitor cerdulatinib demonstrates good tolerability and clinical response in a phase 2a study in relapsed/refractory peripheral T-cell lymphoma and cutaneous T-cell lymphoma. *Blood* 132 (Supplement 1): 1001.

Hu, L., Li, B., Chen, G. et al. (2020). A novel M phase blocker, DCZ3301 enhances the sensitivity of bortezomib in resistant multiple myeloma through DNA damage and mitotic catastrophe. *J. Exp. Clin. Cancer Res.* 39 (1): 105.

Hu, X., Li, J., Fu, M. et al. (2021). The JAK/STAT signaling pathway: from bench to clinic. *Signal Transduct Target Ther.* 6 (1): 402.

Jain, P., Keating, M., Renner, S. et al. (2017). Ruxolitinib for symptom control in patients with chronic lymphocytic leukaemia: a single-group, phase 2 trial. *Lancet Haematol.* 4 (2): e67–e74.

Jerez, A., Clemente, M.J., Makishima, H. et al. (2012). STAT3 mutations unify the pathogenesis of chronic lymphoproliferative disorders of NK cells and T-cell large granular lymphocyte leukemia. *Blood* 120 (15): 3048–3057.

Johnson, D.E., O'Keefe, R.A., and Grandis, J.R. (2018). Targeting the IL-6/JAK/STAT3 signalling axis in cancer. *Nat. Rev. Clin. Oncol.* 15 (4): 234–248.

Kallam, A., Witzig, T.E., Roschewski, M.J. et al. (2019). Phase II multi-center study of ruxolitinib phosphate for the treatment of relapsed or refractory diffuse large B-cell lymphoma (DLBCL) and peripheral T-cell lymphoma (PTCL). *J. Clin. Oncol.* 37 (15): e19063-e19063.

Kaneko, N., Kita, A., Yamanaka, K. et al. (2013). Combination of YM155, a survivin suppressant with a STAT3 inhibitor: a new strategy to treat diffuse large B-cell lymphoma. *Leuk. Res.* 37 (9): 1156–1161.

Keewan, E. and Matlawska-Wasowska, K. (2021). The emerging role of suppressors of cytokine signaling (SOCS) in the development and progression of leukemia. *Cancers (Basel)* 13 (16).

Khan, M.W., Saadalla, A., Ewida, A.H. et al. (2018). The STAT3 inhibitor pyrimethamine displays anti-cancer and immune stimulatory effects in murine models of breast cancer. *Cancer Immunol. Immunother.* 67 (1): 13–23.

Kiel, M.J., Velusamy, T., Rolland, D. et al. (2014). Integrated genomic sequencing reveals mutational landscape of T-cell prolymphocytic leukemia. *Blood* 124 (9): 1460–1472.

Kim, S.J., Yoon, D.H., Kang, H.J. et al. (2019). Ruxolitinib shows activity against Hodgkin lymphoma but not primary mediastinal large B-cell lymphoma. *BMC Cancer* 19 (1): 1080.

Klein, K., Witalisz-Siepracka, A., Maurer, B. et al. (2019). STAT5B(N642H) drives transformation of NKT cells: a novel mouse model for CD56(+) T-LGL leukemia. *Leukemia* 33 (9): 2336–2340.

Kontro, M., Kuusanmaki, H., Eldfors, S. et al. (2014). Novel activating STAT5B mutations as putative drivers of T-cell acute lymphoblastic leukemia. *Leukemia* 28 (8): 1738–1742.

Koppikar, P., Bhagwat, N., Kilpivaara, O. et al. (2012). Heterodimeric JAK-STAT activation as a mechanism of persistence to JAK2 inhibitor therapy. *Nature* 489 (7414): 155–159.

Koskela, H.L., Eldfors, S., Ellonen, P. et al. (2012). Somatic STAT3 mutations in large granular lymphocytic leukemia. *N. Engl. J. Med.* 366 (20): 1905–1913.

Kucuk, C., Jiang, B., Hu, X. et al. (2015). Activating mutations of STAT5B and STAT3 in lymphomas derived from gammadelta-T or NK cells. *Nat. Commun.* 6 (1): 6025.

Kumar, S., Pathania, A.S., Saxena, A.K. et al. (2013). The anticancer potential of flavonoids isolated from the stem bark of Erythrina suberosa through induction of apoptosis and inhibition of STAT signaling pathway in human leukemia HL-60 cells. *Chem. Biol . Interact.* 205 (2): 128–137.

Kuusanmaki, H., Dufva, O., Parri, E. et al. (2017). Drug sensitivity profiling identifies potential therapies for lymphoproliferative disorders with overactive JAK/STAT3 signaling. *Oncotarget* 8 (57): 97516–97527.

Laurent, C., Nicolae, A., Laurent, C. et al. (2020). Gene alterations in epigenetic modifiers and JAK-STAT signaling are frequent in breast implant-associated ALCL. *Blood* 135 (5): 360–370.

Lee, H., Deng, J., Kujawski, M. et al. (2010). STAT3-induced S1PR1 expression is crucial for persistent STAT3 activation in tumors. *Nat. Med.* 16 (12): 1421–1428.

Lee, H., Herrmann, A., Deng, J.H. et al. (2009). Persistently activated Stat3 maintains constitutive NF-kappaB activity in tumors. *Cancer Cell* 15 (4): 283–293.

Lee, S., Park, H.Y., Kang, S.Y. et al. (2015). Genetic alterations of JAK/STAT cascade and histone modification in extranodal NK/T-cell lymphoma nasal type. *Oncotarget* 6 (19): 17764–17776.

Li, X., Wei, Y., and Wei, X. (2020). Napabucasin, a novel inhibitor of STAT3, inhibits growth and synergises with doxorubicin in diffuse large B-cell lymphoma. *Cancer Lett.* 491: 146–161.

Li, Y., Rogoff, H.A., Keates, S. et al. (2015). Suppression of cancer relapse and metastasis by inhibiting cancer stemness. *Proc. Nat.l Acad. Sci. U. S. A.* 112 (6): 1839–1844.

Liu, Y., Deng, J., Wang, L. et al. (2012). S1PR1 is an effective target to block STAT3 signaling in activated B cell-like diffuse large B-cell lymphoma. *Blood* 120 (7): 1458–1465.

Lu, K., Chen, N., Zhou, X.X. et al. (2015). The STAT3 inhibitor WP1066 synergizes with vorinostat to induce apoptosis of mantle cell lymphoma cells. *Biochem. Biophys. Res. Commun.* 464 (1): 292–298.

Lu, K., Li, B., Zhang, H. et al. (2020). A novel silicone derivative of natural osalmid (DCZ0858) induces apoptosis and cell cycle arrest in diffuse large B-cell lymphoma via the JAK2/STAT3 pathway. *Signal Transduct. Target Ther.* 5 (1): 31.

Lyu, M.A., Sung, B., Cheung, L.H. et al. (2010). The rGel/BLyS fusion toxin inhibits STAT3 signaling via down-regulation of interleukin-6 receptor in diffuse large B-cell lymphoma. *Biochem. Pharmacol.* 80 (9): 1335–1342.

Ma, C., Horlad, H., Pan, C. et al. (2017). Stat3 inhibitor abrogates the expression of PD-1 ligands on lymphoma cell lines. *J. Clin. Exp. Hematop.* 57 (1): 21–25.

Majoros, A., Platanitis, E., Kernbauer-Holzl, E. et al. (2017). Canonical and Non-canonical aspects of JAK-STAT signaling: lessons from interferons for cytokine responses. *Front Immunol.* 8: 29.

Mascarenhas, J., Hoffman, R., Talpaz, M. et al. (2018). Pacritinib vs best available therapy, including ruxolitinib, in patients with myelofibrosis: a randomized clinical trial. *JAMA Oncol.* 4 (5): 652–659.

Matsuno, K., Masuda, Y., Uehara, Y. et al. (2010). Identification of a new series of STAT3 inhibitors by virtual screening. *ACS Med. Chem. Let.t* 1 (8): 371–375.

Maude, S.L., Dolai, S., Delgado-Martin, C. et al. (2015). Efficacy of JAK/STAT pathway inhibition in murine xenograft models of early T-cell precursor (ETP) acute lymphoblastic leukemia. *Blood* 125 (11): 1759–1767.

Maurer, B., Nivarthi, H., Wingelhofer, B. et al. (2020). High activation of STAT5A drives peripheral T-cell lymphoma and leukemia. *Haematologica* 105 (2): 435–447.

Meier, J.A. and Larner, A.C. (2014). Toward a new STATe: the role of STATs in mitochondrial function. *Semin. Immunol.* 26 (1): 20–28.

Mesa, R.A., Vannucchi, A.M., Mead, A. et al. (2017). Pacritinib versus best available therapy for the treatment of myelofibrosis irrespective of baseline cytopenias (PERSIST-1): an international, randomised, phase 3 trial. *Lancet. Haematol.* 4 (5): e225-e236.

Meyer, S.C. and Levine, R.L. (2014). Molecular pathways: molecular basis for sensitivity and resistance to JAK kinase inhibitors. *Clin. Cancer Res.* 20 (8): 2051–2059.

Miklossy, G., Hilliard, T.S., and Turkson, J. (2013). Therapeutic modulators of STAT signalling for human diseases. *Nat. Rev. Drug Discov.* 12 (8): 611–629.

Minieri, V., De Dominici, M., Porazzi, P. et al. (2018). Targeting STAT5 or STAT5-regulated pathways suppresses leukemogenesis of Ph+ acute lymphoblastic leukemia. *Cancer Res.* 78 (20): 5793–5807.

Moignet, A., Pastoret, C., Cartron, G. (2021). Ruxolitinib for refractory large granular lymphocyte leukemia. *Am. J. Hematol.* 96 (10): E368-E370.

Moosic, K.B., Paila, U., Olson, K.C. et al. (2019). Genomics of LGL leukemia and select other rare leukemia/lymphomas. *Best Pract. Res. Clin. Haematol.* 32 (3): 196–206.

Mori, R., Wauman, J., Icardi, L. et al. (2017). TYK2-induced phosphorylation of Y640 suppresses STAT3 transcriptional activity. *Sci. Rep.* 7 (1): 15919.

Moser, B., Edtmayer, S., Witalisz-Siepracka, A. et al. (2021). The ups and downs of STAT inhibition in acute myeloid leukemia. *Biomedicines* 9 (8).

Moskowitz, A.J., Ghione, P., Jacobsen, E. et al. (2021). A phase 2 biomarker-driven study of ruxolitinib demonstrates effectiveness of JAK/STAT targeting in T-cell lymphomas. *Blood* 138 (26): 2828–2837.

Ng, S.Y., Yoshida, N., Christie, A.L. et al. (2018). Targetable vulnerabilities in T- and NK-cell lymphomas identified through preclinical models. *Nat. Commun.* 9 (1): 2024.

Nicolae, A., Xi, L., Pittaluga, S. et al. (2014). Frequent STAT5B mutations in gammadelta hepatosplenic T-cell lymphomas. *Leukemia* 28 (11): 2244–2248.

Niu, J., Sun, Y., Chen, B. et al. (2019). Fatty acids and cancer-amplified ZDHHC19 promote STAT3 activation through S-palmitoylation. *Nature* 573 (7772): 139–143.

Ogura, M., Uchida, T., Terui, Y. et al. (2015). Phase I study of OPB-51602, an oral inhibitor of signal transducer and activator of transcription 3, in patients with relapsed/refractory hematological malignancies. *Cancer Sci.* 106 (7): 896–901.

Olson, T.L., Cheon, H., Xing, J.C. et al. (2021). Frequent somatic TET2 mutations in chronic NK-LGL leukemia with distinct patterns of cytopenias. *Blood* 138 (8): 662–673.

Pathania, A.S., Guru, S.K., Ul Ashraf, N. et al. (2015). A novel stereo bioactive metabolite isolated from an endophytic fungus induces caspase dependent apoptosis and STAT-3 inhibition in human leukemia cells. *Eur. J. Pharmacol.* 765: 75–85.

Pavel, A.B., Song, T., Kim, H.J. et al. (2019). Oral Janus kinase/SYK inhibition (ASN002) suppresses inflammation and improves epidermal barrier markers in patients with atopic dermatitis. *J. Allergy Clin. Immunol.* 144 (4): 1011–1024.

Phillips, T.J., Forero-Torres, A., Sher, T. et al. (2018). Phase 1 study of the PI3Kdelta inhibitor INCB040093 ± JAK1 inhibitor itacitinib in relapsed/refractory B-cell lymphoma. *Blood* 132 (3): 293–306.

Reilley, M.J., McCoon, P., Cook, C. et al. (2018). STAT3 antisense oligonucleotide AZD9150 in a subset of patients with heavily pretreated lymphoma: results of a phase 1b trial. *J. Immunother. Cancer* 6 (1): 119.

Ribeiro, D., Melao, A., van Boxtel, R. et al. (2018). STAT5 is essential for IL-7-mediated viability, growth, and proliferation of T-cell acute lymphoblastic leukemia cells. *Blood Adv.* 2 (17): 2199–2213.

Ribrag, V., Lee, S.T., Rizzieri, D. et al. (2021). A phase 1b study to evaluate the safety and efficacy of durvalumab in combination with tremelimumab or danvatirsen in patients with relapsed or refractory diffuse large B-cell lymphoma. *Clin. Lymphoma Myeloma. Leuk.* 21 (5): 309–317, e303.

Rosenquist, R., Bea, S., Du, M.Q. et al. (2017). Genetic landscape and deregulated pathways in B-cell lymphoid malignancies. *J. Intern. Med.* 282 (5): 371–394.

Salas, A., Hernandez-Rocha, C., Duijvestein, M. et al. (2020). JAK-STAT pathway targeting for the treatment of inflammatory bowel disease. *Nat. Rev. Gastroenterol. Hepatol.* 17 (6): 323–337.

Schwartz, D.M., Bonelli, M., Gadina, M. et al. (2016). Type I/II cytokines, JAKs, and new strategies for treating autoimmune diseases. *Nat Rev. Rheumatol.* 12 (1): 25–36.

Schwartz, D.M., Kanno, Y., Villarino, A. et al. (2017). JAK inhibition as a therapeutic strategy for immune and inflammatory diseases. *Nat. Rev. Drug Discov.* 17 (1): 78.

Scuto, A., Kirschbaum, M., Buettner, R. et al. (2013). SIRT1 activation enhances HDAC inhibition-mediated upregulation of GADD45G by repressing the binding of NF-kappaB/STAT3 complex to its promoter in malignant lymphoid cells. *Cell Death Dis.* 4 (5): e635.

Scuto, A., Kujawski, M., Kowolik, C. et al. (2011). STAT3 inhibition is a therapeutic strategy for ABC-like diffuse large B-cell lymphoma. *Cancer Res.* 71 (9): 3182–3188.

Seffens, A., Herrera, A., Tegla, C. et al. (2019). STAT3 dysregulation in mature T and NK cell lymphomas. *Cancers (Basel)* 11 (11).

Sharma, A., Oishi, N., Boddicker, R.L. et al. (2018). Recurrent STAT3-JAK2 fusions in indolent T-cell lymphoproliferative disorder of the gastrointestinal tract. *Blood* 131 (20): 2262–2266.

Shaw, V., Srivastava, S., and Srivastava, S.K. (2021). Repurposing antipsychotics of the diphenylbutylpiperidine class for cancer therapy. *Semin. Cancer Biol.* 68 (5): 75–83.

Simpson, H.M., Furusawa, A., Sadashivaiah, K. et al. (2018). STAT5 inhibition induces TRAIL/DR4 dependent apoptosis in peripheral T-cell lymphoma. *Oncotarget* 9 (24): 16792–16806.

Song, H., Wang, R., Wang, S. et al. (2005). A low-molecular-weight compound discovered through virtual database screening inhibits Stat3 function in breast cancer cells. *Proc. Natl. Acad. Sci. U. S. A.* 102 (13): 4700–4705.

Song, T.L., Nairismagi, M.L., Laurensia, Y. et al. (2018). Oncogenic activation of the STAT3 pathway drives PD-L1 expression in natural killer/T-cell lymphoma. *Blood* 132 (11): 1146–1158.

Spaner, D.E., Luo, Y., Wang, G. et al. (2021). Janus kinases restrain chronic lymphocytic leukemia cells in patients on ibrutinib: results of a phase II trial. *Cancer Med.* 10 (24): 8789–8798.

Spaner, D.E., Wang, G., McCaw, L. et al. (2016). Activity of the Janus kinase inhibitor ruxolitinib in chronic lymphocytic leukemia: results of a phase II trial. *Haematologica* 101 (5): e192–195.

Sun, X., Li, B., Xie, B. et al. (2017). DCZ3301, a novel cytotoxic agent, inhibits proliferation in diffuse large B-cell lymphoma via the STAT3 pathway. *Cell Death Dis.* 8 (10): e3111.

Svoboda, J. (2020). Everolimus plus itacitinib in relapsed/refractory classical Hodgkin lymphoma: results of a phase I/II investigator initiated trial (EVITA Study). 62nd ASH Annual Meeting and Exposition: ASH.

Takeda, K., Kaisho, T., Yoshida, N. et al. (1998). Stat3 activation is responsible for IL-6-dependent T cell proliferation through preventing apoptosis: generation and characterization of T cell-specific Stat3-deficient mice. *J. Immunol.* 161 (9): 4652–4660.

Tasian, S.K., Assad, A., Hunter, D.S. et al. (2018). A phase 2 study of ruxolitinib with chemotherapy in children with philadelphia chromosome-like acute lymphoblastic leukemia (INCB18424-269/AALL1521): dose-finding results from the part 1 safety phase. *Blood* 132 (Supplement 1): 555.

Teramo, A., Gattazzo, C., Passeri, F. et al. (2013). Intrinsic and extrinsic mechanisms contribute to maintain the JAK/STAT pathway aberrantly activated in T-type large granular lymphocyte leukemia. *Blood* 121 (19): 3843–3854, S3841.

Thomas, S., Fisher, K.H., Snowden, J.A. et al. (2015). Methotrexate is a JAK/STAT pathway inhibitor. *Plos One* 10 (7): e0130078.

Tiacci, E., Ladewig, E., Schiavoni, G. et al. (2018). Pervasive mutations of JAK-STAT pathway genes in classical Hodgkin lymphoma. *Blood* 131 (22): 2454–2465.

Uchihara, Y., Komori, R., Tago, K. et al. (2019). Methotrexate significantly induces apoptosis by inhibiting STAT3 activation in NPM-ALK-positive ALCL cells. *Biochem. Pharmacol.* 170: 113666.

Van Den Neste, E., Andre, M., Gastinne, T. et al. (2018). A phase II study of the oral JAK1/JAK2 inhibitor ruxolitinib in advanced relapsed/refractory Hodgkin lymphoma. *Haematologica* 103 (5): 840–848.

Waldmann, T.A. and Chen, J. (2017). Disorders of the JAK/STAT pathway in T cell lymphoma pathogenesis: implications for immunotherapy. *Annu. Rev. Immunol.* 35: 533–550.

Wang, T.T., Yang, J., Zhang, Y. et al. (2019). IL-2 and IL-15 blockade by BNZ-1, an inhibitor of selective gamma-chain cytokines, decreases leukemic T-cell viability. *Leukemia* 33 (5): 1243–1255.

Wingelhofer, B., Maurer, B., Heyes, E.C. et al. (2018). Pharmacologic inhibition of STAT5 in acute myeloid leukemia. *Leukemia* 32 (5): 1135–1146.

Wingelhofer, B., Neubauer, H.A., Valent, P. et al. (2018). Implications of STAT3 and STAT5 signaling on gene regulation and chromatin remodeling in hematopoietic cancer. *Leukemia* 32 (8): 1713–1726.

You, H., Xu, D., Zhao, J. et al. (2020). JAK Inhibitors: prospects in connective tissue diseases. *Clin. Rev. Allergy. Immunol.* 59 (3): 334–351.

Younes, A., Romaguera, J., Fanale, M. et al. (2012). Phase I study of a novel oral Janus kinase 2 inhibitor, SB1518, in patients with relapsed lymphoma: evidence of clinical and biologic activity in multiple lymphoma subtypes. *J. Clin. Oncol.* 30 (33): 4161–4167.

Yu, H., Pardoll, D., and Jove, R. (2009). STATs in cancer inflammation and immunity: a leading role for STAT3. *Nat. Rev. Cancer* 9 (11): 798–809.

Zhang, M., Mathews Griner, L.A., Ju, W. et al. (2015). Selective targeting of JAK/STAT signaling is potentiated by Bcl-xL blockade in IL-2-dependent adult T-cell leukemia. *Proc. Natl. Acad. Sci. U. S. A.* 112 (40): 12480–12485.

Zhang, X., Yue, P., Page, B.D. et al. (2012). Orally bioavailable small-molecule inhibitor of transcription factor Stat3 regresses human breast and lung cancer xenografts. *Proc .Natl. Acad. Sci. U. S. A.* 109 (24): 9623–9628.

Zhao, S., Sedwick, D., and Wang, Z. (2015). Genetic alterations of protein tyrosine phosphatases in human cancers. *Oncogene* 34 (30): 3885–3894.

Zhao, X., Zhang, Z., Moreira, D. et al. (2018). B cell lymphoma immunotherapy using TLR9-targeted oligonucleotide STAT3 Inhibitors. *Mol. Ther.* 26 (3): 695–707.

Zhou, H., Bai, L., Xu, R. et al. (2019). Structure-based discovery of SD-36 as a potent, selective, and efficacious PROTAC degrader of STAT3 protein. *J. Med. Chem.* 62 (24): 11280–11300.

Zhou, H., Bai, L., Xu, R. et al. (2021). SD-91 as A potent and selective STAT3 degrader capable of achieving complete and long-lasting tumor regression. *ACS Med. Chem. Lett.* 12 (6): 996–1004.

Zhou, Q., Peng, C., Du, F. (2018). et al. Design, synthesis and activity of BBI608 derivatives targeting on stem cells. *Eur. J. Med. Chem.* 151: 39–50.

28

Strategies for Targeting MYC

Jemma Longley and Andrew Davies

Southampton Cancer Research UK Centre, Cancer Sciences Unit, Faculty of Medicine, University of Southampton, Centre for Cancer Immunology, Southampton General Hospital, Southampton, SO16 6YD, Hampshire, UK

Take Home Messages

- The use of gene expression profiling in DLBCL has identified a larger cohort of patients with dysregulated MYC expression and poor survival outcomes compared with assessment for FISH rearrangement alone. Further prospective identification of this group and targeted clinical trials are required for further validation.
- Attempts to target MYC directly have so far proven unsuccessful; however, novel agents targeting epigenetic mechanisms and downstream gene expression are encouraging in the pre-clinical and early phase settings.
- Initial intensification of therapy is currently adopted by many centers as standard practice in DHL/THL; however, clinical trials showing the addition of lenalidamide or early escalation to Chimeric Antigen Receptor T-cell therapy (CAR-T) are also encouraging with further follow-up awaited to better define durability of responses.

Introduction

The revised World Health Organization (WHO) histological classification of lymphomas includes a separate group of high-grade B-cell lymphomas (HGBL) characterized by the presence of *MYC*, *BCL2*, and/or *BCL6* rearrangements (double-hit or triple-hit lymphomas, respectively) detected by fluorescence *in situ* hybridization (FISH) (Chen et al. 2018; Jaffe et al. 2017). These subtypes are considered to have an aggressive clinical course and are poorly treated by traditional immunochemotherapy with rituximab, cyclophosphamide, prednisone, vincristine, and doxorubicin (RCHOP), which has led to recent research focusing on improving outcomes for this group of patients (Liu and Barta 2019). These "double-hit" lymphoma (DHL) and "triple-hit" lymphoma (THL) account for 8–12% of all diffuse large B-cell lymphoma (DLBCL) diagnoses, but are over-represented in patients with relapsed/refractory disease, who have a five-year overall survival (OS) and progression-free survival (PFS) rate of 27% and 18%, respectively (Davies 2019). Identification of DHL/THL at diagnosis has allowed for more refined stratification of disease, and the evaluation of intensification of therapy which may improve response rates and PFS though this has not yet translated into an OS benefit (Tylan Magnusson et al. 2021). The negative prognostic significance of MYC rearrangement (MYC-R) in this context is heavily linked to BCL2 and/or BCL6 rearrangements, with studies showing that MYC-R alone has a negligible impact on survival outcomes when compared to cases without MYC-R in DLBCL and therefore does not justify intensification of therapy (Rosenwald et al. 2019). The direct targeting of MYC in this context has historically proven difficult due to its location in the cell nucleus and protein structure, leading to the investigation of alternative methods including the epigenetic regulation of MYC expression itself (Wang et al. 2021).

This chapter will outline the role of MYC in B-cell development and its dysregulation in B-cell lymphomas in conjunction with BCL2 and/or BCL6 rearrangement and the diagnostic challenges faced in DLBCL. We will underscore the difficulties with direct drug targeting of MYC and discuss strategies to overcome this challenge in pre-clinical studies, concluding with published clinical trial data on the treatment of DHL and THL and how this may change practice in the future.

Precision Cancer Therapies: Targeting Oncogenic Drivers and Signaling Pathways in Lymphoid Malignancies: From Concept to Practice, Volume 1, First Edition. Edited by Owen A. O'Connor, Stephen M. Ansell, and John F. Seymour.

Dysregulation of MYC in B-cell Lymphomas

MYC is an essential transcription factor located in the cell nucleus. It is responsible for controlling the expression of up to 15% of the human genome, particularly those genes involved in cell proliferation, apoptosis, DNA damage repair, and metabolism. During B-cell development, MYC is suppressed via transcriptional repression by BCL6 when B-cells enter the germinal center (GC) dark zone where they undergo proliferation and somatic hypermutation of immunoglobulin genes (Nguyen et al. 2017). On re-entry into the light zone, MYC is reactivated and highly expressed in mature B-cells, where they are actively selected for their high-affinity B-cell receptors following exposure to antigen via CD4 positive T helper cells. In addition, these cells are primed for re-entry into the dark zone for further rounds of clonal expansion, thereby maintaining the GC reaction. B-cells within the light zone lack MYC expression exit the GC to form either memory B-cells or plasmablasts. The dysregulation of MYC results in these GC B-cells undergoing uncontrolled re-entry into the GC dark zone independent of antigen selection, which increases the chance of oncogenic mutations leading to the development of B-cell lymphoma (Dang 2012).

The dysregulation of MYC occurs not only in B-cell lymphomas but also in many other malignancies including breast cancer, ovarian cancer and neuroblastoma. Alterations in MYC can arise in a number of ways including copy number gain, chromosomal translocations, point mutations, transcriptional changes, and other epigenetic phenomena including microRNA-mediated dysregulation (Xia and Zhang 2020). MYC dysregulation in DLBCL is primarily a secondary event, as opposed to its role in Burkitt's lymphoma where the classic 8;14 chromosomal translocation results in MYC-R into the intron enhancer of the immunoglobulin (IG) heavy chain locus and contributes to unregulated MYC expression which drives tumor proliferation. In DLBCL, MYC-R alone is more common than other translocations and primarily seen in the context of a complex karyotype which includes BCL2 and/or BCL6 rearrangement (Scott et al. 2018). The translocation position of MYC to either an IG or non-IG locus has been shown by Rosenwald et al. (2019) to be important in determining survival outcomes of DHL/THL in a population of patients treated with RCHOP. These data suggest that MYC-R to an IG translocation partner is associated with inferior survival outcomes in the context of HGBL as opposed to a non-IG partner where outcomes are similar to DLBCL without MYC-R. The outcomes of MYC plus BCL6 rearrangement in DHL have also been controversial, with small cohort sizes limiting clear conclusions, though in the same study there was no OS difference in survival among this group of patients compared to other DHL and THL subtypes, therefore supporting a similar approach with initial intensification of treatment (Rosenwald et al. 2019).

Identifying MYC Rearrangement in the Context of HGBL

In terms of diagnosis, high BCL2 and MYC expression detected by immunohistochemistry (IHC) are present in 20–35% of DLBCL cases; however, these double expressors (DE) do not have gene rearrangements and have improved survival outcomes when compared to HGBL, thus making the initial diagnosis of HGBL challenging (Xia and Zhang 2020). The decision of which biopsies should undergo FISH testing is an area of ongoing debate, with current practices differing across the world, dependent upon resources and the amount of biopsy material available. Overexpression of MYC and BCL2 has been shown to be restricted to patients with disease of the GCG subtype of lymphoma, leading to the conclusion that FISH testing should be performed in patients with GCB-type DLBCL only (Scott et al. 2018). While this approach would test approximately 11–14% of tumors and have a positive predictive value of 30–37%, it would miss up to 35% of HGBL cases, including those activated B-cell (ABC) DLBCL subtypes harboring MYC plus BCL6 rearrangements (Scott et al. 2018). The use of gene signatures to accurately identify HGBL at diagnosis by whole genome sequencing was investigated by Sha et al. (2019) in patients enrolled in the phase 3 REMoDL-B trial, where real-time molecular characterization of tumors was used prospectively to randomize and guide initial therapy. Bortezomib, a selective proteasome inhibitor thought to nullify the affect NF-κB, was added to RCHOP in patients with DLBCL and found to produce no difference in three-year PFS when compared to RCHOP alone (Davies et al. 2019). However, analysis of survival outcomes in this molecular high-grade group, although not statistically significant, showed a trend toward improved three-year PFS with the addition of bortezomib (58% vs. 37%, $p = 0.08$). The molecular high-grade signature (MHG) identified 9% of GCB DLBCL within this poor prognosis group, which was double the number of DHL/THL identified by FISH in the same study (Sha et al. 2019). These MHG lymphomas were enriched for centroblast dark zone GC gene signatures as opposed to the light zone GC as in other GCB DLBCL plus cell cycle/proliferation genes. Frequency of somatic mutations within the epigenetic regulator histone-lysine N-methyltransferase 2D (KMT2D) was higher in the MHG group, along with BCL2, MYC, and DDX3X – an ATP-dependent RNA helicase important in transcription initiation and ribosomal assembly. Interestingly, a small number of MYC-R were identified outside of this MHG group which exhibited survival outcomes similar to other GCB DLBCL, further supporting the concept that the translocation position of MYC may be important when determining which DLBCL are classed as HGBL (Rosenwald et al. 2019; Sha et al. 2019).

Enishi et al. (2019) similarly generated a molecular double-hit signature which included 104 genes differentially expressed in patients with inferior survival outcomes comparable to those in ABC subtypes, which was validated in an independent cohort of patients treated with RCHOP when reduced to a 30-gene model. This gene signature was identified in 27% of tumors of GCB subtype, with only half of those harboring BCL2 and MYC rearrangements as identified by FISH. Therefore, the authors concluded that MYC/BCL2 rearrangement is a surrogate marker for HGBL, representing only a subset of high-grade molecular DLBCL subtypes (Hilton et al. 2019). These tumors displayed a gene expression pattern consistent with intermediate zone GC cell-of-origin, with a high incidence of mutations within chromatin-modifying genes. The analysis of tumor cell morphology revealed low surface receptor expression of major histocompatibility complex class I (MHC-I) and MHC-II with low levels of T-cell infiltration. Hence, it was postulated that this group of patients may benefit from a range of initial treatment approaches including epigenetic modifiers such as enhancer of zeste homolog 2 (EZH2) inhibitors and histone deacetylase (HDAC) inhibitors, enhancing T-cell activation and reducing immune cell evasion by immunomodulatory therapies such as CAR-T cell therapy, lenalidamide, and newer anti-CD20 therapies such as obinutuzumab. These tumor cells have also been shown to be highly metabolically active with increased expression of genes associated with oxidative phosphorylation, providing further evidence that targeting the proteasome with bortezomib may be beneficial in this group of patients (Davies et al. 2019). Further investigation is needed prospectively within the clinical trial setting to validate this gene signature approach to identify HGBL with a focus on practical aspects, including timely availability of results to guide initial treatment decisions to ultimately benefit patients.

Targeting MYC Transcription

Direct targeting of the MYC protein itself has been notoriously difficult in terms of inhibition due to its lack of a ligand-binding domain and cell location, leading to a focus on research targeting alternative pathways to downregulate or inhibit MYC in B-cell lymphomas. The use of bromodomain extra-terminal inhibitors (BETi) which epigenetically downregulate the expression of DLBCL oncogenes such as MYC and BCL6 via targeting of bromodomain 4 (BRD4) has been explored in pre-clinical trials using mouse models and *in vitro* DHL/THL cell lines (Cummin et al. 2020). Histone acetylation results in reduced affinity for DNA binding, promoting gene transcription by the dissociation and unpacking of DNA from its histone proteins. The inhibition of BET proteins including BRD4 blocks recruitment of transcription factors including positive transcription elongation factor beta (PTEF-β) to the acetylated histone sites, preventing RNA polymerase II from binding to its proximal promoter, therefore downregulating oncogene expression at specific points within the genome such as MYC and BCL2 in DLBCL (Figure 28.1) (Shorstova et al. 2021). The use of BET small molecule inhibitors as single agents in phase 1 clinical trials has proved disappointing in a small number of patients with DLBCL, although these lymphomas were not classified as DHL or THL by FISH (Shapiro et al. 2021). However, in the pre-clinical setting, the use of BETi in combination with a BH3 mimetic (BCL2 inhibitor) significantly increased survival in both THL/DHL DLBCL cell lines and in MYC and BCL2 translocated DLBCL xenograft mouse models (Cummin et al. 2020). This mechanism has been demonstrated to be dependent on changes in regulation in the pro-apoptotic protein Bcl-2 Interacting Mediator of cell death (BIM) and subsequent downregulation of miRNA 17~92 cluster in response to MYC inhibition by BETi, which is reversed by combination therapy with the BH3 mimetic venetoclax, leading to enhanced tumor responses (Cummin et al. 2020). Interestingly, the expression of CD47, a cell surface receptor expressed by both normal and tumor cells which downregulates the phagocytic activity of macrophages, was upregulated in DHL/THL and was subsequently reduced following BETi treatment. These findings were replicated in mouse models, where suppression of MYC caused a reduction in CD47 and programmed cell death ligand (PDL1) mRNA and protein expression leading to enhanced anti-tumor responses (Casey et al. 2016). This demonstrates the feasibility of combination therapy of BETi with other immunomodulatory drugs that target both the adaptive and innate immune system in the context of HGBL. Monoclonal antibodies (mAb) directed to CD47 have already been investigated in combination with rituximab in a phase 1 trial in patients with relapsed/refractory non-Hodgkin's lymphoma (NHL) and showed a complete response (CR) in 33% of patients with DLBCL who were ongoing at six months in 91% of patients (Advani et al. 2018). Further clinical trials combining anti-CD47 with other immune checkpoints including programmed cell death 1 (PD1) and PDL1 are ongoing within the relapsed/refractory NHL setting.

EZH2 inhibitors have proven efficacious in patients with both EZH2 gain-of-function mutations and wild-type lymphomas within the clinical trial setting. EZH2 catalyzes the tri-methylation of histone H3 at lysine position 27 (H3K27me3) as part of the polycomb repressive complex (PRC2), epigenetically maintaining transcriptional repression of target genes that negatively regulate the cell cycle and terminal differentiation (Huet et al. 2017) (Figure 28.1). EZH2 activity is reduced by activation of the switch/sucrose non-fermentable (SNF/SWI) multi-chromatin remodeling complex acting in opposition to PCR2 activity and promoting

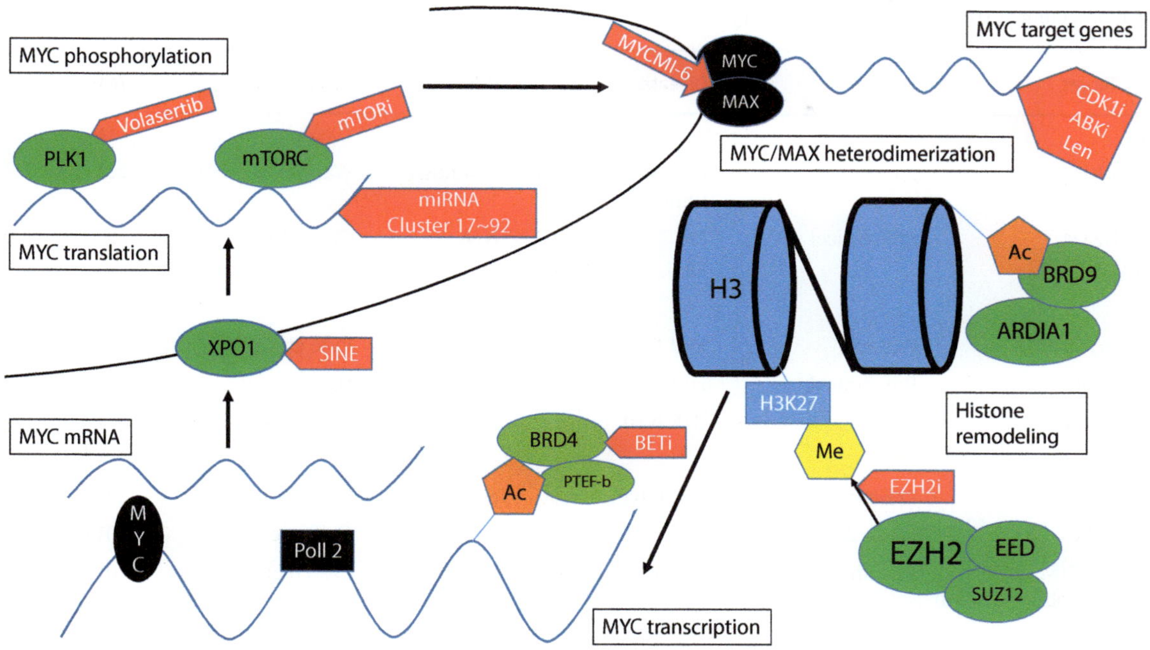

Figure 28.1 Mechanisms of the indirect targeting of MYC.
Abbreviations: CDK1i, cyclin dependant kinase 1 inhibitor; ABKi, Aurora B kinase inhibitor; Len, lenalidomide; Ac, acetylation; H3, histone 3; BRD9, bromodomain containing protein 9; ARDIA1, AT-rich interacting domain-containing protein 1A; H3K27, histone 3 lysine position K27; Me, methylation; EZH2, enhancer of zeste homolog 2; EED, embryonic ectoderm development; SUZ12, suppressor of zeste 12 homolog; BRD4, bromodomain-containing protein 4; BETi, bromodomain and extra-terminal motif inhibitor; Poll 2, RNA polymerase II; MYC, mRNA messenger RNA; XP01, exportin 01; SINE, selective inhibitor of nuclear export; PLK1, polo kinase 1; MYC, MAX heterodimer; MYCMI-6 MYC:MAX protein interactions inhibitor.

terminal differentiation. EZH2 expression in tumor cells downregulates MHC class I and class II expression on their cell surface, resulting in immune evasion by a reduction in tumor antigen presentation (Chowell et al. 2018). The transcriptomic analysis of 347 DLBCL patient samples by Enishi et al. (2019) demonstrated EZH2 mutation enrichment of MHC class I and class II negative lymphomas was associated with a reduced T-cell infiltrate in subsequent studies *in vivo*, which was reversed by EZH2 inhibition. Given this same observation within the tumor microenvironment of HGBL, EZH2 inhibitors may prove efficacious in this subgroup of patients; however, further evidence is needed to explore this option as a future treatment strategy for HGBL (Table 28.1).

Targeting MYC Translation

Protein expression and mRNA translation are tightly regulated by many different proteins including the mammalian target of rapamycin complex 1 (mTORC1), which has been shown to be positively correlated with MYC overexpression in DLBCL patients (Herzog et al. 2021). The initiation of messenger RNA (mRNA) translation is reliant upon phosphorylation of downstream proteins by mTOR1 which is then able to bind RNA helicase (Wang et al. 2021). To date the development of mTOR inhibitors has been limited by toxicity, off-target effects, and the development of resistance mutations during therapy; however, inhibition of downstream proteins including translation initiation factor 4G1 (eIF4G1) which binds capped mRNA has proven beneficial in sensitizing DLBCL cell lines to venetoclax by increasing apoptosis (Eyre et al. 2019; Herzog et al. 2021). Similarly, inhibition of casein kinase 1-e (CK-1e) by the dual phosphoinositide 3-kinase (PI3K) delta inhibitor umbralisib has been shown to inhibit 4EBP1 leading to rapid blockade of MYC translation (Deng et al. 2016).

The export of these translation initiation factors which bind mRNA oncogenes such as MYC from the nucleus to the cytoplasm is mediated by nuclear export proteins including exportin 1 (XPO1), which is upregulated in many different cancers and correlates with poor prognosis (Fischer et al. 2020). The use of selective inhibitors of nuclear export (SINE) compounds including selinexor (KPT-330) and eltanexor (KPT-8602) which target XPO1 in combination with venetoclax in DLBCL has been shown to enhance apoptosis *in vivo* and *in vitro* compared to either single agent alone. A phase 1 trial of selinexor in relapsed/refractory NHL resulted in three of six patients with DLBCL DHL/THL responding to treatment (Kuruvilla et al. 2017). Tumor sample staining revealed decreased expression of MYC, BCL2, and BCL6 proteins by IHC which may account for its therapeutic benefit in those subsets of patients with gene rearrangements.

Table 28.1 Pre-clinical and clinical studies indirectly targeting MYC.

Drug	Target	Status	Disease	ORR	References	Year
MYC transcription						
AZD5153	BRD4	Phase 1	R/R NHL and solid tumors	Unknown	Wang et al.	2019
PLX2583	BRD4	Pre-clinical	MYC-R/ DHL/THL DLBCL	N/A	Cummin et al.	2020
MYC translation						
Vistusertib	mTORC	Phase 2	R/R DLBCL	6%	Eyre et al.	2019
SBI-756	eIF4F	Pre-clinical	DLBCL/MCL	N/A	Herzog et al.	2021
Selinexor	XPO1	Phase 1	R/R NHL	31%	Kuruvilla et al.	2017
MYC stability						
Volasertib	PLK1	Pre-clinical	B-cell lymphoma	N/A	Ren et al.	2018
AZD1152	ABK	Phase 2	R/R DLBCL	20%	Collins et al.	2014
MYCMI-6	MYC/MAX heterodimerization	Pre-clinical	Burkitt's lymphoma	N/A	Castell et al.	2018
MYC downstream gene targets						
Purvanelol A	CDK1	Pre-clinical	MYC-R lymphoma	N/A	Murga-Zamalloa et al.	2017
Lenalidamide	IRF4	Phase 2 (+RCHOP)	MYC-R DLBCL	73%	Chamuleau et al.	2020

Abbreviations: ABK = Aurora B kinase; BRD4 = bromodomain-containing protein 4; CDK1 = cyclin dependant kinase 1; DLBCL = diffuse Large B cell lymphoma; eIF4F = eukaryotic initiation factor 4F; IRF4 = interferon regulatory factor 4; mTORC = mammalian target of rapamycin complex 1; MYC-R = MYC rearrangement; PLK1 = polo-like kinase; R/R = relapsed/refractory; XPO1 = exportin 01.

Targeting MYC Stabilization and Downstream Gene Expression

The phosphorylation of MYC protein by polo-like kinase (PLK1) stabilizes its structure enhancing downstream gene expression. The inhibition of this protein kinase has been shown to downregulate MYC protein expression and in combination with BCL2 antagonists reduced tumor growth of DLBCL cell lines (Ren et al. 2018). The use of volasertib, a PLK1 inhibitor, was assessed in primary DHL samples in an *ex vivo* organotype cell-based platform with a reconstituted lymphoma microenvironment, and found to substantially reduce DHL cell survival (Murga-Zamalloa et al. 2017). This encouraging pre-clinical data has led onto early-phase clinical trials evaluating PLK1 inhibitors in both solid and hematological malignancies.

Another protein kinase, Aurora B kinase (ABK), has been implicated in the stabilization of MYC protein and is frequently overexpressed in a variety of different malignancies. Like PK1, ABK directly phosphorylates MYC protein and is also one of the downstream gene products of MYC transcription factor (Chen et al. 2018). ABK is vital for cell cycle progression and migrates to the centromere spindle and is essential for anaphase to metaphase transition. A phase 2 trial of AZD1152, an ABK inhibitor, was investigated in relapsed/refractory DLBCL, with 40% of patients having undergone previous autologous stem cell transplantation (AutoSCT) (Collins et al. 2015). Unfortunately responses were only seen in 20% of patients and were short in this single-agent study, with no association shown with MYC overexpression (Collins et al. 2015). Difficulty in dosing delivery meant the authors concluded AZD1152 was unlikely to be taken forward in this setting as a single agent, however, proof of principle that ABK-induced responses in heavily pre-treated patients were seen and improvement in pharmacokinetics and dosing schedule may improve responses in combination with other agents such as BCL2 inhibitors in this cohort of patients.

The aberrant downstream gene expression as a result of the MYC oncogene is partly attributed to cell cycle protein kinases responsible for cell cycle entry from G1 phase to the S phase. The cell cyclin-dependant protein kinase 1 (CDK1) is the catalytic subunit of the mitosis (M) phase promoting factor, acting as a checkpoint between the G2 and M phases of the cell cycle (Chen et al. 2018). The use of the small molecule inhibitor purvanelol A, a potent inhibitor of CDK1 in MYC overexpressing human cell lines, resulted in significant cell death independent of p53 expression (Goga et al. 2007). This was replicated in a transgenic Eu-MYC lymphoma mouse model, where survival outcomes were improved with purvanelol A compared with control mice (Goga et al. 2007). Unfortunately, purvanelol A is poorly soluble in aqueous solutions resulting in difficulties with drug delivery, therefore, further studies are awaited to evaluate CDK1 inhibitors as a novel approach in the pre-clinical and clinical trial settings.

The ability of MYC to initiate transcription is dependent upon its heterodimerization with MYC-associated factor X (MAX) and subsequent recruitment of other necessary factors which modify chromatin structure and allow the acetylation of histones resulting in an open chromatin state (Chen et al. 2018). Destabilization of this heterodimer by blocking the MYC–MAX interaction has been investigated to inactivate the function of MYC as a transcription factor and therefore reduce downstream gene expression. To date pre-clinical data has focused on overexpressing MYC cancer cell lines generally and not specifically B-cell lymphomas; however, the small molecule inhibitor MYCMI-6 induced cell death in these cell lines which included Burkitt's Lymphoma and was not cytotoxic to normal human cells (Castell et al. 2018). Subsequent *in vivo* mouse studies involving an MYC-amplified neuroblastoma xenograft model showed increased necrosis, hemorrhage, and reduction of tumor proliferation without serious side effects. These findings correlated significantly with a reduction in MAX MYC binding in tumor tissue itself. Further *in vivo* studies including lymphoma-based murine models are needed to validate these findings within different tumor types that overexpress MYC.

Initial Therapy in MYC-R DLBCL

The initial intensification of therapy for patients with HGBL has included the investigation of dose-adjusted etoposide, prednisolone, vincristine, cyclophosphamide, and doxorubicin plus rituximab (DA EPOCH-R) compared to RCHOP; the addition of lenalidamide to RCHOP; and the use of AutoSCT following first remission and upfront CAR-T cell therapy. In a single-arm phase 2 study in patients with MYC rearrangement alone or in the context of DHL/THL received six cycles of dose-adjusted etoposide phosphate, prednisone, vincristine sulfate, cyclophosphamide, doxorubicin hydrochloride, and rituximab (DA EPOCH-R) plus central nervous system (CNS) prophylaxis consisting of four cycles of intrathecal (IT) methotrexate (Dunleavy et al. 2018). After two years of follow-up, 71% of patients remained event free, which was mirrored in a subgroup analysis in the 24 patients (46% of the cohort) with DHL/THL, with a two-year OS of 82%. Of note seven patients underwent either consolidation radiotherapy, allogenic, or AutoSCT following a complete or partial response, which may have affected results. In contrast to this, a more recent retrospective comparison of patient outcomes receiving initial therapy with RCHOP versus DA EPOCH-R showed no difference in OS rates in THL/DHL (Tylan Magnusson et al. 2021). The four-year OS rate in patients with THL/DHL was 49% in the DA EPOCH-R group (111 patients) versus 54% in the RCHOP group (44 patients), with the majority of deaths occurring within the first two years following diagnosis (89%). It is unclear whether these patients received CNS prophylaxis and therefore CNS relapse may have contributed to poorer outcomes and lack of durability of responses.

Consolidation with AutoSCT in patients with HGBL following attainment of first remission has also been a topic of debate given the dismal prognosis of patients with relapsed disease and the reduced likelihood of long-term responses following treatment with salvage chemotherapy. In a small retrospective study of 36 patients all with DHL, three-year outcomes were similar in patients who underwent AutoSCT versus observation following six cycles of DA EPOCH-R; however, a large proportion of these patients had disease which was refractory to initial chemotherapy and therefore the group that underwent AutoSCT was only 17 patients, with 11 in the observation group (Chen et al. 2018). The three-year PFS and OS were 94% and 79% in both groups, respectively. This analysis did not include single MYC-R as in other studies, which may explain the large proportion of patients who experienced primary refractory disease following DA EPOCH-R. In a subsequent large multicenter retrospective analysis of patients with DHL/THL who achieved first complete or partial remission following immunochemotherapy, Allo or AutoSCT did not provide any further benefit at two-year follow-up in terms of PFS and OS when compared to observation alone; however, the type of induction chemotherapy regime did affect outcome, with higher rates of CR seen with DA EPOCH-R and other intensive regimes compared with RCHOP (Petrich et al. 2014). In a separate retrospective study, patients with DHL/THL achieving a complete remission following initial chemotherapy similarly did not gain any further benefit from subsequent AutoSCT and mirrored the previous study in that the intensity of induction regime did improve survival outcomes, with three-year PFS rates of 56% in those receiving RCHOP compared with 88% in patients receiving intensive therapy including DA EPOCH-R (Landsburg et al. 2017). Although there are no prospective studies comparing AutoSCT versus observation in this specific group of patients, these data do not currently support this approach in patients with HGBL in first remission of their disease.

The addition of the immunomodulatory drug lenalidomide to RCHOP chemotherapy was investigated in the context of HGBL in a phase 2 single-arm study in 82 patients with MYC-R as identified by FISH (Chamuleau et al. 2020). Lenalidomide exposure results in downregulation of MYC and its target genes via cereblon and interferon regulatory factor 4 (IRF4) (Jones et al. 2021). Lenalidomide was commenced with the second cycle of treatment with patients receiving four cycles IT methotrexate prophylaxis. As lenalidomide is able to cross the blood–brain barrier, this makes it an attractive drug to use in the context of HGBL where CNS relapse rates are higher compared with *de novo* DLBCL, further allowing treatment to be completed on an outpatient basis. Indeed, its addition in this study resulted in only one patient experiencing a CNS relapse after 25 months of follow-up and no treatment-related deaths. As a whole cohort, patients had OS outcomes comparable to the DA EPOCH-R single-arm study, with a two-year OS of 73% despite a higher proportion of THL/DHL (65%). Further head-to-head prospective studies are required in this group of HGBL patients to establish any changes in standard of care following these encouraging phase 2 results.

The use of BCL2 inhibitors in combination with chemotherapy in the first-line setting for aggressive B-cell lymphomas has been investigated in early-phase clinical trials. Venetoclax in combination with DA EPOCH-R showed a CR rate of 93% in the frontline setting in patients with aggressive B-cell lymphomas, including 50% of patients with DHL/THL (Rutherford et al. 2021). Of note, those patients with HGBL also had a CR of 93%, of which 71% remained in CR at a median follow-up of 28.1 months, indicating that this regime may produce durable responses; however, longer term follow-up is needed.

The use of CAR-T cell therapy in the DLBCL relapsed/refractory setting is well established; however, its use in the first-line setting in high-risk patients including HGBL has yet to be fully explored. An interim analysis of the single-arm phase 2 ZUMA12 trial using anti-CD19 CAR-T cells (Axi-Cel) in patients with high-risk B-cell lymphoma (60% with DHL or THL) showed an impressive overall response rate (ORR) of 92% and a CR of 75% in 12 response evaluable patients (Neelapu et al. 2019). Further data is awaited regarding durability of these responses; however, median CAR-T cell expansion and CAR-T cell levels were higher in the first-line setting, suggesting that this group of patients may gain most benefit prior to other lines of therapy. This trial included fluorodeoxyglucose (FDG)-positron emission tomography (PET) response-adapted therapy, with patients receiving two cycles of RCHOP prior to interim PET and if positive then treatment escalated to CAR-T cell therapy. This approach spared patients likely to be cured by RCHOP alone the toxicity associated with more intensive regimes while maximizing cure in those with the most aggressive refractory disease. The toxicity of CAR-T cell therapy in the frontline setting in this study revealed a large proportion of patients (80%) experiencing grade 3 and above toxicities, with nearly one-third of patients experiencing grades 3–4 encephalopathy; however, there were no treatment-related deaths. Careful consideration is needed when deciding on which patients may potentially benefit from this approach if adopted as standard practice in the future. Finally, the use of bispecific antibodies (bsAbs) is in its infancy currently in the treatment of DLBCL; however, this approach may prove beneficial in DHL/THL where CAR-T cell therapy has failed to induce durable responses (Salvaris et al. 2021). Currently, there are over 100 bsAbs in development across all malignancies, with CD3/CD20 bsAbs being the most tested in terms of DLBCL in early-phase clinical trials. These antibodies are able to recognize antigen from the patient's own T-cells (CD3) and malignant B-cells (CD20) to enhance immune effector function (Salvaris et al. 2021). This approach may prove useful especially in MYC-R lymphomas where tumor morphology has shown poor infiltration of T-cells secondary to downregulation of MHC class I and class II.

Future Directions

There is no doubt that patients with HGBL require a different initial treatment approach to improve survival outcomes; however, to date, intensification of therapy at diagnosis has not consistently translated in an improvement in OS despite initial improvement in PFS and response rates. The use of immunomodulatory drugs including CAR-T cell therapy and the addition of lenalidomide to RCHOP has proved encouraging in the initial treatment of HGBL; however, further head-to-head phase 3 studies are awaited to guide best practice with longer term follow-up needed. The use of gene profiling upfront to guide initial therapy has identified a larger group of HGBL patients compared to MYC, BCL2, and/or BCL6 rearrangement by FISH, which may guide decisions regarding type of initial therapy for patients in the future. Combining this with a response-adapted approach to identify patients with refractory disease and switching to non-chemotherapy type treatments in the form of immunomodulatory agents early on in the disease course may provide further improvements for patients in this very poor survival group. The use of novel therapies targeting MYC indirectly in combination with other small molecules or immunochemotherapy holds promise to downregulate MYC expression in DHL/THL in the pre-clinical setting; however, early-phase clinical trials are awaited to assess toxicity, dosing, and the feasibility of combination in terms of drug delivery.

Must Read References

Dunleavy, K., Fanale, M.A., Abramson, J.S. et al. (2018). Dose-adjusted EPOCH-R (etoposide, prednisone, vincristine, cyclophosphamide, doxorubicin, and rituximab) in untreated aggressive diffuse large B-cell lymphoma with MYC rearrangement: a prospective, multicentre, single-arm phase 2 study. *Lancet Haematol.* 5 (12): e609–e617.

Rosenwald, A., Bens, S., Advani, R. et al. (2019). Prognostic Significance of MYC Rearrangement and Translocation Partner in Diffuse Large B-Cell Lymphoma: A Study by the

Lunenburg Lymphoma Biomarker Consortium. *J. Clin. Oncol.* 37 (35): 3359–3368.

Wang, C., Zhang, J., Yin, J. et al. 2021). Alternative approaches to target Myc for cancer treatment. *Signal Transduct. Target Ther.* 6 (1): 117.

References

Advani, R., Flinn, I., Popplewell, L. et al. (2018). CD47 blockade by Hu5F9-G4 and Rituximab in Non-Hodgkin's Lymphoma. *N. Engl. J. Med.* 379 (18): 1711–1721.

Casey, S.C., Tong, L., Li, Y. et al. (2016). MYC regulates the antitumor immune response through CD47 and PD-L1. *Science* 352 (6282): 227–231.

Castell, A., Yan, Q., Fawkner, K. et al. (2018). A selective high affinity MYC-binding compound inhibits MYC:MAX interaction and MYC-dependent tumor cell proliferation. *Scientific Rep.* 8 (1): 10064.

Chamuleau, M.E.D., Burggraaff, C.N., Nijland, M. et al. (2020). Treatment of patients with MYC rearrangement positive large B-cell lymphoma with R-CHOP plus lenalidomide: results of a multicenter HOVON phase II trial. *Haematol.* 105 (12): 2805–2812.

Chen, A.I., Leonard, J.T., Okada, C.Y. et al. (2018). Outcomes of DA-EPOCH-R induction plus autologous transplant consolidation for double hit lymphoma. *Leuk. Lymphoma* 59 (8): 1884–1889.

Chen, H., Liu, H., and Qing, G. (2018). Targeting oncogenic Myc as a strategy for cancer treatment. *Signal Transduct. Targeted Ther.* 3 (1): 5.

Chowell, D., Napier, J., Gupta, R. et al. (2018). Modeling the subclonal evolution of cancer cell populations. *Cancer Res.* 78 (3): 830–839.

Collins, G.P., Eyre, T.A., Linton, K.M. et al. (2015). A phase II trial of AZD1152 in relapsed/refractory diffuse large B-cell lymphoma. *Br. J. Haematol.* 170 (6): 886–890.

Cummin, T.E.C., Cox, K.L., Murray, T.D. et al. (2020). BET inhibitors synergize with venetoclax to induce apoptosis in MYC-driven lymphomas with high BCL-2 expression. *Blood Adv.* 4 (14): 3316–3328.

Dang, C.V. (2012). MYC on the path to cancer. *Cell* 149 (1): 22–35.

Davies, A. (2019). Double-hit lymphoma: so what? *Hematol. Oncol.* 37 (S1): 19–23.

Davies, A., Cummin, T.E., Barrans, S. et al. (2019). Gene-expression profiling of bortezomib added to standard chemoimmunotherapy for diffuse large B-cell lymphoma (REMoDL-B): an open-label, randomised, phase 3 trial. *Lancet Oncol.* 20 (5): 649–662.

Deng, C., Lipstein, M.M., Scotto, L. et al. (2016). Silencing of c-Myc Translation through Targeting PI3K delta and CK1 epsilon. *Blood* 129: 88–99.

Dunleavy, K., Fanale, M.A., Abramson, J.S. et al. (2018). Dose-adjusted EPOCH-R (etoposide, prednisone, vincristine, cyclophosphamide, doxorubicin, and rituximab) in untreated aggressive diffuse large B-cell lymphoma with MYC rearrangement: a prospective, multicentre, single-arm phase 2 study. *Lancet Haematol.* 5 (12): e609–e617.

Ennishi, D., Jiang, A., Boyle, M. et al. (2019). Double-hit gene expression signature defines a distinct subgroup of germinal center B-cell-like diffuse large B-cell lymphoma. *J. Clin. Oncol.* 37 (3): 190–201.

Ennishi, D., Takata, K., Béguelin, W. et al. (2019). Molecular and genetic characterization of MHC deficiency identifies EZH2 as therapeutic target for enhancing immune recognition. *Cancer Dis.* 9 (4): 546–563.

Eyre, T.A., Hildyard, C., Hamblin, A. et al. (2019). A phase II study to assess the safety and efficacy of the dual mTORC1/2 inhibitor vistusertib in relapsed, refractory DLBCL. *Hematol. Oncol.* 37 (4): 352–359.

Fischer, M.A., Friedlander, S.Y., Arrate, M.P. et al. (2020). Venetoclax response is enhanced by selective inhibitor of nuclear export compounds in hematologic malignancies. *Blood Adv.* 4 (3): 586–598.

Goga, A., Yang, D., Tward, A.D. et al. (2007). Inhibition of CDK1 as a potential therapy for tumors over-expressing MYC. *Nature Med.* 13 (7): 820–827.

Herzog, L.-O., Walters, B., Buono, R. et al. (2021). Targeting eIF4F translation initiation complex with SBI-756 sensitises B lymphoma cells to venetoclax. *Br. J. Cancer* 124 (6): 1098–1109.

Hilton, L.K., Tang, J., Ben-Neriah, S. et al. (2019). The double-hit signature identifies double-hit diffuse large B-cell lymphoma with genetic events cryptic to FISH. *Blood* 134 (18): 1528–1532.

Huet, S., Xerri, L., Tesson, B. et al. (2017). EZH2 alterations in follicular lymphoma: biological and clinical correlations. *Blood Cancer J* 7 (4): e555–e555.

Jaffe, E.S., Barr, P.M., and Smith, S.M. (2017). Understanding the new WHO classification of lymphoid malignancies: why it's important and how it will affect practice. *Am. Soc. Clin. Oncol. Educ. Book* 37: 535–546.

Jones, J.R., Barber, A., Le Bihan, Y.V. et al. (2021). Mutations in CRBN and other cereblon pathway genes are infrequently associated with acquired resistance to immunomodulatory drugs. *Leukemia* 35 (10): 3017–3020.

Kuruvilla, J., Savona, M., Baz, R. et al. (2017). Selective inhibition of nuclear export with selinexor in patients with non-Hodgkin lymphoma. *Blood* 129 (24): 3175–3183.

Landsburg, D.J., Falkiewicz, M.K., Maly, J. et al. (2017). Outcomes of patients with double-hit lymphoma who achieve first complete remission. *J. Clin. Oncol.* 35 (20): 2260–2267.

Liu, Y. and Barta, S.K. (2019). Diffuse large B-cell lymphoma: 2019 update on diagnosis, risk stratification, and treatment. *Am. J. Hematol.* 94 (5): 604–616.

Murga-Zamalloa, C., Polk, A., Hanel, W. et al. (2017). Polo-like-kinase 1 (PLK-1) and c-myc inhibition with the dual kinase-bromodomain inhibitor volasertib in aggressive lymphomas. *Oncotarget* 8 (70).

Neelapu, S.S., Chavez, J.C., Lin, Y. et al. (2019). ZUMA-12: a phase 2 multicenter study of axicabtagene ciloleucel (axi-cel) as a first-line therapy in patients (pts) with high-risk large B-cell lymphoma (LBCL). *J. Clin. Oncol.* 37 (15_suppl): TPS7574–TPS7574.

Nguyen, L., Papenhausen, P., and Shao, H. (2017). The role of c-MYC in B-cell lymphomas: diagnostic and molecular aspects. *Genes (Basel)* 8 (4): 116.

Petrich, A.M., Gandhi, M., Jovanovic, B. et al. (2014). Impact of induction regimen and stem cell transplantation on outcomes in double-hit lymphoma: a multicenter retrospective analysis. *Blood* 124 (15): 2354–2361.

Ren, Y., Bi, C., Zhao, X. et al. (2018). PLK1 stabilizes a MYC-dependent kinase network in aggressive B cell lymphomas. *J. Clin. Invest.* 128 (12): 5517–5530.

Rosenwald, A., Bens, S., Advani, R. et al. (2019). Prognostic significance of MYC rearrangement and translocation partner in diffuse large B-cell lymphoma: a study by the lunenburg lymphoma biomarker consortium. *J. Clin. Oncol.* 37 (35): 3359–3368.

Rutherford, S.C., Abramson, J.S., Bartlett, N.L. et al. (2021). Venetoclax with dose-adjusted EPOCH-R as initial therapy for patients with aggressive B-cell lymphoma: a single-arm, multicentre, phase 1 study. *Lancet Haematol.* 8(11): E818–E827.

Salvaris, R., Ong, J., and Gregory, G.P. (2021). Bispecific antibodies: a review of development, clinical efficacy and toxicity in B-cell lymphomas. *J. Pers. Med.* 11 (5): 355.

Scott, D.W., King, R.L., Staiger, A.M. et al. (2018). High-grade B-cell lymphoma with MYC and BCL2 and/or BCL6 rearrangements with diffuse large B-cell lymphoma morphology. *Blood* 131 (18): 2060–2064.

Sha, C., Barrans, S., Cucco, F. et al. (2019). Molecular high-grade B-cell lymphoma: defining a poor-risk group that requires different approaches to therapy. *J. Clin. Oncol.* 37 (3): 202–212.

Shapiro, G.I., LoRusso, P., Dowlati, A. et al. (2021). A phase 1 study of RO6870810, a novel bromodomain and extra-terminal protein inhibitor, in patients with NUT carcinoma, other solid tumours, or diffuse large B-cell lymphoma. *Br. J. Cancer* 124 (4): 744–753.

Shorstova, T., Foulkes, W.D., and Witcher, M. (2021). Achieving clinical success with BET inhibitors as anti-cancer agents. *Br. J. Cancer* 124 (9): 1478–1490.

Tylan Magnusson, M.N., Mehta, A., and Goyal, G. (2021). No difference in overall survival between R-chop and R-epoch among patients with advanced stage Myc-rearranged, double hit, or triple hit diffuse large B-cell lymphoma. *EHA Library* 324632 (1).

Wang, C., Zhang, J., Yin, J. et al. (2021). Alternative approaches to target Myc for cancer treatment. *Signal Transduct. Target Ther.* 6 (1): 117.

Xia, Y. and Zhang, X. (2020). The spectrum of MYC alterations in diffuse large B-cell lymphoma. *Acta Haematol.* 143 (6): 520–528.

29

Targeting NOTCH in Lymphoid Malignancies

Deborah Piffaretti[1], Georgia Alice Galimberti[1], and Davide Rossi[1,2,3]

[1] Laboratory of Experimental Hematology, Institute of Oncology Research, Bellinzona, Switzerland
[2] Clinic of Hematology, Oncology Institute of Southern Switzerland, Ente Ospedaliero Cantonale, Bellinzona, Bellinzona, Switzerland
[3] Faculty of Biomedical Sciences, Università della Svizzera Italiana, Lugano, Switzerland

Take Home Messages

- NOTCH, originally described to play a role in fruit fly wing development in 1917, is crucial in regulating cell differentiation and fate.
- NOTCH represents a family of cell membrane surface receptors, with a variety of ligands depending on the specific receptor and cell type that expresses that receptor.
- Perturbation of physiologic NOTCH signaling, through translaocations or mutations, plays in an important role in the initiation and maintenance of the malignant phenotype in a variety of hematologic cancers.
- While drugs have been developed that can impact dysregulated NOTCH signaling, none have been successfully approved in the clinic.

Introduction: NOTCH Signaling

NOTCH was discovered in 1917 by Morgan following John S. Dexter's observation of notched wings (serration at the ends of the wings) in *Drosophila melanogaster* in 1914 (Shen et al. 2021). In metazoa, the regulation of cell differentiation, cell proliferation, cell fate throughout development, and cell death are ascribed to the evolutionarily conserved NOTCH pathway (Kopan 2012). Vertebrates possess four NOTCH receptors: NOTCH1 and NOTCH2, which are the most widely expressed in many tissues at both early developmental stages and in adulthood; NOTCH3, found mainly in vascular smooth muscle and pericytes, and NOTCH4, highly expressed in endothelium (Arruga et al. 2018; Aster et al. 2017). NOTCH are surface receptors, single-pass transmembrane proteins, comprising an N-terminal extracellular portion (NECD) non-covalently bound to a transmembrane (TM) and an intracellular domain (NICD). Newly synthetized NOTCH receptors are glycosylated by the enzymes O-fucosyltransferase (OFUT) or peptide-O-fucosyltransferase (POFUT) and protein O-glucosyltransferase 1 (POGLUT1 also known as Rumi) and then firstly cleaved by PC5/furin convertases at site1 (S1) (Bocci et al. 2020; Gordon et al. 2009; Kopan 2012; Kopan and Ilagan 2009; Logeat et al. 1998) within the endoplasmic reticulum (ER) and Golgi apparatus of signal-receiving cells. Thereafter the mature receptor is exposed on the cell membrane enabling a simple cell–cell communication (Artavanis-Tsakonas et al. 1999; Bray 1998; Henrique and Schweisguth 2019; Kopan and Ilagan 2009). In the canonical pathway, the signaling is initiated through interaction of NECD with the DSL family of TM type I ligands, Delta (or Delta-like: DLL1, DLL3, DLL4) and Serrate (Jagged-like: jagged canonical Notch ligand 1 [JAG1] and jagged canonical Notch ligand 2 [JAG2]) (D'Souza et al. 2010) equipped with DSL (Delta, Serrate, Lag2) domain, on neighboring cells (juxtacrine signaling) (Figure 29.1). Ligand binding induces a conformational change, which exposes the juxtamembrane negative regulatory region (NRR) (Figure 29.1), allowing the enzymatic cleavage of the receptor by ADAM at site2 (S2). S2 cleavage generates a short-lived membrane-bound form of NOTCH, namely, NOTCH extracellular truncated (NEXT), which is then further cleaved by γ-secretase at site 3 and site 4 (S3–S4) followed by the consequent release and activation of NICD (Arruga et al. 2018). Activating interactions between NOTCH and its ligands occur only when these are present on neighboring cells (in *trans* interaction); conversely when they are exposed on the same cell (in *cis* interaction), activation is inhibited (Kopan 2012; Sprinzak et al. 2010). Once activated, NICD transduces the signal and acts as

Precision Cancer Therapies: Targeting Oncogenic Drivers and Signaling Pathways in Lymphoid Malignancies: From Concept to Practice, Volume 1, First Edition. Edited by Owen A. O'Connor, Stephen M. Ansell, and John F. Seymour.

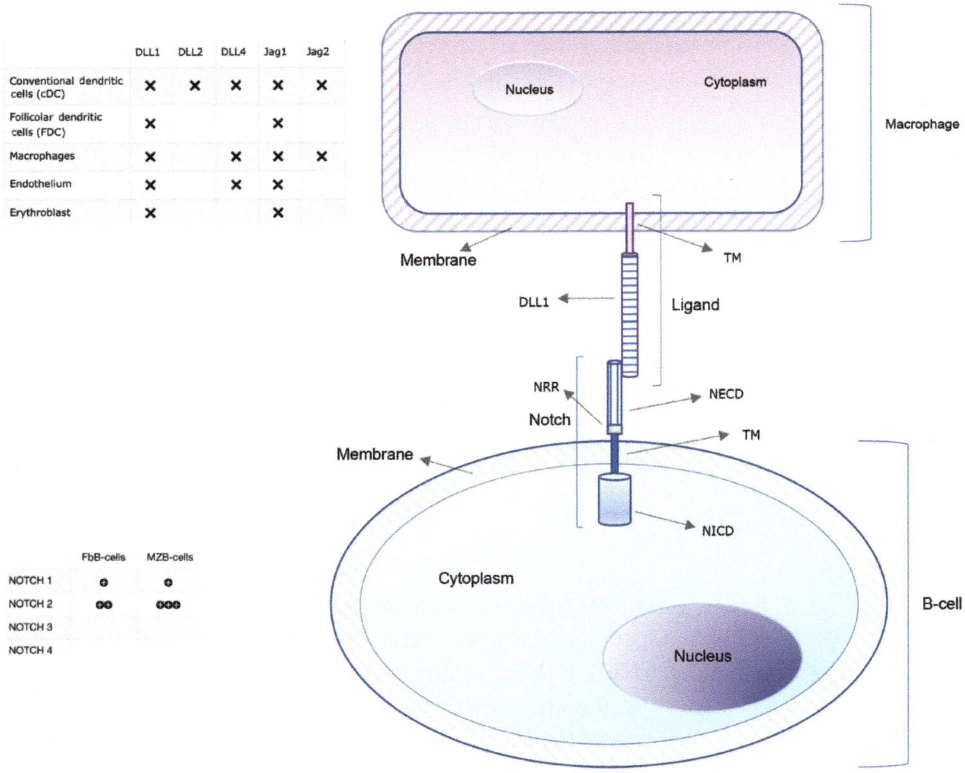

Figure 29.1 Contact between NOTCH and the ligand with a schematic representation of the DSL receptors owned by both signal sending and receiving cells. (1) The extracellular portion (NECD) of NOTCH receptor binds to a DSL ligand, a family of transmembrane (TM) type I ligands, which can be Delta (or Delta-like: DLL1, DLL3, DLL4) and Serrate (Jagged-like: Jag 1, Jag2), of the signal sending cell. (2) The binding induces a conformational change in NOTCH, which exposes the negative regulatory region (NRR) allowing the begin of the signal cascade.

a transcription regulator, traveling and entering the nucleus in order to bind the transcriptional factor CSL (mammals: CBF-1/RBP-J; *D. melanogaster*: Su(H); *Caenorhabditis elegans*: Lag-1) jointly with other transcription cofactors and activate gene transcription (Artavanis-Tsakonas et al. 1999; Henrique and Schweisguth 2019; Kopan 2012; Kopan and Ilagan 2009; Shen et al. 2021). The DNA-binding adaptor CSL can interact either with histone deacetylases (HDAC), that maintains the chromatin in a closed conformation generating repressor complexes, or with histone acetyltransferases (HATs) that conversely open up chromatin. Specifically, in canonical signaling, NCID interacts with the transcription factor RPBJK as core DNA-binding factor, alterating its composition, displacing corepressor molecules (HDAC, SMRT/HDAC1 Associated Repressor Protein (SHARP), Msx2-Interacting Nuclear Target (MINT), Split Ends (SPEN)) (Arruga et al. 2018; Bray 2006; Castel et al. 2013; Hsieh and Hayward 1995), and converting its function from that of a repressor to a transcriptional activator. NICD then recruits transcription coactivators as the adaptor protein Mastermind-like (MAML1, 2, 3) (Arruga et al. 2018; Wu et al. 2000) which in turn recruits HAT p300 (Arruga et al. 2018; Oswald et al. 2001) and other component of the transcription machinery (Kopan 2012; Kopan and Ilagan 2009) as the lysine-specific histone demethylase 1A (LSD1), also known as lysine (K)-specific demethylase 1A (KDM1A), to initiate the transcription of the downstream canonical *NOTCH* target genes including the basic helix-loop-helic (bHLH) class of transcription factors, like hes family bHLH transcription factor 1 (*HES1*) and hes related family bHLH transcription factor with YRPW motif 1 (*HEY1*) (Arruga et al. 2018; Borggrefe and Oswald 2009). The signaling pathway is shut down by phosphorylation of the NICD subunit at proline (P), glutamic acid (E), serine (S), threonine (T)-rich protein sequence (PEST) domain by C/cyclin-dependent kinase 8 (*CDK8*), and subsequent polyubiquitination by E3 ligase complex, which contains F-box and tryptophan-aspartic acid (W-D) repeat domain containing 7 (FBXW7) protein that guides NICD to proteasomal degradation (Figure 29.2). The signaling pathway from cell surface to the genome is then direct and devoid of signaling intermediate and signal amplification. Most *NOTCH*-dependent processes adopt the described core signal transduction known as the canonical pathway. NOTCH receptor activation is dependent on only four known canonical mammalian ligands. This contrasts with the pleiotropic activity of the receptor. The identification of non-canonical ligands devoid of DSL domain broadened the chance of signal activation. Non-canonical ligands can be divided into three categories: membrane-tethered, GPI-linked, and secreted. One of the first reported membrane-tethered non-canonical ligands for NOTCH is Delta-like 1 (DLK1 or PREF1, or FA1) (Bachmann et al. 1996; D'Souza et al. 2010; Laborda et al. 1993; Smas and Sul 1993), which is reported to have a role in the

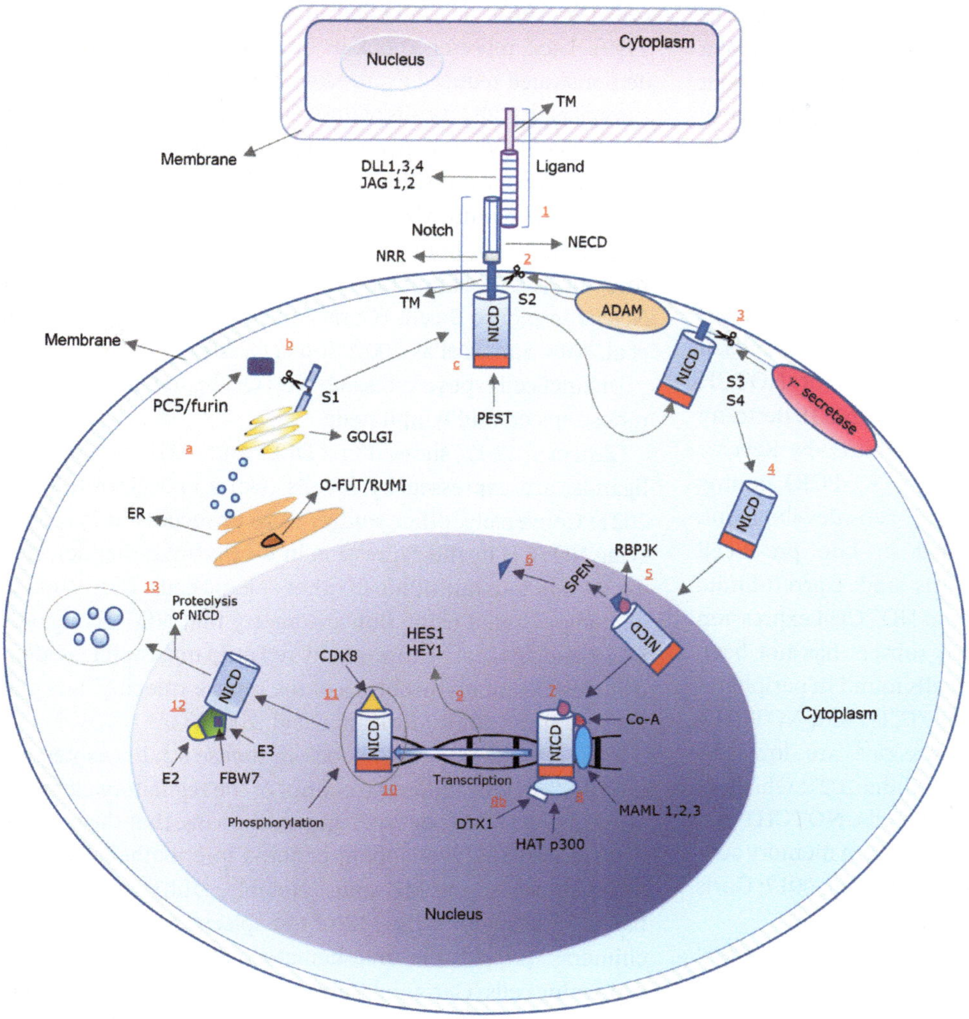

Figure 29.2 Canonical NOTCH signaling. (a) The synthesis of NOTCH begins in the ER and Golgi, where it gets glycosylated by O-FUT and RUMI. (b) Whereupon it undergoes a first cleavage by PC5/furin convertase in S1. (c) At this point the newly synthetized receptor can be exposed on the membrane, where it allows a very simple cell to cell communication. (1) The canonical signaling pathway starts when NOTCH receptor binds to a DSL ligand, inducing a conformational change that leads to the exposure of NRR, (2) allowing the cleavage of the receptor by ADAM at site 2. (3) Once this has happened two further cleavages are carried out by γ-secretase at sites 3 and 4. (4) The intercellular domain (NICD) is now activated and free to enter the nucleus, where it can act as a transcription regulator. (5) Once in the nucleus, the NICD forms a transcriptional complex, first by having RBPJK as core DNA-binding factor. (6) NICD binds to RBPJK altering its composition, displacing corepressor molecules such as SPEN allowing a functional change, transforming RBPJK from being a repressor factor to being a transcriptional factor instead. (7) RBPJK recruits the protein adaptor MAML, which in turn recruits (8) HAT p300 in role to regulate the transcription (9) of the two genes *HES1* and *HEY1*. (8b) It is well known that NOTCH activity has a self-regulating feedback loop, which can be activated by transcriptionally controlling genes encoding cytoplasmic protein that bind to RBPJK, such as DTX1. (10) Once the transcription of NICD-RBJKS complex arrives at NICD's PEST domain, (11) CDK8 binds to NICD subunit and this conducts to the phosphorylation of NICD itself. (12) Phosphorylated NICD undergoes polyubiquitination by E3 ligase complex. (13) The signaling ends with the proteasomal degradation of NICD.

inhibition of adipogenesis (D'Souza et al. 2010; Wang et al. 2006). Another integral membrane-bound NOTCH ligand is Delta/NOTCH-like EGF-related receptor (DNER) (D'Souza et al. 2010; Eiraku et al. 2002). The GPI-linked neural cell adhesion molecules, F3/contactin1 and NB3/contactin6, activate NOTCH signaling inducing oligodendrocyte (OL) differentiation (Cui et al. 2004; D'Souza et al. 2010; Hu et al. 2003). Finally, five secreted non-DSL NOTCH ligands have been reported in vertebrates: connective tissue growth factor/cysteine-rich 61/nephroblastoma overexpressed gene family member (CCN3) (D'Souza et al. 2010; Sakamoto et al. 2002b); microfibril-associated glycoprotein family (MAGP-1 and MAGP-2) (D'Souza et al. 2010; Gibson et al. 1996, 1991); thrombospondin2 (TSP2) (D'Souza et al. 2010; Meng et al. 2009); Y-*box* (YB) protein-1 (D'Souza et al. 2010; Frye et al. 2009; Rauen et al. 2009); and epidermal growth factor-like domain 7 (EGFL7) (D'Souza et al. 2010; Schmidt et al. 2009). In the non-canonical pathway after activation, NCID can bind Rat sarcoma virus-related (RRAS) protein in the cytosol promoting cell adhesion or interact with IKKα one of the catalytic subunits of the IkB kinase (IKK) complexthe core element of

Nuclear factor kappa-light-chain-enhancer of activated B cells (NF-κB) pathway, or LEF1 in the WNT pathway (the name Wnt results from the fusion of the name of the Drosophila segment polarity gene *wingless* and the name of the vertebrate homolog, integrated or *int-1*) (Henrique and Schweisguth 2019).

Role of NOTCH Signaling in B-cell

To define which functions, of the wide variety of processes influenced by NOCTH signaling, may play a role in B-cells, it is crucial to understand which components of NOTCH pathway are expressed in B-cells (He and Pear 2003). Bertrand et al. (2000) analyzed human B-cell progenitors by Reverse transcription polymerase chain reaction (RT-PCR) finding that NOTCH1 is expressed throughout B-cells development, whereas NOTCH2 is only identified in late pre-B-cell compartment ($CD34^{-}CD19^{+}\mu^{lo}$) (Garis and Garrett-Sinha 2021; Hystad et al. 2007). NOTCH3 and NOTCH4 expression in human bone marrow (BM) B-cell subsets has not been examined to date. Human CD20+ B-cells found in peripheral blood (PB) and tonsils express both NOTCH1 and NOTCH2, while NOTCH3 and NOTCH4 expressions are low and absent, respectively (Garis and Garrett-Sinha 2021; Ohishi et al. 2000; Yoon et al. 2009). In tonsillar B-cells, NOTCH1 and NOTCH2 expression was observed in naive and memory subsets but not in germinal center cells (Fabbri et al. 2017; Garis and Garrett-Sinha 2021; Valls et al. 2017).

NOTCH ligand analysis revealed that Delta is either expressed in pro-B ($CD34^{+}CD19^{+}\mu^{-}$), early pre-B ($CD34^{-}CD19^{+}\mu^{-}$), and late pre-B cells; JAG1 is expressed in BM stromal cells, which support B-cell differentiation. NOTCH and Delta coexpression in the same cell led to inhibition of NOTCH signaling.

Different expression patterns of NOTCH receptor were identified during the murine B-cell development, with *Notch2* being highly expressed by cells spanning all stages of adult B-cell development, especially mature B-cells residing in the spleen (Garis and Garrett-Sinha 2021; Saito et al. 2003). Conversely, *Notch1* expression was not detected. Saito and colleagues reported the expression of *Notch1* and *Notch3* in mouse B-cells at all stages, with the highest levels detected in pro- and pre-B-cells in the BM (Garis and Garrett-Sinha 2021; Kitamoto et al. 2005; Radtke et al. 1999; Saito et al. 2003). Walker et al. (2001) demonstrated by flow cytometry that murine BM B220+ cells express both *Notch1* and *Notch2* and that *Notch2* is also expressed in Ig^{+} splenocytes. Subsequently, Moriyama et al. (2008) showed that NOTCH1 and NOTCH2 were both detectable by flow cytometry in B220+ B-cells isolated from the spleen, while NOTCH3 was only barely detectable, and NOTCH4 was undetectable. Additionally, they proved that *Notch2* was expressed at the highest level in marginal zone (MZ) B-cells and in MZ precursors, in accordance with its prominent role in this subset (2008). Furthermore, immunohistochemistry showed that *Jag1* is expressed in BM stromal cells (Walker et al. 2001) and in the splenic MZ (Bash et al. 1999). LacZ reporter knock-in into the mouse *Notch2* locus demonstrated reduced expression of the reporter gene in transitional type I (T1) B-cells of the spleen and in mature follicular B-cells (FOB), while conversely its expression was increased in FOB precursors, transitional type II (T2) B-cells, MZ B-cell precursors, and mature MZ B-cells (Garis and Garrett-Sinha 2021; Tan et al. 2009). Both Lipopolysaccharides (LPS) and B-cell receptor (BCR) stimulation upregulated the expression of *Notch1* in mouse B-cells (Garis and Garrett-Sinha 2021; Kang et al. 2014; Santos et al. 2007; Zhu et al. 2017).

Distinct cell types expressing NOTCH ligand are present in mouse spleen and lymph node.

(Zhu et al. 2017) showed that DLL1 and JAG1, two NOTCH ligands, are expressed by B-cells (Garis and Garrett-Sinha 2021) Conversely, other studies were unsuccessful in identifying NOTCH ligand expression in B-cells but rather detected expression in a multitude of other splenic cells. Moriyama et al. demonstrated using flow cytometry that NOTCH ligands DLL1 and JAG2 are expressed by red pulp macrophages, dendritic cells, and erythroblasts of the mouse spleen (Garis and Garrett-Sinha 2021; Moriyama et al. 2008).

Tan et al. develop LacZ knock-in mouse strains expressing the LacZ enzyme under the control of the regulatory elements of the *DLL1*, *DLL4*, or *JAG1* genes, showing that these genes express partially overlapping patterns in endothelial cells of blood vessels of the MZ sinus. Notably, DLL1 was found in blood vessels within the MZ of the spleen. Additionally, BM chimeras proved the non-hematopoietic origin of LacZ-expressing cells (Garis and Garrett-Sinha 2021; Tan et al. 2009).

NOTCH ligands are also expressed by stromal fibroblastic reticular cell (FRC) subsets, which contribute to NOTCH signaling in B-cells. Depending on localization, gene expression and function FRC can be subdivided into several subsets. One of these subsets is represented by follicular dendritic cell (FDC), which has a fundamental role in organizing B-cell follicles, capturing surface-bound antigen, and stimulating germinal center reactions (Garis and Garrett-Sinha 2021; Perez-Shibayama et al. 2019).

In keeping with this, DLL1 expression in FDC of germinal centers and of the splenic MZ was detected by immunostaining of mouse spleen, while JAG1 was only evident in the MZ (Garis and Garrett-Sinha 2021; Santos et al. 2007). Additionally, this study also proposes that JAG1 versus DLL1 is also expressed by different MZ cells, indeed costaining of the two proteins did not evidenced coexpressing cells. FRC importance in the presentation of NOTCH ligands for MZ B-cell development was highlighted in a study in which DLL1 was detected either in FRC, in CD11c+ DC, or in endothelial cells (Fasnacht et al. 2014; Garis and Garrett-Sinha 2021). DLL1 deletion in FRC, but not in DC and endothelial cells, led to a complete loss of MZ B-cells. Concerning the development of the mouse MZ B-cells, Notch ligand-expressing FRC is essential and may also be implicated in other

B-cell differentiation steps in secondary lymphoid organs. Non-FRC cells such as DC, endothelial cells, and macrophages could also be involved in other B-cell responses.

NOTCH ligand expression was also investigated in human lymphoid tissues, demonstrating that human tonsil tissue and follicular dendritic cells (similarly to mouse FDC) both express DLL1 and JAG1. Furthermore, non-lymphoid cells located in the MZ in the human spleen have been shown to express DLL1 (Descatoire et al. 2014; Garis and Garrett-Sinha 2021). Hence, non-hematopoietic cells are chief expressor of NOTCH ligand either in mice or humans.

Genetic and Microenvironmental Mechanisms of NOTCH Signaling Alteration in CLL and Lymphomas

Genetic Mechanisms

The NOCTH signaling pathway is highly conserved, playing an important role in regulating cell communication, proliferation, differentiation, and apoptosis. *NOTCH* activation is highly dependent on cell type and signal strength (Gu et al. 2016). Considering the multiple roles in a wide assortment of tissues and processes, aberrations ultimately leading to the gain or loss of functions have been associated with a variety of disorders including hematological malignancies (Arruga et al. 2018). Perturbation of the physiological NOTCH signaling takes part in cancer initiation and expansion through different mechanisms. Since the first report of *NOTCH1* chromosomal translocation involvement in T-ALL in early 1990s, *NOTCH* mutations and aberrant signaling have been described in various other hematological malignances, of both myeloid and lymphoid origin either in precursor or mature cells (Gu et al. 2016). *NOTCH1* and *NOTCH2* were reported to be mutated in various mature B-cells malignancies, particularly in chronic lymphocytic leukemia (CLL), mantle cell lymphoma (MCL), and marginal zone lymphoma (MZL) but also diffuse large B-cell lymphomas (DLBCL) (Kridel et al. 2012; Lee et al. 2009; Rossi et al. 2012; Wang et al. 2011).

According to the cancer cell type, *NOTCH* could have an oncogenic or tumor suppressor role (Gu et al. 2016). The advent and systematic application of next-generation sequencing (NGS) to large cohorts of oncologic samples brought to light both known and novel genetic aberrations implicated in different steps of cancer development and progression. Multiple genes, formerly unrecognized, were revelated as recurrently mutated (Arruga et al. 2018). Functional genomic studies are needed to determine how the mutation in a given gene impacts the disease. Diverse B-cell malignancies shared mutations in *NOTCH* family members with different frequencies and mutational patterns. Qualitatively different NOTCH receptor mutations could result in similar effects on protein processing and degradation, leading to an intensified pathway activation and/or reduced protein degradation. Moreover, mutations affecting the downstream actors of NOTCH signaling pathway were described to potentiate positive signals or compromise negative regulators, denotating that multiple mechanisms in neoplastic B-cells cooperate to activate NOTCH pathway. The painted painting prove that NOTCH signaling is finely tuned in cell- and microenvironment-dependent ways. Bear in mind the role of *NOTCH* in normal B-cell development, deeper investigation is crucial to define the orchestration of events directing B-cell transformation. The relevance of NOTCH pathway in leukemia and lymphoma could translate it in an attractive therapeutic target (Arruga et al. 2018).

CLL (NOTCH1)

CLL is a common hematologic malignancy distinguished by clonal expansion of CD5+ B cells (Fabbri and Dalla-Favera 2016; Fabbri et al. 2017; Pekarsky et al. 2010). An exhaustive picture of CLL genome has been defined in the recent years, highlighting a small number of "driver" genes frequently mutated, thus the relatively low burden of genetic lesions. Genetic aberration in CLL involves the *NOTCH1* oncogene, tumor-suppressors *TP53* and *ATM*, the splicing regulator *SF3B1*, and several BCR/Nuclear factor kappa-light-chain-enhancer of activated B cells (NF-κB) regulators, including MYD88, BRRC3, and NFKBIE (Fabbri et al. 2011, 2017; Puente et al. 2011, 2015; Quesada et al. 2011; Wang et al. 2011). At diagnosis *NOTCH1* was revealed as the most commonly mutated among these genes, detected in approximately 4–13% of patients (Fabbri et al. 2011, 2017; Puente et al. 2011, 2015; Quesada et al. 2011; Wang et al. 2011).

The majority of *NOTCH1* mutational events lead to the truncation of the PEST by removing the phosphodegron sequence that is necessary for *FBXW7*-mediated ICN1 (intracellular, cleaved, and active portion of NOTCH1) proteasomal degradation. In a minority of cases, *NOTCH1* point mutation occur in the mRNA at 3′UTR, leading to aberrant splicing that results in PEST domain removal (Fabbri et al. 2011, 2017; Puente et al. 2011, 2015; Quesada et al. 2011; Wang et al. 2011).

NOTCH1 mutations were reported to be associated with poor prognosis in CLL, including a specific subset of patients with disease carrying trisomy 12, immunochemotherapy resistance, disease progression, and transformation to the highly aggressive DLBCL, termed Richter transformation (RT) (Kohlhaas et al. 2021). Unfortunately, the oncogenic role of *NOTCH1* remains poorly defined, so too does the full spectrum of *NOTCH1* controlled genes and their contribution to disease pathogenesis (Arruga et al. 2014; Fabbri et al. 2017; Maura et al. 2015; Puente et al. 2011).

Furthermore, it was reported that independently of *NOTCH1* PEST-truncation CLL cells in the lymph node frequently express ICN1 (Kluk et al. 2013; Onaindia et al. 2015), particularly within proliferation centers, representing pivotal microanatomical sites of both interaction between CLL cells with the accessory cells, and proliferation (Stein et al. 1980). These findings indicate the consequences of microenvironmental stimuli activating *NOTCH1* cascade. Ortega et al. (2015) suggested the existence of a regulatory loop in which not only *NOTCH* induces *MYC* but moreover incurs a bidirectional interaction, where *MYC* by suppressing miR-30a also affects *NOTCH* expression. *In vitro* modeling and primary sample analysis revealed that miR-30a may play a role in regulating *NOTCH* and *MYC* signals. These findings demonstrate that *MYC* can indirectly modulate *NOTCH1/2* levels via miR-30a, exploiting tumor suppressive properties and that in primary samples there is correlation between miR30a levels and *NOTCH1/2* mutational status and expression. Downregulation of miR-30a could lead to upregulation of *NOTCH1* and *NOTCH2* in B-cells malignancies. Anomalous *MYC* activation is common in various B-cells malignancies, and the consequent suppression of miR-30a leading to NOTCH1/2 overexpression may be more frequent then otherwise anticipated. Intriguingly, the consequence of R465C mutation in *FBXW7* gene is the stabilization of *MYC* (King et al. 2013), which contribute to the higher levels of NOTCH expression.

The NOTCH ligand DDL4 was reported to be directly inhibited in endothelial cells by miR-30a, -30b, and -30c (Bridge et al. 2012; Ortega et al. 2015). Additionally, miR-30b was shown to target *NOTCH1* in hematopoietic stem cells and miR-30c was shown to regulate *NOTCH1* expression in the myeloid compartment (Katzerke et al. 2013; Ortega et al. 2015; Su et al. 2013).

Kohlhaas et al. (2021) showed upregulated AKT both in CLL samples with high-risk mutations for RT, namely, those carrying *TP53* and/or *NOTCH1* mutations, and in primary RT samples. Specific *Akt* constitutive activation in B-cells was investigated in combination with Eμ-TCL1 mouse model (Eμ-TCL1Akt-C) resulting in an aggressive lymphoma phenotype with very high disease penetrance, resembling the RT clinical features (slow disease development followed by sudden progression with DLBCL-like morphology). Comparison with lack of cancer-associated mutations in control Cd19-CreAkt-C mice proved that constitutively active *Akt* alone is insufficient to drive leukemia/lymphomagenesis. Multiomics analysis highlighted an increased NOTCH signaling and S100-proteins upregulation in Eμ-TCL1Akt-C cells. Activating *Notch1* mutation is the most frequently acquired aberration in RT patients, accounting for 30% of all mutations (Fabbri and Dalla-Favera 2016; Fabbri et al. 2013; Rossi et al. 2011). S100A4 protein has been implicated in relapsed/refractory (RR) DLBCL (Fornecker et al. 2019) and has been indicated as a potential target in Acute Myeloid Leukemia (AML) (Alanazi et al. 2020), exploiting a functional role in metastasis and cytokine release (Ambartsumian et al. 2019). Furthermore, S100A4 was shown to be regulated by NOTCH and PI3K/AKT signaling in head and neck cancers. In association with NOTCH signaling increased *HES1* (target gene of NOTCH signaling) phosphorylation and expression, along with augmented WEE1 G2 checkpoint kinase (*WEE1*) and *CDK4* (associated with NOTCH signaling activation) activity in RT cells was reported (De Obaldia et al. 2013; Duan et al. 2018; Joshi et al. 2009; Kohlhaas et al. 2021). An *Akt/Notch2IC* synergism was outlined to promote B-cell differentiation toward the MZ compartment (Hampel et al. 2011). In summary, overactivation of NOTCH signaling is directed by constitutive *Akt* activation and vice versa. *Notch1* activation and target gene upregulation were validated only in RT cells. The tumor microenvironment (TME) was taken into account and investigated as a potential source of activating ligands. Here increased DLL1 ligand expression and CD41, FOXP31 specific increase in T cells of Eμ-TCL1Akt-C were identified, improving pro-survival capacity. Constitutive *Akt* activation probably drives a cell–cell interaction program leading to CD41 T-cells expansion and consequent DLL1 overexpression that arouses *Notch1* activation promoting CLL to RT transformation.

Richter's syndrome (RS) represents the evolution of CLL into a more aggressive tumor, most commonly DLBCL. Immunoglobulin heavy locus (IGH) rearrangements analysis indicates whether RS derives from the same B-cell clone or if arises as a secondary independent neoplasia, then if it is clonally related or not to CLL (Arruga et al. 2018; Rossi et al. 2011). The lack of *in vitro* and *in vivo* models severely impaired drug testing resulting in a disease poorly responsive to standard chemoimmunotherapeutic regimen as well as to novel kinase inhibitors. The establishment and genomic characterization of two patient-derived tumor xenograft (PDX) models of RS was reported in a study of Vaisitti et al. (2018), which observed that RS xenografts were genetically, morphologically, and phenotypically stable and similar to the corresponding primary tumor. One of the two PDX model was distinguishable for biallelic *Cdkn2a* and *Tp53* inactivation, monoallelic *Atm* (11q23) deletion, and mutations in *Notch2*, Bruton's tyrosine kinase (*Btk*), *Kras*, and *Egr2*. The second PDX model was characterized by trisomy 12 and mutations in *Notch2*, *Btk*, *Kras*, and *Med12*. Pathway analysis, in accordance with the mutational profile, revealed an overactivation of the BCR, NOTCH, and NF-κB pathways in both PDX models. These two PDX models of RS represent the first *ex vivo* model to investigate the biology of this disease and test novel therapeutic approaches.

Taken together these data suggest that the acquisition of genomic aberrations is not uniquely responsible for the aggressive transformation of indolent lymphomas that could also be initiated by modified functional status of potentially oncogenic signaling pathway supported from the TME (Kohlhaas et al. 2021).

MCL

MCL is an aggressive subtype of B-cell non-Hodgkin's lymphoma (NHL), incurable with standard therapies (Campo and Rule 2015; Fernandez et al. 2010; Hill et al. 2020; Jares et al. 2012; Maddocks 2018; Martin et al. 2009; Pararajalingam et al. 2020; Vose 2017; Yi et al. 2022), with an overall survival (OS) of approximately five years.

In the last decade, the identification of recurrent mutations (*TP53, ATM, NOTCH1/2, HNRNPH1, CCND1, KMT2D*) associated with MCL (Bea et al. 2009, 2013; Delarue et al. 2013; Hill et al. 2020; Pararajalingam et al. 2020; Yi et al. 2022; Zhang et al. 2014) and genetic lesions (del[9p], *ARID1A, SMARCA4*) which increase the resistance to chemoimmunotherapy or targeted therapies (Agarwal et al. 2019; Eskelund et al. 2017; Pararajalingam et al. 2020; Yi et al. 2022; Zhang et al. 2019) was made possible by the advent of massively unbiased parallel sequencing of whole exomes (WES) and RNA-seq of MCL samples. Unfortunately, previous analyses were limited by several restrictions, such as the use of small cohorts in studies utilizing an unbiased approach (Nadeu et al. 2020; Pararajalingam et al. 2020; Yi et al. 2022) that reduced the capability to define and associate patterns of genetic lesions with clinical outcomes, further the limited availability of matched WES, an RNA-seq data, hampered the connection between genotype and phenotype. Finally, the lack of longitudinal samples prevented the evaluation of clonal evolution of MCL in relation of the disease progression to chemoimmunotherapy (Yi et al. 2022). Shuhua et al. performed WES on 152 MCL tumor samples collected from 134 patients, 48 samples had matched RNA-seq data and for 16 patients longitudinal sample collection was faisible. They (Yi et al. 2022) reported that, consistent with other publications (Eskelund et al. 2017; Kridel et al. 2012), *NOTCH1* and/or *TP53* mutations were associated with shorter progression-free survival (PFS). Importantly, their coordinate genetic signatures allowed the identification of genetic subtypes of MCL based on shared genetic features, they applied to 35 recurrent genetic alterations, a non-negative matrix factorization (NMF) consensus clustering algorithm, discovering four clusters with a unique gene expression pattern and different clinical behavior. PFS and OS were significantly different among clusters, patients with C1 subtype had more favorable outcome compared with C2, C3, and C4 subtypes. C1 subtype patients did not reach median PFS, which was 41.2 months for C2, 30.7 months for C3, and 16.1 months for C4. A five-year OS rates for C1–C4 were 100%, 56.7%, 48.7%, and 14.2%, respectively. The 32% of samples enriched in *NOTCH1* mutations were included in C3, which also harbored mutations in *NSD2* (*WHSC1*), *KMT2D*, *SP140*, amp(13q), and del(6q). C3 subtype also showed significant downregulation of genes involved in TNF-α signaling via NF-κB pathway and Interferon-γ (INF-γ) response, but with activated NOTCH signaling. Downregulation in C3 also affected both BCR and IL-2 STAT5 signaling, and *MYC* targets. Cluster analysis results in C1 highly enriched in non-nodal MCL (nnMCL) and C2–C4 are predominantly conventional MCL (cMCL). cMCL presenting similar symptoms were distinguished in three distinct genetic clusters, all characterized by dysregulated cellular pathways. These molecular clusters provide clues for future biomarker-driven clinical trial design aligning treatment with patients most likely to benefit, opening the door to precision medicine creating a connection between genetic discovery and its clinical application (Yi et al. 2022).

FL

Follicular lymphoma (FL) is one of the most common malignant lymphomas, with 80% of cases characterized by the t(14;18)(q32;q21) translocation which plays an important role in lymphomagenesis. Karube et al. reported *NOTCH1* and *NOTCH2* mutations in 6.3% of FL analyzed cases, all of them resulted in protein truncation in the PEST domain, exactly as those identified in other B-cell lymphomas. FL cases affected by *NOTCH* mutations were distinguished by a lower t(14;18)(q32;q21) translocation frequency, a higher incidence of splenic involvement, female predominance, and a more frequent DLBCL component. These results denote that *NOTCH* mutations are uncommon in FL, but can occur in a subset of cases with distinctive clinicopathological features (Karube et al. 2014). The frequency of *NOTCH* mutations in FL is similar to that observed in CLL (4–10%) (Balatti et al. 2012; Fabbri et al. 2011; Karube et al. 2014; Puente et al. 2011; Strefford et al. 2013) and lower compared to MCL (10–12%) (Bea et al. 2009; Karube et al. 2014; Kridel et al. 2012) or splenic marginal zone lymphoma (SMZL) (20–25%) (Karube et al. 2014; Kiel et al. 2012; Rossi et al. 2012). *NOTCH1* and *NOTCH2* mutation ratios differ among these malignancies, with nearly all CLL mutations involving *NOTCH1* with very rare mutations in *NOTCH2* (Fabbri et al. 2013; Karube et al. 2014), conversely about 20% of SMZL shows *NOTCH2* mutations and only 5% has mutation in *NOTCH1* (Karube et al. 2014; Rossi et al. 2012). In MCL, similar frequency of *NOTCH1* and *NOTCH2* mutations was reported (around 5%) (Bea et al. 2013; Karube et al. 2014). In FL, *NOTCH1* was slightly more frequent compared to *NOTCH2*. A subsequent study (Valls et al. 2017) analyzed the gene promoter directly targeted by *BCL6* in human FL. In the aforementioned study, BCL6 repression of NOTCH2 and NOTCH pathway genes was reported. Moreover, they demonstrate an inverse correlation between NOTCH2 and BCL6 pathway gene expression in FL. Comparison of GC B-cells to their naive B-cells precursor resulted in the downregulation of *NOTCH2*, *MAML1*, and several key NOTCH targets. For the development of fully established GCs *NOTCH2* must be silenced. The master regulator of GC formation *BCL6* mediates this downregulation.

They stated that *NOTCH* suppression is a key function of *BCL6* in FL, indeed *BCL6* blockade of induced cell death could be rescued by *NOTCH2* siRNA or antagonist, while *NOTCH2* expression killed FL cells. *NOTCH2* is thus considered a growth suppressor of FL, on the other side *BCL6* mediates FL pathogenesis partially through suppression of NOTCH2 pathway. Vallas et al. (2017) also corroborated these data demonstrating that *Bcl6* inhibitors induced *Notch2* suppressing the FL xenografts growth *in vivo*. The retroinverso BCL6 peptide inhibitor (RI-BPI) is a compound able to block only the N-terminal poxvirus and zinc finger/bric-à-brac, tramtrack and broad complex (POZ/BTB) domain of *Bcl6*, then only affect certain function and does not induce toxicity or inflammation in a long-term treatment of animals, confirming that FL survival is dependent on *Bcl6* recruitment of corepressors to the *Bcl6* POZ/BTB domain.

MZL (NOTCH2)

SMZL is a rare B-cell tumor, of which the pathogenesis remains unknown (Rossi et al. 2012; Trøen et al. 2004). The presence of *TP53* mutation, 7q22–7q31 deletion, or the absence of somatic hypermutations of immunoglobulin genes were correlated with worse prognosis. A first genome-wide gene expression study (Trøen et al. 2004), exploiting the microarray technique on 24 SMZL cases, showed that *NOTCH2* as well as *AP-1* proto-oncogene transcription factors JUN (or c-Jun), JUND, JUNB, and FOS (or c-fos) were specifically upregulated. *NOTCH2* is a transcription factor that induces MZ B-cell differentiation, in which upregulation is indicative for an MZ origin of SMZL (Trøen et al. 2004).

Another study (Rossi et al. 2012) integrating WES and copy number analysis (CNA) showed that SMZL exome carries merely 30 non-silent gene alterations (about 25 non-silent mutations and about 5 CNA per case). Alterations in genes of the NOTCH pathway were highly recurrent (30%) in SMZL, with *NOTCH2* gene most frequently involved (20% of cases). All *NOTCH2* mutations lead to the elimination of C-terminal PEST domain, which is required for proteasomal recruitment, impairing *NOTCH2* degradation (Lee et al. 2009; Rossi et al. 2012) then activating NOTCH2 signaling. In addition to *NOTCH2*, genetic lesions in SMZL are recurrently targeted other modulators or members of the NOTCH pathway, among them *NOTCH1*, *SPEN*, and *DTX1*. Rossi et al. (2012) also reported mutations in other signaling pathways normally involved in MZ B-cell development, indicating that deregulation of MZ B-cell development pathway intervenes in the pathogenesis of about 60% SMZL. Gene expression profiling together with genome-wide DNA-promoter methylation profiling and clinical and biological variables were integrated in a subsequent study (Arribas et al. 2015), where an unsupervised clustering analysis identified two clusters differing in promoter methylation in a test series of 98 samples, then confirmed in an independent validation set of 36 patients. The cluster consisting of patients with higher promoter methylation (high-M) had a shorter OS compared with the cluster with lower promoter methylation (low-M). Interestingly, we showed that the High-M phenotype was related to mutations of the *NOTCH2* gene, IGHV1-02*4 use, loss of 7q31–32, and histologic transformation.

Clonal B-cell expansion has an immunophenotype consistent with MZL, but presents with isolated lymphocytosis and lack of splenic or lymph node enlargements. Xochelli et al. (2014) proposed that in a future classification of B-cell malignancies these lymphoproliferations should be classified as clonal B-cell lymphocytosis with marginal zone features (CBL-MZ). Buscaggin et al. (2014) investigated 16 PB samples of CBL-MZ, identifying according to the criteria defined by Xochelli et al., mutations of *NOTCH1*, *NOTCH2*, *BRAF*, *BIRC3*, *TRAF3*, *TNFAIP3*, *IKBKB*, *MYD88*, *CD79A*, *CD79B*, *CARD11*, and *MAP2K1*. They found mutually exclusive genetic lesions in genes belonging to the program of physiological MZ differentiation in 37% of CBL-MZ cases, a prevalence similar to that described in SMZL. *MYD88* mutations were observed in 25% of cases, *NOTCH2* mutations were reported in 13% of cases, and *TNFAIP3* and *CD79B* mutation in 6% of cases. *NOTCH2* mutations clustered together with cases presenting an intrasinusoidal pattern of BM infiltration, conversely *MYD88* mutations were enriched in cases secreting an IgM monoclonal component, while *MAP2K1* mutations were absent. These results denote that CBL-MZ and SMZL share a similar genotype that could be indicative of a common oncogenic pathway between these disorders. This is consistent with the observation of Xochelli et al. (2014) of recurrent 7q deletion in CBL-MZ, which is also a marker of SMZL (Rinaldi et al. 2011). CBL-MZ presenting in the PB with small B-cell clones harbors mutations of MZ differentiation genes in 43% of cases, indicating that these mutations are early events in the oncogenic process of MZ tumors.

Nodal marginal zone lymphoma (NMZL) is a rare, indolent B-cell neoplasms, differing from SMZL by the dissemination pattern. NMZL is primarily a nodal B-cell tumor with no clinical evidence of splenic or extranodal disease (Arruga et al. 2018; Swerdlow et al. 2008; Thieblemont et al. 2011). The NMZL mutational profile resembles that of SMZL but a distinctive pattern of non-silent somatic lesions in NMZL was identified in a study of Spina et al. (2016) that combined WES, targeted sequencing of tumor-related genes, whole transcriptome sequencing, and analysis of high-resolution single nucleotide polymorphism array. This analysis of 35 cases of NMZL featured 41 recurrently impaired genes (in more than 9% of cases), in particular *KMT2D* (34%), *NOTCH2* and *PTPRD* (20%), and *KLF2* (17%). Although NMZL and SMZL shared a common mutation profile, mutations of *PTPRD*, a receptor protein tyrosine phosphatase involved in cell growth regulation, were only found in NMZL across mature B-cell malignancies and led to loss of PTPRD phosphatase activity ending in cell-cycle transcriptional program deregulation and increased NMZL proliferation index. Shanmugam et al. (2021) screened a wide range of B-cell tumors for *NOTCH* activation by immunohistochemical staining revealing that N2ICD is primarily identified in SMZL, including cases with wild-type (WT) or mutated *NOTCH2*, as for previously reported for *NOTCH1* in CLL. Greater *NOTCH2* activation has been reported in SMZL with *NOTCH2* mutations, in particular within splenic MZ. Conversely, in DLBCL, even in *NOTCH2* mutated cases, scarce evidence of *NOTCH2* activation was described, confining selective pressure for *NOTCH2* activation to low-grade B-cell tumors. On the other hand, in DLBCL with *NOTCH1* mutations its activation was noted.

Finally, a study of Bonfiglio et al. (2022) investigated 303 SMZL spleen samples collected through the IELSG46 multicenter international study taking advantage of a multiplatform approach. Genetic and phenotypic analysis allowed to define self-organized signatures which were then validated in independent primary tumor metadata and finally determined correlation with outcome data. This effort permitted to identify two prominent genetic cluster in SMZL, named NNK- and DMT-SMZLs, with NNK that stand for *NF-κB*, *NOTCH*, and *KLF2* modules, inclusive of 58% of cases, and DMT for DNA-damage response, *MAPK* and *TLR* modules comprising 32% of cases. NNK- and DMT-SMZLs were distinguished not only based on genetic aberrations in multiple genes but also for cytogenetic and immunogenetic features. These genetic clusters not only have differences in gene-expression signatures but also distinct outcomes, with shorter survival in NKK-SMZL. Two distinct types of SMZL immune microenvironment were also defined by digital cytometry and *in situ* profiling, the immune suppressive SMZL, associated with inflammation and immune checkpoint activation in 50% of cases, and the immune-silent SMZL, associated with an immune-excluded phenotype in the other half of cases.

DLBCL (N1 e N2)

DLBCL is the most common lymphoid malignancies in adults and is genetically and phenotypically heterogeneous. Hepatitis C virus (HCV) was shown to be associated with B-cell NHL, particularly with DLBCL and MZL. NOTCH signaling pathway mutations were analyzed in patients enrolled in a study of Arcaini et al. (2015) with 46 cases of DLBCL positive for HCV and 64 patients with DLBCL unrelated to HCV. *NOTCH2* mutations were reported in 20% of HCV-positive patients, while *NOTCH1* mutations only in 4% of HCV-positive cases. Conversely, only one of the HCV-negative samples had a *NOTCH1* or *NOTCH2* mutation. NOTCH pathway lesions were significantly more frequent in HCV-positive patients, resulting in reduced five-year OS, equal to 27% in HCV-positive DLBCL with a mutation in the NOTCH pathway compared to 62% of OS in DLBCL not affected by these genetic lesions. Univariate analysis found an association with shorter OS for age over 60 years, with the presence of *NOTCH2* mutations or any mutation of the NOTCH pathway, which retained an independent significance ($p = 0.029$). They concluded that a subset of DLBCL with positive HCV showed a molecular signature of SMZL and had a worse clinical outcome (Arcaini et al. 2015). Thanks to the gene-expression profiling, subgroups of DLBCL were identified in a following study (Schmitz et al. 2018), named activated B-cell-like (ABC), germinal-center B-cell-like (GCB), and unclassified, according to the cell-of-origin, associated with different response to chemotherapeutic and targeted agents. Schmitz and colleagues (Schmitz et al. 2018) analyzed 574 DLBCL biopsy samples by exome and transcriptome sequencing, array-based DNA CNA, and targeted amplicon resequencing of 372 genes, to determine genes recurrently impaired. They also developed an algorithm to unravel genetic subtypes based on the co-occurrence of genetic lesions. Four prominent genetic clusters were distinguished in DLBCL, namely, MCD (due to the co-occurrence of *MYD88*, *L265P*, and *CD79B*), BN2 (characterized by *BCL6* fusions and *NOTCH2* mutations), N1 (based on *NOTCH1* mutations), and EZB (which stands for *EZH2* mutations and *BCL2* translocations). These subtypes were phenotypically different as demonstrated by differences in gene-expression signatures and immunochemotherapeutic responses; favorable survival was attributed to BN2 and EZB subtypes compared to MCD and N1 subtypes with worst outcomes. MCD and BN2 DLBCL were demonstrated to relay on constitutively active BCR signaling that is sensitive to therapeutic inhibition (Schmitz et al. 2018). Chapuy et al. (2018) carried out a comprehensive genetic analysis on 304 primary DLBCLs identifying low-frequency alterations, recurrent mutations, structural variants (SV), and somatic copy number alterations, defining coordinate signatures in patients having available outcome data.

Consensus clustering was employed to integrate these genetic drivers and permitted the identification of five robust DLBCL subsets: a previously unidentified low-risk ABC-DLBCLs group of extrafollicular/MZ origin; an ABC/GCB-independent group showing biallelic inactivation of *TP53*, with the loss of *CDKN2A* and genomic instability, and two distinct groups of GCB-DLBCLs with targetable alterations and different outcomes. Independent of the clinical International Prognostic Index (IPI), coordinate genetic signatures were able to predict outcome and suggest new treatment combinations possibilities (Chapuy et al. 2018).

Other Genes of the Pathway (FBXW7, SPEN)

The ubiquitin–proteasome system (UPS) takes part in various aspects of cellular process, such as cell cycle progression, differentiation, and survival. *FBXW7*, also known as Sel10, hCDC4, or hAgo, member of the F-box protein family, operates as the substrate recognition component of the SCF E3 ubiquitin ligase. *FBXW7* regulates the degradation of oncoproteins such as NOTCH, C-MYC, cyclin E, MCL-1, mammalian target of rapamycin (mTOR), JUN, and AURKA. The tumor suppressor FBXW7 is one of the most commonly deregulated proteins of the ubiquitin–proteasome system in human tumor. Consistently, *FBXW7* is located at chromosome 4q32, this genomic region is deleted in more than 30% of all human cancers (Yeh et al. 2018). Chapuy et al. (2018) reported that CLUMPS (called EMPRINT) was able to identify mutations clustering at the acceptor groove of *FBXW7*, limiting *CCNE1* recognition and *CUL1/SKP1/FBXW7*-mediated degradation, a tumor suppressor mechanism already reported for other malignancies. High-throughput sequencing of human genetic profiles revealed the high frequency of mutations of *FBXW7* in human cancers, in which function is also inactivated in cancer cells through other mechanisms involving microRNA, long non-coding RNA, and specific oncogenic signaling pathways. *FBXW7* inactivation could open the possibility to selectively target mutant cells through synthetic-lethal mechanism or oncogene dependence. Genes that are selectively essential in cell lines carrying specific driver mutations, but not in healthy cells expressing WT *FBXW7*, could be targeted allowing these mechanisms. Moreover, another study of Yeh et al. (2018) reported that human breast cancer cells experiencing loss of *FBXW7* became hypersensitive to rapamycin (Yeh et al. 2018; Ying et al. 2013), an mTOR inhibitor able to revert the oncogenic effect of *FBXW7* mutation. It was demonstrated that downregulation of *GSK3β* reduces C-MYC T58 phosphorylation, leading to *FBXW7*-mediated C-MYC degradation impairment. Additionally, C-MYC accumulation increases tumor necrosis factor (TNF)-related apoptosis-inducing ligand 5 (*TRAIL5*) expression, which consequently increases death receptor *TRAILR5*-induced apoptosis both *in vitro* and *in vivo* (Yeh et al. 2018; Yumimoto et al. 2015). In the same way, vorinostat, an HDAC inhibitor, induced apoptosis by downregulating MCL-1 and upregulating pro-apoptotic proteins such NOXA and BIM (Greninger et al. 2013; Yeh et al. 2018). Consistently, *FBXW7* mutation in squamous cell carcinoma (SCC) increased *MCL-1* and *BIM* expression, leading to resistance to standard chemotherapy but increased susceptibility to HDAC inhibitors. In conclusion, in *FBXW7*-deficient human colorectal cells a dependency on spindle assembly checkpoint proteins BUBR1, BUB1, and MPS1 was shown, it was also demonstrated that reducing BURB1 in cells deficient for *FBXW7* ultimately leads to cell aneuploidy and overexpression of p53 (Bailey et al. 2015; Yeh et al. 2018). *Fbxw7* not only has cell-autonomous functions in tumor cells, but it was also shown to affect the TME inhibiting tumor metastasis (Yeh et al. 2018; Yumimoto et al. 2015). In detail, *Fbxw7* KO in mouse BM-derived stromal cells upregulates *Notch* expression leading to C-C motif chemokine ligand 2 (*Ccl2*) activation. Upregulation of *Ccl2* in serum leads to monocytic myeloid-derived suppressor cells and macrophages recruitment to the tumor site, thus increasing tumor metastasis. *Ccl2* receptor antagonist may revert the effect of *Fbxw7* depletion, providing a therapeutic strategy to target *FBXW7*-deficient cells in the clinic (Yeh et al. 2018; Yumimoto et al. 2015). *FBXW7* mutations reported are mainly heterozygote, then it is crucial to understand the contribution of both FBXW7 monomers and dimers within a double- or single-mutated unit.

SPEN mutations are reported in a small percentage of SMZL (5%), in 14% NMZL, and also in the BN2 subtype of DLBCL.

The previously cited analysis of Chapuy et al. (2018) on 304 primary DLBCL samples also reported truncating mutations of *SPEN*, the negative regulator of B lymphocyte differentiation into MZ B-cells, which counteract *NOTCH2* activity, (Arruga et al. 2018; Kuroda et al. 2003) associated with cluster 1 (C1) DLBCL, along with *BCL6* and *NF-κB* (Arruga et al. 2018; Chapuy et al. 2018; Schmitz et al. 2018). *SPEN* plays a role in repressing NOTCH signaling by physical interaction and resulting in the repression of *RBPJK* (Arruga et al. 2018; Kuroda et al. 2003; Li et al. 2005; VanderWielen et al. 2011). Actually *SPEN* mutations truncate its C-terminal domain which is implicated in *RBPJK* interaction and is crucial for NOTCH signaling activation.

Inhibitors Tested at the Preclinical Level

Ibrutinib is a small molecule compound able to inhibit B-cell proliferation and survival by irreversible binding to *BTK* and consequent inhibition of BCR pathway, that is commonly aberrantly activated in B-cell tumors. Tumors of the ABC gene expression subgroup of DLBCL depend on chronic active B-cell receptor signaling to survive, this dependency is targetable by ibrutinib. Consistently, a survival advantage was obtained by adding ibrutinib to rituximab, cyclophosphamide, hydroxydaunorubicin hydrochloride (doxorubicin hydrochloride), vincristine (Oncovin) and prednisone (R-CHOP) chemotherapy in younger patients with non-GCB DLBCL in the phase 3 Phoenix clinical trial (NCT01855750). Younger patients of MCD and N1 subtype of DLBCL treated with ibrutinib plus R-CHOP had a three-year event-free survival of 100%, while patients with the same subtype treated just with R-CHOP had significantly inferior event-free survival (42.9% and 50%, respectively) (Wilson et al. 2021). NOTCH1 is strictly connected to various signaling pathways involved in tumorgenesis: they can influence proliferation, immune response, chemosensitivity, apoptosis, and cancer stem cells. Various methods can lead to *NOTCH1* inhibition, most commonly γ-secretase inhibitors are employed, producing a pan-NOTCH inhibition, or the use of *NOTCH1* siRNA or NOTCH1 monoclonal antibodies, producing a more specific blockade. *NOTCH1* downregulation can be adopted alone or in combination with chemotherapy, achieving a synergistic effect and a decrease in chemoresistance, offering an addition to therapeutic strategies adopted for managing cancer harboring high expression levels of *NOTCH1* (Gharaibeh et al. 2020). The role of *NOTCH1* is as heterogeneous as cancer, depending on the type of cancer, its stage and mutations in other relevant genes, *NOTCH1* interacts with different signaling pathways and can behave as tumor suppressor or as oncogene. Regardless its broad role, *NOTCH1* is a valuable target to explore and find new and safer therapeutic options (Gharaibeh et al. 2020). MRK-003 is a potent and selective γ-secretase inhibitor which was evaluated by Mizuma et al. (2012), which was demonstrated to be effective in pancreatic ductal adenocarcinoma (PDAC), a lethal malignancy characterized by aberrant NOTCH pathway activation. The efficacy of MRK-003 was evidenced by nuclear N1ICD downregulation and the consequent inhibition of anchorage-independent growth along with the reduction of tumor-initiating cells able of self-renewal. MRK-003 monotherapy blocked the growing of the tumor in 56% of the xenografts and the combination with gemcitabine showed enhanced anti-tumor effect compared to gemcitabine alone (44%), reducing tumor cell proliferation and inducing apoptosis and intratumoral necrosis. MRK-003 was particularly effective in tumors harboring upregulation of NF-κB pathway components, on the other side upregulation in BCR signaling and nuclear factor erythroid-derived 2-like 2 (NRF2) pathway was connected with response to MRK-003 combination with gemcitabine. These findings support the rationale for small molecule inhibition of NOTCH signaling as potential therapeutic strategy (Kuroda et al. 2003).

Must Read References

Bonfiglio, F., Bruscaggin, A., Guidetti, F., Terzi Di Bergamo, L., Faderl, M., et al. (2022 February 3). Genetic and phenotypic attributes of splenic marginal zone lymphoma. *Blood* 139 (5): 732–747. doi: 10.1182/blood.2021012386. PMID: 34653238.

Chapuy, B., Stewart, C., Dunford, A.J., Kim, J., Kamburov, A. et al. (2018 May). Molecular subtypes of diffuse large B cell lymphoma are associated with distinct pathogenic mechanisms and outcomes. *Nat. Med.* 24 (5): 679–690. doi: 10.1038/s41591-018-0016-8. Epub 2018 Apr 30. Erratum in: Nat Med. 2018 Aug;24(8):1292.Erratum in: Nat Med. 2018 Aug;24(8):1290–1291. PMID: 29713087; PMCID: PMC6613387.

Fabbri, G., Rasi, S., Rossi, D. et al. (2011). Analysis of the chronic lymphocytic leukemia coding genome: role of NOTCH1 mutational activation. *J. Exp. Med.* 208: 1389–1401.

Garis, M., and Garrett-Sinha, L.A. (2021 February 5). Notch signaling in B cell immune responses. *Front Immunol.* 11: 609324. doi: 10.3389/fimmu.2020.609324. PMID: 33613531; PMCID: PMC7892449.

References

Agarwal, R. et al. (2019). Dynamic molecular monitoring reveals that SWI–SNF mutations mediate resistance to ibrutinib plus venetoclax in mantle cell lymphoma. *Nat. Med.* 25 (1): 119–129.

Alanazi, B., Munje, C.R., Rastogi, N. et al. (2020). Integrated nuclear proteomics and transcriptomics identifies S100A4 as a therapeutic target in acute myeloid leukemia. *Leukemia* 34 (2): 427–440.

Ambartsumian, N., Klingelhofer, J., and Grigorian, M. (2019). The multifaceted S100A4 protein in cancer and inflammation. *Methods Mol. Biol.* 1929: 339–365.

Arcaini, L., Rossi, D., Lucioni, M., Nicola, M., Bruscaggin, A. et al. (2015 February). The NOTCH pathway is recurrently mutated in diffuse large B-cell lymphoma associated with hepatitis C virus infection. *Haematol.* 100 (2): 246–252. doi: 10.3324/haematol.2014.116855. Epub 2014 Nov 7. PMID: 25381127; PMCID: PMC4803124.

Arribas, A.J., Rinaldi, A., Mensah, A.A., Kwee, I., Cascione, L. et al. (2015March 19). DNA methylation profiling identifies two splenic marginal zone lymphoma subgroups with different clinical and genetic features. *Blood* 125(12): 1922–1931. doi: 10.1182/blood-2014-08-596247. Epub 2015 Jan 22. PMID: 25612624; PMCID: PMC4416938.

Arruga, F. et al. (2014). Functional impact of NOTCH1 mutations in chronic lymphocytic leukemia. *Leukemia* 28 (5): 1060–1070.

Arruga, F., Vaisitti, T., and Deaglio, S. (2018 November 26). The NOTCH pathway and its mutations in mature B cell malignancies. *Front Oncol.* 8: 550. doi: 10.3389/fonc.2018.00550. PMID: 30534535; PMCID: PMC6275466.

Artavanis-Tsakonas, S., Rand, M.D., and Lake, R.J. (1999 April 30). Notch signaling: cell fate control and signal integration in development. *Science* 284 (5415): 770–776. doi: 10.1126/science.284.5415.770. PMID: 10221902.

Aster, J.C., Pear, W.S., and Blacklow, S.C. (2017 Janauary 24). The varied roles of Notch in cancer. *Annu. Rev. Pathol.* 12: 245–275. doi: 10.1146/annurev-pathol-052016-100127. Epub 2016 Dec 5. PMID: 27959635; PMCID: PMC5933931.

Bachmann, E., Krogh, T.N., Hojrup, P., Skjodt, K., and Teisner, B. (1996). Mouse fetal antigen 1 (mFA1), the circulating gene product of mdlk, pref-1 and SCP-1: isolation, characterization and biology. *J. Reprod. Fertil.* 107: 279–285. [PubMed: 8882295].

Bailey, M.L., Singh, T., Mero, P., Moffat, J., and Hieter, P. (2015 November). Dependence of human Colorectal cells lacking the FBW7 tumor suppressor on the Spindle assembly checkpoint. *Genetics* 201 (3): 885–895. doi: 10.1534/genetics.115.180653. Epub 2015 Sep 8. PMID: 26354767; PMCID: PMC4649658.

Balatti, V., Bottoni, A., Palamarchuk, A. et al. (2012). NOTCH1mutations inCLL associated with trisomy 12. *Blood* 119: 329–331.

Bash, J., Zong, W.X., Banga, S., Rivera, A., Ballard, D.W., Ron, Y. et al. (1999). Rel/NF-kappaB can trigger the Notch signaling pathway by inducing the expression of Jagged1, a ligand for Notch receptors. *EMBO J.* 18: 2803–2811.

Bea, S. et al. (2009). Uniparental disomies, homozygous deletions, amplifications, and target genes in mantle cell lymphoma revealed by integrative high–resolution whole–genome profiling. *Blood* 113 (13): 3059–3069.

Bea, S. et al. (2013). Landscape of somatic mutations and clonal evolution in mantle cell lymphoma. *Proc. Natl. Acad. Sci. U.S.A.* 110 (45): 18250–18255.

Bertrand, F.E., Eckfeldt, C.E., Lysholm, A.S., and LeBien, T.W. (2000). Notch1 and Notch2 exhibit unique patterns of expression in human B-lineage cells. *Leukemia* 14: 2095–2102.

Bocci, F., Onuchic, J.N., and Jolly, M.K. (2020 July 31). Understanding the principles of pattern formation driven by Notch signaling by integrating experiments and theoretical models. *Front Physiol.* 11: 929. doi: 10.3389/fphys.2020.00929. PMID: 32848867; PMCID: PMC7411240.

Bonfiglio, F., Bruscaggin, A., Guidetti, F., Terzi Di Bergamo, L., Faderl, M., et al. (2022 February 3). Genetic and phenotypic attributes of splenic marginal zone lymphoma. *Blood* 139 (5): 732–747. doi: 10.1182/blood.2021012386. PMID: 34653238.

Borggrefe, T. and Oswald, F. (2009). The Notch signaling pathway: transcriptional regulation at Notch target genes. *Cell Mol. Life Sci.* 66: 1631–1646. doi: 10.1007/s00018-009-8668-7.

Bray, S. (1998 December). Notch signalling in Drosophila: three ways to use a pathway. *Semin. Cell Dev. Biol.* 9 (6): 591–597. doi: 10.1006/scdb.1998.0262. PMID: 10075488.

Bray, S.J. (2006). Notch signalling: a simple pathway becomes complex. *Nat. Rev. Mol. Cell Biol.* 7: 678–689. doi: 10.1038/nrm2009.

Bridge, G., Monteiro, R., Henderson, S., Emuss, V., Lagos, D., Georgopoulou, D. et al. (2012 December 13).The microRNA-30 family targets DLL4 to modulate endothelial cell behavior during angiogenesis. *Blood* 120(25):5063–5072. [PubMed: 23086751] 38. Jiang, Q., Lagos-Quintana, M., Liu, D., Shi, Y., Helker, C., Herzog, W., et al. (2013 September). miR-30a regulates endothelial tip cell formation and arteriolar branching. *Hypertension* 62 (3): 592–598. [PubMed: 23817492].

Bruscaggin, A., Monti, S., Arcaini, L., Ramponi, A., Rattotti, S., Lucioni, M., Paulli, M., Gaidano, G., and Rossi, D. (2014December). Molecular lesions of signalling pathway genes in clonal B-cell lymphocytosis with marginal zone features. *Br. J. Haematol.* 167 (5): 718–720. doi: 10.1111/bjh.13052. Epub 2014 Aug 4. PMID: 25088352.

Campo, E. and Rule, S. (2015). Mantle cell lymphoma: evolving management strategies. *Blood* 125 (1): 48–55.

Castel, D., Mourikis, P., Bartels, S.J., Brinkman, A.B., Tajbakhsh, S., and Stunnenberg, H.G. (2013). Dynamic binding of RBPJ is determined by Notch signaling status. *Genes Dev.* 27: 1059–1071. doi: 10.1101/gad.211912.112.

Chapuy, B., Stewart, C., Dunford, A.J., Kim, J., Kamburov, A. et al. (2018 May). Molecular subtypes of diffuse large B cell lymphoma are associated with distinct pathogenic mechanisms and outcomes. *Nat. Med.* 24 (5): 679–690. doi: 10.1038/s41591-018-0016-8. Epub 2018 Apr 30. Erratum in: Nat Med. 2018 Aug;24(8):1292.Erratum in: Nat Med. 2018 Aug;24(8):1290–1291. PMID: 29713087; PMCID: PMC6613387.

Cui, X.Y., Hu, Q.D., Tekaya, M., Shimoda, Y., Ang, B.T. et al. (2004). NB-3/Notch1 pathway via Deltex1 promotes neural progenitor cell differentiation into oligodendrocytes. *J. Biol. Chem.* 279: 25858–25865. [PubMed: 15082708].

D'Souza, B. et al. (2010). Canonical and non-canonical Notch ligands. *Curr. Top. Dev. Bio.* 92: 73–129. doi: 10.1016/S0070-2153(10)92003-6.

D'Souza, B., Meloty-Kapella, L., and Weinmaster, G. (2010). Canonical and non-canonical Notch ligands. *Curr. Top. Dev. Biol.* 92: 73–129. doi: 10.1016/S0070-2153(10)92003-6. PMID: 20816393; PMCID: PMC4286395.

De Obaldia, M.E., Bell, J.J., Wang, X. et al. (2013). T cell development requires constraint of the myeloid regulator C/EBP-a by the Notch target and transcriptional repressor Hes1. *Nat. Immunol.* 14 (12): 1277–1284.

Delarue, R. et al. (2013). CHOP and DHAP plus rituximab followed by autologous stem cell transplantation in mantle cell lymphoma: a phase 2 study from the Groupe d'Etude des Lymphomes de l'Adulte. *Blood* 121 (1): 48–53.

Descatoire, M., Weller, S., Irtan, S., Sarnacki, S., Feuillard, J., Storck, S. et al. (2014). Identification of a human splenic marginal zone B cell precursor with NOTCH2-dependent differentiation properties. *J. Exp. Med* 211 (5): 987–1000. doi: 10.1084/jem.20132203.

Duan, Y., Dong, X., Nie, J. et al. (2018). Wee1 kinase inhibitor MK-1775 induces apoptosis of acute lymphoblastic leukemia cells and enhances the efficacy of doxorubicin involving downregulation of Notch pathway. *Oncol. Lett.* 16 (4): 5473–5481.

Eiraku, M., Hirata, Y., Takeshima, H., Hirano, T., and Kengaku, M. (2002). Delta/notch-like epidermal growth factor (EGF)-related receptor, a novel EGF-like repeat-containing protein targeted to dendrites of developing and adult central nervous system neurons. *J. Biol. Chem.* 277: 25400–25407. [PubMed: 11950833].

Eskelund, C.W. et al. (2017). TP53 mutations identify younger mantle cell lymphoma patients who do not benefit from intensive chemoimmunotherapy. *Blood* 130 (17): 1903–1910.

Fabbri, G. et al. (2011). Analysis of the chronic lymphocytic leukemia coding genome: role of NOTCH1 mutational activation. *J. Exp. Med.* 208 (7): 1389–1401.

Fabbri, G., and Dalla-Favera, R. (2016). The molecular pathogenesis of chronic lymphocytic leukaemia. *Nat. Rev. Cancer* 16 (3): 145–162.

Fabbri, G., Holmes, A.B., Viganotti, M., Scuoppo, C., Belver, L., Herranz, D. et al. (2017). Common nonmutational NOTCH1 activation in chronic lymphocytic leukemia. *Proc. Natl. Acad. Sci. U.S.A.* 114 (14): E2911–E2919. doi: 10.1073/pnas.1702564114.

Fabbri, G., Khiabanian, H., Holmes, A.B. et al. (2013). Genetic lesions associated with chronic lymphocytic leukemia transformation to Richter syndrome. *J. Exp. Med.* 210 (11): 2273–2288.

Fabbri, G., Rasi, S., Rossi, D. et al. (2011). Analysis of the chronic lymphocytic leukemia coding genome: role of NOTCH1 mutational activation. *J. Exp. Med.* 208: 1389–1401.

Fasnacht, N., Huang, H.Y., Koch, U., Favre, S., Auderset, F., Chai, Q. et al. (2014). Specific fibroblastic niches in secondary lymphoid organs orchestrate distinct Notch-regulated immune responses. *J. Exp. Med.* 211 (11): 2265–2279. doi: 10.1084/jem.20132528.

Fernandez, V. et al. (2010). Genomic and gene expression profiling defines indolent forms of mantle cell lymphoma. *Cancer Res.* 70 (4): 1408–1418.

Fornecker, L.M., Muller, L., Bertrand, F. et al. (2019). Multi-omics dataset to decipher the complexity of drug resistance in diffuse large B-cell lymphoma. *Sci. Rep.* 9 (1): 895.

Frye, B.C., Halfter, S., Djudjaj, S., Muehlenberg, P., Weber, S., Raffetseder, U., En-Nia, A., Knott, H., Baron, J.M., Dooley, S. et al. (2009). Y-box protein-1 is actively secreted through a non-classical pathway and acts as an extracellular mitogen. *EMBO Rep.* 10: 783–789. [PubMed: 19483673].

Garis, M., and Garrett-Sinha, L.A. (2021 February 5). Notch signaling in B cell immune responses. *Front Immunol.* 11: 609324. doi: 10.3389/fimmu.2020.609324. PMID: 33613531; PMCID: PMC7892449.

Gharaibeh, L., Elmadany, N., Alwosaibai, K., and Alshaer, W. (2020 November). Notch1 in cancer therapy: possible clinical implications and challenges. *Mol. Pharmacol.* 98 (5): 559–576. doi: 10.1124/molpharm.120.000006. Epub 2020 Sep 10. PMID: 32913140.

Gibson, M.A., Hatzinikolas, G., Kumaratilake, J.S., Sandberg, L.B., Nicholl, J.K., Sutherland, G.R., and Cleary, E.G. (1996). Further characterization of proteins associated with elastic fiber microfibrils including the molecular cloning of MAGP-2 (MP25). *J. Biol. Chem.* 271: 1096–1103. [PubMed: 8557636].

Gibson, M.A., Sandberg, L.B., Grosso, L.E., and Cleary, E.G. (1991). Complementary DNA cloning establishes microfibril-associated glycoprotein (MAGP) to be a discrete component of the elastin-associated microfibrils. *J. Biol. Chem.* 266: 7596–7601. [PubMed: 2019589].

Gordon, W.R., Vardar-Ulu, D., L'Heureux, S., Ashworth, T., Malecki, M.J., Sanchez-Irizarry, C., McArthur, D.G., Histen, G., Mitchell, J.L., Aster, J.C. et al. (2009). Effects of S1 cleavage on the structure, surface export, and signaling activity of human Notch1 and Notch2. *PLoS ONE* 4: e6613.

Greninger, P., Garnett, M.J., McDermott, U., Rothenberg, S.M., Benes, C.H., and Ellisen, L.W. (2013). Mcl-1 and FBW7 control a dominant survival pathway underlying HDAC and Bcl-2 inhibitor synergy in squamous cell carcinoma. *Cancer Discov.* 3: 324–337.

Gu, Y., Masiero, M., and Banham, A.H. (2016). Notch signaling: its roles and therapeutic potential in hematological malignancies. *Oncotarget* 7: 29804–29823.

Hampel, F., Ehrenberg, S., Hojer, C. et al. (2011). CD19-independent instruction of murine marginal zone B-cell development by constitutive Notch2 signaling. *Blood* 118 (24): 6321–6331.

He, Y., and Pear, W.S. (2003 April). Notch signalling in B cells. *Semin. Cell Dev. Biol.* 14 (2): 135–142. doi:10.1016/s1084-9521(02)00182-9. PMID: 12651097.

Henrique, D., and Schweisguth, F. (2019 February 1). Mechanisms of Notch signaling: a simple logic deployed in time and space. *Development* 146 (3): dev172148. doi: 10.1242/dev.172148. PMID: 30709911.

Hill, H.A. et al. (2020). Genetic mutations and features of mantle cell lymphoma: a systematic review and meta–analysis. *Blood Adv.* 4 (13): 2927–2938.

Hsieh, J.J. and Hayward, S.D. (1995). Masking of the CBF1/RBPJ kappa transcriptional repression domain by Epstein-Barr virus EBNA2. *Science* 268: 560–563.

Hu, Q.D., Ang, B.T., Karsak, M., Hu, W.P., Cui, X.Y., Duka, T., Takeda, Y., Chia, W., Sankar, N., Ng, Y.K. et al. (2003). F3/contactin acts as a functional ligand for Notch during oligodendrocyte maturation. *Cell* 115: 163–175. [PubMed: 14567914].

Hystad, M.E., Myklebust, J.H., Bo, T.H., Sivertsen, E.A., Rian, E., Forfang, L. et al. (2007). Characterization of early stages of human B cell development by gene expression profiling. *J. Immunol.* 179 (6): 3662–3671. doi: 10.4049/jimmunol.179.6.3662.

Jares, P. et al. (2012). Molecular pathogenesis of mantle cell lymphoma. *J Clin Invest* 122 (10): 3416–3423.

Joshi, I., Minter, L.M., Telfer, J. et al. (2009). Notch signaling mediates G1/S cell-cycle progression in T cells via cyclin D3 and its dependent kinases. *Blood* 113 (8): 1689–1698.

Kang, J.A., Kim, W.S., and Park, S.G. (2014). Notch1 is an important mediator for enhancing of B-cell activation and antibody secretion by Notch ligand. *Immunology* 143 (4): 550–559. doi: 10.1111/imm.12333.

Karube, K., Martínez, D., Royo, C., Navarro, A., Pinyol, M. et al. (2014 November). Recurrent mutations of NOTCH genes in follicular lymphoma identify a distinctive subset of tumours. *J. Pathol.* 234 (3): 423–430. doi: 10.1002/path.4428. Epub 2014 Sep 18. PMID: 25141821.

Katzerke, C., Madan, V., Gerloff, D., Brauer-Hartmann, D., Hartmann, J.U., Wurm, A.A. et al. (2013 October 3). Transcription factor C/EBP alpha-induced microRNA-30c inactivates Notch1 during granulopoiesis and is downregulated in acute myeloid leukemia. *Blood* 122 (14): 2433–2442. [PubMed: 23974200].

Kiel, M.J., Velusamy, T., Betz, B.L. et al. (2012). Whole-genome sequencingidentifies recurrent somaticNOTCH2mutations in splenic marginalzone lymphoma. *J. Exp. Med.* 209: 1553–1565.

King, B., Trimarchi, T., Reavie, L., Xu, L., Mullenders, J. et al. (2013 June 20). The ubiquitin ligase FBXW7 modulates leukemia-initiating cell activity by regulating MYC stability. *Cell* 153 (7): 1552–1566. doi: 10.1016/j.cell.2013.05.041. PMID: 23791182; PMCID: PMC4146439.

Kitamoto, T., Takahashi, K., Takimoto, H., Tomizuka, K., Hayasaka, M., Tabira, T. et al. (2005). Functional redundancy of the Notch gene family during mouse embryogenesis: analysis of Notch gene expression in Notch3-deficient mice. *Biochem. Biophys. Res. Commun.* 331 (4): 1154–1162. doi: 10.1016/j.bbrc.2005.03.241.

Kluk, M.J. et al. (2013). Gauging NOTCH1 activation in cancer using immunohistochemistry. *PLoS One* 8 (6): e67306.

Kohlhaas, V., Blakemore, S.J., Al-Maarri, M., Nickel, N., Pal, M. et al. (2021 February 4). Active Akt signaling triggers CLL toward Richter transformation via overactivation of Notch1. *Blood* 137 (5): 646–660. doi: 10.1182/blood.2020005734. PMID: 33538798.

Kopan, R. (2012 October 1) Notch signaling. *Cold Spring Harb. Perspect Biol.* 4 (10): a011213. doi: 10.1101/cshperspect.a011213. PMID: 23028119; PMCID: PMC3475170.

Kopan, R. and Ilagan, M.X. (2009 April 17). The canonical Notch signaling pathway: unfolding the activation mechanism. *Cell* 137 (2): 216–233. doi: 10.1016/j.cell.2009.03.045. PMID: 19379690; PMCID: PMC2827930.

Kridel, R., Meissner, B., Rogic, S., Boyle, M., Telenius, A., Woolcock, B. et al. (2012 March 1). Whole transcriptome sequencing reveals recurrent NOTCH1 mutations in mantle cell lymphoma. *Blood* 119 (9): 1963–1971. [PubMed: 22210878]

Kuroda, K., Han, H., Tani, S., Tanigaki, K., Tun, T., Furukawa, T. et al. (2003). Regulation of marginal zone B cell development by MINT, a suppressor of Notch/RBP-J signaling pathway. *Immunity* 18: 301–312. doi: 10.1016/S1074-7613(03)00029-3.

Laborda, J., Sausville, E.A., Hoffman, T., and Notario, V. (1993). dlk, a putative mammalian homeotic gene differentially expressed in small cell lung carcinoma and neuroendocrine tumor cell line. *J. Biol. Chem.* 268: 3817–3820. [PubMed: 8095043].

Lee, S.Y., Kumano, K., Nakazaki, K., Sanada, M., Matsumoto, A., Yamamoto, G. et al. (2009 May). Gain-of-function mutations and copy number increases of Notch2 in diffuse large B-cell lymphoma. *Cancer Science* 100 (5): 920–926. [PubMed: 19445024].

Li, J., Li, J., Yang, X., Qin, H., Zhou, P., Liang, Y., and Han, H. (2005 May 25). The C terminus of MINT forms homodimers and abrogates MINT-mediated transcriptional repression. *Biochim. Biophys. Acta* 1729 (1): 50–56. doi: 10.1016/j.bbaexp.2005.02.001. Epub 2005 Feb 17. PMID: 15777657.

Logeat, F., Bessia, C., Brou, C., LeBail, O., Jarriault, S., Seidah, N.G., and Israël, A. (1998 July 7). The Notch1 receptor is cleaved constitutively by a furin-like convertase. *Proc. Natl. Acad. Sci. U.S.A.* 95 (14): 8108–8112. doi: 10.1073/pnas.95.14.8108. PMID: 9653148; PMCID: PMC20937.

Maddocks, K. (2018). Update on mantle cell lymphoma. *Blood* 132 (16): 1647–1656.

Martin, P. et al. (2009). Outcome of deferred initial therapy in mantle–cell lymphoma. *J. Clin. Oncol.* 27 (8): 1209–1213.

Maura, F. et al. (2015). Insulin growth factor 1 receptor expression is associated with NOTCH1 mutation, trisomy 12 and aggressive clinical course in chronic lymphocytic leukaemia. *PLoS One* 10 (3): e0118801.

Meng, H., Zhang, X., Hankenson, K.D., and Wang, M.M. (2009). Thrombospondin 2 potentiates notch3/jagged1 signaling. *J. Biol. Chem.* 284: 7866–7874. [PubMed: 19147503].

Mizuma, M., Rasheed, Z.A., Yabuuchi, S., Omura, N., Campbell, N.R. et al. (2012 September). The gamma secretase inhibitor MRK-003 attenuates pancreatic cancer growth in preclinical models. *Mol. Cancer Ther.* 11 (9): 1999–2009. doi: 10.1158/1535-7163.MCT-12-0017. Epub 2012 Jul 2. PMID: 22752426; PMCID: PMC3438318.

Moriyama, Y., Sekine, C., Koyanagi, A., Koyama, N., Ogata, H., Chiba, S. et al. (2008). Delta-like 1 is essential for the maintenance of marginal zone B cells in normal mice but not in autoimmune mice. *Int. Immunol.* 20 (6): 763–773. doi: 10.1093/intimm/dxn034.

Nadeu, F. et al. (2020). Genomic and epigenomic insights into the origin, pathogenesis, and clinical behavior of mantle cell lymphoma subtypes. *Blood* 136 (12): 1419–1432.

Ohishi, K., Varnum-Finney, B., Flowers, D., Anasetti, C., Myerson, D., and Bernstein, I.D. (2000). Monocytes express high amounts of Notch and undergo cytokine specific apoptosis following interaction with the Notch ligand,

Delta-1. *Blood* 95 (9): 2847–2854. doi: 10.1182/blood.V95.9.2847.009k19_2847_2854.

Onaindia, A. et al. (2015). Chronic lymphocytic leukemia cells in lymph nodes show frequent NOTCH1 activation. *Haematol.* 100 (5): e200–e203.

Ortega, M., Bhatnagar, H., Lin, A.P., Wang, L., Aster, J.C., Sill, H., and Aguiar, R.C. (2015 April). A microRNA-mediated regulatory loop modulates NOTCH and MYC oncogenic signals in B- and T-cell malignancies. *Leukemia* 29 (4): 968–976. doi: 10.1038/leu.2014.302. Epub 2014 Oct 14. PMID: 25311243; PMCID: PMC4391979.

Oswald, F., Tauber, B., Dobner, T., Bourteele, S., Kostezka, U., Adler, G. et al. (2001). p300 acts as a transcriptional coactivator for mammalian Notch-1. *Mol. Cell Biol.* 21: 7761–7774. doi: 10.1128/MCB.21.22.7761-7774.2001.

Pararajalingam, P., Coyle, K.M., Arthur, S.E., Thomas, N., Alcaide, M. et al. (2020 July 30). Coding and noncoding drivers of mantle cell lymphoma identified through exome and genome sequencing. *Blood* 136 (5): 572–584. doi: 10.1182/blood.2019002385. PMID: 32160292; PMCID: PMC7440974.

Pekarsky, Y., Zanesi, N., and Croce, C.M. (2010). Molecular basis of CLL. *Semin. Cancer Biol.* 20 (6): 370–376.

Perez-Shibayama, C., Gil-Cruz, C., and Ludewig, B. (2019). Fibroblastic reticular cells at the nexus of innate and adaptive immune responses. *Immunol. Rev.* 289 (1): 31–41. doi: 10.1111/imr.12748.

Puente, X.S. et al. (2011). Whole-genome sequencing identifies recurrent mutations in chronic lymphocytic leukaemia. *Nature* 475 (7354): 101–105.

Puente, X.S. et al. (2015). Non-coding recurrent mutations in chronic lymphocytic leukaemia. *Nature* 526 (7574): 519–524.

Quesada, V. et al. (2011). Exome sequencing identifies recurrent mutations of the splicing factor SF3B1 gene in chronic lymphocytic leukemia. *Nat. Genet.* 44 (1): 47–52.

Radtke, F., Wilson, A., Stark, G., Bauer, M., Van Meerwijk, J., Macdonald, H.R. et al. (1999). Deficient T cell fate specification in mice with an induced inactivation of Notch1. *Immunity* 10 (5): 547–558. doi: 10.1016/S1074-7613(00)80054-0.

Rauen, T., Raffetseder, U., Frye, B.C., Djudjaj, S., Muhlenberg, P.J., Eitner, F., Lendahl, U., Bernhagen, J., Dooley, S., and Mertens, P.R. (2009). YB-1 acts as a ligand for Notch-3 receptors and modulates receptor activation. *J. Biol. Chem.* 284: 26928–26940. [PubMed: 19640841].

Rinaldi, A., Mian, M., Chigrinova, E., Arcaini, L., Bhagat, G. et al. (2011). Genome-wide DNA profiling of marginal zone lymphomas identifies subtype-specific lesions with an impact on the clinical outcome. *Blood.* 117(5):1595-604. doi: 10.1182/blood-2010-01-264275. PMID: 21115979.

Rossi, D., Spina, V., Deambrogi, C. et al. (2011). The genetics of Richter syndrome reveals disease heterogeneity and predicts survival after transformation. *Blood* 117 (12): 3391–3401.

Rossi, D., Trifonov, V., Fangazio, M., Bruscaggin, A., Rasi, S., Spina, V. et al. (2012 August 27). The coding genome of splenic marginal zone lymphoma: activation of NOTCH2 and other pathways regulating marginal zone development. *J. Exp. Med.* 209 (9): 1537–1551. [PubMed: 22891273].

Saito, T., Chiba, S., Ichikawa, M., Kunisato, A., Asai, T., Shimizu, K. et al. (2003). Notch2 is preferentially expressed in mature B cells and indispensable for marginal zone B lineage development. *Immunity* 18 (5): 675–685. doi: 10.1016/S1074-7613(03)00111-0.

Sakamoto, K., Yamaguchi, S., Ando, R., Miyawaki, A., Kabasawa, Y., Takagi, M., Li, C.L., Perbal, B., and Katsube, K. (2002b). The nephroblastoma overexpressed gene (NOV/ccn3) protein associates with Notch1 extracellular domain and inhibits myoblast differentiation via Notch signaling pathway. *J. Biol. Chem.* 277: 29399–29405. [PubMed: 12050162].

Santos, M.A., Sarmento, L.M., Rebelo, M., Doce, A.A., Maillard, I., Dumortier, A. et al. (2007). Notch1 engagement by Delta-like-1 promotes differentiation of B lymphocytes to antibody-secreting cells. *Proc. Natl. Acad. Sci. U.S.A* 104 (39): 15454–15459. doi: 10.1073/pnas.0702891104.

Schmidt, M.H., Bicker, F., Nikolic, I., Meister, J., Babuke, T., Picuric, S., Muller-Esterl, W., Plate, K.H., and Dikic, I. (2009). Epidermal growth factor-like domain 7 (EGFL7) modulates Notch signalling and affects neural stem cell renewal. *Nat. Cell Biol.* 11: 873–880. [PubMed: 19503073].

Schmitz, R., Wright, G.W., Huang, D.W., Johnson, C.A., Phelan, J.D. et al. (2018 April 12). Genetics and pathogenesis of diffuse large B-cell lymphoma. *N. Engl. J. Med.* 378 (15): 1396–1407. doi: 10.1056/NEJMoa1801445. PMID: 29641966; PMCID: PMC6010183.

Shanmugam, V., Craig, J.W., Hilton, L.K., Nguyen, M.H., Rushton, C.K., Fahimdanesh, K., Lovitch, S., Ferland, B., Scott, D.W., and Aster, J.C. (2021 January 12). Notch activation is pervasive in SMZL and uncommon in DLBCL: implications for Notch signaling in B-cell tumors. *Blood Adv.* 5 (1): 71–83. doi: 10.1182/bloodadvances.2020002995. PMID: 33570635; PMCID: PMC7805321.

Shen, W., Huang, J., and Wang, Y. (2021 March 26). Biological Significance of NOTCH Signaling Strength. *Front Cell Dev. Biol.* 9: 652273. doi: 10.3389/fcell.2021.652273. PMID: 33842479; PMCID: PMC8033010.

Smas, C.M. and Sul, H.S. (1993). Pref-1, a protein containing EGF-like repeats, inhibits adipocyte differentiation. *Cell* 73: 725–734. [PubMed: 8500166].

Spina, V., Khiabanian, H., Messina, M., Monti, S., Cascione, L. et al. (2016 September 8). The genetics of nodal marginal zone lymphoma. *Blood* 128 (10): 1362–1373. doi: 10.1182/blood-2016-02-696757. Epub 2016 Jun 22. PMID: 27335277; PMCID: PMC5016706.

Sprinzak, D., Lakhanpal, A., LeBon, L., Santat, L.A., Fontes, M.E., Anderson, G.A., Garcia-Ojalvo, J., and Elowitz, M.B.

(2010). Cis-interactions between Notch and Delta generate mutually exclusive signaling states. *Nature* 465: 86–90.

Stein, H. et al. (1980). Immunohistologic analysis of the organization of normal lymphoid tissue and non-Hodgkin's lymphomas. *J. Histochem. Cytochem.* 28 (8): 746–760.

Strefford, J.C., Sutton, L.A., Baliakas, P. et al. (2013). Distinct patterns of novelgene mutations in poor-prognostic stereotyped subsets of chroniclymphocytic leukemia: the case of SF3B1 and subset #2. *Leukemia* 27: 2196–2199.

Su, X., Qian, C., Zhang, Q., Hou, J., Gu, Y., Han, Y. et al. (2013 December 6). miRNomes of haematopoietic stem cells and dendritic cells identify miR-30b as a regulator of Notch1. *Nat. Comm.* 4: 2903.

Swerdlow, S.H. C.E., Harris, N.L., Jaffe, E.S., Pileri, S.A., Stein, H., Thiele, J. et al. (2008). *WHO Classification of Tumors of Haematopoietic and Lymphoid Tissues*, 4e. Copenhagen.

Tan, J.B., Xu, K., Cretegny, K., Visan, I., Yuan, J.S., Egan, S.E. et al. (2009). Lunatic and manic fringe cooperatively enhance marginal zone B cell precursor competition for delta-like 1 in splenic endothelial niches. *Immunity* 30 (2): 254–263. doi: 10.1016/j.immuni.2008.12.016.

Thieblemont, C., Davi, F., Noguera, M.E., and Brière, J. (2011 July). Non-MALT marginal zone lymphoma. *Curr. Opin. Hematol.* 18 (4): 273–279. doi: 10.1097/MOH.0b013e3283477815.

Trøen, G., Nygaard, V., Jenssen, T.K., Ikonomou, I.M., Tierens, A. et al. (2004 November). Constitutive expression of the AP-1 transcription factors c-jun, junD, junB, and c-fos and the marginal zone B-cell transcription factor Notch2 in splenic marginal zone lymphoma. *J Mol Diagn* 6 (4): 297–307. doi:10.1016/S1525-1578(10)60525-9. PMID: 15507668; PMCID: PMC1867488.

Vaisitti, T., Braggio, E., Allan, J.N., Arruga, F., Serra, S. et al. (2018 July 1). Novel Richter Syndrome Xenograft models to study genetic architecture, biology, and therapy responses. *Cancer Res.* 78 (13): 3413–3420. doi: 10.1158/0008-5472.CAN-17-4004. Epub 2018 May 7. PMID: 29735551.

Valls, E., Lobry, A.B., Geng, H., Wang, L., Cardenas, M., Rivas, M. et al. (2017). BCL6 antagonizes NOTCH2 to maintain survival of human follicular lymphoma cells. *Cancer Discov.* 7 (5): 506–521. doi: 10.1158/2159-8290.CD-16-1189.

VanderWielen, B.D., Yuan, Z., Friedmann, D.R., and Kovall, R.A. (2011 April 29). Transcriptional repression in the Notch pathway: thermodynamic characterization of CSL-MINT (Msx2-interacting nuclear target protein) complexes. *J. Biol. Chem.* 286 (17): 14892–14902. doi: 10.1074/jbc.M110.181156. Epub 2011 Mar 3. PMID: 21372128; PMCID: PMC3083192.

Vose, J.M. (2017). Mantle cell lymphoma: 2017 update on diagnosis, risk–stratification, and clinical manage-ment. *Am. J. Hematol.* 92 (8): 806–813.

Walker, L., Carlson, A., Tan-Pertel, H.T., Weinmaster, G., and Gasson, J. (2001). The notch receptor and its ligands are selectively expressed during hematopoietic development in the mouse. *Stem Cells* 19: 543–52.

Wang, L., Lawrence, M.S., Wan, Y., Stojanov, P., Sougnez, C., Stevenson, K. et al. (2011 December 29). SF3B1 and other novel cancer genes in chronic lymphocytic leukemia. *N. Engl. J. Med.* 365 (26): 2497–2506. [PubMed: 22150006].

Wang, Y., Kim, K.A., Kim, J.H., and Sul, H.S. (2006). Pref-1, a preadipocyte secreted factor that inhibits adipogenesis. *J. Nutr.* 136: 2953–2956. [PubMed: 17116701].

Wilson, W.H., Wright, G.W., Huang, D.W., Hodkinson, B., Balasubramanian, S., Fan, Y., Vermeulen, J., Shreeve, M., and Staudt, L.M. (2021 December 13). Effect of ibrutinib with R-CHOP chemotherapy in genetic subtypes of DLBCL. *Cancer Cell* 39 (12): 1643–1653.e3. doi: 10.1016/j.ccell.2021.10.006. Epub 2021 Nov 4. PMID: 34739844; PMCID: PMC8722194.

Wu, L., Aster, J.C., Blacklow, S.C., Lake, R., Artavanis-Tsakonas, S., and Griffin, J.D. (2000). MAML1, a human homologue of Drosophila mastermind, is a transcriptional co-activator for NOTCH receptors. *Nat. Genet.* 26: 484–489. 10.1038/82644.

Xochelli, A., Kalpadakis, C., Gardiner, A., Baliakas, P., Vassilakopoulos, T.P. et al. (2014 February 20). Clonal B-cell lymphocytosis exhibiting immunophenotypic features consistent with a marginal-zone origin: is this a distinct entity? *Blood* 123 (8): 1199–1206. doi: 10.1182/blood-2013-07-515155. Epub 2013 Dec 3. PMID: 24300853.

Yeh, C.H., Bellon, M., and Nicot, C. (2018 August 7). FBXW7: a critical tumor suppressor of human cancers. *Mol. Cancer* 17 (1): 115. doi: 10.1186/s12943-018-0857-2. PMID: 30086763; PMCID: PMC6081812.

Yi, S., Yan, Y., Jin, M., Bhattacharya, S., Wang, Y. et al. (2022 February 1). Genomic and transcriptomic profiling reveals distinct molecular subsets associated with outcomes in mantle cell lymphoma. *J. Clin. Invest.* 132 (3): e153283. doi: 10.1172/JCI153283. PMID: 34882582; PMCID: PMC8803323.

Ying, C.Y., Dominguez-Sola, D., Fabi, M., Lorenz, I.C., Hussein, S. et al. (2013 October). MEF2B mutations lead to deregulated expression of the oncogene BCL6 in diffuse large B cell lymphoma. *Nat. Immunol.* 14 (10): 1084–1092. doi: 10.1038/ni.2688. Epub 2013 Aug 25. PMID: 23974956; PMCID: PMC3954820.

Yoon, S.O., Zhang, X., Berner, P., Blom, B., and Choi, Y.S. (2009). Notch ligands expressed by follicular dendritic cells protect germinal center B cells from apoptosis. *J. Immunol.* 183 (1): 352–358. doi: 10.4049/jimmunol.0803183.

Yumimoto, K., Akiyoshi, S., Ueo, H., Sagara, Y., Onoyama, I. et al. (2015 February). F-box protein FBXW7 inhibits cancer metastasis in a non-cell-autonomous manner. *J. Clin. Invest.* 125 (2): 621–635. doi: 10.1172/JCI78782. Epub 2015 Jan 2. PMID: 25555218; PMCID: PMC4319427.

Zhang, J. et al. (2014). The genomic landscape of mantle cell lymphoma is related to the epigenetically determined chromatin state of normal B cells. *Blood* 123 (19): 2988–2996.

Zhang, L. et al. (2019). Metabolic reprogramming toward oxidative phosphorylation identifies a therapeutic target for mantle cell lymphoma. *Sci. Transl. Med.* 11 (491): eaau1167.

Zhu, G., Wang, X., Xiao, H., Liu, X., Fang, Y., Zhai, B. et al. (2017). Both Notch1 and its ligands in B cells promote antibody production. *Mol. Immunol.* 91: 17–23. doi: 10.1016/j.molimm.2017.08.021.

30

Targeting NF-κB in Oncology, an Untapped Therapeutic Potential

Matko Kalac

Precision Immunology Institute, Tisch Cancer Center, Icahn School of Medicine at Mount Sinai, New York, NY, USA

Take Home Messages

- Since its discovery in the 1980s and more recently, strong evidence of its crucial role in lymphomagenesis, NF-κB has been at the focal point of oncology drug development.
- Despite extensive efforts, the result has been only one of moderate success at finding NF-κB targeting anti-cancer drugs.
- Experience with targeting upstream molecules of NF-κB, such as inhibitors of BTK, has had a transformative effect in hematologic malignancies.
- Further research is therefore needed to fully utilize NF-κB's enormous potential as a target in oncology.

Introduction

Nuclear factor-kappaB (NF-κB) is a family of transcription factors that plays a crucial role in lymphocyte development and activation (Liu et al. 2017; Yu et al. 2020). By serving as a key regulator of both the innate and the adaptive immunity, the NF-κB protein family controls inflammation by stimulating cell proliferation and secretion of pro-inflammatory cytokines, cell migration, and angiogenesis (Sun 2017). NF-κB is also known to play an important role in carcinogenesis, since tumors can modulate NF-κB's vast control over cell survival to their advantage (Coussens and Werb 2002; Taniguchi and Karin 2018).

Numerous processes such as infections (viral and bacterial), products of cell death (necrotic cells, DNA fragments), oxidative stress, and inflammation can rapidly activate NF-κB, which quickly reverts to its baseline status after the induction signal is gone (Karin and Greten 2005). In the case of malignant transformation and tumor progression however, both malignant cells and surrounding non-malignant inflammatory cells constitutively activate NF-κB and promote tumorigenesis (Staudt 2010). Malignant cells co-opt NF-κB through disruption of the delicate regulation between inhibitors of NF-κB (family of IκB proteins, A20, CYLD) and its activators (NF-κB activating cytokines such as TNFα and IL-1) (Ben-Neriah and Karin 2011).

The NF-κB family consists of five structurally related member proteins (p105/p50, p65, c-Rel, RelB, and p100/p52) that participate within two well-described activation pathways – canonical (classical) and non-canonical (alternative) NF-κB pathways (Sen and Baltimore 1986; Zhang et al. 2017). All of these proteins share a conserved REL homology domain and form homo- or heterodimers which can, following activation, move to the nucleus and regulate gene transcription (Perkins 2012).

Various external stimuli that are responsible for the canonical NF-κB pathway activation merge at the crucial step of IκB kinase (IKKs) activation. IKK activation is a phosphorylation-dependent event that leads to phosphorylation of one of the NF-κB inhibitory units called IκBs. IκB phosphorylation results in their ubiquitination and degradation by the proteasome. Importantly, IκB degradation releases the NF-κB dimer, which can then translocate to the nucleus and bind to DNA (Oeckinghaus and Ghosh 2009).

Activation of the non-canonical pathway is mediated by distinct number of tumor necrosis factor (TNF) superfamily receptors, potentially suggesting a more specific function of this pathway. A crucial role is played in this context by the NF-κB inducing kinase (NIK). Upon activation of the non-canonical pathway, there is an accumulation of NIK in the cytoplasm (by way of degradation of its inhibitor tumor necrosis family receptors [TNFR]-associated factor 3). NIK, together with IKKα induces cleavage of p100 to a shorter protein named p52. Following the cleavage of p100, p52 together with its

Precision Cancer Therapies: Targeting Oncogenic Drivers and Signaling Pathways in Lymphoid Malignancies: From Concept to Practice, Volume 1, First Edition. Edited by Owen A. O'Connor, Stephen M. Ansell, and John F. Seymour.

heterodimer partner RelB can translocate to the nucleus and exert its transcription factor activity (Ghosh and Hayden 2008).

In this chapter, the regulatory details of NF-κB pathway activation will be discussed in the context of lymphoid malignancies and other tumors. There will be a special focus on targetable points within the pathway with a review of existing, Food and Drug Administration (FDA)-approved drugs targeting NF-κB, and also novel therapeutic approaches currently under pre-clinical and clinical investigation. Furthermore, a focus will be directed at NF-κB mediators and their crosstalk with other oncogenic pathways.

Historical Perspective for the Role of NF-κB in Malignancy

The first connection between chronic inflammation and cancer was postulated as early as the nineteenth century by Rudolph Virchow (Balkwill and Mantovani 2010). Early experiments in animal models showed that carcinomas can be induced by chemical or biologic irritants (Fujiki 2014). The full importance of chronic inflammation in carcinogenesis was elucidated in the 1990s through detailed molecular studies clarifying the role of cytokines, inflammatory cells, and growth factors in cancer-related inflammation (Coussens and Werb 2002). NF-κB was discovered in 1986 by David Baltimore's group as a B-cell specific transcription factor (Sen and Baltimore 1986). Its important role in carcinogenesis was discovered in colitis-associated colon cancer and hepatocellular carcinoma in 2004 (Greten et al. 2004; Pikarsky et al. 2004).

Further support for the role of inflammation in cancer development came from epidemiological studies showing that chronic infections (such as hepatitis B virus [HBV], hepatitis C virus [HCV], human papilloma virus, *Helicobacter pylori*), autoimmune conditions, and exposure to noxious chemicals result in increased risk of developing cancer (Kuper et al. 2000). It is now estimated that persistent infections and chronic inflammation are associated with at least 15–20% of cancer deaths worldwide (Plummer et al. 2016), and that obesity-associated inflammation might be responsible for another 15% of the death toll of cancer (Calle et al. 2003).

Chronic inflammation supports cancer progression even after the initial malignant transformation. Constitutive NF-κB activation in this setting occurs through several mechanisms including tumor's ability to induce inflammation (necrosis due to insufficient blood flow or microbial invasion into a poorly vascular tumor tissue) or by iatrogenic factors (such as chemotherapy and radiotherapy which induce necrotic death with reactive oxygen species production and DNA damage). The end result of all these changes can be the development of chemotherapy resistance and the compromise of the anti-tumor immunity (Grivennikov et al. 2010).

NF-κB has been at the focal point of oncology drug development research since its discovery. Despite extensive efforts, the result has been only one of moderate success at finding NF-κB targeting anti-cancer drugs. Further research is therefore needed to fully utilize NF-κB's enormous potential as a target in oncology (Ramadass et al. 2020).

Canonical NF-κB Pathway

Prototypical NF-κB proteins in the canonical pathway are p65 (also known as RelA) and p50. In the absence of an activating stimulus, p65 and p50 are sequestered in the cytoplasm by their inhibitor proteins known commonly as IκB (Sun 2017; Vallabhapurapu and Karin 2009). IκB family consists of three groups of molecules: (i) the typical IκB proteins (IκBα, IκBβ, and IκBε); (ii) NF-κB precursor proteins (p100 and p105); and (iii) the atypical IκB proteins (IκBζ, BCL-3, and IκBNS) (Hoffmann et al. 2006; Sun et al. 1993; Tam and Sen 2001; Whiteside et al. 1997). The central event in the activation of the canonical NF-κB pathway is phosphorylation of IκBs by IKK. IKK consists of two homologous catalytic subunits IKKα (IKK1) and IKKβ (IKK2), as well as a regulatory subunit IKKγ (NEMO – NF-κB essential modulator). IKKβ is responsible for IκB phosphorylation while IKKα participates mostly in the non-canonical pathway (Häcker and Karin 2006; Rao et al. 2010). Numerous surface signals lead to IKK activation (Figure 30.1, highlighted square in red) and phosphorylation of IκB. Phosphorylation of the IκB protein leads to its K48-linked ubiquitination and subsequent degradation in the proteasome (Hayden and Ghosh 2008). Following this event, the p50-p65 dimer is released and able to translocate to the nucleus and drive target gene transcription (Whiteside et al. 1997). Cell surface signals, including those transmitted via T-cell receptor (TCR), B-cell receptor (BCR), inflammatory cytokines, and innate pattern-recognition receptors (PRR), can quickly activate the canonical NF-κB (Takeuchi and Akira 2010).

Lipopolysaccharides (LPS) are a classical example of innate immunity-mediated NF-κB activation (Cao 2016). Recognition of LPS as well as other activators such as microbial pathogen associated molecular patterns or damaged tissue-associated molecular patterns (PAMPs and DAMPs, respectively) by the innate immune cells such as dendritic cells or macrophages leads to production of TNF-α, IL-1, IL-6 and other proinflammatory cytokines. PRRs such as Toll-like receptors (TLRs) serve as proinflammatory signal mediators on the surface of the cell as well as downstream. TLR4 is a transmembrane receptor that recruits MyD88 following LPS stimulation which subsequently leads to recruitment of IRAK4 and IRAK1 (IL-1 receptor-associated kinase 4 and 1), TRAF6 and TAK1 (TGF-β-activated kinase 1). TRAF6 possesses E3-ligase function which mediates autoubiquitination, phosphorylation and activation of TAK1. Activated TAK1 then leads to IKK activation and downstream NF-κB activation (Figure 30.1) (Akira and Takeda 2004; Kawagoe et al. 2008; Xia et al. 2009).

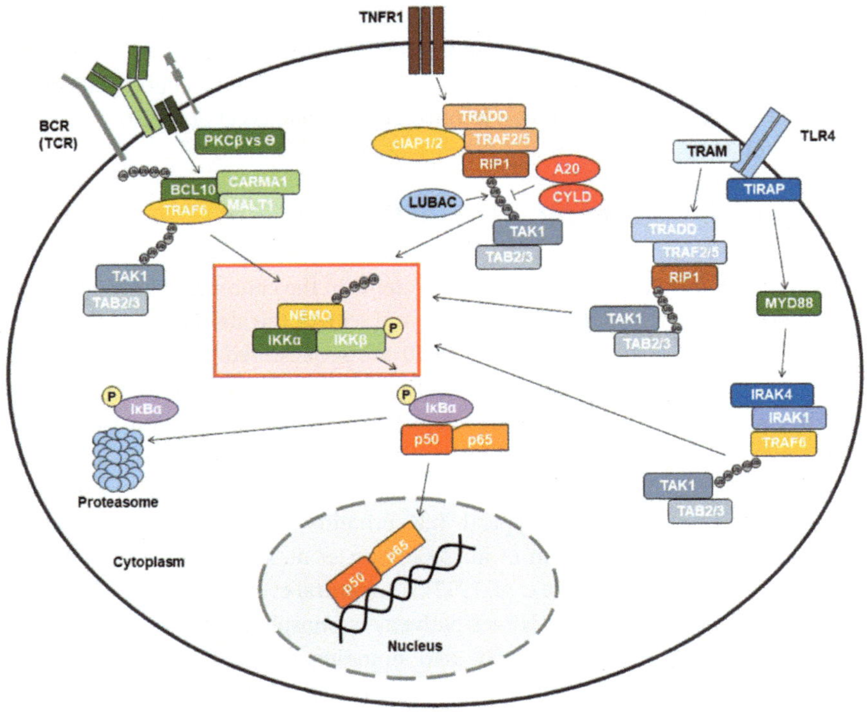

Figure 30.1 Canonical NF-κB pathway. Signals downstream of BCR (or TCR), TNFR1 and TLR4 lead to IKK activation, IκBα phosphorylation and degradation with p50-p65 dimer translocation to the nucleus.

Canonical NF-κB activation can additionally occur following interaction between TNF and its receptor TNFR1. TNFR1 forms a complex with TRADD (tumor necrosis factor receptor type 1-associated DEATH domain protein) through its cytoplasmic death domain and is responsible for the assembly of E3 ubiquitin ligases cIAP1 and cIAP2. Subsequently, this complex recruits TRAFs (TRAF2 and TRAF5) and protein kinase RIP1. This assembly results in RIP1 K63-ubiquitination and its recruitment to NEMO, formation of TAK1-IKK complex, and activation of IKK with downstream NF-κB activation (Baker et al. 2011; Hsu et al. 1996; Michallet et al. 2008).

DNA damage can also activate the canonical NF-κB. This process is mediated via activation of ATM (ataxia teleangiectasia mutated) and post-translational modifications of NEMO which are crucial for signal transduction (Bartek and Lukas 2006).

Adoptive immune response in B- and T-cells is regulated by their receptors, BCR and TCR, respectively. Downstream NF-κB activation in both pathways revolves around the activation of CBM complex (consisting of CARD11, BCL10 and MALT1). CBM activation is mediated by protein kinase C Θ (PKCΘ) in T-cells, and PKCβ in B-cells. Both of these enzymes phosphorylate CARD11 (also known as CARMA-1), which results in the conformational change of CARD11 and the recruitment of BCL10 and MALT1 into CBM complex (Pomerantz et al. 2002; Sun et al. 2004). MALT1 subsequently recruits TRAF6 which mediates K63 ubiquitination of BCL10 and activation of TAK1 leading to IKK-mediated NF-κB activation (Hu and Sun 2016; Li and Rudensky 2016; Thome 2004). Crucial step in PKC-Θ and -β activation is the generation of diacylglycerol (DAG). In TCR pathway, DAG is created via ZAP70 and phospholipase Cγ1 (PLCγ1) (Bi et al. 2001; Li et al. 2005). In BCR signaling pathway however, SRC family of kinases including LYN, FYN, and BLK activates SYK (cytosolic tyrosine kinase) and Bruton's tyrosine kinase (BTK), which in turn activates PLCγ2 leading to DAG production (Shinohara et al. 2005; Su et al. 2002).

Because of NF-κB's rapid activation as well as its important role in the activation of numerous genes responsible for cellular division and proliferation, its aberrant activation can lead to chronic inflammation, autoimmunity, and cancer (Yu et al. 2020). As such, NF-κB is strictly controlled by negative and positive regulation. Negative regulation of p50 and p65 is mediated by its inhibitors, IκB proteins, which sequester NF-κB in the cytoplasm. One of the NF-κB target genes are those encoding IκBs, leading to rapid inactivation of NF-κB (Sun et al. 1993). Additional negative regulation is provided by the degradation of the NF-κB dimers at the transcriptional level (Li et al. 2005). Deubiquitination is another important level of control exerted upstream of IKK. Deubiquitinases A20 and CYLD serve to remove K63-linked ubiquitin chains of RIP1, TRAF6, and NEMO leading to disassembly of the IKK complex (Hymowitz and Wertz 2010; Xu et al. 2020). Positive regulation of NF-κB is mediated by ubiquitinases downstream of TNFR: TRAF-mediated polyubiquitination and LUBAC (linear ubiquitin chain assembly complex) mediated linear ubiquitination. TRAF6 polyubiquitinates NEMO which leads to the activation of TAK1 and IKK. Similarly, linear K63 ubiquitination of TAK1 mediated by LUBAC also leads to IKK activation (Chen 2012; Chiang and Gack 2017). Crucial downstream TNFR signaling molecule is RIP1 which has a bipolar function with regards to NF-κB activation. When ubiquitinated by cIAP1/2 it serves as an activator of NF-κB, while its deubiquitination by CYLD leads to NF-κB inactivation (Xu et al. 2020).

Non-canonical NF-κB Pathway

NIK (NF-κB inducing kinase) is a central enzyme responsible for non-canonical NF-κB activation (Sun 2017). In resting lymphocytes, NIK is constitutively targeted for degradation in the proteasome. This degradation is mediated by cIAP1/2 and TRAF2/3 which polyubiquitinate NIK (Yu et al. 2020). NF-κB activation signals, mediated by the members of TNFR superfamily (e.g. Cyclin-dependent kinase 4 [CD40], transmembrane activator and CAML interactor [TACI], or B-cell activating factor receptor [BAFF-R]), lead to TRAF2/3 degradation which then abrogates interaction between NIK and cIAP1/2 (Figure 30.2). Non-canonical NF-κB pathway activation can also occur by the endosome-dependent activation of MAC (complement membrane attack complex) induced by human PRA (panel reactive antibody) (Sun 2017).

Following the upstream activation, NIK accumulates in the cytoplasm where it associates with and phosphorylates IKKα. The principle NF-κB proteins involved in the non-canonical pathway are p100/p52 and RelB. Like IκBα, p100 serves as an inhibitory molecule and its cleavage to p52 allows for p52-RelB dimer to translocate to the nucleus. C-terminal of p100 contains NIK responsive sequence consisting of two serine residues that serve as a direct target for phosphorylation.

Phosphorylation of p100 leads to E3 ligase ubiquitination and subsequent degradation in the proteasome (Xiao et al. 2001). This process is counteracted by a deubiquitinase Otub1, an enzyme leading to stabilization of p100 (Li et al. 2019). Additional negative regulation of the non-canonical pathway is mediated by deubiquitinase OTUD7B, similarly to the way A20 negatively regulates CBM complex in the canonical pathway (Evans et al. 2001; Mevissen et al. 2016).

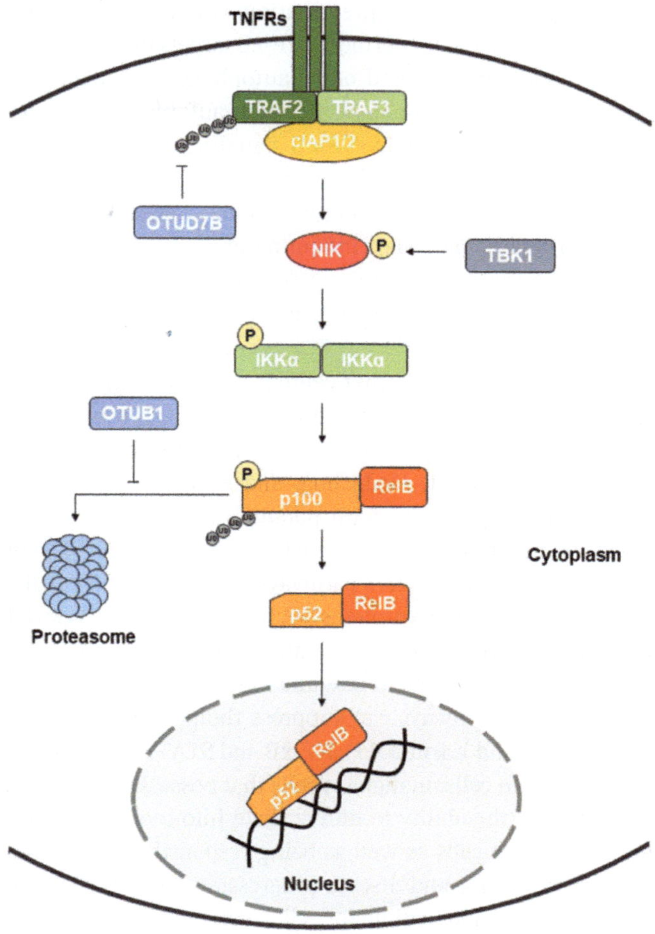

Figure 30.2 Non-canonical NF-κB pathway. NIK is a crucial mediation in the non-canonical NF-κB activation. The accumulation of NIK leads to IKKα activation and cleavage of p100 to p52 which results in p52-RelB translocation to the nucleus.

NF-κB in Tumorigenesis and Promotion of Malignant Cell Growth

NF-κB is known to affect a wide range of cellular processes including those responsible for cell survival and growth (Sun 2017). Pro-tumorigenic cytokines such as TNF and IL-6 are direct NF-κB targets and their levels are elevated in numerous malignancies, frequently correlating with a poor prognosis (Balkwill 2009; Taniguchi and Karin 2014). TNF is also a crucial participant in a positive NF-κB loop as it directly promotes NF-κB activation (Balkwill 2009). Depending on the cellular context and ubiquitination status of the RIP1, TNF can have a somewhat bipolar effect by either inducing cellular death or by promoting survival. Numerous examples suggest that malignant cells can co-opt NF-κB to promote its survival (Chen 2012; Xu et al. 2020).

IL-6 is responsible for the activation of other pro-oncogenic pathways including JAK/STAT3, RAS/MAPK, and PI3K/AKT pathways which further support oncogenic activation and metastasis in crosstalk with NF-κB. TNF, IL-6, and other cytokines, as well as CC chemokines and CX chemokines, stimulate primary tumor growth, growth factor synthesis, angiogenesis, and metastasis (Taniguchi and Karin 2018).

Autophagy and senescence are important cellular processes which have a delicate interplay with NF-κB since both have anti- and pro-tumorigenic effect (Taniguchi et al. 2016; White et al. 2010). Autophagy serves as an anti-tumor process by either inhibiting tumor-stimulating inflammation or by increasing tumor immunogenicity through more efficient antigen processing and presentation (Zhong et al. 2016; Zhong et al. 2016). Furthermore, NF-κB targets include beclin 1 (BECN1), SQSTM1, and other autophagy-associated proteins to enhance autophagy, whereas autophagy degrades IKK subunits and inhibits NF-κB signaling (Balkwill 2009). Senescence is a process of irreversible cellular inactivation that is observed in normal and malignant tissues. While this would in general mean less inflammation, senescent cells are still able to secrete pro-tumorigenic cytokines such as IL-1, IL-6, and IL-8 and stimulate tumor growth (Taniguchi and Karin 2018).

NF-κB interacts with other cellular pathways important in the regulation of cell survival: JAK/STAT3, p53, c-Jun NH2-Terminal Kinase (JNK), WNT/β-catenin, interferon regulatory factor (IRF), Notch1, Hedgehog, and others. Activation of many of these pathways with potential for pro-tumorigenic effect is inflammation (Taniguchi and Karin 2018). For example, NF-κB and STAT3 pathways cooperate in the regulation of pro-oncogenic proteins such as MYC and CyclinD1 and stimulate the expression of anti-apoptotic proteins such as Bcl-X_L and Bcl2 (Grivennikov and Karin 2010). Additionally, both of these pathways can suppress the production of p53 (Ben-Neriah and Karin 2011). NF-κB and STAT3 are activated in cancer stem cells, malignant cells that possess self-renewal capacity and the ability to differentiate into more differentiated malignant cells as well as being responsible for chemotherapy resistance and disease progression. Both NF-κB and STAT3 can promote malignant cell development and maintenance by way of production of SLUG, TWIST1, and SNAIL. IKKβ directly phosphorylates p53 which leads to its polyubiquitination and degradation in the proteasome. Cells with mutated p53 exhibit chronic activation of NF-κB (Gudkov and Komarova 2016; Xia et al. 2009). Furthermore, IKKβ can phosphorylate IRF3 which leads to decreased expression of TNFα required for NF-κB (Covert et al. 2005; Taniguchi and Karin 2018). Activation of Notch1 can induce NF-κB activation and its inhibition leads to decreased NF-κB activity. Equally, NF-κB can serve as an important activator of Notch1 (Ang and Tergaonkar 2007).

NF-κB can directly promote tumor initiation as it controls the production of reactive oxygen species as well as reactive nitrogen species, molecules responsible for DNA damage and potential somatic mutations (Grivennikov et al. 2010). Additionally, NF-κB is responsible for stimulating the cell entry into cell cycle when one of the DNA strands has acquired mutation, which ensures subsequent incorporation of the mutation in both DNA strands of the daughter cells (Joyce et al. 2001; Kiraly et al. 2015). Malignant cell initiation is stimulated by chronic inflammation and constitutive NF-κB activation through aneuploidy, chromosomal instability, and epigenetic changes in the cells (Nakshatri et al. 2015; Ren et al. 2011; Vento-Tormo et al. 2014). Chronic inflammation furthermore leads to induction of the cancer stem cells and inactivation of p53 (Gudkov et al. 2011). Another important example of NF-κB in cancer initiation is the induction of apolipoprotein B mRNA-editing enzyme, catalytic polypeptide-like (APOBEC) family of DNA-modifying enzymes such as activation-induced deaminase (AID) (Park 2012). AID is an enzyme which deaminates cytosine residues resulting in cytosine-to-thymine transitions and is well described as tumor initiator in lymphomas and gastrointestinal cancers. NF-κB is also a crucial regulator of the epithelial-to-mesenchymal transition (EMT), invasive behavior, and angiogenesis (Wu and Zhou 2009). It does so by activating previously mentioned SLUG, TWIST1, and SNAIL which initiate the EMT process. Furthermore, matrix-degrading enzymes such as MMP9 are the target of NF-κB and responsible for early extravasation into blood and lymphatics (Huang et al. 2001; Pires et al. 2017; Scheel and Weinberg 2012). Chronic inflammation additionally supports angiogenesis by way of production of reactive oxygen species which stimulate inflammatory cells such as macrophages to produce VEGF 9 (Grivennikov et al. 2010).

Oncogenic Alterations in Lymphoma and Other Hematologic Malignancies

NF-κB is crucial for normal development and activation of lymphocytes. It is therefore understandable that a variety of lymphoid malignancies are characterized by NF-κB overactivation, frequently due to genetic alterations in its regulators in the upstream signaling pathways (Grondona et al. 2018). Genetic alterations in NF-κB member proteins themselves are rare and instead overactivation of NF-κB occurs in genetic alterations upstream (Grondona et al. 2018). First report of chronic NF-κB activation and its implication in lymphoma development came from animal studies with viral oncogene v-Rel (Beug et al. 1981). Subsequently, genetic lesions driving constitutive NF-κB activation have been described in numerous lymphomas including adult T-cell leukemia/lymphoma (ATLL), diffuse large B-cell lymphoma (DLBCL), primarily of the activated B-cell type (ABC), classical Hodgkin's lymphoma (cHL), Waldenstrom's macroglobulinemia (WM), chronic lymphocytic leukemia (CLL), mantle cell lymphoma (MCL), mucosa-associated lymphoid tissue (MALT) lymphomas, and multiple myeloma (MM) (Annunziata et al. 2007; Bargou et al. 1996; Davis et al. 2001; Grondona et al. 2018; Ni et al. 2001; Rahal et al. 2014; Savage et al. 2003; Xu et al. 2020).

MyD88 is an important downstream signaling molecule for the TLRs. Following TLRs activation by PAMPs or DAMPs the Myddosome is created (MyD88 homodimers) which interacts and activates IRAKs and TRAF6 (Dossang et al. 2016; Vollmer et al. 2017). TRAF6-mediated phosphorylation of TAK1 leads to IKK activation (Ngo et al. 2011; Takaesu et al. 2000). MyD88 is frequently mutated in lymphoid neoplasms, as up to 40% of ABC subtype DLBCL cases have MYD88 mutations. MyD88 mutations represent the most frequently mutated oncogene in this lymphoma. The most common activating mutation is L265P which is also observed in WM, CLL, and MALT-lymphoma (Ngo et al. 2011; Puente et al. 2011; Treon et al. 2012; Yan et al. 2012). The importance of these activating mutations is demonstrated through experiments in germinal center B-cell like (GCB) DLBCL, which exhibit substantially less NF-κB dependency then ABC DLBCL. Ectopic expression of $MyD88^{L265P}$ in GCB DLBCL cells leads to NF-κB activation independently of TLRs (Avbelj et al. 2014). Additionally, mouse experiments have shown that expression of $MyD88^{L265P}$ leads to formation of ABC-like lymphoproliferative disorders (Knittel et al. 2016).

Chronic BCR signaling has an important role in overactivation of NF-κB in B-cell lymphomas, particularly in those of post-germinal origin, such as ABC DLBCL or CLL (Grondona et al. 2018). In a normal lymphocyte, an immunoglobulin molecule, together with CD79A/B signals downstream via ITAMs (Johnson et al. 1995). This leads to recruitment of several enzymes including LYN, SYK, FYN, BLK and BTK, all of which results in PLCγ2 activation and DAG production (Harwood and Batista 2010). Increased DAG and Ca^{2+} levels activate PKCβ which is responsible for CARMA1 phosphorylation and NF-κB translocation to the nucleus (Thome et al. 2010). Chronic BCR signaling in B-cell lymphomas has been reported through chronic antigen stimulation, either by infectious agents (such as HBC, HCV, and *H. pylori*) (Quinn et al. 2001) or self-antigens (necrotic cellular by-products) or by genetic lesions driving the activation (Young et al. 2015). The toxicity of small molecule inhibitors and knockout models of the various members of the BCR pathway such as CD79A/B, SYK, PLCγ2, or BTK in ABC DLBCL and CLL further exemplifies the importance of continuous activation of this pathway for malignant cell survival (Davis et al. 2010; Grondona et al. 2018; Ngo et al. 2006). CD79B was found to be mutated in approximately 20% of primary ABC DLBCL samples, usually by way of substitution of the membrane-proximal ITAM tyrosine (Y196) (Davis et al. 2010). While this mutation alone is not sufficient to enhance the NF-κB mediated B-cell proliferation (Wan et al. 2017), dual mutation with MyD88 does lead to malignant transformation and currently CD79B/MyD88 mutated DLBCL represents a distinct subtype of the disease with adverse outcomes compared to other distinct genetic subtypes (Schmitz et al. 2018). Loss of LYN in WM (which can have dual effect on BCR pathway by both activating it and inhibiting it) and overexpression of SYK (in MCL) have been reported as additional events responsible for chronic BCR and NF-κB activation (Hunter et al. 2014).

The hallmark of NF-κB and lymphocyte activation is the creation of high molecular weight complex comprised of CARMA1, BCL10, and MALT1 (CBM complex) (Thome 2004; Grondona et al. 2018). MALT1 is responsible for the recruitment of TRAF6, which polyubiquitinates MALT1, BCL10, and TRAF6 itself (Oeckinghaus et al. 2007). These TRAF6-added polyubiquitin chains serve as docking sites for the IKK complex (Sun et al. 2004). Linear ubiquitin chain assembly complex (LUBAC) is also recruited to the CBM complex and in turn promotes activation of the IKK by mediating its linear ubiquitination (Rahighi et al. 2009). Polyubiquitination also results in the recruitment of TAK1, ultimately responsible for IKK phosphorylation (Adhikari et al. 2007). Recurrent gain-of-function mutations in the genes encoding for CBM proteins result in constitutive NF-κB activation and have been described in a wide range of lymphomas including ABC DLBCL, MCL, MALT lymphoma, ATLL, and cutaneous T-cell lymphoma (CTCL) (Davis et al. 2001; Da Silva Almeida et al. 2015; Grondona et al. 2018; Xu et al. 2020). The toxicity of RNAi-mediated silencing of either CARMA1, BCL10, or MALT1 expression observed in ABC DLBCL cell lines further demonstrates the importance of CBM-mediated signaling in this tumor entity. As a result, there is an ongoing interest in CBM complex blockade (Fontan et al. 2018), including evaluation of MALT1 inhibitors in clinical studies (Lu et al. 2019).

Oncogenic CARMA1 mutations are well described in ABC DLBCL and other lymphomas. These mutations reduce the autoinhibitory function of CARMA1 and lead to constitutive NF-κB activation, independently of the upstream signaling (Lenz et al. 2008).

Translocations involving MALT1 and resulting in MALT1-BCL10 overexpression or a creation of a fusion protein of MALT1 with cellular inhibitor of apoptosis protein 2 (cIAP2) have been well described in MALT lymphomas (Dierlamm et al. 1999; Willis et al. 1999). cIAP2-MALT1 can activate both the canonical (via the MALT1-dependent recruitment of TRAF6 and proteolytic inactivation of A20) and non-canonical NF-κB pathways (by cleavage of CYLD and subsequent ubiquitination of RIP1) drive the growth of MALT lymphomas and numerous others such as DLBCL and ATLL (Noels et al. 2007). As such targeting MALT1 overactivation represents a promising therapeutic approach (Ferch et al. 2009).

A20 is characterized as a tumor suppressor in B-cell lymphomas and its inactivation by inactivating mutations or epigenetic silencing have been well described in several lymphoma subtypes (Honma et al. 2009). A20 exerts its negative control of the NF-κB by deubiquitination of the CBM complex. Its inactivation alone is not sufficient for lymphomagenesis, instead it is frequently found with other pro-oncogenic mutations such as CD79B or MyD88 (Chu et al. 2011; Grondona et al. 2018).

LUBAC is a ubiquitin ligase complex consisting of HOIP, HOIL-1, and SHARPIN that has important regulatory function in NF-κB pathway, as mentioned above. Single nucleotide polymorphism in HOIP that results in increased LUBAC activity has been described. Furthermore, knockdown experiments silencing LUBAC in ABC DLBCL cells lead to inhibition of NF-κB and cell death (Dubois et al. 2014; Yang et al. 2014).

MM and cHL harbor genetic alterations which lead to constitutive activation of the non-canonical NF-κB pathway (Otto et al. 2012; Ranuncolo et al. 2012). Since NIK is the central point of this pathway, any changes that result in overexpression of NIK or its stability from degradation will result in its activation. Examples include copy number gains in the MAP3K14 gene (which encodes NIK) or chromosomal translocations placing MAP3K14 under the control of immunoglobulin enhancer elements. A NIK fusion protein which lacks the TRAF3-binding domain has also been reported. This fusion protein exhibits increased stability due to its resistance to TRAF3-dependent proteasomal degradation. Additionally, inactivating changes affecting negative regulators of NIK such cIAP2 have been described in MCL and DLBCL, and TRAF3 in MM, cHL, and DLBCL. Overactivation of TNFR family members (BAFF-R, RANK, LTβR, and CD40) also results in accelerated TRAF3 clearance and NIK activation and is described in MM and several lymphomas (Grondona et al. 2018; Liao et al. 2004).

Viral infections can overactivate the non-canonical NF-κB pathway and serve as an oncogenic signal. Epstein–Barr Virus (EBV) can, via its latent membrane protein 1 (LMP-1), induce non-canonical NF-κB pathway and serve as an oncogene. Similar pro-oncogenic effect is observed with Tax, a viral protein of human T-cell leukemia virus 1 (HTLV-1), responsible for ATLL (Ishikawa et al. 2015; Kimura et al. 2013).

Genetic changes in the NFKB2 gene locus itself can result in the disruption of the inhibitory ankyrin repeats at the C-terminus of the precursor p100. Such altered gene produces truncated, constitutively active p100 protein, which does not require NIK for activation. The deubiquitinase CYLD has been identified as a tumor suppressor due to its negative control of NF-κB. Mutations or transcriptional silencing of CYLD have been described on MM (Grondona et al. 2018).

Additional mechanisms of NF-κB activation are the changes that cause the aberrant expression of IκB proteins. In cHL, various genetic lesions have been described that result in the generation of truncated IκBα isoforms which lack part of the ankyrin repeats and are thus unable to sequester the NF-κB dimers in the cytoplasm. Similar changes have been reported with IκBε, again resulting in increased nuclear presence of NF-κB proteins, as well as with atypical IκBs such as BCL3 and IκBζ (Grondona et al. 2018; Nogai et al. 2013).

Role of NF-κB in Solid Malignancies

Unlike genetic alterations driving constitutive NF-κB activation in lymphoid malignancies, mutations of NF-κB pathway genes are rarely seen in solid malignancies (Taniguchi and Karin 2018). As previously mentioned, acute and chronic inflammation, as well as obesity-related inflammation plays an important role in carcinogenesis (Taniguchi and Karin 2018). One of the first studies implicating NF-κB in malignant transformation was described in colitis-associated colorectal cancer (CAC) (Greten et al. 2004). Inflammatory bowel disease (IBD) and gastritis can greatly increase the risk of cancer by way of chronic inflammation-associated NF-κB and STAT3 activation and production of pro-tumorigenic cytokines (TNF, IL-1, IL-6, IL-17A, and IL-23) (Grivennikov et al. 2010). In CAC, NF-κB has a dual pro-oncogenic role as a crucial mediator in both epithelial cells as well as in myeloid cells. In epithelial cells, NF-κB prevents apoptosis while in myeloid cells it stimulates the production of pro-inflammatory cytokines (Greten et al. 2004). There is numerous additional data to support the role of chronic inflammation in the development of sporadic colon cancer. First, most cases of sporadic colorectal cancer are associated with an increased production of pro-inflammatory cytokines. Second, elevated expression of these cytokines in patients who have been diagnosed with stage II colorectal cancer predicts high risk of progression to metastatic disease (Schetter et al. 2009). Third, long-term intake of non-steroidal anti-inflammatory drugs such as aspirin and indomethacin results in 20–40% reduction in the risk of colonic adenomas and colorectal cancer in individuals at average risk (Ulrich et al. 2006). Gut microbiota has also been implicated in tumorigenesis, where microbial products are recognized by PRRs, and lead to NF-κB activation and inflammation. Gut microbiota can furthermore affect tumorigenesis, metastasis, and the effectiveness and toxicity of chemotherapy (Routy et al. 2018; Roy and Trinchieri 2017).

Hepatocellular carcinoma (HCC) is another example of malignancy that is highly dependent on inflammation (Mittal and El-Serag 2013; Taniguchi and Karin 2018). There is a clear link between chronic inflammation mediated by viral hepatitis (both HBV and HCV) and HCC. Additionally, growing incidence of non-alcoholic steatohepatitis (NASH) together with alcoholic steatohepatitis further supports the role of NF-κB in this malignancy (Mittal and El-Serag 2013). One of the first reports implicating NF-κB in tumorigenesis came from HCC models that used multidrug resistance protein 2 (MRD2) deficient mice. Hepatocytes in these animals cannot secrete phospholipids into bile, which results in inflammatory cholangitis, eventually progressing to HCC. While this process is not fully understood, the hypothesis is that TNF secreted from Kupffer cells stimulates NF-κB activation. Inhibition of TNF signaling suppresses the expression of NF-κB-dependent pro-survival genes, resulting in enhanced hepatocyte apoptosis (Mauad et al. 1994). Additionally, overexpression of hepatocyte-specific IκBα mutant with super-repressor activity induces the death of pre-malignant cells and blocks HCC development. Subsequent studies further demonstrated the important role of NF-κB in liver malignancy. This is in part due to the fact that surrounding myeloid cells can secrete pro-inflammatory cytokines aiding in the process of malignant transformation. Metabolic syndrome and obesity are associated NASH and chronic inflammation with increased production of TNF and IL-6 leading to augmented risk of HCC formation (Park et al. 2010).

A predominant type of pancreatic cancer is pancreatic ductal adenocarcinoma (PDAC), which is characterized by KRAS activating mutations such as KRAS G12D mutation. KRAS G12D leads to IL-1α expression through AP1 activation, which in turn activates NF-κB. This NF-κB activation stimulates the expression of IL-1α and SQSTM1, therefore creating an IL-1α–SQSTM1 feedforward loop which maintains NF-κB activation (Bryant et al. 2014; Ling et al. 2012). NF-κB cooperates with other oncogenic pathways such as Notch to stimulate PDAC development (Maniati et al. 2011). Similarly, in lung cancer, tobacco smoke was found to promote KRAS G12D mutation leading to NF-κB overexpression (Takahashi et al. 2010).

There are numerous other solid and hematological malignancies such as prostate cancer, breast cancer, melanoma, thyroid cancer, and acute myeloid leukemia (AML) where NF-κB was found to be important in disease initiation, progression, and metastasis or in resistance to available therapeutics and therefore adverse outcomes (Sfanos and De Marzo 2012; Taniguchi and Karin 2018).

NF-κB Targeted Therapies

Approved Drugs

While almost 20 years of research has been dedicated to the role of NF-κB in cancer, the search for direct NF-κB inhibitors has not been successful (Ramadass et al. 2020). A potential explanation for this can be found in the widespread influence NF-κB exhibits on numerous physiological processes (Herscovitch and Gilmore 2006). A sobering example is the IKK inhibitors which were once touted as "treasure trove for drug development" in oncology and rheumatology (Karin et al. 2004). They were evaluated in phases 1 and 2 clinical studies in rheumatology and oncology; however, their further development was discontinued because of toxicity and for underwhelming efficacy. Some of the studies evaluating IKK inhibitors did not report the reason behind discontinuation of further clinical development (Herrington et al. 2016).

The focus has since transitioned to the development of drugs that exhibit either a peripheral effect on NF-κB or its upstream and downstream modulators. One of the first drugs developed and approved for the use in clinic were proteasome inhibitors (PI). PI such as bortezomib, carfilzomib, and ixazomib form the backbone of anti-myeloma therapy and have significant efficacy in other lymphoid malignancies such as mantle cell lymphoma (Ramadass et al. 2020). Bortezomib prevents degradation of IκBα in the proteasome and therefore increases the total available IκBα protein which in turn inhibits NF-κB translocation to the nucleus. The effect on IκBα is not selective since bortezomib reversibly inhibits chymotrypsin like activity of the 26S proteasome. Due to this non-selective inhibition of the proteasome, bortezomib affects a wide array of other proteins, including those important in apoptosis such as activated caspases. Furthermore, several studies on proteasome inhibition in MM cells demonstrated that accumulation of unfolded proteins in the endoplasmic reticulum (ER), so called ER stress, triggers pro-apoptotic signals and causes cellular stress by way of ROS accumulation. This is now considered to be the main mechanism of action by which bortezomib induces apoptosis in MM, rather than its effect on NF-κB. Several additional factors have been identified as predictors of bortezomib treatment through this mechanism. Low levels of XBP1, ATF3, and ATF4 proteins that regulate UPR and ER stress-induced were found in patients who responded poorly to bortezomib treatment (Ri 2016).

A major shift in the management of certain hematologic malignancies occurred with the introduction of BTK inhibitors (Wen et al. 2021). These agents inhibit BCR signaling and thereby downregulate the NF-κB pathway. Once difficult to treat, high-risk patients with CLL associated with certain adverse genetic characteristics (such as loss of TP53) exhibited outcomes that were equal to those patients without adverse genetic characteristics. Additionally, these patients could avoid getting aggressive chemotherapy with all of its toxicities (Wen et al. 2021). While the majority of patients treated with BTK inhibitors did not achieve complete remission (CR), very good disease control by way of partial remissions meant that CLL requiring treatment could be managed as a chronic condition. First approved BTK inhibitor was ibrutinib (Byrd et al. 2014; Farooqui et al. 2015), and several other compounds were developed including FDA-approved molecules such as acalabrutinib (Sharman et al. 2020) or zanubrutinib (https://library.ehaweb.org/eha/2021/eha2021-virtual-congress/330170/peter.hillmen.first.interim.analysis.of.alpine.study.results.of.a.phase.3.html?f=listing%3D0%2Abrowseby%3D8%2Asortby%3D1%2Asearch%3Dalpine; Song et al. 2020). Additional modifications of newer molecules such as non-covalent BTK inhibition (pirtobrutinib) allow for the use of these drugs even in patients whose lymphomas has acquired resistance to the covalent molecules (Mato et al. 2021). BTK inhibitors have now been approved in other lymphomas including marginal zone lymphoma (MZL), MALT lymphomas, MCL, and WM and have shown promising results in DLBCL of the ABC subtype (Wen et al. 2021).

While the PI3K pathway and its inhibitors form a separate pro-oncogenic pathway, there are interconnections with the NF-κB pathway that warrant discussion (Romashkova and Makarov 1999). AKT is a serine/threonine kinase that is a key downstream mediator of the PI3K pathway with numerous targets important in cellular survival including NF-κB (Sizemore et al. 1999). Main control is via degradation of IκBα by phosphorylated and activated AKT (Gustin et al. 2004). Several PI3K inhibitors have been developed and approved for the use in hematologic malignancies such as idelalisib (Gopal et al. 2014). Their use remains low due to their toxicity profile (autoimmune manifestations such as pneumonitis, colitis, and opportunistic infections) as well as low efficacy. PI3K isoform specific compounds have been developed in an effort to improve the adverse event (AE) profile and allow for combination with other drugs used in the treatment of B-cell malignancies. These include copanlisib (alpha and delta isoform), duvelisib (gamma and delta isoform), and umbralisib (delta isoform) (Vanhaesebroeck et al. 2021).

Dysregulation of NF-κB and pro-inflammatory cytokines represents a central point in pathophysiology of autoimmune disease and as such several of the agents used in rheumatology have been studied in inflammation-associated cancers or lymphomas as well. As such tumor necrosis factor receptor super family (TNFRSF) inhibitors have been well studied. Receptor activator of NF-κB ligand (RANKL) inhibitor denosumab is approved for, among other indications, metastases to bone, multiple myeloma, and hypercalcemia due to malignancy (Novack et al. 2003; https://www.amgen.com/media/news-releases/2014/12/fdaapproves-amgens-xgeva-denosumab-for-the-treatment-of-hypercalcemia-of-malignancy-refractory-tobisphosphonate-therapy/).

Anti-inflammatory agents such as NSAIDs were previously discussed in the context of prevention of colorectal cancer. Aspirin and other NSAIDs such as COX2 inhibitors and sulindac were shown to be associated with a 20–40% reduction in the incidence of colorectal adenomas and cancer in individuals of average risk (Dubé et al. 2007).

Low-dose methotrexate (MTX) remains the disease modifying anti-rheumatic drug of choice in rheumatoid arthritis (Willkens and Watson 1982). Same weekly low doses of MTX are used as immunosuppressive therapy in large granular leukemia (LGL) (Lamy and Loughran 2011) and CTCL (Zackheim et al. 1996).

The JAK/STAT pathway cross-communicates with NF-κB via phosphorylated AKT and therefore can exert important influence. Numerous JAK inhibitors have been developed and explored both in autoimmune disease and hematologic malignancies. Tofacitinib was the first approved drug that is used in rheumatoid arthritis. Ruxolitinib is a JAK1/JAK2 inhibitor that is approved for the use in myeloproliferative disorders and is used in graft versus host disease (Verstovsek et al. 2010; Zeiser et al. 2020).

Albeit molecules such as CD79 and CD19 cooperate with BCR in antigen recognition and therefore can influence the activity of NF-κB in B-cell malignancies, novel drugs targeting these molecules such as polatuzumab vedotin (Sehn et al. 2020) (antibody drug conjugate targeting CD79b) and chimeric antigen receptor T-cells (Neelapu et al. 2020) and bispecific antibodies (targeting CD19) are not considered NF-κB inhibitors due to their unique mechanisms of action. It is, however, intriguing that polatuzumab vedotin has a particularly notable effect in previously untreated patients with ABC subtype of DLBCL (Tilly et al. 2022).

Epigenetic drugs such as hypomethylating agents and histone deacetylase (HDAC) inhibitors have a broad reaching effect as they post-translationally modify many cellular targets. Because the state of specific acetylation of p65 greatly affects its ability to bind to DNA and drive the transcription of its target genes, it is understandable how HDAC inhibitors could have a significant effect on NF-κB. For example, acetylation of specific lysine residue Lys122 and Lys123 decreases DNA binding of NF-κB p65, whereas Lys221 and Lys218 acetylation enhances the DNA binding of NF-κB p65. Additionally, hypomethylating agents and HDAC inhibitors can directly reduce the phosphorylation of IKKα/β and result in muted NF-κB activation (Ramadass et al. 2020).

Crucial regulation of p65 within the nucleus resides on proteins regulating their translocation across the nuclear membrane, called importins and exportins. Improtins and exportins shuttle various proteins between the nucleus and the cytoplasm and their inhibition has been explored in preclinical and clinical level. Selinexor, an exportin inhibitor, is FDA approved for use in DLBCL and MM (Chari et al. 2019). Ivermectin, an anti-protozoal drug, was shown to have importin inhibitory activity (Wagsta et al. 2012).

In Development

NF-κB pathway and its inhibition remain at the forefront of scientific interest in the times when we are experiencing a revolution in the approach to treatment of malignancies. Particular interest remains in therapeutic approaches that could alter the tumor microenvironment and therefore allow immunotherapy to achieve better effect. These and other experimental therapies are discussed below (Ramadass et al. 2020).

While broad IKKα/β inhibitors (such as SAR-113945 or MLN-0415) failed to advance within the clinical studies due to their broad effect on physiological processes controlled by NF-κB, some investigators believe that development of more selective and non-ATP competitive inhibitors will lead to more clinical success. For example, sulfasalazine, an anti-inflammatory drug used in inflammatory bowel disease (IBD) (Weber et al. 2000) and some NSAIDs (Yin et al. 1998) exert their anti-NF-κB activity in part by antagonizing the ATP binding to IKKs. Additional venues for drug development include molecules that would specifically block IKKγ (NEMO), IKKε, TBK1, and NIK (Ramadass et al. 2020). One example of a drug that has been approved is amlexanox, a TBK1 inhibitor that was used for aphthous ulcers but is no longer available in the United States. It is, however, still used in Japan for asthma and allergic rhinitis (Bell 2005). NIK inhibition was explored in multiple myeloma due to its crucial role in the control of non-canonical NF-κB pathway. Research with small molecule inhibitor of NIK, JNJ-64290694, has not advanced beyond pre-clinical stage (https://traconpharma.gcs-web.com/news-releases/news-release-details/traconpharmaceuticals-reports-fourth-quarter-and-year-end-2018).

IRAK is a downstream molecule of IL1R and TLR1 and cooperates with MYD88 leading to NF-κB activation. Due to frequentgeneticalterationsofMYD88inlymphoidmalignancies, IRAK inhibition represents an attractive target. Pacritinib is a JAK2 and Fms-like tyrosine kinase 3 (FLT3) inhibitor that also inhibits IRAK1 (Singer et al. 2018). IRAK-specific inhibitors such as PF-06650833 (Danto et al. 2019), CA-4948 (Younes et al. 2019), and R-835 (Lamagna et al. 2000) have been explored in clinical studies in patients with autoimmune diseases or myeloid malignancies. KT-474 is an orally available, a first-in-class IRAK4 PROTAC (proteolysis targeting chimera) mediates ubiquitination and degradation of the target protein, is in clinical studies in patients with rheumatoid arthritis and other autoimmune disorders. Additional studies are planned in patients with hematological malignancies (https://investors.kymeratx.com/news-releases/news-release-details/kymera-discloses-new-kt-474-clinical-data-unveils-new).

Other upstream inhibitors of BCR signaling including SYK, LYN, PKCβ, and MALT1 are at various stage of clinical development and their clear role in the therapeutic algorithm for B-cell lymphomas has yet to be fully clarified (Ramadass et al. 2020).

Mitogen-activated protein kinase (MAPK) pathway is another broad reaching cellular signaling pathways that can affect cellular proliferation and survival via its downstream molecules ERK, p38, and JNK. It also interacts with other signaling pathways, including NF-κB. The inhibitors of MAPK effector proteins, such as ulixertinib (ERK inhibitor), have been explored extensively in clinical studies focusing on patients with autoimmune disease and cancer (Braicu et al. 2019).

cIAP inhibitors have also been explored in the clinical arena based on that cIAP1, cIAP2, and XIAP represent critical regulators of NF-κB through the TNFR pathway. Notable examples include ASTX660, a cIAP1/2/XIAP inhibitor with efficacy in PTCL and CTCL (Mita et al. 2020) and second mitochondria-derived activators of caspase (SMAC) mimetics with cIAP/XIAP inhibitory function, AT406, and APG-1387 with activity in various solid malignancies (Pan et al. 2018).

Inhibition of the proteasome-ubiquitin system has been discussed above in the section on proteasome inhibitors and other drugs that could affect the process of ubiquitination. The role of deubiquitination (DUB) inhibitors or NEDD8 activating enzyme (NAE) inhibitors has yet to be fully elucidated. A phase study of a DUB inhibitor VLX1570 has been discontinued due to pulmonary toxicity observed in patients with multiple myeloma (Rowinsky et al. 2020). NEDD8 is a ubiquitin-like protein that can post-translationally modify various cellular targets, including NEDDylation of the Cullin-RING-E3 ubiquitin ligases. This process leads to the activation of these ligases, a critical step in the process of the proteasome-mediated protein degradation. This broad intervention to a slew of cellular products could result in adverse effects which prevented the use of higher doses of a first in class drug, pevonedistat in clinical studies (Swords et al. 2017). Pevonedistat showed promising activity in early phase clinical studies in myeloid malignancies but failed to provide a benefit is a phase 3 study (https://www.takeda.com/newsroom/newsreleases/2021/takeda-provides-update-on-phase-3-panther-pevonedistat-3001-trial).

In the context of microenvironment and the role of NF-κB, it is widely recognized that chemotherapy, surgical resection, and radiotherapy could potentially contribute to tumor progression because of increased inflammation and genotoxic stress (Taniguchi and Karin 2018). The same process could also increase the expression of increase PD-L1 on malignant tissue and allow for more efficacy of checkpoint inhibitors. Inhibition of NF-κB can furthermore alter the T-cell population within the malignant tissue so it can be if crucial importance to understand how to achieve this balance that would allow for more efficacy of the immunotherapy (Karin and Greten 2005).

Recently discovered novel approach in NF-κB inhibition includes stabilization of IκB to p50-p65 dimer, sequestering it in the cytoplasm and preventing its binding to DNA (Kalac et al. 2020).

Summary

As we discuss above, NF-κB has a tremendous, untapped potential as a novel drug target in oncology. Because of its implication in wide array physiologic and pathophysiologic processes, innovative ways of controlling this pathway are needed. This is in order to use as an anti-cancer target, avoiding excessive toxicity. Modern lymphoma therapy has been transformed by development of inhibitors that act on targets upstream of NF-κB. Replicating similar effect directly on NF-κB therefore represents an exciting and worthy challenge.

Must Read References

Liu, T., Zhang, L., Joo, D. et al. (2017). NF-κB signaling in inflammation. *Signal Transduct. Target Ther.* 2: 17023. doi: 10.1038/sigtrans.2017.23.

Taniguchi, K., Karin, M. (2018). NF-κB, inflammation, immunity and cancer: coming of age. *Nat. Rev. Immunol.* 18: 309–324.

Yu, H., Lin, L., Zhang, Z. et al. (2020). Targeting NF-κB pathway for the therapy of diseases: mechanism and clinical study. *Signal Transduct. Target Ther.* 5: 209.

References

Adhikari, A., Xu, M., and Chen, Z.J. (2007). Ubiquitin-mediated activation of TAK1 and IKK. *Oncogene* 26: 3214–3226.

Akira, S. and Takeda, K. (2004). Toll-like receptor signalling. *Nat. Rev. Immunol.* 4: 499–511.

Ang, H.L. and Tergaonkar, V. (2007). Notch and NFkappaB signaling pathways: do they collaborate in normal vertebrate brain development and function? *Bioessays* 29: 1039–1047.

Annunziata, C.M., Davis, R.E., Demchenko, Y. et al. (2007). Frequent engagement of the classical and alternative NF-κB pathways by diverse genetic abnormalities in multiple myeloma. *Cancer Cell.* 12: 115–130.

Avbelj, M., Wolz, O.O., Fekonja, O. et al. (2014). Activation of lymphoma-associated MyD88 mutations via allostery-induced TIR-domain oligomerization. *Blood* 124: 3896–3904.

Baker, R.G., Hayden, M.S., and Ghosh, S. (2011). NF- κB, inflammation, and metabolic disease. *Cell Metab.* 13: 11–22.

Balkwill, F. (2009). Tumour necrosis factor and cancer. *Nat. Rev. Cancer.* 9: 361–371.

Balkwill, F. and Mantovani, A. (2010). Inflammation and cancer: back to virchow? *Lancet* 357: 539–545.

Bargou, R.C., Leng, C., Krappmann, D. et al. (1996). High-level nuclear NF-κB and Oct-2 is a common feature of cultured Hodgkin/reed-sternberg cells. *Blood.* 87: 4340–4347.

Bartek, J. and Lukas, J. (2006). Cell biology. the stress of finding NEMO. *Science* 311: 1110–1111.

Bell, J. (2005). Amlexanox for the treatment of recurrent aphthous ulcers. *Clin. Drug Investig.* 25: 555–566.

Ben-Neriah, Y. and Karin, M. (2011). Inflammation meets cancer, with NF-κB as the matchmaker. *Nat. Immunol.* 12: 715–723.

Beug, H., Muller, H., Grieser, S. et al. (1981). Hematopoietic cells transformed in vitro by REVT avian reticuloendotheliosis virus express characteristics of very immature lymphoid cells. *Virology* 115: 295–309.

Bi, K., Tanaka, Y., Coudronniere, N. et al. (2001). Antigen-induced translocation of PKC-theta to membrane rafts is required for T cell activation. *Nat. Immunol.* 2: 556–563.

Braicu, C., Buse, M., Busuioc, C. et al. (2019). A comprehensive review on MAPK: a promising therapeutic target in cancer. *Cancers (Basel).* 11: 1618.

Bryant, K.L., Mancias, J.D., Kimmelman, A.C. et al. (2014). KRAS: feeding pancreatic cancer proliferation. *Trends. Biochem. Sci.* 39: 91–100.

Byrd, J.C., Brown, J.R., O'Brien, S. et al. (2014). Ibrutinib versus ofatumumab in previously treated chronic lymphoid leukemia. *N. Engl. J. Med.* 371: 213–223.

Calle, E.E., Rodriguez, C., Walker-Thurmond, K. et al. (2003). Overweight, obesity, and mortality from cancer in a prospectively studied cohort of U. S. adults. *N. Engl. J. Med.* 348: 1625–1638.

Cao, X. (2016). Self-regulation and cross-regulation of pattern-recognition receptor signalling in health and disease. *Nat. Rev. Immunol.* 16: 35–50.

Chari, A., Vogl, D.T., Gavriatopoulou, M. et al. (2019). Oral selinexor-dexamethasone for triple-class refractory multiple myeloma. *N. Engl. J. Med.* 381: 727–738.

Chen, Z.J. (2012). Ubiquitination in signaling to and activation of IKK. *Immunol. Rev.* 246: 95–106.

Chiang, C. and Gack, M.U. (2017). Post-translational control of intracellular pathogen sensing pathways. *Trends. Immunol.* 38: 39–52.

Chu, Y., Vahl, J.C., Kumar, D. et al. (2011). B cells lacking the tumor suppressor TNFAIP3/A20 display impaired differentiation and hyperactivation and cause inflammation and autoimmunity in aged mice. *Blood* 117: 2227–2236.

Coussens, L.M. and Werb, Z. (2002). Inflammation and cancer. *Nature* 420: 860–867.

Covert, M.W., Leung, T.H., Gaston, J.E. et al. (2005). Achieving stability of lipopolysaccharide-induced NF-kappaB activation. *Science* 309: 1854–1857.

Da Silva Almeida, A.C., Abate, F., Khiabanian, H. et al. (2015). The mutational landscape of cutaneous T cell lymphoma and Sézary syndrome. *Nat. Genet.* 47: 1465–1470.

Danto, S.I., Shojaee, N., Singh, R.S.P. et al. (2019). Safety, tolerability, pharmacokinetics, and pharmacodynamics of PF-06650833, a selective interleukin-1 receptor-associated kinase 4 (IRAK4) inhibitor, in single and multiple ascending dose randomized phase 1 studies in healthy subjects. *Arthritis. Res. Ther.* 21: 269.

Davis, R.E., Brown, K.D., Siebenlist, U. et al. (2001). Constitutive nuclear factor κB activity is required for survival of activated B cell-like diffuse large B cell lymphoma cells. *J. Exp. Med.* 194: 1861–1874.

Davis, R.E., Ngo, V.N., Lenz, G. et al. (2010). Chronic active B-cell-receptor signalling in diffuse large B-cell lymphoma. *Nature* 463: 88–92.

Dierlamm, J., Baens, M., Wlodarska, I. et al. (1999). The apoptosis inhibitor gene API2 and a novel 18q gene, MLT, are recurrently rearranged in the t(11;18)(q21;q21) associated with mucosa-associated lymphoid tissue lymphomas. *Blood* 93: 3601–3609.

Dossang, A.C., Motshwene, P.G., Yang, Y. et al. (2016). The N-terminal loop of IRAK-4 death domain regulates ordered assembly of the Myddosome signalling scaffold. *Sci. Rep.* 6: 37267.

Dubé, C., Rostom, A., Lewin, G. et al. (2007). U.S. preventive services task force. the use of aspirin for primary prevention of colorectal cancer: a systematic review prepared for the U.S. preventive services task force. *Ann. Intern. Med.* 146: 365.

Dubois, S.M., Alexia, C., Wu, Y. et al. (2014). A catalytic-independent role for the LUBAC in NF-κB activation upon antigen receptor engagement and in lymphoma cells. *Blood.* 123: 2199–2203.

Evans, P.C., Taylor, E.R., Coadwell, J. et al. (2001). Isolation and characterization of two novel A20-like proteins. *Biochem. J.* 357: 617–623.

Farooqui, M.Z.H., Valdez, J., Martyr, S. et al. (2015). Ibrutinib for previously untreated and relapsed or refractory chronic lymphocytic leukaemia with TP53 aberrations: a phase 2, single-arm trial. *Lancet* 16: 169–176.

Ferch, U., Kloo, B., Gewies, A. et al. (2009). Inhibition of MALT1 protease activity is selectively toxic for activated B cell-like diffuse large B cell lymphoma cells. *J. Exp. Med.* 206: 2313–2320.

Fontan, L., Qiao, Q., Hatcher, J.M. et al. (2018). Specific covalent inhibition of MALT1 paracaspase suppresses B cell lymphoma growth. *J. CLin. Invest.* 128: 4397–4412.

Fujiki, H. (2014). Gist of Dr. Katsusaburo Yamagiwa's papers entitled "Experimental study on the pathogenesis of epithelial tumors" (I to VI reports). *Cancer Sci.* 105: 143–149.

Ghosh, S. and Hayden, M.S. (2008). New regulators of NF-κB in inflammation. *Nat. Rev. Immunol.* 8: 837–848.

Gopal, A.K., Kahl, B.S., de Vos, S. et al. (2014). PI3Kδ inhibition by idelalisib in patients with relapsed indolent lymphoma. *N. Engl. J. Med.* 370: 1008–1018.

Greten, F.R., Eckmann, L., Greten, T.F. et al. (2004). IKKbeta links inflammation and tumorigenesis in a mouse model of colitis-associated cancer. *Cell.* 118: 285–296.

Grivennikov, S.I., Greten, F.R., and Karin, M. (2010). Immunity, inflammation, and cancer. *Cell* 140: 883–899.

Grivennikov, S.I. and Karin, M. (2010). Dangerous liaisons: STAT3 and NF-kappaB collaboration and crosstalk in cancer. *Cytokine. Growth Factor Rev.* 21: 11–19.

Grondona, P., Bucher, P., Schulze-Ostoff, K. et al. (2018). κB activation in lymphoid malignancies: genetics, signaling, and targeted therapy. *Biomedicines* 6: 38.

Gudkov, A.V., Gurova, K.V., and Komarova, E.A. (2011). Inflammation and p53: a tale of two stresses. *Genes Cancer.* 2: 503–516.

Gudkov, A.V. and Komarova, E.A. (2016). p53 and the carcinogenicity of chronic inflammation. *Cold Spring Harb. Perspect. Med.* 6: a026161.

Gustin, J.A., Ozes, O.N., Akca, H. et al. (2004). Cell type-specific expression of the IkappaB kinases determines the significance of phosphatidylinositol 3-kinase/Akt signaling to NF-kappa B activation. *J. Biol. Chem.* 279: 1615–1620.

Häcker, H. and Karin, M. (2006). Regulation and function of IKK and IKK-related kinases. *Science STKE*2006: re13.

Harwood, N.E. and Batista, F.D. (2010). Early events in B cell activation. *Annu. Rev. Immunol.* 28: 185–210.

Hayden, M.S. and Ghosh, S. (2008). Shared principles in NF-kappaB signaling. *Cell* 132: 344–362.

Herrington, F.D., Carmody, R.J., and Goodyear, C.S. (2016). Modulation of NF-κB signaling as a therapeutic target in autoimmunity. *J. Biomol. Screen.* 21: 223–242.

Herscovitch, M. and Gilmore, T.D. (2006). Inhibitors of NF-kB signaling: 785 and counting. *Oncogene* 25: 6887–6899.

Hoffmann, A., Natoli, G., and Ghosh, G. (2006). Transcriptional regulation via the NFkappaB signaling module. *Oncogene* 25: 6706–6716.

Honma, K., Tsuzuki, S., Nakagawa, M. et al. (2009). TNFAIP3/A20 functions as a novel tumor suppressor gene in several subtypes of non-Hodgkin lymphomas. *Blood* 114: 2467–2475.

Hsu, H., Huang, J., Shu, H.B. et al. (1996). TNF-dependent recruitment of the protein kinase RIP to the TNF receptor-1 signaling complex. *Immunity* 4: 387–396.

Hu, H. and Sun, S.C. (2016). Ubiquitin signaling in immune responses. *Cell Res.* 26: 457–483.

Huang, S., Pettaway, C.A., Uehara, H. et al. (2001). Blockade of NF-kappaB activity in human prostate cancer cells is associated with suppression of angiogenesis, invasion, and metastasis. *Oncogene* 20: 4188–4197.

Hunter, Z.R., Xu, L., Yang, G. et al. (2014). The genomic landscape of Waldenstrom macroglobulinemia is characterized by highly recurring MYD88 and WHIM-like CXCR4 mutations, and small somatic deletions associated with B-cell lymphomagenesis. *Blood* 123: 1637–1646.

Hymowitz, S.G. and Wertz, I.E. (2010). A20: from ubiquitin editing to tumour suppression. *Nat. Rev. Cancer.* 10: 332–341.

Ishikawa, C., Senba, M., and Mori, N. (2015). Induction of IκB-ζ by Epstein–Barr virus latent membrane protein-1 and CD30. *Int. J. Oncol.* 47: 2197–2207.

Johnson, S.A., Pleiman, C.M., Pao, L. et al. (1995). Phosphorylated immunoreceptor signaling motifs (ITAMs) exhibit unique abilities to bind and activate Lyn and Syk tyrosine kinases. *J. Immunol.* 155: 4596–4603.

Joyce, D., Albanese, C., Steer, J. et al. (2001). NF-kappaB and cell-cycle regulation: the cyclin connection. *Cytokine. Growth Factor Rev.* 12: 73–90.

Kalac, M., Mangone, M., Rinderspacher, A. et al. (2020). N-quinoline-benzenesulfonamide derivatives exert potent anti-lymphoma effect by targeting NF-κB. *iScience* 23: 101884.

Karin, M. and Greten, F.R. (2005). NF-κB: linking inflammation and immunity to cancer development and progression. *Nat. Rev. Immunol.* 5: 749–759.

Karin, M., Yamamoto, Y., and Wang, Q.M. (2004). The IKK NF-κB system: a treasure trove for drug development. *Nat. Rev. Drug Discov.* 3: 17–26.

Kawagoe, T., Sato, S., Matsushita, K. et al. (2008). Sequential control of Toll-like receptor-dependent responses by IRAK1 and IRAK2. *Nat. Immunol.* 9: 684–691.

Kimura, R., Senba, M., Cutler, S.J. et al. (2013). Human T cell leukemia virus type I tax-induced IκB-ζ modulates tax-dependent and tax-independent gene expression in T cells. *Neoplasia* 15: 1110–1124.

Kiraly, O., Gong, G., Olipitz, W. et al. (2015). Inflammation-induced cell proliferation potentiates DNA damage-induced mutations in vivo. *PLoS Genet.* 11: e1004901.

Knittel, G., Liedgens, P., Korovkina, D. et al. (2016). B-cell-specific conditional expression of Myd88p.L252P leads to the development of diffuse large B-cell lymphoma in mice. *Blood* 127: 2732–2741.

Kuper, H., Adami, H.O., and Trichopoulos, D. (2000). Infections as a major preventable cause of human cancer. *J. Intern. Med.* 248: 171–183.

Lamagna, C., Gundel, C., Chan, M. et al. (2000). R835, a novel IRAK1/4 dual inhibitor in clinical development, blocks TLR4 signaling in human and mouse. *Ann. Rheumat. Dis.* 79 (Suppl_1): FRI0016.

Lamy, T. and Loughran, J.T.P. (2011). How I treat LGL leukemia. *Blood* 117: 2764–2774.

Lenz, G., Davis, R.E., Ngo, V.N. et al. (2008). Oncogenic CARD11 mutations in human diffuse large B cell lymphoma. *Science* 319: 1676–1679.

Li, M.O. and Rudensky, A.Y. (2016). T cell receptor signalling in the control of regulatory T cell differentiation and function. *Nat. Rev. Immunol.* 16: 220–233.

Li, Q., Lu, Q., Bottero, V. et al. (2005). Enhanced NF-kappaB activation and cellular function in macrophages lacking IkappaB kinase 1 (IKK1). *Proc. Natl. Acad. Sci. U. S. A.* 102: 12425–12430.

Li, Y., Sedwick, C.E., Hu, J. et al. (2005). Role for protein kinase ctheta (PKCtheta) in TCR/CD28-mediated signaling through the canonical but not the noncanonical pathway for NF-kappaB activation. *J. Biol. Chem.* 280: 1217–1223.

Li, Y., Yang, J.Y., Xie, X. et al. (2019). Preventing abnormal NF-κB activation and autoimmunity by Otub1-mediated p100 stabilization. *Cell Res.* 29: 474–475.

Liao, G., Zhang, M., Harhaj, E.W. et al. (2004). Regulation of the NF-κB-inducing kinase by tumor necrosis factor receptor-associated factor 3-induced degradation. *J. Biol. Chem.* 279: 26243–26250.

Ling, J., Kang, Y., Zhao, R. et al. (2012). KrasG12D-induced IKK2/β/NF-κB activation by IL-1α and p62 feedforward loops is required for development of pancreatic ductal adenocarcinoma. *Cancer Cell* 21: 105–120.

Liu, T., Zhang, L., Joo, D. et al. (2017). NF-κB signaling in inflammation. *Signal Transduct. Target Ther.* 2: 17023. doi: 10.1038/sigtrans.2017.23.

Lu, T., Connolly, P.J., Philippar, U. et al. (2019). Discovery and optimization of a series of small-molecule allosteric inhibitors of MALT1 protease. *Bioorg Med. Chem. Lett.* 29: 126743.

Maniati, E., Bossard, M., Cook, N. et al. (2011). Crosstalk between the canonical NF-κB and Notch signaling pathways inhibits Pparγ expression and promotes pancreatic cancer progression in mice. *J. Clin. Invest.* 121: 4685–4699.

Mato, A.R., Shah, N.N., Jurczak, W. et al. (2021). Pirtobrutinib in relapsed or refractory B-cell malignancies (BRUIN): a phase 1/2 study. *Lancet* 397: 892–901.

Mauad, T.H., van Nieuwkerk, C.M., Dingemans, K.P. et al. (1994). Mice with homozygous disruption of the mdr2 P-glycoprotein gene. A novel animal model for studies of nonsuppurative inflammatory cholangitis and hepatocarcinogenesis. *Am. J. Pathol.* 145: 1237–1245.

Mevissen, T.E.T., Kulathu, Y., Mulder, M.P.C. et al. (2016). Molecular basis of Lys11-polyubiquitin specificity in the deubiquitinase Cezanne. *Nature* 538: 402–405.

Michallet, M.C., Meylan, E., Ermolaeva, M.A. et al. (2008). TRADD protein is an essential component of the RIG-like helicase antiviral pathway. *Immunity* 28: 651–661.

Mita, M.M., LoRusso, P.M., Papadopoulos, K.P. et al. (2020). A phase I study of ASTX660, an antagonist of inhibitors of apoptosis proteins, in adults with advanced cancers or lymphoma. *Clin. Cancer Res.* 26: 2819–2826.

Mittal, S. and El-Serag, H.B. (2013). Epidemiology of hepatocellular carcinoma: consider the population. *J. Clin. Gastroenterol.* 47 (Suppl(0)): S2–6.

Nakshatri, H., Appaiah, H.N., Anjanappa, M. et al. (2015). NF-κB-dependent and -independent epigenetic modulation using the novel anti-cancer agent DMAPT. *Cell. Death Dis.* 6: e1608.

Neelapu, S.S., Jacobson, C.A., Oluwole, O.O. et al. (2020). Outcomes of older patients in ZUMA-1, a pivotal study of axicabtagene ciloleucel in refractory large B-cell lymphoma. *Blood* 135: 2106–2109.

Ngo, V.N., Davis, R.E., Lamy, L. et al. (2006). A loss-of-function RNA interference screen for molecular targets in cancer. *Nature* 441: 106–110.

Ngo, V.N., Young, R.M., Schmitz, R. et al. (2011). Oncogenically active MYD88 mutations in human lymphoma. *Nature* 470: 115–119.

Ni, H., Ergin, M., Huang, Q. et al. (2001). Analysis of expression of nuclear factor kappa B (NF-κB) in multiple myeloma: downregulation of NF-κB induces apoptosis. *Br. J. Haematol.* 115: 279–286.

Noels, H., van Loo, G., Hagens, S. et al. (2007). A novel TRAF6 binding site in MALT1 defines distinct mechanisms of NF-κB activation by API2middle dotMALT1 fusions. *J. Biol. Chem.* 282: 10180–10189.

Nogai, H., Wenzel, S.S., Hailfinger, S. et al. (2013). IκB-ζ controls the constitutive NF-κB target gene network and survival of ABC DLBCL. *Blood* 122: 2242–2250.

Novack, D.V., Yin, L., Hagen-Stapleton, A. et al. (2003). The IkappaB function of NF-kappaB2 p100 controls stimulated osteoclastogenesis. *J. Exp. Med.* 198: 771–781.

Oeckinghaus, A. and Ghosh, S. (2009). The NF-κB family of transcription factors and its regulation. *Cold Spring Harb. Perspect. Biol.* 1: a000034.

Oeckinghaus, A., Wegener, E., Welteke, V. et al. (2007). Malt1 ubiquitination triggers NF-κB signaling upon T-cell activation. *EMBO J.* 26: 4634–4645.

Otto, C., Giefing, M., Massow, A. et al. (2012). Genetic lesions of the TRAF3 and MAP3K14 genes in classical Hodgkin lymphoma. *Br. J. Haematol.* 157: 702–708.

Pan, W., Luo, Q., Yan, X. et al. (2018). A novel SMAC mimetic APG-1387 exhibits dual antitumor effect on HBV-positive hepatocellular carcinoma with high expression of cIAP2 by inducing apoptosis and enhancing innate anti-tumor immunity. *Biochem. Pharmacol.* 154: 127–135.

Park, E.J., Lee, J.H., Yu, G.Y. et al. (2010). Dietary and genetic obesity promote liver inflammation and tumorigenesis by enhancing IL-6 and TNF expression. *Cell* 140: 197–208.

Park, S.R. (2012). Activation-induced Cytidine Deaminase in B Cell Immunity and Cancers. *Immune Netw.* 12: 230–239.

Perkins, N.D. (2012). The diverse and complex roles of NF-κB subunits in cancer. *Nat. Rev. Cancer.* 12: 121–132.

Pikarsky, E., Porat, R.M., Stein, I. et al. (2004). NF-kappaB functions as a tumour promoter in inflammation-associated cancer. *Nature* 431: 461–466.

Pires, B.R., Mencalha, A.L., Ferreira, G.M. et al. (2017). NF-kappaB is involved in the regulation of EMT genes in breast cancer cells. *PLoS One* 12: e0169622.

Plummer, M., de Martel, C., Vignat, J. et al. (2016). Global burden of cancers attributable to infections in 2012: a synthetic analysis. *Lancet Glob. Health* 4: e609–16.

Pomerantz, J.L., Denny, E.M., and Baltimore, D. (2002). CARD11 mediates factor-specific activation of NF-kappaB by the T cell receptor complex. *EMBO J.* 21: 5184–5194.

Puente, X.S., Pinyol, M., Quesada, V. et al. (2011). Whole-genome sequencing identifies recurrent mutations in chronic lymphocytic leukaemia. *Nature* 475: 101–105.

Quinn, E.R., Chan, C.H., Hadlock, K.G. et al. (2001). The B-cell receptor of a hepatitis C virus (HCV)-associated non-Hodgkin lymphoma binds the viral E2 envelope protein, implicating HCV in lymphomagenesis. *Blood* 98: 3745–3749.

Rahal, R., Frick, M., Romero, R. et al. (2014). Pharmacological and genomic profiling identifies NF-κB-targeted treatment strategies for mantle cell lymphoma. *Nat. Med.* 20: 87–92.

Rahighi, S., Ikeda, F., Kawasaki, M. et al. (2009). Specific recognition of linear ubiquitin chains by NEMO is important for NF-κB activation. *Cell* 136: 1098–1109.

Ramadass, V., Vaiyapuri, T., and Tergaonkar, V. (2020). Small molecule NF-κB pathway inhibitors in clinic. *Int. J. Mol. Sci.* 21: 5164.

Ranuncolo, S.M., Pittaluga, S., Evbuomwan, M.O. et al. (2012). Hodgkin lymphoma requires stabilized NIK and constitutive RelB expression for survival. *Blood* 120: 3756–3763.

Rao, P., Hayden, M.S., Long, M. et al. (2010). IkappaBbeta acts to inhibit and activate gene expression during the inflammatory response. *Nature* 466: 1115–1119.

Ren, J., Wang, Y., Gao, Y. et al. (2011). FAT10 mediates the effect of TNF-α in inducing chromosomal instability. *J. Cell Sci.*124: 3665–3675.

Ri, M. (2016). Mechanism of action of bortezomib in multiple myeloma therapy. *Int. J. Myeloma.* 6: 1–6.

Romashkova, J.A. and Makarov, S.S. (1999). NF-kappaB is a target of AKT in anti-apoptotic PDGF signalling. *Nature* 401: 86–90.

Routy, B., Le Chatelier, E., Derosa, L. et al. (2018). Gut microbiome influences efficacy of PD-1-based immunotherapy against epithelial tumors. *Science* 359: 91–97.

Rowinsky, E.K., Paner, A., Berdeja, J.G. et al. (2020). Phase 1 study of the protein deubiquitinase inhibitor VLX1570 in patients with relapsed and/or refractory multiple myeloma. *Invest. New Drugs* 38: 1448–1453.

Roy, S. and Trinchieri, G. (2017). Microbiota: a key orchestrator of cancer therapy. *Nat Rev Cancer.* 17: 271–285.

Savage, K.J., Monti, S., Kutok, J.L. et al. (2003). The molecular signature of mediastinal large B-cell lymphoma differs from that of other diffuse large B-cell lymphomas and shares features with classical Hodgkin lymphoma. *Blood* 102: 3871–3879.

Scheel, C. and Weinberg, R.A. (2012). Cancer stem cells and epithelial-mesenchymal transition: concepts and molecular links. *Semin. Cancer Biol.* 22: 396–403.

Schetter, A.J., Nguyen, G.H., Bowman, E.D. et al. (2009). Association of inflammation-related and microRNA gene expression with cancer-specific mortality of colon adenocarcinoma. *Clin. Cancer Res.* 15: 5878–5887.

Schmitz, R., Wright, G.W., Huang, D.W. et al. (2018). *N. Eng. J. Med.* 378: 1396–1407.

Sehn, L.H., Herrera, A.F., Flowers, C.R. et al. (2020). Polatuzumab vedotin in relapsed or refractory diffuse large B-cell lymphoma. *J. Clin. Oncol.* 38: 155–165.

Sen, R. and Baltimore, D. (1986). Multiple nuclear factors interact with the immunoglobulin enhancer sequences. *Cell* 46: 705–716.

Sfanos, K.S. and De Marzo, A.M. (2012). Prostate cancer and inflammation: the evidence. *Histopathology* 60: 199–215.

Sharman, J.P., Egyed, M., Jurczak, W. et al. (2020). Acalabrutinib with or without obinutuzumab versus chlorambucil and obinutuzumab for treatment-naïve chronic lymphocytic leukaemia (ELEVATE-TN): a randomised, controlled, phase 3 trial. *Lancet* 395: 1278–1291.

Shinohara, H., Yasuda, T., Aiba, Y. et al. (2005). PKC beta regulates BCR-mediated IKK activation by facilitating the interaction between TAK1 and CARMA1. *J. Exp. Med.* 202: 1423–1431.

Singer, J.W., Fleischman, A., Al-Fayoumi, S. et al. (2018). Inhibition of interleukin-1 receptor-associated kinase 1 (IRAK1) as a therapeutic strategy. *Oncotarget* 9: 33416–33439.

Sizemore, N., Leung, S., and Stark, G.R. (1999). Activation of phosphatidylinositol 3- kinase in response to interleukin-1 leads to phosphorylation and activation of the NF-kappaB p65/RelA subunit. *Mol. Cell. Biol.* 19: 4798–4805.

Song, Y., Zhou, K., Zou, D. et al. (2020). Treatment of patients with relapsed or refractory mantle–cell lymphoma with zanubrutinib, a selective inhibitor of bruton's tyrosine kinase. *Clin. Cancer Res.* 26: 4216–4224. https://investors.kymeratx.com/news-releases/news-release-details/kymera-discloses-new-kt-474-clinical-data-unveils-new

Staudt, L.M. (2010). Oncogenic activation of NF-κB. *Cold Spring Harb. Perspect. Biol.* 2: a000109.

Su, T.T., Guo, B., Kawakami, Y. et al. (2002). PKC-beta controls I kappa B kinase lipid raft recruitment and activation in response to BCR signaling. *Nat. Immunol.* 3: 780–786.

Sun, L., Deng, L., Ea, C.K. et al. (2004). The TRAF6 ubiquitin ligase and TAK1 kinase mediate IKK activation by BCL10 and MALT1 in T lymphocytes. *Mol. Cell* 14: 289–301.

Sun, S.C. (2017). The non-canonical NF-κB pathway in immunity and inflammation. *Nat. Rev. Immunol.* 17: 545–558.

Sun, S.C., Ganchi, P.A., Ballard, D.W. et al. (1993). NF-kappa B controls expression of inhibitor I kappa B alpha: evidence for an inducible autoregulatory pathway. *Science* 259: 1912–1915.

Swords, R.T., Watts, J., Erba, H.P. et al. (2017). Expanded safety analysis of pevonedistat, a first-in-class NEDD8-activating enzyme inhibitor, in patients with acute myeloid leukemia and myelodysplastic syndromes. *Blood Cancer J.* 7: e520.

Takaesu, G., Kishida, S., Hiyama, A. et al. (2000). TAB2, a novel adaptor protein, mediates activation of TAK1 MAPKKK by linking TAK1 to TRAF6 in the IL-1 signal transduction pathway. *Mol. Cell.* 5: 649–8.

Takahashi, H., Ogata, H., Nishigaki, R. et al. (2010). Tobacco smoke promotes lung tumorigenesis by triggering IKKbeta- and JNK1-dependent inflammation. *Cancer Cell.* 17: 89–97.

Takeuchi, O. and Akira, S. (2010). Pattern recognition receptors and inflammation. *Cell* 140: 805–820.

Tam, W.F. and Sen, R. (2001). IkappaB family members function by different mechanisms. *J. Biol. Chem.* 276: 7701–7704.

Taniguchi, K. and Karin, M. (2014). IL-6 and related cytokines as the critical lynchpins between inflammation and cancer. *Semin. Immunol.* 26: 54–74.

Taniguchi, K. and Karin, M. (2018). NF-κB, inflammation, immunity and cancer: coming of age. *Nat. Rev. Immunol.* 18: 309–324.

Taniguchi, K., Yamachika, S., He, F. et al. (2016). p62/SQSTM1 –dr. Jekyll and Mr. Hyde that prevents oxidative stress but promotes liver cancer. *FEBS Lett.* 590: 2375–2397.

Thome, M. (2004). CARMA1, BCL-10 and MALT1 in lymphocyte development and activation. *Nat. Rev. Immunol.* 4: 348–359.

Thome, M., Charton, J.E., Pelzer, C. et al. (2010). Antigen receptor signaling to NF-κB via CARMA1, BCL10, and MALT1. *Cold Spring Harb. Perspect Biol.* 2: a003004.

Tilly, H., Morschauser, F., Sehn, L.H. et al. (2022). Polatuzumab vedotin in previously intreated diffuse large B-cell lymphoma. *N. Eng. J. Med.* 386: 351–363.

Treon, S.P., Xu, L., Yang, G. et al. (2012). MYD88 L265P somatic mutation in Waldenstrom's macroglobulinemia. *N. Engl. J. Med.* 367: 826–833.

Ulrich, C.M., Bigler, J., and Potter, J.D. (2006). Non-steroidal anti-inflammatory drugs for cancer prevention: promise, perils and pharmacogenetics. *Nat. Rev. Cancer* 6: 130–140.

Vallabhapurapu, S. and Karin, M. (2009). Regulation and function of NF-kappaB transcription factors in the immune system. *Annu. Rev. Immunol.* 27: 693–733.

Vanhaesebroeck, B., Perry, M.W.D., Brown, J.R. et al. (2021). PI3K inhibitors are finally coming of age. *Nat. Rev. Drug Discov.* 20: 741–769.

Vento-Tormo, R., Rodríguez-Ubreva, J., Lisio, L.D. et al. (2014). NF-κB directly mediates epigenetic deregulation of common microRNAs in Epstein–Barr virus-mediated transformation of B-cells and in lymphomas. *Nucleic Acids Res.* 42: 11025–11039.

Verstovsek, S., Kantarjian, H., Mesa, R.A. et al. (2010). Safety and efficacy of INCB018424, a JAK1 and JAK2 inhibitor, in myelofibrosis. *N. Engl. J. Med.* 363: 1117–1127.

Vollmer, S., Strickson, S., Zhang, T. et al. (2017). The mechanism of activation of IRAK1 and IRAK4 by interleukin-1 and Toll-like receptor agonists. *Biochem J.* 474: 2027–2038.

Wagsta, K.M., Sivakumaran, H., Heaton, S.M. et al. (2012). Ivermectin is a specific inhibitor of importin/-mediated nuclear import able to inhibit replication of HIV-1 and dengue virus. *Biochem. J.* 443: 851–856.

Wan, J.Q., Jeelall, Y.S., Humburg, P. et al. (2017). Synergistic cooperation and crosstalk between MYD88(L265P) and mutations that dysregulate CD79B and surface IgM. *J. Exp. Med.* 214: 2759–2776.

Weber, C.K., Liptay, S., Wirth, T. et al. (2000). Suppression of NF-kappaB activity by sulfasalazine is mediated by direct inhibition of IkappaB kinases alpha and beta. *Gastroenterology* 119: 1209–1218.

Wen, T., Wang, J., Shi, Y. et al. (2021). Inhibitors targeting Bruton's tyrosine kinase in cancers: drug development advances. *Leukemia* 35: 312–332.

White, E., Karp, C., Strohecker, A.M. et al. (2010). Role of autophagy in suppression of inflammation and cancer. *Curr. Opin. Cell Biol.* 22: 212–217.

Whiteside, S.T., Epinat, J.C., Rice, N.R. et al. (1997). I kappa B epsilon, a novel member of the I kappa B family, controls RelA and cRel NF-kappa B activity. *EMBO J.* 16: 1413–1426.

Willis, T.G., Jadayel, D.M., Du, M.Q. et al. (1999). Bcl10 is involved in t(1;14)(p22;q32) of MALT B cell lymphoma and mutated in multiple tumor types. *Cell* 96: 35–45.

Willkens, R.F. and Watson, M.A. (1982). Methotrexate: a perspective of its use in the treatment of rheumatic diseases. *J. Lab. Clin. Med.* 100: 314–321.

Wu, Y. and Zhou, B.P. (2009). Inflammation: a driving force speeds cancer metastasis. *Cell Cycle.* 8: 3267–3273.

Xia, Y., Padre, R.C., De Mendoza, T.H. et al. (2009). Phosphorylation of p53 by IkappaB kinase 2 promotes its degradation by beta-TrCP. *Proc. Natl. Acad. Sci. U. S. A.* 106: 2629–2634.

Xia, Z.P., Sun, L., Chen, X. et al. (2009). Direct activation of protein kinases by unanchored polyubiquitin chains. *Nature* 461: 114–119.

Xiao, G., Harhaj, E.W., and Sun, S.C. (2001). NF-κB-inducing kinase regulates the processing of NF-κB2 p100. *Mol. Cell.* 7: 401–409.

Xu, X., Kalac, M., Markson, M. et al. (2020). Reversal of CYLD phosphorylation as a novel therapeutic approach for adult T-cell leukemia/lymphoma (ATLL). *Cell Death Dis.* 11: 94.

FDA approves amgens XGEVA denosumab for the treatment of hypercalcemia of malignancy refractory to bisposphonate therapy. Available online: https://www.amgen.com/media/news-releases/2014/12/fdaapproves-amgens-xgeva-denosumab-for-the-treatment-of-hypercalcemia-of-malignancy-refractory-tobisphosphonate-therapy

https://library.ehaweb.org/eha/2021/eha2021-virtual-congress/330170/peter.hillmen.first.interim.analysis.of.alpine.study.results.of.a.phase.3.html?f=listing%3D0%2Abrowseby%3D8%2Asortby%3D1%2Asearch%3Dalpine

Yan, Q., Huang, Y., Watkins, A.J. et al. (2012). BCR and TLR signaling pathways are recurrently targeted by genetic changes in splenic marginal zone lymphomas. *Haematologica* 97: 595–598.

Yang, Y., Schmitz, R., Mitala, J. et al. (2014). Essential role of the linear ubiquitin chain assembly complex in lymphoma revealed by rare germline polymorphisms. *Cancer Discov.* 4: 480–493.

Yin, M.J., Yamamoto, Y., and Gaynor, R.B. (1998). The anti-inflammatory agents aspirin and salicylate inhibit the activity of I(kappa)B kinase-beta. *Nature* 396: 77–80.

Younes, A., Nowakowski, G., Rosenthal, A.C. et al. (2019). Phase 1 dose-finding study investigating CA-4948, an IRAK4 kinase inhibitor, in patients with R/R NHL: report of initial efficacy and updated safety information. *Blood* 134 (Suppl_1): 5327.

Young, R.M., Wu, T., Schmitz, R. et al. (2015). Survival of human lymphoma cells requires B-cell receptor engagement by self-antigens. *Proc. Natl. Acad. ScI. U.S.A.* 112: 13447–13454.

Yu, H., Lin, L., Zhang, Z. et al. (2020). Targeting NF-κB pathway for the therapy of diseases: mechanism and clinical study. *Signal Transduct. Target Ther.* 5: 209.

TRACON pharmaceuticals reports fourth quarter and year-end 2018 financial results and provides corporate update. Available online: https://traconpharma.gcs-web.com/news-releases/news-release-details/traconpharmaceuticals-reports-fourth-quarter-and-year-end–2018

Zackheim, H.S., Kashani-Sabet, M., and Hwang, S.T. (1996). Low-dose methotrexate to treat erythrodermic cutaneous T-cell lymphoma: results in twenty-nine patients. *J. Am. Acad. Dermatol.* 34: 626–631.

Zeiser, R., von Bubnoff, N., Butler, J. et al. (2020). REACH2 trial group ruxolitinib for glucocorticoid-refractory acute graft-versus-host disease. *N. Engl. J. Med.* 382: 1800–1810.

Zhang, Q., Lenardo, M.J., and Baltimore, D. (2017). 30 Years of NF-κB: a blossoming of relevance to human pathobiology. *Cell* 168: 37–57.

Zhong, Z., Sanchez-Lopez, E., and Karin, M. (2016). Autophagy, inflammation, and immunity: a troika governing cancer and its treatment. *Cell* 166: 288–298.

Zhong, Z., Umemura, A., Sanchez-Lopez, E. et al. (2016). NF-κB restricts inflammasome activation via elimination of damaged mitochondria. *Cell* 164: 896–910.

https://www.takeda.com/newsroom/newsreleases/2021/takeda-provides-update-on-phase-3-panther-pevonedistat-3001-trial

31

Targeting the Cell Cycle and Cyclin-dependent Kinases

Chiara Tarantelli[1] *and Francesco Bertoni*[1,2]

[1] *Institute of Oncology Research, Faculty of Biomedical Sciences, USI, Bellinzona, Switzerland*
[2] *Oncology Institute of Southern Switzerland, Ente Ospedaliero Cantonale, Bellinzona, Switzerland*

Take Home Messages

- Deregulation of CDKs is a frequent event in lymphoid malignancies.
- No compound directly targeting CDKs is currently used for the management of patients with lymphoma or CLL.
- Clinical anti-lymphoma activity, including some complete remissions, has been observed in early clinical trials.
- Newer generations of compounds, improved patient selection, and study designs may allow better targeting of individual CDKs.

Introduction

Cyclin-dependent kinases (CDKs) are a class of serine/threonine kinases playing a central role in the control of cell cycle progression. They are characterized by their functional dependence on a regulatory subunit, a cyclin, that regulates their enzymatic activity (Malumbres 2014). They were discovered in the 1970s–1980s, and their importance in gene transcription and cell division modulation has been thoroughly defined in the ensuing years. The co-ordination of the activity of CDKs within the cell cycle is regulated by the CDKs transient association with cyclins, different protein inhibitors, and post-transcriptional modification, by which specific substrates are activated in a time-dependent progression (Obaya and Sedivy 2002).

CDK Family and Cyclins

The catalytic subunit, the CDK, must associate with a concordant regulatory subunit, the cyclin, the expression of which is modulated during the cell cycle (Figure 31.1). This oscillation in protein production determined the adoption of "cyclins" as the protein family name. In fact, while CDKs are ubiquitously expressed throughout the cell cycle, cyclins are synthetized periodically and degraded at specific phases of the cell cycle, in a way that cell cycle progresses in a regulated and ordered manner (Obaya and Sedivy 2002). Pioneering studies on the genetic and biochemical features of CDKs were initially conducted in yeasts and frogs. In the budding yeast *Saccharomyces cerevisiae*, cell cycle regulatory CDKs comprise two components and up to 10 cyclins. CDKs belonging to this group can phosphorylate multiple substrates. Interestingly, the number of CDKs increased during evolution, such that 20 CDKs and 30 cyclin can be expressed in human cells (Cao et al. 2014).

According to their function, CDKs can be classified into two main groups: cell cycle- and transcription-related. CDKs belonging to the first group can bind more than one cyclin, while a single cyclin regulates the kinases of the second group. **CDK1, CDK2, CDK3, CDK4, CDK5,** and **CDK6** are the most important cell cycle-related proteins, while **CDK7, CDK8, CDK19,** and **CDK9** are transcription-related kinases (Figure 31.2 and Table 31.1). CDK1 is necessary for normal progression of the cell cycle (Santamaria et al. 2007), while CDK2 and CDK3 are redundant (Ortega et al. 2003). CDK4 and CDK6 are both regulated by cyclin D. CDK5 is activated by non-cyclin

Precision Cancer Therapies: Targeting Oncogenic Drivers and Signaling Pathways in Lymphoid Malignancies: From Concept to Practice, Volume 1, First Edition. Edited by Owen A. O'Connor, Stephen M. Ansell, and John F. Seymour.

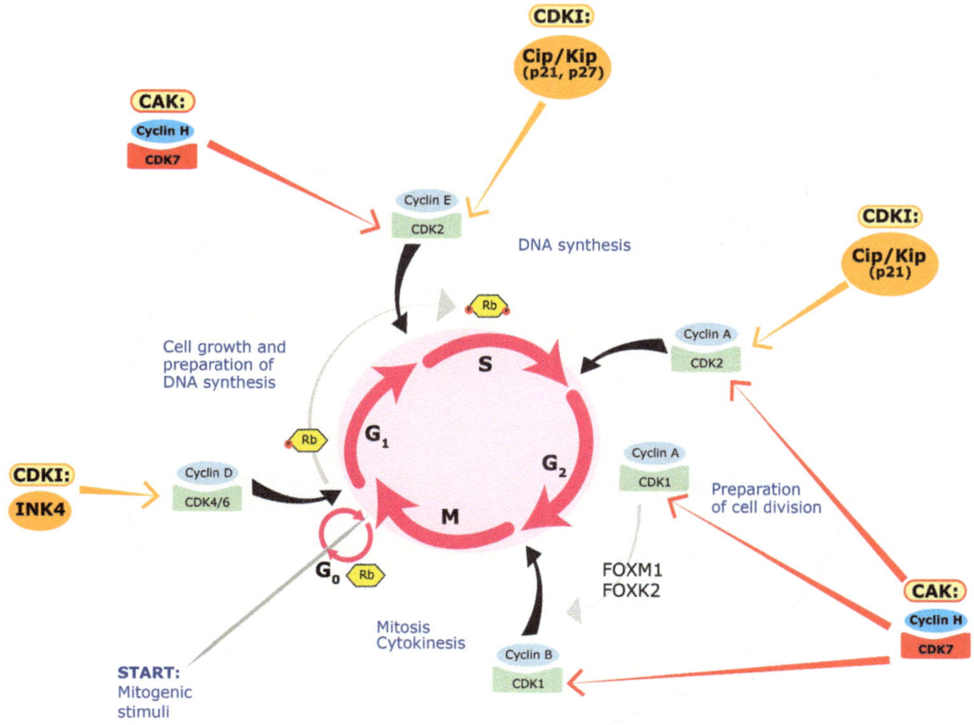

Figure 31.1 Cell cycle pathways and CDK/cyclins actors. Schematic representation of cell cycle regulation.

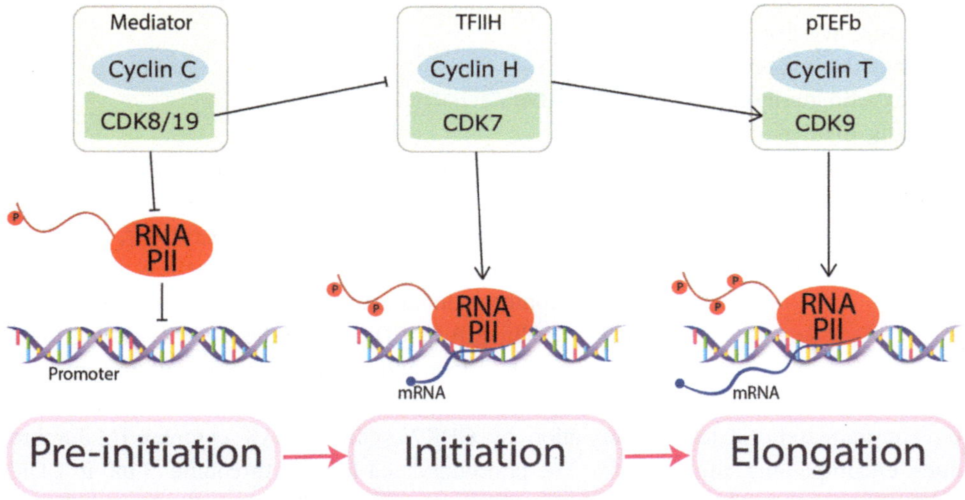

Figure 31.2 Regulation of transcription by CDK/cyclins. CDK/Cyclin complexes regulate different phases of transcription, from pre-initiation to elongation.

proteins, as CDK5R1 (p35) and CDK5R2 (p39). Among transcriptional CDKs, CDK7 is a subunit of the transcription factor II human (TFIIH) and regulates transcription initiation step at gene promoter region, where CDK7 phosphorylates the Ser5 residue of the RNA polymerase II (RNAPII) carboxy-terminal domain (CTD). CDK7 is also a CDK-activating kinase (CAK). CDK8 and the other member of this family CDK19 are kinases in the Mediator complex, responsible for regulating RNAPII during transcription (Carlsten et al. 2013). CDK9 is the catalytic subunit of the positive transcription elongation factor b (pTEFb), and also functions in the DNA damage response when complexed with cyclin K (Yu et al. 2010). Protein levels of cyclin subunits of the transcriptional CDKs, but not of cell cycle-related CDKs, do not periodically oscillate during cell cycle, suggesting post-translational regulation (Carlsten et al. 2013).

Table 31.1 Summary of CDKs/cyclin functions in cell cycle and transcription regulation.

		Function	
CDKs	**Cyclins**	**Cell cycle**	**Transcription**
CDK1	Cyclin A	G2/M transition	
	Cyclin B	Mitosis	
CDK2	Cyclin E	G1/S transition	
	Cyclin A	S/G2 transition	
CDK3	Cyclin C	G0/G1 transition	
CDK4	Cyclin D	G1 phase	
CDK6		G1 phase	
CDK7	Cyclin H	CDK-activating (CAK)	Initiation (TFIIH complex)
CDK8	Cyclin C		Pre-initiation (Mediator complex)
CDK9	Cyclin T		Elongation (pTEFb complex)
CDK11	Cyclin L		Transcriptional regulator
CDK12	Cyclin K, L		Alternative splicing
CDK13	Cyclin L		Alternative splicing

Abbreviations: CAK = CDK-activating kinase; pTEFb = positive transcription elongation factor b; TFIIH = transcription factor II human.

As a protein family, cyclins are characterized by containing a "cyclin box," a domain that folds in five α-helices and serves for CDKs binding (Malumbres 2014). Two cyclin boxes are present in many cyclins, the one at the C-terminal is necessary for the correct folding of the molecule, while the box present at N-terminal serves for CDK binding. The cyclin family comprises approximately 29 proteins in humans, divided among different subfamilies. Cyclins belonging to classes A (A1 and A2), B, D (D1, D2 and D3), and E (E1 and E2) are devoted to control cell cycle progression. Cyclins of classes C, H, K, L, and T are the major partners of transcriptional CDKs.

CDKs Structure

CDKs are proteins ranging in size from approximately 250 to more than 1500 amino acid residues encompassing the central protein kinase domain, in which the amino- and/or carboxy-terminal domains have variable lengths (Malumbres 2014). The amino-terminal extension contains beta-sheets, while the carboxy-terminal lobe is rich in α-helices. Between the two lobes, the catalytic site is positioned. The N-terminal contains a glycine-rich inhibitory element (G-loop), while the C-lobe includes the activation segment with the phosphorylation-sensitive residue in the T-loop. In the cyclin-free inactivated form, the CDK catalytic domain is closed by the T-loop and the activation segment in the C-terminal is disordered, ensuring that the catalytic pocket is inaccessible.

As mentioned, the periodic oscillation in levels of CDK/cyclin activities is tightly regulated by a number of different mechanisms, namely, cyclin synthesis, activation of CDKs by CAK, inhibition of CDKs by CDK inhibitors (CDKIs), and ubiquitin-dependent proteasomal degradation of cyclins.

CDKs Activation

CDK activity is regulated not only by cyclin binding but also by CDK phosphorylation status. CDK phosphorylation by CAK is responsible for activating the kinase; in particular, CDK7 and cyclin H represent physiologic CAK (Larochelle et al. 2007). An ordered conformational activation loop starts with binding of cyclins (cyclin E/A in CDK2/1) to the C-helix, leading to the exposure of the T-loop and opening of the activation segment, so that the phospho-acceptor Ser/Thr becomes accessible for phosphorylation by CDK7/cyclin H CAK complex (Malumbres 2014). The phosphorylated form of threonine (T160 in CDK2 and T161 in CDK1) serves to stabilize the active form of the heterodimer, making the catalytic pocket accessible for enzymatic activity. Contact between CDK4 and cyclin D occurs in the N-terminal and an open conformation is not seen after heterodimer binding. Cdc25 phosphatase can also induce activation of the cell cycle by removing inhibitory signals in CDKs.

CDKs Inhibition

Phosphorylation of residues located in the glycine-rich region (G-loop) of the CDKs N-terminal (T14 and Y15 in CDK2) represents an inhibitory signal for the kinase activity. Deactivating phosphorylations are performed by the kinases Wee and Myt1, and CDK-inactivating phosphorylation can be removed by Cdc25 phosphatases to ensure activation of CDKs and cell cycle progression (Boutros et al. 2007).

Cell cycle-related CDKs and CDK-cyclin complexes can be inhibited by the interaction with molecules known as CDKIs. They are divided into two families, known as INK4 and Cip/Kip. The INK4 family comprises $p15^{INK4a}$, $p16^{INK4b}$, $p18^{INK4c}$, and $p19^{INK4}$ (Sherr and Roberts 1999), proteins able to block the progression in G1 through inhibition of cyclin D-CDK4 and cyclin D-CDK6 interaction. INK4 proteins are specific for CDK4 and CDK6 and interact with monomeric CDKs. They prevent the activation of CDK4 and CDK6 provided by cyclin D or by CAK by conformational changes in the cyclin interface and the ATP-binding pocket (Jeffrey et al. 2000). Specific INK4 proteins are activated by different signals. p15 expression is induced by anti-mitogenic factors such as transforming growth factor (TGF)-β (Reynisdottir et al. 1995); p16 is induced by Ras activation and as a consequence of RB1/p105 and p53 inactivation (Serrano et al. 1997). Cip/Kip family is composed by p21, p27, and p57 proteins, encoded by the genes *CDKN1A*, *CDKN1B*, and *CDKN1C*, respectively (Sherr and Roberts 1999). These proteins exert their inhibitory activity by interacting with both CDK and cyclin components of the CDK-cyclin complex. p21 has specific target inhibition to CDK2-cyclin E and CDK2-cyclin A, while p27 preferentially binds CDK2-cyclin E. Different signals can also activate specific Cip/Kip proteins. p21 is activated mainly in presence of DNA damage (Karimian et al. 2016). p27 is devoted to keep cells in quiescent status (Besson et al. 2006), while p57 has an important role in embryonic cell cycle (Andrews et al. 2007).

The cell cycle is also controlled by regulated degradation of cyclins by E3 ubiquitin ligases, namely, the Skp1-Cul1-F box protein (SCF) complex and the APC/C ubiquitinases (Santo et al. 2015). The first ubiquitinates cyclins from late G_1 to early M phase, while the latter degrades cyclins from anaphase till the end of G1 phase.

CDKs Function

Cell Cycle-related CDK-cyclin Complexes

Adult tissues are maintained in a quiescent state, called G_0. In certain cell types, such as neurons and skeletal muscle cells, this state is irreversible, and these cells cannot progress through the cell cycle. Other cell types stay in quiescent phase transiently and can re-enter from G_0 to early G_1 depending on phosphorylation status of retinoblastoma protein (Rb) (Rubin 2013). Mitogenic stimuli induce the activation of Ras, mitogen-activated protein kinase (MAPK), and phosphatidyl inositol 3 kinase (PI3K)-AKT signaling pathways, and genes encoding for D-type cyclins are upregulated. Once cyclin D is transcribed, the complex with the highly homologous CDK4 or CDK6 can be formed and activated, indeed cell cycle can progress (Malumbres and Barbacid 2001). In particular, the two CDKs can phosphorylate and inactivate the Rb protein (Rubin 2013). Inactivation of Rb protein by CDK4/CDK6 represents a key stage known as restriction point: extracellular mitogenic stimuli are uninfluential in the progression of the cell cycle (Bartek et al. 1996). Rb phosphorylation by cyclin D and CDK4 or CDK6 results in Rb inactivation and transcription activating of genes responsible for DNA synthesis (S phase) or mitosis, such as cyclin E and cyclin A (Malumbres and Barbacid 2001). Cyclin E can now assemble CDK2-cyclin E complex: Rb is further phosphorylated to assure its inactivation (Harbour et al. 1999), chromosome de-condensation through histone synthesis and centrosome duplication at the G_1-S boundary occur, and DNA is replicated (Santo et al. 2015). At late stages of the S phase, CDK2 assembles with cyclin A to boost the transition to the G_2 phase. In the G_2 phase, CDK1 is activated by cyclin A and cyclin B, and phosphorylation of the transcription factors FOXM1 and FOXK2 activates genes responsible for mitotic entry (Laoukili et al. 2008; Marais et al. 2010). CDK1/cyclin B complex activation leads to centrosome maturation, chromosome condensation and mitosis entry after breaking nuclear envelope, regulating the two first phases of mitosis (prophase and metaphase) (Ubersax et al. 2003). Anaphase progression depends on degradation of cyclin B, achieved by anaphase-promoting complex/cyclosome (APC/C), and the full depletion of CDK1 marks mitotic exit (Nigg 2001). Cell division terminates with completion of mitosis and cytokinesis.

Compensatory roles and more complex interaction exist between CDKs and cyclins. For example, CDK2 can substitute Ckd4/6 for cyclin D binding, CDK1 can bind cyclin E or D in absence of CDK2 and CDK4/6.

Transcription-related CDK-cyclin Complexes

CDKs are also important regulators of gene transcription by reversible phosphorylation of the CTD of RNAPII. The phosphorylation status of RNAPII CTD oscillates between a hypophosphorylated state, which is able to enter the preinitiation complex, and a hyperphosphorylated form responsible for transcriptional elongation (Egloff et al. 2012). The CTD can be phosphorylated by some cell cycle-related CDKs (CDK1 or CDK2) and especially from transcriptional CDKs such as CDK7, CDK8, CDK19, and CDK9. CDK7/cyclin H is an activator of transcription and a member of the TFIIH; the complex phosphorylates the CTD of RNAPII and activates CDK9, the catalytic subunit of the pTEFb, to promote transcriptional elongation (Santo et al. 2015). The activated form of CDK9/cyclin T can now allow productive elongation by phosphorylation of the negative elongation factor (NELF) and then promote progressive transcription by phosphorylation of the CTD of RNAPII (Santo et al. 2015). Transcription termination ends with dephosphorylation of RNAPII, making it accessible for another cycle of transcript initiation. CDK8 (or CDK19)/cyclin C are subunits of the Mediator complex, which phosphorylates cyclin H to block the activity of TFIIH and phosphorylates the CTD of RNAPII to prevent its binding to gene promoter (Santo et al. 2015). The CDK11/cyclin L complex and CDK12-13/cyclin K control the RNAPII transcription at different stages (Aleem and Arceci 2015).

DNA Damage and Repair

Cell cycle progression is a highly controlled process, in which "cell cycle checkpoints" permit proper cellular duplication events. Sensing and repair of possible genetic defects allow the transition to the next phase, or cell senescence, or apoptosis. Transitions from G_1 to S and from G_2 to M are strictly regulated. In G_1 to S, DNA damage is sensed by ataxia telangiectasia mutated (ATM) and AMT- and Rad3-related (ATR), which detect double-strand and single-strand DNA brakes, respectively (DDB and SSDNA) (Abraham 2001; Santo et al. 2015). ATM and ATR phosphorylate and activate Chk2 and Chk1, respectively. The kinase Chk2 or Chk1 inactivate Cdc25A phosphatase, which is not able to remove inhibitory phosphates from CDK2, leading to G_1/S arrest. In this stage, p53 induces $p21^{Cip1}$ transcription and high p53 levels lead to permanent inhibition of cell cycle progression with induction of senescence or, when even more highly expressed, to apoptosis (Fridman and Lowe 2003; Ventura and Giordano 2019). In G_2/M checkpoint, the ATM-Chk2-Cdc25 or ATR-Chk1-Cdc25 pathways recognize unrepaired DNA damage in G_2 and inhibit the mitotic complex CDK1/cyclin B by downregulation of Cdc25 phosphatase and upregulation of Wee1 (Mailand et al. 2002; Santo et al. 2015). Therefore, inactivated phosphorylation of CDK1 is achieved. This signaling cascade leads to cell cycle arrest in G_2/M.

Cell cycle progression, and propagation of integral genetic material from the parental to the daughter cells, is ensured by checkpoint activation and as a convergent outcome to CDKs inhibition. For this reason, CDKs are considered drivers of cell cycle progression and target for anti-tumoral treatments.

CDK-cyclin Deregulation in Cancer

Uncontrolled proliferation seen in human cancer is associated with deregulation of CDK/cyclin proteins. Loss of cell cycle inhibition can be mediated by activating mutation of CDKs, cyclins, and CAK, and inactivating mutations of checkpoint regulators, tumor suppressor genes, or CDKI. Alterations of CDK- or cyclin-expressing genes can also be due to their amplification and translocation, or protein overexpression. In lymphoid tumors, the best examples are perhaps provided by cyclin D1 and p16 (CDKN2A) (Aleem and Arceci 2015). The presence of chromosomal translocations juxtaposing the *CCND1* gene, coding cyclin D1, to the immunoglobulin heavy chain genes represents the genetic hallmark of mantle cell lymphoma (MCL) (Swerdlow et al. 2017). Inactivation of p16, via genetic losses (including homozygous deletions) or promoter methylation of its *CDKN2A* coding gene, is a frequent event, mainly associated with aggressive diseases and histologic transformation (Chigrinova et al. 2013; Lenz et al. 2008; Pasqualucci et al. 2014; Swerdlow et al. 2017). Inactivation, via DNA losses and/or somatic mutation, of genes coding checkpoint proteins such as ATM is common, for example in MCL and in chronic lymphocytic leukemia (CLL) (Carrassa et al. 2020).

A tumorigenic role has been established for certain cell cycles regulators, and inhibition of components of this finely regulated environment results in cell cycle arrest, transcriptional arrest, and apoptosis, preventing malignant cell proliferation. Several inhibitors are under development pre-clinically, in early-phase studies and some have been recently approved for treatment in cancer.

Targeting CDKs in Lymphoid Malignancies

As highlighted in the previous sections, CDKs represent very important therapeutic targets, and much effort has been applied by academics and the pharmaceutical industry to produce compounds able to inhibit them. Due to the high homologies among the different CDKs, it is very difficult to develop highly specific inhibitors.

CDK4/6 Inhibitors

So far, the pharmacological inhibition of CDK4/6 has been the most successful story among the efforts toward targeting CDKs, as shown by multiple drugs of this class already approved by the regulatory agencies. CDK4/6 inhibitors interfere in the progression form the G_1 to S phase of the cell cycle. CDK4 and CDK6 belong to the same subfamily of proteins due to their high homology and they are required by different tissues and in different development stages. CDK6 is fundamental during hematopoiesis, and mice lacking CDK6 show transient growth arrest and impaired production of blood cells components precursor cells (Aleem and Arceci 2015). Indeed, neutropenia is one of the most common adverse effects of CDK6 inhibitors clinically, associated with dose-limiting toxicity (Dickson 2014; Richter et al. 2021). In MCL, the translocation t(11;14) induces deregulated cyclin D1 expression, leading to CDK4/6 upregulation (Lee et al. 2020).

Pre-clinical activity as single agents has been reported in lymphoma models for various CDK4/6 inhibitors (Bisi et al. 2017, 2017; Hee et al. 2018; Hoareau-Aveilla et al. 2019; Ishio et al. 2022; Kim et al. 2018; Marzec et al. 2006; Tanaka et al. 2020; Tarantelli et al. 2020). So far, the most studied compounds are **palbociclib** (PD0332991) (Gong et al. 2017; Hoareau-Aveilla et al. 2019; Ishio et al. 2022; Kim et al. 2018; Marzec et al. 2006; Tarantelli et al. 2020), **ribociclib** (LEE011) (Hee et al. 2018; Kim et al. 2018), and **abemaciclib** (LY2835219) (Gong et al. 2017; Kim et al. 2018; Tanaka et al. 2020), all Food and Drug Administration (FDA) approved for breast cancer patients. In the phase 1, among 16 patients with relapsed/refractory (R/R) MCL, palbociclib led to an overall response rate (ORR) of 18.7% with one complete response (CR; 6%), and reduction of Rb phosphorylation and Ki-67 expression after treatment (Leonard et al. 2012). In a phase 2 of abemaciclib, the ORR was 36% with 7% of CR (Morschhauser et al. 2021) in 28 patients with R/R MCL. No responses were observed in the seven patients with R/R MCL enrolled in the ribociclib phase 1 trial (Infante et al. 2016).

CDK4/6 amplifications or translocations and direct D-cyclin deregulation are in general associated with higher sensitivity to CDK4/6 inhibitors, while RB1 loss is associated with decreased sensitivity (Asghar et al. 2022; Gong et al. 2017; Kim et al. 2018). Consequently, various basket trials for solid tumors and lymphoma, adult and pediatric patients currently exploring targeted agents in genetically defined subgroups of patients have incorporated palbociclib for cases with tumors bearing amplification of CCND1/2/3 or CDK4/6 with maintained Rb expression: the MATCH Screening Trial, (NCT02465060), the SMMART/PRIME Trial, (NCT03878524), the CAPTUR (NCT03297606), and The Pediatric MATCH Screening Trial (NCT03155620).

The use of CDK4/6 inhibitors has also been explored in combinations, pre-clinically (Chaturvedi et al. 2019; Chiron et al. 2014, 2013; Hee et al. 2018; Kozaki et al. 2018; Sun et al. 2015; Tarantelli et al. 2020) and clinically (Martin et al. 2019a, 2019b). The vast majority of data are with palbociclib: combinations with PI3K inhibitors (idelalisib [Chiron et al. 2013] and copanlisib [Tarantelli et al. 2020]), BTK inhibitors (ibrutinib [Chiron et al. 2014] and tirabrutinib [Kozaki et al. 2018]), and epigenetic agents (HDAC inhibitor vorinostat [Chaturvedi et al. 2019] and BET inhibitor JQ1 [Sun et al. 2015]) show higher anti-tumor activity than monotherapies in various lymphoma models. A phase 2 study (NCT03478514) is testing the combination of palbociclib and ibrutinib in R/R MCL, based on the 67% of ORR and 37% of CR reported in the phase 1 with 27 patients with R/R MCL (Martin et al. 2019a). A phase 1 study has tested palbociclib in combination with the proteasome inhibitor bortezomib in 19 patients with R/R MCL, showing signs of clinical activity with one CR (5%) (Martin et al. 2019b).

Specific Inhibitors

CDK9 is part of the elongation complex and phosphorylates the CTD of the RNAPII promoting transcription, thus acting a transcriptional regulator. Among the most impacted transcripts are those with a high mRNA turnover rate, such as MCL1 and MYC, and indeed CDK9 inhibitors are sometimes represented or "advertised" as potential indirect MCL1 inhibitors.

AZD4573 is a CDK9 inhibitor, with potent activity against hematological cancer models in vivo and in vitro (Cidado et al. 2020; Roderick et al. 2021; Thieme et al. 2021), as well in combination with venetoclax in models resistant to the BCL2 inhibitor alone (Cidado et al. 2020), and with acalabrutinib, also in models resistant to the BTK inhibitor (Roderick et al. 2021). Apoptosis induction through MCL1 depletion was recognized as a mechanism of cellular cell death. Its activity was investigated also in vivo as single agent or in combination with venetoclax. A phase 1 trial has enrolled 44 patients with a range of R/R hematological cancers (NCT03263637), but results have not yet been presented. A phase 1/2 trial is now recruiting patients with R/R diffuse large B-cell lymphoma (DLBCL), MCL, and marginal zone lymphoma (MZL) to study AZD4573 plus acalabrutinib (NCT04630756).

CDKI-73 (LS-007) is a selective CDK9 inhibitor, which has shown the ability to induce caspase-dependent apoptosis in CLL and DLBCL cells as a single agent (Richter et al. 2021; Walsby et al. 2013; Xie et al. 2020). Downregulation of MCL1 and Xiap by CDKI-73 are the proposed mechanisms of the synergism observed with fludarabine in CLL cells (Walsby et al. 2013), while the synergism with enhancer of zester homolog 2 (EZH2) inhibitors (EPZ6438 and GSK126) appears due the capacity of these agents to counteract the increase in H3K27me3 levels otherwise caused by CDK9 inhibition (Xie et al. 2020). No trials have clinically explored the use of CDKI-73.

Atuveciclib (BAY 1143572) is a pTEFb/CDK9 inhibitor, with anti-tumor activity in various pre-clinical B- and T-cell lymphoma models (Kinoshita et al. 2018; Narita et al. 2017; Tarantelli et al. 2020), mediated via downregulation of MCL1, and MYC (Kinoshita et al. 2018; Narita et al. 2017). Synergism with copanlisib has also been reported but only in a minority of the cell lines treated with the combination (Tarantelli et al. 2020). Atuveciclib has entered early clinical assessment, but no data is yet available from the phase 1 study (NCT01938638).

The atuveciclib-derivative CDK9 inhibitor **VIP152** (BAY 1251152) has proven pre-clinical activity in CLL models (Sher et al. 2021). CR was achieved in two (28%) of the first seven patients with R/R high-grade B-cell lymphoma with MYC and BCL2/BCL6 translocations treated within the still ongoing phase 1 (NCT02635672) (Diamond et al. 2022). VIP152 is also being evaluated in additional phase 1/2 studies for patients with R/R CLL patients and Richter's syndrome (NCT04978779) and in other patients with R/R lymphoma (NCT05371054). VIP152 has received orphan drug designation for DLBCL.

The newer generation novel CDK9 inhibitors **GFH 009** and **KB 0742** (KI-ARv-03) have just entered early clinical evaluation for patients with R/R lymphoma and CLL (NCT04588922, NCT04718675, respectively).

CDK7 Inhibitors

CDK7 is involved in regulation of both the cell cycle, phosphorylating the T-loops of cell cycle CDKs CDK1/2/4/6, and of transcription, phosphorylating the RNAPII CTD and many important oncogenic transcription factors such as c-Myc (Marineau et al. 2022). Different CDK7 inhibitors have entered the early clinical evaluation Among the CDK7 inhibitors, **SY-5609** has available data in lymphomas. SY-5609 exerts anti-tumor activity against MCL cell lines as a single agent and in combination with the BTK inhibitor acalabrutinib (Johannessen et al. 2021), also leading to downregulation of cyclin D1 and of E2F1. Early trials are ongoing but not for lymphoma patients.

Inhibitors Targeting Multiple CDKs

As above mentioned, due to the high homology among CDKs many available compounds and drugs inhibit multiple CDKs. A number of compounds have been evaluated in lymphoma or CLL, but the clinical activity as single agent has been generally modest and, for most of them, their clinical development has been halted.

The CDK2 and 9 inhibitor **fadraciclib** (CYC-065) has pre-clinical anti-tumor activity in DLBCL, with downregulation of MYC and MCL1 levels, as well synergism with venetoclax and BET inhibitors (Frame et al. 2016). No data is available for the ongoing phase 1/2 with fadraciclib as a single agent for patients with R/R solid tumors or lymphoma (NCT04983810). Another phase 1 has been designed to explore the combination with venetoclax in patients with R/R CLL (NCT03739554).

Voruciclib (P1446A) is an orally available pan-CDKI with demonstrated pre-clinical activity in lymphoma (DLBCL) and CLL, as a single agent and in combination with venetoclax (Dey et al. 2017; Lesnick et al. 2020; Paiva et al. 2015). As for other compounds inhibiting CDK9, the capacity to downregulate transcripts such as MCL1 or MYC plays an important role in their anti-tumor effect (Dey et al. 2017). No objective responses have been reported so far in the initial 14 patients with lymphoma (DLBCL, n = 7) enrolled in the still ongoing voruciclib phase 1 (NCT03547115) (Konopleva et al. 2021).

Alvocidib (flavopiridol, DSP-2033; HL-275, IND 46211, L-86-8275, MDL-107826A, NSC 649890) is a first-generation pan-CDKI that inhibits CDK1, 2, 4, 6, 7, and 9, with proven anti-tumor activity in lymphoma and CLL models (Arguello et al. 1998; Bonvini et al. 2009; Chen et al. 2005; Lam et al. 2001; Pepper et al. 2003). The effect appears due to CDK9 inhibition and pTEFb inactivation, leading to a transcription globally unpaired, affecting especially high turnover rate mRNA, as cell cycle and apoptosis genes (Chen et al. 2005; Lam et al. 2001). Modest activity was observed in the clinical setting, when flavopiridol was given as single agent. The ORR was 11%, with no CR, both in patients with R/R MCL (n = 28) and R/R CLL (n = 36) enrolled in phase 2 studies with flavopiridol given as one-hour bolus daily for three days repeated every three weeks (Byrd et al. 2005; Kouroukis et al. 2003). Two other studies (phase 1 [Jones et al. 2014] and phase 1/2 [Miljkovic et al. 2019]) have been done with flavopiridol given as 30-minute loading dose followed by a four-hour continuous infusion for four consecutive weeks every six weeks: the ORR was 11% in 43 patients with pretreated lymphoma (Jones et al. 2014) and 3.8% in 26 patients with R/R lymphoma, mostly MCL (n = 15) and DLBCL (n = 10) (Miljkovic et al. 2019). No responses were seen when flavopiridol was given as a 72-hour infusion every two weeks in patients with R/R MCL (n = 10) or R/R CLL (n = 15) (Byrd et al. 2005; Lin et al. 2002). Higher activity has been observed with flavopiridol given in combination with other agents. A phase 1 study investigated flavopiridol (one-hour infusion) combined with fludarabine, and rituximab in 38 patients, with mostly MCL (n = 10), CLL (n = 10), or follicular lymphoma (n = 9) (Lin et al. 2010). The ORR was 82%, with 50% of CR, with no differences between untreated (n = 22) and pretreated (n = 16) patients (Lin et al. 2010). In another phase 1, nine lymphoma patients (MCL, n = 6) were treated with flavopiridol plus the proteasome inhibitor bortezomib achieving an ORR of 33% (CR, 11%) (Holkova et al. 2014). No trials are currently running for lymphoma or CLL patients.

Dinaciclib (SCH727965, MK-7965; PS-095760) is a CDK1, 2, 5, and 9 inhibitor and has a potent activity in reducing cell viability and cell cycle arrest. Its efficacy is not only due to the ATP-competitive CDKs interaction but also to the interplay with the acetyl-lysine recognition site of bromodomains (Martin et al. 2013). Dinaciclib has pre-clinical activity in lymphoma and CLL models (Chen et al. 2016; Gregory et al. 2015; Horing et al. 2017; Johnson et al. 2012; Zhao et al. 2019). Dinaciclib reduces MCL1 transcript in aggressive MYC-driven lymphomas and in CLL, and prolongs survival in mice bearing Eμ-Myc and IG-Myc translocated lymphoma (Gregory et al. 2015; Johnson et al. 2012). The anti-leukemic effect of dinaciclib on CLL cells is blocked when tumor cells are co-cultured with stromal cells or fibronectin, but the addition of PI3Kα inhibitor overcomes the induced resistance (Johnson et al. 2012). In MCL cells, the combination of fatty acid synthase inhibitor with dinaciclib is synergistic in inducing apoptosis by NOXA stabilization and MCL1 reduction (Horing et al. 2017). Various trials have assessed dinaciclib both as single agent (Fabre et al. 2014; Gregory et al. 2022) and in combination (Flynn et al. 2015; Ghia et al. 2017). ORR in R/R CLL was 54% in a larger phase 1 with 52 patients with no CR (Flynn et al. 2015). The compound also entered a phase 3 for R/R CLL compared with the anti-CD20 antibody ofatumumab, which however was terminated due to program prioritization (Ghia et al. 2017). The ORR was 40% in the 20 patients enrolled, with no CR (Ghia et al. 2017). One of four patients with R/R CLL enrolled in the phase 1 exploring the combination of dinaciclib and rituximab achieved CR (25%) (Fabre et al. 2014). The combination of dinaciclib with the PD-1 inhibitor pembrolizumab achieved an ORRs of 29.4% dinaciclib in R/R CLL (n =) and 21.1% in R/R DLBCL (n = 38) (Gregory et al. 2022). Dinaciclib has received orphan drug designation for CLL, but no trials are currently ongoing for lymphoma or CLL.

AT7519 is another multi-cyclin-dependent kinase inhibitor that potently inhibits CDK1, 2, 4, 5, 6, and 9 (Squires et al. 2009). It mainly acts by blocking RNAPII phosphorylation (Santo et al. 2010). In the phase 1, enrolling patients with either solid tumors or lymphoma, none of the latter achieved responses (ORR, 0%) (Chen et al. 2014). In the phase 2, none of four patients with R/R CLL attained a disease response (ORR, 0%), while 2/12 patients with R/R solid tumors attained a PR (ORR, 17%) (Seftel et al. 2017). No additional trials are currently running with AT7519.

Riviciclib (P276-00) is a CDK1, 4, and 9 inhibitor. Pre-clinical data is available in MCL, in which the compound decreases cyclin D1 and MCL1 levels and synergizes with bortezomib and doxorubicin (Shirsath et al. 2012). No objective responses were seen in the 13 patients with R/R MCL enrolled in a phase 2 (Cassaday et al. 2015). No additional trials are currently running with riviciclib.

Roniciclib (BAY 1000394) is an inhibitor of CDK1, 2, 4, 6, 7, and 9 and it is active pre-clinically in various B- and T-cell lymphoma models (Tarantelli et al. 2020). It also shows a synergism or an additive effect with the PI3K inhibitor copanlisib in half of the cell lines exposed to the combination (Tarantelli et al. 2020). However, no objective responses were seen in the seven patients with lymphoma from the roniciclib phase 1 (Bahleda et al. 2017).

Seliciclib (CYC202, R-roscovitine) inhibits CDK1, 2, 5, 7, and 9 and has shown pre-clinical anti-tumor activity in MCL (Lacrima et al. 2005), DLBCL (Lacrima et al. 2007), and CLL models (Alvi et al. 2005; Hahntow et al. 2004; Lacrima et al. 2007; Weingrill et al. 2007). Cyclin D1 and MCL1 proteins are also downregulated in MCL (Lacrima et al. 2005). No clinical data for patients with lymphoma is available from the phase 1. Seliciclib is currently in phase 2 (NCT03774446) for non-oncological indications (Cushing's disease).

Anti-tumor activity has been reported with the CDK7, 12, and 13 inhibitor **THZ1** in various peripheral T-cell lymphoma models as a single agent and in combination with BCL2 inhibitors, especially the pan-BH3 inhibitor obatoclax (Cayrol et al. 2017).

SNS-032 (BMS-387032) is a CDK2, 7, and 9 inhibitor with anti-tumor activity in DLBCL, MCL, and CLL models (Chen et al. 2010, 2009; Jiang et al. 2022). No clinical activity was seen in the 19 patients with R/R CLL treated in the phase 1 trial (Tong et al. 2010).

Among other compounds, with no data available in the lymphoma setting, we can mention some that are in clinical development: the CDK8 and 19 inhibitor **RVU120** (SEL120) (Pakulska et al. 2021), currently in phase1 trial for patients with R/R acute myeloid leukemia (AML) and high-risk myelodysplastic syndrome (NCT04021368); the CDK2, 4, and 6 inhibitor **ebvaciclib** (PF-06873600) (Freeman-Cook et al. 2021), in phase 2 for breast cancer patients (NCT03519178).

Pre-clinical activity in CLL models has been described with the multikinase inhibitor **zotiraciclib** (TG02, SB-1317), which targets CDK1, 2, 5, and 9, and also, among others, JAK2 and FLT3 (Chen et al. 2021). No results are available for the 16 patients with R/R CLL enrolled in the phase 1 (NCT01699152).

Resistance

No drugs belonging to the class of the CDKIs are in routine clinical use in patients with lymphoma beyond the early-phase clinical trials presented above. Thus, there is no data describing the mechanisms of resistance in the clinical setting. The only reliable data available is for the resistance to CDK4/6 inhibitors that are used more commonly in the solid tumors field. We have already stated that CDK4/6 and D-cyclin amplifications/translocations correlate with higher sensitivity, while RB1 inactivation with decreased sensitivity. The first lesions are commonly detected in lymphomas such as DLBCL and MCL, suggesting potential activity of these drugs. However, the RB1 loss is also recurrent in the same lymphoma types (Ferrero et al. 2020; Mian et al. 2012), and suggests that resistance to single agents can also be frequent, in line with the limited activity seen in the early clinical trials (Infante et al. 2016; Leonard et al. 2012; Morschhauser et al. 2021). Moreover, also *CDKN2A* inactivation, also frequent in MCL and DLBCL (Ferrero et al. 2020; Lenz et al. 2008), could also predict low sensitivity to CDK4/6 inhibitors (Asghar et al. 2022). Activation of CDK2 is another mechanism of resistance to CDK4/6 inhibitors in solid tumors as well in AML pre-clinical models, and it could be overcome adding CDK2 inhibitors (Berthet et al. 2007; Freeman-Cook et al. 2021). Induction of autophagy, endoplasmic reticulum stress, and upregulation of anti-apoptotic proteins have been observed as possible mechanisms of resistance to flavopiridol (Mahoney et al. 2012; Richter et al. 2021; Yeh et al. 2015).

Future Directions

Despite the strong rationale underlying their use and the encouraging pre-clinical data, no drugs targeting CDKs have, so far, become part of the treatment landscape for patients with lymphoma or CLL. Less benefit than expected has been seen with the most advanced class of compounds, the CDK4/6 inhibitors (Infante et al. 2016; Leonard et al. 2012; Morschhauser et al. 2021), while more promising data is emerging from the clinical trials with CDK9 inhibitors (Diamond et al. 2022). There are many potential explanations that can justify these results. While lesions associated with sensitivity are certainly enriched in, for example MCL, they are also often concurrent with lesions that, in solid tumors, correlate with resistance to the drugs. Detailed genetic analyses of tumor specimens taken at the time of the study enrollment could help in identifying the patients who might benefit the most. Up to now, almost all the drugs that have entered the clinical evaluation are not highly selective for a specific CDK, as mentioned, due to high homology among the proteins. The selectivity might be improved with novel approaches to target CDKs, including the use of proteolysis targeting chimeras (PROTAC) and molecular glues (Rana et al. 2021), which can lead to the increased binding of an inhibitor for a specific target protein. It is also important to underline the difficulties in comparing the antitumor activity or the toxicity profiles of the different CDKIs based on the reported kinome selectivity data, since these are not obtained using the same experimental conditions or using the same assays. The toxicity, mainly hematologic and gastrointestinal for CDK4/6 inhibitors (Dickson 2014; Infante et al. 2016; Morschhauser et al. 2021; Richter et al. 2021), is another issue since it leads to treatment interruptions. Compounds with higher specificity and optimization of the treatment schedules might help in overcoming this issue. Moreover, determining the optimal administration schedules and the use in combination with other agents will also be important in determining the clinical efficacy, as suggested by the studies with flavopiridol (Byrd et al. 2005; Kouroukis et al. 2003; Lin et al. 2002).

In conclusions, CDKs provide a very wide range of potential targets and therapeutic modalities that have not yet been effectively exploited for patients affected by lymphoid malignancies. We can expect more in the future with newer generations of compounds, improved patient selection, and study designs.

Must Read References

Marzec, M., Kasprzycka, M., Lai, R. et al. (2006). Mantle cell lymphoma cells express predominantly cyclin D1a isoform and are highly sensitive to selective inhibition of CDK4 kinase activity. *Blood* 108 (5): 1744–1750.

Chiron, D., Di Liberto, M., Martin, P. et al. (2014). Cell-cycle reprogramming for PI3K inhibition overrides a relapse-specific C481S BTK mutation revealed by longitudinal functional genomics in mantle cell lymphoma. *Cancer Discov.* 4 (9): 1022–1035.

Diamond, J.R., Boni, V., Lim,E. et al. (2022). First-in-human dose-escalation study of cyclin-dependent kinase 9 inhibitor VIP152 in patients with advanced malignancies shows early signs of clinical efficacy. *Clin. Cancer Res.* 28 (7): 1285–1293.

References

Abraham, R.T. (2001). Cell cycle checkpoint signaling through the ATM and ATR kinases. *Genes. Dev.* 15 (17): 2177–2196.

Aleem, E. and Arceci, R.J. (2015). Targeting cell cycle regulators in hematologic malignancies. *Front. Cell. Dev. Biol.* 3 (16): 16.

Alvi, A.J., Austen, B., Weston, V.J. et al. (2005). A novel CDK inhibitor, CYC202 (R-roscovitine), overcomes the defect in p53-dependent apoptosis in B-CLL by downregulation of genes involved in transcription regulation and survival. *Blood* 105 (11): 4484–4491.

Andrews, S.C., Wood, M.D., Tunster, S.J. et al. (2007). Cdkn1c (p57Kip2) is the major regulator of embryonic growth within its imprinted domain on mouse distal chromosome 7. *BMC Dev. Biol.* 7: 53.

Arguello, F., Alexander, M., Sterry, J.A. et al. (1998). Flavopiridol induces apoptosis of normal lymphoid cells, causes immunosuppression, and has potent antitumor activity In vivo against human leukemia and lymphoma xenografts. *Blood* 91 (7): 2482–2490.

Asghar, U.S., Kanani, R., Roylance, R. et al. (2022). Systematic review of molecular biomarkers predictive of resistance to CDK4/6 inhibition in metastatic breast cancer. *JCO. Precis. Oncol.* 6 (6): e2100002.

Bahleda, R., Grilley-Olson, J.E., Govindan, R. et al. (2017). Phase I dose-escalation studies of roniciclib, a pan-cyclin-dependent kinase inhibitor, in advanced malignancies. *Br. J. Cancer* 116 (12): 1505–1512.

Bartek, J., Bartkova, J., and Lukas, J. (1996). The retinoblastoma protein pathway and the restriction point. *Curr. Opin. Cell. Biol.* 8 (6): 805–814.

Berthet, C., Rodriguez-Galan, M.C., Hodge, D.L. et al. (2007). Hematopoiesis and thymic apoptosis are not affected by the loss of Cdk2. *Mol. Cell. Biol.* 27 (14): 5079–5089.

Besson, A., Gurian-West, M., Chen, X. et al. (2006). A pathway in quiescent cells that controls p27Kip1 stability, subcellular localization, and tumor suppression. *Genes. Dev.* 20 (1): 47–64.

Bisi, J.E., Sorrentino, J.A., Jordan, J.L. et al. (2017). Preclinical development of G1T38: a novel, potent and selective inhibitor of cyclin dependent kinases 4/6 for use as an oral antineoplastic in patients with CDK4/6 sensitive tumors. *Oncotarget.* 8 (26): 42343–42358.

Bonvini, P., Zorzi, E., Mussolin, L. et al. (2009). The effect of the cyclin-dependent kinase inhibitor flavopiridol on anaplastic large cell lymphoma cells and relationship with NPM-ALK kinase expression and activity. *Haematologica.* 94 (7): 944–955.

Boutros, R., Lobjois, V., and Ducommun, B. (2007). CDC25 phosphatases in cancer cells: key players? good targets? *Nat. Rev. Cancer* 7 (7): 495–507.

Byrd, J.C., Peterson, B.L., Gabrilove, J. et al. (2005). Treatment of relapsed chronic lymphocytic leukemia by 72-hour continuous infusion or 1-hour bolus infusion of flavopiridol: results from cancer and leukemia group B study 19805. *Clin. Cancer. Res.* 11 (11): 4176–4181.

Cao, L., Chen, F., Yang, X. et al. (2014). Phylogenetic analysis of CDK and cyclin proteins in premetazoan lineages. *BMC Evol. Biol.* 14: 10.

Carlsten, J.O., Zhu, X., and Gustafsson, C.M. (2013). The multitalented mediator complex. *Trends Biochem. Sci.* 38 (11): 531–537.

Carrassa, L., Colombo, I., Damia, G. et al. (2020). Targeting the DNA damage response for patients with lymphoma: preclinical and clinical evidences. *Cancer Treat Rev.* 90: 102090.

Cassaday, R.D., Goy, A., Advani, S. et al. (2015). A phase II, single-arm, open-label, multicenter study to evaluate the efficacy and safety of P276-00, a cyclin-dependent kinase inhibitor, in patients with relapsed or refractory mantle cell lymphoma. *Clin. Lymphoma. Myeloma. Leuk.* 15 (7): 392–397.

Cayrol, F., Praditsuktavorn, P., Fernando, T.M. et al. (2017). THZ1 targeting CDK7 suppresses STAT transcriptional activity and sensitizes T-cell lymphomas to BCL2 inhibitors. *Nat. Commun.* 8: 14290.

Chaturvedi, N.K., Hatch, N.D., Sutton, G.L. et al. (2019). A novel approach to eliminate therapy-resistant mantle cell lymphoma: synergistic effects of vorinostat with palbociclib. *Leuk. Lymphoma.* 60 (5): 1214–1223.

Chen, E.X., Hotte, S., Hirte, H. et al. (2014). A phase I study of cyclin-dependent kinase inhibitor, AT7519, in patients with advanced cancer: NCIC clinical trials group IND 177. *Br. J. Cancer* 111 (12): 2262–2267.

Chen, R., Chubb, S., Cheng, T. et al. (2010). Responses in mantle cell lymphoma cells to SNS-032 depend on the biological context of each cell line. *Cancer Res.* 70 (16): 6587–6597.

Chen, R., Keating, M.J., Gandhi, V. et al. (2005). Transcription inhibition by flavopiridol: mechanism of chronic lymphocytic leukemia cell death. *Blood* 106 (7): 2513–2519.

Chen, R., Tsai, J., Thompson, P.A. et al. (2021). The multi-kinase inhibitor TG02 induces apoptosis and blocks B-cell receptor signaling in chronic lymphocytic leukemia through dual mechanisms of action. *Blood Cancer J.* 11 (3): 57.

Chen, R., Wierda, W.G., Chubb, S. et al. (2009). Mechanism of action of SNS-032, a novel cyclin-dependent kinase inhibitor, in chronic lymphocytic leukemia. *Blood* 113 (19): 4637–4645.

Chen, Y., Germano, S., Clements, C. et al. (2016). Pro-survival signal inhibition by CDK inhibitor dinaciclib in chronic lymphocytic leukaemia. *Br. J. Haematol.* 175 (4): 641–651.

Chigrinova, E., Rinaldi, A., Kwee, I. et al. (2013). Two main genetic pathways lead to the transformation of chronic lymphocytic leukemia to Richter syndrome. *Blood* 122 (15): 2673–2682.

Chiron, D., Di Liberto, M., Martin, P. et al. (2014). Cell-cycle reprogramming for PI3K inhibition overrides a relapse-specific C481S BTK mutation revealed by longitudinal functional genomics in mantle cell lymphoma. *Cancer Discov* 4 (9): 1022–1035.

Chiron, D., Martin, P., Di Liberto, M. et al. (2013). Induction of prolonged early G1 arrest by CDK4/CDK6 inhibition reprograms lymphoma cells for durable PI3Kdelta inhibition through PIK3IP1. *Cell Cycle* 12 (12): 1892–1900.

Cidado, J., Boiko, S., Proia, T. et al. (2020). AZD4573 is a highly selective CDK9 inhibitor that suppresses MCL-1 and induces apoptosis in hematologic cancer cells. *Clin. Cancer Res.* 26 (4): 922–934.

Dey, J., Deckwerth, T.L., Kerwin, W.S. et al. (2017). Voruciclib, a clinical stage oral CDK9 inhibitor, represses MCL-1 and sensitizes high-risk diffuse large B-cell lymphoma to BCL2 inhibition. *Sci. Rep.* 7 (1): 18007.

Diamond, J.R., Boni, V., Lim, E. et al. (2022). First-in-human dose-escalation study of cyclin-dependent kinase 9 inhibitor VIP152 in patients with advanced malignancies shows early signs of clinical efficacy. *Clin. Cancer Res.* 28 (7): 1285–1293.

Dickson, M.A. (2014). Molecular pathways: CDK4 inhibitors for cancer therapy. *Clin. Cancer Res.* 20 (13): 3379–3383.

Egloff, S., Dienstbier, M., and Murphy, S. (2012). Updating the RNA polymerase CTD code: adding gene-specific layers. *Trends Genet.* 28 (7): 333–341.

Fabre, C., Gobbi, M., Ezzili, C. et al. (2014). Clinical study of the novel cyclin-dependent kinase inhibitor dinaciclib in combination with rituximab in relapsed/refractory chronic lymphocytic leukemia patients. *Cancer Chemother. Pharmacol.* 74 (5): 1057–1064.

Ferrero, S., Rossi, D., Rinaldi, A. et al. (2020). KMT2D mutations and TP53 disruptions are poor prognostic biomarkers in mantle cell lymphoma receiving high-dose therapy: a FIL study. *Haematologica* 105 (6): 1604–1612.

Flynn, J., Jones, J., Johnson, A.J. et al. (2015). Dinaciclib is a novel cyclin-dependent kinase inhibitor with significant clinical activity in relapsed and refractory chronic lymphocytic leukemia. *Leukemia* 29 (7): 1524–1529.

Frame, S.M., Pohler, E., MacKay, C. et al. (2016). Abstract 1309: CYC065, a novel CDK2/9 inhibitor, is an effective inducer of cell death and synergizes with BCL2 and BET inhibitors in B-cell lymphoma, including double-hit lymphomas. *Cancer Res.* 76 (14_Supplement): 1309-1309.

Freeman-Cook, K.D., Hoffman, R.L., Behenna, D.C. et al. (2021). Discovery of PF-06873600, a CDK2/4/6 Inhibitor for the treatment of cancer. *J. Med. Chem.* 64 (13): 9056–9077.

Fridman, J.S. and Lowe, S.W. (2003). Control of apoptosis by p53. *Oncogene* 22 (56): 9030–9040.

Ghia, P., Scarfo, L., Perez, S. et al. (2017). Efficacy and safety of dinaciclib vs ofatumumab in patients with relapsed/refractory chronic lymphocytic leukemia. *Blood* 129 (13): 1876–1878.

Gong, X., Litchfield, L.M., Webster, Y. et al. (2017). Genomic aberrations that activate D-type cyclins are associated with enhanced sensitivity to the CDK4 and CDK6 inhibitor abemaciclib. *Cancer Cell* 32 (6): 761–776. e766.

Gregory, G.P., Hogg, S.J., Kats, L.M. et al. (2015). CDK9 inhibition by dinaciclib potently suppresses Mcl-1 to induce durable apoptotic responses in aggressive MYC-driven B-cell lymphoma in vivo. *Leukemia* 29 (6): 1437–1441.

Gregory, G.P., Kumar, S., Wang, D. et al. (2022). Pembrolizumab plus dinaciclib in patients with hematologic malignancies: the phase 1b KEYNOTE-155 study. *Blood Adv.* 6 (4): 1232–1242.

Hahntow, I.N., Schneller, F., Oelsner, M. et al. (2004). Cyclin-dependent kinase inhibitor Roscovitine induces apoptosis in chronic lymphocytic leukemia cells. *Leukemia* 18 (4): 747–755.

Harbour, J.W., Luo, R.X., Dei Santi, A. et al. (1999). Cdk phosphorylation triggers sequential intramolecular interactions that progressively block Rb functions as cells move through G1. *Cell* 98 (6): 859–869.

Hee, Y.T., Yan, J., Nizetic, D. et al. (2018). LEE011 and ruxolitinib: a synergistic drug combination for natural killer/T-cell lymphoma (NKTCL). *Oncotarget* 9 (61): 31832–31841.

Hoareau-Aveilla, C., Quelen, C., Congras, A. et al. (2019). miR-497 suppresses cycle progression through an axis involving CDK6 in ALK-positive cells. *Haematologica* 104 (2): 347–359.

Holkova, B., Kmieciak, M., Perkins, E.B. et al. (2014). Phase I trial of bortezomib (PS-341; NSC 681239) and "nonhybrid" (bolus) infusion schedule of alvocidib (flavopiridol; NSC 649890) in patients with recurrent or refractory indolent B-cell neoplasms. *Clin. Cancer Res.* 20 (22): 5652–5662.

Horing, E., Montraveta, A., Heine, S. et al. (2017). Dual targeting of MCL1 and NOXA as effective strategy for treatment of mantle cell lymphoma. *Br. J. Haematol.* 177 (4): 557–561.

Infante, J.R., Cassier, P.A., Gerecitano, J.F. et al. (2016). A phase I study of the cyclin-dependent kinase 4/6 inhibitor ribociclib (LEE011) in patients with advanced solid tumors and lymphomas. *Clin. Cancer Res.* 22 (23): 5696–5705.

Ishio, T., Kumar, S., Shimono, J. et al. (2022). Genome-wide CRISPR screen identifies CDK6 as a therapeutic target in adult T-cell leukemia/lymphoma. *Blood* 139 (10): 1541–1556.

Jeffrey, P.D., Tong, L., and Pavletich, N.P. (2000). Structural basis of inhibition of CDK-cyclin complexes by INK4 inhibitors. *Genes. Dev.* 14 (24): 3115–3125.

Jiang, L., Wen, C., Zhou, H. et al. (2022). Cyclin-dependent kinase 7/9 inhibitor SNS-032 induces apoptosis in diffuse large B-cell lymphoma cells. *Cancer Biol. Ther.* 23 (1): 319–327.

Johannessen, L., Henry, S., Sawant, P. et al. (2021). SY5609, a potent and selective CDK7 Inhibitor, potentiates BTK inhibitor activity in mantle cell lymphoma preclinical models. *Blood* 138: 1205.

Johnson, A.J., Yeh, Y.Y., Smith, L.L. et al. (2012). The novel cyclin-dependent kinase inhibitor dinaciclib (SCH727965) promotes apoptosis and abrogates microenvironmental cytokine protection in chronic lymphocytic leukemia cells. *Leukemia* 26 (12): 2554–2557.

Jones, J.A., Rupert, A.S., Poi, M. et al. (2014). Flavopiridol can be safely administered using a pharmacologically derived schedule and demonstrates activity in relapsed and refractory non-Hodgkin's lymphoma. *Am. J. Hematol.* 89 (1): 19–24.

Karimian, A., Ahmadi, Y., and Yousefi, B. (2016). Multiple functions of p21 in cell cycle, apoptosis and transcriptional regulation after DNA damage. *DNA Repair (Amst)* 42: 63–71.

Kim, S., Tiedt, R., Loo, A. et al. (2018). The potent and selective cyclin-dependent kinases 4 and 6 inhibitor ribociclib (LEE011) is a versatile combination partner in preclinical cancer models. *Oncotarget* 9 (81): 35226–35240.

Kinoshita, S., Ishida, T., Ito, A. et al. (2018). Cyclin-dependent kinase 9 as a potential specific molecular target in NK-cell leukemia/lymphoma. *Haematologica* 103 (12): 2059–2068.

Konopleva, M., Brander, D.M., Patel, K. et al. (2021). A phase 1 dose-escalation study of the oral CDK inhibitor voruciclib in patients with relapsed/refractory B-cell malignancies or acute myeloid leukemia (AML): preliminary results of the completed dose escalation stage in AML. *Blood* 138 (Supplement 1): 3423-3423.

Kouroukis, C.T., Belch, A., Crump, M. et al. (2003). Flavopiridol in untreated or relapsed mantle-cell lymphoma: results of a phase II study of the national cancer institute of canada clinical trials group. *J. Clin. Oncol.* 21 (9): 1740–1745.

Kozaki, R., Vogler, M., Walter, H.S. et al. (2018). Responses to the selective Bruton's tyrosine kinase (BTK) inhibitor tirabrutinib (ONO/GS-4059) in diffuse large B-cell lymphoma cell lines. *Cancers (Basel)* 10 (4).

Lacrima, K., Rinaldi, A., Vignati, S. et al. (2007). Cyclin-dependent kinase inhibitor seliciclib shows in vitro activity in diffuse large B cell lymphomas. *Leuk. Lymphoma.* 48 (1): 158–167.

Lacrima, K., Valentini, A., Lambertini, C. et al. (2005). In vitro activity of cyclin-dependent kinase inhibitor CYC202 (Seliciclib, R-roscovitine) in mantle cell lymphomas. *Ann. Oncol.* 16 (7): 1169–1176.

Lam, L.T., Pickeral, O.K., Peng, A.C. et al. (2001). Genomic-scale measurement of mRNA turnover and the mechanisms of action of the anti-cancer drug flavopiridol. *Genome. Biol.* 2 (10): RESEARCH0041.

Laoukili, J., Alvarez, M., Meijer, L.A. et al. (2008). Activation of foxM1 during G2 requires cyclin A/Cdk-dependent relief of autorepression by the FoxM1 N-terminal domain. *Mol. Cell Biol.* 28 (9): 3076–3087.

Larochelle, S., Merrick, K.A., Terret, M.E. et al. (2007). Requirements for Cdk7 in the assembly of Cdk1/cyclin B and activation of Cdk2 revealed by chemical genetics in human cells. *Mol. Cell* 25 (6): 839–850.

Lee, C., Huang, X., Di Liberto, M. et al. (2020). Targeting CDK4/6 in mantle cell lymphoma. *Ann. Lymphoma.* 4.

Lenz, G., Wright, G.W., Emre, N.C. et al. (2008). Molecular subtypes of diffuse large B-cell lymphoma arise by distinct genetic pathways. *Proc. Natl. Acad. Sci. U. S. A.* 105 (36): 13520–13525.

Leonard, J.P., LaCasce, A.S., Smith, M.R. et al. (2012). Selective CDK4/6 inhibition with tumor responses by PD0332991 in patients with mantle cell lymphoma. *Blood* 119 (20): 4597–4607.

Lesnick, C., Wood, J., Parikh, S.A. et al. (2020). Voruciclib plus venetoclax show high efficacy for CLL b cells on human stromal cells. *J Clin Oncol* 38 (15): e20009–e20009.

Lin, T.S., Blum, K.A., Fischer, D.B. et al. (2010). Flavopiridol, fludarabine, and rituximab in mantle cell lymphoma and indolent B-cell lymphoproliferative disorders. *J. Clin. Oncol.* 28 (3): 418–423.

Lin, T.S., Howard, O.M., Neuberg, D.S. et al. (2002). Seventy-two hour continuous infusion flavopiridol in relapsed and refractory mantle cell lymphoma. *Leuk. Lymphoma.* 43 (4): 793–797.

Mahoney, E., Lucas, D.M., Gupta, S.V. et al. (2012). ER stress and autophagy: new discoveries in the mechanism of action and drug resistance of the cyclin-dependent kinase inhibitor flavopiridol. *Blood* 120 (6): 1262–1273.

Mailand, N., Podtelejnikov, A.V., Groth, A. et al. (2002). Regulation of G(2)/M events by Cdc25A through phosphorylation-dependent modulation of its stability. *EMBO J.* 21 (21): 5911–5920.

Malumbres, M. (2014). Cyclin-dependent kinases. *Genome. Biol.* 15 (6): 122.

Malumbres, M. and Barbacid, M. (2001). To cycle or not to cycle: a critical decision in cancer. *Nat. Rev. Cancer* 1 (3): 222–231.

Marais, A., Ji, Z., Child, E.S. et al. (2010). Cell cycle-dependent regulation of the forkhead transcription factor FOXK2 by CDK.cyclin complexes. *J. Biol. Chem.* 285 (46): 35728–35739.

Marineau, J.J., Hamman, K.B., Hu, S. et al. (2022). Discovery of SY-5609: a selective, noncovalent inhibitor of CDK7. *J. Med. Chem.* 65 (2): 1458–1480.

Martin, M.P., Olesen, S.H., Georg, G.I. et al. (2013). Cyclin-dependent kinase inhibitor dinaciclib interacts with the acetyl-lysine recognition site of bromodomains. *ACS Chem. Biol.* 8 (11): 2360–2365.

Martin, P., Bartlett, N.L., Blum, K.A. et al. (2019a). A phase 1 trial of ibrutinib plus palbociclib in previously treated mantle cell lymphoma. *Blood* 133 (11): 1201–1204.

Martin, P., Ruan, J., Furman, R. et al. (2019b). A phase I trial of palbociclib plus bortezomib in previously treated mantle cell lymphoma. *Leuk Lymphoma* 60 (12): 2917–2921.

Marzec, M., Kasprzycka, M., Lai, R. et al. (2006). Mantle cell lymphoma cells express predominantly cyclin D1a isoform and are highly sensitive to selective inhibition of CDK4 kinase activity. *Blood* 108 (5): 1744–1750.

Mian, M., Scandurra, M., Chigrinova, E. et al. (2012). Clinical and molecular characterization of diffuse large B-cell lymphomas with 13q14.3 deletion. *Ann. Oncol.* 23 (3): 729–735.

Miljkovic, M.D., Roschewski, M., Dunleavy, K., and Wilson, W.H. (2019). Hybrid dosing of the cyclin-dependent kinase (CDK) inhibitor flavopiridol in relapsed/refractory mantle cell lymphoma and diffuse large B-cell lymphoma. *Leuk. Lymphoma.* 60 (13): 3320–3323.

Morschhauser, F., Bouabdallah, K., Stilgenbauer, S. et al. (2021). Clinical activity of abemaciclib in patients with relapsed or refractory mantle cell lymphoma – a phase II study. *Haematologica* 106 (3): 859–862.

Narita, T., Ishida, T., Ito, A. et al. (2017). Cyclin-dependent kinase 9 is a novel specific molecular target in adult T-cell leukemia/lymphoma. *Blood* 130 (9): 1114–1124.

Nigg, E.A. (2001). Mitotic kinases as regulators of cell division and its checkpoints. *Nat. Rev. Mol. Cell Biol.* 2 (1): 21–32.

Obaya, A.J. and Sedivy, J.M. (2002). Regulation of cyclin-Cdk activity in mammalian cells. *Cell Mol. Life Sci.* 59 (1): 126–142.

Ortega, S., Prieto, I., Odajima, J. et al. (2003). Cyclin-dependent kinase 2 is essential for meiosis but not for mitotic cell division in mice. *Nat. Genet.* 35 (1): 25–31.

Paiva, C., Godbersen, J.C., Soderquist, R.S. et al. (2015). Cyclin-dependent kinase inhibitor P1446A induces apoptosis in a JNK/p38 MAPK-dependent manner in chronic lymphocytic leukemia B-cells. *PLoS One* 10 (11): e0143685.

Pakulska, U., Adamczyk, E., Dziedzic, K. et al. (2021). Abstract 1018: SEL120, a CDK8/CDK19 inhibitor, possesses strong multilineage differentiation potential in AML. *Cancer Res.* 81 (13_Supplement): 1018-1018.

Pasqualucci, L., Khiabanian, H., Fangazio, M. et al. (2014). Genetics of follicular lymphoma transformation. *Cell Rep.* 6 (1): 130–140.

Pepper, C., Thomas, A., Fegan, C. et al. (2003). Flavopiridol induces apoptosis in B-cell chronic lymphocytic leukaemia cells through a p38 and ERK MAP kinase-dependent mechanism. *Leuk. Lymphoma.* 44 (2): 337–342.

Rana, S., Mallareddy, J.R., Singh, S. et al. (2021). Inhibitors, PROTACs and molecular glues as diverse therapeutic modalities to target cyclin-dependent kinase. *Cancers. (Basel)* 13 (21).

Reynisdottir, I., Polyak, K., Iavarone, A. et al. (1995). Kip/Cip and Ink4 Cdk inhibitors cooperate to induce cell cycle arrest in response to TGF-beta. *Genes. Dev.* 9 (15): 1831–1845.

Richter, A., Schoenwaelder, N., Sender, S. et al. (2021). Cyclin-dependent kinase inhibitors in hematological malignancies-current understanding, (pre-)clinical application and promising approaches. *Cancers (Basel)* 13 (10).

Roderick, J., Boiko, S., Andersen, C.L. et al. (2021). AZD4573 effectively induces apoptosis in r/r MCL as a monotherapy or in combination with acalabrutinib. *Blood* 138 (Supplement 1): 2255-2255.

Rubin, S.M. (2013). Deciphering the retinoblastoma protein phosphorylation code. *Trends Biochem. Sci.* 38 (1): 12–19.

Santamaria, D., Barriere, C., Cerqueira, A. et al. (2007). Cdk1 is sufficient to drive the mammalian cell cycle. *Nature* 448 (7155): 811–815.

Santo, L., Siu, K.T., and Raje, N. (2015). Targeting cyclin-dependent kinases and cell cycle progression in human cancers. *Semin. Oncol.* 42 (6): 788–800.

Santo, L., Vallet, S., Hideshima, T. et al. (2010). AT7519, A novel small molecule multi-cyclin-dependent kinase inhibitor, induces apoptosis in multiple myeloma via GSK-3beta activation and RNA polymerase II inhibition. *Oncogene* 29 (16): 2325–2336.

Seftel, M.D., Kuruvilla, J., Kouroukis, T. et al. (2017). The CDK inhibitor AT7519M in patients with relapsed or refractory chronic lymphocytic leukemia (CLL) and mantle cell lymphoma. A phase II study of the canadian cancer trials group. *Leuk. Lymphoma.* 58 (6): 1358–1365.

Serrano, M., Lin, A.W., McCurrach, M.E. et al. (1997). Oncogenic ras provokes premature cell senescence associated with accumulation of p53 and p16INK4a. *Cell* 88 (5): 593–602.

Sher, S., Beaver, L., Williams, K. et al. (2021). VIP152 is a novel CDK9 inhibitor with efficacy in chronic lymphocytic leukemia. *Blood* 138 (Supplement 1): 270-270.

Sherr, C.J. and Roberts, J.M. (1999). CDK inhibitors: positive and negative regulators of G1-phase progression. *Genes. Dev.* 13 (12): 1501–1512.

Shirsath, N.P., Manohar, S.M., and Joshi, K.S. (2012). P276-00, a cyclin-dependent kinase inhibitor, modulates cell cycle and induces apoptosis in vitro and in vivo in mantle cell lymphoma cell lines. *Mol. Cancer* 11: 77.

Squires, M.S., Feltell, R.E., Wallis, N.G. et al. (2009). Biological characterization of AT7519, a small-molecule inhibitor of cyclin-dependent kinases, in human tumor cell lines. *Mol. Cancer Ther.* 8 (2): 324–332.

Sun, B., Shah, B., Fiskus, W. et al. (2015). Synergistic activity of BET protein antagonist-based combinations in mantle cell lymphoma cells sensitive or resistant to ibrutinib. *Blood* 126 (13): 1565–1574.

Swerdlow, S.H., Campo, E., Seto, M. et al. (2017). Mantle cell lymphoma. In: *WHO Classification of Tumours of Haematopoietic and Lymphoid Tissues – Revised*, 4e (S.H. Swerdlow, E Campo, NL Harris et al. ed.), 285–290. Lyon, France: IARC Press.

Tanaka, Y., Momose, S., Tabayashi, T. et al. (2020). Abemaciclib, a CDK4/6 inhibitor, exerts preclinical activity against aggressive germinal center-derived B-cell lymphomas. *Cancer Sci.* 111 (2): 749–759.

Tarantelli, C., Lange, M., Gaudio, E. et al. (2020). Copanlisib synergizes with conventional and targeted agents including venetoclax in B- and T-cell lymphoma models. *Blood Adv.* 4 (5): 819–829.

Thieme, E., Sun, D., Sharma, G.G. et al. (2021). Transcriptional reprogramming of super-enhancer associated oncogenes following inhibition of cyclin-dependent kinase-9 (CDK9) in aggressive non-Hodgkin lymphoma (NHL). *Blood* 138 (Supplement 1): 3493-3493.

Tong, W.G., Chen, R., Plunkett, W. et al. (2010). Phase I and pharmacologic study of SNS-032, a potent and selective Cdk2, 7, and 9 inhibitor, in patients with advanced chronic lymphocytic leukemia and multiple myeloma. *J. Clin. Oncol.* 28 (18): 3015–3022.

Ubersax, J.A., Woodbury, E.L., Quang, P.N. et al. (2003). Targets of the cyclin-dependent kinase Cdk1. *Nature* 425 (6960): 859–864.

Ventura, E. and Giordano, A. (2019). *Cell Cycle*. Reference Module in Life Sciences, Elsevier.

Walsby, E., Pratt, G., Shao, H. et al. (2013). A novel Cdk9 inhibitor preferentially targets tumor cells and synergizes with fludarabine. *Oncotarget* 5 (2).

Weingrill, E., Wölfler, A., Strunk, D. et al. (2007). Roscovitine in B-chronic lymphocytic leukemia cells: high apoptosis-inducing efficacy and synergism with alemtuzumab independent of the patients' pretreatment status. *Haematologica* 92 (9): 1286–1288.

Xie, S., Wei, F., Sun, Y.M. et al. (2020). EZH2 inhibitors abrogate upregulation of trimethylation of H3K27 by CDK9 inhibitors and potentiate its activity against diffuse large B-cell lymphoma. *Haematologica* 105 (4): 1021–1031.

Yeh, Y.Y., Chen, R., Hessler, J. et al. (2015). Up-regulation of CDK9 kinase activity and Mcl-1 stability contributes to the acquired resistance to cyclin-dependent kinase inhibitors in leukemia. *Oncotarget* 6 (5): 2667–2679.

Yu, D.S., Zhao, R., Hsu, E.L. et al. (2010). Cyclin-dependent kinase 9-cyclin K functions in the replication stress response. *EMBO Rep.* 11 (11): 876–882.

Zhao, H., Li, S., Wang, G. et al. (2019). Study of the mechanism by which dinaciclib induces apoptosis and cell cycle arrest of lymphoma Raji cells through a CDK1-involved pathway. *Cancer Med.* 8 (9): 4348–4358.

Index

Precision Cancer Therapies: Targeting Oncogenic Drivers and Signaling Pathways in Lymphoid Malignancies: From Concept to Practice, Volume 1, First Edition. Edited by Owen A. O'Connor, Stephen M. Ansell, and John F. Seymour.

C

d

e

f

g

h

i

j